Liver Disease in Children

Fourth Edition

Liver Disease in Children

Fourth Edition

Edited by

Frederick J. Suchy, MD
Chief Research Officer and Director,
Children's Hospital Colorado Research Institute, Children's Hospital Colorado;
Professor of Pediatrics and Associate Dean for Child Health Research,
University of Colorado School of Medicine, Aurora, CO, USA

Ronald J. Sokol, MD
Professor and Vice Chair of Pediatrics;
Section Head, Gastroenterology, Hepatology and Nutrition;
Director, Colorado Clinical and Translational Sciences Institute; and Arnold Silverman MD Chair in Digestive Health,
University of Colorado School of Medicine and Children's Hospital Colorado, Aurora, CO, USA

William F. Balistreri, MD
Director Emeritus,
Pediatric Liver Care Center; Medical Director Emeritus, Liver Transplantation;
Dorothy M. M. Kersten Professor of Pediatrics, Division of Gastroenterology, Hepatology and Nutrition,
Cincinnati Children's Hospital Medical Center, University of Cincinnati College of Medicine, Cincinnati, OH, USA

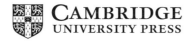

CAMBRIDGE
UNIVERSITY PRESS

CAMBRIDGE
UNIVERSITY PRESS

University Printing House, Cambridge CB2 8BS, United Kingdom

Published in the United States of America by Cambridge University Press, New York

Cambridge University Press is part of the University of Cambridge.

It furthers the University's mission by disseminating knowledge in the pursuit of education, learning and research at the highest international levels of excellence.

www.cambridge.org
Information on this title: www.cambridge.org/9781107013797

Fourth edition © Cambridge University Press 2014
Third edition © Cambridge University Press 2007
Second edition © Lippincott, Williams & Wilkins 2001
First edition © Mosby 1994

Fourth edition first published 2014
Third edition first published 2007
Second edition first published 2001
First edition first published 1994

Printed in the United Kingdom by Bell and Bain Ltd

A catalogue record for this publication is available from the British Library

Library of Congress Cataloging-in-Publication Data
Liver disease in children. – Fourth edition / edited by Frederick J. Suchy, MD, chief research officer, and director, The Children's Hospital Research Institute, Children's Hospital Colorado, professor of pediatrics and associate dean for Child Health Research, University of Colorado School of Medicine, Aurora, CO, USA, Ronald J. Sokol, MD, professor and vice chair of pediatrics, section head, Gastroenterology, Hepatology and Nutrition, director, Colorado Clinical and Translational Sciences Institute; and Arnold Silverman MD, chair in digestive health, University of Colorado School of Medicine and Children's Hospital Colorado, Aurora, CO, USA, William F. Balistreri, MD, director emeritus, Pediatric Liver Care Center, medical director emeritus, Liver Transplantation, and Dorothy M. M. Kersten, professor of pediatrics, Division of Gastroenterology, Hepatology and Nutrition, Cincinnati Children's Hospital Medical Center, University of Cincinnati College of Medicine, Cincinnati, OH, USA.
        pages cm
ISBN 978-1-107-01379-7 (Hardback)
1. Liver–Diseases.   2. Pediatric gastroenterology.   I. Suchy, Frederick J., editor of compilation.   II. Sokol, Ronald J., editor of compilation.   III. Balistreri, William F., editor of compilation.
RJ456.L5L575 2014
618.92′362–dc23   2013021438

ISBN 978-1-107-01379-7 Hardback

Contents

Contributors

Estella M. Alonso MD
Professor, Department of Pediatrics, Northwestern University, Chicago, and Director of Hepatology, Department of Gastroenterology, Hepatology and Nutrition, Children's Memorial Hospital, Chicago, IL, USA

Maria H. Alonso MD
Associate Professor of Surgery and Pediatrics, Department of Surgery, University of Cincinnati College of Medicine, Cincinnati, OH, USA

Fernando Alvarez MD
Chief, Division of Gastroenterology, Hepatology and Nutrition, CHU Saint Justine Medical Centre, and Professor, Department of Pediatrics and Deaprtment of Microbiology and Immunology, University of Montreal, Montreal, Quebec, Canada

Rana F. Ammoury MD
Assistant Professor, Department of Gastroenterology and Nutrition, Steele Children's Research Center, University of Arizona, Tucson, AZ, USA

Karl E. Anderson MD FACP
Associate Director, General Research Center, and Director, Division of Human Nutrition, Department of Preventive Medicine and Community Health, University of Texas Medical Branch, Galveston, TX, USA

Ronen Arnon MD
Associate Professor, Departments of Pediatrics, Hepatology and Surgery, Medical Director of Pediatric Hepatology and Liver Transplantation, Mount Sinai School of Medicine, New York, NY, USA

William F. Balistreri MD
Director Emeritus, Pediatric Liver Care Center, Medical Director Emeritus, Liver Transplantation and Dorothy M. M. Kersten Professor of Pediatrics, Division of Gastroenterology, Hepatology and Nutrition, Cincinnati Children's Hospital Medical Center, University of Cincinnati College of Medicine, Cincinnati, OH, USA

Manisha Balwani MD MS
Assistant Professor, Department of Genetics and Genomic Studies and Department of Medicine, Mount Sinai School of Medicine, New York, NY, USA

Mark Bartlett
Fellow in Pediatric Gastroenterology, University of Minnesota, Minneapolis, MN, USA

Jorge A. Bezerra MD
Director, Pediatric Liver Care Center; Professor of Pediatrics, The William and Rebecca Balistreri Chair of Pediatric Hepatology, Division of Gastroenterology, Hepatology and Nutrition, University of Cincinnati College of Medicine and Cincinnati Children's Hospital Medical Center, Cincinnati, OH, USA

Kevin E. Bove MD
Professor, Division of Pediatric Pathology, University of Cincinnati Department of Pediatrics, Cincinnati Children's Hospital Medical Center, Cincinnati, OH, USA

T. Andrew Burrow MD
Assistant Professor of Clinical Genetics, Cincinnati Children's Hospital Medical Center, Cincinnati, OH, USA

Kathleen M. Campbell MD
Assistant Professor, Department of Pediatrics, Division of Gastroenterology, Hepatology and Nutrition, University of Cincinnati College of Medicine and Cincinnati Children's Hospital Medical Center, Cincinnati, OH, USA

Stephen Cederbaum MD
Professor Emeritus, Psychiatry, Pediatrics and Human Genetics, University of California Los Angeles, Los Angeles, CA, USA

Mei-Hwei Chang MD
Department of Pediatrics and Hepatitis Research Center, National Taiwan University Hospital, College of Medicine, Taipei, Taiwan

Robert J. Desnick MD
Dean for Genetics and Genomic Medicine; Professor and Chairman Emeritus, Genetic and Genomic Sciences; Professor

of Pediatrics; Professor of Oncological Sciences; and Professor of Obstetrics, Gynecology, and Reproductive Science, Mount Sinai School of Medicine, New York, NY, USA

Frank W. DiPaola MD
Clinical Fellow, Pediatric Gastroenterology, Division of Gastroenterology, Hepatology and Nutrition, Cincinnati Children's Hospital Medial Center and University of Cincinnati College of Medicine, Cincinnati, OH, USA

Josée Dubois MD
Professor of Medical Imaging, CHU Saint Justine Medical Centre, University of Montreal, Montreal, Quebec, Canada

Amy Feldman MD
Fellow, Department of Gastroenterology, Hepatology and Nutrition, University of Colorado School of Medicine and Children's Hospital Colorado, Aurora, CO, USA

Andrew P. Feranchak MD
Willis C. Maddrey MD Professorship in Liver Disease, Department of Pediatrics, UT Southwestern Medical Center and Children's Medical Center, Dallas, TX, USA

Milton J. Finegold MD
Professor, Department of Pathology and Immunology and Department of Pediatrics, Baylor College of Medicine, Houston, TX, USA

Joshua R. Friedman MD PhD
Assistant Professor of Pediatrics, Perelman School of Medicine at the University of Pennsylvania, Division of Gastroenterology, Hepatology, and Nutrition, Children's Hospital of Philadelphia, Philadelphia, PA, USA

Fayez K. Ghishan MD
Professor and Chair, Department of Pediatrics; Director of the Steele Children's Research Center, University of Arizona, Tucson, AZ, USA

Melanie B. Gillingham PhD
Department of Molecular and Medical Genetics, Oregon Health and Science University, Portland, OR, USA

Glenn R. Gourley MD
Professor, Department of Pediatrics, University of Minnesota, Minneapolis, MN, USA

Gregory A. Grabowski MD
Professor of Pediatrics and Molecular Genetics, Biochemistry and Microbiology, Cincinnati Children's Hospital Medical Center, Cincinnati, OH, USA

Nikita A. Gupta MD
Assistant Professor of Pediatric Gastroenterology, Emory University School of Medicine, and Pediatric Hepatologist, Children's Healthcare of Atlanta, GA, USA

Nedim Hadžić MD
Professor of Paediatric Hepatology, King's College Medical School, London, UK

James E. Heubi MD
Director, Clinical Translational Research Center, and Professor, Department of Pediatrics, Cincinnati Children's Hospital Medical Center and University of Cincinnati College of Medicine, Cincinnati, OH, USA

Evelyn K. Hsu MD
Assistant Professor of Pediatrics, Division of Gastroenterology and Hepatology, Seattle Children's Hospital, University of Washington School of Medicine, Seattle, WA, USA

M. Kyle Jensen MD MS
Assistant Professor of Pediatric Gastroenterology and Hepatology, University of Utah, Primary Children's Medical Center, Salt Lake City, UT, USA

Maureen M. Jonas MD
Senior Associate in Medicine, Division of Gastroenterology, Hepatology and Nutrition, Children's Hospital Boston, and Professor of Pediatrics, Harvard Medical School, Boston, MA, USA

Binita M. Kamath MD MRCP
Assistant Professor, Department of Paediatrics, University of Toronto; Staff Physician, Division of Gastroenterology, Hepatology and Nutrition, Hospital for Sick Children, Toronto, Ontario, Canada

Saul J. Karpen MD PhD
Emory University School of Medicine, Department of Pediatric Gastroenterology, Hepatology and Nutrition, Atlanta, GA, USA

Nanda Kerkar MD
Associate Professor of Pediatrics, Division of Gastroenterology, Hepatology and Nutrition, Pediatric Liver Disease/Liver Transplant Program, Mount Sinai School of Medicine, New York, NY, USA

Rohit Kohli MBBS MS
Associate Professor, Department of Pediatrics, University of Cincinnati College of Medicine, and Co-Director, Cincinnati Children's Steatohepatitis Center, Cincinnati Children's Hospital Medical Center, Cincinnati, OH, USA

Richard L. Kradin MD
Gastrointestinal Pathology Service and Department of Pathology, Massachusetts General Hospital; and Department of Pathology, Harvard Medical School, Boston, MA, USA

Gregory Y. Lauwers, MD
Gastrointestinal Pathology Service and Department of Pathology, Massachusetts General Hospital; and Department of Pathology, Harvard Medical School, Boston, MA, USA

Dolores Lopez-Terrada MD PhD
Professor of Pathology and Pediatrics, Baylor College of Medicine, Houston, TX, USA

Cara L. Mack MD
Associate Professor of Pediatrics, Section of Pediatric Gastroenterology, Hepatology and Nutrition, Digestive Health Institute, Children's Hospital Colorado, University of Colorado School of Medicine, Aurora, CO, USA

Alexander G. Miethke MD
Assistant Professor, Division of Gastroenterology, Hepatology and Nutrition, Department of Pediatrics, University of Cincinnati College of Medicine, and Pediatric Liver Care Center, Children's Hospital Medical Center, Cincinnati, OH, USA

Grant Mitchell MD
Professor, Medical Genetic Division, Department of Pediatrics Saint Justine Medical Centre, University of Montreal, Montreal, Quebec, Canada

Karen F. Murray MD
Professor of Pediatrics, Division Chief, Gastroenterology and Hepatology, Seattle Children's Hospital, University of Washington School of Medicine, Seattle, WA, USA

Michael R. Narkewicz MD
Professor of Pediatrics, Section of Gastroenterology, Hepatology and Nutrition, Children's Hospital Colorado, University of Colorado School of Medicine, Aurora, CO, USA

Jaimie D. Nathan MD
Assistant Professor of Surgery and Pediatrics, Department of Surgery, University of Cincinnati College of Medicine, Cincinnati, OH, USA

Vicky Lee Ng MD FRCPC
Associate Professor of Paediatrics, University of Toronto, and Medical Director, Liver Transplant Program, Division of Gastroenterology, Hepatology and Nutrition, SickKids Transplant Centre, Hospital for Sick Children, Toronto, Ontario, Canada

Donald A. Novak MD
Department of Pediatrics, University of Florida, and Division of Pediatric Gastroenterology, Shands Hospital, Gainesville, FL, USA

Antonio R. Perez-Atayde MD
Director of Speical Techniques and Staff Pathologist, Department of Pathology, Boston Children's Hospital and Harvard Medical School, Boston, MA, USA

David H. Perlmutter MD
Physician-in-Chief and Scientific Director, Vira I. Heinz Professor of Pediatrics, and Chair, Department of Pediatrics, University of Pittsburgh School of Medicine, Children's Hospital of Pittsburgh of UPMC, Pittsburgh, PA, USA

David A. Piccoli MD
Chief, Division of Gastroenterology, Hepatology and Nutrition, Fred and Suzanne Biesecker Professor of Pediatrics, Perelman School of Medicine at the University of Pennsylvania, Children's Hospital of Pennsylvania, Philadelphia, PA, USA

Piero Rinaldo, MD PhD
Professor of Laboratory Medicine and Pathology, Department of Laboratory Medicine and Pathology, Department of Laboratory Genetics, and Department of Pediatric and Adolescent Medicine, Mayo Clinic, Rochester, MN, USA

Eve A. Roberts, MD MA FRCP
Adjunct Associate Professor, Departments of Medicine, Paediatrics and Gastroenterology, University of Toronto, and Hepatologist, Division of Gastroenterology and Nutrition, Hospital for Sick Children, Toronto, Ontario, Canada

Philip Rosenthal MD
Professor of Pediatrics and Surgery; Director Pediatric Hepatology Director Pediatric Clinical Research, Departments of Pediatrics and Surgery and the Liver Center, the University of California, San Francisco, CA, USA

Pierre A. Russo MD
Chief, Anatomic Pathology, Children's Hospital of Philadelphia, Philadelphia, PA, USA

Frederick C. Ryckman MD
Professor of Surgery and Pediatrics, Director of Pediatric Surgery Training Program, Pediatric Liver Care Center, Cincinnati Children's Hospital, Cincinnati, OH, USA

Meghana Sathe MD
Assistant Professor, Department of Pediatrics, University of Texas Southwestern and Children's Medical Center, Dallas, TX, USA

Kathleen B. Schwarz MD
Professor of Pediatrics, Johns Hopkins University School of Medicine, and Chief, Pediatric Liver Center, Johns Hopkins Hospital, Baltimore, MD, USA

Kenneth D. R. Setchell PhD
Department of Pathology and Laboratory Medicine, Cincinnati Children's Hospital Medical Center and Department of Pediatrics, University of Cincinnati College of Medicine, Cincinnati, OH, USA

Benjamin L. Shneider MD
Director, Pediatric Hepatology, Professor of Pediatrics University of Pittsburgh, Children's Hospital of Pittsburgh of UPMC, Pittsburgh, PA, USA

Jason Soden MD

Associate Professor, Department of Gastroenterology, Hepatology, and Nutrition, University of Colorado School of Medicine and Children's Hospital Colorado, Aurora, CO, USA

Ronald J. Sokol MD

Professor and Vice Chair of Pediatrics; Section Head, Gastroenterology, Hepatology and Nutrition; Director, Colorado Clinical and Translational Sciences Institute; and Arnold Silverman MD Chair in Digestive Health, University of Colorado School of Medicine and Children's Hospital Colorado, Aurora, CO, USA

Nancy B. Spinner PhD

Professor of Pathology and Genetics, Chief, Division of Genomic Diagnostics, and Evelyn Willing Bromley Chair of Pediatric Pathology, Department of Pathology Perelman School of Medicine at the University of Pennsylvania, Children's Hospital of Pennsylvania, Pittsburgh, PA, USA

Robert H. Squires MD

Clinical Director, Pediatric Gastroenterology, Hepatology and Nutrition, Children's Hospital of Pittsburgh of UPMC, and Professor of Pediatrics, University of Pittsburgh, Pittsburgh, PA, USA

Robert D. Steiner MD FAAP FACMG

Credit Unions for Kids Professor of Pediatric Research, Vice Chair for Research in Pediatrics, Department of Pediatrics, Medical and Molecular Genetics and Program in Molecular and Cellular Biosciences, Oregon Health and Science University, Portland, OR, USA

Frederick J. Suchy MD

Chief Research Officer, and Director, Children's Hospital Colorado Research Institute, Children's Hospital Colorado; Professor of Pediatrics and Associate Dean for Child Health Research, University of Colorado School of Medicine, Aurora, CO, USA

Shikha S. Sundaram MD MSc

Assistant Professor of Pediatrics, Section of Gastroenterology, Hepatology and Nutrition, Children's Hospital Colorado and University of Colorado School of Medicine, Aurora, CO, USA

Riccardo A. Superina MD

Professor, Department of Surgery, Northwestern University Feinberg School of Medicine, and Ann and Robert G. Lurie Children's Hospital of Chicago, Siragusa Transplant Center, Chicago, IL, USA

Gregory M. Tiao MD

Attending Surgeon, Division of Pediatric General and Thoracic Surgery, Associate Professor of Surgery and Pediatrics, and, Surgical Director of Liver Transplantation, Cincinnati Children's Hospital Medical Center, Cincinnati, OH, USA

Paul A. Watkins MD PhD

Professor of Neurology, Johns Hopkins University School of Medicine, Kennedy Krieger Institute, Baltimore, MD, USA

Peter F. Whittington MD

Professor of Pediatrics and Medicine, Northwestern University Feinberg School of Medicine, and Director, Siragusa Transplantation Center, Ann and Robert H. Lurie Children's Hospital of Chicago, Chicago, IL, USA

Derek Wong MD

Assistant Professor of Pediatrics, Division of Medical Genetics, David Geffen School of Medicine at University of California Los Angeles, CA, USA

Stavra A. Xanthakos MD MS

Assistant Professor, Division of Gastroenterology, Hepatology and Nutrition, University of Cincinnati Department of Pediatrics, Cincinnati Children's Hospital Medical Center, Cincinnati, OH, USA

Yiwei Zong PhD

Associate Project Manager, Department of Strategic Management, China Resources, China

Preface

Seven years have passed since the publication of the third edition of *Liver Disease in Children*. This text continues to be the premier, comprehensive reference on pediatric liver disease. Pediatric hepatology continues to grow and evolve as a distinct discipline and so it remains a challenge to provide comprehensive coverage without markedly increasing the length of this text. To keep the size of this textbook within limits, the number of references for each chapter has been limited to classical and the most relevant current citations. The editors felt that this was a reasonable compromise, since ready access to the literature is possible through resources such as PubMed.

We have appreciated the contributions of so many of our colleagues over the past two decades, but to ensure a fresh perspective and to involve experts who have emerged in the field, 11 of the chapters are written by authors contributing to this textbook for the first time. These contributors have provided particular expertise in areas such as liver development, autoimmune liver disease, intestinal failure-associated liver disease, fatty liver disease, and inborn errors of metabolism. There is also expanded coverage of liver transplantation.

As has been the case with its predecessors, this fourth edition presents a critical review of pediatric hepatology and its scientific underpinnings by recognized experts in the field. Major advances have occurred, notably in the understanding of liver development, molecular physiology of the liver and biliary tract, and molecular virology. Our ability to diagnose and treat children with liver disease has continued to improve. Genome-wide association studies are defining new risk factors for disorders such as non-alcoholic fatty liver disease, hepatitis B and C infection, biliary atresia, hepatic malignancy, and autoimmune liver disease. The ability to diagnose previously enigmatic disorders or identify modifier genes through whole exome or whole genome sequencing is becoming more common. The correlation of phenotype with genotype is sometimes possible. Genetic determinants of liver fibrosis are also being identified. Variants in genes involved in drug metabolism, drug transport, and the immune response have been linked to the risk of some adverse drug reactions. Emerging technologies are bearing fruit as new therapeutics for liver disease and hepatic fibrosis are becoming available, and these will need detailed evaluation in children. There is increasing emphasis on the notion of personalized medicine in which thorough phenotyping of patients is correlated with a wealth of genomic data to better understand and treat our patients.

We are grateful to all of our contributing authors for their efforts in crafting the fourth edition of *Liver Disease in Children*. We are confident that it will remain an essential reference for all physicians involved in the care of children with liver disease.

Frederick J. Suchy MD
Ronald J. Sokol MD
William F. Balistreri MD

Liver development

Yiwei Zong and Joshua R. Friedman

Introduction

Liver development requires two linked processes: differentiation of the various hepatic cell types from their embryonic progenitors and the arrangement of those cells into structures that permit the distinctive circulatory, metabolic, and excretory functions of the liver.

Primarily through the use of rodent, fish, and frog model systems, many essential regulators of liver development have been identified. These include extracellular signaling molecules, intracellular signal transduction pathways, and transcription factors. In recent years, transcriptional regulation by microRNA has also been implicated in liver development. In addition, a class of biliary diseases associated with defects in the cholangiocyte cilium has highlighted the importance of this structure in bile duct morphology and cellular polarity.

This chapter describes the stages of liver development in conjunction with their associated molecular pathways. Whenever relevant, links to pediatric liver disease will be indicated.

One important insight that has emerged from the study of liver development is that the process is not complete at birth, because bile duct remodeling is ongoing (see below). In addition, it has become clear that many of the molecular pathways that direct liver development are reactivated during the course of liver regeneration. Therefore insights derived from the embryonic and fetal liver may be relevant in the context of liver injury at any age.

Overview of liver development

Following gastrulation, all animal embryos are composed of three germ layers: the ectoderm, mesoderm, and endoderm. In humans, gastrulation occurs at approximately day 16 of gestation (embryonic day 7 in the mouse). The major epithelial cells of the liver – hepatocytes and cholangiocytes – are derived from the endoderm (Figure 1.1). However, these cells represent only about two-thirds of the liver volume. The remaining one-third consists of a variety of cells derived primarily from

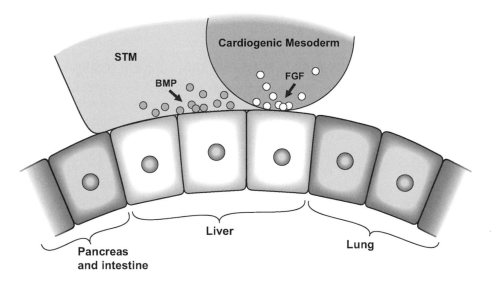

Figure 1.1 Liver specification. Liver specification occurs when the ventral foregut endoderm receives inductive signals from the adjacent cardiogenic mesoderm and the septum transversum mesenchyme (STM). BMP, bone morphogenetic protein; FGF, fibroblast growth factor.

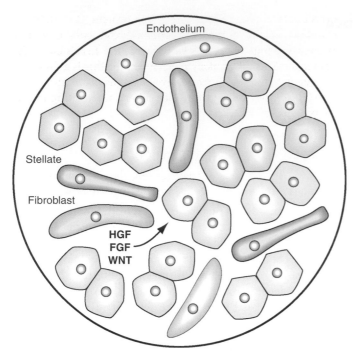

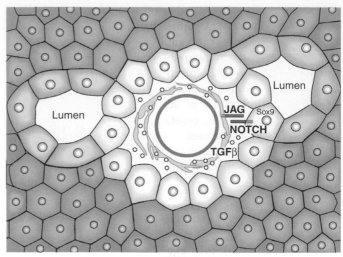

Figure 1.3 The ductal plate. In response to transforming growth factor-β (TGFβ), hepatoblasts in a ring surrounding the portal vein differentiate to form the ductal plate. In a process dependent on JAGGED/NOTCH signaling and regulated by SOX9, the periportal ductal plate cells induce cholangiocyte differentiation in more peripheral hepatoblasts, resulting in ductules.

Figure 1.2 The liver bud. Proliferation and expansion of hepatoblasts into the septum transversum mesenchyme requires signals from endothelium and mesenchymal cells, resulting in formation of the liver bud. FGF, fibroblast growth factor; HGF, hepatocyte growth factor.

the mesoderm, including vascular cell types: Kupffer cells, stellate cells, fibroblasts, and leukocytes. Therefore, liver development requires the coordinated integration of these cells from distinct embryonic layers into a single whole.

The first stage of liver development is *specification*, during which endoderm cells adjacent to the cardiogenic mesoderm begin to differentiate into hepatoblasts, as indicated by the expression of proteins such as albumin and α-fetoprotein (Figure 1.1). This is followed by *liver bud formation* and *expansion*: the hepatoblasts proliferate and penetrate the endoderm basement membrane to form the liver bud (Figure 1.2). In humans, this occurs at approximately day 25 (E9 in the mouse). The liver bud then expands in size, intercalating into the adjacent septum transversum mesenchyme (STM), in the process surrounding angioblasts that will ultimately give rise to the portal veins. Other mesenchymal cells are integrated into the liver at this stage and will differentiate into fibroblasts and stellate cells [1].

During the *epithelial differentiation* stage, hepatoblasts mature into hepatocytes or differentiate into cholangiocytes. The differentiation of cholangiocytes occurs in a distinctive spatial pattern, first indicated by the expression of cytokeratin 19 in a sheath of cells surrounding each portal vein branch; this structure is called the *ductal plate* (Figure 1.3). At one or two points along the circumference of the ductal plate, some adjacent hepatoblasts are also induced to differentiate into cholangiocytes, forming a tubular lumen between these cells and the first layer of ductal plate cells. These structures develop into the bile ducts, while the remainder of the ductal plate is lost, most likely via transdifferentiation into periportal hepatocytes [2]. Several congenital diseases are associated with defects in the development and maturation of the ductal plate; collectively, these are referred to as *ductal plate malformations* (see below and Chapter 41). The hepatic artery is the last component of the *portal triad* (portal vein, bile duct(s), and hepatic artery) to appear, and it is dependent on preceding bile duct development [3]. Although the process of hepatic arteriogenesis is not fully characterized, it is likely to involve signaling between the bile ductules and angioblasts in the periportal zone.

Liver specification

Importance of signals from adjacent tissues

In the mouse embryo, the endoderm at E8 comprises approximately 500 cells. Of these, only a few cells in the ventral foregut endoderm will be specified as hepatoblasts (Figure 1.1). This is the combinatorial effect of signals transmitted by the adjacent cardiac mesoderm (CM) and STM, both of which are required for the initial stages of liver development [4–6]. Initially, the endoderm in contact with the CM is stimulated by fibroblast growth factor (FGF) released by the CM. The dose of FGF received is critical, because exposure to higher levels of FGF results in the differentiation of the endoderm to lung rather than liver, and lower levels of FGF result in pancreatic differentiation [7]. Further development of the embryo places the ventral foregut endoderm in contact with the STM, from which the endoderm receives secreted bone morphogenic proteins (BMPs). Both FGF and BMP signals are required for liver specification [4–6].

The secreted glycoproteins of the WNT family also play an essential role in liver development, as indicated by studies in zebrafish and frog (*Xenopus*) models. At the earliest stages, in the zebrafish the Wnt pathway must be repressed to allow the establishment of the foregut endoderm following gastrulation [8,9]. Later, the Wnt family members Wnt2bb and Wnt2 are required for liver specification and expansion of the liver bud [10]. This example illustrates the general pattern that *regulators often function at multiple stages of organogenesis* (Table 1.1). As a result, genetic defects may affect multiple aspects of liver development.

Transcription factors in liver specification

Members of the Foxa (forkhead box A) family of transcription factors are the earliest known endoderm-specific proteins required for liver specification in the mouse [11], and members of the Gata transcription factor family are required shortly thereafter [12]. Both Foxa and Gata proteins are bound to liver-specific genes such as *Alb* (encoding albumin) in the endoderm *before* these genes are expressed; in fact, Foxa and Gata are bound to liver-specific genes in broad regions of the endoderm that will give rise to intestine and never express *Alb*. Collectively, this indicates that a broad region of the embryonic endoderm is developmentally competent to respond to inductive signals (such as FGF or BMP) by virtue of transcription factor binding to tissue-specific genes. Known as "pioneer factors," the Foxa and Gata proteins have the ability to establish a "pre-pattern" of chromatin modifications that permits the binding of other transcription factors and the activation of cell type-specific gene expression [7,13]. A third transcription factor, hepatocyte nuclear factor-1β (HNF1β), is also required for liver specification; loss of Hnf1β in the zebrafish embryo results in liver bud agenesis through to a failure of the endoderm to respond to FGF [14]. However, it is not known if HNF1β can function as a pioneer factor in binding and releasing repressive chromatin structure.

As might be expected from the essential nature of both the liver itself and its role in fetal hematopoiesis, no human disorders have been linked to defects in liver specification, as these would be expected to result in early fetal loss.

Formation and expansion of the liver bud
Transcription factors in the liver bud

Once they are specified within the endoderm, liver progenitor cells differentiate into hepatoblasts. In order to form the liver bud, the normal cell–cell contacts of the endoderm must be released so that the hepatoblasts can migrate into the adjacent mesenchyme. This also requires disruption of the basement membrane underlying the endoderm layer. Finally, the hepatoblasts must proliferate to rapidly increase the liver mass. Several transcription factors have been linked to these processes. The homeobox protein HHEX is a target of GATA6, and hepatoblasts lacking either GATA6 or HHEX are properly specified but fail to form the liver bud [12,15]. Two other linked transcription factors are required for expansion of the

hepatoblasts into the STM. The T-box protein Tbx3 activates expression of the homeobox protein Prox1, and in mouse embryos lacking either Tbx3 or Prox1, the hepatoblasts fail to enter the STM. The likely mechanism for this is a failure to downregulate the cell junction proteins, thus preventing hepatoblasts from separating from each other and adopting migratory properties [16,17].

Inductive signaling in the liver bud

As is the case for hepatic specification, the liver bud stage of liver development depends on intrinsic signals as well as signals from outside the liver primordium. The STM into which the hepatoblasts migrate includes endothelial cells that have not yet been incorporated into blood vessels. In mouse embryos that lack endothelial cells, the hepatoblasts do not enter the STM and no liver bud is formed [18]. The function of the STM endothelium is likely to be mediated in part by the secretion of WNT ligands by the endothelium. These ligands are also secreted by stellate cells in the liver bud, although these are not sufficient to support liver bud development. The requirement for STM-derived signals is also illustrated by the absence of liver bud growth in mice lacking the homeobox protein Hlx, a transcription factor expressed in the STM but not in hepatoblasts [19].

Additional findings confirm the central importance of WNT/β-catenin signaling in liver bud development. β-Catenin is a protein with dual roles: it plays both a structural role as an adapter in bridging the actin cytoskeleton and E-cadherin at the apical junction and a separate regulatory role in transducing WNT signals. The binding of WNT ligands to their receptors on hepatoblasts results in translocation of the transcriptional activator β-catenin to the nucleus and the expression of target genes. Overall, there is a peak of β-catenin activation during liver bud expansion in the mouse, and loss of β-catenin in hepatoblasts leads to severe defects in liver bud growth and differentiation [20]. As in FGF signaling, liver development is sensitive to the magnitude of WNT pathway activity, as artificial β-catenin activation in hepatoblasts results in liver hypoplasia and defective differentiation.

A hypoplastic liver phenotype is also observed in mouse embryos lacking hepatocyte growth factor (HGF), which is released by mesenchymal fibroblasts and binds to the c-Met receptor on hepatoblasts [21]. Furthermore, HGF and Wnt signaling are linked in the mouse, as β-catenin is bound to c-Met at the cell membrane, and the binding of HGF to c-Met results in β-catenin activation [22]. Interestingly, β-catenin also mediates FGF signaling in the liver bud, as FGF released by stellate cells leads to β-catenin activation upon binding to FGF receptors on hepatoblasts [23].

While cell–cell adhesion by hepatoblasts must be decreased to permit expansion of the liver bud into the STM, at later stages hepatoblasts must adhere to each other as a normal aspect of their epithelial nature. The signaling protein transforming growth factor-β (TGFβ) functions in part to promote

Table 1.1 Major regulatory factors in liver development

Human gene or gene family	Protein type	Function
Hepatic specification		
FGF family	Secreted proteins	Specification of endoderm to hepatoblast fate
BMP family	Secreted proteins of the TGFβ superfamily	Specification of endoderm to hepatoblast fate
FOXA family	Forkhead box transcription factors	Specification of endoderm to hepatoblast fate
GATA4 and *GATA6*	Zinc-finger transcription factors	Specification of endoderm to hepatoblast fate
HNF1B	Homeodomain transcription factor β	Specification of endoderm to hepatoblast fate
WNT	Secreted proteins	Specification of endoderm to hepatoblast fate
Liver bud formation and growth		
HHEX	Homeodomain transcription factor	Liver bud formation
PROX1	Prospero-type homeodomain transcription factor	Liver bud expansion into the STM
TBX3	T-box transcription factor	Liver bud expansion into STM
ONECUT family (HNF6 and OC1)	Onecut transcription factors	Stage-specific effects on liver growth
WNT	Secreted signaling proteins	Stage-specific effects on liver growth
CTNNB1	β-Catenin; nuclear effector of WNT signaling	Effector of WNT signaling
HGF	Secreted signaling protein	Fetal liver growth
MET	Hepatocyte growth factor receptor	Fetal liver growth
Ductal plate formation and morphogenesis		
TGFB	Secreted signaling proteins of the TGFβ superfamily	Ductal plate specification
ONECUT family	Onecut transcription factors	Establishment of TGFβ gradient
JAG	Membrane-bound signaling proteins	Biliary differentiation and morphogenesis
NOTCH	Membrane-bound receptors for JAG ligands	Biliary differentiation and morphogenesis
SOX9	SRY-related HMG-box transcription factor	Biliary differentiation and morphogenesis
miR-30 family	MicroRNA	Biliary morphogenesis
Hepatocyte and cholangiocyte differentiation		
HNF4A	Orphan nuclear receptor HNF4α	Hepatocyte differentiation
HNF1A	Homeodomain transcription factor HNF1α	Hepatocyte differentiation
HNF1B	Homeodomain transcription factor HNF1β	Bile duct morphogenesis
FOXA family	Forkhead box transcription factors	Bile acid metabolism, bile duct growth
ONECUT family	Onecut transcription factors	Cholangiocyte and hepatocyte differentiation
NR5A2	Liver receptor homologue 1 (LRH1), a nuclear receptor family transcription factor	Multiple hepatocyte metabolic pathways
OSM	Secreted signaling protein	Hepatoctye differentiation
Extrahepatic bile duct development		
SOX17	SRY-related HMG-box transcription factor	EHBD formation
HES1	Basic helix-loop-helix (bHLH) transcription factor	EHBD formation
HHEX	Homeodomain transcription factor	EHBD differentiation
HNF6	Onecut transcription factor	EHBD differentiation, gallbladder formation
HNF1B	Homeodomain transcription factor HNF1β	EHBD differentiation

EHBD, extrahepatic bile duct; STM, septum transversum mesenchyme; TGF, transforming growth factor expression of the adhesion proteins E-cadherin and β_1-integrin in the liver bud. Cell–cell adhesion and liver bud growth are defective in mouse embryos lacking Smad2 and Smad3, two proteins essential for TGFβ signal transduction [24].

The fetal liver is also highly populated with hematopoietic cells, and beginning at approximately 6 weeks of human gestation it is the major source of blood cells. The hematopoietic cells and the fetal liver cells are mutually dependent. Absence of the liver bud results in death from anemia [11]. Conversely, the developing hepatocytes express the receptor for oncostatin M, a signaling molecule that is released by the hematopoietic cells, and loss of this receptor leads to incomplete hepatocyte differentiation [25].

Overall, hepatoblasts receive a variety of signals from the surrounding mesenchyme that promote the migration, proliferation, and cell–cell interactions necessary for establishment of the liver bud. The STM cells differentiate into non-epithelial cell types of the liver, such as stellate cells and perivascular mesenchymal cells [26].

Differentiation of hepatoblasts into hepatocytes and cholangiocytes

The epithelial cell population of the liver comprises hepatocytes and cholangiocytes. Hepatocytes perform the metabolic and synthetic functions of the liver, as well as the excretory function of bile synthesis. Cholangiocytes modify the bile and form the bile ducts that serve as the conduit of bile to the small intestine. At approximately week 9 of human gestation (E13 in the mouse embryo), differentiation of hepatoblasts into cholangiocytes and hepatocytes begins. This process continues through approximately 6 months of age, and thus cholestatic disorders of infancy appear in the context of a developing hepatobiliary tree. Macroscopically, the differentiation begins at the hilum and proceeds toward the periphery. Microscopically, cholangiocyte differentiation is restricted to cells surrounding the portal vein branches, forming a structure known as the ductal plate, which in three dimensions more closely resembles a cylindrical sheath) (Figure 1.3).

Hepatocyte differentiation

In differentiating hepatocytes, TBX3 is a positive regulator of hepatocyte-specific transcription factors, including HNF4α and the CCAAT/enhancer binding protein-α (C/EBPα). Genome-wide studies have shown that HNF4α and C/EBPα are bound to large sets of genes that define the hepatocyte phenotype, including those responsible for glycogen, triglyceride, and protein metabolism [27,28]. In addition, TBX3 represses the cholangiocyte transcription factor HNF6 [16]. Another hepatocyte-specific transcription factor is the POU-homeobox protein HNF1α; deficiency of HNF1α results in phenylketonuria through loss of *PAH* expression (encoding phenylalanine hydroxylase) [29]. Several other key liver-specific proteins, such as albumin, α1-antitrypsin, and

fibrinogen, are also downregulated in the absence of HNF1α [29]. The importance of HNF1α is highlighted by the finding that exogenous expression of *Hnf1A*, *Gata4*, and *Foxa3* in mice is both necessary and sufficient to convert adult fibroblasts to a hepatocyte-like state [30].

In addition to its role in hepatic specification, FOXA2 is important in the mature hepatocyte, where it regulates bile acid metabolism and is bound to many other metabolic genes [31]. FOXA1 and FOXA2 also function in the cross-talk between differentiating hepatocytes and cholangiocytes. Conditional deletion of Foxa1 and Foxa2 at E14.5 in the mouse liver leads to biliary hyperplasia, associated with excess interleukin-6 signaling from hepatocytes to cholangiocytes. Interleukin-6 acts as a growth factor for cholangiocytes, so that under normal circumstances, FOXA-mediated repression of interleukin-6 production by hepatocytes halts the growth of cholangiocytes after sufficient ducts have been formed [32]. Following differentiation, both hepatocytes and cholangiocytes proliferate to achieve the proper liver size, in a process that is controlled by Yap1 in mice, a component of the Hippo signaling pathway [33]. The Hippo/Yap1 pathway controls organ size in different tissues through effects on cell growth and apoptosis.

Other factors that define the hepatocyte cell type include several nuclear hormone receptors whose function is to respond to metabolites and xenobiotics, such as farsenoid X receptor (encoded by *NR1H4*), pregnane X receptor (*NR1I2*), constitutive androstane receptor (*NR1I3*), and liver receptor homologue-1 (*NR5A2*). Each of these genes is expressed as the hepatoblast differentiates into a hepatocyte.

Cholangiocyte differentiation and intrahepatic bile duct morphogenesis

As in earlier stages of liver development, extracellular signals are key determinants of hepatoblast differentiation (Figure 1.4). The portal vein endothelium and/or the portal mesenchyme secrete members of the TGFβ protein family (activin and TGFβ1–3), so that the periportal hepatoblasts are exposed to higher levels than more distant hepatoblasts [34]. This signal induces the differentiation of the periportal hepatoblasts into CK19-positive cholangiocyte precursors, forming the ductal

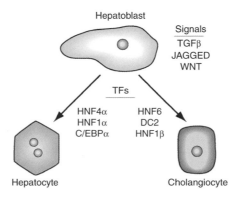

Figure 1.4 Hepatoblast differentiation. The differentiation of hepatoblasts into cholangiocytes and hepatocytes is controlled by inductive signals and transcription factor networks. C/EBP, CCAAT/ enhancer binding protein; DC2, dendritic cells type 2; HNF, hepatocyte nuclear factor; TGFβ, transforming growth factor-β.

plate. Antibody-mediated blockade of TGFβ in the E10.5 mouse embryo inhibits cholangiocyte differentiation, and in ex vivo cultures of liver bud tissue exogenous TGFβ is sufficient to induce biliary differentiation [34]. Signaling through WNT and FGF signaling is also important in hepatoblast differentiation, by promoting a cholangiocyte cell fate over the hepatocyte cell fate. Activation of WNT signaling *after* liver bud formation results in a loss of hepatocytes, whereas biliary differentiation is maintained; conversely, loss of WNT pathway function in hepatoblasts leads to biliary hypoplasia.

Two members of the ONECUT family of transcription factors named HNF6 (OC1) and OC2 link transcriptional regulation to TGFβ signaling in the periportal region. In the absence of both HNF6 and OC2, the gradient of TGFβ activity surrounding the portal vein is lost. Both cholangiocyte and hepatocyte differentiation are affected by the loss of the TGFβ gradient. There is a loss of bile duct development in *Hnf6/Oc2*-deficient mice, while the parenchymal hepatocytes have a mixed hepatocyte/cholangiocyte phenotype [34,35]. This establishes HNF6 and OC2 as key promoters of cholangiocyte differentiation.

The JAGGED (JAG)/NOTCH signaling pathway is also essential in biliary development. Unlike secreted ligands such as WNT, FGF, and TGFβ, the JAGGED ligands and their NOTCH receptors are integral membrane proteins. Therefore JAGGED/NOTCH signaling requires direct cell–cell contact. In the mouse liver bud, *Jag1* is expressed in the periportal mesenchyme, resulting in Notch activation exclusively in a sheath of cells surrounding the portal vein. These ductal plate cells are identified by the expression of the biliary cytokeratin CK19. In mice lacking Jag1 in the periportal mesenchyme, the initial biliary specification occurs, but the subsequent formation of biliary tubules fails[36], most likely because Notch activity in the initial ductal plate cells results in *Jag1* expression in these same cells – thereby transmitting the signal of Notch activation one cell layer further away from the portal vein (Figure 1.3). At one or two points around the ductal plate circumference, this results in a primitive ductule comprising two layers surrounding a lumen [37]. The remaining portions of the ductal plate do not form bile ducts; instead they become periportal hepatocytes, cells of the canals of Hering linking the canaliculi to the bile ducts, and cholangiocyte-like progenitor cells [2]. Bile duct tubulogenesis is regulated in part by the transcription factor SOX9, as conditional deletion of Sox9 in the fetal mouse liver results in a delay in duct formation. The importance of Notch signaling in controlling biliary differentiation is further supported by studies in the mouse showing that ectopic Notch activity in the liver results in excessive biliary differentiation, while loss of Notch activity leads to a loss of bile ducts [38,39].

In humans, mutations in one allele of *JAG1* or *NOTCH2* results in a syndrome of intrahepatic biliary hypoplasia, facial, cardiovascular, and vertebral anomalies known as Alagille syndrome (Chapter 14) [40]. The multisystem manifestations of JAG/NOTCH haploinsufficiency highlight the widespread importance of this pathway and its sensitivity to cellular levels of ligand or receptor.

Both cholangiocyte and hepatocyte differentiation are controlled by networks of transcription factors (Figure 1.4). Conditional deletion of *Hhex* in the mouse liver bud results in abnormal bile ducts and decreased expression of *Hnf6* and the homeodomain transcription factor HNF1β, thereby placing Hhex above these factors in the regulatory hierarchy [41]. Mice in which *Hnf1B* is deleted in the liver bud have a nearly complete lack of mature bile ducts, although the ductal plate forms normally [42]. This implicates HNF1β in the maturation of the ductal plate cells. The function of HNF1β is not strictly limited to cholangiocytes, as the expression of several hepatocyte-specific genes is also disrupted in this mouse model. Loss of *Hnf6* results in significantly decreased HNF1β levels, whereas *Hnf6* expression is normal in livers lacking *HnF1β* [34,35,42]. In zebrafish, forced expression of *hnf1b* rescues biliary defects in larvae in which *hnf6* is knocked down, supporting hnf1b as downstream of hnf6. This implies that the pathway proceeds from HHEX activation of HNF6 to HNF6-mediated activation of HNF1β in cholangiocytes. The importance of HNF1β in bile duct development is supported by the description of an infant with cholestatic jaundice and intrahepatic bile duct paucity associated with a mutation in *HNF1B* [43].

The role of microRNA

As detailed above, numerous transcription factors and signaling pathways have been implicated in hepatobiliary development. Recently, investigators have examined more novel mechanisms involved in development, including the role of microRNAs in liver development. MicroRNAs are short (approximately 22 nucleotides) non-coding RNAs that function as post-transcriptional repressors by RNA-induced silencing. Members of the miR-30 family are expressed in ductal plate and juvenile bile ducts, and inhibition of miR-30a in the zebrafish larva results in functional and structural biliary defects [44]. In cultured hepatoblasts, miR-30 regulated the TGFβ receptor ligand activin. Therefore, miR-30 may function in biliary development partly by regulating TGFβ signaling. The miR-23b cluster is predominantly expressed in hepatoblasts outside the portal area, and like miR-30 it can regulate TGFβ signaling, in this case by targeting ASMAD proteins downstream of the TGFβ receptor. Two other miRNAs, miR-495 and miR-218, may also participate in hepatocyte differentiation by repressing HNF6 and OC2. The study of microRNA in liver development is a young field and it is likely that more regulatory pathways involving microRNAs will be discovered in the future.

Diseases of ductal plate malformation

Defects in ductal plate development result in a class of cholangiopathy known as ductal plate malformations (Chapter 41). Ductal plate malformations are characterized by the retention of ductal plate-like structures in the postnatal and adult liver, often associated with biliary cysts and/or progressive fibrosis. While the $Hnf6^{-/-}$ mouse shows evidence of ductal plate malformation with cysts, no human equivalent disease has been related to *HNF6* mutations. However, haploinsufficiency for HNF1β causes bile duct paucity and ductal plate malformation in humans [45]. In addition, several congenital disorders are linked by ductal plate malformation and defects of the cholangiocyte cilium. These include autosomal recessive polycystic kidney disease, congenital hepatic fibrosis, Caroli disease, Meckel syndrome, Joubert syndrome, and others. In these diseases, cholangiocyte differentiation and initial formation of the primitive periportal ductules proceed normally, but they fail to develop mature bile ducts and the ductal plate structure is retained. This is associated with a failure to establish normal cholangiocyte apical–basal polarity. A unifying feature of these diseases is structural or functional defects of the cholangiocyte cilium. The ductal plate malformations (and their associated genes) illustrate the central importance of cholangiocyte polarity, with a basal region resting on the extracellular matrix and an apical region with a functional cilium (see Chapter 41).

Extrahepatic biliary system development

The extrahepatic bile duct system comprises the left and right hepatic ducts, the common hepatic duct, the cystic duct, the gallbladder, and the common bile duct. The cholangiocytes of the extrahepatic ducts are larger than their intrahepatic counterparts but are otherwise very similar morphologically and as measured by gene expression. The transcription factors HHEX, HNF6, and HNF1β regulate both intra- and extrahepatic bile duct development. In *Hhex*-deficient mice, the extrahepatic bile duct epithelium is converted to an intestinal morphology, whereas loss of *Hnf6* results in gallbladder agenesis and abnormal extrahepatic bile duct differentiation [35,41]. While the gallbladder is present in HNF1β-deficient mice, its epithelium is dysplastic [42].

Despite having these regulators in common, the intra- and extrahepatic systems have distinct embryologic origins. While the intrahepatic ducts are derived from liver bud hepatoblasts, as described above, the extrahepatic bile duct system originates from a distinct foregut region distinguished by the presence of the transcription factors PDX1 and SOX17. This region also gives rise to the ventral pancreas [46]. The Notch target gene *Hes1* in the mouse is activated by Sox17 and then completes a negative feedback loop by repressing *Sox17* expression in the pancreatic precursors. Through an unknown mechanism, *Sox17* and *Hes1* expression are maintained exclusively in the

bile duct precursors. Loss of *Hes1* in mice results in extrahepatic bile duct agenesis and ectopic pancreatic tissue in the biliary domain [46,47]. Conditional deletion of *Sox17* results in replacement of the extrahepatic biliary structures with ectopic pancreas tissue. If *Sox17* is ectopically expressed in the mouse, Hhex, HNF6, and HNF1β are upregulated and the ventral pancreas is replaced by bile duct tissue [46]. Collectively, these results depict a pathway in which SOX17 promotes biliary differentiation through several biliary transcription factors, while a negative feedback loop involving HES1 prevents biliary differentiation in the pancreatic zone.

It is not known how continuity is assured between the intra- and extrahepatic biliary systems, given their distinct embryonic origins.

Maintaining the developed liver

As summarized above, hepatoblasts are the precursors for the hepatocytes and cholangiocytes that are present at birth. This differentiation is apparently complete in the sense that no cells remain in a hepatoblast state (as determined by the expression of markers such as CK19 and α-fetoprotein) beyond the neonatal period. This raises the question as to what cells are utilized to derive cholangiocytes and hepatocytes and permit growth and liver regeneration after injury.

In the uninjured or mildly injured liver, it is clear that mature hepatocytes are the source of new hepatocytes, and a similar process is likely to generate new bile ducts [48]. However, a variety of experimental toxic or cholestatic liver injury models have demonstrated that a non-hepatocyte population can also supply new hepatocytes. Known as oval cells in rodents and liver progenitor cells in humans, their exact nature has not yet been fully defined. They arise from cells in or near the canals of Hering; while several marker genes have been associated with the liver progenitor cell, it is not clear if these reflect a single cell type or distinct multipotent cell populations. A recent advance in the field is the use of genetic tools to perform lineage tracing in a conditional manner, thereby allowing cells to be "marked" *prior* to any injury. The marked cells and their progeny can then be detected over the course of an injury response. This approach has revealed that cells morphologically similar to cholangiocytes and positive for the transcription factor Sox9 are capable of giving rise to hepatocytes and cholangiocytes under some conditions in the mouse. Overall, the epithelial cells of the liver can arise from different cell types depending on the presence of hepatic injury, and even the type and degree of injury [49,50].

References

1. Asahina K, Tsai SY, Li P, *et al.* Mesenchymal origin of hepatic stellate cells, submesothelial cells, and perivascular mesenchymal cells during mouse liver development. *Hepatology* 2009;**49**:998–1011.

2. Carpentier R, Suner RE, van Hul N, *et al.* Embryonic ductal plate cells give rise to cholangiocytes, periportal hepatocytes, and adult liver progenitor cells. *Gastroenterology* 2011;**141**:1432–1438, 8 e1–e4.

3. Clotman F, Libbrecht L, Gresh L, *et al.* Hepatic artery malformations associated with a primary defect in intrahepatic bile duct development. *J Hepatol* 2003;**39**:686–692.

4. Rossi JM, Dunn NR, Hogan BL, Zaret KS. Distinct mesodermal signals,

including BMPs from the septum transversum mesenchyme, are required in combination for hepatogenesis from the endoderm. *Gene Dev* 2001;**15**:1998–2009.

5. Gualdi R, Bossard P, Zheng M, *et al.* Hepatic specification of the gut endoderm in vitro: cell signaling and transcriptional control. *Gene Dev* 1996;**10**:1670–1682.

6. Jung J, Zheng M, Goldfarb M, Zaret KS. Initiation of mammalian liver development from endoderm by fibroblast growth factors. *Science* 1999;**284**:1998–2003.

7. Zaret KS. Regulatory phases of early liver development: paradigms of organogenesis. *Nat Rev* 2002;**3**:499–512.

8. McLin VA, Rankin SA, Zorn AM. Repression of Wnt/beta-catenin signaling in the anterior endoderm is essential for liver and pancreas development. *Development* 2007;**134**:2207–2217.

9. Goessling W, North TE, Lord AM, *et al.* APC mutant zebrafish uncover a changing temporal requirement for wnt signaling in liver development. *Dev Biol* 2008;**320**:161–174.

10. Poulain M, Ober EA. Interplay between Wnt2 and Wnt2bb controls multiple steps of early foregut-derived organ development. *Development* 201;**138**:3557–3568.

11. Lee CS, Friedman JR, Fulmer JT, Kaestner KH. The initiation of liver development is dependent on Foxa transcription factors. *Nature* 2005;**435** (7044):944–947.

12. Zhao R, Watt AJ, Li J, *et al.* GATA6 is essential for embryonic development of the liver but dispensable for early heart formation. *Mol Cell Biol* 2005;**25**:2622–2631.

13. Xu CR, Cole PA, Meyers DJ, *et al.* Chromatin "prepattern" and histone modifiers in a fate choice for liver and pancreas. *Science* 2011;**332** (6032):963–966.

14. Lokmane L, Haumaitre C, Garcia-Villalba P, *et al.* Crucial role of vHNF1 in vertebrate hepatic specification. *Development* 2008;**135**:2777–2786.

15. Bort R, Signore M, Tremblay K, Martinez Barbera JP, Zaret KS. *Hex* homeobox gene controls the transition of the endoderm to a pseudostratified, cell emergent epithelium for liver bud development. *Dev Biol* 2006;**290**:44–56.

16. Ludtke TH, Christoffels VM, Petry M, Kispert A. Tbx3 promotes liver bud expansion during mouse development by suppression of cholangiocyte differentiation. *Hepatology* 2009;**49**:969–978.

17. Sosa-Pineda B, Wigle JT, Oliver G. Hepatocyte migration during liver development requires Prox1. *Nat Genet* 2000;**25**:254–255.

18. Matsumoto K, Yoshitomi H, Rossant J, Zaret KS. Liver organogenesis promoted by endothelial cells prior to vascular function. *Science* 2001;**294** (5542):559–563.

19. Hentsch B, Lyons I, Li R, *et al.* Hlx homeo box gene is essential for an inductive tissue interaction that drives expansion of embryonic liver and gut. *Gene Dev* 1996;**10**:70–79.

20. Tan X, Yuan Y, Zeng G, *et al.* Beta-catenin deletion in hepatoblasts disrupts hepatic morphogenesis and survival during mouse development. *Hepatology* 2008;**47**:1667–1679.

21. Schmidt C, Bladt F, Goedecke S, *et al.* Scatter factor/hepatocyte growth factor is essential for liver development. *Nature* 1995;**373**(6516):699–702.

22. Monga SP, Mars WM, Pediaditakis P, *et al.* Hepatocyte growth factor induces Wnt-independent nuclear translocation of beta-catenin after Met-beta-catenin dissociation in hepatocytes. *Cancer Res* 2002;**62**:2064–2071.

23. Berg T, Rountree CB, Lee L, *et al.* Fibroblast growth factor 10 is critical for liver growth during embryogenesis and controls hepatoblast survival via beta-catenin activation. *Hepatology* 2007;**46**:1187–1197.

24. Weinstein M, Monga SP, Liu Y, *et al.* Smad proteins and hepatocyte growth factor control parallel regulatory pathways that converge on beta1-integrin to promote normal liver development. *Mol Cell Biol* 2001;**21**:5122–5131.

25. Kamiya A, Kinoshita T, Ito Y, *et al.* Fetal liver development requires a paracrine action of oncostatin M through the gp130 signal transducer. *EMBO J* 1999;**18**:2127–2136.

26. Asahina K, Zhou B, Pu WT, Tsukamoto H. Septum transversum-derived mesothelium gives rise to hepatic stellate cells and perivascular mesenchymal cells in developing mouse liver. *Hepatology* 2011;**53**:983–995.

27. Odom DT, Zizlsperger N, Gordon DB, *et al.* Control of pancreas and liver gene expression by HNF transcription factors. *Science* 2004;**303** (5662):1378–1381.

28. Friedman JR, Larris B, Le PP, *et al.* Orthogonal analysis of C/EBPbeta targets in vivo during liver proliferation. *Proc Natl Acad Sci USA* 2004;**101**:12986–12991.

29. Pontoglio M, Barra J, Hadchouel M, *et al.* Hepatocyte nuclear factor 1 inactivation results in hepatic dysfunction, phenylketonuria, and renal Fanconi syndrome. *Cell* 1996;**84**:575–585.

30. Sekiya S, Suzuki A. Direct conversion of mouse fibroblasts to hepatocyte-like cells by defined factors. *Nature* 2011;**475**(7356):390–393.

31. Bochkis IM, Rubins NE, White P, *et al.* Hepatocyte-specific ablation of Foxa2 alters bile acid homeostasis and results in endoplasmic reticulum stress. *Nat Med* 2008;**14**:828–836.

32. Li Z, White P, Tuteja G, *et al.* Foxa1 and Foxa2 regulate bile duct development in mice. *J Clin Invest* 2009;**119**:1537–1545.

33. Zhang N, Bai H, David KK, *et al.* The Merlin/NF2 tumor suppressor functions through the YAP oncoprotein to regulate tissue homeostasis in mammals. *Dev Cell* 2010;**19**:27–38.

34. Clotman F, Jacquemin P, Plumb-Rudewiez N, *et al.* Control of liver cell fate decision by a gradient of TGF beta signaling modulated by Onecut transcription factors. *Gene Dev* 2005;**19**:1849–1854.

35. Clotman F, Lannoy VJ, Reber M, *et al.* The onecut transcription factor HNF6 is required for normal development of the biliary tract. *Development* 2002;**129**:1819–1828.

36. Hofmann JJ, Zovein AC, Koh H, *et al.* Jagged1 in the portal vein mesenchyme regulates intrahepatic bile duct development: insights into Alagille syndrome. *Development* 2010;**137**:4061–4072.

37. Antoniou A, Raynaud P, Cordi S, *et al.* Intrahepatic bile ducts develop according to a new mode of tubulogenesis regulated by the transcription factor SOX9. *Gastroenterology* 2009;**136**:2325–2333.

38. Tchorz JS, Kinter J, Muller M, *et al.* Notch2 signaling promotes biliary

epithelial cell fate specification and tubulogenesis during bile duct development in mice. *Hepatology* 2009;**50**:871–879.

39. Zong Y, Panikkar A, Xu J, *et al*. Notch signaling controls liver development by regulating biliary differentiation. *Development* 2009;**136**:1727–1739.

40. Li L, Krantz ID, Deng Y, *et al*. Alagille syndrome is caused by mutations in human JAGGED1, which encodes a ligand for NOTCH1. *Nat Genet* 1997;**16**:243–251.

41. Hunter MP, Wilson CM, Jiang X, *et al*. The homeobox gene *Hhex* is essential for proper hepatoblast differentiation and bile duct morphogenesis. *Dev Biol* 2007;**308**:355–367.

42. Coffinier C, Gresh L, Fiette L, *et al*. Bile system morphogenesis defects and liver dysfunction upon targeted deletion of HNF1beta. *Development* 2002;**129**:1829–1838.

43. Beckers D, Bellanne-Chantelot C, Maes M. Neonatal cholestatic jaundice as the first symptom of a mutation in the hepatocyte nuclear factor-1beta gene (HNF-1beta). *J Pediatr* 2007;**150**:313–314.

44. Hand NJ, Master ZR, Eauclaire SF, *et al*. The microRNA-30 family is required for vertebrate hepatobiliary development. *Gastroenterology* 2009;**136**:1081–1090.

45. Raynaud P, Tate J, Callens C, *et al*. A classification of ductal plate malformations based on distinct pathogenic mechanisms of biliary dysmorphogenesis. *Hepatology* 2011;**53**:1959–1966.

46. Spence JR, Lange AW, Lin SC, *et al*. Sox17 regulates organ lineage segregation of ventral foregut progenitor cells. *Dev Cell* 2009;**17**:62–74.

47. Sumazaki R, Shiojiri N, Isoyama S, *et al*. Conversion of biliary system to pancreatic tissue in Hes1-deficient mice. *Nat Genet* 2004;**36**:83–87.

48. Friedman JR, Kaestner KH. On the origin of the liver. *J Clin Invest* 2011;**121**:4630–4633.

49. Malato Y, Naqvi S, Schurmann N, *et al*. Fate tracing of mature hepatocytes in mouse liver homeostasis and regeneration. *J Clin Invest* 2011;**121**:4850–4860.

50. Furuyama K, Kawaguchi Y, Akiyama H, *et al*. Continuous cell supply from a Sox9-expressing progenitor zone in adult liver, exocrine pancreas and intestine. *Nat Genet* 2011;**43**:34–41.

Functional development of the liver

Frederick J. Suchy

Introduction

The liver attains its highest relative size at about 10% of fetal weight at the ninth week of gestation. Early in gestation the liver is the primary site for hematopoiesis. At 7 weeks of gestation, hematopoietic cells outnumber hepatocytes. Primitive hepatocytes are smaller than mature cells and are deficient in glycogen. As the fetus nears term, hepatocytes predominate and enlarge with expansion of the endoplasmic reticulum and accumulation of glycogen. Hepatic blood flow, plasma protein binding, and intrinsic clearance by the liver (reflected in the maximal enzymatic and transport capacity of the liver) also undergo significant postnatal maturation. These changes correlate with an increased capacity for hepatic metabolism and detoxification. At birth, the liver constitutes about 4% of body weight compared with 2% in the adult. Liver weight doubles by 12 months of age and increases three-fold by 3 years of age.

The functional development of the liver that occurs in concert with growth requires a complicated orchestration of changes in hepatic enzymes and metabolic pathways that result in the mature capacity of the liver to undertake metabolism, biotransformation, and vectorial transport. Greengard has established a paradigm for hepatic development based on a group of several hepatic enzymes studied in the rat and less extensively in humans. In one pattern of hepatic development, enzymatic activity is high in a fetus and falls during postnatal development. Examples would include thymidine kinase and ornithine decarboxylase [1]. The activities of other enzymes are expressed initially during early fetal development and continue to increase progressively after birth. Examples include glutamate dehydrogenase, fructose-1,6-diphosphatase, and aspartate aminotransferase [1]. Another group of enzymes is expressed perinatally and continues to increase progressively after birth. These enzymes include phosphoenolpyruvate carboxykinase (PEPCK) and uridine 5'-diphosphate glucuronyltransferase (UGT). A final pattern of development occurs with enzymes that are expressed significantly after birth and peak at weaning, including alanine aminotransferase and alcohol dehydrogenase.

The stepwise appearance of new groups of enzymes during development may be related causally to sequential changes in the level of circulating hormones [1]. For example, total serum thyroxine and triiodothyronine levels of the human fetus undergo a sudden increase between the ninth and tenth weeks of gestation. Similarly, fetal plasma concentrations of cortisol and cortisone are as high by the third month of gestation as at term. There is also a sudden increase in plasma glucagon at birth, which may influence the expression of the neonatal cluster of enzymes in rat liver. The final steps of biochemical differentiation, including the synthesis of enzymes necessary to process a solid diet, occur just before weaning in the rat. A natural surge in cortisone and thyroxine at this time may be important in mediating this change.

With advances in cellular and molecular biology, mechanisms underlying these developmental changes have been found to be extremely complicated and regulated at transcriptional, translational, and post-translational levels. A complete discussion of this topic is beyond the scope of this review. Only selected examples of developmental changes in the functional capacity of the liver are discussed, particularly those with relevance to understanding susceptibility to liver disease.

Hepatic energy metabolism in the fetus and neonate

There is increasing epidemiological and experimental evidence that perturbations of perinatal energy homeostasis including maternal diabetes, maternal obesity or malnutrition, and intrauterine growth retardation can predispose to obesity and the metabolic syndrome later in life. Therefore, non-alcoholic fatty liver disease (NAFLD), the most common liver disorder in adults and children and a feature of the metabolic syndrome, in part has its origin in the fetus. Recent findings indicate that epigenetic methylation of critical genes involved in metabolism detected in human fetal tissues at birth is strongly associated with childhood total and central body adiposity, factors repeatedly found in patients with NAFLD [2].

Carbohydrate metabolism

Glucose is the primary fuel for the fetus and accounts for 50–80% of energy consumption. The fetus is completely dependent upon the mother for the continuous transfer of glucose across the placenta [3]. Maternal glucose production increases by approximately 15–30% in late gestation. The availability of glucose to the fetus is also enhanced by maternal insulin resistance. At birth the neonate must rapidly transition to independent control of glucose homeostasis. The tenuous nature of perinatal–neonatal glucose metabolism is exemplified by the multiplicity of disorders associated with neonatal hypoglycemia, including many liver diseases [3].

Glycogen synthesis begins in the fetus at about the ninth week of gestation, with glycogen stores rapidly accumulating near term, at which time the fetal liver contains an amount of glycogen two to three times higher than that in the adult liver (40–60 mg/g liver) [3]. These large stores of hepatic glycogen are important for maintenance of blood glucose levels during the perinatal period before other energy sources are available and before the onset of hepatic gluconeogenesis. Since efficient regulation of the synthesis, storage, and degradation of glycogen develops only near the end of a full-term gestation, there is propensity to hypoglycemia in preterm infants. Other sources of carbohydrates, particularly galactose, are converted to glucose, but there is substantial dependence on glucogenesis for supplies of glucose early in life, particularly if glycogen stores are low. There is significant reaccumulation of glycogen around the second postnatal week and stores reach adult levels at about 3 weeks in normal full-term infants [3]. The blood glucose concentration in the neonate can be maintained for about a 10- to 12-hour fast by glycogenolysis until hepatic glycogen is reduced to <12 mg/g liver. The mechanisms underlying the initiation of hepatic glycogenolysis postnatally are not defined completely, but a number of features are known to occur:

- accumulation of glycogen in fetal liver (to levels two- to three-fold higher than in the adult by term)
- low rates of gluconeogenesis by fetal liver
- low rates of glucose use by fetal liver
- amino acids forming an important energy source for fetal liver (extensive transamination and oxidative degradation)
- high capacity of fetal liver for fatty acid synthesis
- rapid induction of ability to oxidize fatty acids during first days of life
- fatty acid oxidation critical to support of hepatic gluconeogenesis
- rapid increase in hepatic ketogenesis after birth.

Another important feature of fetal hepatic carbohydrate metabolism is a deficiency of glucose-6-phosphatase activity [4]. This enzyme, which is present in liver and kidney, is a microsomal enzyme that is involved in the last step of hepatic glucose synthesis. Gluconeogenic flux is directed into hexose and pentose phosphate pools and to glycogen formation, with minimal fetal glucose production in the liver [4]. The level of glucose-6-phosphatase increases to near adult levels at term and rises further after birth. Gluconeogenesis, the synthesis of glucose from lactate, amino acids, and other small molecules, does not occur at significant rates in the fetal liver [3]. Fetuses are hyperinsulinemic, and insulin is known to behave as an inhibitor of the gluconeogenic gene expression program. In animal studies, fetal glucose utilization has been shown to be approximately equal to umbilical glucose uptake over a wide variety of maternal glucose concentrations. The enzymes necessary for hepatic gluconeogenesis are present in the near-term fetus. However, the level of activity of the rate-limiting enzyme of gluconeogenesis, PEPCK, is extremely low in the late-gestation fetus and increases rapidly after birth [3].

Changes in several other hepatic enzymes underlie differences in carbohydrate metabolism between the fetus and neonate [5]. For example, there is a deficiency of hepatic glucokinase, a high K_m glucose-phosphorylating enzyme, until the time of weaning. In contrast, the amount of activity of hexokinase I, a low K_m glucose-phosphorylating enzyme, is high in fetal liver and declines at the end of gestation. Hepatic glucose uptake may be limited by the ability to phosphorylate glucose in the fetal and neonatal liver. The activity of hepatic galactokinase, the enzyme that phosphorylates galactose, the other major hexose in the neonatal diet, rapidly increases near term, probably to assimilate the large intake of galactose in the newborn diet. Glucose may be taken up by the fetal liver, but this process is inhibited by lactate, amino acids, and fatty acids and is not stimulated by insulin as it is postnatally. Glucose utilization by the fetal liver is low, owing to the use of alternative fuels such as amino acids and lactate. A mechanism possibly available to increase hepatic glucose uptake is an increase in glycolytic flux resulting from a decrease in the hepatic concentration of glucose 6-phosphate [4]. The levels of activity of several key enzymes that can decrease glucose 6-phosphate, including glucokinase and pyruvate kinase, are low in fetal liver, impairing the ability of the fetal liver to increase glucose uptake by decreasing the hepatic concentration of glucose 6-phosphate.

There appears to be little hepatic glucose uptake in the neonate [5]. Animal studies have shown preferential hepatic uptake of galactose and lactate after a meal, with incorporation of galactose into glycogen or its conversion to glucose. Glucose appears to be delivered for use by peripheral tissues; galactose is used preferentially by the liver for carbohydrate synthesis.

After birth and before the onset of suckling there is a time lapse in which the newborn undergoes a unique kind of starvation [3]. During this period, glucose is scarce and ketone bodies are not available, because of the delay in ketogenesis. Under these circumstances, the newborn is supplied with another metabolic fuel, lactate, which is utilized as a source of energy and carbon skeletons [3]. Neonatal rat lung, heart, liver, and brain utilize lactate for energy production and lipogenesis. Recent studies using stable isotopes have shown that gluconeogenesis from lactate and pyruvate is established by

4–6 hours after birth. Gluconeogenesis from pyruvate contributes as much as 30% to total glucose production in healthy term babies between 5 and 6 hours after a feed. Both glycogenolysis and gluconeogenesis are stimulated by the surges of serum catecholamines and glucagon associated with birth.

After the initiation of suckling, plasma insulin levels fall and glucagon and catecholamines rise. Theses hormones activate hepatic glycogen phosphorylase, which induces glycogenolysis, maintaining glucose levels immediately after birth [3]. When liver stores of glycogen are exhausted after 12 hours, gluconeogenesis is then required. The low blood glucose levels and increased cortisol levels activate hepatic glucose 6-phosphatase, and PEPCK is induced by the reversal of the insulin/glucagon ratio. Together these adaptations lead to increased hepatic glucose release from gluconeogenesis. The molecular mechanisms underlying this dramatic change have not been completely elucidated, but PEPCK, which catalyzes the initial step in hepatic gluconeogenesis, is tightly regulated by glucagon, glucocorticoids, thyroid hormone, insulin, and glucose. A number of transcription factors that bind to the *PEPCK* gene promoter appear be important in the process, including the glucocorticoid receptor, the retinoic acid receptor, the retinoid X receptor, the forkhead box family members, CCAAT/enhancer binding protein (C/EBPα), cAMP response element-binding protein (CREB), COUP transcription factor 2, and hepatocyte nuclear factor (HNF) 4α [6]. The peroxisome proliferator-activated receptor-coactivator 1α (PGC1α) is a transcriptional coactivator thought to be a master regulator of liver energy metabolism through its capacity to activate genes involved in gluconeogenesis including those for HNF4α and GR. Another transcription factor, FOXO1, has also been shown to be required for the gluconeogenic action of PGC1α. However, PGC1α is expressed at much higher levels in rat fetal than adult liver. After birth, PGC1α is not induced further unless the animals are fasted, even as gluconeogenesis is markedly induced. It is unknown why PGC1α seems to be partially disassociated from regulation of gluconeogenesis in the fetus and newborn [6]. These data give some sense of the complexity of the changes that occur in gene expression that allow maintenance of blood glucose concentrations after birth.

Amino acid metabolism

There is a high rate of hepatic uptake of all of the essential and most of the non-essential amino acids by the fetal liver including all of the gluconeogenic amino acids. In the fetus, the carbon from these amino acids is released primarily as glutamate and pyruvate with a smaller amount of hepatic release of serine, ornithine, and aspartate [7]. In contrast to after birth, the carbon from these amino acids is released from the liver solely as glucose. Amino acids are an important source of energy for the fetus. Amino acids as a metabolic fuel provide an amount of energy for the fetus equivalent to that provided by glucose. Even essential amino acids are oxidized for energy in the fetus. In animal studies, amino acids account for approximately one-third of fetal carbon uptake and over 40% of fetal energy requirements [7]. In rodent studies, the uptake of glutamine, alanine, and lysine by the liver is much greater than their incorporation into protein. The large uptake of amino acids by the liver and the increase in hepatic concentrations of free amino acids during gestation, which decline after birth, likely contribute to the synthesis of other substrates, such as glycogen and glucose. Interorgan cycling between the fetal liver and placenta has been proposed for non-essential amino acids like glycine and serine.

Most of the enzymes required for regulation of amino acid metabolism are expressed at birth. However, there may be delayed appearance of the activity of p-hydroxyphenylpyruvate oxidase, a key enzyme in the degradation of tyrosine. A relative deficiency of this enzyme is thought to cause transient neonatal tyrosinemia.

The use of amino acids by the fetal liver may differ significantly from that by the adult [8]. For example, there is preferential use of the β-carbon of serine for DNA synthesis by fetal liver and for RNA synthesis by adult liver. The high concentration of free amino acids in fetal liver may have a key role in regulation of hepatic growth. For example, high concentrations of free amino acids suppress intralysosomal proteolysis.

Many amino acids are transported actively by the placenta through specific carrier mechanisms. Net flux of amino acids from placenta to fetus has been demonstrated for all essential amino acids and most non-essential amino acids except for aspartate, glutamate, and serine. Most amino acids also are taken up avidly by the fetal liver [8]. There is evidence for net production of serine, glutamate, and aspartate by the fetal liver, with no umbilical uptake. Studies in the pregnant sheep model indicate that maternal serine is not transferred to the fetus but is metabolized, in large part to glycine, which is transferred to the fetus and taken up by the fetal liver [8]. Fetal serine requirements are largely met by production in the liver via the action of serine hydroxymethyltransferase and the glycine cleavage system. The uptake of some neutral and basic amino acids by the placenta is in considerable excess of the estimated growth requirements, providing further evidence that some amino acids undergo extensive transamination and oxidative degradation in the fetus.

Human fetal amino acid metabolism was recently studied in healthy pregnant women before elective cesarean section at term, using continuous stable isotope infusions of the essential amino acids [9]. Fetuses showed significant leucine, valine, and methionine uptake and turnover rates. There was net transport of α-keto-isocaproate, but not α-keto-isovalerate (the leucine and valine ketoacids, respectively) from the fetus to the placenta. The data suggested high oxidation rates of leucine and valine, up to half of net uptake. The results are consistent with high rates of protein breakdown and synthesis, comparable with, or even slightly higher than, that in premature infants. The relatively large uptakes of total leucine and valine carbon also suggest high fetal oxidation rates of these essential branched-chain amino acids.

The hepatic uptake of glutamine in the fetus appears to be greater than that of any other amino acid [10]. The placenta is a major source of the glutamine that enters the fetal circulation. Net flux of glutamine from the maternal circulation into the placenta, large in comparison to the net fluxes of other amino acids, occurs and is augmented by placental glutamine synthesis. After glutamine transport into the fetal circulation, the fetal liver is the primary site for its uptake and for glutamate production and, as such, determines the glutamate supply to the placenta [10]. Glutamine is converted to glutamine and ammonia by glutaminase. The placenta can also produce glutamate by branched-chain amino acid transamination. Although glutamine is a gluconeogenic amino acid, its uptake by the fetal liver is not coupled with a significant amount of fetal hepatic gluconeogenesis. The fetal liver releases glutamate, which is taken up by the placenta and for the most part rapidly oxidized. A significant proportion of the remaining glutamine that is not metabolized to glutamate in the liver and transported to the placenta is used by the fetal tissues for growth.

The distribution and zonation of enzymes involved in glutamine metabolism during development have been evaluated extensively [10]. Glutamine synthetase catalyzes the reaction of glutamate and α-ketoglutarate with the production of glutamine. This ammonia-scavenging pathway has been studied in developing rodent liver. In adult liver, glutamine synthetase protein and mRNA are localized exclusively to the hepatocytes immediately adjacent to central veins. This restricted localization correlates with hepatic uptake of metabolic precursors used by glutamate synthetase, such as glutamate and α-ketoglutarate. Ornithine aminotransferase also is colocalized to this area. In contrast, in fetal mouse liver, glutamine synthetase mRNA is expressed in all fetal hepatocytes at mid-gestation and at term, but the enzyme protein is not detectable [11]. The shift to the adult pattern of glutamine synthetase localization in the perivenous hepatocytes occurs postnatally. This mature pattern of perivenous expression is a permanent feature of the adult liver. There is no regression to the fetal pattern with liver injury or with regeneration.

The capacity for urea synthesis by the fetal liver is well established by mid-gestation, and the liver serves as the major site for ammonia clearance in the fetus. There is significant endogenous fetal ammonia production by peripheral tissues, with hepatic clearance. Owing to a mature complement of urea cycle enzymes by mid to late gestation, there is a capacity to increase urea production with increased ammonia and nitrogen uptake.

The transulfuration pathway is an aspect of amino acid metabolism that has been well studied and has important implications for nutrition of the infant. A low level of cystathionase activity in the fetus impairs the trans-sulfuration pathway by which dietary methionine is converted to cysteine. After birth there is a rapid increase in cystathionase activity in the human liver. Moreover, stable-isotope studies in term human neonates confirms robust trans-sulfuration of methionine, confirming that cysteine is not a conditionally essential amino acid in the neonatal period [12]. The level of cysteine is 50% higher than that of methionine in human milk, supporting the notion that a sufficient quantity of this amino acid must be provided to the neonate. Similar dietary requirements may exist for other sulfur-containing amino acids, such as taurine.

Taurine is considered a "conditionally" essential amino acid, particularly in the neonate, and is not incorporated into proteins [13]. Although taurine accounts for only 3% of the free amino acid pool in plasma, it accounts for 25% of this pool in liver. In addition to its defined role in the bile salt conjugation, taurine is also involved in membrane stabilization, osmoregulation, modulation of calcium flux, antioxidation, neuromodulation, cell proliferation, and immune regulation. Cysteine sulfinic acid decarboxylase is a rate-limiting enzyme for taurine biosynthesis in the human. Another key enzyme for cysteine metabolism, cysteine dioxygenase, has a critical role in determining the flux of cysteine between cysteine catabolism/taurine synthesis and glutathione synthesis. Preterm infants are particularly dependent on an adequate dietary intake to maintain plasma taurine levels because renal immaturity impairs tubular reabsorption and an immature enzymatic pathway limits biosynthesis.

Lipid metabolism

After the first third of gestation, enhanced lipolytic activity in maternal adipose tissue related to estrogen stimulation and insulin resistance contributes to hyperlipidemia; there is an increase in plasma triacylglycerol concentrations as well as smaller rises in phospholipid and cholesterol concentrations [14]. The catabolic state of pregnancy favors maternal tissue lipid use as energy sources, thus sparing glucose and amino acids for the fetus. Maternal hypertriglyceridemia contributes to fetal growth and development and serves as an energy depot for maternal dietary fatty acids [15]. Triglycerides do not cross the placental barrier, but the presence of lipoprotein receptors in the placenta, along with lipoprotein lipase, phospholipase A2, and intracellular lipase activities, lead to the release to the fetus of polyunsaturated fatty acids transported as triglycerides in maternal plasma lipoproteins [16].

Maternal cholesterol is essential for fetal use as components of cell membranes and as precursor of bile acids and steroid hormones. Although the fetus relies on maternal cholesterol during early gestation, during late pregnancy fetal tissues have a high capacity to synthesize cholesterol [15].

Free fatty acids oxidized in the maternal liver as ketone bodies provide an alternative fuel for the fetus, augmenting glycogenolysis and gluconeogenesis [16]. The fetus obtains fatty acids through de novo synthesis, passive diffusion of non-esterified fatty acids across the placenta, and selective maternofetal placental transport for certain fatty acids, particularly physiologically important long-chain, polyunsaturated fatty acids [15]. The modest amounts of free fatty acids transferred across the placenta are stored in the liver and adipose tissue and are not used by peripheral tissues. The capacity for fatty acid synthesis by the fetal liver is high, peaking in mid-gestation [17]. In rodent models, the level of acetyl CoA carboxylase, the rate-limiting enzyme for fatty acid synthesis in adult liver, is low, suggesting an alternative mechanism for provision of CoA derivatives [15]. Maternally derived ketones and glucose may be precursors for fatty acid synthesis by the fetal liver [15].

Although some fatty acids can passively diffuse across the placenta, much less is known about transport of other lipids. Recent studies have found that mRNAs for apolipoprotein B (apoB) and microsomal triglyceride transfer protein are expressed in the human placenta [18]. Term placental tissue was found to produce and secrete apoB-100 particles in vitro. The apoB-containing lipoproteins carry cholesterol and triglyceride as well as fat-soluble vitamins and glycoproteins. The term placenta weighs approximately four times more than the fetal liver so is likely to make a significant contribution to the fetal plasma pool of apoB-containing lipoproteins.

Fat that accumulates in the fetal liver is mobilized soon after birth, not for export of free fatty acids but for local utilization [18]. The oxidation of fat results in significant generation of adenosine triphosphate (ATP) for energy and ketone body formation for use by peripheral tissue [16]. Similar to adult liver, a lysosomal acid lipase mediates the breakdown of triacylglycerols. There is rapid maturation of the ability of the liver to oxidize fatty acids during the first days of life. The liver is the main source for synthesis of ketone bodies used by other tissues. The concentrations of ketone bodies, including acetoacetate, 3-hydroxybutyrate, and acetone, increase in the blood during the first 24 hours after birth. In the liver, the postnatal development of long-chain fatty acid oxidation and ketogenesis is regulated by pancreatic hormones, the levels of which change markedly at birth, with a fall in insulin and a rise in glucagon levels [19].

The postnatal increase in hepatic fatty acid oxidation is critically important in supporting hepatic gluconeogenesis [18]. Milk feedings provide the major source for calories postnatally; this high-fat, low-carbohydrate diet supports active gluconeogenesis to maintain levels of blood glucose [17]. Both long- and medium-chain fatty acids from the diet stimulate gluconeogenesis by increasing the hepatic supply of gluconeogenic precursors and activating hepatic gluconeogenesis. In rodent models, the rate of hepatic lipogenesis decreases just prior to birth, as a result of a reduction in the activity of lipogenic enzymes. The large amounts of non-esterified free fatty acids present during the suckling period may underlie the inhibition of acetyl CoA carboxylase activity. At weaning, the lipogenic capacity of the liver increases in response to a high-carbohydrate diet. The specific activity and amount of mRNA for fatty acid synthase and acetyl CoA carboxylase increase significantly in the liver [18].

There is a marked increase in plasma free fatty acid concentrations after birth in infants [14]. Fatty acids varying in their chain length and degree of saturation have very specific roles in metabolism. Short-chain fatty acids may act as local growth factors in the intestine; medium- and saturated long-chain fatty acids are important sources of energy; polysaturated long-chain fatty acids are involved in metabolic regulation; and very-long-chain fatty acids are important structural components of membranes [18]. Free fatty acids may supply approximately 42 kJ/kg daily of energy for the newborn. Fat stores complementing gluconeogenesis in a newborn may be particularly important for the infant who is small for gestational age [20]. The induction of fatty acid oxidation that occurs at birth is part of a coordinate increase in hepatic gluconeogenesis that occurs after birth in an effort to adapt to an alteration in energy supply.

Biotransformation

The liver is the main site for metabolism of drugs and xenobiotics, and therefore is unusually susceptible to structural and functional injury following exposure to drugs and toxins. Infants and children may be more or less vulnerable to toxic liver injury than adults. Immaturity of pathways for biotransformation may prevent efficient degradation and elimination of a toxic compound; in other circumstances, the same immaturity may limit the formation of a reactive metabolite [21].

Many variables influence drug metabolism, including liver size, liver blood flow, plasma protein binding, and intrinsic clearance (a product of the enzymatic and transport capacity of the liver) [21]. Infants and young children actually have a greater liver-to-body mass ratio than adults, but many of the functions of the hepatocyte involving detoxification, energy metabolism, and excretion of wastes require significant pre- and postnatal maturation to attain adult capacity. The underlying pharmacogenetics may also influence either the affinity or the capacity of an enzyme responsible for biotransformation of a drug or toxin. The development of the array of mechanisms involved in the process for the most part is not completely defined [22].

Three general stages of drug metabolism occur in the liver: phase I reactions (oxidations–reductions and hydrolyses), phase II reactions (synthetic conjugations with sulfate, acetate, glucuronic acid, glycine, and glutathione), and phase III processes (export out of the liver via transporters on the sinusoidal and canalicular membranes) [21]. Many phase I and phase II enzymes that are critically important for drug metabolism are polymorphically expressed, developmentally regulated, and subject to considerable inducibility because of exposure to drugs, xenobiotics, and environmental factors. This has a number of effects:

● decreased capacity of the neonatal liver to metabolize, detoxify, and excrete many drugs
● deficiency of many enzymes required for oxidative, reductive, hydrolytic, and conjugation reactions
● early production of many cytochrome P450 (CYP) enzymes in the embryo and fetus, such as CYP3A7, which is involved in steroid metabolism

- delayed expression of other CYP enzymes, such as CYP1A2, important in drug metabolism
- reduced activity of many phase II enzymes, including uridine diphosphate glucuronyltransferases in fetus and neonate.

There have been many recent advances in understanding of the mechanisms that regulate the expression of genes encoding the enzymes and transporters involved in drug metabolism. However, owing to the difficulty in obtaining liver tissue from human fetuses and children, there are many gaps in our understanding of these pathways during early life. Perinatal expression of the relevant proteins may occur at the transcriptional, translational, and/or post-translational level so measurements of mRNA, protein, and enzyme activity may eventually be required to provide a complete representation.

The xenobiotic nuclear receptors (NRs), the pregnane X receptor (PXR, also known as the steroid and xenobiotic receptor), the constitutive androstane receptor (CAR), and the aryl hydrocarbon receptor (AhR) coordinately induce genes involved in the three phases of xenobiotic metabolism, including oxidative metabolism, conjugation, and transport [23]. Many xenobiotics are ligands for the orphan NRs, CAR and PXR, which both heterodimerize with the retinoid X receptor (RXR) and transcriptionally activate the promoters of many genes involved in drug metabolism. Similarly, the AhR, which dimerizes with the AhR nuclear translocator in response to many polycyclic aromatic hydrocarbons, regulates genes for the CYP enzymes. Immunoreactivity for AhR can be detected in human fetal liver, but there is little else known about its development. Both PXR and CAR are expressed at low (and highly variable) levels in pre- and neonatal human liver relative to liver tissue derived from older children, with CAR expressed at higher levels relative to PXR in prenatal liver. In contrast, mRNA expression of the heterodimer partner RXRα was less variable and did not differ appreciably between pre- and postnatal liver samples. Information is lacking about expression of the many coactivators and histone-modifying enzymes that are attracted to the gene promoters upon ligand binding and needed for the activity of NRs.

The CYP enzymes perform the majority of phase I reactions. In humans, approximately 59 CYP enzymes have been identified and these are classified into families according to sequence homology [24]. Overall levels are highest in the liver, but significant and even exclusive expression can be found for some CYPs in other tissues. Developmental expression of CYP enzymes is one of the key factors determining the pharmacokinetic status pre- and postnatally [21]. Drug-metabolizing CYP enzymes, the major phase I enzymes, are active in human liver at very early stages of intrauterine development, albeit at much lower concentrations than in the adult. The liver of the human fetus and even the embryo possesses relatively well-developed metabolism of xenobiotics. For example, there is experimental evidence for the presence of CYP1A1, CYP1B1, CYP2C8, CYP2D6, CYP2E1, CYP3A4,

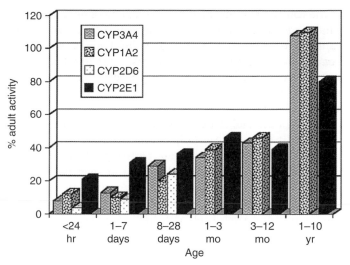

Figure 2.1 Development of cytochrome P450 enzymes. (Data compiled from references 21,22,24,25.)

CYP3A5, and CYP3A7 in the fetal liver after the embryonic phase (approximately 8 to 9 weeks of gestation) [25]. Significant xenobiotic metabolism also occurs during organogenesis (before 8 weeks of gestation). The major increase in both activity and number of different enzymes takes place after birth, probably during the first year of life. Information concerning these developmental changes in the human is incomplete [25]. Figure 2.1 shows the postnatal development of several of the more important CYP450 enzymes.

CYP1A1 is also present during organogenesis, and metabolizes exogenous toxins, some of which are procarcinogens [24]. Production of CYP1A1 declines with age and it is not detectable in adult liver. CYP1A2, important in its metabolism of caffeine and theophylline, is not produced significantly in fetal liver, exists at a very low level in the neonate, but reaches adult levels by the fourth or fifth postnatal month [25]. CYP1A2 was also not detectable in fetal liver samples (gestation 14 to 40 weeks). A progressive increase in CYP1A2 catalytic activity and protein levels has been measured: in neonatal samples at 4–5% of adult levels, in samples from infants aged 1–3 months at 10–15%, in samples from children aged 3–12 months at 20–25%, and in samples from children aged 1–9 years at 50–55% [25].

The CYP2C subfamily metabolizes many clinically important drugs: CYP2C9 is the major hepatic CYP2C enzyme, followed by CYP2C19 and CYP2C8, and these together are responsible for the oxidative metabolism of approximately one-third of clinically important drugs [25]. Both CYP2C8 and CYP2C9 are minimally expressed in fetal liver [24]. CYP2C9, which metabolizes phenytoin, achieves adult activity by 1–6 months postnatally and exceeds adult activity by 3–10 years of age. Eleven polymorphisms of CYP2C9 have been detected and this adds a further layer of complexity in considering the therapeutic efficacy or potential for toxicity of drugs such as ibuprofen and indomethacin, which are used in the neonate and are substrates for this enzyme. Protein and catalytic activity for CYP2C19 that were 12–15% of mature values were observed as early as 8 weeks of gestation and were similar throughout the prenatal period. CYP2C19 expression did not change at birth, increased linearly over the first 5 postnatal months, and varied 21-fold from 5 months to 10 years. Adult CYP2C19 protein and activity values were observed in samples from children older than 10 years [25].

CYP2E1 is present in some second-trimester fetuses and is involved in metabolism of organic solvents including alcohol and is the primary enzyme involved in the generation of *N*-acetyl-*p*-benzoquinone-imine, the hepatotoxic metabolite of acetaminophen. CYP2E1 activity is low in the fetus, reaches 30–40% of adult levels by 1 year, and is fully expressed by age 10 years [21]. After birth, hepatic CYP2D6 becomes active. CYP2D6 has many genetic polymorphisms leading to differing capacities to metabolize exogenous drugs, including psychotropic drugs and antihypertensives [25].

The CYP3A subfamily is the most abundant of the CYP enzymes and is involved in the metabolism of approximately 50% of commonly used medications [21]. CYP3A7, the major fetal hepatic cytochrome (30–50% of total liver P450), is uniquely present during organogenesis and is involved in steroid metabolism. Expression declines after the first postnatal week and is undetectable in most livers by 1 year of age. Variably detectable in the fetus, CYP3A5 is expressed at significant levels in about half of all children [25]. CYP3A4 is the major functional member of the CYP3A subfamily expressed postnatally and metabolizes over 75 drugs. CYP3A4 expression is low in the fetus and newborn but reaches 50% of adult values between 6 and 12 months of age [25]. CYP3A4 is induced by many drugs, including phenytoin and rifampin, and can be inhibited by erythromycin, cimetidine, and many other commonly used agents.

The flavin-containing monooxygenases (FMOs), encoded by six genes, mediate the NADPH-dependent oxidative metabolism of a wide variety of drugs, such as chlorpromazine and promethazine, as well as environmental toxins [26]. The development of FMO isoforms 1, 2, 3, 4, and 5 has been studied in human tissues. A comparison between fetal liver and adult liver showed that FMO1 was the only FMO that was low; all other FMOs had greater amounts of mRNA than in adult liver; FMO5 was the most prominent FMO form detected in fetal liver.

The development of phase II enzymes, including glucuronosyl transferases, sulfotransferases (SULTs), glutathione *S*-transferases (GSTs), *N*-acetyltransferases (NATs), and methyl transferases, has been studied less well than the CYP system. Sufficient information is available to indicate that important differences in the activities of these enzymes exist between children and adults and that each phase II enzyme for which data are known follows a distinct pattern of development.

An important group of conjugation reactions are catalyzed by the UGTs. There are more than 10 known isoforms; these are involved not only in the glucuronidation of many hydrophobic drugs such as morphine and acetaminophen but also in the biotransformation of important endogenous substrates, including bilirubin and ethinylestradiol. However, isoform specificity for these substrates has not been fully characterized. Serious adverse events associated with inadequate glucuronidation of chloramphenicol in the neonate have highlighted the importance of developmental changes in UGT activity [24]. There are significant isoform-specific differences, which preclude a generalization of a simple developmental pattern for UGT activity. UGT2B7 is the only UGT isoform that has been characterized during ontogeny, both in vitro and in vivo, using morphine as the probe drug [25]. Glucuronidation of morphine in fetuses aged 15–27 weeks is only 10–20% that of the adult. Morphine metabolism usually reaches adult capacity between 2 and 6 months after birth but may not fully mature in some individuals until 30 months of age. Genetic polymorphisms have been identified for the UGT family, not only affecting UGT1A, which glucuronidates bilirubin, but also three other UGT isoforms. Mutations of *UGT1A* lead to Crigler–Najjar and Gilbert syndromes, inherited forms of hyperbilirubinemia. The impact of these genetic differences on drug metabolism remains to be established because of overlapping isoform specificity of the drugs studied as well as a lack of specific probe substrates to test the activity of individual UGT isoforms in relation to these mutations.

The GST family is a group of dimeric enzymes that conjugate glutathione to a wide variety of electrophilic compounds. The eight different GST classes demonstrate considerable overlap in substrate specificity [27]. The developmental expression of these enzymes is not well defined. Hepatic GSTA1 and GSTA2 have been detected at 10 weeks of gestation and attain adult levels by 1–2 years of age [28]. Although *GSTM*, encoding GSTμ, is minimally expressed in the fetus, it dramatically increases to adult levels after birth. In contrast, GSTP1 is highly expressed in the first trimester and decreases progressively through gestation. Enzyme activity is still detectable in the neonate but is absent from adult liver. The functional significance of these ontogenic changes remains unknown.

The development of NAT2 has been studied in human fetal liver. Genetic variation in the *NAT2* locus accounts for the rapid or slow acetylator status of individuals that is important in metabolism of isoniazid. Acetylation activity by this enzyme was absent during the first 14 weeks of gestation, with some activity detected by 16 weeks. All infants between 0 and 55 days of age were phenotypically slow acetylators, whereas 50% of infants aged 122–224 days and 62% of those aged 225–342 days were found to be fast acetylators. Activity of NAT2 seemed to be fully determined by 3 years of age, with 50% expressing the slow acetylation phenotypes, similar to the adult population [29].

The SULT family catalyze the transfer of a sulfuryl group to a plethora of drugs, endogenous substrates, and xenobiotics. There are at least 11 isoforms with overlapping substrate specificity. The pattern and extent of expression of the various SULT isoforms during development are not well defined [24].

Several isoforms have been studied in detail. Hepatic SULT2A1, important for steroid metabolism, is at low levels at 25 weeks of gestation and increases to near adult levels in the neonate. Hepatic SULT1A3 is involved in catecholamine metabolism and is highly expressed in early gestation and progressively declines through the late fetal and neonatal periods. The enzyme cannot be detected in adult liver. SULT1E1, a cardinal estrogen-inactivating enzyme, achieved the highest levels of expression during the earliest periods of gestation in prenatal male livers, indicating a requisite role for estrogen inactivation in the developing male. Overall, fetal and neonatal livers have significant capacity for sulfation at a time when other phase II enzymes critical for detoxification, particularly UGTs, are poorly developed.

Epoxide hydroxylase is an enzyme critical to the hydrolysis of epoxide metabolites produced by phase I reactions [25]. Microsomal (EPHX1) and cytosolic (EPHX2) forms exist. Substrates for microsomal epoxide hydroxolase include arene oxide intermediates of several aromatic anticonvulsants, such as phenytoin and carbamazepine. In human fetal liver, microsomal epoxide hydroxylase activity has been found to be correlated weakly with both increasing gestational age and protein concentration. After 22 weeks of gestation, fetal activity is approximately 50% of that observed in adult liver. There is less known about the ontogeny of the cytosolic form. Enzyme activity can be detected in fetal liver at 14 weeks of gestation and by 27 weeks is about 20% of activity in adult liver [25].

There is limited information about the development of membrane transport proteins that participate in phase III of drug metabolism. The multidrug resistance gene 1 (*MDR1*) encodes a critical efflux pump, P-glycoprotein, located on the canalicular membrane of hepatocytes. MDR1 mRNA was very low in human fetal and neonatal livers in comparison with young adults [30]. The multidrug resistance-related protein 2 (MRP2, gene *ABCC2*) is an ATP-dependent transport protein mediating the excretion of multivalent anionic molecules including glutathione conjugates and glucuronidated compounds. The mRNA for MRP2 has recently been studied in human fetal livers at gestational age 14–20 weeks and was present at 50% of the amount found in adult livers. Moreover, MRP2 showed mainly canalicular localization, which was indistinct compared with adult liver [31].

Hepatobiliary function during development

Knowledge of the capacity for hepatic bile formation and excretory function during human development is incomplete and is derived largely from indirect evidence [32]:

- synthesis of unusual bile acids in the fetus and neonate
- decreased bile acid pool size
- low intraluminal bile acid concentrations in the intestine and gallbladder
- inefficient ileal bile acid readsorption
- low rate of bile acid clearance from portal blood
- elevated serum bile acid concentrations in the neonate.

Biliary bile acid concentrations are low during fetal and neonatal development and increase progressively in response to maturation of pathways for bile acid biosynthesis and with increasing capacity for transport within the intestinal and hepatic limbs of the enterohepatic circulation. Colombo *et al.* found that total bile acid concentrations were extremely low (<0.05 mmol/L) in human fetal bile before 17 weeks of gestation but increased 20-fold between 16 and 20 weeks, reflecting a surge in bile acid synthesis [33]. Even at birth in the full-term infant, however, biliary bile acid concentrations remain relatively low in comparison with those in the older child and adult. The ability of the fetal and neonatal gallbladder to concentrate bile acids also appears to be less developed than that of the adult. In several studies involving human neonates, intraluminal bile acid concentrations of 1–2 mmol/L have been found after meal stimulation and exhibit little variation throughout the day [34]. In the term neonate, cholic acid pool size measured by isotopic dilution methods was smaller ($290 \pm 236\,\text{mg/m}^2$) than that of the adult ($605 \pm 122\,\text{mg/m}^2$) [35]. Total pool size was even smaller in premature infants and correlated directly with extremely low intraluminal bile acid concentrations measured in the duodenum postprandially [36]. Bile secretion and bile acid output appear to function near a maximum during early life and cannot be stimulated further by the hormonal milieu of the postprandial period. Bile acid synthesis, bile acid pool size, intraluminal bile acid concentrations, and presumably bile secretion increase gradually during the first year of life in the human [32].

The factors that control the development of the enterohepatic circulation of bile acids remain largely unexplored. It has been demonstrated that infants whose mothers were treated with dexamethasone before birth to induce lung maturation in the fetus also exhibited a significant increase in intraluminal bile acid concentrations during meals, which averaged 5.3 mmol/L in infants of treated mothers compared with 1.8 mmol/L in infants of untreated mothers [36]. This marked increase in intraluminal bile acid concentrations was associated with a four-fold increment in bile acid pool size. Therefore, corticosteroids probably have a role in influencing the development of bile acid synthesis.

Bile acid synthesis and metabolism in the liver of human fetus and neonate are significantly different from that occurring in the liver of adult [37]. The presence of relatively high proportions of hyocholic acid (often greater than cholic acid) and several 1β-hydroxycholanoic acid isomers indicates that C-1, C-4, and C-6 hydroxylation are important pathways in bile acid synthesis during development [37]. Relatively large amounts of unusual bile acids are detected during infancy, particularly during the period up to 1 month of age. At that time, 1β,3α,7α,12α-tetrahydroxy-5β-cholan-24-oic, 7α,12α-dihydroxy-3-oxo-5β-chol-1-en-24-oic, and 7α,12α-dihydroxy-3-oxo-4-cholen-24-oic acids are predominant among the unusual urinary bile acids present [34]. These bile acids are unlikely to be good substrates for transport by basolateral and canalicular transporters and may not be ligands for the NR

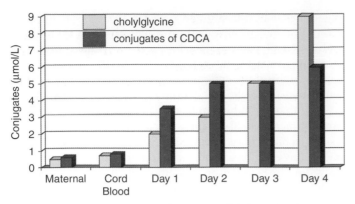

Figure 2.2 Serum concentrations of conjugates of cholic acid and chenodeoxycholic acid (CDCA) in normal newborns. (Redrawn from Suchy *et al.*, 1981 [38], with permission.)

farsenoid X receptor (FXR), which is critical for regulation of bile acid homeostasis.

The development of hepatic excretory function in the infant has been followed using serum bile acid concentrations as a measure of the efficiency of hepatic transport [38]. Uptake of bile acids by the adult liver is extremely efficient, with a high first-pass extraction rate. The fractional extraction varies considerably according to bile acid structure but may exceed 90% for conjugates of cholic acid. The serum level of bile acids for a healthy human fetus is determined by spillover reaching the liver from the intestine. In the human fetus, it has been shown that the bile acid concentrations are lower in serum from the umbilical artery than from the umbilical vein, indicating that fetal serum bile acid concentrations are maintained at a relatively low level by net transport across the placenta to the mother [39]. Specific transport mechanisms of brush border and basal membranes of the human placental syncytiotrophoblast mediate the bidirectional transfer of bile acids between the fetal and maternal circulations [32]. After birth, the conjugates of the primary bile acids cholate and chenodeoxycholate increase progressively in serum to reach concentrations during the first week of life that are significantly higher than in normal older children and adults and similar to patients with cholestatic liver disease (Figure 2.2). Unlike the transient physiologic hyperbilirubinemia of the newborn, serum bile acids levels remain elevated to a degree similar to that in infants 6–8 weeks of age. A gradual decline to adult level occurs only after 6 months of life [38]. It is important to recognize that serum bile acids are an enterohepatic "entity" with levels being determined not only by hepatic uptake but also by intestinal absorption. The rate of intestinal absorption of bile acids is determined by the load, by the intrahepatic concentrations, and by the kinetics of passive and active absorption from the intestine. The high levels observed in the serum of infants are remarkable because of the lower bile acid pool size and the immature mechanisms for intestinal reabsorption that also have been documented during this time of life [40]. The elevation of serum bile acid concentrations during the first

year of life has been referred to in the literature as physiologic cholestasis or physiologic hypercholanemia of infancy [38].

Hepatocellular transport of a number of other organic anions, including the xenobiotics digoxin, eosin, indocyanine green, and bromosulfophthalein, has been studied during mammalian development [41]. The hepatic uptake of these compounds is decreased in developing compared with mature animals. Bromosulfophthalein, a substrate for the plasma membrane carrier used by bilirubin, has been examined in several studies to evaluate the hepatic excretory function in normal human infants. Tested at birth, full-term and premature infants demonstrated delayed clearance of bromosulfophthalein from serum compared with adults if given a dose comparable on the basis of body weight. Decreased uptake of bromosulfophthalein, as well as an altered volume of distribution, has been noted in the neonatal period. The ability to remove bromosulfophthalein from the circulation improved during the first month of life. The clearance of indocyanine green also was decreased in a group of normal full-term neonates [41]. The low rate of indocyanine green elimination and the low affinity constant compared with older children and adults were attributed to a possible altered hepatic blood flow or a decreased intrinsic capacity of the liver to extract this anion from the portal circulation.

Bile secretion starts at the beginning of the fourth month of gestation in the human, and thereafter the biliary system constantly contains bile, which is secreted into the gut and colors its contents (meconium) a dark green. There is little additional information about the maturation of the process of bile formation in the human fetus and neonate. Owing to technical difficulties in performing physiologic studies in the fetus, there also is limited information about the process in animal models. Available studies indicate that the process is immature in the near-term fetus in comparison with the adult. For example, Little *et al.* [42] have demonstrated in the term fetal rhesus monkey that the sum of radiolabeled taurocholate recovered in fetal gallbladder plus intestinal contents averaged only 34% of a dose infused intravenously. A substantial proportion (18–40%) was excreted across the placenta and was recovered in maternal bile. Immaturity of hepatic organic anion transport was demonstrated further by the failure of the fetal monkey liver to excrete unconjugated or conjugated [14C]-bilirubin into bile [43]. Spontaneous bile flow also was found to be significantly lower in near-term fetal sheep and dogs in comparison with that observed in adult animals, even though these species are thought to be precocious with respect to the maturation of hepatic excretory function [44].

Studies in neonatal and, to a lesser extent, fetal animals indicate that rates of bile secretion, bile acid excretion, and bile acid excretion in response to an exogenous infusion of bile acids are decreased in comparison with the adult [44,45]. Bile flow is lowest in the most immature animals and increases progressively with postnatal age. There are significant differences among species as to how much of this developmental change is related to bile flow stimulated by bile acids – the so-called bile acid-dependent fraction of bile flow. In both the rabbit and dog models, there was an increased biliary clearance of inulin in infant animals, suggesting increased entry at the level of the canalicular membrane or through the paracellular pathway. It is possible that an increase in biliary permeability in the immature animal may allow greater excretion of water and electrolytes to maintain low rates of bile flow despite reduced bile salt secretion and a low rate of bile salt-independent flow. In keeping with the concept of a period of physiologic cholestasis in a neonate, the increase in biliary track permeability frequently is observed in experimental models of cholestasis.

In the rat, there is evidence that a developmentally related increase in bile flow rate was principally a result of the increase in bile acid-independent flow. Hepatic glutathione was low in the fetus but increased to approximate adult levels by 7 days postnatally. In contrast, significant efflux of glutathione and its constituent amino acids into bile did not occur until weaning (21 days of age). During weaning, there was a five-fold increase in biliary glutathione and a two-fold increase in bile flow rate. Biliary bile acid concentration remained constant throughout this period of development, with only a 30–50% increase in its secretion rate [46].

Factors such as hormones and second messenger systems regulate bile flow but have not been studied extensively during development [45]. In dogs studied during the first 3 days of life, the administration of secretin or glucagon failed to stimulate bile flow or produced only a minimal choleretic effect [45]. In these animals, biliary bicarbonate excretion in response to secretin increased with age and in parallel with the stimulation of bile flow. High plasma levels of these secretagogues have been detected in the young of other species. One interpretation of these findings is that spontaneous bile secretion in neonatal animals such as the dog is stimulated maximally by these hormones, and so exogenous administration no longer produces a choleretic effect. The age-related choleresis may indicate maturation of receptors for these hormones on the surface membrane of hepatocytes or biliary epithelial cells or of the postreceptor response to agonist binding.

Bile flow into the duodenum depends on bile acid secretion determined by hepatic secretory function and also on active contraction of the main biliary storage organ, the gallbladder. Recent studies have examined the volume and contractility of the gallbladder in neonates [47]. Term neonates more readily showed significant gallbladder contraction. In preterm infants, significant contraction was observed after conceptual age 31 weeks or with body weight >1300 g. In enterally fed term neonates, a 50% reduction in gallbladder volume was observed 15 minutes after starting the feeding, with return to a baseline volume by 90 minutes. In other studies, preterm infants of more than 33 weeks of gestation showed a gallbladder response to feeding with a contraction index of at least 50%. Very preterm infants (gestational age 27–32 weeks) showed no postprandial gallbladder contraction, or the contraction index was under 50%. In a follow-up study of nine very preterm infants, the contraction index exceeded 50% at a postconceptual age of 29–32 weeks [48]. The contraction index in these preterm infants was dependent on gestational age at birth and on the bolus volume of feeding.

The mechanical performance of the gallbladder in its ability to attain adequate intraluminal pressures has been examined in newborn piglets [49]. The intraluminal pressure was found to be lower at similar gallbladder volumes, and the increase in pressure subsequent to stimulation by cholecystokinin was less in neonatal than in adult gallbladders. In situ, neonatal gallbladders were found to be 3- to 12-fold less compliant than in the adult. Additional studies indicated that the neonatal gallbladder smooth muscle was responsive to both histamine and cholecystokinin; however, sufficient smooth muscle mass may not be present to lead to an appreciable change in gallbladder compliance. These data suggest that adequate intraluminal pressures probably are not generated in this neonatal model to overcome the resistances offered by the common bile duct and sphincter of Oddi.

Cellular mechanisms of bile formation during development

Similar to the process in mature animals, bile formation during development is critically dependent on the functional capacity of the basolateral sodium pump as well as on the ontogenesis of specific carriers for bile acids and other ions on the plasma membrane [32]. Almost all of the information about the cellular mechanisms of hepatic transport are derived from studies using isolated hepatocytes and domain-specific plasma membrane vesicles in experimental animals.

The ontogenesis of Na^+/K^+-ATPase activity, which provides the driving force for many membrane transport processes involved in ion uptake and excretion, has been studied in rodent liver and differs somewhat from other tissues, such as intestine and kidney. Enzyme activity was significantly lower in basolateral membranes from late fetal (day 21 or 22 of gestation) and neonatal (day 1) rat liver compared with membranes from the adult [50]. Kinetic analysis of Na^+/K^+-ATPase activity at various concentrations of ATP revealed that the maximum velocity of the enzyme reaction was 70% and 90% of adult activity in the fetus and neonate, respectively. These differences in enzyme activity were statistically significant, but it is not known whether they are of biologic importance because of the large reserve capacity of this transporter for ion pumping. Measurements of enzyme activity and protein content in membrane fractions in vitro may not correlate directly with the capacity of intact hepatocytes for cation pumping. In keeping with this concept, another study demonstrated greater ouabain-inhibitable uptake of Rb+ (a substrate for the sodium-potassium pump) by hepatocytes isolated from neonatal compared with mature rats [51]. Available studies indicate that the activity of Na^+/K^+-ATPase is unlikely to be rate limiting during development in providing the driving forces for the transport system involved in bile formation.

Bile acid transport across the basolateral plasma membrane of the hepatocyte occurs largely through an Na$^+$-dependent cotransport mechanism. Studies in hepatocytes and basolateral plasma membrane vesicles isolated from fetal and neonatal rats indicate that this process is developmentally regulated [50]. Transport activity is absent through much of gestation but is expressed just prior to birth. There is a progressive increase in transport activity during postnatal development. Adult rates of bile acid uptake are attained just after the time of weaning. Analysis of transport kinetics reveals no change in K_m, a possible reflection of carrier affinity for bile acids, but a four-fold increase in maximum velocity between 7 and 56 days of life [50].

The mechanisms for the intracellular transport of bile acids and other organic anions from the sinusoidal to the canalicular domain remain poorly understood in developing and mature liver. Possible age-related changes in intracellular compartmentalization have been demonstrated in isolated hepatocytes loaded with labeled taurocholate. In these studies, after preloading with radiolabeled plus cold bile acid (5–100 µmol/L), total taurocholate efflux, estimated by the decrease in cell taurocholate content, was unexpectedly greater from suckling than from adult rat hepatocytes [52]. Insight into why intracellular sequestration of bile acids is less effective in the developing animal in comparison with the adult has been evaluated further by assessing the activity of a cytosolic bile acid-binding peptide. The activity of the bile acid-binding protein was found to be decreased markedly in fetal and neonatal rat liver in comparison with older age groups [53]. The concentration of the protein did not approach adult levels until 14 days postnatally. In addition, mRNA for the hepatic AKR1C4, the major bile binder in rat liver, was detectable on fetal day 20 and increased progressively after birth. Development of the capacity to bind bile acids within the cell seems to parallel the maturation of mechanisms for bile acid uptake, synthesis, and canalicular excretion.

Preliminary studies have also been carried out to define developmental changes in bile acid transport across the canalicular plasma membrane. An ATP-dependent process with properties virtually identical to that described in the adult also was present in 7-day-old rat liver canalicular membrane vesicles (FJ Suchy, M Ananthanarayanan, unpublished observations). The maximum velocity for ATP-dependent transport was approximately 60% of that determined in adult liver; K_m was similar at both ages. An ATP-dependent system is functional in neonatal liver and may be sufficient for biliary secretion of bile acids at a time when other components of the enterohepatic circulation of bile acids (including synthesis, pool size, ileal absorption, basolateral transport, and potential dependent canalicular excretion) are immature.

The molecular bases of developmental changes in anion transporters are being elucidated. Detailed studies on the basolateral sodium taurocholate cotransporting polypeptide (Ntcp)

in rat liver have shown that Ntcp mRNA is absent throughout much of gestation and is first detected at day 20 of fetal life, reaching adult levels at day 7 after birth [54]. In addition, Ntcp protein is detected shortly after birth in a partially glycosylated form that persists up to 4 weeks of age. The level of transcription of *Ntcp*, as assessed by nuclear run-on studies, is relatively low up to day 21 of gestation, with an abrupt increase at day 1 and reaching adult levels by 1 week of life. It is not known how critical transcription factors, including HNF4α and the NRs RXR/RARα, which regulate transcription of *NTCP*, are involved in the developmental expression of this transporter [55]. Transcriptional and post-transcriptional mechanisms seem to be involved in the developmental regulation of Ntcp expression in the rat.

The development of the bile salt export pump (BSEP; encoded by *ABCB11*) has been studied in the rat at the level of transcription and by quantification of Bsep mRNA and protein in fetal and neonatal rats [56]. There was minimal expression of Bsep mRNA in the near-term fetus but it increased abruptly to 50% of adult levels on postnatal day 1 and further to 90% of adult values by 1 week of life [56]. There was minimal levels of Bsep protein before birth, with an increase to 40% of the adult on the first day of life; levels increased to 90% of the adult value by 1 week of life and further increased to adult values by 4 weeks of life. The patterns of Bsep mRNA and protein are quite similar prenatally and postnatally in two other studies. There was minimal transcription of *Bsep* assessed by nuclear run-on assays at the fetal age, with an abrupt increase in transcription on the first day of life. Transcription rates in adult nuclei were not significantly different from nuclei from 1-week-old rat livers [56].

Zinchuk *et al.* [57] have localized Bsep in developing rat liver using immunofluorescence microscopy. Similar to the Western blotting results, Bsep immunofluorescence was not detected in fetal liver. In the newborn animals, the staining of bile canaliculi was indistinct, whereas in adults it was very compact and sharply defined. In livers of 1-week-old but not adult rats, fluorescence was frequently seen in subapical areas of hepatocytes possibly belonging to the so-called subapical vesicular compartment.

The development of BSEP has recently been studied in human fetal liver samples at gestational age 14–20 weeks [31]. The mean expression levels of BSEP mRNA were 30% of adult values. The immunohistochemical localization of BSEP in fetal liver differed from the adult liver. In the adult liver, there was sharp-linear staining of bile canaliculi for BSEP. However, in fetal liver, BSEP showed a partially intracellular and partially canalicular pattern. These findings suggested decreased expression of BSEP and inefficient targeting of BSEP to the canalicular membrane in the fetus [31]. MRP2 transports conjugated bilirubin and glutathione conjugates. In the rat, Mrp2 mRNA levels were low through most of rat gestation, increased to about 30% of adult levels just after birth and reached adult levels by 1 week of age.

Nuclear run-on assays confirmed low transcription of *Mrp2* in the fetus and adult rats by 1 week of age. There was minimal Mrp2 protein detected at the fetal stages (at fetal days 20 and 21), with an abrupt increase at postnatal day 1. At 1 week of life, Mrp2 protein reached 35% of the adult level, and it was up to 70% of the adult level by 4 weeks of age.

Bile salts can regulate the expression of transport systems through the action of critical NRs that are transcription factors binding bile acids as ligands [58]. The most important of these receptors, FXR, is a member of the NR1 family of NRs and binds to an inverted repeat motif as a heterodimer with RXRα. Genes for bile salt transporters that are directly or indirectly regulated by FXR include *BSEP*, *MRP2*, rat *Ntcp*, *OATP-C*, and *OATP8* in hepatocytes, and *I-BABP* and *ASBT* (apical sodium-dependent transporter) in the intestine. Activation of the bile salt efflux pumps BSEP and MRP2 by bile acids is an important adaptive mechanism by which hydrophobic bile acids can promote their own excretion into bile [58]. Repression of the genes for bile salt transporters by FXR occurs indirectly. Rat *Ntcp*, human *OATP-C*, and mouse *ASBT* are transcriptionally repressed by bile salts through FXR-mediated induction of the small heterodimer partner (SHP). This is an NR (NR0B2) that does not bind ligands but interacts with other NRs to inhibit their effects on gene expression [58].

Because of the central role of several NRs in regulating bile acid homeostasis and other transport systems that contribute to bile formation, development of the most important NRs has recently been studied For the purposes of this review, only the data related to FXR and SHP are discussed [55]. Real-time polymerase chain reaction analysis of hepatic NR expression from fetal day 17 through adult revealed that steady-state mRNA levels for all NRs were low during the embryonic period [55]; FXR mRNA was barely detected at 1.5–5.9% of adult levels between embryonic days 17 and 21. However, on postnatal day 1, mRNA rose to 13.6%, and on day 7 there was a further rise to 101% of adult values. The level remained between 104% and 117% for the next 14 days but increased to 144% by day 21 of life. In contrast to FXR, the RXRα mRNA remained relatively low, between 4.4% and 35% of adult values, between embryonic day 17 and postnatal day 7 and reached 69.9% during postnatal week 4. These data suggest that different mechanisms of transcriptional regulation are operative for FXR and RXRα.

The NR SHP is a non-DNA-binding protein that acts as a strong repressor of many genes, including rat *cyp7a1* and *Ntcp*. The expression of SHP mRNA is low throughout the embryonic period in the rat (days 17–20), remaining at 0.25–0.35% of the adult. On embryonic day 21, SHP mRNA was 8.3% of the adult level but increased and was maintained at 60% of adult values between postnatal days 1 and 14. The amount of mRNA reached adult levels by day 21 [55].

The amount of FXR protein was at 16.8% of adult values on embryonic days 20 and postnatal day 7 in the rat. However, because FXR mRNA was at 100% of adult level on postnatal day 7, post-transcriptional regulatory mechanisms are likely involved in determining FXR expression in the postnatal period. At 4 weeks of age, protein levels rose to 75.2% of the adult [55].

There was also significant disparity between mRNA and protein levels with regard to RXRα in the developing liver. Whereas the mRNA levels remained at 32.8–69.9% at postnatal days 7–28, protein levels were at 113.6% and 96.5% at days 7 and 28, respectively. Because RXRα heterodimerizes with all of the type II NRs, its availability, possibly enhanced by a long half-life [55], may not be limiting the activity of these receptors in the postnatal period.

Despite the extremely low levels of SHP mRNA during embryonic days 17–20 (0.25–0.35% of adult) in the rat, SHP protein was 8.4% of the adult level at embryonic day 20. However, during the postnatal period, there was good correlation between the mRNA and protein levels for this potent repressor of cyp7a1 and Ntcp. On the basis of these data, it is likely that the repressive effect of SHP on transporter gene expression is significant only during the postnatal period [55].

The functional expression of FXR/RXRα was also assessed by electromobility shift assay [55]. The complex formed by binding of FXR to its inverted repeat IR-1 element was 32% of the adult amount on embryonic day 20 and reached adult levels by postnatal day 28. Comparison of the degree of FXR binding in this assay with the amount of its mRNA demonstrates more activity than can be accounted for by the level of mRNA, implying additional levels of post-transcriptional control. However, in the postnatal period, the temporal pattern seen in the electromobility shift assay compares well with mRNA levels (full activity at day 28), indicating transcriptional regulation as the major mechanism of control.

The clinical implications of immature hepatic excretory function are well known to pediatricians. Liver dysfunction in the neonate, regardless of the cause, commonly is associated with a failure of bile secretion and cholestatic jaundice. It is not uncommon to observe cholestasis in association with Gram-negative infections during a parenteral nutrition and during the initial presentation of a variety of inborn errors of metabolism. Increasing numbers of reports of biliary sludge formation and gallstones in critically ill infants may be a reflection of immature hepatic excretory function, particularly in regard to the excretion of bile acids. It is likely that additional forms of inherited cholestasis will be proven eventually to represent exaggeration or persistence of a developmental deficit in hepatic ion transport or bile acid metabolism. Profound cholestasis and progressive liver failure can occur in infants with several inherited defects in the pathway for the biosynthesis of bile acids. In these disorders, the lack of primary bile acids critical for generating canalicular bile flow and the toxicity of abnormal bile acid precursors lead to cholestasis and progressive liver injury.

References

1. Greengard O. Effects of hormones on development of fetal enzymes. *Clin Pharmacol Ther* 1973;**14**:721–726.

2. Godfrey KM, Sheppard A, Gluckman PD, *et al.* Epigenetic gene promoter methylation at birth is associated with child's later adiposity. *Diabetes* 2011;**60**:1528–1534.

3. Beardsall K, Diderholm BM, Dunger DB. Insulin and carbohydrate metabolism. Best practice and research. *Clin Endocrinol Metab* 2008;**22**:41–55.

4. Hay WW, Jr. Placental-fetal glucose exchange and fetal glucose metabolism. *Trans Am Clin Climatol Assoc* 2006;**117**:321–339; discussion 39–40.

5. Kalhan SC, Parimi P, Van Beek R, *et al.* Estimation of gluconeogenesis in newborn infants. *Am J Physiol Endocrinol Metab* 2001;**281**:E991–E997.

6. Yubero P, Hondares E, Carmona MC, *et al.* The developmental regulation of peroxisome proliferator-activated receptor-gamma coactivator-1alpha expression in the liver is partially dissociated from the control of gluconeogenesis and lipid catabolism. *Endocrinology* 2004;**145**:4268–4277.

7. Van den Akker CH, van Goudoever JB. Recent advances in our understanding of protein and amino acid metabolism in the human fetus. *Curr Opin Clin Nutr* 2010;**13**:75–80.

8. van den Akker CH, Schierbeek H, Dorst KY, *et al.* Human fetal amino acid metabolism at term gestation. *Am J Clin Nutr* 2009;**89**:153–160.

9. van den Acer CH, Schierbeek H, Minderman G, *et al.* Amino acid metabolism in the human fetus at term: leucine, valine, and methionine kinetics. *Pediatr Res* 2011;**70**:566–571.

10. Battaglia FC. Glutamine and glutamate exchange between the fetal liver and the placenta. *J Nutr* 2000;**130**(4S Suppl):974S–977S.

11. Shiojiri N, Wada JI, Tanaka T, *et al.* Heterogeneous hepatocellular expression of glutamine synthetase in developing mouse liver and in testicular transplants of fetal liver. *Lab Invest* 1995;**72**:740–747.

12. Thomas B, Gruca LL, Bennett C, *et al.* Metabolism of methionine in the newborn infant: response to the parenteral and enteral administration of nutrients. *Pediatr Res* 2008;**64**:381–386.

13. Bouckenooghe T, Remacle C, Reusens B. Is taurine a functional nutrient? *Curr Opin Clin Nutr* 2006;**9**:728–733.

14. Ghio A, Bertolotto A, Resi V, Volpe L, Di Cianni G. Triglyceride metabolism in pregnancy. *Adv Clin Chem* 2011;**55**:133–153.

15. Herrera E, Amusquivar E, Lopez-Soldado I, Ortega H. Maternal lipid metabolism and placental lipid transfer. *Horm Res* 2006;**65**(Suppl 3):59–64.

16. Herrera E. Lipid metabolism in pregnancy and its consequences in the fetus and newborn. *Endocrine* 2002;**19**:43–55.

17. Herrera E, Lopez-Soldado I, Limones M, Amusquivar E, Ramos MP. Lipid metabolism during the perinatal phase, and its implications on postnatal development. *Int J Vitam Nutr Res* 2006;**76**:216–224.

18. Girard J, Ferre P, Pegorier JP, Duee PH. Adaptations of glucose and fatty acid metabolism during perinatal period and suckling-weaning transition. *Physiol Rev* 1992;**72**:507–562.

19. Pegorier JP, Prip-Buus C, Duee PH, Girard J. Hormonal control of fatty acid oxidation during the neonatal period. *Diabetes Metab* 1992;**18**:156–160.

20. Haggarty P. Effect of placental function on fatty acid requirements during pregnancy. *Eur J Clin Nutr* 2004;**58**:1559–1570.

21. Kearns GL, Abdel-Rahman SM, Alander SW, *et al.* Developmental pharmacology: drug disposition, action, and therapy in infants and children. *N Engl J Med* 2003;**349**:1157–1167.

22. Leeder JS, Kearns GL, Spielberg SP, van den Anker J. Understanding the relative roles of pharmacogenetics and ontogeny in pediatric drug development and regulatory science. *J Clin Pharmacol* 2010;**50**:1377–1387.

23. Vyhlidal CA, Gaedigk R, Leeder JS. Nuclear receptor expression in fetal and pediatric liver: correlation with CYP3A expression. *Drug Metab Dispos* 2006;**34**:131–137.

24. Blake MJ, Castro L, Leeder JS, Kearns GL. Ontogeny of drug metabolizing enzymes in the neonate. *Semin Fetal Neonat Metab* 2005;**10**:123–138.

25. Hines RN. The ontogeny of drug metabolism enzymes and implications

for adverse drug events. *Pharmacol Ther* 2008;**118**:250–267.

26. Zhang J, Cashman JR. Quantitative analysis of *FMO* gene mRNA levels in human tissues. *Drug Metab Dispos* 2006;**34**:19–26.

27. Josephy PD. Genetic variations in human glutathione transferase enzymes: significance for pharmacology and toxicology. *Hum Genomics Proteomics* 2010;**2010**:876–940.

28. Hein DW, Doll MA, Fretland AJ, *et al.* Molecular genetics and epidemiology of the NAT1 and NAT2 acetylation polymorphisms. *Cancer Epidemiol Biomarkers Prev* 2000;**9**:29–42.

29. Myllynen P, Immonen E, Kummu M, Vahakangas K. Developmental expression of drug metabolizing enzymes and transporter proteins in human placenta and fetal tissues. *Expert Opin Drug Metab Toxicol* 2009;**5**:1483–1499.

30. Miki Y, Suzuki T, Tazawa C, Blumberg B, Sasano H. Steroid and xenobiotic receptor (SXR), cytochrome P450 3A4 and multidrug resistance gene 1 in human adult and fetal tissues. *Mol Cell Endocrinol* 2005;**231**(1–2):75–85.

31. Chen HL, Liu YJ, Feng CH, *et al.* Developmental expression of canalicular transporter genes in human liver. *J Hepatol* 2005;**43**:472–477.

32. Arrese M, Ananthananarayanan M, Suchy FJ. Hepatobiliary transport: molecular mechanisms of development and cholestasis. *Pediatr Res* 1998;**44**:141–147.

33. Colombo C, Zuliani G, Ronchi M, *et al.* Biliary bile acid composition of the human fetus in early gestation. *Pediatr Res* 1987;**21**:197–200.

34. Balistreri WF, Heubi JE, Suchy FJ. Immaturity of the enterohepatic circulation in early life: factors predisposing to "physiologic" maldigestion and cholestasis. *J Pediatr Gastroenterol Nutr* 1983;**2**:346–354.

35. Watkins JB, Ingall D, Szczepanik P, Klein PD, Lester R. Bile-salt metabolism in the newborn. Measurement of pool size and synthesis by stable isotope technique. *N Engl J Med* 1973;**288**:431–434.

36. Watkins JB, Szczepanik P, Gould JB, Klein P, Lester R. Bile salt metabolism in the human premature infant. Preliminary observations of pool size

and synthesis rate following prenatal administration of dexamethasone and phenobarbital. *Gastroenterology* 1975;**69**:706–713.

37. Setchell KD, Dumaswala R, Colombo C, Ronchi M. Hepatic bile acid metabolism during early development revealed from the analysis of human fetal gallbladder bile. *J Biol Chem* 1988;**263**:16637–16644.

38. Suchy FJ, Balistreri WF, Heubi JE, Searcy JE, Levin RS. Physiologic cholestasis: elevation of the primary serum bile acid concentrations in normal infants. *Gastroenterology* 1981;**80**:1037–1041.

39. Itoh S, Onishi S, Isobe K, Manabe M, Inukai K. Foetomaternal relationships of serum bile acid pattern estimated by high-pressure liquid chromatography. *Biochem J* 1982;**204**:141–145.

40. Balistreri WF. Immaturity of hepatic excretory function and the ontogeny of bile acid metabolism. *J Pediatr Gastr Nutr* 1983;**2**(Suppl 1):S207–S214.

41. Klinger W. Biotransformation of drugs and other xenobiotics during postnatal development. *Pharmacol Ther* 1982;**16**:377–429.

42. Little JM, Smallwood RA, Lester R, Piasecki GJ, Jackson BT. Bile-salt metabolism in the primate fetus. *Gastroenterology* 1975;**69**:1315–1320.

43. Bernstein RB, Novy MJ, Piasecki GJ, Lester R, Jackson BT. Bilirubin metabolism in the fetus. *J Clin Invest* 1969;**48**:1678–1688.

44. Smallwood RA, Lester R, Plasecki GJ, *et al*. Fetal bile salt metabolism. II. Hepatic excretion of endogenous bile salt and of a taurocholate load. *J Clin Invest* 1972;**51**:1388–1397.

45. Tavoloni N, Jones MJ, Berk PD. Postnatal development of bile secretory physiology in the dog. *J Pediatr Gastroenterol Nutr* 1985;**4**:256–267.

46. Mohan P, Ling SC, Watkins JB. Ontogeny of hepatobiliary secretion: role of glutathione. *Hepatology* 1994;**19**:1504–1512.

47. Ho ML, Chen JY, Ling UP, Su PH. Gallbladder volume and contractility in term and preterm neonates: normal values and clinical applications in ultrasonography. *Acta Paediatr* 1998;**87**:799–804.

48. Jawaheer G, Pierro A, Lloyd DA, Shaw NJ. Gall bladder contractility in neonates: effects of parenteral and enteral feeding. *Arch Dis Child Fetal* 1995;**72**:F200–F202.

49. Kaplan GS, Bhutani VK, Shaffer TH, *et al*. Gallbladder mechanics in newborn piglets. *Pediatr Res* 1984;**18**:1181–1184.

50. Suchy FJ, Bucuvalas JC, Goodrich AL, Moyer MS, Blitzer BL. Taurocholate transport and Na⁺-K⁺-ATPase activity in fetal and neonatal rat liver plasma membrane vesicles. *Am J Physiol* 1986;**251**(5 Pt 1):G665–C673.

51. Bellemann P. Amino acid transport and rubidium-ion uptake in monolayer cultures of hepatocytes from neonatal rats. *Biochem J* 1981;**198**:475–483.

52. Belknap WM, Zimmer-Nechemias L, Suchy FJ, Balistreri WF. Bile acid efflux from suckling rat hepatocytes. *Pediatr Res* 1988;**23**:364–367.

53. Stolz A, Sugiyama Y, Kuhlenkamp J, *et al*. Cytosolic bile acid binding protein in rat liver: radioimmunoassay, molecular forms, developmental characteristics and organ distribution. *Hepatology* 1986;**6**:433–439.

54. Hardikar W, Ananthanarayanan M, Suchy FJ. Differential ontogenic regulation of basolateral and canalicular bile acid transport proteins in rat liver. *J Biol Chem* 1995;**270**: 20841–20846.

55. Balasubramaniyan N, Shahid M, Suchy FJ, Ananthanarayanan M. Multiple mechanisms of ontogenic regulation of nuclear receptors during rat liver development. *Am J Physiol Gastriointest Liver Physiol* 2005;**288**: G251–G260.

56. Tomer G, Ananthanarayanan M, Weymann A, Balasubramanian N, Suchy FJ. Differential developmental regulation of rat liver canalicular membrane transporters Bsep and Mrp2. *Pediatr Res* 2003;**53**: 288–294.

57. Zinchuk VS, Okada T, Akimaru K, Seguchi H. Asynchronous expression and colocalization of Bsep and Mrp2 during development of rat liver. *Am J Phys - Gastr L*. 2002;**282**: G540–G548.

58. Wagner M, Zollner G, Trauner M. Nuclear receptors in liver disease. *Hepatology* 2011;**53**: 1023–1034.

Mechanisms of bile formation and cholestasis

Nikita A. Gupta and Saul J. Karpen

Cholestatic disorders comprise a large group of conditions affecting infants and children. Damage to the liver occurs from multiple effects of the various retained biliary constituents, including various lipids, toxins, and bile acids. Therefore impairments in bile flow and secretion – cholestasis – particularly in the infant liver, drive the development and progression of liver disease. With the recent findings of genetic causes of cholestasis (see Chapter 13), many of the previously labeled "indeterminate" or "idiopathic" forms of cholestasis have now been properly assigned to specific impairments in critical genes involved in the formation of bile, including a primary focus on genes for the canalicular transporters [1,2]. In a similar vein, exploration of the effects of various endogenous and exogenous factors on the expression and function of these same essential genes has led to a greater molecular understanding of acquired forms of cholestasis. It is now becoming increasingly possible to assign genetic contributors to both genetic and acquired forms of liver disease. In addition, we have an increased understanding of how these gene products are engaged in the response and adaptation to cholestasis, and, intriguingly, why these processes may not be fully adequate to protect the liver. In particular, see Stapelbroek *et al.* [1], Mullenbach and Lammert [2], and Karpen and Trauner [3], who discuss our increasing knowledge of the expression, structure, and regulation of these genes and gene products in the underlying processes that lead to cholestasis. It is now accepted that the processes of bile formation, cholestasis, and adaptation are inherently intertwined with structural, developmental, biochemical, intercellular communication, subcellular organization, cell signaling pathways, and physiological components of the liver and liver function. In this chapter, attention will focus upon the basic mechanisms of bile formation, as well as the *genetic* and *acquired* pathways that lead to cholestasis.

Summary of the physiology of bile formation

Bile constituents

Bile is an aqueous fluid produced in the liver by a number of interweaving processes, molecules, and pathways that engage intracellular and membrane protein functions in both hepatocytes and cholangiocytes [1,4–6]. In particular, membrane ATP-binding cassette (ABC) transporters play essential and, surprisingly, modifiable roles in bile formation since these are the means to deliver specific molecules into bile [4]. Of the solutes, bile acids form the major component while phospholipids, cholesterol and bilirubin conjugates, heavy metals, and a variety of detoxified and modified metabolites constitute the remainder [6,7]. In essence, the composition and nature of the substances in bile are thus under direct control of membrane transporter function, since these are the final "gatekeepers" that either permit or do not permit their delivery into bile.

Bile formation physiology

Bile formation occurs mainly via the secretion of solutes and water from both hepatocytes and cholangiocytes [8]. Among the many functions of bile, and maintenance of its flow, is to fulfill the role of the liver as an excretory organ, with the endpoint of delivery being the intestinal lumen, and ultimately, fecal elimination. In general, toxic substances, drugs, endobiotics, and xenobiotics that are modified and detoxified by hepatocytes are efficiently excreted into bile to provide an overall survival benefit for the organism. Moreover, the role of intestinal luminal bile acids as a principal aid for the absorption of long-chain fats and fat-soluble vitamins inherently links bile acid flux across the hepatocyte with nutrition and overall health. This has particular relevance for the growth impairments seen in children with many different forms of neonatal cholestasis since the health of infants is particularly susceptible to any impediments to normal growth.

Bile flow dynamics: receptors and disease

The main driving force for bile flow is the secretion and recirculation of bile acids [7]. Bile acids are efficiently taken up from the portal circulation via several resident transporter proteins, primarily the Na^+-dependent bile acid importer (NTCP, or SLC10A1), and various organic anion transporters (members of the organic anion transporter family) [9,10]. Bile acids are rapidly transported across the cytoplasm of

---

Liver Disease in Children, Fourth Edition, ed. Frederick J. Suchy, Ronald J. Sokol, and William F. Balistreri. Published by Cambridge University Press. © Cambridge University Press 2014.

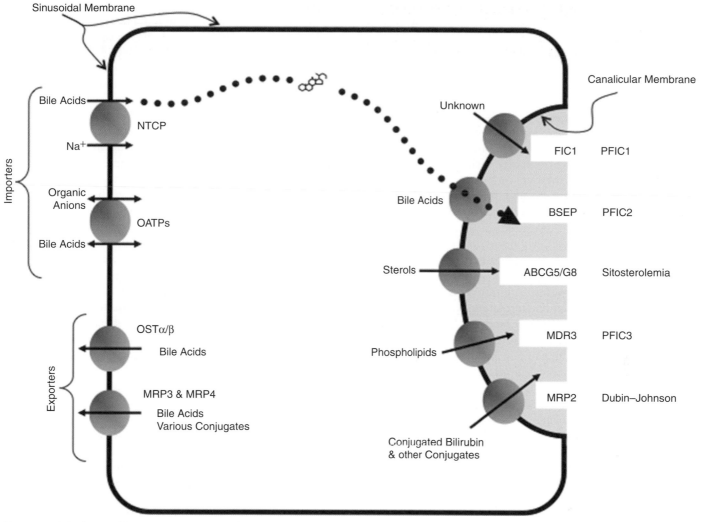

Figure 3.1 Roles for critical hepatic transporters in the formation of bile and adaptation to cholestasis. The sinusoidal surface is shown on the left and the canalicular surface on the right. Diseases associated with defects in specific genes for canalicular transporters are given on the right. Note that bile acids have several means of transport across the sinusoidal membrane, both import and export, while there is one canalicular bile acid transporter, the bile salt export pump (BSEP). These transporters allow for fine tuning of intracellular bile acid concentrations as a means to adapt to a variety of cholestatic conditions. The dotted line shows the principal means for bile acid flux across the hepatocyte. NTCP, Na$^+$/taurocholate cotransporting polypeptide; OATP, organic acid-transporting polypeptide; OST, organic solute transporter; MRP, multidrug resistance-associated protein; FIC1, familial intrahepatic cholestasis 1; MDR, multidrug-resistance protein. Official gene designations: FIC1 (*ATP8B1*), BSEP (*ABCB11*), MDR3 (*ABCB4*), MRP2 (*ABCC2*).

hepatocytes mainly via unknown mechanisms, and efficiently secreted into the canalicular lumen via an ATP cassette transporter, known as the bile salt export pump (BSEP; encoded by *ABCB11*) [11,12]. It is the secretion of bile acids against a steep concentration gradient that is the ultimate, rate-limiting step of bile secretion (Figure 3.1). As expected, when this transporter is mutated, bile acid flow is reduced and bile acids are retained within hepatocytes, leading to the liver disease known as progressive familial intrahepatic cholestasis (PFIC) type 2 (see Chapter 13). The other main solutes in bile, phospholipids, cholesterol, and bilirubin conjugates, are also secreted into bile via substrate-specific ABC transporters. Phospholipids are secreted via a "floppase," the multidrug resistance-associated protein 3 (MDR3; encoded by *ABCB4*), which, when mutated, leads to the disease PFIC3 [2,13,14].

Cholesterol is secreted via two half-transporters combined of the ABC family (encoded by *ABCG5* and *ABCG8*, respectively); if either gene is mutated, this leads to the disease sitosterolemia, and perhaps to liver disease [15]. Finally, conjugated bilirubin appears to be excreted into bile primarily via the multidrug resistance-associated protein 2 (MRCP2, encoded by *ABCC2*); mutation of this gene leads to Dubin–Johnson syndrome [16]. Recent studies have given further insight into the pathogenesis of these defects. It is now known that in single gene defects there may be aberrant pre-mRNA splicing and/or abnormal protein processing/functioning, opening up therapeutic opportunities for targeted mutation-specific therapies [17,18]. These discoveries and assignments of specific genes to specific biliary transport functions have led to an exciting and expanding understanding of the molecular determinants of bile formation, but have also led to a greater understanding of how these physiological processes can be suppressed with either mutations or alterations in gene expression and protein activity. For a detailed discussion of roles for FIC1, BSEP, and MDR3 and their genes, and the diseases caused by mutations, see Chapter 13.

Of clinical interest is the molecular distinction between bile acid flux across the hepatocyte and the export conjugated bilirubin, although clinically, the two are generally considered linked events during cholestasis. But since the two substances are transported by distinct transporters with different substrate affinities and regulation, there are certainly situations where an individual can be cholestatic and have normal conjugated bilirubin flux, and times where elevated conjugated bilirubin levels are a marker for impaired MRP2 production (e.g. Dubin–Johnson syndrome), while bile flow is normal. This is just one indication of the evolving nature of information about bile formation over the past few years, with an expectation that these discoveries will continue to improve our understanding of the molecular nature of bile formation.

In addition to flux of these solutes, bile formation is dependent upon ion flux in both hepatocytes and cholangiocytes. In humans, up to 40% of bile formation is derived from bile ducts [6], and a main determinant of bile flow is the secretion of chloride, which is primarily determined by the apical positioning of the cystic fibrosis transmembrane conductance regulator in cholangiocytes [8]. In diseases where bile duct development is impaired, as in Alagille syndrome (see Chapter 14) cholestasis is a common clinical feature.

General principles of cholestasis and hepatic adaptation

The definition of cholestasis as a blockage or severe impairment in the flow of bile is true in a few disease states that affect the overall "plumbing" of the liver (e.g. biliary atresia, common bile duct obstruction), but with more sophisticated recent genetic understanding of bile formation, it is clear that cholestasis can occur without frank ductal obstruction when there is impaired functioning of the proteins necessary for the formation of bile. Bile is composed of numerous substances, but the main solutes (salts, bile acids, phospholipids, cholesterol, bilirubin) each have a particular molecular method of becoming part of bile, mainly via substrate-specific canalicular transporters [6]. The main components of bile are bile acids, and it is the flux/recirculation of bile acids that is the main driving force to bile formation. The liver, and in particular the polarized hepatocyte, is the primary tissue that is responsible for the synthesis and transport of bile acids, and thus is most likely to be damaged by bile acid retention when bile flow is reduced. Bile acid concentration in peripheral circulation is generally <10 μmol/L, while that in portal blood varies from low 10–20 μmol/L between meals to upwards of 100 μmol/L postprandially, while there is a significant gradient of concentrations in bile itself up to 3–30 mmol/L [19]. Therefore, the

highest concentration of bile acids is in the canalicular lumen, and it is the intracellular retention of bile acids that appears to be the most important disease-producing consequence of cholestasis, and is the focus of adaptation. If bile flow is obstructed either downstream (e.g. Alagille syndrome-associated bile duct paucity or biliary atresia), or right at the canalicular membrane (e.g. PFIC2), bile acid concentrations will rise within hepatocytes. Bile acids are both detergents and signaling molecules and, when retained within hepatocytes, lead to altered membrane composition and function, derangements of subcellular organelles, and broad changes in cell signaling pathways and gene expression [20]. Some of these changes lead to attempts at adaptation by reducing either the toxicity or concentration of retained bile acids by P450-based mechanisms or sinusoidal export, respectively [21]. Prolonged retention of bile acids within the liver leads to activation of Kupffer cells, stellate cells, and myofibroblasts, with consequent increased production of cytokines and progression of fibrosis. Therefore, the overall effects of cholestasis, perhaps even long term, can in a broad way be ascribed to the effects of retained bile acids. Finally, little is known about the actual molecular causes of the enhanced susceptibility of the infant liver to cholestatic insults, although an immaturity of bile acid flux is present [22,23].

Over the past few years, much has been understood about how the hepatocyte responds to, and adapts to, retained bile acids. Less is known about cholangiocytes. The hepatocyte is poised to respond to retained bile acids with a coordinated approach that treats retained bile acids as if they were a dangerous, foreign compound: that is, high levels of retained bile acids as xenotoxic endobiotics. Multiple processes, both transcriptional (mainly nuclear receptor mediated) and post-transcriptional, are engaged in the hepatocyte [5,21,24] with the overall concept being to reduce concentration by suppressing bile acid import and synthesis, reduce toxicity with hydroxylation and conjugation, and to increase export by sinusoidal, and to a lesser extent, canalicular efflux. At the transcriptional level, bile acids are activators of at least three members of the nuclear receptor (NR) superfamily – the constitutive androstane receptor (CAR), the pregnane X receptor (PXR), and the farsenoid X receptor (FXR) – and these three gene regulators are the primary means for effecting the transcriptional reprogramming of the hepatocyte in cholestasis. Genetically modified mice with mutations in any of these genes are essentially normal, except when exposed to cholestatic conditions. In cholestasis, mice without any one or more of these three regulators rapidly develop hepatocyte apoptosis and necrosis, all apparently by an inability to adapt to retained bile acids. Some of the other receptors which have been implicated include the vitamin D receptor [25], the glucocorticoid receptor [26] and liver receptor homolog-1 [27]. These receptors have been a target for several drugs such as ursodeoxycholic acid and budesonide, both of which have been used in primary biliary cirrhosis, with mixed results. Another cell membrane receptor, TGR5, has been alluded to as having a crucial role in mediating the systemic actions of bile acids [28]. Importantly, in genetically normal mice, these NR-regulated adaptive mechanisms can be enhanced with small molecules that bind to the NR, lending an exciting prospect for future treatment paradigms (see below). Although the expression of some NRs has been studied in humans and experimental animals with various forms of cholestasis, there is little information on how assembly of coregulators and histone-modifying enzymes that regulate the function of NRs are involved in perpetuating and adapting to cholestasis. There are a number of possible mechanisms: (1) the production of coactivators and histone-modifying enzymes may be impaired or induced in cholestasis, (2) their recruitment to the nucleosome may be disrupted by alterations in chromatin structure, and (3) there may be active recruitment of corepressors and histone deacetylases to the promoters of critical genes.

Genetic mechanisms of cholestasis and development of bile formation

There are multiple genetic mechanisms that lead to cholestasis, most involving mutations in genes for critical hepatobiliary transporter or formation/structure of bile ducts. An impaired ability to transport essential biliary substances across the canalicular membrane of the hepatocyte leads to obligate retention of that substance within hepatocytes (e.g. PFIC2, bile acids) or a deficiency of a substance in the biliary lumen (e.g. PFIC3, phospholipids), leading to bile acid induced damage in hepatocytes or cholangiocytes, respectively [4]. It is readily understood that an inability to export bile acids is an important factor. However, although increasing evidence points to various other factors such as aberrant pre-mRNA splicing and defective protein levels and function [18], exactly why mutations in select gene products leads to disease is not always clear,

Acquired mechanisms of cholestasis

In addition to the single gene defects noted above that can lead to cholestasis, it is generally more prevalent that multifactorial, or structural, mechanisms are the main participants. Of these, drug-induced, total parenteral nutrition (TPN) or sepsis/inflammation induced mechanisms are now being recognized to have molecular underpinnings.

Sepsis-associated cholestasis

Osler was among the first to describe the association of non-hepatitic infections leading to a functional impairment in bile flow; "toxemic jaundice" [29]. It has been well known, but poorly understood, that such cholestasis does not result from damage or destruction of hepatocytes but is a functional impairment from either bacterial products (e.g. endotoxin), or inflammation-induced cytokines. Infants in particular are more susceptible to the effects of sepsis on bile flow, perhaps

due to immaturity of bile formation or adaptive mechanisms [30,31]. Sepsis-associated cholestasis is a principal cause of cholestasis in adults as well, although it is not usually at the top of the list of differential diagnoses. Administration of endotoxin (bacterial lipopolysaccharides from Gram-negative bacteria) to nearly all animal models leads to a rapid and sustained impairment in bile flow [32,33]. These effects appear to be caused by the release of endotoxin-induced cytokines from resident hepatic macrophages, Kupffer cells, which, in turn, act upon receptors in the sinusoidal membrane of neighboring hepatocytes to induce cell signaling changes that lead to reduced bile formation. The inflammatory milieu causes stimulation of a proinflammatory signaling cascade, which leads to reduced expression and activity of a large number of nuclear transcriptional regulators many of which are essential for maintenance of hepatobiliary transporter gene expression [32].

It is also likely the endotoxin may act directly upon hepatocytes and cholangiocytes, since these cells have cell surface receptors for endotoxin and other microbial products [31]. In addition, the liver is a central player in the hepatic response to infection and injury – the acute phase response – of which one may reasonably include sepsis-associated cholestasis as a component. The hepatic acute phase response is a coordinated transcriptional reprogramming and prioritization of liver function as a means to restore homeostasis and help with injury repair and infection throughout the body. When activated by mediators of inflammation such as endotoxin, the liver changes gene expression to increase secretion of many substances and enzymes to restore homeostasis (e.g. protease inhibitors), fight infection (e.g. complement, C-reactive peptide), and direct amino acids and lipids to the periphery; this is all coordinated via intracellular complex and overlapping cell signaling pathways initiated by endotoxin and cytokines such as tumor necrosis factor-α and interleukins 1β and 6 [34]. These same cytokines that activate the expression of secretory substances from the liver during the acute phase response are also involved in the suppression of function and expression of critical hepatobiliary transporters.

When exposed to lipopolysaccharide (LPS), bile flow is rapidly and profoundly reduced via a combination of molecular targeting of cell signaling pathways at existing membrane transporter proteins and control of transporter gene transcription in the nucleus [35]. Within 15–60 minutes after exposure to LPS, membrane localization of both BSEP and MRP2 are significantly reduced, apparently through both degradation and trafficking from canalicular membranes into submembrane vesicles [36,37]. Variable effects on FIC1, and MDR3 proteins have been seen in several experimental and human models. In the medium to long term, LPS and LPS-induced cytokines, primarily by activating members of the family of mitogen-activated protein kinases, lead to marked alterations in the activity of several gene regulators of a broad number of transporters, namely those that are activated by members of the NR family [32]. Molecular cross-talk between bile acid-activated NRs and proinflammatory nuclear mediators may provide new means of understanding adaptive processes within the liver. Inflammation-induced cholestasis and the effects of retained molecules in cholestasis on inflammatory signals are interwoven in the liver, providing potential opportunities for research and therapeutics [32].

Drug-induced cholestasis

It is well known that many drugs can lead to damage of liver parenchymal cells (e.g. acetaminophen), while some interfere with the basic mechanisms of the formation of bile [38–40]. Cholestasis as a component of drug-related hepatotoxicity can involve a variety of mechanisms including direct cholangiocyte toxicity and necrosis, impairments in bile acid transport, and thickening of biliary secretions [20].

Infants and young children have reduced detoxification pathways compared with older children and adults, suggesting that there is an enhanced susceptibility to cholestatic effects of certain drugs [41]. This enhanced susceptibility is not fully understood but appears to involve developmentally regulated expression of detoxification and transport genes, immature protective measures against apoptosis/necrosis, and a role for altered inflammatory responses to damaged tissues. With the availability of genome-wide association studies since the mid 1990s, there has been a shift toward their application to personalized components in liver pathobiology. With drug-induced liver injury, the focus is shifting to the interaction between the environment (such as the drug) and genetic correlates and predispositions [40,42,43].

Total parental nutrition-associated cholestasis

Among the more prevalent associations of the rapid progression to end-stage liver disease is the setting of neonates with intestinal failure, who are dependent upon TPN, leading to a condition known as TPN-associated cholestasis. This entity was seen soon after the introduction of TPN in neonates, yet the underlying cause, or more likely causes, are unknown [44,45]. The typical clinical situation is a premature infant who has damaged or resected small intestine and is unable to advance feeds. Development of TPN-associated cholestasis can occur as soon as 2 weeks, with hepatomegaly and conjugated hyperbilirubinemia, while cirrhosis has been reported in as little as 2 months. Moreover, the cholestasis and injury can resolve, if patients are weaned off TPN, attesting to the timeliness and confluence of these damaging factors in early infancy. Therefore, there is an inherent susceptibility in this clinical setting that is not readily replicated in older children or adults with TPN dependence.

There appear to be four main contributors to TPN-associated cholestasis: immaturity, infection, inadequate gut function, and a toxic/missing component in the TPN [45,46]. Despite TPN being administered for nearly 40 years, we still have little evidence as to which one of these four contributors are most relevant. Support for all four components has been provided, yet the molecular, or cellular, etiologies remain elusive. The inherent immaturity of bile formation and flow – the "physiologic cholestasis of the newborn" [23] – and drug metabolism pathways [41] support the concept that premature infant livers may be more susceptible to any cholestatic insult, although neither function has been adequately quantified in these babies. The scenario of infection and inflammation contributing to cholestasis in these infants is seen quite often, whereby bouts of infection are often heralded by elevations in serum levels of conjugated bilirubin [30]. Inadequate oral intake reduces the nutritional and hormonal input from the gut to liver function and bile flow, with evidence of an immaturity and impairment of certain gut hormones in intestinal failure and TPN dependence [47]. Decreased bile acid synthesis has also been seen in TPN-associated cholestasis. Finally, many components of the TPN solution have been implicated as cholestatic (minerals, amino acids, sterols, fatty acids to name a few) or absent but, to date, none has been definitively associated with causing cholestasis. In one of the few epidemiological studies, adults on TPN had lower hepatic complications on lower lipid infusions than higher, suggesting that there may be a component in the lipids that is cholestatic [48]. Among more recent cell culture and animal studies, data include molecular pathways that implicate inflammatory cascades as well as phytosterols; however, more work needs to be performed to identify the actual molecular targets [49,50].

Adaptation to cholestasis

The hepatocyte adapts to cholestasis by engaging broadly acting protective measures at the membrane, in the cytoplasm, and by a reprogramming of transcription in the nucleus. In addition to changes within hepatocytes, cell-to-cell communication, balancing immunologic responses to infected or damaged cells, with the endogenous capacity of the liver to regenerate, is an additional component to the liver's response to cholestasis. Over the past few years, it has become apparent that this coordination of response to cholestatic injury is multilayered, integrative, and quite complex, but on a practical front, it may be amenable to therapeutic intervention.

In general, the primary location of effecting a response to cholestasis resides within hepatocytes, likely because of this cell's role in handling bile acids, which can abruptly and profoundly rise in intracellular concentrations with all forms of cholestasis. Reducing the inherent toxicity of retained bile acids within hepatocytes is a major goal of the hepatocyte's response to cholestasis [3]. When bile acid concentrations rise within cells, there are profound effects on cell signaling and integrity of membranes and subcellular structures. As detergents, bile acids affect membrane fluidity and protein structure, while as cell signaling molecules, bile acids affect

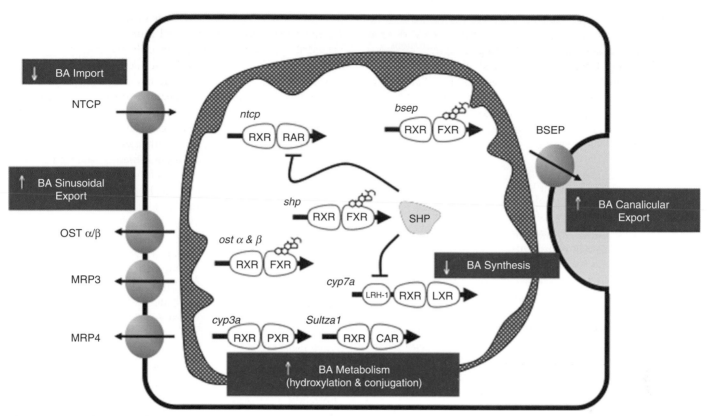

Figure 3.2 General overview of the nuclear adaptive response of the hepatocyte to bile acid (BA) retention. The hepatocyte engages multiple processes in order to reduce retention of intracellular BAs. In addition to those shown here, there are direct effects on resident metabolic pathways and transporter and proteins. The overall process functionally involves reduction of sinusoidal import and synthesis, engagement of P450-mediated hydroxylation and conjugation pathways for detoxification, and increased canalicular export. Shown are a few key target genes and members of the nuclear receptor superfamily whose activation by ligands (e.g. bile acids for the farnesoid X receptor (FXR)) leads to these adaptive changes in gene expression. Relevant regulatory promoter regions are shown, although the list of target genes, and transcriptional regulators, is much more extensive [3,51]. RXR, retinoid X receptor; RAR, retinoic acid receptor; CAR, constitutive androstane receptor; PXR, pregnane X receptor; LXR, liver X receptor; SHP, small heterodimer partner.

kinase pathways, initiate apoptosis, and alter gene expression, among many other critical cellular functions [4,5,51]. Over the past few years, the essential components of the hepatocyte's response to retained bile acids is coordinated to reduce sinusoidal import and synthesis, increase canalicular export, and engage P450-based xenobiotic metabolism pathways (hydroxylation and conjugation) as a means to reduce intracellular concentrations and toxicity. In addition, recent evidence suggests that at least two sinusoidal transporters are activated to export retained bile acids across the sinusoidal membrane (see Figure 3.1). These responses to bile acid overload are, in general, related to bile acids acting as gene regulators – as ligands for several NR family members (mainly CAR, FXR, PXR), which then act as transcriptional activators for target genes whose proteins function to effect the changes noted above (Figure 3.2). This is an evolving avenue of research that overall indicates that the hepatocyte has adaptive responses in place to handle cholestasis, and that these pathways may be amenable to pharmacological therapies [3,21,52,53].

Future expectations

Although we have seen new identifications of genes associated with genetic forms of cholestasis (e.g. PFIC), it is still evident to practitioners that much remains to be discovered, including genes that are modifiers of cholestatic liver disease. On a diagnostic front, it is anticipated that we will be able to explore diagnostics as well as genotype–phenotype correlations as more and more of these disease-causing genes become available for commercial testing (see www.genetests.org for current lists), or are discovered as part of ongoing multicenter clinical trials (e.g. ChILDREN [www.childrennetwork.org]). Nutritional and therapeutic means of enhancing the response of the liver to cholestasis [3,24], as well as knowledge about the roles of immaturity, inflammation, and diet-derived substances that may, in fact, exacerbate ongoing cholestasis, are expected to be revealed. Finally, with the discovery of the roles for inflammation and NR-mediated means of adaptation to cholestasis, anticholestatic therapeutic agents are expected to be available for testing, given the frank paucity of available agents at present [3,24,52,54].

References

1. Stapelbroek JM, van Erpecum KJ, Klomp LW, *et al.* Liver disease associated with canalicular transport defects: current and future therapies. *J Hepatol* 2010;**52**:258–271.

2. Mullenbach R, Lammert F. An update on genetic analysis of cholestatic liver diseases: digging deeper. *Digest Dis* 2011;**29**:72–77.

3. Karpen SJ, Trauner M. The new therapeutic frontier: nuclear receptors and the liver. *J Hepatol* 2010;**52**:455–462.

4. Nicolaou M, Andress E, Zolnerciks J, *et al.* Canalicular ABC transporters and liver disease. *J Pathol* 2011:doi 10.

5. Kosters A, Karpen SJ. Bile acid transporters in health and disease. *Xenobiotica* 2008;**38**:1043–1071.

6. Nathanson MH, Boyer JL. Mechanisms and regulation of bile secretion. *Hepatology* 1991;**14**:551–566.

7. Hofmann AF. Biliary secretion and excretion in health and disease: current concepts. *Ann Hepatol* 2007;**6**:15–27.

8. Feranchak AP, Sokol RJ. Cholangiocyte biology and cystic fibrosis liver disease. *Semin Liver Dis* 2001;**21**:471–488.

9. Dawson PA, Lan T, Rao A. Bile acid transporters. *J Lipid Res* 2009;**50**:2340–2357.

10. Stieger B. The role of the sodium-taurocholate cotransporting polypeptide (NTCP) and of the bile salt export pump (BSEP) in physiology and pathophysiology of bile formation. In Page CP, Rosenthal W, Michel MC, *et al.* (eds.) *Handbook of Experimental Pharmacology.* Heidelberg: Springer, 2011, pp. 205–259.

11. Suchy FJ, Ananthanarayanan M. Bile salt excretory pump: biology and pathobiology. *J Pediatr Gastroenterol Nutr* 2006;**43**(Suppl 1):S10–S16.

12. Stieger B. Recent insights into the function and regulation of the bile salt export pump (ABCB11). *Curr Opin Lipidol* 2009;**20**:176–181.

13. Davit-Spraul A, Gonzales E, Baussan C, *et al.* The spectrum of liver diseases related to *ABCB4* gene mutations: pathophysiology and clinical aspects. *Semin Liver Dis* 2010;**30**:134–146.

14. Colombo C, Vajro P, Degiorgio D, *et al.* Clinical features and genotype-phenotype correlations in children with progressive familial intrahepatic cholestasis type 3 related to *ABCB4* mutations. *J Pediatr Gastroenterol Nutr* 2011;**52**:73–83.

15. Miettinen TA, Klett EL, Gylling H, *et al.* Liver transplantation in a patient with sitosterolemia and cirrhosis. *Gastroenterology* 2006;**130**:542.

16. Keitel V, Nies AT, Brom M, *et al.* A common Dubin–Johnson syndrome mutation impairs protein maturation and transport activity of MRP2 (*ABCC2*). *Am J Physiol Gastrointest Liver Physiol* 2003;**284**:G165–174.

17. Mullenbach R, Lammert FC. The transporter "variome": the missing link between gene variants and bile salt transporter function. *Hepatology* 2009;**49**:352–354.

18. Byrne JA, Strautnieks SS, Ihrke G, *et al.* Missense mutations and single nucleotide polymorphisms in ABCB11 impair bile salt export pump processing and function or disrupt pre-messenger RNA splicing. *Hepatology* 2009;**49**:553–567.

19. Hofmann AF. The enterohepatic circulation of bile acids in man. *Clin Gastroenterol* 1977;**6**:3–24.

20. Jaeschke H, Gores GJ, Cederbaum AI, *et al.* Mechanisms of hepatotoxicity. *Toxicol Sci* 2002;**65**:166–176.

21. Wagner M, Zollner G, Trauner M. Nuclear receptor regulation of the adaptive response of bile acid transporters in cholestasis. *Semin Liver Dis* 2010;**30**:160–177.

22. Watkins JB, Szczepanik P, Gould JB, *et al.* Bile salt metabolism in the human premature infant. Preliminary observations of pool size and synthesis rate following prenatal administration of dexamethasone and phenobarbital. *Gastroenterology* 1975;**69**:706–713.

23. Suchy FJ, Balistreri WF, Heubi JE, *et al.* Physiologic cholestasis: elevation of the primary serum bile acid concentrations in normal infants. *Gastroenterology* 1981;**80**:1037–1041.

24. Trauner M, Halilbasic E. Nuclear receptors as new perspective for the management of liver diseases. *Gastroenterology* 2011;**140**:1120–1125.

25. Zollner G, Trauner M. Nuclear receptors as therapeutic targets in cholestatic liver diseases. *Br J Pharmacol* 2009;**156**:7–27.

26. Khan AA, Chow EC, van Loenen-Weemaes AM, *et al.* Comparison of effects of VDR versus PXR, FXR and GR ligands on the regulation of CYP3A isozymes in rat and human intestine and liver. *Eur J Pharm Sci* 2009;**37**:115–125.

27. Lee JM, Lee YK, Mamrosh JL, *et al.* A nuclear-receptor-dependent phosphatidylcholine pathway with antidiabetic effects. *Nature* 2011;**474**:506–510.

28. Pols TW, Noriega LG, Nomura M, *et al.* The bile acid membrane receptor TGR5: a valuable metabolic target. *Digest Dis* 2011;**29**:37–44.

29. Osler WH. *Principles and Practice of Medicine*, 4th edn. New York: Appleton, 1901.

30. Dunham EC. Septicemia in the newborn. *Am J Dis Children* 1933;**45**:229–253.

31. Zimmerman HJ, Fang M, Utili R, *et al.* Jaundice due to bacterial infection. *Gastroenterology* 1979;**77**:362–374.

32. Kosters A, Karpen SJ. The role of inflammation in cholestasis: clinical and basic aspects. *Semin Liver Dis* 2010;**30**:186–194.

33. Bolder U, Tonnu HT, Schteingart CD, *et al.* Hepatocyte transport of bile acids and organic anions in endotoxemic rats: impaired uptake and secretion. *Gastroenterology* 1997;**112**:214–225.

34. Moshage H. Cytokines and the hepatic acute phase response. *J Pathol* 1997;**181**:257–266.

35. Trauner M, Wagner M, Fickert P, *et al.* Molecular regulation of hepatobiliary transport systems: clinical implications for understanding and treating cholestasis. *J Clin Gastroenterol* 2005;**39**:S111–S124.

36. Bolder U, Jeschke MG, Landmann L, *et al.* Heat stress enhances recovery of hepatocyte bile acid and organic anion transporters in endotoxemic rats by multiple mechanisms. *Cell Stress Chaperones* 2006;**11**:89–100.

37. Saeki J, Sekine S, Horie T. LPS-induced dissociation of multidrug resistance-associated protein 2 (Mrp2) and radixin is associated with Mrp2 selective internalization in rats. *Biochem Pharmacol* 2011;**81**:178–184.

38. Padda MS, Sanchez M, Akhtar AJ, *et al.* Drug-induced cholestasis. *Hepatology* 2011;**53**:1377–1387.

39. Tujios S, Fontana RJ. Mechanisms of drug-induced liver injury: from bedside to bench. *Nat Rev Gastroenterol* 2011;**8**:202–211.

40. Stieger B, Geier A. Genetic variations of bile salt transporters as predisposing factors for drug-induced cholestasis, intrahepatic cholestasis of pregnancy and therapeutic response of viral hepatitis. *Expert Opin Drug Metab Toxicol* 2011;**7**:411–425.

41. Kearns GL, Abdel-Rahman SM, Alander SW, *et al.* Developmental pharmacology: drug disposition, action, and therapy in infants and children. *N Engl J Med* 2003;**349**:1157–1167.

42. Russmann S, Jetter A, Kullak-Ublick GA. Pharmacogenetics of drug-induced liver injury. *Hepatology* 2010;**52**:748–761.

43. Zollner G, Wagner M, Trauner M. Nuclear receptors as drug targets in cholestasis and drug-induced hepatotoxicity. *Pharmacol Ther* 2010;**126**:228–243.

44. Abernathy CO, Utili R, Zimmerman HJ. Immaturity of the biliary excretory system predisposes neonates to intrahepatic cholestasis. *Med Hypoth* 1979;**5**:641–647.

45. Carter BA, Shulman RJ. Mechanisms of disease: update on the molecular etiology and fundamentals of parenteral nutrition associated cholestasis. *Nat Clin Pract Gastrol* 2007;**4**:277–287.

46. Carter BA, Karpen SJ. Intestinal failure-associated liver disease: management and treatment strategies past, present, and future. *Semin Liver Dis* 2007;**27**:251–258.

47. Teitelbaum DH, Han-Markey T, Drongowski RA, *et al.* Use of cholecystokinin to prevent the development of parenteral nutrition-associated cholestasis. *J Parenter Enteral Nutr* 1997;**21**:100–103.

48. Colomb V, Jobert-Giraud A, Lacaille F, *et al.* Role of lipid emulsions in cholestasis associated with long-term parenteral nutrition in children. *J Parenter Enteral Nutr* 2000;**24**:345–350.

49. El Kasmi KC, Anderson AL, Devereaux MW, *et al.* Toll like receptor 4 dependent Kupffer cell activation and liver injury in a novel mouse model of parenteral nutrition. *Hepatology* 2012;**55**:1518–1528.

50. Kurvinen A, Nissinen MJ, Andersson S, *et al.* Parenteral plant sterols and intestinal failure associated liver disease in neonates: a prospective nationwide study. *J Pediatr Gastroenterol Nutr* 2012;**54**:803–811.

51. Wagner M, Zollner G, Trauner M. Nuclear receptors in liver disease. *Hepatology* 2011;**53**:1023–1034.

52. Boyer JL. Nuclear receptor ligands: rational and effective therapy for chronic cholestatic liver disease? *Gastroenterology* 2005;**129**:735–740.

53. Trauner M, Baghdasaryan A, Claudel T, *et al.* Targeting nuclear bile acid receptors for liver disease. *Digest Dis* 2011;**29**:98–102.

54. Karpen SJ. Exercising the nuclear option to treat cholestasis: CAR and PXR ligands. *Hepatology* 2005;**42**:266–269.

Chapter

4

Acute liver failure in children

Robert H. Squires and Estella M. Alonso

Introduction

Pediatric acute liver failure (ALF) is not a single diagnosis. Rather, pediatric ALF is a complex, rapidly progressive clinical syndrome that is the final common pathway for many disparate conditions; some known and others yet to be identified [1,2]. The estimated frequency of ALF in all age groups in the USA is about 17 cases per 100 000 population per year, but the frequency in children is unknown. In the USA, ALF accounts for 10–15% of pediatric liver transplants performed annually. Management requires a multidisciplinary team involving the hepatologist, critical care specialist, and liver transplant surgeon.

Acute liver failure is a rapidly evolving clinical condition. The absence of adequately powered studies to inform diagnostic algorithms, to assess markers of disease severity and trajectory, and to guide liver transplant decisions transfers a significant burden to the clinician. Constructing a diagnostic approach and individualized management strategy that may include the decision to pursue liver transplantation is challenging. There are a number of pressing clinical questions faced when children with pediatric ALF first present. Does the patient have a condition that is treatable? What is the risk of deterioration or improvement on each day the child is alive with his/her native liver? Is a living related or deceased liver transplant necessary for patient survival? Is full recovery possible without a liver transplant? Are associated morbidities recoverable or irreversible?

Clinical characterization

The "definition" of pediatric ALF is in evolution. In adults, the strict definition requires the onset of hepatic encephalopathy (HE) less than 8 weeks after the first signs of hepatic dysfunction. While HE is a required element for adults with liver failure, it is acknowledged that it is difficult to assess in children and may not be clinically apparent until the terminal stages of the disease process [3]. Current encephalopathy scores were developed for adults with cirrhosis and portal hypertension and not ALF. In the setting of ALF, mental status changes caused by infection, metabolic derangements, or anxiety associated with acute illness may confound assessment of mental status changes attributed to a liver-based encephalopathy. The "onset of jaundice" is a time point that is difficult to define as it is dependent on clinical observation by individuals with disparate expertise in assessing jaundice. Jaundice may go undetected for a period of time. The interval between the apparent onset of jaundice and HE has been used to characterize various "subtypes" of pediatric ALF such as "hyperacute," "acute," and "subacute" pediatric ALF, and yet the first day of the illness is all but impossible to define. There are currently no validated alternatives to these imperfect subjective measures to distinguish categories of patients with acute severe liver injury from ALF or to distinguish ALF that is recoverable without liver transplant from those who would die without liver transplant.

Recognizing the difficulty in assessing encephalopathy in children, recent studies of pediatric ALF have included children without clinical encephalopathy [4]. Entry criteria for the longitudinal cohort study by the Pediatric Acute Liver Failure Study Group were developed by a consensus of experts who served as the site principal investigators [1]. Those entry criteria are (1) children with no known evidence of chronic liver disease, (2) biochemical evidence of acute liver injury, and (3) coagulopathy not corrected by vitamin K. The presence of encephalopathy is required if the prothrombin time (PT) is between 15 and 19.9 seconds or the international normalized ratio (INR) is between 1.5 and 1.9; however, if the PT is at least 20 seconds or the INR 2.0 or more, patients were enrolled with or without HE.

In the era before liver transplantation, the dynamic natural history of pediatric ALF was for children to either survive or die and a worsening clinical course did not preclude a favorable outcome (Figure 4.1). A previously healthy patient typically experiences a non-specific prodrome of variable duration with features that might include abdominal discomfort and malaise with or without fever. Symptoms may persist or wax and wane for days or weeks before the child is brought to medical attention. In the absence of jaundice or other clinically evident sign of liver dysfunction, the child may receive empiric

Liver Disease in Children, Fourth Edition, ed. Frederick J. Suchy, Ronald J. Sokol, and William F. Balistreri. Published by Cambridge University Press. © Cambridge University Press 2014.

Table 4.1 Etiology of acute liver failure in 653 children from the Pediatric Acute Liver Failure Study Group 2000–2007

Final diagnosis	Number (%) at various ages					
	<4 weeks	4–8 weeks	9 weeks to <1 year	1–5 years	6–10 years	>10 years
Indeterminate	28 (37.8)	9 (40.9)	37 (45.1)	116 (67.4)	46 (62.2)	74 (32.3)
Acetaminophen	0 (0)	1 (4.6)	4 (4.9)	7 (4.1)	2 (2.7)	67 (29.3)
Metabolic	12 (16.2)	6 (27.3)	16 (19.5)	8 (4.7)	6 (8.1)	20 (8.7)
Autoimmune	0 (0)	0 (0)	5 (6.1)	12 (7.0)	4 (5.4)	22 (9.6)
Viral hepatitis	16 (21.6)	0 (0)	3 (3.7)	8 (4.7)	2 (2.7)	11 (4.8)
Shock/ischemia	3 (4.1)	2 (9.1)	5 (6.1)	4 (2.3)	5 (6.8)	6 (2.6)
Drug induced	0 (0)	0 (0)	1 (1.2)	2 (1.2)	3 (4.1)	16 (7.0)
Neonatal iron storage disease	10 (13.5)	3 (13.6)	1 (1.2)	0 (0.0)	0 (0.0)	0 (0.0)
Veno-occlusive disease	0 (0)	0 (0)	3 (3.7)	1 (0.6)	1 (1.4)	4 (1.8)
Hemophagocytic syndrome	1 (1.4)	0 (0)	5 (6.1)	3 (1.7)	0 (0)	1 (0.4)
Budd–Chiari syndrome	0 (0)	0 (0)	0 (0)	0 (0)	1 (1.4)	1 (0.4)
Other diagnosis	4 (5.4)	1 (4.6)	1 (1.2)	6 (3.5)	1 (1.4)	4 (1.8)
Multiple diagnosis	0 (0)	0 (0)	1 (1.2)	5 (2.9)	3 (4.1)	3 (1.3)
Total	74	22	82	172	74	229

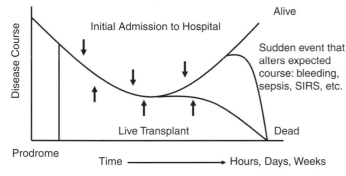

Figure 4.1 The clinical trajectory of a child with acute liver failure is difficult to predict. Liver transplantation interrupts the natural history of acute liver failure. Improved assessment and estimate of the clinical trajectory will enhance transplant decisions in the future. SIRS, systemic inflammatory response syndrome.

treatment to relieve symptoms. However, if there are clinical signs of liver injury or encephalopathy, or if blood work is obtained that reveals hepatic dysfunction, the clinical syndrome of pediatric ALF can be recognized.

With the exception of acute ingestions (e.g. mushrooms, acetaminophen), the precise onset of disease is rarely identified. Patient outcome is reflected, in part, by the interaction among etiology, disease severity, supportive management, and treatment. Yet, outcomes vary among children with seemingly similar etiology, disease severity, and treatment; therefore, additional factors are likely involved to explain these variations. Modifying factors likely include the inflammatory milieu, end-organ damage, immune activation, potential for liver regeneration, and management interventions. Medical

and liver transplant decisions require reliable repeated assessments of the probability of survival with native liver from one time interval to the next.

Liver transplant decisions for children with ALF, which must include the risks associated with living organ donation, are made difficult given the uncertainty of patient outcome. The uncertainty regarding where the patient resides along the "natural course" of the disease at the time of initial presentation or at any point thereafter requires considerable clinical judgment. Liver transplant arbitrarily interrupts the natural course of pediatric ALF and it is accepted that some patients who receive a liver transplant may have survived without one. Given the insufficient number of organs to satisfy patient needs, the field would be well served if there were a more precise method to identify those patients who will survive without a liver transplant, as well as those who will die despite liver transplant.

Etiology

Specific etiologies can be broadly categorized as infectious, immunologic, metabolic, and toxin/drug related. Currently, a specific diagnosis is not established in over 50% of pediatric ALF and these children are categorized as indeterminate. Table 4.1 details the causes of ALF in 653 children enrolled in the Pediatric Acute Liver Failure Study from 19 pediatric liver transplant centers in the USA, Canada, and the UK between 2000 and 2007. In developing countries, the etiologies are similar but are dominated by infectious etiologies, with hepatitis A virus (HAV) being the most common (Table 4.2). This brief summation of diseases that can cause pediatric ALF is supplemented by other chapters detailing each specific disease state.

Table 4.2 Etiologies in developing countries

Etiology	No.							Total (%)
	Brazil 1992–1999	North Brazil 1984–2002	Argentina 1982–2002	Kolkata 1986–2003	North India 1997–2000	Hong Kong 1993–2002	Chile 1995–2003	
Indeterminate	6	1	68		4	6	12	97 (23)
Hepatitis A	37	3	128	15	34		10	227 (55)
Hepatitis B	2	4	2	7	5			20 (5)
Hepatitis C								0
Hepatitis E				13	17			30 (7)
Hepatitis A/E					7			7 (2)
Hepatitis B/D		11						11 (3)
Hepatitis A/C	1							1
Hepatitis A/B		1						1
Hepatitis B/C		1						1
Autoimmune			5				3	8 (2)
Drugs			3			2	2	7 (2)
Wilson disease			2					2
Yellow fever	2							2
Other			2					2
Total	46	23	210	35	67	8	27	416

Acetaminophen

Acetaminophen (N-acetyl-p-aminophenol (paracetamol)) is widely used in children for management of fever and pain. It is available without prescription and is commercially available as a single formulation or can be compounded with decongestants or narcotics. Acetaminophen is safe and well tolerated when dosing instructions are strictly followed. However, it has a low therapeutic index, and in certain individuals or clinical scenarios, chronic administration of therapeutic dosages of acetaminophen can result in significant hepatotoxic effects [5,6]. Two clinical scenarios are associated with acetaminophen hepatotoxicity.

The most common scenario follows an intentional single ingestion of a hepatotoxic dose that is >100 mg/kg. Plasma acetaminophen at 4 and 24 hours after a single ingestion will assist in determining the relative toxicity of the ingestion [7]. Females over 10 years of age represent the most common demographic associated with intentional overdose in children, but it should be considered in all age groups outside the newborn period [1]. Immediately following ingestion, patients may experience non-specific symptoms of nausea and vomiting. While a liver biopsy is not generally indicated in the setting of known acetaminophen overdose, centrilobular hepatic necrosis is the hallmark finding and should raise the consideration of acetaminophen toxicity even without a clear history of exposure. N-Acetylcysteine given enterally or intravenously can successfully reverse the toxic injury if given as soon after the ingestion as possible, ideally within 24 hours. If treatment is delayed beyond 24 hours following ingestion, the patient is at increased risk of having irreversible liver injury. Regardless of the interval between ingestion and presentation, N-acetylcysteine should be administered where a toxic ingestion occurred. Serum aminotransferase levels can reach over 10 000 IU/mL and the total bilirubin is generally lower than might be expected given the degree of liver injury, typically <10 mg/dL. If treatment is not initiated, jaundice develops within 48 to 72 hours, with death occurring in the most severe cases by 5 to 7 days following the ingestion.

Therapeutic misadventures or unintentional exposure to a single hepatotoxic dose of acetaminophen or chronic exposure at daily doses of <100 mg/kg can also result in hepatotoxicity. Risk factors for developing severe hepatotoxicity include concomitant use of other medicines that alter hepatic metabolism, delayed medical care, younger age, and prolonged periods of fasting [5,8]. The presence of acetaminophen adducts in the serum may indicate unsuspected acetaminophen hepatotoxicity [9]. Although the magnitude of this clinical problem in children is not well defined, 48% of acetaminophen-induced ALF in adults in the USA results from unintentional overdosing, reinforcing the concept that accidental misuse of this medication leading to serious liver injury is relatively common [10]. Similar to children with a single intentional overdose, alanine aminotransferase levels can reach into the many thousands with a relatively low total bilirubin level. The therapeutic benefit of *N*-acetylcysteine in patients with chronic acetaminophen exposure is untested and uncertain.

Medication (non-acetaminophen) or toxin

Liver injury caused by drugs, herbals, or toxins other than acetaminophen was identified in less than 3% of cases in the Pediatric Acute Liver Failure Study Group registry, the vast majority occurring in children over 10 years of age [1]. The list of xenobiotics associated with liver failure is extensive and expanding, a partial list is found in Table 4.3. Hepatotoxic agents, such as industrial solvents and mushroom toxin, are dose dependent and will predictably result in liver injury or failure. The diagnosis of hepatotoxic liver injury is based upon the interval between drug ingestion and the onset of symptoms, the known hepatotoxicity of the offending agent, serum drug levels (if available), and liver biopsy findings [11]. However, idiosyncratic drug reactions are more common. The diagnosis of idiosyncratic drug-related liver failure is based upon largely circumstantial evidence, so a degree of skepticism should be maintained regarding the role of drug exposure in causing the hepatic injury [6,12]. Exposure to drugs with a strong history of idiosyncratic liver injury – so-called black box drugs because of the warning for liver injury posted in US Food and Drug Administration required drug information – should be considered strongly. These include isoniazid, propylthiouracil, and halothane.

A careful history of exposure to hepatotoxins should be obtained from the family of any child presenting in ALF, including prescription and non-prescription drugs in the home that could have been ingested accidentally. In teenagers, a history should include evidence of depression, recreational drug use (e.g. cocaine, ecstasy), or solvent sniffing. Any exposure to hepatotoxic drugs, chemicals, or herbals should be considered possibly related to the liver injury. Ingestion of the *Amanita* mushroom is clearly traced to ALF.

Liver biopsy can assist in diagnosis of drug-induced idiosyncratic liver injury. The histologic pattern of injury observed should be that expected from the drug to which the patient has been exposed. The patterns seen are hepatitis (hepatocellular necrosis), cholestasis, mixed cholestasis and hepatitis, and steatosis. Drugs that cause hepatitis (e.g. isoniazid, propylthiouracil, and halothane) have the greatest potential for causing pediatric ALF. Drugs associated with steatosis (e.g. sodium valproate, amiodarone) may also cause liver failure. Drugs that cause cholestasis (oxacillin) rarely produce liver failure, whereas drugs that cause mixed cholestasis and hepatitis (sulfa drugs) sometimes do. If histology differs from that expected by the drug in question, another cause should be

Table 4.3 Medications and toxins associated with acute liver failure

Type	Xenobiotics
Anti-infective	Clavulanic acid/amoxicillin Trimethoprim–sulfamethoxazole Isoniazid Minocycline/doxycycline Quinolone (ciprofloxacin, norfloxacin) Voriconazole Macrolide (erythromycin, clarithromycin, azithromycin) Others
Anticonvulsants	Phenytoin Valproic acid Carbamazepine Others
Immunomodulators/ anti-inflammatory	Methotrexate Azathioprine Non-steroidal anti-inflammatory drugs Acetaminophen Biological (i.e. infliximab, basiliximab, etc.) Others
Recreational drugs	Ecstasy Cocaine Others
Complementary, alternative or herbal medication	Pyrrolizidine alkaloids Germander Ma huang Chaparral Black cohosh root Pennyroyal Kava Others
Toxin/industrial solvents	Amatoxin (mushrooms from *Amianita* spp.) Carbon tetrachloride Tricholorethylene 2-Nitropropane 1,2,3-Trichloropropane

sought. Exposure to a drug or toxin should not preclude a thorough search for other causes of liver injury.

Valproic acid, phenytoin, carbamazepine, and felbamate are the most common offenders in children [1]. Valproic acid, when used to control seizures in children with unsuspected mitochondrial disease, may precipitate ALF. Antimicrobial agents such as isoniazid, ampicillin-clavulanic acid, roxithromycin, and nitrofurantoin as well as a number of antiviral agents used in the treatment of HIV have been reported to cause pediatric ALF. Chemotherapeutic agents such as cyclophosphamide and dacarbazine, are associated with hepatic vein injury resulting in veno-occlusive disease and pediatric ALF. Other potential medications that should be considered in the proper clinical setting include halothane (anesthetic), amiodarone (antiarrhythmic), propylthiouracil (hyperthyroidism), and trazodone (antidepressant). Recreational drug use, particularly cocaine and methylene-dioxyamphetamine ("ecstasy"), is associated with pediatric ALF in teenagers and even younger children who live in environments where these compounds are accessible. Complementary or alternative medical therapies are utilized with increased frequency. Examples of herbal remedies associated with liver failure include pyrrolizidine alkaloids, germander, Chinese herbal medicine, ma huang, chaparral, black cohosh root, pennyroyal, and kava [13].

Immune dysregulation

Autoimmune marker positive

The serological markers associated with autoimmune liver disease, which include anti-nuclear antibody (ANA), anti-smooth muscle antibody (ASMA), and anti-liver–kidney microsomal (ALKM) antibody are detected in about 7% of children with ALF [1]. The true frequency of positive auto-immune markers in pediatric ALF is not known as all three markers were obtained in only 55% of patients in the Pediatric Acute Liver Failure Study Group, while 21% of children showed no markers [14]. Autoimmune-marker positive pediatric ALF occurred in 7–10% of children over 1 year of age and in just over 4% of children between 9 weeks and 12 months of age. Therefore, this condition should be considered in all age groups outside of early infancy.

The significance of autoantibodies in pediatric ALF is not clear as they can be found in patients with other known causes of liver failure such as Wilson disease and drug-induced liver failure. Elevated serum globulins may not be present and the condition appears to be evenly distributed among males and females. Histologic features show evidence of immune activation with the presence of a plasma cell-enriched portal tract infiltrate, central perivenulitis, and lymphoid follicles with evidence of massive hepatic necrosis [15]. However, there should be no evidence of chronicity on the initial biopsy. Corticosteroids can interrupt the liver injury in many patients. Some children appear to tolerate weaning corticosteroids without recurrence of their disease, while recurrent disease may be more common in adults.

Hemophagocytic lymphohistiocytosis

Hemophagocytic lymphohistiocytosis is an enigmatic condition characterized by fever, hepatosplenomegaly, marked elevation in serum aminotransferase levels, cytopenias, hypertriglyceridemia, hyperferritinemia, and hypofibrinogenemia [16]. Additional diagnostic criteria now include low or absent natural killer (NK) cell activity, serum ferritin $\geq 500\,\mu g/L$, and soluble CD25 (soluble interleukin-2 receptor) $\geq 2400\,U/mL$ [16]. It can present from infancy through adolescence, although it is most commonly diagnosed in the first 5 years of life.

Neonatal hemochromatosis

Neonatal hemochromatosis results from an intrauterine alloimmune liver injury. Maternal immunoglobulin G appears to activate fetal complement, which leads to the formation of the membrane attack complex and results in liver cell injury [17]. The degree of liver injury can be so profound that death from liver failure can occur within the first few weeks of life. Therefore, liver failure associated with neonatal hemochromatosis is technically a terminal event of a chronic intrauterine liver disease. However, the phenotype of a family's index case of neonatal hemochromatosis confronting the clinician is one of ALF and thus deserves to be included in this section for clinical purposes.

Characteristic clinical features include refractory hypoglycemia, severe coagulopathy, hypoalbuminemia, elevated serum ferritin ($>1000\,\mu g/L$), and ascites. Strikingly, serum aminotransferase levels are normal or near normal and should alert the clinician to the possibility of neonatal hemochromatosis. Extrahepatic iron deposition is a hallmark finding. Hemosiderin deposition in the minor salivary glands obtained by a buccal mucosal biopsy is often seen. Alternatively, MRI of the abdomen would suggest the diagnosis with the finding of reduced T_2-weighted intensity of the liver and/or the pancreas relative to the spleen. Exchange transfusion and high-dose intravenous immunoglobulin is the preferred treatment for neonatal hemochromatosis [18].

Inherited metabolic disease

Metabolic diseases may not fit the definition of ALF precisely as the condition was certainly present prior to presentation. However, a number of conditions will present acutely in a child who is not known to have the condition until the diagnosis is established during the first episode of ALF. Overall, metabolic diseases account for just over 10% of pediatric ALF [2]. While some conditions, such as mitochondrial disease, may present at any age, many metabolic conditions presenting as liver failure segregate within age groups. Metabolic conditions that should be considered in these age groups are listed in Table 4.4. Details of the specific conditions can be found in other sections of this textbook. Highlighting those which have been associated with a presentation of ALF is the purpose of this section.

Metabolic conditions affecting infants in the first few months of life include galactosemia, tyrosinemia, Niemann–Pick type C, mitochondrial hepatopathies, and urea cycle defects [19]. Galactosemia should be considered in a child consuming breast milk or other lactose-containing formulae and developing liver failure associated with reducing substances in the urine. Tyrosinemia can present with a profound coagulopathy and normal or near normal serum aminotransferase levels. Both galactosemia and tyrosinemia can present in association with Gram-negative sepsis. Niemann–Pick type C is a lysosomal storage disease and marked splenomegaly is often noted. Mitochondrial hepatopathies are increasingly

Table 4.4 Metabolic disease presenting as acute liver failure

Age	Condition
<6 months	Galactosemia Niemann–Pick type C Tyrosinemia Glycosylation defect Mitochondrial disease[a]
7 months to 4 years	Mitochondrial disease[a] Tyrosinemia α$_1$-Antitrypsin deficiency Hereditary fructose intolerance Urea cycle defects
5 years to 18 years	Wilson disease Mitochondrial disease[a] Fatty liver of pregnancy

[a] Fatty acid oxidation defects, respiratory chain defects, mitochondrial DNA depletion.

recognized as an important cause of liver failure due to deficiencies in respiratory complexes I, III or IV or mitochondrial DNA depletion. With rare exceptions, mitochondrial hepatopathies have associated systemic mitochondrial dysfunction characterized by progressive neurologic deficiencies or cardiomyopathy or myopathy. Multisystem mitochondrial dysfunction serves as a contraindication to liver transplant. However, patients who do not have extrahepatic manifestations of their disease may have isolated hepatic mitochondrial dysfunction amenable to liver transplantation [20]. Unfortunately, multisystem involvement may not be apparent at the time of liver transplant, placing the child at risk for developing symptoms in the future. Lactic acidosis and an elevated molar ratio of lactate to pyruvate (>25 mol/mol) should alert the clinician to the possibility of a mitochondrial hepatopathy. Defects in fatty acid oxidation, a primary function of mitochondria, may become clinically apparent during a period of fasting, as a consequence of anorexia associated with an acute illness, or when the infant begins to sleep through the night.

In older infants and young children up to 5 years of age, mitochondrial diseases, tyrosinemia, hereditary fructose intolerance, and urea cycle defects can be identified [1]. Mitochondrial hepatopathies, particularly disorders of fatty acid oxidation, occur commonly in this age group [21]. Hereditary fructose intolerance presents only after the introduction of fructose and/or sucrose. Urea cycle defects typically present with hyperammonemia, mental status changes and seizures, but without liver synthetic dysfunction. However, pediatric ALF has been associated with arginosuccinate synthetase deficiency (citrullinemia type 1) and ornithine transcarbamylase deficiency, although the mechanism of liver injury is uncertain.

Wilson disease is the most common metabolic condition associated with pediatric ALF in children over 5 years of age [1]. The presence of a Coombs-negative hemolytic anemia, marked hyperbilirubinemia, low serum ceruloplasmin, and a low serum alkaline phosphatase should prompt consideration of Wilson disease, but confirming the diagnosis remains a challenge. Findings in a predominately adult population suggests that the combination of an alkaline phosphatase to total bilirubin ratio of <4 and an aspartate aminotransferase to alanine aminotransferase ratio of >2.2 provided a rapid and accurate method for diagnosis of Wilson disease presenting as ALF [22]. However, these findings have not yet been confirmed in a pediatric population. Fatty acid oxidation defects can also present with ALF in older children and adolescents.

Infectious diseases

A non-specific prodrome consisting of fever, nausea, vomiting, and abdominal discomfort will precede many cases of ALF in children regardless of etiology. Therefore, it is not surprising that early accounts of ALF often attributed the cause to a virus or infection. As the ability to identify specific infectious agents through serology, culture, and polymerase chain reaction technology has been applied, the common hepatitis viruses have not often been found in ALF unless they were endemic to the region or in association with a community outbreak. Although an as yet unidentified infectious agent may account for some unexplained cases of ALF in children, efforts to identify rare infectious agents in adults have not been fruitful. Therefore, a reasonable alternative is to classify as indeterminate any patient without an identifiable cause for the ALF until such time as a more specific diagnosis can be established.

Hepatitis viruses

Acute HAV infection accounts for up to 80% of pediatric ALF in developing countries [23]. In the Pediatric Acute Liver Failure Study, which reflects the introduction of the HAV vaccine in 1995, only 0.8% of children had HAV and ALF [1]. Less than 1% of children with symptomatic HAV develop ALF.

Acute hepatitis B virus (HBV) infection resulting in ALF is uncommon in pediatric series from Western Europe and North America, where HBV is not endemic. Among the first 653 patients in the Pediatric Acute Liver Failure Study, HBV was not reported as a final diagnosis. However, in areas where it is endemic, HBV accounts for 40–70% of pediatric ALF. Death occurs more commonly in older patients and in individuals who acquired HBV following a blood transfusion. Mutations in the HBV genome appear to be a risk factor in the development of ALF [24].

Hepatitis C virus infection has rarely been identified as the cause for ALF, and ALF has not been observed in large studies of transfusion-acquired hepatitis C virus infection [25]. Hepatitis C virus RNA has not been detected in the serum of patients with sporadic fulminate hepatitis without defined cause [26].

Hepatitis E virus infection is documented by association with epidemics of water-borne diseases not caused by HAV or by the presence of anti-hepatitis E virus antibody in serum. Most experience with hepatitis E virus comes from the Indian subcontinent, where 38% of pediatric ALF cases were caused by hepatitis E virus alone or in combination with HAV [27]. The case fatality rate from ALF among pregnant women in one study was 10.1%, with women in the third trimester particularly at risk. A higher incidence of hepatitis E virus-associated pediatric ALF may be documented if the frequency of serologic testing for the virus increases in the evaluation of pediatric ALF [14].

Infection with viruses other than hepatitis viruses

The viruses in the herpes family are highly cytopathic and can cause severe hepatic necrosis, often in the absence of significant inflammation. Herpes simplex virus, human herpesvirus 6 (HHV-6), varicella–zoster virus, cytomegalovirus, and Epstein–Barr virus have been reported to cause ALF in both immunocompromised and immunocompetent hosts [2]. Herpes simplex virus most commonly affects infants and newborns while Epstein–Barr virus is the virus most frequently implicated in older children and adolescents. As herpes simplex virus is a sexually transmitted disease, it should also be considered in sexually active adolescents. Human herpesvirus 6 was detected in the explanted livers of patients who underwent liver transplant for ALF of unknown cause. However, this virus is so prevalent as a latent infection in humans that causality may be difficult to prove in cases of ALF. Little is known about the incidence or case fatality rates among children with ALF secondary to herpesvirus infection. However, early detection utilizing newer diagnostic techniques, such as real-time polymerase chain reaction, and early institution of specific therapy may improve survival [28].

Parvovirus B19 routinely infects children, causing one of the common childhood exanthemas [2]. It rarely can cause severe bone marrow depression and has been associated with mild hepatitis. Its role as a cause of pediatric ALF is controversial as it is often associated with other viruses known to cause pediatric ALF. This virus has been sought and not found in other studies involving larger numbers of patients with ALF and aplastic anemia.

Syncytial giant cell hepatitis with ALF was associated with paramyxovirus infection in a series from Toronto [29]. This infection is more likely to result in chronic progressive hepatitis or late-onset hepatic failure than ALF but should be considered in all three circumstances. Other viruses associated with ALF include adenovirus, dengue fever, and members of the enterovirus family such as echovirus [11,21] and coxsackie A and B.

Non-viral infectious hepatitis

Infectious agents other than viruses only rarely have been recorded as producing ALF. Despite the rarity of occurrence, they should be considered carefully in every case because they are potentially treatable.

Systemic sepsis occasionally presents in a manner that is virtually indistinguishable from ALF. Reported infectious etiologies include *Neisseria meningitides* infection, septic shock and intra-abdominal abscesses, and portal sepsis with enteric organisms. Spirochetal infection can affect liver function and produce severe hepatitis, even hepatic failure. Congenital syphilis has rarely been determined as a cause of ALF but should be excluded carefully in any neonate with severe hepatitis. Leptospirosis very rarely causes hepatic failure. Finally, in endemic areas, *Brucella* spp. (brucellosis), *Coxiella burnetii* (Q fever), *Plasmodium falciparum*, and *Entamoeba histolytica* infections have presented as ALF.

Other rare causes

Liver failure may be the presenting manifestation of a systemic condition. For example, leukemia can present as liver failure [1]. Cardiovascular shock associated with systemic hypotension, as seen in patients with trauma, sepsis, hemorrhage, cardiomyopathy or left heart failure (e.g. hypoplastic left heart), or following cardiac bypass may also develop liver failure. Liver failure may be the presenting feature of celiac disease and, if recognized, is potentially treatable following institution of a gluten-free diet [30].

Indeterminate failure

A specific diagnosis is not identified in approximately 50% of children with pediatric ALF [1]. Historically, indeterminate pediatric ALF has been classified as non-A non-B hepatitis, neonatal hepatitis, or non-A–E hepatitis. Such nomenclature may imply the etiology is an undetected or yet to be discovered virus. Efforts to identify novel or unexpected hepatotropic viruses have not yet been rigorously undertaken in children, but such searches in adults were unrevealing [31]. While the clinical relevance is uncertain, 12% of children with indeterminate pediatric ALF were found to harbor acetaminophen-cysteine adducts without a clear toxic exposure to acetaminophen [9]. This raises the possibility that unsuspected acetaminophen toxicity may be present in some children with indeterminate ALF; alternatively, this finding may just represent acetaminophen exposure without any relation to the pathogenesis of the ALF.

Indeterminate pediatric ALF likely consists of multiple patient subgroups (Figure 4.2). One subgroup reflects an incomplete diagnostic evaluation, occurring for a variety of reasons including variation in diagnostic prioritization or premature interruption of the planned diagnostic tests by death, liver transplantation, or clinical improvement in which further diagnostic studies are abandoned. For example, children with indeterminate ALF were incompletely evaluated for autoimmune hepatitis with only 79% undergoing any testing for autoimmune hepatitis and only 55% had all three autoantibodies determined [14]. Another subgroup likely comprises patients with an undefined pathophysiological injury that is not identified using our current diagnostic

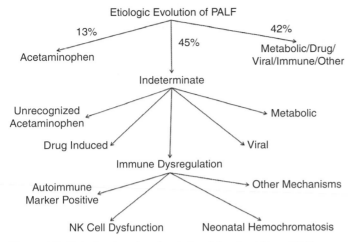

Etiologic Evolution of PALF

13% — Acetaminophen

45% — Indeterminate

42% — Metabolic/Drug/Viral/Immune/Other

Indeterminate:
- Unrecognized Acetaminophen
- Drug Induced
- Immune Dysregulation
- Metabolic
- Viral

Immune Dysregulation:
- Autoimmune Marker Positive
- NK Cell Dysfunction
- Neonatal Hemochromatosis
- Other Mechanisms

Figure 4.2 Etiologic categories of acute liver failure in children (PALF). A portion of the indeterminate group likely constitutes incomplete evaluation because of death, liver transplant, or clinical improvement. In addition, the indeterminate cohort may include unexpected acetaminophen toxicity, a novel or unrecognized virus, metabolic/xenobiotic injury, or undiagnosed immune dysregulation. A prioritized diagnostic algorithm will reduce the number of indeterminate cases and identify potentially treatable conditions as well as those patients where liver transplantation would be futile. Reduced morbidity and mortality and a more informed liver transplantation decision may result from improved diagnostic strategies.

strategies. Again with autoimmune hepatitis as an example, 5 of 62 patients with a final diagnosis of autoimmune hepatitis had no positive markers for the disorder reported and were deemed to have "marker negative" autoimmune hepatitis. One could speculate that such cases may reflect an ill-defined immune dysregulation that is pathophysiologically distinct from autoimmune disease but clinically responsive to similar treatment strategies.

"Recurrent" liver failure

In rare instances, a child will appear to recover completely from an episode of indeterminate pediatric ALF only to experience a second or even third episode. Conditions associated with recurrent pediatric ALF include metabolic disease, particularly fatty acid oxidation defects and respiratory chain disorders, and re-exposure to an unsuspected drug or herbal remedy.

Diagnostic approach

The diagnostic evaluation of children with ALF can be challenged by many factors. These include the volume of blood needed to complete diagnostic tests, a rapid clinical trajectory ending in death or liver transplantation prior to a complete evaluation, a differential diagnosis that is incomplete or not prioritized, or clinical improvement that mitigates diagnostic curiosity. In pediatric ALF, nearly 50% of patients are left with an indeterminate diagnosis. Given the rarity of pediatric ALF, an age-based diagnostic approach is useful to improve

diagnostic yield. If a specific diagnosis can be secured, an effective treatment could alter the natural history of the disease.

A detailed history and physical examination cannot be overlooked or abbreviated [2]. The history should include the onset of symptoms such as jaundice, change in mental status, easy bruising, vomiting, and fever. Exposure to contacts with infectious hepatitis, history of blood transfusions, a list of prescription and over-the-counter medications in the home, intravenous drug use, or a family history of Wilson disease, α_1-antitrypsin deficiency, infectious hepatitis, infant deaths, or autoimmune conditions might lead to a specific diagnosis. Evidence of developmental delay and/or seizures should prompt an early assessment for metabolic disease. Pruritus, ascites, or growth failure might suggest a chronic liver condition with an acute presentation.

Physical assessment should include evaluation of growth, development, and nutrition status; evidence of jaundice, bruises, or bleeding following venopuncture; and petechiae. Hepatomegaly alone or with splenomegaly, ascites, and peripheral edema can be present. Kayser–Fleischer rings are present in only 50% of patients with Wilson disease who present with ALF. Fetor hepaticus is a sweet distinctive aroma to the breath associated with HE but is rarely present. Findings suggestive of chronic liver disease include digital clubbing, palmar erythema, cutaneous xanthoma, and prominent abdominal vessels, suggesting long-standing portal hypertension. Altered mental status should be assessed but may be difficult to assess in infants and young children.

Laboratory tests for diagnosis will necessarily compete with other studies required to assess the health of the patient and the severity of liver injury. Therefore, laboratory studies needed for management and diagnosis should be prioritized into three areas: (1) general tests to assess hematological, renal, pancreatic, and electrolyte abnormalities; (2) liver-specific tests to assess the degree of inflammation, injury, and function; and (3) diagnostic tests. As over 30% of children with ALF are under 3 years of age, limitations on the volume of blood that can be drawn demands a knowledgeable prioritization of tests. In addition, required blood work in preparation for a liver transplant also competes for this limited resource. Proactive coordination of laboratory and diagnostic tests is helpful to ensure high priority tests are performed expeditiously.

The distribution of diagnoses varies greatly within the pediatric age group. While some conditions such as herpes simplex virus can occur within all age categories, others such as neonatal hemochromatosis and Wilson disease are found within a more narrow age range. Therefore, age-based diagnostic prioritization would serve to enhance the likelihood of establishing a diagnosis as quickly as possible. Table 4.5 lists diagnostic tests that would be most useful for children of different ages based upon the expected diagnoses. Diagnostic tests should not be limited to those listed, but should take a high priority when testing is initiated.

Table 4.5 Age-specific diagnostic prioritization

Age	Tests
< 3 months of age	Herpes blood PCR (or other testing: HSV IgM, viral culture of blood or CSF, CSF PCR)
	Enterovirus blood PCR (or other testing)
	Lactate, pyruvate (mitochondrial screen)
	Plasma acylcarnitine profile (fatty acid oxidation defects)
	Ferritin (neonatal iron storage disease screen)
	Serum amino acid profile (urea cycle and metabolic)
	Echocardiography (cardiac dysfunction)
	Abdominal ultrasound with Doppler (vascular and anatomic dysfunction)
	Confirm newborn screen results (galactosemia)
	Confirm maternal hepatitis B serology
3 months to 4 years	HBsAg, HAV IgM, EBV (VCA IgM or EBV PCR)
	Lactate, pyruvate (mitochondrial screen)
	Autoimmune markers: ANA, ASMA, ALKM, IgG
	Drug history, acetaminophen level
	Plasma acylcarnitine profile (fatty acid oxidation defects)
	Serum amino acids
	Abdominal ultrasound with Doppler (vascular and anatomic)
5 years to 18 years	HBsAg, HAV IgM, EBV (EBV VCA IgM or PCR)
	Autoimmune markers: ANA, ASMA, ALKM, IgG
	Ceruloplasmin
	Drug history, acetaminophen level
	Lactate, pyruvate (mitochondrial screen)
	Plasma acylcarnitine profile (fatty acid oxidation defects)
	Serum amino acids
	Abdominal ultrasound with Doppler (vascular and anatomic)
Additional diagnostic screening tests to consider directed by history and clinical course	Infectious causes:
	blood culture
	viral PCR in blood for adenovirus, enterovirus, EBV, human herpesvirus 6, parvovirus
	nasal wash for influenza (infections)
	hepatitis E antibody
	Soluble interleukin-2 receptor, ferritin in older patients, triglycerides (hemophagocytic lymphohistiocytosis)
	Echocardiography (cardiac)
	MRI for tissue iron (neonatal iron storage)
	Urine succinyl acetone (tyrosinemia)
	Urine orotic acid (urea cycle defects)
	Urine organic acids (metabolic)
	Liver copper, Wilson gene mutation analysis (Wilson disease)
	Liver biopsy for histology, culture, electron microscopy

ALKM, anti-liver–kidney microsome antibody; ANA, anti-nuclear antibody; ASMA, anti-smooth muscle antibody; CSF, cerebrospinal fluid; EBV, Epstein–Barr virus; HAV, hepatitis A virus; HBV, hepatitis B virus; HBsAg, HBV surface antigen; HSV, herpes simplex virus; PCR, polymerase chain reaction; VCA, EBV viral capsid antigen.

Identification of those conditions that are amenable to specific therapy would be relevant to subsequent pregnancies, or would be a contraindication to liver transplantation, should take priority [2]. Acute acetaminophen toxicity, herpes simplex, and hemophagocytic lymphohistiocytosis have targeted treatments that can be life saving. Autoimmune hepatitis, a potentially treatable cause of ALF in children of all ages, should be considered early in the evaluation process to enable prompt initiation of treatment. However, autoimmune markers are found in conditions other than autoimmune hepatitis, thus necessitating subjective clinical judgment to

influence the final diagnosis and treatment strategy [14]. Acute liver failure may be the initial symptom associated with metabolic defects related to carbohydrate, fatty acid, and protein metabolism in which dietary management serves as treatment. Identifying an index case of neonatal hemochromatosis will provide an opportunity to treat the mother during subsequent pregnancies with intravenous immunoglobulin and prevent the condition in subsequent pregnancies. Recovery from the acute liver injury in tyrosinemia can be accomplished with nitisinone (2(2-nitro-4-fluoromethylbenzoyl)-1,3-cyclohexanedione). A patient with a systemic mitochondrial disease presenting as ALF, either independent of or associated with valproate intake, will not benefit from liver transplant as outcome is uniformly poor. Characterization of underlying mechanisms of liver injury associated with immune dysregulation, metabolic disorders, and unsuspected acetaminophen exposure will identify patients who may be amenable to targeted treatment strategies.

Pathogenesis

The liver is remarkably tolerant and unperturbed despite its engagement with "first-pass" exposure to xenobiotics, foreign proteins, endotoxins, and other potential hepatotoxic substances. The initiation, potentiation, resolution, and recovery of liver injury is efficient, complex, enigmatic, and redundant. How and why patients within the same diagnostic category, such as autoimmune hepatitis, can have myriad presentations ranging from asymptomatic elevations of serum aminotransferases to fatal liver failure is yet to be determined. At the heart of most models of liver injury rests an aberrant or exuberant inflammatory or immune response. It will be through this prism that the discussion on pathogenesis will be viewed.

Hepatic immunology

The liver has a unique, integrated immune system [32]. In addition to hepatocytes, an estimated 20–40% of the liver cell mass consists of endothelial cells, Kupffer cells, or hepatic macrophages, lymphocytes, biliary cells, and stellate cells. The immunologic milieu that exists within the liver is notably different than that of the peripheral blood compartment. The balance between CD8 and CD4 T-cells favors CD8 cells with effector/memory cells more frequent in liver parenchyma than peripheral blood. Natural killer T-cells (NKT-cells) as well as NK cells are more abundant in the liver where there is also a large source of gamma–delta T-cells. Antigen-presenting cells may be conventional (e.g. Kupffer cells, liver sinusoidal endothelial cells, and dendritic cells) or unconventional (e.g. hepatocytes).

Both innate and adaptive immune responses are generated within the liver. However, given the hepatic enrichment by NK cell, NKT-cells, and Kupffer cells, it is not surprising that the innate immune response predominates [33]. Under normal circumstances, the lymphocyte-driven innate response provides a nimble but temperate reaction to pathogens that present to the liver. Kupffer cells and other immune cells express pattern-recognition receptors that detect and bind pathogen-associated molecular patterns expressed on the presumptive pathogen, which is then phagocytosed and quietly eliminated. Activated CD8 cells residing in the liver direct the immune response against bacterial and viral invasion. Priming of intrahepatic T-cells may occur within the liver without having to circulate through draining lymph nodes, thus expediting the immune response [34]. Hepatic NK cells serve to modulate the inflammatory response by mediating the balance between proinflammatory (T helper 1) and anti-inflammatory (T helper 2) cytokines that are generated.

Adaptive immune responses involve both B- and T-cells. Very few B-cells reside in the normal liver and thus little is known about their role except under pathologic conditions such as HBV and hepatitis C infections. Antigen-specific CD8 T-cells generate an effector response that includes rapid proliferation coupled with the production of proinflammatory cytokines as well as initiation of cytolytic mechanisms such as perforin and granzyme [32]. Not unexpectedly, the redundancy of the human immune response cannot be easily divided into separate and distinct components. For example, recent findings suggest that NK cells may have features associated with the adaptive immune response such as "memory," with rapid secondary expansion upon re-exposure to antigen that is associated with degranulation and cytokine production [35]. Therefore, while missteps in the livers' overall tolerance of real or perceived pathogens rarely result in liver failure, understanding these events will provide opportunities to extend our knowledge of the interactions between the liver and its environment.

Drug- and toxin-induced injury

Drug-induced liver injury causes approximately 15% of pediatric ALF, with acetaminophen toxicity accounting for 80% of the drug-induced cases. The mechanisms by which drugs cause liver injury vary [11]. Acetaminophen toxicity resulting from ingestion of a single overdose has been the most extensively investigated. An overdose of acetaminophen overwhelms cellular mechanisms that safely metabolize the compound, leaving reactive acetaminophen oxygen species that, after depleting glutathione stores, covalently bind to intracellular proteins and likely disrupt critical intracellular structures, resulting in features of both apoptotic and necrotic cell death mediated in part by c-Jun N-terminal kinase [36,37]. Necrotic hepatocytes may release high-mobility group box-1, which stimulates resident Kupffer cells through toll-like receptor 4 to release proinflammatory cytokines coupled by recruitment and activation of neutrophils [38]. Therefore, both toxic injury and the following intense mixed inflammatory response contribute to the liver injury. Interestingly, hepatic progenitor cells or oval cells appear to be resistant to acetaminophen toxicity [39] and this property may account, in part, for improved survival in appropriately treated patients with acute acetaminophen toxicity.

Mitochondrial injury is an increasingly recognized mechanism by which drugs can cause pediatric ALF [40]. Injury to mitochondria can take a number of different pathways either singly or in combination, which include mitochondrial DNA depletion or damage (fialuridine, stavudine), direct inhibition of the mitochondrial respiratory chain (acetaminophen, amiodarone), uncoupling of oxidative phosphorylation (diclofenac, ibuprofen), direct inhibition of mitochondrial fatty acid oxidation (valproic acid, tamoxifen), and opening of mitochondrial permeability transition pores (valproic acid, disulfiram).

Naturally occurring liver toxins are rare but do occur. Amatoxins are bicyclic octapeptides found in nine species of *Amanita* mushrooms. Amatoxins remain intact even after cooking or prolonged storage, have a low median lethal dose, and the amount present in a single mushroom can be fatal. RNA polymerase II is inhibited by amatoxins, resulting in global interruption of protein synthesis and cell death [41]. Kava is an extract of the Pacific Island plant *Piper methysticum*. The mechanism of liver injury is uncertain but it is speculated that it inhibits cytokine P450 enzymes or depletes glutathione. Other herbal hepatotoxins that have been associated with liver failure include Margosa oil, Noni juice, *Atractylis gummifera*, and green tea extract.

Vascular injury

Acute liver failure can result from reduced or absent arterial blood flow to the liver. The insult can occur as a consequence of hemorrhagic shock, trauma, sepsis, coarctation of the aorta, congenital heart defects associated with low cardiac output, congestive heart failure, and liver transplant. Myriad processes are initiated following liver ischemia that include the release of pro- and anti-inflammatory cytokines and chemokines, complement activation, along with the activation of both the innate and the adaptive immune response. Mitochondrial injury resulting in ATP depletion and surge in toxic reactive oxygen species contribute to the injury.

Liver failure associated with acute obstruction of hepatic outflow is rare but has been described in patients later found to have a coagulation disorder leading to a hypercoagulable state; in patients with Behçet syndrome or idiopathic Budd–Chiari syndrome; and in women immediately postpartum [2].

Immune/inflammatory injury

The extent to which hepatic immune dysregulation in general or immune-mediated liver injury in particular, together with the systemic inflammatory response syndrome, is involved in the pathogenesis of pediatric ALF is not known [42–44]. And yet, given the rich and varied hepatic immunologic environment, it would be expected that immune and inflammatory mechanisms are involved in both the initiation and perpetuation of pediatric ALF in most, if not all, cases. Liver cell injury associated with viral hepatitis is not caused by direct injury from the virus but rather from "collateral damage" associated with a vigorous immune response to clear the virus from the liver. Drug-induced liver injury may result in the formation of neoantigens, consisting of reactive metabolites of the offending drug coupled with cellular constituents that induce an immune response.

The inflammatory response encompasses both injury and healing through a dynamic duet between pro- and anti-inflammatory responses [45]. Proinflammatory responses are generated by immune effector cells, such as Kupffer cells, B- and T-lymphocytes, and neutrophils, releasing a host of proportioned chemokines, adhesins, and cytokines. The compensatory anti-inflammatory response is initiated almost simultaneously to disengage the inflammatory response through anti-inflammatory cytokines interleukin-4, interleukin-10, transforming growth factor-β and others to deactivate the cellular immune function and reduce antigen-presenting capability. Exaggeration or dysregulation of either the pro- or anti-inflammatory responses can result in increased mortality and susceptibility to sepsis and multiorgan dysfunction.

Liver cell regeneration

Following acute liver injury, survival and recovery is dependent at least in part on the remarkable ability of the liver to regenerate from injury [46]. Low rates of spontaneous recovery in adults with idiopathic and drug-induced ALF have been attributed, in part, to diminished capacity for regeneration. Elucidation of the mechanisms that govern hepatic regeneration in the setting of ALF could lead to the development of agents that promote regeneration and the recognition of biomarkers with which to assess the degree of regeneration. Each of these would be of great benefit in clinical hepatology. Biological markers of liver regeneration would be particularly useful in the decision to proceed to liver transplantation in pediatric ALF. Those with a profile predicting little or no regenerative ability may best be served by transplantation, while those with a vigorous regenerative response would hold some hope of recovery.

Liver histology in acute liver failure

Liver cell necrosis is characteristic of ALF resulting from viral infections, most toxic and ischemic injuries, and some metabolic diseases. The degree of hepatocellular necrosis and its histologic pattern vary by cause and by individual case. Establishing a pathologic diagnosis by liver biopsy has not been considered critical in patient management, largely because of the associated risks and, at times, the disappointing impact histology has in altering the treatment strategy or establishing the diagnosis. Recently, the transvenous (e.g. transjugular) approach to obtain liver tissue has so markedly reduced the risks of obtaining a liver biopsy in this population that many more biopsies are being performed in the setting of ALF. As a consequence, much should be learned about the value of biopsy in this setting.

Most liver samples from children with ALF show massive confluent or multilobular necrosis (Figure 4.3). In many specimens, it is difficult to identify any remaining viable hepatocytes. The reticulin framework of the lobule is collapsed, and the mass of the liver is small. A moderate inflammatory infiltrate, usually consisting mainly of neutrophils, may be evident. In some patients, no evidence of regeneration can be found [47]; in others, there is proliferation of duct-like structures that probably results from attempts at regeneration. Occasionally, if orthotopic liver transplantation is performed early in the course of rapidly progressive ALF, the gross surgical and microscopic appearances of the liver are relatively normal. The lobular structure and framework may be intact, including a normal cord pattern, but the hepatocytes are necrotic. Inflammation is absent. This lesion suggests widespread,

(a)

(b)

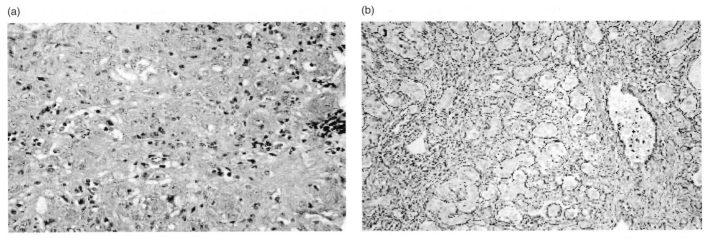

Figure 4.3 Liver histopathology from a patient with indeterminate acute liver failure. (a) Transjugular biopsy at time of presentation shows confluent necrosis with a little parenchymal inflammation. There were no viable hepatocytes evident in any of the several cores. This section shows some tubular structures thought to represent attempted regeneration. (Hematoxylin & eosin, original magnification 200×.) (b) This reticulin stain shows focal collapse. The distance between the central vein and portal area on the left is diminished, and the reticulin framework between is condensed. (Reticulin stain, original magnification 100×.)

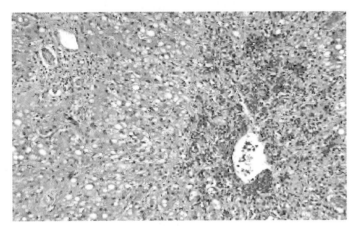

Figure 4.4 Hepatactomy specimen from a teenager who overdosed on acetaminophen. The specimen showed extensive sublobular necrosis throughout the liver. The central orientation of the necrosis is evident in this section because of the hemorrhage in and around the central vein on the right. The periportal zone is relatively spared, with a narrow rim of viable hepatocytes seen around the portal triad in the upper left. Between the frank necrosis and the rim of viable hepatocytes is a zone of hepatocyte injury notable by steatosis and ballooning of marginally viable hepatocytes. (Hematoxylin & eosin, original magnification 100×.)

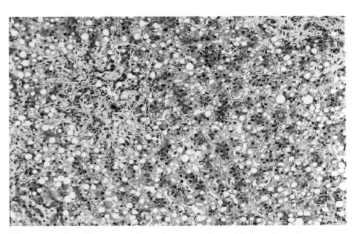

Figure 4.5 Liver biopsy specimen from an infant with hereditary fructose intolerance and hepatic failure. There is both diffuse hepatocyte necrosis and steatosis, mainly macrovesicular. Other findings include pseudotubule formation and condensation of organelles and cytoplasmic elements within hepatocytes. Interlobular bile ducts also are injured, with irregular shape of cholangiocytes and some vacuolization. The patient recovered normal liver function within 5 days of eliminating fructose from the diet. (Hematoxylin & eosin, original magnification 200×.)

simultaneous lethal injury of hepatocytes. Much less commonly, the pathologic specimen demonstrates lesser degrees of necrosis. Diffuse hepatocellular necrosis, with patchy loss of hepatocytes throughout the lobule, may be seen in viral hepatitis. Non-icteric fulminant failure, some drug-induced liver disease (e.g. acetaminophen), and hypoxic–ischemic hepatitis are characterized by sublobular necrosis, with orientation of necrosis around central veins (Figure 4.4) [48,49].

Diffuse hepatic steatosis is observed rarely in ALF in children. This lesion is characterized by hepatocellular fat in a microvesicular pattern and is identical at a light-microscopic level to the hepatic lesion of Reye syndrome. In adults, it is seen most often in fatty liver of pregnancy; in

children, it is seen in association with toxic injury or inborn errors of metabolism (see Etiology). The absence of cell necrosis in association with failure of liver function implies organelle failure as the cause. Hepatomegaly is often evident. Serum aminotransferase levels usually are elevated, but only to a mild to moderate degree (usually <400 IU/L). Jaundice is minimal (serum bilirubin concentration usually <10 mg/dL), which suggests that certain organelle functions remain intact and also that bilirubin production probably is not increased. Full histologic recovery is the rule if the patient survives.

A third lesion, characterized by diffuse swelling of hepatocytes with condensation of organelles and cytoplasmic elements (Figure 4.5), is seen in association with some inborn errors of metabolism. Hepatocyte necrosis is spotty and usually not prominent. Macrovesicular fat with displacement of nuclei is seen in a variable proportion of hepatocytes, sometimes a majority. This lesion suggests organelle injury that is severe enough to cause the death of some hepatocytes. Aminotransferase levels and serum bilirubin levels are elevated moderately. Full histologic recovery is the rule if the metabolic injury can be controlled.

Finally, the histologic picture may be dominated by a mixed inflammatory infiltrate consisting primarily of lymphocytes with a scattering of plasma cells, neutrophils, and eosinophils in conjunction with hepatic necrosis. Fibrosis, which would suggest chronic disease, is not present. The inflammatory infiltrate is not limited to the portal tracks but can be found within the lobule and around the central vein. Serum autoimmune markers may be present, but often are not, and the underlying cause for the liver injury is often not determined.

Complications and management

General management principles

Close collaboration between gastroenterology/hepatology, intensive care, neurology, neurosurgery, nephrology, metabolic disease specialists as well as transplant surgeons will afford the child the best opportunity to survive. After the initial characterization of the patient presentation, proper patient management needs to be conducted along multiple parallel paths: (1) monitor and support the patient and organ systems, (2) identify and treat complications, (3) develop an age-appropriate diagnostic prioritization strategy, and (4) treat the patient to maximize health and survival [2].

Admission to a highly skilled nursing environment, which, in most cases, will be an intensive care unit is essential and allows frequent monitoring of mental status. A cardiorespiratory and oxygen saturation monitor should not substitute for careful and frequent bedside assessment by an experienced nurse or clinician. Input and output should be strictly monitored. Care-givers must carefully examine the child multiple times during the day and night to assess evidence of changing mental status or HE, increased respiratory effort, changing heart rate or changes in blood pressure which might be signs of infection, increasing cerebral edema, or electrolyte imbalance.

Laboratory monitoring should include a complete blood count, electrolytes, renal function tests, glucose, calcium, phosphorus, ammonia, coagulation profile, total and direct bilirubin, and blood cultures. Diagnostic laboratory studies should be prioritized. While arterial ammonia measurement is ideal, it is not practical in children with stage 0–II HE; venous ammonia obtained from a free-flowing catheter and promptly placed on ice and transported to the laboratory may be a suitable substitute. Placement of arterial and central catheters should be reserved for patients who show signs of clinical deterioration to late-stage II or stage III HE.

In the absence of the need for volume resuscitation, total intravenous fluids should initially be restricted to between 85 and 95% of maintenance fluids to avoid overhydration yet still provide sufficient glucose and phosphorus to achieve normal serum values. Adjustment in fluid rates are based upon the clinical conditions, but relative fluid restriction should be an underlying principle. Nutritional support, including protein, should be provided if the patient can eat safely or with intravenous nutritional support. Some protein restriction may be necessary, but it should not be eliminated.

Central nervous system
Encephalopathy

Hepatic encephalopathy is a neuropsychiatric syndrome associated with hepatic dysfunction. Changes in behavior, cognition, neurological examination, and electroencephalography (EEG) are used to characterize the patient as having one of five clinical stages of HE ranging from stage 0 with minimal or no evidence of neurological dysfunction to stage IV coma (Table 4.6) [50]. Clinical staging of HE was originally developed to assess patients with cirrhosis and not ALF, but in the absence of a better clinical tool, use of the current scoring system has been found to have important clinical and prognostic implications. The role of other modalities to assess neurological function, such a visual evoked potentials, transcranial Doppler, cerebral near-infrared spectroscopy, and biomarkers in the detection of HE are unclear at the present time. While neurologic morbidity remains a major determinant of outcome following pediatric ALF, further studies are needed to improve early detection of neurologic injury, standardize management of seizures and HE, and to determine whether such interventions improve outcomes.

Occurrence of HE is not always clinically apparent in infants and young children. However, some degree of encephalopathy is present on admission in 50% of children with ALF entering the Pediatric Acute Liver Failure Study, but encephalopathy was identified in 65% within the first 7 days following entry into the study [1]. The patient should be assessed frequently as neurological deterioration can be devastatingly rapid. Distinguishing hepatic-based encephalopathy from other causes of an altered mental status such as sepsis, hypotension, electrolyte disturbances, anxiety or "intensive care unit psychosis" is difficult for all age groups. Hyperammonemia plays a central role in the development of HE in most cases. However, a specific level of ammonia does not result in a predictable degree of encephalopathy. Initial treatment would include minimizing excess stimulation, reducing protein intake, treating suspected sepsis, and removing sedative medications that would affect mental status. Medical therapy with lactulose is used empirically but lacks evidence of efficacy. Bowel "decontamination" with rifaximin or neomycin can be used as a second-tier treatment, but ototoxicity and nephrotoxicity are potential risks when neomycin is used. Sodium benzoate has been used adults with cirrhosis, but concerns about increasing blood ammonia with this treatment have been raised.

Table 4.6 Stages of hepatic encephalopathy

Stage	Clinical	Reflexes	Neurologic signs	Electroencephalography changes
0	None	Normal	None	Normal
I	*Infant/child*: inconsolable crying, inattention to task, not acting like self to parents	Normal or hyper-reflexic	Difficult or impossible to test adequately	Difficult or impossible to test adequately
	Adult: confused, mood changes, altered sleep habits, forgetful	Normal	Tremor, apraxia, impaired hand-writing	Normal or diffuse slowing to theta rhythm, triphasic waves
II	*Infant/child*: inconsolable crying, inattention to task, not acting like self to parents	Normal or hyper-reflexic	Difficult or impossible to test adequately	Difficult or impossible to test adequately
	Adult: drowsy, inappropriate behavior, decreased inhibitions	Hyper-reflexic	Dysarthria, ataxia	Abnormal, generalized slowing, triphasic waves
III	*Infant/child*: somnolence, stupor, combativeness	Hyper-reflexic	Difficult or impossible to test adequately	Difficult or impossible to test adequately
	Adult: stuporous, obeys simple commands	Hyper-reflexic, (+) Babinski	Rigidity	Abnormal, generalized slowing, triphasic waves
IV	*Infant/child*: comatose, arouses with painful stimuli (IVa) or no response (IVb)	Absent	Decebrate or decorticate	
	Adult: comatose, arouses with painful stimuli (IVa) or no response	Absent	Decebrate or decorticate	Abnormal, very slow, delta activity

Not all patients with HE develop a clinically important increase in intracranial pressure. However, those that do can experience devastating consequences. Direct intracranial pressure monitoring is the most sensitive and specific test compared with less invasive neuroradiographic procedure, such as cranial CT. Monitoring of intracranial pressure remains controversial because of the associated complications of the procedure and no evidence of improved survival for those who were monitored.

Both generalized and focal seizures may occur in children with ALF. The frequency of non-convulsive (electrographic) seizures in this population has not been studied in detail. However, convulsive or non-convulsive seizures are known to occur during a critical illness. In most cases, treatment begins with phenytoin, but practices are variable and there is no definitive standard of care. For seizures that are refractory to phenytoin, therapeutic options may include midazolam infusion, phenobarbital, levitaracetam, or topiramate. The selection of drug will depend on the patient's mental status, physiologic stability, availability of EEG monitoring to titrate drug infusions, and institutional experience.

Cerebral edema

Cerebral edema is a life-threatening complication of ALF [51]. It occurs most commonly in those with advanced encephalopathy (grade III or IV) and can be rapidly progressive. Detection of cerebral edema in the early stages is difficult as non-invasive assessment with clinical assessment or radiographic studies may not be sufficiently sensitive. The most sensitive test requires surgical placement of an intracranial pressure (ICP) monitor which carries its own risk for the patient with an uncorrectable coagulopathy and carries a risk of bleeding between 10–20%, although it is often minimal [52]. Use of activated factor VII in recent years has made placement of ICP monitors somewhat safer. However, once in place and properly functioning, intracranial pressure monitoring is useful to assess response to treatment of increased cerebral pressure and during surgical procedures, including liver transplantation, to gauge fluid and medical management of the unconscious patient.

The pathogenesis of cerebral edema is complex involving the interaction among ammonia, cerebral blood flow, and inflammation [53]. Elevated levels of ammonia are generated as a consequence of the failing liver which leads to increased intracerebral concentrations. Ammonia enters the astrocyte which is rich in glutamine synthetase. Conversion of ammonia and glutamate to glutamine, a potent intracellular osmolyte, results in an osmotic gradient that favors astrocyte swelling that contributes to cerebral edema and intracranial hypertension. The tight regulation of cerebral blood flow is tested in the setting of ALF. Alterations in systemic and intracranial vascular resistance, coupled with restrictions to blood flow due to edema makes estimates of an "ideal" cerebral perfusion pressure (mean arterial pressure minus intracranial pressure) difficult. Changes in the inflammatory milieu, sepsis, fluid or blood product administration and other factors can result in a sudden and often unanticipated increase in intracranial pressure and its consequences.

Management of cerebral edema involves meticulous supportive management to maintain oxygen saturation above 95%, fluid restriction between 85 and 90% of maintenance, diastolic pressure >40 mmHg, adequate sedation, head elevation of 20° to 30° and neutral head position, and consideration of empiric broad spectrum antibiotics to minimize the development of bacterial infection [53]. Therapies targeted specifically to improve cerebral edema have not met scientific rigor, but they include hypertonic saline to maintain serum sodium between 145 meq/L and 150 meq/L, and mannitol keeping serum osmolarity <320 mOsm/L to create a more favorable osmotic gradient to extract water from the brain. Hypothermia has been used in adults with ALF with some success.

Hematologic system

Coagulopathy

Both PT and INR are used in virtually all prognostic schemes to assess the severity of liver injury in the setting of ALF and are also assumed to be markers for the risk of bleeding in these patients. In patients with ALF, both procoagulant proteins (e.g. factors V, VII, and X and fibrinogen) and anticoagulant proteins (e.g. antithrombin, protein C, and protein S) are reduced [2]. This balanced reduction in the pro- and anticoagulant proteins may account for the relative infrequency of clinically important bleeding in the patient with ALF in the absence of a provocative event such as infection or increased portal hypertension. Therefore, the PT/INR may reasonably reflect the reduction of some of the liver-based coagulation proteins but not the relative risk of bleeding. Efforts to "correct" the PT/INR with fresh frozen plasma or other procoagulation products such as recombinant factor VII should occur primarily in the setting of active bleeding or in anticipation of an invasive surgical procedure. Assurance of adequate vitamin K can be accomplished by intravenous infusion.

Aplastic anemia

Bone marrow failure, characterized by a spectrum of features ranging from mild pancytopenia to aplastic anemia, occurs in a significant minority of children with ALF [54]. It is identified most commonly in the setting of indeterminate ALF and may not be clinically evident until after emergency liver transplantation. Treatment includes immunomodulatory medications such as corticosteroids, cyclosporine A, anti-lymphocyte or anti-thymocyte globulin as well as hematopoietic stem cell transplant.

Gastrointestinal system

Ascites

Ascites develops in some but not all patients. Precipitating factors include hypoalbuminemia, excessive fluid administration, and infection. The primary treatment is fluid restriction. Diuretics should be reserved for patients with respiratory compromise or generalized fluid overload. Overly aggressive diuresis may precipitate hepatorenal syndrome.

Bleeding

Gastrointestinal bleeding occurs surprisingly infrequently given the degree of coagulopathy. Prophylactic use of acid-reducing agents is often initiated when the patient is admitted, but their usefulness is difficult to assess. Causes for bleeding include gastric erosions or ulcers due to use of non-steroidal anti-inflammatory medications, or idiopathic gastroduodenal ulceration. Infection can precipitate bleeding in this vulnerable population, so blood cultures and initiation of antibiotics should also be considered when bleeding develops. Administration of platelets, blood, and plasma is necessary if bleeding is hemodynamically significant.

Pancreatitis

Biochemical and clinical pancreatitis is increasingly recognized as a condition associated with multisystem failure in critically ill children. In patients who develop pancreatitis in the setting of ALF, glucose and fluid management may become even more challenging.

Renal system

Evidence of renal insufficiency and ALF on admission should be assessed for evidence of a medication or toxin as the precipitating cause. Prerenal azotemia can develop if fluid restriction is too excessive for the patient's needs. Acute deterioration of renal function after presentation with ALF may result from systemic hypotension in sepsis or hemorrhage. Hepatorenal syndrome is a feared renal complication associated with ALF, although it occurs more commonly in the setting of chronic liver disease with established cirrhosis. Hepatorenal syndrome can progress rapidly over the course of 2 weeks (type I) or more slowly (type II) [2]. The diagnosis is suspected when there is evidence of deteriorating renal function in the absence of bleeding, hypotension, sepsis, or nephrotoxic medications and in association with failure to improve with volume expansion. Urine sodium is typically low. Renal replacement therapy with continuous venovenous hemofiltration or dialysis may be necessary in some patients, but only liver transplantation can reverse hepatorenal syndrome. Patients who present simultaneously with both ALF and renal dysfunction may have sustained a toxic injury (e.g. acetaminophen, solvent, drug) or have Wilson disease.

Metabolic disorders

Hypoglycemia results from impaired gluconeogenesis and depleted glycogen stores. Glucose infusion rates as high as 10–15 mg/min per kg body weight may be required to achieve stable serum glucose levels and will require a central venous catheter for hypertonic glucose solutions. Hypokalemia may occur secondary to dilution from volume overload, ascites, or renal wasting. Serum phosphorus should be monitored frequently as hypophosphatemia can be profound. Acid–base disturbances can be complicated with respiratory alkalosis from hyperventilation, respiratory acidosis from respiratory failure, metabolic alkalosis from hypokalemia, and metabolic acidosis from hepatic necrosis, shock, and increased anaerobic metabolism.

Infections

Patients with ALF have an enhanced susceptibility to bacterial infection and sepsis from immune system dysfunction [2]. Evidence of infection may be subtle, such as tachycardia, intestinal bleeding, reduced renal output, or changes in mental status. Fever may not be present. Blood cultures should be obtained with any evidence of clinical deterioration and antibiotics initiated with a clinical concern for sepsis due to Gram-positive or Gram-negative organisms.

Cardiopulmonary system

Excessive fluid administration contributes to pulmonary edema and should be avoided. Careful fluid restriction and discrete use of diuretics may be needed in some instances, but should be used with caution. Central venous pressure monitoring may assist in assessing volume needs for the child. Ionotropic support may be needed to maintain perfusion of vital organs.

Nutrition

Nutrition support should be maintained to avoid a catabolic state. If it is not safe for the child to receive oral or enteral feeding, intravenous alimentation should be initiated to provide at least 1 g/kg protein daily. Adjustment in the protein allotment may be needed based on the serum ammonia. Micronutrients such as copper and manganese should be reduced or eliminated in patients with liver disease while chromium, molybdenum, and selenium should be reduced or eliminated if renal disease is also present.

Liver support

Plasmapheresis/plasma exchange

Plasmapheresis facilitates the removal of suspected toxins in the blood to facilitate a milieu in which the liver might recover or regenerate. Evidence of its usefulness in children with ALF is sparse, and while coagulation profiles may improve, the procedure has not been shown to improve neurologic outcome or ability of the liver to recover spontaneously. One potential disadvantage of this procedure is the non-selective removal of potentially helpful substances such as hepatocyte growth factor. The use of selective filters to facilitate retention of this potentially beneficial substance would make this therapy more attractive.

Membrane adsorbent recirculating system

The membrane adsorbent recirculating system is an elaborate detoxification system in which a membrane with albumin-related binding sites separates the patients' blood from an albumin dialysate. Albumin-bound substances, such as bilirubin, aromatic amino acids, and endogenous benzodiazepine-like substances, can be transferred to the membrane-binding sites and then to the albumin within the dialysate for removal. Unbound, free low-molecular-weight molecules, such as ammonia, can pass freely down a concentration gradient into the dialysate. The system has been used to treat children with mushroom poisoning and as a bridge for retransplantation. However, in the absence randomized trials, its relevance in the overall treatment of ALF is uncertain.

Disease severity assessment

Once pediatric ALF is identified, there are currently no reliable tools to predict survival or death. Biochemical tests (lactate, total bilirubin, phosphorus, INR, PT, ammonia, vitamin D-binding protein (Gc-globulin)), clinical features (encephalopathy, cerebral edema), diagnosis (acetaminophen) or combinations of the three have been tried without reliable success.

Existing liver failure scoring systems, including the Kings College Hospital Criteria, the Clichy Score, the Model for End-Stage Liver Disease Score, and Pediatric End-Stage Liver Disease Score, fall well short of the ideal prognostic tool [2]. Recently, the Liver Injury Unit Score developed specifically for pediatric ALF was proposed [55]. Utilizing the registry of the Pediatric Acute Liver Failure Study to test the validity of the Liver Injury Unit Score showed that the predictive accuracy for discriminating death from survival without liver transplant had 61–69% sensitivity and 65–72% specificity, depending on whether admission or peak values was used, and whether PT or INR was used [56]. Sensitivity and specificity of the King's College Hospital Criteria for death versus survival without liver transplant for non-acetaminophen-induced pediatric ALF were 61% and 56%, respectively. Using the Pediatric Acute Liver Failure Study Registry data to modify the cut-points of the components of these criteria to improve sensitivity and specificity improved sensitivity to nearly 74% and specificity to 80%. Although better, there is still room for improvement. We believe the ideal scoring system should reflect the dynamic nature of pediatric ALF and incorporate periodic clinical changes into deriving the likelihood of death or survival.

Liver transplant

Liver transplant decisions

Liver transplantation is often life saving when a condition without specific therapy is irreversible or fails to respond to treatment. At the same time, liver transplant is also irreversible and has profound consequences both on organ allocation as well as the recipient and family. The high frequency of liver transplant when the diagnosis is uncertain, coupled with children removed from the liver transplant list through clinical improvement before an organ became available, raises the possibility that liver transplant may proceed in situations in which spontaneous recovery may have occurred. Long-term outcomes following liver transplant for pediatric ALF are less favorable than when liver transplant is performed for chronic liver diseases such as biliary atresia. This is likely because of multiple factors including the severity of illness at the time of transplant and the possibility that the transplant was performed in circumstances in which death was inevitable regardless of the intervention. A more reliable modeling scheme is needed to readily and effectively distinguish the patient who would die from the one who would survive without liver transplant and to recognize when it would be futile to proceed with liver transplant.

Organ allocation in the setting of acute liver failure

Organ allocation for children with ALF remains an evolving process. In the late 1980s, highest priority went to those individuals who were expected to die within 24 hours. In 1991, the concept of a "status 1" patient was extended to both adults and children with a life expectancy of fewer than 7 days regardless of etiology; however, this approach disadvantaged children given the overwhelming number of adults with decompensated, chronic liver disease; a status 2A category was established for the latter adult group. In 1999, the Institute of Medicine issued a report that established disease severity scores for adults (Model for End-Stage Liver Disease) and children (Pediatric End-stage Liver Disease) with chronic liver disease. The status 1 category was preserved, however. Currently, a pediatric candidate can be listed as status 1A or 1B. In both categories, the child must be in an intensive care unit. Status 1A has four diagnostic categories: (1) fulminate liver failure, (2) primary non-function following liver transplantation, (3) hepatic artery thrombosis, and (4) acute decompensated Wilson disease. Status 1B is given to children in intensive care with chronic liver disease. To qualify for status 1A for fulminate liver failure, the United Network for Organ Sharing has defined fulminate liver failure as the onset of hepatic encephalopathy within 8 weeks of the first symptoms of liver disease in the absence of pre-existing liver disease, and one of the following three criteria: (1) ventilator dependence; (2) need for dialysis or continuous venovenous hemofiltration or continuous venovenous hemodialysis; or (3) INR >2.0. Children who are classified as status 1A will revert to their Pediatric End-stage Liver Disease Scores after 7 days unless an attending physician re-lists the patient as a status 1A.

In the future, the transplant decision process may include mathematical models that provide quantitative representations of the anticipated clinical trajectory, the likelihood of a successful outcome with liver transplant (whether from a deceased donor or living), and the likelihood of a successful outcome (recovery) in the absence of liver transplant. Early iterations of these models have been constructed in adults [57]. These models combine accurate understanding of (1) the risk of death in the absence of transplantation, (2) the expected survival after transplantation given the characteristics at transplant, and (3) the natural history of the disease, which is represented by the expected change in the predictors of pre-transplant death and post-transplant survival. These issues, particularly the risk of death and the natural history of the disease, will require better characterization in pediatric ALF.

Liver transplantation

Liver transplantation has improved overall survival for children with ALF. A deceased-donor whole, split, or cut-down liver transplant was used in nearly 86% of all transplants for ALF in children in a recent report from the Studies of Pediatric Liver Transplant consortium [58]. Living donor liver transplant for children with ALF and concurrent multiorgan failure is associated with improved 30-day and 6-month survival compared with recipients of a deceased donor liver allograft [59]. Improved outcome for patients receiving a living donor liver transplant is likely related to a reduced cold ischemia time and wait time, resulting in a more expeditious time to transplant for these seriously ill children. Auxiliary liver transplant has been used as a "bridge" to provide needed time for the native liver to regenerate, but challenges remain as to the timing for withdrawal of immunosuppression and involution of the transplanted graft [60].

Liver cell transplant

The role of hepatocyte transplantation in pediatric ALF is yet to be determined and may be an area of investigation in the future [61]. Hepatocyte transplantation may serve as a bridge to transplant or, perhaps, a "cure" for some children with metabolic diseases. It has been used in a small number of children with ALF. However, technical challenges as well as lack of a readily available source for hepatocytes have limited the opportunity for this procedure at most centers.

Outcomes

In the pre transplant era and an adult definition of ALF, spontaneous survival occurred in 28% of patients overall, and only 4% of those with stage IV coma [62]. More recently, with improvements in management of critically ill children coupled with a more lenient definition of pediatric ALF, outcomes have improved [1,2,19].

Findings from the Pediatric Acute Liver Failure Study revealed that 21-day outcome varied by diagnosis, age, and degree of encephalopathy [1,19]. Spontaneous survival or survival with their native liver was highest amongst those with ALF caused by acetaminophen (94%). Spontaneous survival occurred less frequently for those with ALF caused by metabolic disease (44%) or drugs other than acetaminophen (41%), and in indeterminate ALF (45%). As might be expected, those with higher coma scores had lower spontaneous survival. Unexpectedly, 21% of patients with a peak coma score of 0 either died or received a liver transplant. Therefore, many with minimal or no clinical evidence of encephalopathy do not survive with their native liver. For children with an established diagnosis, the percentage of those receiving a liver transplant ranged between 20 and 33%. However, liver transplant occurred in 46% of those patients with an indeterminate diagnosis. Therefore, children who do not have a specific diagnosis are more likely to receive a liver transplant. Only 2% of children with acetaminophen-induced ALF received a liver transplant in this cohort. The major causes of death for all who do not receive a liver transplant include multiorgan system failure, cerebral edema and herniation, and sepsis.

Both early and late graft loss and death is higher among children who undergo liver transplantation for ALF than for those with chronic liver disease [63]. Reasons for these findings are uncertain, but one possibility is the immune dysregulation that may be associated with pediatric ALF, which could lead to increased susceptibility to infection or graft rejection.

References

1. Squires RH, Jr., Shneider BL, Bucuvalas J, *et al.* Acute liver failure in children: the first 348 patients in the pediatric acute liver failure study group. *J Pediatr* 2006;**148**:652–658.

2. Squires RH, Jr. Acute liver failure in children. *Semin Liver Dis* 2008;**28**:153–166.

3. Rivera-Penera T, Moreno J, Skaff C, *et al.* Delayed encephalopathy in fulminant hepatic failure in the pediatric population and the role of liver transplantation. *J Pediatr Gastroenterol Nutr* 1997;**24**:128–134.

4. Lee WS, McKiernan P, Kelly DA. Etiology, outcome and prognostic indicators of childhood fulminant hepatic failure in the United Kingdom. *J Pediatr Gastroenterol Nutr* 2005;**40**:575–581.

5. Heubi JE, Barbacci MB, Zimmerman HJ. Therapeutic misadventures with acetaminophen: hepatoxicity after multiple doses in children. *J Pediatr* 1998;**132**:22–27.

6. Watkins PB, Seeff LB. Drug-induced liver injury: summary of a single topic clinical research conference. *Hepatology* 2006;**43**:618–631.

7. Rumack BH. Acetaminophen overdose in children and adolescents. *Pediatr Clin North Am.* 1986;**33**:691–701.

8. Rivera-Penera T, Gugig R, Davis J, *et al.* Outcome of acetaminophen overdose in pediatric patients and factors contributing to hepatotoxicity. *J Pediatr* 1997;**130**:300–304.

9. James LP, Alonso EM, Hynan LS, *et al.* Detection of acetaminophen protein adducts in children with acute liver failure of indeterminate cause. *Pediatrics* 2006;**118**:e676–e681.

10. Larson AM, Polson J, Fontana RJ, *et al.* Acetaminophen-induced acute liver failure: results of a United States multicenter, prospective study. *Hepatology* 2005;**42**:1364–1372.

11. Abboud G, Kaplowitz N. Drug-induced liver injury. *Drug Saf* 2007;**30**:277–294.

12. Reuben A, Koch DG, Lee WM. Drug-induced acute liver failure: results of a US multicenter, prospective study. *Hepatology* 2010;**52**:2065–2076.

13. Stickel F, Patsenker E, Schuppan D. Herbal hepatotoxicity. *J Hepatol* 2005;**43**:901–910.

14. Narkewicz MR, Dell Olio D, Karpen SJ, *et al.* Pattern of diagnostic evaluation for the causes of pediatric acute liver failure: an opportunity for quality improvement. *J Pediatr* 2009;**155**: 801–806.

15. Stravitz RT, Lefkowitch JH, Fontana RJ, *et al.* Autoimmune acute liver failure: proposed clinical and histological criteria. *Hepatology* 2011;**53**:517–526.

16. Henter JI, Horne A, Arico M, *et al.* HLH-2004: diagnostic and therapeutic guidelines for hemophagocytic lymphohistiocytosis. *Pediatr Blood Cancer* 2007;**48**:124–131.

17. Pan X, Kelly S, Melin-Aldana H, Malladi P, Whitington PF. Novel mechanism of fetal hepatocyte injury in congenital alloimmune hepatitis involves the terminal complement cascade. *Hepatology* 2010;**51**:2061–2068.

18. Rand EB, Karpen SJ, Kelly S, *et al.* Treatment of neonatal hemochromatosis with exchange transfusion and intravenous immunoglobulin. *J Pediatr* 2009;**155**:566–571.

19. Sundaram SS, Alonso EM, Narkewicz MR, Zhang S, Squires RH. Characterization and outcomes of young infants with acute liver failure. *J Pediatr* 2011;**159**:813–818.

20. Sokal EM, Sokol R, Cormier V, *et al.* Liver transplantation in mitochondrial respiratory chain disorders. *Eur J Pediatr* 1999;**158**(Suppl 2):S81–S84.

21. Shneider BL, Rinaldo P, Emre S, *et al.* Abnormal concentrations of esterified carnitine in bile: a feature of pediatric acute liver failure with poor prognosis. *Hepatology* 2005;**41**:717–721.

22. Korman JD, Volenberg I, Balko J, *et al.* Screening for Wilson disease in acute liver failure: a comparison of currently available diagnostic tests. *Hepatology* 2008;**48**:1167–1174.

23. Moreira-Silva SF, Frauches DO, Almeida AL, Mendonca HF, Pereira FE. Acute liver failure in children: observations in Vitoria, Espirito Santo State, Brazil. *Rev Soc Bras Med Trop* 2002;**35**:483–486.

24. Bartholomeusz A, Locarnini S. Hepatitis B virus mutants and fulminant hepatitis B: fitness plus phenotype. *Hepatology* 2001;**34**:432–435.

25. Farci P, Alter HJ, Shimoda A, *et al.* Hepatitis C virus-associated fulminant hepatic failure. *N Engl J Med* 1996;**335**:631–634.

26. Liang TJ, Jeffers L, Reddy RK, *et al.* Fulminant or subfulminant non-A, non-B viral hepatitis: the role of hepatitis C and E viruses. *Gastroenterology* 1993;**104**:556–562.

27. Poddar U, Thapa BR, Prasad A, Singh K. Changing spectrum of sporadic acute viral hepatitis in Indian children. *J Trop Pediatr* 2002;**48**:210–213.

28. Verma A, Dhawan A, Zuckerman M, *et al.* Neonatal herpes simplex virus infection presenting as acute liver failure: prevalent role of herpes simplex virus type I. *J Pediatr Gastroenterol Nutr* 2006;**42**:282–286.

29. Phillips MJ, Blendis LM, Poucell S, *et al.* Syncytial giant-cell hepatitis. Sporadic hepatitis with distinctive pathological features, a severe clinical course, and paramyxoviral features. *N Engl J Med* 1991;**324**:455–460.

30. Stevens FM, McLoughlin RM. Is coeliac disease a potentially treatable cause of liver failure? *Eur J Gastroenterol Hepatol* 2005;**17**:1015–1017.

31. Umemura T, Tanaka E, Ostapowicz G, *et al*. Investigation of SEN virus infection in patients with cryptogenic acute liver failure, hepatitis-associated aplastic anemia, or acute and chronic non-A-E hepatitis. *J Infect Dis* 2003;**188**:1545–1552.

32. Racanelli V, Rehermann B. The liver as an immunological organ. *Hepatology* 2006;**43**(Suppl 1):S54–S62.

33. Gao B, Jeong WI, Tian Z. Liver: an organ with predominant innate immunity. *Hepatology* 2008;**47**:729–736.

34. Crispe IN. The liver as a lymphoid organ. *Annu Rev Immunol* 2009;**27**:147–163.

35. Paust S, Senman B, von Andrian UH. Adaptive immune responses mediated by natural killer cells. *Immunol Rev* 2010;**235**:286–296.

36. Gunawan BK, Liu ZX, Han D, *et al*. c-Jun N-terminal kinase plays a major role in murine acetaminophen hepatotoxicity. *Gastroenterology* 2006;**131**:165–178.

37. Kon K, Kim JS, Jaeschke H, Lemasters JJ. Mitochondrial permeability transition in acetaminophen-induced necrosis and apoptosis of cultured mouse hepatocytes. *Hepatology* 2004;**40**:1170–1179.

38. Liu ZX, Han D, Gunawan B, Kaplowitz N. Neutrophil depletion protects against murine acetaminophen hepatotoxicity. *Hepatology* 2006;**43**:1220–1230.

39. Kofman AV, Morgan G, Kirschenbaum A, *et al*. Dose- and time-dependent oval cell reaction in acetaminophen-induced murine liver injury. *Hepatology* 2005;**41**:1252–1261.

40. Begriche K, Massart J, Robin MA, Borgne-Sanchez A, Fromenty B. Drug-induced toxicity on mitochondria and lipid metabolism: mechanistic diversity and deleterious consequences for the liver. *J Hepatol* 2011;**54**:773–794.

41. Karlson-Stiber C, Persson H. Cytotoxic fungi: an overview. *Toxicon* 2003;**42**:339–349.

42. Antoniades CG, Berry PA, Wendon JA, Vergani D. The importance of immune dysfunction in determining outcome in acute liver failure. *J Hepatol* 2008;**49**:845–861.

43. Eksteen B, Afford SC, Wigmore SJ, Holt AP, Adams DH. Immune-mediated liver injury. *Semin Liver Dis* 2007;**27**:351–366.

44. Adams DH, Ju C, Ramaiah SK, Uetrecht J, Jaeschke H. Mechanisms of immune-mediated liver injury. *Toxicol Sci* 2010;**115**:307–321.

45. Mi Q, Li NY, Ziraldo C, *et al*. Translational systems biology of inflammation: potential applications to personalized medicine. *Per Med* 2010;**7**:549–559.

46. Michalopoulos GK. Liver regeneration. *J Cell Physiol* 2007;**213**:286–300.

47. Ichai P, Roque-Afonso AM, Sebagh M, *et al*. Herpes simplex virus-associated acute liver failure: A difficult diagnosis with a poor prognosis. *Liver Transplant* 2005;**11**:1550–1555.

48. Alonso EM, Sokol RJ, Hart J, *et al*. Fulminant hepatitis associated with centrilobular hepatic necrosis in young children. *J Pediatr* 1995;**127**: 888–894.

49. Ussery XT, Henar EL, Black DD, Berger S, Whitington PF. Acute liver injury after protracted seizures in children. *J Pediatr Gastroenterol Nutr* 1989;**9**:421–425.

50. Whitington PF, Alonso AE. Fulminant hepatitis and acute liver failure. In Kelly DA (ed.) *Paediatric Liver Disease*. Oxford: Blackwell, 2003, pp. 107–126.

51. Wendon J, Lee W. Encephalopathy and cerebral edema in the setting of acute liver failure: pathogenesis and management. *Neurocrit Care* 2008;**9**:97–102.

52. Stravitz RT, Kramer AH, Davern T, *et al*. Intensive care of patients with acute liver failure: recommendations of the US Acute Liver Failure Study Group. *Crit Care Med* 2007;**35**:2498–2508.

53. Shawcross DL, Wendon JA. The neurological manifestations of acute liver failure. *Neurochem Int* 2012;**60**:662–671.

54. Hadzic N, Height S, Ball S, *et al*. Evolution in the management of acute liver failure-associated aplastic anaemia in children: a single centre experience. *J Hepatol* 2008;**48**:68–73.

55. Liu E, MacKenzie T, Dobyns EL, *et al*. Characterization of acute liver failure and development of a continuous risk of death staging system in children. *J Hepatol* 2006;**44**:134–141.

56. Lu BR, Zhang S, Narkewicz MR, *et al*. Evaluation of the liver injury scoring system to predict survival in a multinational study of pediatric acute liver failure. *J Pediatr* 2013;**162**: 1010–1016.

57. Alagoz O, Maillart L, Schaefer A, Roberts MS. Determining the acceptance of cadaveric livers using an implicit model of the waiting list. *Operations Res* 2007;**55**:24–36.

58. Baliga P, Alvarez S, Lindblad A, Zeng L. Posttransplant survival in pediatric fulminant hepatic failure: the SPLIT experience. *Liver Transplant* 2004;**10**:1364–1371.

59. Mack CL, Ferrario M, Abecassis M, *et al*. Living donor liver transplantation for children with liver failure and concurrent multiple organ system failure. *Liver Transplant* 2001;**7**:890–895.

60. Girlanda R, Vilca-Melendez H, Srinivasan P, *et al*. Immunosuppression withdrawal after auxiliary liver transplantation for acute liver failure. *Transplant Proc* 2005;**37**:1720–1721.

61. Soltys KA, Soto-Gutierrez A, Nagaya M, *et al*. Barriers to the successful treatment of liver disease by hepatocyte transplantation. *J Hepatol* 2010;**53**:769–774.

62. Psacharopoulos HT, Mowat AP, Davies M, *et al*. Fulminant hepatic failure in childhood: an analysis of 31 cases. *Arch Dis Child* 1980;**55**:252–258.

63. Soltys KA, Mazariegos GV, Squires RH, Sindhi RK, Anand R. Late graft loss or death in pediatric liver transplantation: an analysis of the SPLIT database. *Am J Transplant* 2007;**7**:2165–2171.

Chapter

5

Cirrhosis and chronic liver failure

Evelyn K. Hsu and Karen F. Murray

Introduction

The word "cirrhosis" comes from the Greek *kirrhos*, meaning yellowish, tawny, and describes the gross pathology of the diseased liver. Since the late 1980s, however, clinicians have used the definition provided by the World Health Organization, which defines cirrhosis as a diffuse liver process where fibrosis has resulted in a conversion of the liver architecture into structurally abnormal nodules [1]. This distortion of liver architecture leads to compression of hepatic vascular and biliary structures, creating a further imbalance in the delivery of nutrients, oxygen, and metabolites. Even after the original insult has been controlled or stopped, the cirrhotic state persists. Although the causes of chronic liver disease encompass a wide spectrum of pathophysiological processes, cirrhosis is a common outcome [2].

Classification

Schemes for categorizing fibrosis and cirrhosis have been developed based upon gross morphology, microscopic histology (Figures 5.1–5.3), etiology, and clinical presentation. Categorization based upon gross morphology and histology has limited utility because it does not distinguish between the original pathogenic mechanisms of disease. The more commonly used pathologic staging systems (developed for the histopathologic description of the viral hepatitides), META-VIR and Ishak, stage fibrosis by varying degrees of presence of fibrosis, ranging from portal expansion to cirrhosis.

Within cirrhosis, many liver diseases have specific histologic patterns (e.g. biliary cirrhosis, hepatocellular cirrhosis, and cardiac cirrhosis) early in the cirrhosis progression; however, as cirrhosis advances, the patterns merge, rendering broad

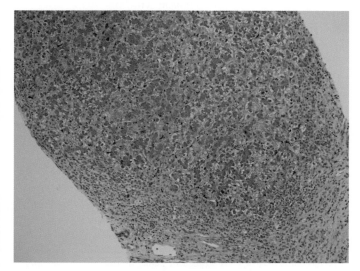

Figure 5.1 Autoimmune hepatitis showing expanded and fibrotic portal tract at bottom with piecemeal necrosis at the limiting plate. (Trichrome stain, magnification ×100.) (Courtesy of Dr. Kathleen Patterson, Seattle Children's Hospital.)

Figure 5.2 Biliary cirrhosis in a patient with biliary atresia, showing bile duct proliferation and bile plugging in the bile ducts. (Hematoxylin & eosin stain, magnification ×40.) (Courtesy of Dr. Kathleen Patterson, Seattle Children's Hospital.)

Liver Disease in Children, Fourth Edition, ed. Frederick J. Suchy, Ronald J. Sokol, and William F. Balistreri. Published by Cambridge University Press. © Cambridge University Press 2014.

Figure 5.3 Biliary cirrhosis in a patient with biliary atresia, showing proliferating bile ducts with bile plugging plus cholestasis in hepatocytes. (Hematoxylin & eosin, magnification ×100.) (Courtesy of Dr. Kathleen Patterson, Seattle Children's Hospital.)

Table 5.1 Diseases potentially resulting in cirrhosis

Type	Disorders
Metabolic disorders	α₁-Antitrypsin deficiency
	Cystic fibrosis
	Fructosemia
	Galactosemia
	Gaucher disease
	Glycogen storage disease, type III and type IV
	Hemochromatosis
	Indian childhood cirrhosis
	Histiocytosis X
	Niemann–Pick disease type C
	Tyrosinemia
	Wilson disease
	Wolman disease
Infectious diseases	Cytomegalovirus
	Chronic hepatitis B ± delta agent
	Chronic hepatitis C
	Herpes simplex virus
	Rubella
	Ascending cholangitis
	Recurrent neonatal sepsis
Inflammatory diseases	Autoimmune hepatitis
	Primary sclerosing cholangitis
Biliary malformations	Biliary atresia
	Arteriohepatic dysplasia (Alagille syndrome)
	Intrahepatic biliary hypoplasia
	Choledochal cyst
	Congenital hepatic fibrosis
	Intrahepatic cystic biliary dilatation (Caroli disease)
Vascular lesions	Budd–Chiari syndrome
	Congestive heart failure
	Congestive pericarditis
	Veno-occlusive liver disease
	Venocaval web
Toxic disorders	Toxins found in nature (mushrooms)
	Organic solvents
	Hepatotoxic drugs (e.g. methotrexate)
Nutritional disorders	Hypervitaminosis A
	Total parenteral alimentation
	Malnutrition
Idiopathic diseases	Cerebrohepatorenal syndrome (Zellweger syndrome)
	Progressive familial intrahepatic cholestasis
	Idiopathic neonatal hepatitis

pathological classifications unhelpful. Table 5.1 has a list of disorders that progress to cirrhosis to provide a framework for the diagnostic investigation of cirrhosis, a basis for prognosis determination, and a foundation for genetic counseling.

Cirrhosis is now increasingly defined by clinical outcomes rather than pathologic staging systems. When synthetic function of the liver is maintained, the term *compensated* cirrhosis is used. Within the compensated group, there is a distinctly different prognosis based on the absence or presence of varices. Over time, compensated patients can progress to *decompensated* cirrhosis, which is defined as the loss of normal synthetic ability of the liver and the development of jaundice or the clinical complications of portal hypertension such as ascites, variceal hemorrhage, and hepatic encephalopathy (HE). The more severe stage of decompensated cirrhosis include the patients who have developed life-threatening complications of their disease, such as recurrent variceal hemorrhage, refractory ascites, hyponatremia, and/or renal failure.

Pathophysiology

Cirrhosis represents a fluid, dynamic state, wherein the forces of cell injury (necrosis), cellular activation response to injury (fibrosis), and regeneration (nodule formation) compete. It is the derangement of the balance of these three processes that leads to cirrhosis.

Extracellular matrix, fibrogenesis and regeneration

Extracellular matrix (ECM) proteins have both mechanical and functional roles, contributing to strength of the membrane, modifying vascular flow, and controlling the movement of cells while also serving as ligands and receptors in the cellular signaling pathways. Hepatic fibrosis is a wound healing response characterized by the accumulation of ECM following liver injury. This injury may occur as a result of almost any insult, including viral invasion, immunological dysregulation, ischemia, and toxin exposure. Whereas in the normal liver, there is a tightly regulated balance between ECM protein synthesis and breakdown, sustained hepatocellular injury leads to chronic inflammation, excessive ECM protein synthesis, and consequently the development of scar tissue in the liver parenchyma.

The most important and well-characterized structural ECM proteins in the liver are collagen, proteoglycans, laminin, fibronectin, and matricellular proteins [3]. In a normal liver, the ECM makes up less than 3% of the area on a tissue slide section and 0.5% of the weight of the liver, primarily in the subendothelial space of Disse, primary vascular structures (portal tracts and central veins), and the liver capsule. Following liver injury, the normal matrix of the space of Disse is converted from a collagen IV/VI composition to a matrix composed of collagens I and III and fibronectin. This alteration in compositional structure results in *capillarization* of the sinusoids and creates an obstruction of flow of plasma between the sinusoidal lumen and hepatocytes, greatly affecting function. These altered sinusoids form conduits from portal to central veins, which shunt blood from the terminal portal veins and hepatic arteries to the central hepatic veins with little direct contact with hepatocytes. As the connective tissue network advances, connective tissue bands form, which run between portal triads or between portal triads and central veins. These septa may impede blood flow to entire hepatic lobules, resulting in further ischemic damage and cell dropout.

The reduction in the amount of viable, well-vascularized hepatic tissue leads to compensatory hepatocellular growth and nodule formation. These hepatic nodules increasingly impede blood flow to the lobules by directly compressing hepatic arterial and venous blood flow. This cycle becomes self-sustaining and can persist independently of the initial insult.

In addition to producing structural molecules, ECM also regulates cellular activity through the production of growth factors and matrix metalloproteinases. Several ECM components bind integral signaling cytokines such as transforming growth factor (TGF)-β, tumor necrosis factor-α, platelet-derived growth factor, hepatocyte growth factor, and interleukin-2. These cytokines activate intracellular signaling pathways that regulate and propagate fibrosis. The principal factor implicated in liver fibrosis is TGFβ, which is produced by monocytes and macrophages.

In a fibrotic liver, ECM proteins can increase up to eight-fold over those in normal liver [4]. If stimulated by inflammatory cells or by various cytokines, hepatocytes and their supportive cells secrete an altered ECM. The ECM is vital to the survival and proper function of each cell and provides a stable environment within tissue compartments. In order to understand fibrosis, and ultimately to identify new therapies to reverse the disease process, it is important to understand the changes in the proteins and the cells that synthesize them.

The most important cell in the pathogenesis of fibrosis is the myofibroblast, which works to synthesize and deposit ECM. This is a contractile secretory cell that produces α-smooth muscle actin. Prior research has concentrated upon the hepatic stellate cell, which, after transformation to a myofibroblast, indeed plays an important role in liver fibrosis. Exciting advances since the late 1990s, however, have led to a greater appreciation of the spectrum of cells that can become precursors to myofibroblasts in the damaged liver. It is unclear whether resident or extrahepatic stem cells become or differentiate into the non-parenchymal cells. Endothelial cells (through epithelial to mesenchymal transition), portal fibroblasts, Kupffer cells, and bone marrow-derived myofibroblasts have all been implicated as precursors.

Three conditions are necessary for cells to differentiate into myofibroblasts: (1) high levels of TGFβ, (2) fibronectin splice variant extra domain A, and (3) increased local mechanical tension. These factors act on potential precursors of myofibroblasts to cause them to differentiate. In normal liver, platelet-derived serotonin promotes liver regeneration through the interaction with the 5-HT_{2A} subclass of receptor for serotonin, which are expressed on hepatocytes. In contrast, expression of the 5-HT_{2B} receptor is relatively low in healthy liver but is highly expressed in the activated hepatic stellate cells associated with fibrotic liver. Consequently, these hepatic stellate cells suppress hepatocyte proliferation through their stimulation by serotonin, an act that increases production of TGFβ1, a powerful suppressor of hepatocyte proliferation. Therefore, the regenerative properties of serotonin acting through 5-HT_{2A} receptors on hepatocytes are opposed by the antiregenerative effects of 5-HT_{2B} receptors on hepatic stellate cells [5].

In vitro studies of the liver have shown that mechanical forces at the cellular level can impact cell function, motility, adhesion, contractility, and, most importantly, differentiation state [6]. Mechanical stiffness leads to activation of hepatic stellate cells and expression of α-smooth muscle actin, as well as myofibroblastic differentiation of portal fibroblasts, thus propagating a vicious cycle of increased deposition of stiff matrix leading to increased differentiation, and so on. Mature scars rich in ECM cross-links and elastin are self-propagating and are more difficult to remodel. The clinical correlation is seen in animal models of fibrosis and in patients with chronic hepatitis C infection, where MR elastography studies have shown that hepatitis C-infected livers with no detectable fibrosis can be stiffer than the liver in uninfected patients, and that perhaps liver stiffness precedes fibrosis.

As understanding of the mechanisms underlying hepatic fibrosis increases, effective antifibrotic therapy will be the ultimate goal, although there are no antifibrotic agents currently known to be effective in humans. Possible antifibrogenic therapies fall into four categories: (1) those directed at inflammation and immune response, (2) those directed toward antagonizing ECM-producing cells and their profibrogenic properties, (3) those directing ECM-producing cells to the proapoptotic pathway, and (4) those increasing degradation of fibrillar ECM [2]. The most well-described antifibrogenic agents to date are colchicine, corticosteroids, interleukin-10, alpha-tocopherol, and silymarin. Fibrosis in human chronic liver disease generally has such slow evolution that testing in clinical trials is difficult. Additionally, liver biopsy, the gold standard for assessment of liver fibrosis, is not ideal as it is not a rapid, safe, and reproducible way to monitor progression of fibrosis and subsequently the effectiveness of antifibrotic therapy in the liver. The search is ongoing for an ideal serum and/ or imaging marker of liver fibrosis.

The continual regeneration of the liver against the background of altered ECM composition and chronic inflammation predisposes to the development of hepatocellular carcinoma. As management of portal hypertension and other complications of cirrhosis have improved, hepatocellular carcinoma has become a more common clinical event in the adult population as well as the pediatric group [7].

Studies of liver regeneration have largely utilized the two-thirds partial hepatectomy model in rodents to examine the molecular and cellular mechanisms of liver regeneration [8]. Interestingly, in the resection model, regeneration is compensatory hyperplasia controlled by the metabolic needs of the organism. A great deal of work has examined these mechanisms. Because of the extent of cell proliferation and upregulation needed to restore liver mass following resection, and the importance of the liver for survival, hundreds of pathways have been implicated in regeneration; they are highly conserved and redundant.

Epidermal growth factor receptor and its ligands (epidermal growth factor, TGFα, amphiregulin, and heparin-binding epidermal growth factor-like growth factor) and hepatocyte growth factor have been most thoroughly studied. Matrix metalloproteinases have been shown to be important in the processing and release of growth factors from the ECM. The WNT/β-catenin pathway has also been implicated in liver regeneration. Studies have largely been directed toward transplantation (small-for-size and segmental grafts) and have not yet identified a target in these factors or inhibitors to modify the progression of cirrhosis.

Clinical features of cirrhosis and portal hypertension

The clinical presentation of cirrhosis depends on the causative underlying liver disease as well as on the pace of progression of hepatocellular dysfunction and fibrosis. Many children and adolescents present with findings discovered incidentally during routine physical examinations, or as a result of an investigation of an unrelated condition. In others, the discovery of chronic liver disease may be sudden and dramatic, such as with the onset of hematemesis, encephalopathy, ascites, or infection. Compensated cirrhosis, with its preservation of hepatic function despite the cirrhosis, is in contrast to decompensated cirrhosis, where patients suffer from progressive complications of liver disease (fatigue, ascites, variceal

bleeding, HE) with associated hepatic dysfunction. Measurement of the hepatic venous pressure gradient is increasingly used to stratify risk of complications of portal hypertension, with a value of >10–12 mmHg representing a critical threshold beyond which features of portal hypertension are generally found [7]. The clinical manifestations of cirrhosis affect children and adults similarly, with the exception of growth failure uniquely affecting children. It is unusual to find all, or even a majority, of these signs in any particular patient, however, and rarely cirrhotic patients can lack any obvious physical or laboratory evidence of their condition. Signs of systemic illness such as failure to thrive, anorexia, easy fatigability, muscle weakness, and nausea and vomiting may be present. Examination of the abdomen may reveal a firm nodular liver edge and the spleen may be enlarged in the setting of portal hypertension.

Ascites is often associated with hypoalbuminemia, steatorrhea secondary to cholestasis, and reduced bile acid availability for fat absorption in the intestine. A history of epistaxis, hematemesis, and hematochezia may be related to coagulopathy of liver disease or to portal hypertension with esophageal and rectal varices. Pallor may be present without bleeding because of the anemia of chronic liver disease. Cyanosis and digital clubbing are often present and are related to chronic hypoxemia secondary to pulmonary–systemic collateral circulation and ventilation–perfusion mismatching (hepatopulmonary syndrome (HPS)). Skin and extremity changes include jaundice, although it is not always discernible by the patient or the patient's family. Other skin manifestations of chronic liver disease include spider angiomata and palmar erythema. Spider angiomata are easily recognizable as small, raised, dark lesions with radially distributed convoluted vascular branches, and their pathogenesis is related to elevated systemic levels of estrogen secondary to the liver's inability to detoxify it from the circulation. Although it is not unusual to have several spider angiomata, the presence of more than five in the body region drained by the superior vena cava is abnormal and is suggestive of chronic liver disease. Palmar erythema is similarly related to the vasoactive effects of elevated systemic hormones [9]. White nails (terry nails) are often seen in cirrhotic patients, where the nail beds are white with a loss of the lunula and a dark band at the tip. The exact pathogenesis is not known, but biopsies of the nail bed have shown increased connective tissue and decreased vascularity.

The encephalopathy of liver disease may be prominent, or it may present in subtle forms such as deterioration of school performance, reversal of the sleep–wake cycle, depression, or emotional outbursts. It can be difficult to discern in a child, particularly the very young, and often neurocognitive evaluation is required. A neurologic examination can reveal asterixis (rhythmic hand flapping on wrist extension), a prolonged relaxation phase of deep tendon reflexes, and a positive Babinski sign. Table 5.2 shows physical findings associated with chronic liver disease and cirrhosis.

Table 5.2 Physical findings associated with cirrhosis and portal hypertension

Body region	Findings
General	Poor growth, malnutrition, fever, muscle wasting, fatigue, decreased exercise tolerance, cyanosis
Skin and extremities	Jaundice, flushing or pallor, palmar erythema, spider angiomata, digital clubbing, terry nails
Abdomen	Distension, caput medusa, ascites, shrunken liver, large spleen, rectal varices
Central nervous system	Asterixis, positive Babinski reflex, prolonged relaxation phase of deep tendon refluxes, mental status changes
Miscellaneous	Gynecomastia, testicular atrophy, feminization, delayed puberty

Extrahepatic complications of cirrhosis

Patients with cirrhosis may be predisposed to developing pigmented gallstones, which may be related to a decreased bile acid pool, bile stasis, and estrogen-like feminization. The preponderance of pigment stones, however, suggests that hemolysis (secondary to hypersplenism) and abnormal bilirubin metabolism play a primary role in stone formation.

Pulmonary manifestations

The development of arteriovenous shunts in the lungs has the primary clinical features of respiratory complaints associated with chronic liver disease, HPS. Dyspnea on exertion is the most common complaint. Platypnea (shortness of breath worsened by sitting up) and orthodeoxia (hypoxemia worsened when in the upright position) are the classic findings and result from gravitational increase in the blood flow through the dilated shunts in the bases of the lungs. Other factors that should increase suspicion for HPS are the presence of digital clubbing, development of cough, and decreased oxygen saturation.

Increased lung vascular endothelial endothelin B receptor expression and increased circulating levels of endothelin-1 are thought be central to the development of the intrapulmonary vasodilatation observed in HPS. The onset of HPS may be triggered by endothelin-1 activation of the endothelin B receptor leading to increased nitric oxide production by the endothelial nitric oxide synthase in the pulmonary endothelium. Pulmonary vascular remodeling through angiogenesis is also likely to play a role [10].

Orthotopic liver transplantation is the current preferred treatment for HPS, increasing 5-year survival from 23% to 76% [11]. Resolution of HPS following transplant can take up to 2 years. Garlic therapy has been implicated in improving pulmonary vasodilatation; however, treatment in children has not been shown to change outcomes [12]. Transjugular intrahepatic portosystemic shunting (TIPS) has been implemented in a limited capacity in children without sufficient results to recommend its use in children with HPS.

In addition to HPS, there is true pulmonary artery hypertension caused by the increased resistance to blood flow that occurs in the setting of chronic liver disease. Diagnosis of portopulmonary hypertension is defined by elevated mean pulmonary artery pressure (at rest >25 mmHg), increased pulmonary vascular resistance, and normal pulmonary artery occlusion pressure in the setting of liver disease and portal hypertension. It is diagnosed by right heart catheterization, and prevalence is difficult to predict, although in adult liver transplantation candidates, it has been reported to be as high as 8%. Its pathogenesis is incompletely understood, but it is likely related to an imbalance of vascular mediators that favor vasoconstriction, excessive pulmonary blood flow leading to endothelial damage, vascular remodeling, and microvascular thrombosis. On autopsy, the vascular changes have been described as medial hypertrophy and endothelial/smooth muscle cell proliferation in the small pulmonary arteries, and are not related to severity of liver disease or degree of portal hypertension [13].

There is a paucity of prospective randomized placebo-controlled trials in portopulmonary hypertension to establish clinical guidelines. Conventional management has included diuretics and fluid limitation to avoid fluid overload. Beta-blockers, often used for control of bleeding esophageal varices, are contraindicated as they often worsen exercise capacity and pulmonary hemodynamics. Liver transplant is contraindicated because of the high risk of cardiopulmonary mortality related to perioperative right ventricular dysfunction [14]; however, patients who show clinical improvement of mean pulmonary artery pressure with medical treatment such as prostaglandin analogues (epoprostenol), phosphodiesterase-5 inhibitors (sildenafil), or endothelin receptor antagonists (bosentan, ambrisentan) may benefit from orthotopic liver transplantation with improvement or resolution of portopulmonary hypertension [15,16].

Hematologic manifestations

Hematologic changes associated with cirrhosis include anemia and coagulopathy. The anemia of cirrhosis may be multifactorial in cause, including blood loss via the gastrointestinal tract, hemolysis secondary to hypersplenism, iron and folic acid deficiency secondary to malabsorption, malnutrition associated with malabsorption and anorexia, and dilution of red blood cell volume as a result of sodium and water retention. The coagulopathy of cirrhosis also is multifactorial, with a decrease in the synthesis of liver-derived clotting proteins, including prothrombin and factors VII and IX, and increased consumption of clotting factors through increased fibrinolysis and disseminated intravascular coagulation. Malnutrition, vitamin K deficiency, and thrombocytopenia as a result of hypersplenism may exacerbate the problem.

Table 5.3 Stages of encephalopathy

	Stage I	Stage II	Stage III	Stage IV
Mental status	Alert, oriented, irritable; sleep rhythm reversal	Lethargic, confused, combative	Stupor, marked confusion	Comatose; may respond to painful stimuli
Motor	Obeys commands; tremor, poor handwriting	Purposeful movement, grimacing, tremor	Local response to pain, intention tremor	Abnormal reflexes, no motor activity
Asterixis	Uncommon	Usually present	Present, if cooperative	Unable to elicit
Muscle tone	Normal	Increased	Increased	Increased or flaccid
Reflexes	Normal	Hyper-reflexic	Hyper-reflexic	Hyper-reflexic/absent
Respiratory effort	Normal/hyperventilation	Hyperventilation	Hyperventilation	Irregular
Eyes	Spontaneous opening	Open with verbal stimuli	Open with verbal stimuli	Sluggish or fixed; may open eyes with noxious stimuli
Electroencephalography	No gross abnormality	Grossly abnormal with slower rhythms	Theta activity and triphasic waves	Delta waves present

Decreased blood flow through the portal vein predisposes patients toward portal vein thrombosis.

Cardiovascular manifestations

Cardiovascular manifestations of cirrhosis include a high cardiac output state related to changes in systemic vascular resistance, with peripheral vasodilation, pulmonary vascular resistance, and hepatic blood flow (portal hypertension). The sustained increase in cardiac output results in the flushed appearance of patients with cirrhosis. Systemic hypertension is not common in cirrhosis.

Endocrine manifestations

Endocrine manifestations of cirrhosis result from failure of the liver to conjugate or metabolize hormones and include diabetes mellitus, which may present as subtle hyperinsulinemia without overt signs; hypothyroidism; syndrome of inappropriate secretion of antidiuretic hormone, presenting as hyponatremia; and feminization, including gynecomastia (benign proliferation of the glandular tissue of the male breast) and decreased axillary hair. Gynecomastia results from both the increased production of androstenedione and the increased circulating levels of estradiol. Delayed puberty is common in children with chronic liver disease. Cirrhotic patients also demonstrate relative adrenal insufficiency, where there is an inappropriate plasma cortisol response to adrenocorticotropic hormone [17].

Neurologic manifestations

Occurrence of HE in chronic liver disease is grouped into stages, as shown in Table 5.3. Changes in consciousness include hypersomnia, reversal of sleep pattern, apathy, slowed speech, decreased spontaneous movement, and eventually coma. Personality changes commonly seen in chronic liver disease include irritability, inability to cooperate, and childishness. These personality changes can be normal reactions to chronic disease in children, and their true cause may not be understood until frank encephalopathy is present. Intellectual deterioration with slight or gross confusion may be present. Focal defects in visual spatial skills also may appear, even if confusion is not present. The neuropsychological testing that is often used in adults, such as tests of constructional apraxia or the Reitan trail-making test, may be difficult to administer if the child is at too early a developmental stage.

The most characteristic sign of CNS dysfunction is asterixis, a flapping tremor that is demonstrated if the patient's arms are outstretched and wrists are hyperflexed for 30 seconds. The tremor is absent at rest and present during voluntary movement. Asterixis also is seen in uremia, congestive heart failure, and respiratory failure. Deep tendon reflexes may be exaggerated in early encephalopathy, but in late stages the muscles become flaccid and the reflexes disappear.

Minimal HE (MHE), in which patients lack obvious signs and symptoms of encephalopathy but may have subtle symptoms and impairment on neuropsychiatric evaluation, is an entity that has been examined in depth in the adult population, affecting up to 70% of cirrhotic patients. Its incidence in children is unknown. Although MHE is thought to be of little consequence in adults, there is increasing concern that early diagnosis and treatment may be important for preservation of brain function, particularly in children, who may be more vulnerable because of their potential brain growth and development. In contrast with patients with onset of liver disease in adulthood, deficits in global intellectual measures in children persist even after liver transplantation [18]. One uncontrolled small study demonstrated the utility of MR spectrography in the detection of MHE in children.

Immunologic manifestations

Cirrhosis is an immunocompromised state that increases susceptibility to infections, which account for a significant portion of mortality. The most common infections in cirrhotic patients are spontaneous bacterial peritonitis (SBP), urinary tract infections, and pneumonia [19]. Cirrhosis-associated immune dysfunction syndrome is a state of systemic immune dysfunction that results in an attenuated response to clearing cytokines, bacteria, and endotoxins from the circulation because of liver insufficiency. In addition to these factors, phagocytic activity and neutrophil mobility are impaired in cirrhosis through the decreased responsiveness to cytokine signaling. Innate immunity is additionally hampered by a decreased bactericidal and opsonization capacity. The liver is host to key reticuloendothelial cells that play an important role in clearing bacteria from the bloodstream. Loss of normal parenchyma and portosystemic shunting, where blood is directed away from the liver, contribute to overall decreased blood and toxins reaching the liver.

Renal manifestations

Renal and fluid complications often seen in cirrhosis result from decreased portal flow with compensatory maladaptive splanchnic vascular vasodilatation and decreased effective arterial blood volume, which then leads to activation of the renin–angiotensin system, with increased sodium and water retention. In the setting of hypoalbuminemia and portal hypertension, ascites formation further exacerbates the decreased effective arterial blood volume, feeding back into the cycle of further activation of the renin–angiotensin system [20]. Adults with hepatorenal syndrome (HRS) are at a higher risk of waitlist mortality.

Nutritional issues

Malnutrition in cirrhosis results from anorexia, with consequent inadequate calorie and protein intake; malabsorption; steatorrhea; and fat-soluble vitamin deficiencies. Malnutrition is a common complication of liver disease and is particularly relevant in the infant population. Standard measures of weight, height and body mass index underestimate the extent of malnutrition in children, particularly in those with advancing hepatosplenomegaly and ascites; triceps skinfold thickness is a more accurate assessment of nutritional status. Inadequate nutritional intake related to anorexia or the general malaise that accompanies chronic liver disease is further exacerbated by increased metabolic demand. Malabsorption of ingested foods, particularly fats, is also common in advanced liver disease. Deficiencies of fat-soluble vitamins can exacerbate other complications of cirrhosis, such as coagulopathy. Failure of linear growth secondary to chronic malnutrition is often observed in children with advanced liver disease and is associated with poor outcomes both before and after liver transplantation [21].

Orthopedic manifestations

Hepatic osteodystrophy (liver-associated bone disease) is a significant issue in the pediatric population with chronic liver disease and is related to poor nutrition, malabsorption of vitamin D, and systemic inflammation. Fractures are increasingly common in cirrhotic patients, and patients should be screened for decreased bone mineral density with dual energy X-ray absorptiometry [22].

Evaluation

Evaluation of a patient with liver dysfunction and suspected cirrhosis should focus on determining both the cause and the stage of liver disease. Table 5.4 lists the diagnostic tests that should be considered in evaluating a child with liver disease. Serologic testing for infectious diseases should include screens for hepatitis B and C viruses. In appropriate clinical situations (fever in the setting of previous biliary tree surgery), bacterial cultures of blood and possibly liver tissue should be obtained.

Tests for metabolic liver disease should include quantification of serum α_1-antitrypsin with determination of phenotype by protein isoelectric focusing, fasting blood sugar (glycogen storage disease), and sweat chloride test (for cystic fibrosis). Evaluation for galactosemia (urinary reducing substances) and tyrosinemia (serum amino acids with urinary organic acids) could be considered, although these conditions usually present more acutely. In older children, the diagnoses Wilson disease and autoimmune hepatitis should be considered. The initial evaluation for Wilson disease includes serum ceruloplasmin, a 24-hour urine collection for copper, and a slit-lamp ophthalmologic examination. Direct sequencing of *ATP7B* is widely available and is now the standard for molecular diagnosis [23]. Screening for autoimmune hepatitis uses anti-smooth muscle antibody, anti-mitochondrial antibody, anti-liver–kidney-microsomal antibody, and anti-nuclear antibody, as well as total IgG level.

An abdominal ultrasound examination aids in the evaluation of gallstones, choledochal cyst, Caroli disease (cystic dilatation of the intrahepatic biliary tree), and spleen size. A Doppler ultrasound should be done to evaluate the anatomy and blood flow of the hepatic arterial and venous system. In infants in whom the consideration of extrahepatic biliary atresia is paramount, a biliary scintiscan should be done. In patients with suspected extrahepatic biliary tree obstruction, endoscopic retrograde cholangiopancreatography could provide additional information regarding etiology. The timing of liver biopsy in the investigation of suspected cirrhosis in children remains a matter of clinical judgment. A biopsy may be critical to confirm the presence of cirrhosis suspected on clinical grounds, to verify an etiology, or if the investigations outlined here fail to reveal the cause of the chronic liver disease.

Table 5.4 Diagnostic tests in chronic liver disease and cirrhosis

Disorder	Diagnostic test
Infections	
Hepatitis B	Hepatitis B surface antigen, heptatitis B e antigen/antibody, viral DNA with PCR
Hepatitis C	Hepatitis C antibody, RNA antigen, viral DNA with PCR
Cytomegalovirus	Serology and urine for virus, viral DNA with PCR
Epstein–Barr virus	Serology, heterophile antibody
Bacterial cholangitis	Blood and liver tissue culture
Autoimmune chronic active hepatitis	Anti-nuclear antibodies, anti-smooth muscle antibody, anti-mitochondrial antibody, anti-liver–kidney-microsomal antibody, total IgG level
Metabolic disorders	
α_1-Antitrypsin deficiency	Serum α_1-antitrypsin, protein isoelectric focusing
Glycogen storage disease	Lactic acid, fasting blood sugar, uric acid, liver and muscle tissue enzyme level
Galactosemia	Urinary non-glucose reducing sugar, red blood cell galactose-1-phosphate uridyltransferase level
Tyrosinemia	Serum amino acid levels, urine organic acids
Neonatal hemochromatosis	Buccal biopsy, MRI for iron deposition in pancreas
Cystic fibrosis	Sweat chloride test, genotype analysis
Wilson disease	Serum copper, serum ceruloplasmin, 24-hour urinary collection for copper, slit-lamp examination, liver copper concentration, Wilson genetics

PCR, polymerase chain reaction.

Assessment of liver function and prognosis in cirrhosis

An ideal test of liver function should be able to indicate whether irreversible and potentially fatal changes have occurred early in the patient's course, and it should be practical and pose minimal risk to the patient. The standard measurements of hepatic function involve a number of tests, few of which actually measure functional capacity of the liver.

Serum presence of liver proteins

The hepatic aminotransferases, aspartate aminotransferase and alanine aminotransferase, are sensitive indicators of hepatocellular injury. These proteins are intracellular enzymes that are normally present in low concentrations systemically but are released from the hepatocyte into the circulation when hepatocellular necrosis occurs. High serum aminotransferase levels suggest acute hepatocellular disease, whereas moderate elevations suggest chronic liver disease. In fulminant hepatic failure, decreasing or low serum aminotransferases can either herald complete destruction of the liver or demonstrate liver recovery. Aspartate aminotransferase is not specific to the liver, and elevations can occur in cardiac disease (myocardial infarction, pericarditis, myocarditis), muscle disease (muscular dystrophy, myositis), and hemolysis (hemolytic anemia or red cell injury caused by traumatic phlebotomy). Alanine aminotransferase is more specific to the hepatocyte. Since aminotransferases in serum are an indicator of hepatocellular injury, the most serious shortcomings are its lack of prognostic value and its inability to quantitatively measure liver function or synthetic capacity.

Hyperbilirubinemia may be associated with hepatocellular dysfunction, the obstruction of bile flow, or extrahepatic diseases such as hemolytic anemia. In obstructive biliary disease, serum alkaline phosphatase and gamma-glutamyltransferase usually are elevated along with bilirubin, because these enzymes are localized in the cellular membranes of canalicular cells. Both of these enzymes are not specific to the liver and can be elevated in other disease processes. In the hepatic disorders of childhood, these tests generally have poor prognostic value; that is, although greatly elevated levels may be associated with poor prognosis, mildly elevated levels provide no reassurance that there is not serious and progressive liver disease.

Investigations that reflect hepatic synthetic capacity are better predictors of survival. Hypoalbuminemia and clotting factor deficiencies have been associated with liver failure, and it has been suggested that decreased synthesis of these proteins by injured hepatocytes is responsible for these deficiencies. Serum albumin concentrations alone are not reliable indicators of liver function or prognosis as they reflect albumin distribution and degradation as well as liver-derived synthesis. Because albumin has a serum half-life of 21 days, serum levels often do not represent current albumin production, particularly in the presence of ascites. Albumin is a component of ascitic fluid, and serum albumin slowly equilibrates with albumin in the ascitic fluid. The liver supplies essentially the entire intravascular pool of albumin and, with progressive ascites, an increasingly large extravascular albumin pool as well. Measurements of albumin synthetic rates have shown normal, decreased, or increased rates of albumin synthesis.

Because of their short half-lives, clotting factors in serum have been studied as indices of liver function, particularly in acute settings. It is generally agreed that increased prothrombin time unresponsive to vitamin K implies poor hepatic synthetic capacity and decompensated hepatocellular disease. Because of its short half-life (6 hours), factor VII has been evaluated as a prognostic indicator in acute liver failure. As is often the case, single determinations of serum factor VII levels are not as helpful as serial determinations over time, since it is a static variable. Low levels of factors V, VII, and XIII or plasminogen are associated with poor prognoses. Studies of serum clotting factor activities are confounded by alterations in the degradation rates of the proteins. The presence of disseminated intravascular coagulation, for example, aggravates the clotting factor deficiency resulting from liver disease. Additionally, the prognostic value of clotting factor levels in early or milder forms of liver disease is not known. Isolated changes in the serum concentration of liver-derived proteins are non-specific (changes may reflect extrahepatic disease) and insensitive (changes may lag behind changes in protein synthesis rates).

Dynamic tests

Dynamic tests relate to the function of the liver in metabolizing or eliminating defined substances. These tests have the advantage of being able to quantify the functional status at the time point of assessment. Indocyanine green is an infrared-absorbing and fluorescent agent that is nearly exclusively eliminated by the liver into the bile following intravenous injection. It does not undergo enterohepatic recirculation. Its clearance can be measured non-invasively at the bedside using a transcutaneous system, with results obtained within 6 to 8 minutes [24]. Side effects are rare (1 in 40 000), but indocyanine green contains iodine and so should not be used in patients with an iodine allergy or thyrotoxicosis. Its prognostic value has been shown to be superior to standard tests in critically ill patients, as well as in predicting long-term survival after liver resection [25].

Bromosulfophthalein is extracted exclusively by the liver following intravenous injection but is inferior to indocyanine green clearance in determining hepatic functional reserve and also is associated with severe systemic reactions.

Caffeine is metabolized by the liver to paraxanthine, theobromine, and theophylline by hepatic microsomal systems, and elimination takes significantly longer in patients with cirrhosis than in healthy volunteers. Serum metabolite/caffeine ratios can be measured using laboratory equipment (high-performance liquid chromatography) and is limited in practicality. The caffeine breath test measures plasma clearance and exhalation of labeled carbon dioxide following injection of labeled caffeine and has correlated with bromosulfophthalein clearance.

Amino acid clearance, galactose elimination capacity, the monoethylglycinxylidide test, and the aminopyrine breath test have been studied as tests of liver function but are limited by cumbersome administration and potentially dangerous side effects.

Assessment of pretransplant mortality

Since the 1980s, dramatic improvements in surgical technique and the use of effective immunosuppression have made hepatic transplantation a widely used procedure for children with end-stage liver disease, and with this has come a shortage in the availability of cadaveric organs. In February of 2002, in response to a mandate from the US Federal Government, the United Network for Organ Sharing implemented changes in liver allocation system in both children and adults from a waiting time-based system to one that incorporated an objective score that predicts pretransplant mortality. In children over 12 and adults, the Model for End-stage Liver Disease (MELD) score, a model initially developed as a short-term predictor of mortality in patients under going TIPS procedure, was shown to effectively predict 3- and 6-month mortality in patients with end-stage liver disease from a variety of diagnoses [26]. Based on the Studies in Pediatric Liver Transplantation (SPLIT) database, a multicenter database of 779 children of various diagnoses listed for liver transplant, 17 different variables were analyzed to create a model that incorporated five objective factors (serum bilirubin, serum albumin, international normalized ratio, presence of growth failure, and age) to predict mortality at 3 and 6 months [27]. This Pediatric End-stage Liver Disease (PELD) score is now used to determine liver allocation to children under 12 years of age.

Management of the chronic complications of cirrhosis

In many patients, the chronic complications of cirrhosis can be prevented, or at least ameliorated, by early detection. The physician must carefully and compulsively monitor patients with cirrhosis, even if it appears to be compensated. Ascites, bleeding, infection, and encephalopathy are serious and occasionally life threatening in patients with advancing liver disease.

Coagulopathy

Chronic liver disease has long been the model of acquired bleeding disorders, although an emerging school of thought has posited that, in fact, because of decreased production of both procoagulant and anticoagulant factors, a new balance is achieved [28]. The current basic tests that are used to assess coagulation do not reflect the true ability to clot. Under usual conditions, a complex balance among coagulation, direct inhibition of coagulation, platelets, and fibrinolysis maintains hemostasis. The liver plays an important role in the maintenance of all aspects of this balance.

Basic laboratory tests for coagulation (measurement of prothrombin time and activated partial thromboplastin time) are used to assess risk of hemorrhage and guide transfusion in patients with cirrhosis, but they are poorly correlated with onset/duration of both bleeding from surgical/invasive procedures and gastrointestinal bleeding [28]. Thrombin in the plasma of cirrhotic patients is similar to that in healthy subjects, reflecting an even reduction of procoagulant and anticoagulant factors. Although there are decreased liver-associated coagulation factors, there is also a concomitant decrease in procoagulatory factors such as protein C. The prothrombin time expressed as international normalized ratio is used in the PELD/MELD score to prioritize patients for liver transplantation, but it was not originally validated for use in patients with chronic liver disease [29].

Platelet number and function can be affected by liver disease. In normal conditions, platelets interact with von Willebrand factor to adhere to damaged vessel walls, promote aggregation, and for a primary hemostatic plug. Cirrhotic patients have lower levels of a plasma metalloprotease (ADAMTS 13) that acts as an inhibitory factor for von Willebrand factor, and hence patients with advanced chronic liver disease have very high levels of von Willebrand factor. In the setting of cirrhosis and portal hypertension, thrombocytopenia may result from splenic sequestration. In healthy people, the spleen stores 30% of the platelet pool; in those with portal hypertension, this increases to 90%. In patients with chronic liver disease, however, the very high levels of von Willebrand factor can restore platelet adhesion in sites of vascular injury.

Fibrinolysis is highly regulated and is initiated immediately upon deposition of fibrin within the vasculature; the proenzyme plasminogen is converted into active enzyme plasmin, which then degrades fibrin. In normal physiologic conditions, this conversion is regulated by tissue plasminogen activator, urokinase plasminogen activator, and activated factor XII. Opposition of these profibrinolytic factors is carried out by plasminogen activator inhibitor, plasmin inhibitor, and thrombin-activatable fibrinolysis inhibitor. Contrasting results have been reported, but the parallel quantitative and qualitative changes in profibrinolytic and antifibrinolytic factors likely restore the balance in patients with liver disease.

The in vitro procoagulant imbalance associated with chronic liver disease and cirrhosis sheds new light on the management of these patients, particularly in the unrestricted use of plasma infusion to correct the results of conventional coagulation tests that may not reflect the true homeostatic state, and also in the evaluation of risk of prothrombotic events such as portal vein thrombosis and peripheral vein thrombosis.

Ascites: pathophysiology, diagnosis and management

Chronic liver disease is implicated in the majority of cirrhotic infants and children with hepatic ascites. The accumulation of fluid is multifactorial and represents a breakdown of the normal intravascular volume homeostasis.

Patients with cirrhosis and ascites have abnormal renal sodium retention. Total body sodium is dependent upon the balance between sodium intake, sodium excreted in the urine, and relatively fixed non-renal sodium losses. The peripheral arterial vasodilation theory of ascites formation in chronic liver disease predicts that sodium and water retention in response to peripheral vasodilatation increases plasma volume enough to cause ascites formation. Nitric oxide has been implicated, although the mechanism is not yet well understood. Vasodilatation leads to effective hypovolemia, which is sensed by the kidneys, activating the renin–angiotensin–aldosterone system and leading to increased antidiuretic hormone and free water retention. The compensatory free sodium and water retention are not sufficient to achieve systemic homeostasis and further worsen portal hypertension and increased mesenteric blood volume. Portal hypertension acts to increase hydrostatic pressure across the mesenteric circulation, which leads to the increase of intestinal lymph; this outpaces lymphatic drainage capacity and directly accumulates in the peritoneum as ascites [30].

Additionally, decreased plasma colloid oncotic pressure results from the hypoalbuminemia associated with synthetic liver failure. The osmotic gradient that normally draws interstitial fluid into the intravascular space is decreased, allowing for increased fluid accumulation in the peritoneum and decreased effective intravascular volume, which continues to activate the renin–angiotensin–aldosterone system.

The onset of ascites may be slow and insidious, or its appearance may be rapid. Sudden onset of ascites is associated with an acute insult to the liver such as hemorrhage, shock, infection, or occlusion of the portal vein. Slowly progressive liver failure is associated with an insidious onset. The presentation of ascites in children may differ from that in adults. The first indication may be inappropriate weight gain and abdominal distension. On physical examination, "shifting" dullness to percussion may be present. A fluid wave is more difficult to detect in a child than in an adult. As more fluid accumulates, the presence of ascites becomes more obvious. Abdominal distension, scrotal distension in males, and ballotable intra-abdominal organs (early) may be present. Prominence of the abdominal wall veins indicative of portosystemic collaterals often occurs. Worsening of umbilical, femoral, inguinal, and incisional hernias result from increased intra-abdominal pressure. Pleural effusions and respiratory distress can result.

Ultrasound is a fairly sensitive technique to detect ascites but is limited by obesity and the presence of complex loculated fluid collections. Plain radiography can show displacement of the colon, centrally located floating small bowel loops, and separation of bowel loops (Figure 5.4). Cross-sectional imaging with CT and MRI, although not commonly used, are good for detection of fluid in the abdominal peritoneal cavity.

Abdominal paracentesis functions to diagnosis the presence of infection of the ascitic fluid, SBP. Cell count and culture aid in the diagnosis of SBP, and albumin is used to calculate the serum-to-ascites albumin gradient, a more reliable measure than total protein in the ascitic fluid. A high gradient value (>1.1 g/dL) indicates ascites from portal hypertension, whereas a low gradient value (<1.1 g/dL) suggests an alternative diagnosis (serositis, peritoneal carcinomatosis, tuberculous peritonitis, pancreatic ascites, biliary leak ascites, nephrotic syndrome).

Treatment should be considered in patients who have tense ascites resulting in abdominal discomfort or respiratory compromise. Small amounts of fluid only detected on ultrasound

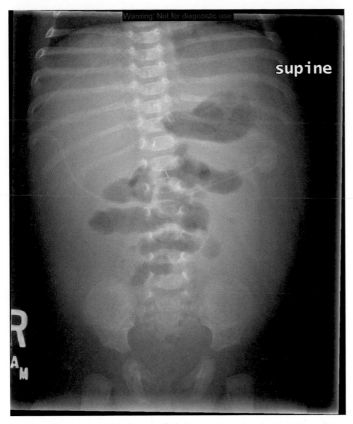

Figure 5.4 Abdominal radiograph of infant with ascites showing centrally loops of "floating" bowel and bulging flanks. (Courtesy of Dr. Jonathan Swanson, Seattle Children's Hospital.)

can be followed and managed conservatively. In most patients, restriction of sodium intake and diuretic administration works well to create a negative sodium balance that potentiates the mobilization of ascitic fluid. Patients who are diuretic resistant can be treated with large-volume paracentesis or TIPS as a bridge to orthotopic liver transplantation.

Restriction of dietary sodium is often unpalatable and difficult in a pediatric population where growth and development prioritize increased caloric intake, but it can be effective in limiting ascites. Restriction of sodium to 2 mEq/kg body weight per day facilitates reduced ascites formation. Restriction of water intake is usually not required or recommended unless serum sodium falls below 125 mEq/L.

Diuretics can be used to promote sodium excretion, with the goal of diuretic treatment being a negative fluid balance limited to 10 mL/kg daily in children. Faster diuresis can result in intravascular volume depletion. Spironolactone is an aldosterone antagonist that spares renal potassium excretion by acting on the cortical and medullary collectin tubules. In infants and young children, the starting dosage of spironolactone is 1 mg/kg daily, with the dose increased in increments of 1 mg/kg daily to a maximum dose of 6 mg/kg daily. In older children and adolescents, the starting dose of 100–200 mg/day can be increased 100 mg every 3 to 4 days up to a maximum

dose of 600 mg. Adverse effects can include azotemia, hyperkalemia, and volume contraction.

A loop diuretic such as furosemide acts to inhibit sodium reabsorption in the loop portion of the nephron. When used in conjunction with spironolactone, it will promote potassium loss and alleviate hyperkalemia. The starting dosage in older children and adolescents is 40 mg/day, increased gradually to a maximum dose of 240 mg. Infants and young children should be started at 1 mg/kg daily, with a maximum dose of 6 mg/kg daily. Side effects include ototoxicity and nephrocalcinosis. Thiazide diuretics act at the cortical diluting site and proximal tubule to promote sodium excretion. They are a good maintenance diuretic after initial diuresis with spironolactone. In older children and adolescents, the dosage is 50 to 100 mg/day, while in infants, doses start at 2 to 3 mg/kg daily. Side effects associated with thiazides are: hypokalemia, hyperglycemia, hyperuricemia, and pancreatitis. With any diuretic therapy, serum electrolytes, creatinine, and blood urea nitrogen should be measured frequently until stable.

Diuretic therapy is usually effective, and large-volume therapeutic paracentesis is usually not necessary. It can, however, be indicated in patients with refractory ascites or respiratory compromise, with up to 100 mL/kg removed at one time if combined with intravenous infusion of 1 g/kg of 25% albumin (1 g/kg).

Placement of an intrahepatic fistula between the hepatic veins and the portal system, TIPS, can be used to relieve symptoms related to portal hypertension such as ascites and esophageal variceal bleeding. Particularly in patients with severe liver dysfunction, however, it can cause worsening liver failure, and HE can occur as a result of the shunting. There are currently indications and guidelines for placement in adults, but utilization in children is not as common, likely secondary to a general perception of increased risk. Several limited studies have shown comparable success and efficacy of TIPS placed in children, as long as attention is paid to the technical challenges inherent in the pediatric population such as stent selection, anticipation of growth, encroachment on the main portal vein in the case of future transplantation, and limitations of contrast material [31].

Peritoneovenous shunting (LeVeen and Denver shunts) allow for unidirectional flow through a catheter of ascitic fluid to the venous system. The insertion of this shunt can resolve ascites; however, complications are frequent, including shunt obstruction, coagulopathy, pulmonary embolism, and sepsis. Additionally, in adults, duration of survival was not prolonged in patients with a shunt.

Spontaneous bacterial peritonitis

Spontaneous bacterial peritonitis refers to bacterial infection of ascitic fluid not associated with gut perforation or other intraabdominal source. Diagnosis depends upon positive culture of ascitic fluid or absolute polymorphonuclear cell count >250 cells/μL. In patients with chronic liver disease who have

Table 5.5 Differential ascitic fluid findings in spontaneous bacterial peritonitis and peritonitis secondary to intestinal perforation

Assay	Spontaneous bacterial peritonitis	Intestinal perforation peritonitis
Polymorphonuclear cell count	>250 cells/μL	>250 cells/μL
Total protein	<1 g/dL	>1 g/dL
Glucose	>50 mg/dL	<50 mg/dL
Lactate dehydrogenase	Serum levels	>Serum levels
Culture results	Single bacterial organism	Polymicrobial

Box 5.1 New diagnostic criteria of hepatorenal syndrome in cirrhosis

Cirrhosis with ascites

Serum creatinine >1.5 mg/dL (133 μmol/L)

No improvement of serum creatinine (decrease to <1.5 mg/dL) after at least 2 days with diuretic withdrawal and volume expansion with albumin; the recommended dose of albumin is 1 g/kg body weight per day up to a maximum of 100 g/day

Absence of shock

No current or recent treatment with nephrotoxic drugs

Absense of parenchymal kidney disease as indicated by proteinuria >500 mg/day, microhematuria (>50 red blood cells per high-power field), and/or abnormal renal ultrasonography

Source: from Salerno *et al.*, 2007 [36].

bowel edema resulting from portal hypertension, intestinal permeability is enhanced, favoring the translocation of bacteria into mesenteric lymph nodes and overflow into the circulation. Once in the circulation, the bacteria colonize ascitic fluid and remain uncleared because of deficiencies in immunity, opsonization, and neutrophil function [32].

Although SBP is usually monomicrobial, and usually a result of Gram-negative enteric bacteria, most commonly *Escherichia coli*, *Klebsiella* species, and *Enterococcus faecalis*, a different spectrum of organisms may be responsible for SBP in young children, with reported instances of *Streptococcus pneumoniae* in addition to enteric organisms such as *Klebsiella pneumoniae* and *Hemophilus influenzae* [33]. Polymicrobial infections suggest bowel perforation and secondary peritonitis.

A patient with ascites with concurrent fever, abdominal pain, or elevated white blood cell count should be assessed for SBP. Common symptoms in children include increasing abdominal distension, fever, abdominal pain, vomiting, and diarrhea. In younger infants, symptoms can include poor feeding and lethargy. Almost one-third of adults with SBP can be asymptomatic at the time of diagnosis, and the management of patients with chronic liver disease and ascites includes initial diagnostic paracentesis at time of admission to the hospital. Ascitic fluid obtained at paracentesis should immediately be inoculated into blood culture bottles at the bedside to increase the sensitivity of detection [34]. The bacterial concentration in infected ascitic fluid is usually low, and success and increased diagnostic yield requires inoculation of at least 10 mL of sample into blood culture bottles at the bedside. Every ascitic fluid sample should be tested for protein, albumin, glucose and lactate dehydrogenase, and ascitic fluid cell count should be performed. Table 5.5 reviews the findings in ascitic fluid in patients with SBP compared with those with intestinal perforation.

The mortality rate associated with SBP is as high as 55% in adults, with fewer data in children. Mortality rate decreases with earlier diagnosis and aggressive treatment with broad-spectrum intravenous antibiotics. The recurrence rate for SBP is high, and oral antibiotic prophylaxis with either norfloxacin or ciprofloxacin has reduced recurrence [32]. Because of concerns for the emergence of resistant organisms with long-term use of antibiotics, primary prophylaxis is not currently recommended.

Hepatorenal syndrome

The annual incidence of HRS in adults with end-stage liver disease is as high as 8% [35]. It is a diagnosis of compromised renal function that is difficult to make as there are no specific diagnostic markers. This is evident particularly in patients with cirrhosis, where other causes of renal failure are fairly common, such as hypovolemia-induced renal failure, parenchymal renal disease, and drug-induced renal failure. Current studies and consensus statements have introduced specific diagnostic criteria where these other diagnoses are excluded [20,36] (Box 5.1). In patients who are not on diuretic therapy, urinary and serum electrolytes can be informative in distinguishing between causes of renal failure (Table 5.6).

Hepatorenal syndrome is typically characterized by intense renal vasoconstriction, resulting in low renal perfusion, decreased glomerular filtration rate, and profoundly decreased renal ability to excrete sodium and free water. The pathophysiology of HRS is not completely understood. Portal hypertension contributes to decreased systemic vascular resistance through primary arterial vasodilatation in the splanchnic circulation, which is thought to result from increased production and activity of multiple vasodilatory factors (nitric oxide, carbon monoxide, and endogenous cannabinoids). In early cirrhosis, increased cardiac output can compensate for modest decreases in systemic vascular resistance; however, with advanced cirrhosis and cardiac dysfunction, cardiac output can no longer compensate, and there is underfilling of the arterial circulation. This underfilling leads to activation of vasoconstrictor systems such as the renin–angiotensin system and the sympathetic nervous system, which helps to maintain effective arterial blood volume but causes profound

Table 5.6 Important differential urinary findings in acute azotemia in patients with liver disease

	Prerenal azotemia	Hepatorenal syndrome	Acute tubular necrosis
Urinary sodium concentration (mEq/L)	<10	<10	>30
Urinary osmolality (mOsm)	>100; >plasma osmolality	>100; >plasma osmolality	Equal to plasma osmolality
Urine:plasma creatine	>30:1	>30:1	<20:1
Fractional excretion of sodium (%)	<1	<1	>2
Urinary sediment	Normal	Normal	Casts, debris
Response to volume expansion	Sustained diuresis	Brief or no diuresis	No diuresis

dysfunction in the ability of the kidney to regulate sodium and free water retention. Abnormally increased sodium and free water retention contribute to fluid overload, ascites, and edema, and further intrarenal vasoconstriction and decreased perfusion lead to renal failure.

Histologic changes are minimal, although autopsy findings in subjects who have undergone liver transplantation show a universal occurrence of glomerular changes including glomerulosclerosis and membranoproliferative glomerulonephritis – changes that are reversible after liver transplantation.

Bacterial translocation may worsen circulatory dysfunction by stimulating an inflammatory response, with the production of proinflammatory cytokines in the splanchnic circulation. Additionally, SBP can often lead to renal failure in patients with end-stage liver disease, with prolonged increased levels of vasoactive mediators and cytokines in the splanchnic system [37]. Administration of albumin 1.5 g/kg at diagnosis of SBP and 1 g/kg 48 hours later can reduce the risk of HRS in cirrhotic patients, and is thought to exert a helpful effect on circulatory function and bind the excess vasoactive mediators and cytokines. Antibiotic administration can ameliorate circulatory abnormalities in cirrhotic patients by either reducing the incidence of SBP or by selective intestinal decontamination [38].

The clinical presentation of HRS varies in both rapidity of onset and severity. Its incidence in children has not been well described. It is categorized in two forms: type 2 is characterized by moderate and steadily worsening renal function, accompanied by refractory ascites; type 1 is more severe in presentation, creatinine levels doubling or increasing to >2.5 mg/dL within 2 weeks of onset. Type 1 usually presents with rapidly progressive renal failure following a precipitating event and often is accompanied by impairment of other organ systems (heart, liver, adrenals, brain). Its natural prognosis is poor, with average survival of 1 month. The MELD scoring system was developed to prioritize candidates for liver transplant based on renal dysfunction and has, since its implementation, led to decreased mortality rates on the adult waitlist without decreasing 3-year post-transplant survival [39].

Recent advances have been made with vasoconstrictor therapy, which has shown improved survival in responders to therapy in comparison with those who do not respond. Larger

studies are required to assess whether the use of vasoconstrictors improves survival overall.

Clinical management

The most important principle underlying the management of HRS is the discovery and aggressive treatment of reversible causes of renal failure, particularly prerenal azotemia and urinary tract obstruction. Nephrotoxic drugs such as aminoglycosides should be avoided in patients with severe liver failure; infections such as SBP should be treated with cefotaxime or other antibiotics unlikely to aggravate kidney function. Dehydration, gastrointestinal hemorrhage, and septicemia should be addressed promptly to minimize the ensuing increased risk of HRS. Hypovolemia should be identified and treated immediately. Diuretics should be discontinued as spironolactone therapy is contraindicated in the setting of renal failure because of the risk of hyperkalemia and loop diuretics are often ineffective. It is crucial to avoid excessive intravenous fluid administration in the setting of sodium and free-water retention, as this can precipitate fluid overload, hyponatremia, ascites, and edema. Large-volume ascites exacerbating respiratory distress or discomfort should be treated with infusion of albumin and large-volume paracentesis [20].

Despite the renal vasoconstriction that occurs in HRS, treatment with renal vasodilators such as dopamine or prostaglandins has been shown to be ineffective. The current best approach is the administration of vasoconstrictor therapy. Several studies (only in adults with type 1 HRS) have shown that vasopressin analogues can be effective in almost half of patients with HRS and should be first-line therapy. Other vasoconstrictors, such as the alpha-adrenergic agonist midodrine, can be effective, but evidence on their use is more limited. A number of patients (~12%) can develop cardiovascular complications. No studies have looked at the administration of vasoconstrictors for treatment of HRS in the pediatric population.

Hemodialysis or continuous venovenous hemofiltration as renal replacement therapy has been used in patients with HRS awaiting liver transplant, but it remains unclear whether or not prognosis is improved in those patients who are not candidates for liver transplant [40]. Available data supporting the use of portosystemic shunts in HRS do not yet support this approach, although it may be effective in certain select patients.

Hepatic encephalopathy

Hepatic encephalopathy refers to a range of neuropsychiatric abnormalities seen in patients with cirrhosis. Effects include disturbed consciousness and coma, personality changes, intellectual deterioration, and speech and motor dysfunction. The sudden onset and rapid reversibility of encephalopathy in liver disease suggest that it is metabolic in origin. Although it is not completely understood, particularly in children, several theories have been put forward and have gained and lost favor over time. The pathophysiology of HE is thought to result from portosystemic shunting contributing to increased ammonia, increased endogenous benzodiazepines and increased GABA-ergic tone, and increased manganese deposition in the brain; all are potentiated by increased permeability of the blood–brain barrier.

In the setting of severe liver disease, blood from the intestine is shunted around the liver through collateral vessels or through the liver as the blood passes by damaged or necrotic hepatocytes. Potentially neurotoxic nitrogenous intestinal metabolites such as ammonia, which would be usually removed by the healthy liver, are found in the circulation in patients with liver dysfunction. Shunting and hepatocyte dysfunction have a synergistic effect in the development of HE.

The blood–brain barrier serves to isolate the brain from potentially toxic substances in the systemic circulation. In liver failure, neurotoxins such as ammonia and mercaptans may directly mediate the changes in blood–brain barrier permeability. Ammonia is an important factor related to the pathogenesis of encephalopathy, and therapeutic measures targeting the formation of ammonia have been widely used to treat HE. Serum ammonia is generated from both exogenous and endogenous sources, with ingested protein accounting for nearly half of circulating ammonia. Digestion of amino acids by gut bacterial urease releases ammonia. In the healthy state, most of the serum ammonia is removed and detoxified by the liver, with up to 90% removed through "first pass" metabolism from the gut [41]. The liver than detoxifies the ammonia through the urea cycle or through the transamination by glutaminase of α-ketoglutarate to glutamate or glutamine. Glutaminase also is found in skeletal muscle and the brain. In individuals with chronic liver disease and skeletal muscle wasting, reduction of ammonia levels through synthesis of glutamine is diminished [42]. There are data linking worsening encephalopathy to high serum ammonia levels; however, ammonia alone may not be the main mediator of HE, as there is poor correlation between blood ammonia levels and stage of HE. Cerebrospinal fluid glutamine concentrations, which reflect differences in intracerebral metabolism of ammonia, have improved correlation with the degree of encephalopathy in cirrhosis.

The false neurotransmitter hypothesis posits that "false" (not normally present in normal systemic or neurologic circulation) inhibitory neurotransmitters may accumulate in the brain and cause HE. Octopamine, tryptophan, and other aromatic amino acids are found in high serum concentrations in the setting of acute liver failure, but in vivo studies have not supported this hypothesis and it has fallen out of favor. The amino acid gamma-aminobutyric acid is an additional inhibitory neurotransmitter produced in the brain by the decarboxylation of glutamic acid, and it has been implicated as a major mediator of hepatic encephalopathy because of its role in CNS inhibition [43]. Brain gamma-aminobutyric acid content is increased in patients with HE because of the increased permeability of the blood–brain barrier. Inhibition of neurotransmission from increased GABA-ergic tone can lead to further neurologic compromise.

Increased cerebral concentration of manganese has been correlated with increased T_1-weighted MRI signaling in the basal ganglia/globus pallidus complex of the brain, which could possibly account for extrapyramidal signs in patients with HE. Liver transplantation reverses this finding.

Astrocytes play an important role in neuronal function, and there are characteristic pathologic findings in patients with HE, particularly the presence of "Alzheimer type II astrocytosis." Increased intracellular metabolism of ammonia leads to the production of glutamine, which exerts an osmotic effect on astrocytes, causing increased intracellular water and cell swelling. This contributes to cerebral edema and increases the risk of brain herniation. When ammonia is chronically high, as in chronic liver disease, cerebral edema is less of a concern because of the activation of brain osmoregulatory mechanisms and the production of myoinositol to counter the osmotic effect of ammonia upon astrocytes [41].

Diagnosis is based upon clinical presentation, and few tests have been used outside of the realm of research to classify and identify HE. Some diagnostic algorithms exist for adults, but have not been widely tested and verified in children. Electroencephalography can aid in diagnosis, with characteristic slowing from the normal alpha-range frequency to the delta range. Stimuli such as opening the eyes fail to reduce the abnormal background activity, and the trace may show relatively typical "triphasic" waves. These abnormalities may even precede biochemical changes as well as behavioral changes. Neuropsychological testing with the Psychometric Hepatic Encephalopathy Score (PHES), a battery of tests evaluating memory and neuromotor function, has been used in studying mild encephalopathy. Neuroimaging with single-photon emission CT (SPECT) shows correlation between deficits in memory, psychomotor speed, and efficiency with changes in blood flow on SPECT. Use of MR spectroscopy has revealed a large increase in glutamine plus glutamate concentration and decrease in myoinositols even in patients with MHE [43]. This was also found in children with HE, correlating with levels of branched-chain amino acids [18], which is even more concerning given the fact that children with liver disease and liver failure display deficits in global intellectual measures as well as in neuropsychiatric testing with persistence of symptoms even after liver transplantation.

In most patients, HE is initiated by a precipitating event, such as gastrointestinal hemorrhage, infection, the administration of sedatives, or dehydration after overaggressive diuresis. The clinical course of HE fluctuates and is variable. Frank encephalopathy is often preceded by MHE, the mild cognitive impairment of patients who have cirrhosis and portosystemic shunts. Minimal HE has gained recognition as clinically significant as it can impact on quality of life and functions of daily living such as driving and executing complex tasks [42].

The first step in treatment of HE is to identify and treat any precipitating factors. Sedatives should be avoided as they can precipitate or worsen the HE. If sedation is needed, benzodiazepines and opioids should be avoided. Measures such as diet control, increased gut transit, acidification of the gut, and antimicrobial therapy directed at decreasing serum ammonia are commonly implemented. Standard therapy for chronic HE includes restriction of protein to 40 g/day. This is difficult in children, where restriction of protein can result in growth failure, and it should only be undertaken carefully and with attention to overall nutritional state.

The ratio of serum concentration of aromatic amino acids (such as phenylalanine, tyrosine, and tryptophan) to the serum concentration of branched-chain amino acids (leucine, isoleucine, and valine) is increased in adults with cirrhosis and HE. Reported effects of intravenous or oral supplementation with branched-chain amino acids have been variable. One large randomized controlled trial using long-term (2 years) supplementation found improvements in a number of complications and in quality of life in the treatment group [44]. Branched-chain amino acids have been used as an enteral protein supplement in children with advanced cirrhosis and malnutrition, but studies have not explored their use in the treatment of HE in children [45]. Benzodiazepines [46] and dopaminergic agonists [47] do not have sufficient data to support treatment.

Lactulose (β-galactosidofructose), a semisynthetic disaccharide, is a primary treatment for hepatic encephalopathy. When taken by mouth, this disaccharide reaches the colon where gut bacteria cleave it to its basic sugars, galactose and fructose, and further metabolize the sugars to lactic acid, acetic acid, and various organic acids. The acidification of the fecal contents trap ammonia in its less absorbable form, ammonium. The adult dose is 10–30 mL (lactulose 10 g/15 mL) three times each day. Pediatric dosages are 0.3–0.4 mL/kg two to three times daily to attain three soft acidic stools per day. It can cause bloating, flatulence, and severe and unpredictable diarrhea. Lactitol (β-galactoside sorbitol) is another synthetic disaccharide used in the treatment of HE. Its mode of action is identical to that of lactulose, with its main advantage being that it is available in powdered form and is more palatable than its liquid syrup counterpart.

Antibiotic therapy with neomycin, vancomycin, and metronidazole, directed toward reduction of ammonia production from gut bacteria, has been used, with or without non-absorbable disaccharides such as lactulose, in patients with HE with benefit [48]. Long-term use is complicated, however, because of ototoxicity, renal damage, and the development of peripheral neuropathy. A recent double-blind randomized placebo-controlled trial over 6 months comparing rifaximin (a minimally absorbed oral antimicrobial agent with broad-spectrum activity against Gram-positive and Gram-negative aerobic and anaerobic enteric bacteria) with placebo in adults with HE showed significant reduced risk of HE episodes in the treatment group with no significant difference in adverse effects [49].

Malnutrition and chronic liver disease

Chronic liver disease may interfere with nutritional status by interrupting a key metabolic process or allowing the persistence of a metabolic imbalance. The liver plays a key role in the homeostasis of various serum proteins (e.g. albumin and coagulation factors), gluconeogenesis (and thus the maintenance of safe blood glucose levels), and lipid balance (as an important site of cholesterol synthesis, by controlling the metabolism of fatty acids and by contributing to fat absorption through the production and secretion of bile). All of these processes require energy, substrate, and control mechanisms; interruption of any of these processes may result in a diminished state of nutrition.

Malnutrition is common in children with chronic liver disease and cirrhosis, and may result from a variety of factors. Fat malabsorption is seen in patients with cholestasis, and such patients will present with weight loss or failure to thrive. Alternatively, they can present with symptoms specific to fat-soluble vitamin deficiency, such as coagulopathy or vitamin D-deficiency rickets. The caloric intake of many patients with chronic liver disease is insufficient to maintain positive energy balance. Increasing the caloric density via supplementation or nasogastric tube feedings has been shown to improve nitrogen balance.

Children with liver disease should be weighed and measured carefully at each clinic visit, and any changes in anthropometrics should prompt a careful re-evaluation of their nutritional state. Impaired nutritional state may result in increased morbidity and mortality rates after transplantation; growth assessment plays a primary role in the care and evaluation of children with cirrhosis. Although the specific benefits of improved dietary intake may be difficult to measure, there is evidence that improved nutrition may result in overall improvements in state of health. Administration of enteral feedings in adults is well tolerated and associated with decreases in mortality rate.

Most children with cirrhosis have fat-soluble vitamin deficiency, and supplementation of these vitamins as well as medium-chain triglycerides may be necessary to achieve optimal growth. If a child is unable to take adequate protein and calories, there should be a low threshold to initiate night-time nasogastric tube feeding. Parenteral nutrition support should only be considered in failure of all supplementary enteral feeds. The nutritional assessment and care of children with cirrhosis is complicated and requires a multi-disciplinary approach including pediatric dietitian, physician, and feeding specialists.

Conclusions

Cirrhosis is a potential consequence of many acute and chronic liver disorders affecting the child. As the molecular biology of fibrogenesis is better understood, the pathogenesis of cirrhosis is becoming clearer. The complications of advancing liver disease are better understood, and the management of these infants and children can be planned on a rational basis. Ultimately, the compromise of hepatic function that accompanies the irreversible course of cirrhosis and chronic liver disease leads to liver transplantation for the majority of patients. Hope for new antifibrogenic agents and therapy for the complications of advanced liver disease will change this course for our patients in the future.

References

1. Garcia-Tsao G, Friedman S, Iredale J, Pinzani M. Now there are many (stages) where before there was one: in search of a pathophysiological classification of cirrhosis. *Hepatology* 2010;**51**:1445–1449.

2. Pinzani M, Rombouts K. Liver fibrosis: from the bench to clinical targets. *Dig Liver Dis* 2004;**36**:231–242.

3. Hernandez-Gea V, Friedman SL. Pathogenesis of liver fibrosis. *Annu Rev Pathol* 2011;**6**:425–456.

4. Wells RG. Cellular sources of extracellular matrix in hepatic fibrosis. *Clin Liver Dis* 2008;**12**:759–768.

5. Ebrahimkhani MR, Oakley F, Murphy LB, *et al.* Stimulating healthy tissue regeneration by targeting the 5-HT(2B) receptor in chronic liver disease. *Nat Med* 2011;**17**:1668–1673.

6. Wells RG. The role of matrix stiffness in regulating cell behavior. *Hepatology* 2008;**47**:1394–1400.

7. Pinzani M, Rosselli M, Zuckermann M. Liver cirrhosis. *Best Pract Res Clin Gastroenterol* 2011;**25**:281–290.

8. Riehle KJ, Dan YY, Campbell JS, Fausto N. New concepts in liver regeneration. *J Gastroenterol Hepatol* 2011;**26**(Suppl 1):203–212.

9. Satapathy SK, Bernstein D. Dermatologic disorders and the liver. *Clin Liver Dis* 2011;**15**:165–182.

10. Sussman NL, Kochar R, Fallon MB. Pulmonary complications in cirrhosis. *Curr Opin Organ Transplant* 2011;**16**:281–288.

11. Swanson KL, Wiesner RH, Krowka MJ. Natural history of hepatopulmonary syndrome: impact of liver transplantation. *Hepatology* 2005;**41**:1122–1129.

12. Willis AD, Miloh TA, Arnon R, *et al.* Hepatopulmonary syndrome in children: is conventional liver transplantation always needed? *Clin Transplant* 2011;**25**:849–855.

13. Ridaura-Sanz C, Mejia-Hernandez C, Lopez-Corella E. Portopulmonary hypertension in children. A study in pediatric autopsies. *Arch Med Res* 2009;**40**:635–639.

14. Mukhtar NA, Fix OK. Portopulmonary hypertension. *J Clin Gastroenterol* 2011;**45**:703–710.

15. Savale L, O'Callaghan DS, Magnier R, *et al.* Current management approaches to portopulmonary hypertension. *Int J Clin Pract Suppl* **169**:11–18.

16. Laving A, Khanna A, Rubin L, *et al.* Successful liver transplantation in a child with severe portopulmonary hypertension treated with epoprostenol. *J Pediatr Gastroenterol Nutr* 2005;**41**:466–468.

17. Maheshwari A, Thuluvath PJ. Endocrine diseases and the liver. *Clin Liver Dis* 2011;**15**:55–67.

18. Foerster BR, Conklin LS, Petrou M, Barker PB, Schwarz KB. Minimal hepatic encephalopathy in children: evaluation with proton MR spectroscopy. *AJNR Am J Neuroradiol* 2009;**30**:1610–1613.

19. Bonnel AR, Bunchorntavakul C, Reddy KR. Immune dysfunction and infections in patients with cirrhosis. *Clin Gastroenterol Hepatol* 2011;**9**:727–738.

20. Gines P, Schrier RW. Renal failure in cirrhosis. *N Engl J Med* 2009;**361**:1279–1290.

21. Utterson EC, Shepherd RW, Sokol RJ, *et al.* Biliary atresia: clinical profiles, risk factors, and outcomes of 755 patients listed for liver transplantation. *J Pediatr* 2005;**147**:180–185.

22. Wibaux C, Legroux-Gerot I, Dharancy S, *et al.* Assessing bone status in patients awaiting liver transplantation. *Joint Bone Spine.* 2011;**78**:387–391.

23. Schilsky ML, Ala A. Genetic testing for Wilson disease: availability and utility. *Curr Gastroenterol Rep.* 2010;**12**:57–61.

24. Sakka SG. Assessing liver function. *Curr Opin Crit Care.* 2007;**13**:207–214.

25. Ohwada S, Kawate S, Hamada K, *et al.* Perioperative real-time monitoring of indocyanine green clearance by pulse spectrophotometry predicts remnant liver functional reserve in resection of hepatocellular carcinoma. *Br J Surg* 2006;**93**:339–346.

26. Kamath PS, Wiesner RH, Malinchoc M, *et al.* A model to predict survival in patients with end-stage liver disease. *Hepatology* 2001;**33**:464–470.

27. McDiarmid SV, Anand R, Lindblad AS. Development of a pediatric end-stage liver disease score to predict poor outcome in children awaiting liver transplantation. *Transplantation* 2002;**74**:173–181.

28. Tripodi A, Mannucci PM. The coagulopathy of chronic liver disease. *N Engl J Med* 2011;**365**:147–156.

29. Tripodi A, Chantarangkul V, Mannucci PM. The international normalized ratio to prioritize patients for liver transplantation: problems and possible solutions. *J Thromb Haemost* 2008;**6**:243–248.

30. Giefer MJ, Murray KF, Colletti RB. Pathophysiology, diagnosis, and management of pediatric ascites. *J Pediatr Gastroenterol Nutr* 2011;**52**:503–513.

31. Lorenz JM. Placement of transjugular intrahepatic portosystemic shunts in children. *Tech Vasc Interv Radiol* 2008;**11**:235–240.

32. Koulaouzidis A, Bhat S, Saeed AA. Spontaneous bacterial peritonitis. *World J Gastroenterol* 2009;**15**:1042–1049.

33. Haghighat M, Dehghani SM, Alborzi A, *et al.* Organisms causing spontaneous bacterial peritonitis in children with

liver disease and ascites in Southern Iran. *World J Gastroenterol* 2006;**12**:5890–5892.

34. Caruntu FA, Benea L. Spontaneous bacterial peritonitis: pathogenesis, diagnosis, treatment. *J Gastrointest Liver Dis* 2006;**15**:51–56.

35. Arroyo V, Fernandez J, Gines P. Pathogenesis and treatment of hepatorenal syndrome. *Semin Liver Dis* 2008;**28**:81–95.

36. Salerno F, Gerbes A, Gines P, Wong F, Arroyo V. Diagnosis, prevention and treatment of hepatorenal syndrome in cirrhosis. *Gut* 2007;**56**:1310–1318.

37. Grange JD, Amiot X. Nitric oxide and renal function in cirrhotic patients with ascites: from physiopathology to practice. *Eur J Gastroenterol Hepatol* 2004;**16**:567–570.

38. Rasaratnam B, Kaye D, Jennings G, Dudley F, Chin-Dusting J. The effect of selective intestinal decontamination on the hyperdynamic circulatory state in cirrhosis. A randomized trial. *Ann Intern Med* 2003;**139**:186–193.

39. Gonwa TA, McBride MA, Anderson K, *et al*. Continued influence of preoperative renal function on outcome of orthotopic liver transplant (OLTX) in the US: where will MELD lead us?. *Am J Transplant* 2006;**6**:2651–2659.

40. Capling RK, Bastani B. The clinical course of patients with type 1 hepatorenal syndrome maintained on hemodialysis. *Ren Fail* 2004;**26**:563–568.

41. Mas A. Hepatic encephalopathy: from pathophysiology to treatment. *Digestion* 2006;**73**(Suppl 1):86–93.

42. Stewart CA, Smith GE. Minimal hepatic encephalopathy. *Nat Clin Pract Gastroenterol Hepatol* 2007;**4**:677–685.

43. Ross BD, Jacobson S, Villamil F, *et al*. Subclinical hepatic encephalopathy: proton MR spectroscopic abnormalities. *Radiology* 1994;**193**:457–463.

44. Charlton M. Branched-chain amino acid enriched supplements as therapy for liver disease. *J Nutr* 2006; **136**(1 Suppl):295S–298S.

45. Charlton CP, Buchanan E, Holden CE, *et al*. Intensive enteral feeding in advanced cirrhosis: reversal of malnutrition without precipitation of hepatic encephalopathy. *Arch Dis Child* 1992;**67**:603–607.

46. Als-Nielsen B, Gluud LL, Gluud C. Benzodiazepine receptor antagonists for hepatic encephalopathy. *Cochrane Database Syst Rev* 2004;(2): CD002798.

47. Als-Nielsen B, Gluud LL, Gluud C. Dopaminergic agonists for hepatic encephalopathy. *Cochrane Database Syst Rev* 2004;(4):CD003047.

48. Morgan MY, Blei A, Grungreiff K, *et al*. The treatment of hepatic encephalopathy. *Metab Brain Dis* 2007;**22**:389–405.

49. Bass NM, Mullen KD, Sanyal A, *et al*. Rifaximin treatment in hepatic encephalopathy. *N Engl J Med* 2010;**362**:1071–1081.

Chapter

6

Portal hypertension

Benjamin L. Shneider

Introduction

A portal system is one, which by definition, begins and ends with capillaries. The major portal system in humans is one in which the capillaries originate in the mesentery of the intestines and spleen and end in the hepatic sinusoids. Capillaries of the superior mesenteric and splenic veins supply the portal vein with a nutrient- and hormone-rich blood supply (Figure 6.1) [1]. The partially oxygenated portal venous blood supplements the oxygenated hepatic arterial flow to give the liver unique protection against hypoxia. Blood flow from the hepatic artery and portal vein is well coordinated to maintain consistent flow and explains the ability of the liver to withstand thrombosis of either of these major vascular structures. This well-regulated blood flow, in conjunction with the very low resistance found in the portal system, results in a low baseline portal pressure in healthy individuals.

Portal hypertension, defined as an elevation of portal blood pressure above 5 mmHg, is one of the major causes of morbidity and mortality in children with liver disease. The high prevalence of biliary tract disease in pediatric liver disorders (e.g. biliary atresia), compared with adult liver disorders, predisposes to the expression of portal hypertension earlier in the clinical course of liver disease relative to the manifestation of the sequelae of hepatic insufficiency. Portal hypertension is a complication of a wide variety of pediatric liver disorders (Table 6.1). Its complications are some of the leading indications for liver transplant. Systematic investigations of the pathophysiology and treatment of portal hypertension have been performed primarily in adults. Since the earlier edition of this book, there has been a continued growth in the investigation of portal hypertension in children [2–6]. As before, caution needs to be exercised in the extrapolation of the results of randomized trials in adults to the care of children. Current approaches to the care of children with portal hypertension appear to be variable and are in large part adapted from experience in adults to meet the needs of children [7].

Portal hypertension in general is the result of a combination of increased portal resistance and/or increased portal blood flow. The signs and symptoms of portal hypertension

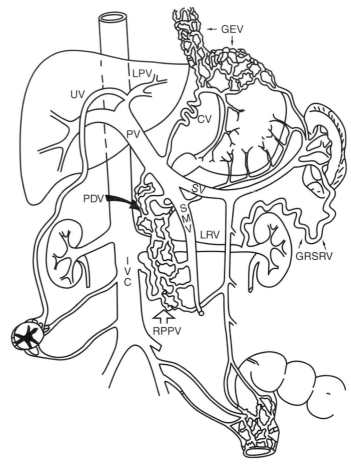

Figure 6.1 Portal venous anatomy and common portosystemic collaterals. PV, portal vein; IVC, inferior vena cava; SMV, superior mesenteric vein; SV, splenic vein; LPV, left branch of the portal vein; UV, umbilical vein (to caput medusae); CV, coronary vein plus short gastric veins lead to gastroesophageal varices (GEV); GRSRV, gastrorenal–splenorenal veins; RPPV, retroperitoneal-paravertebral veins; PDV, pancreatico-duodenal veins. Internal rectal hemorrhoids are unlabeled at the bottom of the diagram. (Reprinted with permission from Subramanyam et al., 1983 [1].)

are primarily a result of decompression of this supraphysiologic venous pressure via portosystemic collaterals and can be best understood by examination of the portal venous anatomy (Figure 6.1). Splenomegaly and its associated hypersplenism

Table 6.1 Pediatric diseases associated with portal hypertension

Anatomic level	Disorder
Extrahepatic disorders	Venous obstruction Splenic vein thrombosis Portal vein thrombosis/cavernous transformation Budd–Chiari syndrome Inferior vena cava obstruction
Intrahepatic disorders	Biliary tract disease Extrahepatic biliary atresia Cystic fibrosis Choledochal cyst Sclerosing cholangitis Intrahepatic cholestasis syndromes Alagille syndrome Byler disease Bile duct hypoplasia Congenital hepatic fibrosis Caroli disease
Hepatocellular disease	Autoimmune hepatitis Hepatitis B and C Wilson disease α_1-Antitrypsin deficiency Glycogen storage type IV Toxins Ethanol Methtrexate 6-Mercaptopurine
Miscellaneous	Chronic congestive heart failure Arteriovenous fistula Splenomegaly

result from splenic congestion, whereas esophageal and rectal varices form from decompression through portosystemic collaterals. Hemorrhage from esophageal varices is the major cause of morbidity and mortality associated with portal hypertension. Decompression of portal hypertension via portosystemic collaterals by definition leads to portosystemic shunting and results in related complications, including primarily hepatic encephalopathy and hepatopulmonary syndrome. Portal hypertension plays a key role in the pathogenesis of the development of ascites and complications related to ascites, including bacterial peritonitis and hepatorenal syndrome. This chapter will review experimental models of portal hypertension, the pathophysiology of portal hypertension, its clinical presentation, and strategies for evaluation and treatment of its sequelae. Where appropriate, important differences between adult and pediatric disease will be highlighted.

Experimental models of portal hypertension

Animal models of portal hypertension have been critical in the study of its pathophysiology. The clinical applicability of the results of these studies may be directly dependent on the experimental method used to induce the portal hypertension. Two commonly used techniques are bile duct ligation and partial stenosis of the portal vein. Bile duct ligation involves ligation and transection of the common bile duct. Transection is essential because of the finding of recanalization of the common bile duct when simple ligation is performed. Bile duct ligation would appear to be most applicable to diseases characterized by high-grade cholestasis, particularly biliary atresia. An important proviso is the fact that bile duct ligation models are relatively short term secondary to the degree of illness of the animal. The portal vein stenosis model involves ligature constriction of the portal vein to a set diameter (usually based on a catheter size) and is akin to portal vein obstruction. Varying the size of the catheter permits generation of graded degrees of portal hypertension. Other techniques of generating animal models of portal hypertension include hepatotoxin (e.g. carbon tetrachloride) exposure and infection with *Schistosomiasis mansoni*. In all of these approaches, in vivo monitoring is performed with pressure gauges and thermodilution catheters, and by radioactive microsphere distribution. This allows for accurate direct measurement of important parameters of portal hypertension, including heart rate, arterial and portal blood pressures, portal venous and hepatic artery blood flow, and portosystemic shunting [8]. Cardiac output and systemic and portal resistances can be calculated from these direct measurements. The role of endogenous physiologic mediators and the effect of a variety of pharmacologic agents on these parameters can thus be carefully assessed. Application of these models to genetically modified mice has permitted assessment of individual gene products in the pathophysiology of portal hypertension [9].

Pathophysiology of portal hypertension

Fluid mechanics are useful in understanding the pathophysiology of portal hypertension. Pressure is directly proportional to both blood flow through the portal system and resistance to that flow. In most circumstances it appears that the initial abnormality in the development of portal hypertension is an increase in the vascular resistance to flow of blood between the splanchnic bed and the right atrium. The etiology of this increased resistance is variable but usually involves compromise of the vascular lumen. Because resistance is inversely related to the radius of the lumen raised to the fourth power, small changes in the vasculature can result in large changes in pressure. The anatomic level of the vascular change can be prehepatic, intrahepatic, or posthepatic. It is clear that changes in resistance cannot completely explain the picture of portal hypertension. Portosystemic shunting should decompress the system and return portal pressures toward normal, yet this is not the case. A hyperdynamic state is clinically apparent in most patients with portal hypertension and has been well documented in a variety of animal models of portal hypertension [8]. This is manifested by tachycardia and decreased systemic vascular resistance and was first identified in adults in the 1950s [10]. These hemodynamic changes lead to an overall increase in portal venous flow and thus maintenance of portal hypertension. Decreased responsiveness of the mesenteric vasculature to physiologic levels of endogenous vasoconstrictors contributes to the overall increase in portal blood flow. A variety of hypotheses exist to explain the development of the hyperdynamic circulation that occurs in advanced liver disease. The changes in vascular resistance and hemodynamic state are also referred to as the backward and forward flow theories of portal hypertension and in some combination account for the increased portal blood pressure seen in advanced liver disease.

Increased vascular resistance

The portal and hepatic venous systems are low-resistance systems in healthy individuals. It is useful to divide the increased vascular resistance seen in portal hypertension into intra- and extrahepatic sources. Long-standing passive congestion of blood in the liver has been associated with the development of cirrhosis, which leads to increased resistance by other mechanisms and is becoming a major issue in the long-term follow-up of children who have undergone Fontan procedures. The suprahepatic vena cava and/or hepatic veins can be partially or totally obstructed by membranes or thrombosis leading to a syndrome often referred to as Budd–Chiari syndrome. This can be an acute or chronic process. The pathophysiology of the obstruction is typically related to compression by a mass, often a tumor, or thrombosis related to myeloproliferative disease or a hypercoagulable state [11]. Vasculopathies such as Behçet disease can also predispose to thrombosis of the hepatic veins. The pediatric manifestations of Budd–Chiari syndrome have been reviewed [12]. Portal pressure was elevated in 19 of 20 children studied, and esophageal varices were present in 11. A clear etiology for the obstruction could be demonstrated in only 5 of the children.

One of the more common pediatric causes of increased extrahepatic resistance is obstruction of the portal vein. In a review of the treatment of esophageal varices at a major referral center, 33% of the children had portal vein obstruction [13]. Although the etiology is obscure in most instances, neonatal umbilical vein catheterization, omphalitis, or trauma has been associated with portal vein obstruction. A variety of congenital malformations also have been associated with portal vein obstruction, including cardiac and urinary tract anomalies. As in Budd–Chiari syndrome, hypercoagulable states may predispose to the development of portal vein thrombosis. These conditions include deficiencies in protein S, protein C, and antithrombin III, and specific mutations in factor V, factor II, and methyltetrahydrofolate reductase. Systemic conditions such as paroxysmal nocturnal hemoglobinuria also can contribute. Cavernous transformation is the appearance of the recanalization of, or collaterals around, a thrombosed portal vein. These lesions lead to portal hypertension directly because portal resistance is markedly elevated.

Compression of the biliary system by the cavernoma may lead to biliary disease [14]. In general, hepatic function is intact and the major morbidity and mortality are a direct result of complications stemming from the associated portal hypertension, particularly esophageal varix hemorrhage. Effective management of these complications can be especially rewarding because of the absence of ongoing liver disease. Results of the study of the portal vein stenosis model of portal hypertension may be particularly applicable to this subgroup of children. Splenic vein obstruction can result in portal hypertension, although this is uncommon in children. Identification of splenic vein thrombosis as the cause of portal hypertension is very important, because splenectomy can be curative.

Intrahepatic causes of increased portal resistance constitute the remainder of the diseases associated with pediatric portal hypertension. The mechanisms of increased resistance are more varied than the extrahepatic etiologies. In many pediatric forms of chronic liver disease, resistance is increased secondary to impingement on the intrahepatic portal venule lumen as opposed to sinusoidal effects seen in adults. Hepatocyte swelling and hyperplasia in combination with portal tract inflammation and fibrosis are the major factors involved. Collagen deposition in the space of Disse also may contribute to increased intrahepatic resistance, although this has not been well studied in pediatric diseases. One of the major clinical differences from the extrahepatic etiologies of portal hypertension, particularly in portal vein obstruction, is the presence of ongoing hepatocellular injury. Biliary tract disease is a common cause of significant liver disease in children. Biliary atresia and its sequelae after hepatoportoenterostomy make up a large percentage of clinical series of advanced pediatric liver disease [13]. Other relatively common pediatric disorders that primarily involve the biliary tract include cystic fibrosis, choledochal cysts, sclerosing cholangitis, total parenteral hyperalimentation-related cholestasis, Alagille syndrome, chronic rejection, congenital hepatic fibrosis associated with autosomal recessive polycystic kidney disease, and the progressive intrahepatic cholestasis syndromes (particularly diseases with dysfunction of the bile salt export pump (BSEP) and multidrug resistance-associated protein 3 (MDR3)). These diseases, which primarily involve the biliary system, lead to bile duct proliferation, portal inflammation, and fibrosis. These processes all result in compromise of the portal venules and with more advanced disease compromise of the sinusoidal lumen (akin to adult primarily hepatocellular disease), leading to increased resistance to portal flow. Early in the course of disease, hepatocyte function is preserved, resulting in the expression of manifestations of portal hypertension to a greater extent and at an earlier time than the manifestations related to hepatocellular dysfunction. Therefore, therapeutic interventions directed at preventing complications of portal hypertension in children with biliary disease may be relatively more meaningful, given the potential long-term function of the liver. In fact, successful management of variceal hemorrhage in children with biliary atresia may postpone the need for liver transplant for extended periods of time [15]. This is in contrast to adults, where variceal hemorrhage is often a harbinger of poor short-term prognosis [16]. The greater prevalence of biliary tract disease in children (e.g. biliary atresia) relative to adults (e.g. alcoholic liver disease, hepatitis C and fatty liver disease) makes the complications of portal hypertension relatively more significant in pediatric than in adult liver disease. Adult therapeutic approaches should not necessarily be directly applied to children because of the difference in underlying liver function and the different pathophysiologies of the underlying diseases relative to the development of portal hypertension. Bile duct obstruction models of portal hypertension may be more applicable to the majority of pediatric diseases, although the utility of this model is significantly compromised by the clinical instability and shortened lifespan of animals with complete bile duct obstruction. Genetic models of biliary disease (e.g. Alagille syndrome, cystic fibrosis, autosomal recessive polycystic kidney disease, MDR3 deficiency) may be interesting new systems for the study of portal hypertension.

In most types of liver disease, vasoactive substances may play an important role in regulating intrahepatic resistance to blood flow [17,18]. In contrast to the peripheral vasodilatation seen in cirrhosis, intrahepatic resistance is increased. The ability of the hepatic sinusoidal endothelial cells to secrete and respond to vasodilators is impaired. Local levels of nitric oxide may be reduced in the liver and novel means of increasing these levels may yield new avenues for the treatment of portal hypertension. Levels of endothelin-1, a potent vasoconstrictor, have been found to be elevated in chronic liver disease associated with cirrhosis. Liver injury appears to induce increased release of endothelin-1 from either endothelial or stellate cells in the liver. This endothelin acts locally to cause vasoconstriction of the preterminal portal venules and thus significant elevations in portal pressure.

Primarily hepatocellular disorders are also common in children and can lead to portal hypertension. Included in this group of diseases are chronic hepatitis (particularly autoimmune hepatitis and hepatitis B and C), Wilson disease, α_1-antitrypsin deficiency, and a variety of metabolic and toxin-related disorders. In these disorders, changes in hepatic architecture and cirrhotic nodule formation lead to increases in portal resistance. In addition, in those disorders that are characterized by significant portal inflammation (e.g. autoimmune hepatitis and Wilson disease), the portal tract inflammation can lead to a pathophysiology similar to that seen in primary biliary tract disease. The ultimate effect is a compromise of the sinusoidal lumen. In addition, postsinusoidal resistance is most likely increased because of fibrosis and architectural changes. The end result is more similar to chronic liver diseases in adults as there is a greater degree of liver dysfunction present at the time of the manifestation of portal hypertension. Therefore, for these diseases, extrapolations of the results of adult clinical series are more realistic.

A variety of rare disorders exist that lead to portal hypertension but do not fit into the schema of intrahepatic (primary biliary tract or hepatocellular) or extrahepatic etiologies of portal hypertension. These diseases are not common in children and are included as examples of other pathophysiologies involved in the development of portal hypertension. The theory that increased portal inflow alone can lead to portal hypertension is supported by the finding of portal hypertension in patients with splanchnic arteriovenous fistulas or splenomegaly. Veno-occlusive disease of the hepatic venule and hepatoportal sclerosis may increase portal resistance by sclerosis of the venous vessels as opposed to extrinsic compression. Veno-occlusive disease is most commonly associated with chemotherapy but has been reported to be reversible when it is related to pyrrolizidine-containing tea. Defibrotide prophylaxis may prevent chemotherapy-related venoocclusive disease and has reduced the prevalence of this problem in bone marrow transplant recipients. Hepatoportal sclerosis is an enigmatic disorder that is manifest by portal hypertension in the face of normal to near-normal liver function test results, patent hepatic and portal veins, and portal fibrosis without evidence of either cirrhosis or nodule formation [19]. Nodular regenerative hyperplasia of the liver is another poorly understood disorder that is associated with non-cirrhotic portal hypertension. It is seen in the setting of the use of medications such as 6-thioguanine, but it can be an isolated idiopathic phenomenon. Schistosomiasis, one of the leading causes of portal hypertension in the world, is uncommon in the pediatric age range. Portal tract inflammation results from the host response to the parasitic egg in the hepatic venule, leading to compromise of the intrahepatic portal vein lumen. The degree of fibrosis seen in schistosomiasis may have a genetic basis. Pharmacologic treatment of the schistosomiasis may ameliorate the related portal hypertension.

Hemodynamic changes

Increased resistance to portal blood flow may be the primary event in the development of portal hypertension, but it is clear that various hemodynamic changes contribute to and amplify the increased portal blood pressure that is observed. Both clinical studies and animal models have demonstrated the hemodynamic events that occur. Most of these investigations have not been performed in children or pediatric models, so the findings should be interpreted with caution. A recent careful examination of cardiac function in children with biliary atresia who were listed for liver transplantation revealed features of cardiomyopathy and some features of hyperdynamic circulation [5]. The hyperdynamic circulatory state is characterized by increased cardiac output, decreased splanchnic arteriolar tone, and decreased splanchnic vascular vasoconstrictor responsiveness. The net result is increased portal inflow, which directly contributes to portal hypertension. A variety of factors may be involved in the development of this hyperdynamic state, and dissection of their relative contributions to the resulting hyperdynamic circulation is important, but difficult at best.

Increased cardiac output in advanced liver disease is the result of increased venous return to the heart and diminished cardiac afterload. Arteriolar vasodilatation is one of the key elements of this process. Parabiotic models indicate that humoral mediators are involved. When the output of the carotid artery of a portal hypertensive rat is infused into the superior mesenteric vein of a normal rat, total vascular resistance of the mesentery is reduced in the recipient rat. Similar studies in which the donated blood is subjected to hepatic metabolism do not show this effect. Consequently, portosystemic shunting may be important for the development of this vasodilatation.

A variety of mediators have been proposed to contribute to this vasodilatation, although the focus of recent studies has been primarily on the role of nitric oxide. Glucagon causes vasodilatation and is increased in advanced liver disease. This is partly the result of portosystemic shunting and bypassing of normal hepatic metabolism, but in addition pancreatic output of glucagon is elevated. Bile acids also have been proposed to cause vasodilatation, although experimental models have yielded contradictory results. It is clear that very high levels of bile acids will result in vasodilatation, but these levels may only be seen in severe cholestasis. In a portal vein stenosis model of portal hypertension, cholestyramine therapy, which reduced serum bile acid levels to normal, did not affect portal pressure. In a similar study, serum bile acid levels were reduced to subphysiologic levels by bile duct diversion. This led to an increase in splanchnic resistance and a decrease in both portal venous inflow and pressure. Neither of these studies is particularly relevant to cholestatic disorders, where serum bile acids are much higher. It is also important to realize that luminal concentrations of bile salts are often diminished in cholestasis. Therefore, the issue of the role of bile acids remains speculative. Prostaglandins, adenosine, calcitonin gene-related peptide, carbon monoxide, and endocannabanoids also have been thought to mediate the vasodilation in cirrhosis.

One of the most important mediators of vasodilatation may be nitric oxide [20]. An inhibitor of nitric oxide production, N^{γ}-monomethyl-L-arginine, decreased cardiac output and increased splanchnic and peripheral vascular resistance in a portal vein stenosis model. Portal venous inflow was decreased, but portocollateral resistance was increased, yielding an end result of no change in portal pressure. N^{ω}-Nitro-L-arginine, another nitric oxide synthetase blocker, corrects the vascular hyporeactivity observed in portal hypertensive rats. In the portal vein ligation model, one of the first responses to the portal hypertension is actually vasoconstriction of the superior mesenteric artery. This leads to sheer stresses with subsequent release of nitric oxide by endolethial nitric oxide synthase. The effects of nitric oxide in the splachnic bed are dominant and ultimately lead to vasodilatation. There are likely to be multiple pathways that mediated this effect, since mice that lack both inducible and endothelial nitric oxide synthase still develop a hyperdynamic state in portal hypertensive models. Although nitric oxide synthetase blockers would not appear to be useful agents to treat portal hypertension, their effect suggests a role of nitric oxide in the generation of the vasodilatation associated with portal hypertension. Nitric oxide release in severe liver diseases may be mediated in part through the effects of elevated levels of tumor necrosis factor-α. Thalidomide, which inhibits production of this cytokine, ameliorates the hyperdynamic circulation in rats with portal vein ligation-induced portal hypertension. An expanded intravascular volume is also an important part of the pathophysiology of the hyperdynamic circulation, via an increase in venous return and preload. Vasodilatation alone or associated with advanced liver disease is primarily responsible for increased sodium retention and increased vascular volume. This is the result of the renal response to vasodilatation and effective diminished perfusion. Sodium restriction in a portal vein stenosis model decreased plasma volume and thus normalized cardiac output and decreased portal pressure. Therefore, sodium restriction and/or diuretic therapy might be useful in the management of all patients with significant portal hypertension.

It has recently become clear that, in addition to the factors described above, alterations in serotonergic and sympathetic tone play a part in the pathogenesis of portal hypertension. Clonidine, a central alpha-adrenergic antagonist, decreases postsinusoidal resistance and thus decreases portal blood pressure. Carvedilol, which combines non-specific blockade of β- and α_1-adrenoceptors, has been shown to have enhanced activity in the treatment of portal hypertension [21]. Two serotonergic antagonists have been studied for effects on portal hypertension. Ketanserin, a serotonin and alpha-adrenergic antagonist, reduced portal pressure to an extent greater than its alpha-adrenergic blockade. Ritanserin, a more specific serotonergic blocker, decreased portal pressure without affecting mean arterial pressure. It is hypothesized that this effect was secondary to a decrease in portocollateral resistance. Although the side effects of hypotension and encephalopathy may limit their clinical usefulness, the effects of these antagonists suggest a role for abnormal serotonergic tone in the pathophysiology of portal hypertension. Decreased responsiveness of the mesenteric vasculature to endogenous vasconstrictors plays an additional important role in the pathogenesis of portal hypertension.

In addition to the vascular changes seen in response to chronic liver disease, there are intrinsic cardiac responses. Cirrhotic cardiomyopathy includes left ventricular hypertrophy, abnormalities in conduction and relaxation, and reduced response to stress. These changes have been modeled in a mouse model of biliary fibrosis using 3,5-diethoxycarbonyl-1,4-dihydroxychollidine. Cardiac abnormalities have been described in infants and children with biliary atresia and may have clinical consequences, particularly after liver transplantation [5].

Overall, a complex cycle of events leads to the hyperdynamic circulation, which is responsible for the forward flow portion of the pathophysiology of portal hypertension.

A baseline state of liver disease and increased portal resistance initiates the process. Hepatocellular dysfunction and portosystemic shunting result in the generation of a variety of humoral factors, which lead to vasodilatation, enhanced cardiac output, and increased plasma volume. Splanchnic arteriolar vasodilatation and mesenteric venodilatation leads to increased portal inflow and elevated portal pressure. This leads to further portosystemic shunting and increased levels of circulating vasodilators, and it may lead to worsened hepatocellular injury. The self-perpetuating cycle of portal hypertension and portosystemic shunting continues until a state of equilibrium is reached, which consists of increased portal pressure and a hyperdynamic circulation. Ultimately, this results in decreased portal perfusion of the injured liver. Intriguing studies in rabbits, whose liver disease is induced by a high-cholesterol diet, appear to indicate that mechanical augmentation of portal blood flow paradoxically reduced portal pressures and vascular resistance. Liver function apparently was also improved and was related to an increase in hepatic oxygenation.

Clinical manifestations

The clinical presentation of portal hypertension can be dramatic because it can be the first symptom of long-standing silent liver disease. In several large series of children with portal hypertension, approximately two-thirds presents with hematemesis or melena, usually from rupture of an esophageal varix [13,22,23]. Gastrointestinal hemorrhage can also be associated with bleeding from portal hypertensive gastropathy, gastric antral vascular ectasia, or from gastric, duodenal, peristomal, or rectal varices. Variceal hemorrhage is the result of increased pressure within the varix, which leads to changes in the diameter of the varix and increased wall tension.

When the wall tension exceeds the variceal wall strength, physical rupture of the varix occurs. Given the high blood flow and pressure in the portosystemic collateral system, coupled with the lack of a natural mechanism to tamponade variceal bleeding, the rate of hemorrhage can be striking and life threatening. Almost all of the patients reported in the above series had splenomegaly at the time of hemorrhage; thus, the combination of gastrointestinal hemorrhage and splenomegaly should be suggestive of portal hypertension until proven otherwise. The sentinel bleeding episode in these children occurred at a wide range of ages, starting as early as 2 months of age. No particular peak age of presentation has been demonstrated. Many of the episodes of hemorrhage that have been reported have been associated with upper respiratory tract infections, fever, or aspirin ingestion. It is possible that increases in abdominal pressure from coughing associated with respiratory infections and increases in cardiac output from the tachycardia associated with fever may result in increases in portal pressure and increased tendency to hemorrhage. Aspirin ingestion is associated with platelet dysfunction and gastrointestinal mucosal damage, both of which would predispose to hemorrhage. Other physiologic factors have been associated with increased portal pressures, which might increase the risk of variceal hemorrhage. These factors include physical exercise, blood or food in the stomach, and normal circadian rhythms.

The next most common presentation of portal hypertension is splenomegaly. In many instances, this is first discovered on routine physical examination. Many patients will have been aware of a vague fullness in the left upper quadrant for many years. Occasionally manifestations of hypersplenism, including thrombocytopenia, leukopenia, petechiae, or ecchymoses, will prompt evaluation, leading to the discovery of portal hypertension. Extensive hematologic evaluations, including bone marrow biopsies, may have been undertaken before portal hypertension is considered. Therefore, the hematologist should include a liver profile and potentially Doppler ultrasonography in the evaluation of any child with thrombocytopenia, particularly if there is the simultaneous finding of leukopenia. Rarely will the associated cytopenias lead to clinically relevant disease. Although splenomegaly is a common finding in patients with portal hypertension, splenic size does not seem to correlate well with portal pressure [22].

Certain cutaneous vascular patterns are specific to portal hypertension. Prominent vascular markings on the abdomen are the result of portocollateral shunting through subcutaneous vessels. The direction of flow through these veins can be indicative of the site of obstruction. When the inferior vena cava is occluded, drainage is usually cephalad, although it is caudad below the umbilicus if the inferior vena cava is patent. Decompression of portal hypertension through the umbilical vein results in prominent periumbilical collaterals, which have been referred to as a caput medusa. An audible venous hum, the Cruveilhier–Baumgarten murmur, can occasionally be appreciated through these vessels. Caput medusae are rarely seen in children, partly because of the high prevalence of portal vein obstruction associated with umbilical vein obliteration. Portal hypertensive rectopathy or rectal varices may be more common than generally appreciated. In children with short gut, stomal varices, which are a site of low resistance, are often easily observed and a common site of hemorrhage.

Hepatopulmonary syndrome (pulmonary arteriovenous shunting) is an important clinical manifestation of portal hypertension [24]. In this condition, there is intrapulmonic right-to-left shunting of blood, which results in systemic desaturation. The mechanisms involved in the development of hepatopulmonary syndrome are not known, but they are likely to include many of the vasoactive substances involved in the genesis of the hyperdynamic circulation, including nitric oxide and endothelin-1. One of the best-described animal models of hepatopulmonary syndrome is bile duct ligation, which is particularly relevant given the high prevalence of this problem in biliary atresia. Interestingly, hepatopulmonary syndrome can occur in the absence of intrinsic liver disease and has been described as a sequelae of congenital portosystemic shunting. Therefore portosystemic shunting may be the key pathologic event leading to hepatopulmonary syndrome. The prevalence of hepatopulmonary syndrome in chronic pediatric liver disease is not well characterized and depends on the method of diagnosis. Symptomatic hepatopulmonary syndrome (e.g. shortness of breath, exercise intolerance, and digital clubbing) is typically a late manifestation and thus series that depend on symptomatic presentation likely underestimate the true prevalence of this complication. Agitated saline echocardiography is a very sensitive measure of intrapulmonic shunting and can easily detect asymptomatic disease [25]. Positive echocardiographic studies were reported in 64% of children with biliary atresia who were prospectively studied [26]. The clinical relevance of this finding is not known, as the natural history of mild shunting is not well described. Macroaggregated albumin scanning can be used to quantify the degree of shunting, which can be useful in clinical decision making and in follow-up of hepatopulmonary syndrome. In a large pediatric series, 26 of 1116 children with chronic liver disease had clinically significant pulmonary arteriovenous shunting [27]. A variety of medical treatments have been tried and not found to be effective in treating this unusual complication of portal hypertension. Liver transplantation is very effective in reversing hepatopulmonary syndrome but theoretically may have limited efficacy in children with very severe disease. Full reversal of the shunting may take many months. Efficacy of transplantation is primarily limited by the ability of a particular patient to tolerate the perioperative cardiopulmonary stress of surgery. Screening for hepatopulmonary syndrome should be included in the evaluation and treatment of any child with portosystemic shunting, cirrhosis, and/or portal hypertension. In light of the orthodeoxia associated with this condition, measurement of peripheral oxygen saturation in children who are upright at the time of testing should be an effective screen. Any children with oxygen saturations persistently below 97% should undergo further testing, including agitated saline echocardiography and/or macroaggregated albumin scanning, to assess the presence or absence of hepatopulmonary syndrome and its severity.

Pulmonary hypertension is pathophysiologically related to hepatopulmonary syndrome [24]. It is an unusual but worrisome manifestation of pediatric liver disease [28]. The exact pathophysiology of the development of this pulmonary hypertension is unclear, but it seems to be associated with the presence of portal hypertension. Decreased hepatic clearance and portosystemic shunting of humoral mediators is hypothesized to be involved in this process. Routine screening for this rare complication is recommended in adults but not typically in children, although it has been described in both adults and children. Endothelin-1 receptor antagonists, prostacyclin analogues and sildenafil may be effective in some cases of portopulmonary hypertension. In addition, liver transplantation may need to be considered as an urgent intervention in order to prevent the development of irreversible disease. Severe portopulmonary hypertension, defined by a pulmonary artery pressure >50 mmHg is a contraindication to liver transplantation due to perioperative mortality. Unlike hepatopulmonary syndrome, portopulmonary hypertension does not typically reverse after isolated liver transplantation, although anecdotal reports of reversal in children have been reported [29]. This is likely because the disease is the result of obliteration of the lumen of the pulmonary artery. Definitive treatment for severe portopulmonary hypertension may need to include liver, heart, and lung transplantation.

The other major manifestations of portal hypertension impact on the kidney and brain. Renal-related complications include ascites and hepatorenal syndrome. Sodium retention, which is probably initiated by the already discussed systemic vasodilatation, may lead to ascites as an initial presentation of portal hypertension. The elevated portal blood pressure increases the Starling forces, which drive fluids out of the intravascular space into the peritoneum. In addition, impaired lymphatic drainage contributes to the development of ascites. Portal hypertension predisposes to bacterial translocation in the intestine and bacterial peritonitis. Very-late-stage cirrhosis is associated with enhanced free-water retention and hyponatremia. Hepatorenal syndrome is a particularly ominous complication of the renal disease associated with portal hypertension. Type I hepatorenal syndrome is an acute form of renal failure that cannot be ascribed to other causes of renal failure (e.g. infection, nephrotoxic medications, shock, or other forms of nephropathy). Short-term mortality is very high in patients with acute hepatorenal syndrome, although recently described treatment strategies have improved this outlook somewhat. There is little published experience with the diagnostic criteria and management of hepatorenal syndrome in children [30]. Hepatic encephalopathy is a complication associated with portosystemic shunting typically in the setting of advanced liver disease and relatively significant hepatocellular dysfunction. Subtle hepatic encephalopathy may exist in children with portal vein thrombosis, where there is minimal liver dysfunction [2]. Therefore, the clinician needs to consider this problem in children with chronic liver disease and behavioral disorders. Diagnosis of hepatic encephalopathy in children, particularly in its milder forms, is problematic at best.

Natural history

An accurate description of the natural history of portal hypertension in children is essential for a rigorous assessment of the efficacy of traditional and novel forms of therapy. A variety of complex and relatively accurate modeling systems of portal hypertension in adults have been developed [16]. Unfortunately, the natural history of pediatric portal hypertension is difficult to accurately assess because of the wide range of disorders that result in portal hypertension in children. Many of these disorders have unique pathophysiologies and clinical courses. The most confounding problem in attempting to describe the natural history of portal hypertension retrospectively in children is the wide variety of therapeutic interventions that have been applied in a non-controlled manner. In addition, there are only a few distinct diagnostic entities in which the prevalence of portal hypertension is high enough to generate clinically significant series. Extrahepatic portal vein obstruction and biliary atresia represent two entities where clinically meaningful series of untreated patients exist and can be used as a guide to the natural history of pediatric portal hypertension.

Extrahepatic portal vein obstruction

Portal vein obstruction is a useful example of the natural history of portal hypertension in the setting of slowly progressive liver disease. The presentation in children is usually one of gastrointestinal hemorrhage or the incidental discovery of splenomegaly. In two retrospective series, 167 patients presented from the ages of 10 days to 75 years [22,23]. In most cases, it was not possible to date the event leading to portal vein obstruction. As a result, it is unclear if the wide age range can be used as evidence for long-standing clinically benign disease. In 21 patients with presumed neonatal portal venous obstruction, presentation by hemorrhage was gradual over a period of as long as 12 years. Although the vast majority of the patients at some time in their life experienced gastrointestinal hemorrhage, a significant number of patients never bled. Four patients had fatal first hemorrhage episodes, although three of these instances were blamed on insufficient blood supplies. Sixty-one patients received medical management alone. The four described above died during their initial bleeding episode. Of the remainder, eight (13%) subsequently died of gastrointestinal hemorrhage. A minority of patients had no further episodes of hemorrhage. Most had several more episodes of bleeding, with a general observation of decreased frequency and severity after puberty. This phenomenon of apparently "out-growing" portal hypertension may be the result of recanalization of the portal vein or the development of collaterals and spontaneous portosystemic shunts through sites other than the gastroesophageal varices. Ascites and end-stage liver disease is unusual in portal vein thrombosis. Subtle hepatic encephalopathy may be more prevalent than previously thought [2]. Failure to thrive, pubertal delay, and a form of biliary disease that has cystic features and manifestations akin to sclerosing cholangitis have been reported in long-term follow-up. It has been hypothesized that the biliary disease is the result of partial obstruction from the cavernoma associated with the portal vein obstruction. In summary, portal vein obstruction is associated with potentially, but not usually, life-threatening gastrointestinal hemorrhage. The time from portal vein obstruction to hemorrhage appears to be quite variable, as is the clinical course. Minimal ongoing hepatic injury makes portal vein obstruction a more benign form of portal hypertension. Treatment recommendations must be tailored to the individual on a case-by-case basis with an understanding of the expertise of the treating center and physicians. Accumulating reports of the success of mesentericoportal (meso Rex) bypass surgery needs to be incorporated into the clinical decision making in the management of individuals with portal vein thrombosis [31]. The physiologic restoration of normal portal flow after this procedure has profound implications in its role in the management of portal vein thrombosis (see below) and will likely change the natural history of this disease.

Biliary atresia

Biliary atresia is the leading cause of significant pediatric liver disease and the single most common indication for liver transplantation in children [32]. Unlike portal vein obstruction, this is an example of a disease where portal hypertension is associated with ongoing and progressive liver disease. Biliary atresia is universally fatal in early childhood unless operative intervention is undertaken. At the time of portoenterostomy, portal hypertension has been documented, and its subsequent natural history is complicated by the variable results of portoenterostomy [33]. In general, the complications of portal hypertension are more prevalent in patients with poor biliary drainage or postoperative cholangitis [33]. Variceal hemorrhage is a common problem in children with biliary atresia and can occur as early as the first year of life [15,34,35]. The importance of bile flow, as manifest by total serum bilirubin, in the prognosis after variceal hemorrhage is reflected in reported experiences from Denver and Hong Kong [15,35]. Survival without liver transplantation after first variceal hemorrhage is significantly greater in children with total serum bilirubin <4 mg/dL [15]. In most circumstances, variceal bleeding appears to be life threatening and recurrent unless some intervention is undertaken. Variceal hemorrhage in these patients requires intervention, which must be tempered with the prospect of possible liver transplantation in the future. Given the progressive nature of portal hypertension associated with biliary atresia, the effects of interventions, both medical and surgical, are more easily discerned.

Diagnostic evaluation

Portal hypertension should be suspected in any child with significant gastrointestinal hemorrhage or unexplained splenomegaly. Physical examination should be directed at assessing for evidence of chronic liver disease. Care should be taken to look for growth failure or cutaneous lesions consistent with chronic liver disease (e.g. telangiectasia, palmar erythema). The combination of gastrointestinal hemorrhage and splenomegaly is highly suggestive of portal hypertension until proven otherwise. Laboratory studies should be aimed at evaluation of liver function. In addition, white blood cell and platelet counts may give evidence of hypersplenism. Thrombocytopenia in the setting of clinically suspected portal hypertension is a reasonable predictor of the potential for the presence of esophageal varices [6]. In children with portal vein thrombosis or Budd–Chiari syndrome, investigation of thrombophilia or myeloproliferative disease is potentially indicated.

A wide variety of diagnostic tests are available to document and quantify portal hypertension. Most have been well studied in adults but not in children. Many of the quantitative studies are invasive and most useful in a research setting to study response to treatment and in some cases to predict risk of gastrointestinal hemorrhage. In the pediatric age range, a combination of ultrasonography and flexible fiberoptic endoscopy can usually determine if portal hypertension or esophageal varices are present or absent. Recent advances in the use of multidetector CT and hepatic venous pressure gradient (HVPG) measurement in children may change approaches to the assessment of portal hypertension in children in the future [3,36].

Ultrasonography

Advances in ultrasonography, most specifically Doppler flow studies, have made this the investigation of choice in children. Its non-invasive nature is ideally suited for this age group. A great deal of data can be obtained in 30–60 minutes. As with many other procedures, the information that is obtained is directly dependent on the skill and experience of the operator. An abdominal survey can yield important information, including hepatic size and echogenicity. A small liver in the setting of portal hypertension is a potentially worrisome finding. Increased echogenicity is commonly seen in cirrhosis. Intrahepatic bile ducts can be assessed for evidence of dilatation consistent with extrahepatic obstruction or Caroli disease. Spleen size can be easily measured and will give indirect evidence about the presence or absence of portal hypertension. Unfortunately, spleen size does not appear to correlate directly with portal pressure and is not a highly accurate predictor of the presence or absence of varices. Renal abnormalities, associated with portal vein thrombosis and congenital hepatic fibrosis/Caroli disease, can easily be detected. Finally, ascites, which may not be evident on physical examination, can be demonstrated.

Doppler sonography of the hepatic and mesenteric vasculature affords an even greater amount of important information. The presence or absence of patent vessels can be determined in addition to vessel diameter, direction of blood flow in the vessel, and the presence or absence of echogenic material within the blood vessel. Vascular anomalies are usually readily detected. In children, normal non-fasting portal blood flow as assessed by Doppler examination is hepatopedal at 10 to 30 cm/s, although considerable variability exists in this measurement. Portal vein velocity decreases in severe portal hypertension as intrahepatic resistance increases. Hepatofugal flow in the left gastric, paraduodenal, or paraumbilical veins is consistent with portal hypertension, although this may be a relatively late finding. Reversal of flow in the superior mesenteric vein or splenic vein may be indicative of spontaneous mesentericocaval or splenorenal shunts, respectively. Hepatic arterial flow is often increased in portal hypertension as part of the normal compensation for diminished portal venous inflow. In selected studies in adults, careful analysis of either portal venous blood flow or superior mesenteric artery flow velocity has revealed a correlation with portal pressure. Unfortunately,

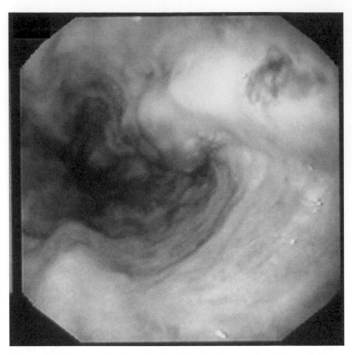

Figure 6.2 Endoscopic view of varices. Three columns of varices are seen.

these quantitative ultrasound studies have not been universally useful and have not been characterized in children.

Endoscopy

Flexible fiberoptic endoscopy can be used for the definitive determination of the presence of esophageal varices (Figure 6.2). This examination is particularly useful in determining if gastrointestinal hemorrhage in a child with chronic liver disease is secondary to variceal rupture. The differential diagnosis includes gastric or duodenal ulcers, gastritis, Mallory–Weiss tears, and portal hypertensive gastropathy. In 22 children with cirrhosis and upper gastrointestinal hemorrhage, eight had gastric or duodenal ulcers [37]. In adults, the endoscopic appearance of varices can be predictive of the risk of future hemorrhage. The red wale sign and cherry-red spot are particularly associated with increased risk of hemorrhage. Variceal size may be the most important prognostic finding. These findings have been systematically assessed in one group of children, those with biliary atresia. In this group, esophageal red markings and gastric varices along the cardia are predictive of an increased risk of subsequent variceal hemorrhage [4]. Intravariceal pressure can be measured by upper endoscopy, although this requires a very cooperative patient and once again has not been performed in children. Indirect variceal pressure measurement using an endoscopic pressure gauge might be more plausible for investigation in children. Capsule endoscopy can be used to look for esophageal varices, although the cost-effectiveness and feasibility of this approach with current equipment/approaches is open to question. Size issues and the ability of a young child to swallow the capsule also limits the applicability of capsule endoscopy in pediatrics.

Other investigations

A variety of other diagnostic investigations exist for the assessment of portal hypertension. Most of these studies have not been extensively characterized in children secondary to their invasive nature. Selective angiography of the celiac axis, superior mesenteric artery, and splenic vein can be particularly useful in assessing the extrahepatic vascular anatomy. In particular, these studies are helpful in suspected portal vein thrombosis and are essential for surgical decompression of this lesion. These studies may be essential for the diagnosis and appropriate therapy of splenic vein thrombosis. A combination of ultrasonography, inferior cavography, CT with intravenous contrast, or magnetic resonance venography can be used to document the vascular lesions associated with Budd–Chiari syndrome [12]. Portal pressure can be directly measured by examination of splenic pulp pressure during splenoportography, although this is primarily an historical technique. The HVPG is one of the classic measurements used in assessing portal hypertension in adults [38]. A balloon-tipped catheter is inserted into the antecubital vein and advanced to the hepatic vein, where free and wedged hepatic vein pressures can be measured. The wedged hepatic vein pressure is usually a good index of portal vein pressure when the main lesion in the hepatic vasculature is limited to the sinusoidal area. The difference between the free and wedged hepatic vein pressures is the HVPG. An HVPG <12 mmHg appears to be needed for variceal hemorrhage to occur. In addition, the HVPG is a reproducible measurement for studying the effects of a variety of medical and surgical interventions. Growing evidence in adults indicates the potential importance of HVPG measurements. Responses of HVPG to pharmacotherapy may be predictive of future chances of recurrent variceal hemorrhage. Given the relatively invasive nature of this measurement, there is limited well-documented pediatric experience with it outside of that associated with the placement of transjugular intrahepatic portosystemic shunts. In a single study, it appears that HVPG measurements are feasible in children and yield results similar to adults [3]. An important caveat is the unexpected finding of intrahepatic venovenous collaterals in biliary atresia, which can influence the accuracy of this measurement. In addition, HVPG measurements are not as accurate in presinusoidal liver disease, which is the case for many of the prevalent pediatric forms of chronic liver disease (e.g. biliary atresia, portal vein thrombosis). Given the growing data indicating that assessment of portal pressures is predictive of both the risk of hemorrhage and the potential response to therapy, development of a practical and reliable pediatric measure is of great importance.

Therapy

The therapy of portal hypertension is primarily directed at the management of its most dramatic manifestation: variceal hemorrhage. Variceal hemorrhage is a medical emergency, and patients with chronic liver disease should be instructed to seek immediate medical attention for any signs or symptoms of variceal hemorrhage. The management of variceal hemorrhage can be divided into preprimary prophylaxis, prophylaxis (primary) of the first episode of bleeding, emergency therapy, and prophylaxis (secondary) of subsequent bleeding episodes. As with many other aspects of the science of portal hypertension, almost all of the modes of therapy are based on trials in adults. Many of these trials are controlled randomized double-blinded studies, yielding comprehensive meta-analyses and consensus statements [39–41]. The literature of the management of pediatric variceal hemorrhage is mostly descriptive or anecdotal and there are fundamental issues in the conduct of randomized trials involving children [42]. As a result, there have only been two randomized trials of therapies for portal hypertension in children [43,44]. Because of the difficulties in obtained evidenced-based approaches, expert opinions have been advanced [7].

Preprimary prophylaxis

The concept of preprimary prophylaxis is that early treatment of portal hypertension has the potential to delay or prevent the development of esophageal varices or other manifestations of portal hypertension. In an *S. mansoni* mouse model of portal hypertension, the administration of propranolol 5 weeks into the infection resulted in a significant reduction in the development of portal hypertension, portosystemic shunting, and portal venous inflow. A randomized trial of timolol, a nonselective beta-blocker, on the development of varices in adults unfortunately did not show a significant effect. Consequently, at present, preprimary prophylaxis remains an interesting concept, but one that is not applicable in clinical practice.

Primary prophylaxis

The issue of prophylaxis of the first episode of variceal hemorrhage in children is controversial and is predicated on experience with adults, who primarily have alcoholic cirrhosis [42]. Surveillance endoscopy in children with liver disease and stigmata of portal hypertension is primarily justified if the clinician anticipates recommending a prophylactic regimen, although there may be value in surveillance for patients who live in remote areas far from medical care. Given the unpredictability of the timing of the first episode of variceal hemorrhage, primary prophylaxis regimens need to be associated with relatively low potential morbidity and mortality. As such, beta-blockade has been much more extensively used in this setting. The improved risk–benefit ratio of endoscopic ligation therapy relative to sclerotherapy has led to reassessment of its role in primary prophylaxis. The technical details of endoscopic ligation therapy will be discussed below. Uncontrolled preliminary pediatric experience with the use of propranolol in the primary prophylaxis of variceal hemorrhage has recently been reported [45,46].

Beta-blocker therapy of portal hypertension is optimal with non-selective agents. The primary effect may be blockade of

β_2-adrenoceptors of the splanchnic bed, leaving unopposed α-adrenoceptor stimulation and thus decreased splanchnic and portal perfusion. An additional important mechanism involves decreasing heart rate by β_1-adrenoreceptor blockade, thus lowering cardiac output and portal perfusion. Finally, evidence exists for a specific effect of propranolol that decreases collateral circulation (e.g. azygous vein blood flow). Therapeutic doses in adults are expected to decrease the pulse rate by at least 25%, although these guidelines are somewhat problematic in children, where baseline and follow-up measures may be difficult. A wide dosing range (0.6 to 8.0 mg/kg daily divided into two to four doses) has been required in children in order to observe a "therapeutic effect" [45]. The major adverse effects associated with the use of propranolol are heart block and exacerbation of asthma. Beta-blockade will inhibit treatment of asthma with beta-adrenergic agents. Beta-blockade also has the potential to interfere in the physiologic response to hypoglycemia; thus, these agents should be avoided in children with diabetes.

Beta-blockers have been consistently shown to reduce the frequency of bleeding episodes, and in some trials they have improved long-term survival in patients with esophageal varices. Initial randomized trials demonstrated efficacy in patients who have had a previous bleeding episode. Subsequently, propranolol was shown to be effective in patients with varices who had never bled. In a study of 230 patients randomized to propranolol or placebo, the incidence of hemorrhage and mortality over a 14-month period was reduced by almost 50%. The successful results of numerous trials of propranolol have been summarized by meta-analyses [41]. It is clear that a goal of at least a 25% reduction in resting heart rate needs to be achieved to see these effects. In those patients, where HVPG fell below 12 mmHg, subsequent variceal hemorrhage appears to be unlikely. Unfortunately, propranolol often does not reduce HVPG to this extent, a possible threshold for hemorrhage. Therefore combinations of beta-blockade and vasodilation therapy are now under investigation. Isosorbide-5-mononitrate, a long-acting vasodilator, may potentiate the effects of propranolol on the HVPG. Combination pharmacologic agents, such as carvedilol, may have enhanced efficacy [21]. Unfortunately, there is little if any prospective data on the safety or feasibility of beta-blockade in children with portal hypertension. Furthermore, there are few data indicating that beta-blockade is effective for primary prophylaxis in children. Consequently, this approach should be considered investigational in children.

Endoscopic band ligation therapy has been used with greater frequency in adults with high-risk varices [47]. As with beta-blockade, endoscopic band ligation therapy cannot be recommended for routine use in children with varices. In fact, a small randomized trial of prophylactic endoscopic sclerotherapy in children showed no survival benefit [43]. Given the invasive nature of the technique, selected application of this approach may be appropriate only in children with apparently high-risk varices who live in remote locations. In biliary atresia, varices with red markings or those found in association with gastric varices on the cardia may be at increased risk of bleeding, although a survival benefit from primary prophylaxis of these varices has not been demonstrated [4].

Emergency therapy for variceal hemorrhage

The initial management of variceal hemorrhage is stabilization of the patient. Vital signs, particularly tachycardia or hypotension, can be particularly helpful in assessing blood loss. Patients taking beta-blockers may not manifest the usual compensatory tachycardia and are at higher risk of developing hemodynamically significant hypotension. Fluid resuscitation, in the form of crystalloid initially followed by red blood cell transfusion, is critical. These fluids need to be administered carefully to avoid overfilling the intravascular space and increasing portal pressure. Optimal hemoglobin levels in adults with variceal hemorrhage are between 7 and 8 g/dL. Nasogastric tube placement is safe and may be an essential part of the management of these patients. It allows for documentation of the rate of ongoing bleeding and removal of blood, a protein source that may precipitate encephalopathy. In addition, blood in the stomach increases splanchnic blood flow and potentially could worsen portal hypertension and ongoing hemorrhage. Platelets should be administered when platelet levels are $<50 \times 10^9$/L, and coagulopathy should be corrected with vitamin K or fresh frozen plasma, the former being particularly relevant in patients with cholestasis. The value of recombinant factor VIIa has recently been questioned, as it may predispose to vascular thromboses. In fact, while patient with end-stage liver disease often have abnormal prothrombin times, global assessment of clotting does not reveal a predisposition to hemorrhage apart from in severe thrombocytopenia [48]. Intravenous antibiotic therapy should be strongly considered for all patients with variceal hemorrhage in light of the high risk of potentially fatal infectious complications. Once the patient is stabilized, endoscopy should be performed to document that the hemorrhage is indeed from variceal rupture. Signs of recent hemorrhage include visualization of ongoing hemorrhage, the presence of a fresh clot, or the presence of varices with fresh blood in the stomach and no other source of bleeding. Continued hemorrhage at the time of diagnostic endoscopy is a finding that portends a poor prognosis. Care should be taken to avoid disrupting fresh clot formation. A significant percentage of both children and adults with chronic liver disease and gastrointestinal hemorrhage will have sources of bleeding other than varices, including duodenal or gastric ulceration [37]. As such, diagnostic endoscopy is an integral part of the emergency management of acute gastrointestinal hemorrhage in the child with portal hypertension. Pharmacotherapy of acute hemorrhage need not be withheld until endoscopy can be performed. In fact, adequate pharmacotherapy may facilitate an endoscopic approach. At the time of diagnostic endoscopy, initial management in the form of sclerotherapy or ligation can commence.

Many episodes of variceal hemorrhage will spontaneously terminate, and supportive therapy is all that is required. Unfortunately, some episodes can become life threatening and require urgent therapy. Acute measurement of an HVPG >20 mmHg in adults predicts patients who will have an eventful evolution after the initial bleeding episode. Hemorrhage that persists for more than 6 hours or requires more than one red blood cell transfusion necessitates further intervention. A wide range of potential therapeutic approaches exists. Documentation of their efficacy in adults is fairly convincing, whereas the data in children are scanty at best. In general, a clinical decision is made that the risk of further blood product administration and potential hemodynamic compromise outweighs the side effects associated with further therapy. As in children in general, the most benign therapies are frequently the most favorable initial modalities of treatment.

Emergency pharmacologic therapy

The pharmacologic therapy of acute variceal bleeding typically consists of the use of terlipressin, vasopressin, or somatostatin (or their respective analogues). Vasopressin has the longest history of usage and acts by increasing splanchnic vascular tone and thus decreasing portal blood flow. Its use is often limited by the side effects of this vasoconstriction, which include left ventricular failure, bowel ischemia, angina, and chest and abdominal pain. Only a limited number of studies have compared vasopressin therapy with supportive care alone. In these studies, vasopressin leads to more rapid control of gastrointestinal hemorrhage, but no significant effect on mortality was seen. Of 215 children with acute variceal hemorrhage, 184 had bleeding arrested by the combined use of fluid support and vasopressin [49]. Vasopressin has a half-life of 30 minutes and is usually administered as a bolus followed by a continuous infusion. The recommended doses for children are 0.33 U/kg as a bolus over 20 minutes followed by a continuous infusion of the same amount hourly or a continuous infusion of 0.2 U/min per 1.73 m^2. The continuous infusion can be increased to up to three times its initial rate. These recommendations are apparently empiric, based on clinical practice and most likely derived from extrapolation of adult dosages. Terlipressin, a long-acting synthetic analogue of vasopressin, has shown similar effects and does not require continuous infusion. Side effects appear to be reduced relative to vasopressin. A potential significant advantage of terlipressin is its favorable effect on both control of hemorrhage and mortality. Unfortunately, terlipressin has not been approved for use in the USA, and there are limited data regarding its use in children.

Alternatives to vasopressin have been investigated because of its poor side effect profile. Somatostatin and its synthetic homologue octreotide have also been shown to decrease splanchnic blood flow. This effect is presumably mediated by blockade of secretion of vasoactive peptides by the intestine. Its effects on acute variceal hemorrhage appear to be similar to those of vasopressin, with fewer side effects. Like vasopressin, the dosing of these agents in children is empiric. Our own unpublished experience and the published experience in other pediatric centers indicates that intravenous octreotide appears to be relatively well tolerated by sick infants and children [50]. Continuous infusions of octreotide at 1.0–5.0 μg/h per kg body weight appear to be effective but may need to be initiated by the administration of a bolus of 1 hour's worth of the infusion. There is a critical need for better safety and efficacy data on these agents in infants and children.

Emergency endoscopic therapy

As noted above, approximately 15% of children will have persistent hemorrhage despite conservative management plus some form of splanchnic vasoconstriction. The most commonly used second approach is endoscopic sclerotherapy or endoscopic band ligation. This therapy is very effective in controlling bleeding, although it may be technically challenging in the individual with rapid hemorrhage. An extensive experience with emergency sclerotherapy exists in children, and it is rare for additional therapy to be required [13]. A variety of methods are used that chemically cause the varices to clot off and fibrose. Sclerosants, chemically irritating compounds such as ethanolamine or tetradecyl sulfate, are injected either intra- or paravariceally, until bleeding has stopped. Sclerotherapy is associated with a series of complications of its own, which will be discussed below. In the setting of emergency sclerotherapy, it is important to be aware of the significant incidence of associated bacteremia and to consider prophylaxis in nearly all patients. The major drawback of an endoscopic approach to treating acute hemorrhage is that the bloody field that is frequently encountered makes the procedure technically challenging. Endoscopic band ligation of varices may be a preferable approach because it is easier and safer to perform in an obscured field. In this approach the entire varix is drawn into the endoscope and an elastic band snares the vessel (Figures 6.3 and 6.4) [51]. A randomized trial of ligation versus sclerotherapy in adults demonstrated similar control of active bleeding and recurrence of hemorrhage, with significantly lower overall complications and mortality in the patients treated with endoscopic ligation. A potential concern in the application of this technique in small children, where the esophageal wall is thinner than in adults, is entrapment of the full thickness of the esophageal wall by the rubber band and subsequent ischemic necrosis and perforation. In addition, there may be technical difficulties in performing band ligation in children younger than 2 years of age because of difficulties in passing the endoscope. In most cases, a combination of conservative management, splanchnic vasoconstriction, and endoscopic sclerotherapy or band ligation will stop acute variceal hemorrhage.

Emergency mechanical therapy

The Sengstaken–Blakemore tube was designed to stop hemorrhage by mechanically compressing esophageal and gastric varices. The device consists of a rubber tube with

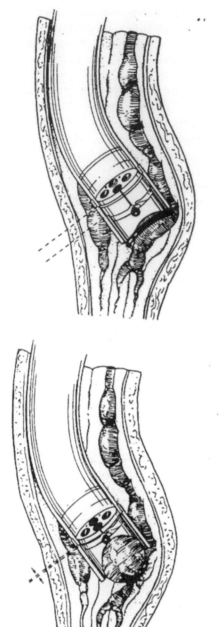
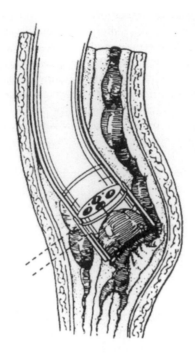
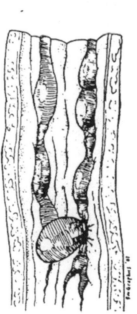

Figure 6.3 Technique of endoscopic ligation of esophageal varices. The endoscopic tip is positioned over a variceal column in the distal esophagus (upper left). Suction is applied to draw the esophageal mucosa and varix up into the dead space with the ligating device (upper right). The tripwire is pulled and the O-ring slipped around the aspirated tissue (lower left). (Reprinted with permission from Stiegmann, 1988 [51].)

at least two balloons. It is passed into the stomach where the first balloon is inflated and pulled up snug against the gastroesophageal junction. Once the tube is secured in place, the second balloon is inflated in the esophagus at a pressure (60–70 mmHg) that compresses the varices without necrosing the esophagus. A channel in the rubber tube allows gastric contents to be sampled for evidence of bleeding. This therapy is very effective in controlling hemorrhage acutely. Unfortunately, it is associated with a significant number of complications and a high incidence of rebleeding when the tube is removed. Most patients find this treatment uncomfortable, and its use in children requires significant sedation. Obstruction of the esophagus by the apparatus increases the risk of aspiration pneumonia, which can be a devastating complication in an individual with liver failure. Rebleeding has been reported in 33% to 60% of patients. Given these problems, the Sengstaken–Blakemore tube is reserved for severe uncontrollable hemorrhage and generally serves as a temporizing measure until a more definitive procedure can be performed. Intubation and heavy sedation is typically recommended for children requiring this approach.

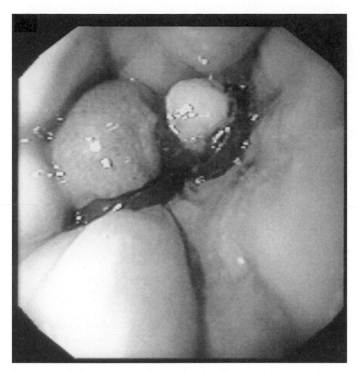

Figure 6.4 Endoscopic view of banded varices. Two bands are seen after placement on a varix.

Emergency surgical and interventional radiology

Surgical therapy is usually a last resort for acute variceal hemorrhage. Many of the patients with recalcitrant hemorrhage will be found to have gastric varices. The reluctance to perform emergency surgery partly stems from its associated high mortality but also from concerns of increased incidence of encephalopathy and greater difficulty of subsequent liver transplantation. The variety of surgical procedures that have been performed for intractable hemorrhage can be divided into transection, devascularization, and portosystemic shunting. Portosystemic shunting will be discussed in greater detail below. The techniques of esophageal transection and devascularization are rarely used and work by interrupting blood flow through the esophagus. Obviously significant morbidity can be associated with esophageal transection. Liver transplantation can be an effective means of treating esophageal varix hemorrhage, if an acceptable organ can be procured quickly enough. Esophageal varix embolization via a percutaneous transhepatic or trans-splenic approach has been advocated by some as another method of controlling acute hemorrhage. Transjugular intrahepatic portosystemic shunt placement (TIPS) may be the optimal approach for intractable hemorrhage. It does not require surgery or puncture of an organ that is predisposed to hemorrhage. A catheter is inserted into the jugular vein and is advanced into the hepatic vein, where a needle is used to form a tract between the portal vein and the hepatic vein (Figure 6.5) [52]. This tract is expanded with a balloon angioplasty catheter, and a stent is then placed, forming the permanent portosystemic shunt. The experience

with this procedure in children as an emergency procedure is somewhat limited. Given the high risks associated with either Sengstaken–Blakemore tube or emergency surgical approaches, TIPS may be the treatment of choice in this setting, particularly when liver transplantation is imminent. Size limitations and local expertise may be the limiting factor in some cases.

In summary, the approach to acute variceal hemorrhage in the pediatric patient is a stepwise progression from least invasive to most invasive. An adequate trial of conservative medical management is recommended, although evidence of significant bleeding (i.e. requiring transfusion of >10 mL/kg to maintain a hemoglobin between 7 and 8 g/dL) is an indication for more aggressive treatment. Intravenous antibiotic therapy should be strongly considered. Pharmacotherapy in the acute setting includes terlipressin or octreotide. Endoscopic band ligation is generally effective in those few patients who remain unresponsive and/or should be implemented soon after control of bleeding as part of secondary prophylaxis (see below). Use of TIPS should be reserved for patients with unresponsive hemorrhage and serves as an excellent bridge to transplantation. The ultimate long-term prognosis for the patient and the particular strengths of the team caring for the patient are key factors in choosing the particular approach for a given patient in a given institution.

Secondary prophylaxis

The decision making in the long-term management of the patient with portal hypertension and a previous episode of variceal hemorrhage is very complex. The first level of consideration involves the natural history of portal hypertension and more importantly the natural history of the underlying liver disease. As discussed above, there are significant differences in the natural history of portal hypertension in the setting of minimal and inactive versus active and progressive hepatic disease. As a result, certain individuals might have the possibility to outgrow their portal hypertension through the development of spontaneous portosystemic shunts, whereas others might be expected to develop end-stage liver disease and ultimately be candidates for liver transplant. Another important issue relates to the presence or absence of systemic manifestations of the underlying disease. Decision making in cystic fibrosis and congenital hepatic fibrosis/autosomal recessive polycystic kidney disease need to incorporate the prognosis of the pulmonary and renal diseases, respectively [53,54]. Complexity also stems from the great diversity in therapeutic modalities. The physiologic goal of pharmacologic therapy varies from program to program (i.e. change in heart rate, hepatic portal venous gradient pressure, etc.). Sclerotherapy can be administered with a wide variety of sclerosing agents and by two different techniques (intra- or paravariceal). Endoscopic band ligation offers an important and generally safer alternative to sclerotherapy. At least six different portosystemic shunting procedures have been described, all with their own

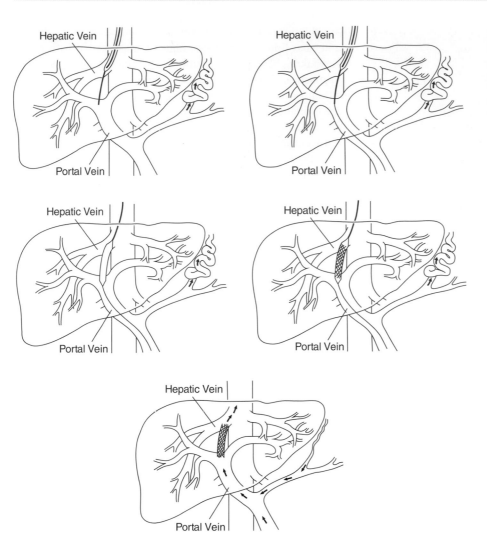

Figure 6.5 Technique of transjugular intrahepatic portosystemic shunting (TIPS). A catheter is inserted into the jugular vein and is advanced into the hepatic vein, where a needle is used to form a tract between the portal vein and the hepatic vein. This tract is expanded with a balloon angioplasty catheter, and a stent is then placed, forming the permanent portosystemic shunt. (Reprinted with permission from Zemel *et al.*, 1991 [52].)

advantages and disadvantages. A final level of complexity results from the varying results of randomized and non-randomized trials in adults. The trials are difficult enough to compare in adults and cannot necessarily be extrapolated to children, in whom alcoholic liver disease and end-stage hepatitis C are rare. Given these complex issues, the major modalities of long-term secondary prophylactic therapy of portal hypertension will be reviewed: endoscopic therapy, portosystemic shunting, and liver transplantation. The rationale for beta-blockade has been discussed as possible primary prophylaxis. It may also be used for secondary prophylaxis or as an adjunctive approach to endoscopic therapy. In particular, the rationale, effectiveness, and complications of these treatments will be stressed. Randomized trials will be reviewed and the pediatric experiences highlighted.

Secondary prophylaxis: sclerotherapy and ligation therapy

Sclerotherapy and band ligation therapy work by physical obliteration of esophageal varices. Hemorrhage may occur during the several weeks required to complete the obliteration, and there is a tendency for the vessels to recanalize. Most

importantly, the principal problem of portal hypertension is not addressed, and there is the risk of bleeding from varices elsewhere in the gastrointestinal tract, notably the stomach. Despite these problems, endoscopic therapy has been a mainstay of the treatment of esophageal varices. In addition, there is a significant amount of clinical experience with these approaches in children [13,43,44,55,56].

The effectiveness of sclerotherapy has been studied for prevention of initial bleeding and for subsequent bleeding episodes. Sclerotherpy, which has in general been supplanted by band ligation, is reviewed here for completeness. In addition, in very young children, band ligation therapy may not be feasible and sclerotherapy may be required. Intravariceal, paravariceal, and some combination injection protocols have been used. A wide variety of sclerosant agents have been used without a clear-cut difference in their efficacy or adverse effects. Several randomized trials have demonstrated that sclerotherapy, initiated after the first bleeding episode, reduces long-term morbidity and mortality. A meta-analysis of seven studies and 748 patients revealed mortality rates of 47% in the sclerotherapy group and 61% in the conservatively managed group [57]. Successful results of sclerotherapy in children have been reported, although no randomized trials have shown survival benefits in pediatrics [13].

A variety of complications are associated with sclerotherapy. Retrosternal pain, bacteremia, and fever after treatment are common. Esophageal ulceration may occur after sclerotherapy, and the associated symptoms may be ameliorated with carafate slurry therapy. Stricture formation can be managed by dilatation therapy. As noted above, the primary problem of portal hypertension is not addressed by this therapy, and recurrent varices are not unexpected. Occasional reports of esophageal perforation, aspiration pneumonia, spinal cord paralysis, mediastinitis, septicemia, bronchoesophageal fistulas, and cardiac tamponade exist. In children, abnormal esophageal manometry may be seen after sclerotherapy.

The range of potential complications associated with endoscopic sclerotherapy has prompted the development of alternative endoscopic methods of treatment, including variceal ligation and clipping therapy. Endoscopic ligation therapy is a derivative of rubber band ligation of hemorrhoids. The technique involves suctioning of a varix into the end of an endoscope so that a rubber band can be placed around the varix, leading to thrombosis (Figures 6.3 and 6.4). Multiple ligators have circumvented early problems of repeated esophageal intubations [56]. Direct comparisons of endoscopic sclerotherapy and variceal ligation in adults have yielded results in favor of ligation. Similar findings have been reported in a randomized trial of sclerotherapy versus ligation therapy in children [44]. The major advantage of variceal ligation is avoidance of needle injection of varices. This appears to reduce the rate of complications. In addition, variceal ligation apparently leads to obliteration in fewer sessions and is associated with a lower rate of early rebleeding. The latter may be related to milder esophageal ulcers in ligation compared with sclerotherapy. Review of uncontrolled published pediatric experience and the single randomized pediatric study with these techniques appears to indicate that these principles apply to children. Endoscopic variceal ligation using a clipping apparatus is an approach that involves application of metal clips as opposed to rubber bands. The technique has the advantage of using a standard endoscope and does not require multiple intubations because the clips can be passed through the biopsy channel. Published experience with this apparatus in children is limited.

Secondary prophylaxis: portosystemic shunting

A variety of procedures have been used to divert portal blood flow and decrease portal blood pressure (Figure 6.6) [58]. The portacaval shunt diverts nearly all of the portal blood flow into the subhepatic inferior vena cava. This very effectively decompresses the portal system but also diverts a significant amount of blood from its normal hepatic metabolism, predisposing to the development of hepatic encephalopathy. Decreased hepatic blood flow theoretically also may lead to worsening of underlying liver disease. An intermediate shunt can be made by

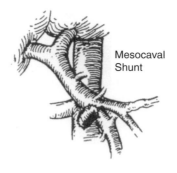

Mesocaval Shunt

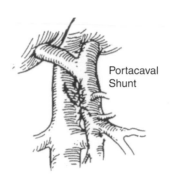

Portacaval Shunt

Distal Splenorenal Shunt

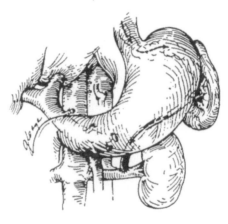

Figure 6.6
Portosystemic shunting procedures. The mesocaval shunt is formed with insertion of a graft between the superior mesenteric vein and the inferior vena cava. The portacaval shunt is formed by side-to-side anastomosis of the portal vein and the inferior vena cava. A distal splenorenal shunt is formed by end-to-side anastomosis of the splenic vein and the left renal vein. (Reprinted with permission from Brems *et al.*, 1989 [58].)

placing a graft between the mesenteric or portal vein and the vena cava. This decompresses the portal system while allowing a greater amount of portal blood to flow into the liver. The use of grafts unfortunately is associated with increased risk of thrombosis, and many times with worsening retrograde flow in the portal vein and greater diversion of portal flow through the shunt. Another approach involves diversion of splenic blood flow into the left renal vein, which can be done non-selectively (central) or semiselectively (distal splenorenal shunt).

A substantial pediatric experience with surgical portosystemic shunting has been accumulated over the past 20 years [59,60]. The results are clearly different in patients with extra- or intrahepatic portal hypertension. In general, responses are favorable with extrahepatic portal hypertension, with low rates

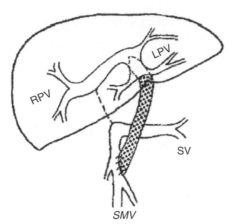

Figure 6.7 Meso Rex bypass. A graft (stippled) is interposed between the superior mesenteric vein (SMV) and the intrahepatic left portal vein (LPV). SV, splenic vein; RPV, right portal vein. (With permission from de Ville de Goyet et al., 1998 [61].)

of mortality and encephalopathy. Minimal encephalopathy may be a more prevalent problem than realized and requires specialized testing for its identification [2]. The response to portosystemic shunting with intrahepatic liver disease is very dependent upon the stage of the underlying liver disease and the near-term prognosis of that liver disease. Outcomes are generally poor in advanced liver disease, with the development of progressive liver disease and encephalopathy. When available liver transplantation is likely, it is preferable to shunting when decompensated liver disease exists. In contrast, outcome can be quite excellent in the child with compensated liver disease and portosystemic shunting is likely underutilized in this setting in pediatrics.

An alternative shunting procedure for children with extrahepatic portal vein thrombosis is the meso Rex bypass (Figure 6.7) [31,61]. This procedure involves placement of an autologous venous graft from the mesenteric vasculature to the left intrahepatic portal vein. The procedure was originally devised to treat portal vein thrombosis seen in pediatric liver transplant recipients. It was subsequently applied to treat patients with extrahepatic portal vein thrombosis. One of the major advantages of this approach is the restoration of normal portal blood flow, which eliminates the risk of hepatic encephalopathy and should preserve hepatic function. Recent studies indicate that children with extrahepatic portal vein thrombosis may have subtle features of encephalopathy, which are ameliorated by the meso Rex bypass [2]. As such, the criteria for candidacy for this procedure, both from the perspective of clinical indication and surgical feasibility, are not clear and some have advocated that this procedure be considered in all children with portal vein thrombosis and a cavernoma. Standard diagnostic imaging studies may not clearly indicate whether there is patency of the intrahepatic portal vein and retrograde or transhepatic portography may be required. The absence of the intrahepatic portal vein by angiography does not necessarily preclude successful completion of a meso Rex bypass. The potential for hypercoagulable states in these children must be kept in mind, particularly in light of the risk for postoperative thrombosis. Standard functional assessments of

coagulation may be abnormal in the presence of portal vein thrombosis; therefore, protein and molecular assays may be required to confirm a true hypercoagulable state.

In stark contrast to these excellent results in portal vein thrombosis, there are generally poor results for portosystemic shunting in children with decompensated liver disease secondary to intrahepatic diseases. The incidence of recurrent bleeding and death (both from recurrent hemorrhage and progressive liver dysfunction) in this group approaches 50%. Hepatic encephalopathy is a serious and not infrequent complication of portosystemic shunting in decompensated liver disease. The prevalence of this complication in children with intrahepatic disease is not well documented. Finally, portosystemic shunting has not been shown to improve long-term survival in patients with intrahepatic disease. Ultimately, most children with decompensated progressive liver disease and medically resistant esophageal varices will need to undergo orthotopic liver transplantation. In a group of 85 children who underwent transplantation for advanced liver disease and had a clear history of esophageal varix bleeding, long-term survival was far better than with any other available mode of therapy [62]. Prior portosystemic shunting can make orthotopic liver transplantation technically more difficult, requiring a significantly greater number of transfusions. In addition, prior splenectomy may increase the risk of sepsis and, therefore, appropriate immunizations against encapsulated organisms should be considered for the child who may require splenectomy. Overall, surgical portosystemic shunting is an excellent approach to the long-term management of children with intractable variceal hemorrhage in the setting of compensated cirrhosis. In addition, significant gastric variceal hemorrhage in children may be an indication to consider surgical shunting, since there is minimal data on the safety and efficacy of and limited local experience with endoscopic injection of N-butyl cyanoacrylate in children. An alternative shunting procedure for children with refractory variceal hemorrhage is TIPS, and this may serve as an effective bridge to transplantation [63]. The procedure is typically feasible, with published success in infants as small as 5 kg, although special procedural modifications must be undertaken for small children [64]. Long-term problems with shunt occlusion limit the overall application of this efficacious therapy, although newer data with coated stents may improve the long-term patency rates for TIPS.

Summary of the clinical approach to portal hypertension

Management of the child with clinical stigmata of portal hypertension who has not experienced variceal hemorrhage is complex and unclear at the present time. Surveillance endoscopy is predicated on the availability of an efficacious primary prophylactic therapy. Beta-blocker therapy is accepted as such in adults, and endoscopic ligation therapy is also gaining acceptance. Pilot data in children appear to indicate that this approach is feasible, but sufficient data do not exist to make a firm recommendation in favor of primary prophylaxis. Therefore, surveillance endoscopy and primary prophylaxis does not generally appear to be indicated in children with portal hypertension who have not had variceal hemorrhage. Certain special medical and social circumstances, where an initial bleeding episode is particularly risky, would justify application of adult approaches, including annual to biannual surveillance endoscopy and prophylactic beta-blocker therapy. The question of primary prophylaxis is one of the most important and difficult areas for future investigative trials in pediatric hepatology [42].

Management of acute variceal hemorrhage is more straightforward. Initial interventions should include stabilization of the patient, placement of a nasogastric tube, and institution of intravenous antibiotic therapy. Diagnostic or therapeutic endoscopy should be scheduled as soon as is safe and feasible. In the interim, pharmacologic treatment with either octreotide or terlipressin is indicated and may facilitate endoscopic therapy. Intractable and severe hemorrhage should be treated by TIPS.

The long-term approach to prevention of recurrent variceal hemorrhage in children must be adapted for the type of liver disease, presence or absence of systemic disease, the needs of a specific patient, and the particular skills of the institution. The approach to extrahepatic portal vein obstruction is evolving. In general, the unpredictability of the timing of the sentinel bleeding episode and the low incidence of fatality associated with that episode make prophylactic therapy inadvisable. Enthusiasm for utilization of the meso Rex bypass is increasing because of the physiologic nature of the procedure. It may be possible that this procedure should be considered for all children with portal vein thrombosis and a cavernoma. Certainly, in the patient with persistent problems with variceal hemorrhage, bypass is the procedure of choice. Endoscopic approaches and distal splenorenal shunting may need to be considered in patients where bypass is not feasible. The long-term management of portal hypertension in the child with biliary atresia is more complex. In those patients with incomplete bile drainage, liver transplantation appears to be inevitable and should be the major focus of therapeutic intervention. Temporizing measures for these children may include band ligation therapy or TIPS. Those patients who have a more successful response to portoenterostomy, as manifest by improvement in serum total bilirubin levels, have a more favorable long-term outlook. Variceal hemorrhage may be followed by relatively long-term survival with medical intervention. The potential risks and benefits of beta-blocker therapy are unknown and should be the subject of a multicenter trial. Endoscopic therapy in this group is an excellent initial approach. Recurrent hemorrhage might be amenable to portosystemic shunting as opposed to transplantation.

The approach to patients with more slowly progressive intrahepatic diseases is more difficult to generalize. The approach to patients with slowly progressive disease and compensated cirrhosis should be similar to the child with biliary atresia and a functioning hepatoportoenterostomy. The child with more rapidly progressive disease and/or decompensated cirrhosis will likely need to be considered for liver transplantation, with either endoscopic treatment or TIPS as a temporizing measure.

The study of portal hypertension has become very sophisticated in adults, but is in its infancy in children. Well-conceived and creatively designed multicenter trials will be required to determine if the principles that have been developed in adults can be extrapolated to children. Particular care will be required in choosing a homogeneous and representative patient population with a significant risk of complications of portal hypertension.

References

1. Subramanyam B, Balthazar E, Madamba M, *et al.* Sonography of portosystemic venous collaterals in portal hypertension. *Radiology* 1983;**146**:161–166.

2. Mack CL, Zelko FA, Lokar J, *et al.* Surgically restoring portal blood flow to the liver in children with primary extrahepatic portal vein thrombosis improves fluid neurocognitive ability. *Pediatrics* 2006;**117**:e405–412.

3. Miraglia R, Luca A, Maruzzelli L, *et al.* Measurement of hepatic vein pressure gradient in children with chronic liver diseases. *J Hepatol* 2010;**53**:624–629.

4. Duche M, Ducot B, Tournay E, *et al.* Prognostic value of endoscopy in children with biliary atresia at risk for early development of varices and bleeding. *Gastroenterology* 2010;**139**:1952–1960.

5. Desai MS, Zainuer S, Kennedy C, *et al.* Cardiac structural and functional alterations in infants and children with biliary atresia, listed for liver transplantation. *Gastroenterology* 2011;**141**:1264–1272.

6. Gana JC, Turner D, Mieli-Vergani G, *et al.* A clinical prediction rule and platelet count predict esophageal varices in children. *Gastroenterology* 2011;**141**:2009–2016.

7. Shneider B, Bosch J, De Franchis R, *et al.* Portal hypertension in children: expert pediatric opinion on the report of the Baveno V consensus workshop on the methodology of diagnosis and therapy in portal hypertension. *Pediatr Transplant* 2012; **16**:426–437.

8. Vorobioff J, Bredfeldt JE, Groszmann RJ. Increased blood flow through the portal system in cirrhotic rats. *Gastroenterology* 1984;**87**:1120–1126.

9. Iwakiri Y, Cadelina G, Sessa WC, Groszmann RJ. Mice with targeted deletion of eNOS develop hyperdynamic circulation associated with portal hypertension. *Am J Physiol Gastrointest Liver Physiol* 2002;**283**:G1074–1081.

10. Kowalski HJ, Abelmann WH. The cardiac output at rest in Laennec's cirrhosis. *J Clin Invest* 1953;**32**:1025–1033.

11. Janssen HL, Garcia-Pagan JC, Elias E, *et al.* Budd–Chiari syndrome: a review by an expert panel. *J Hepatol* 2003;**38**:364–371.

12. Gentil-Kocher S, Bernard O, Brunelle F, *et al.* Budd–Chiari syndrome in children: report of 22 cases. *J Pediatr* 1988;**113**:30–38.

13. Howard ER, Stringer MD, Mowat AP. Assessment of injection sclerotherapy in the management of 152 children with oesophageal varices. *Br J Surg* 1988;**75**:404–408.

14. Gauthier-Villars M, Franchi S, Gauthier F, *et al.* Cholestasis in children with portal vein obstruction. *J Pediatr* 2005;**146**:568–573.

15. Miga D, Sokol RJ, Mackenzie T, *et al.* Survival after first esophageal variceal hemorrhage in patients with biliary atresia. *J Pediatr* 2001;**139**:291–296.

16. D'Amico G, De Franchis R. Upper digestive bleeding in cirrhosis. Post-therapeutic outcome and prognostic indicators. *Hepatology* 2003;**38**:599–612.

17. Rockey D. The cellular pathogenesis of portal hypertension: stellate cell contractility, endothelin, and nitric oxide. *Hepatology* 1997;**25**:2–5.

18. Iwakiri Y. Endothelial dysfunction in the regulation of cirrhosis and portal hypertension. *Liver Int* 2012;**32**:199–213.

19. Okuda K, Kono K, Ohnishi K, *et al.* Clinical study of eighty-six cases of idiopathic portal hypertension and comparison with cirrhosis with splenomegaly. *Gastroenterology* 1984;**86**:600–610.

20. Pizcueta MP, Pique JM, Bosch J, Whittle BJ, Moncada S. Effects of inhibiting nitric oxide biosynthesis on the systemic and splanchnic circulation of rats with portal hypertension. *Br J Pharmacol* 1992;**105**:184–190.

21. Tripathi D, Hayes PC. The role of carvedilol in the management of portal hypertension. *Eur J Gastroenterol Hepatol* 2010;**22**:905–911.

22. Webb LJ, Sherlock S. The aetiology, presentation and natural history of extra-hepatic portal venous obstruction. *Q J Med* 1979;**48**:627–639.

23. Mitra SK, Kumar V, Datta DV, *et al.* Extrahepatic portal hypertension: a review of 70 cases. *J Pediatr Surg* 1978;**13**:51–57.

24. Kochar R, Fallon MB. Pulmonary diseases and the liver. *Clin Liver Dis* 2011;**15**:21–37.

25. Abrams GA, Jaffe CC, Hoffer PB, Binder HJ, Fallon MB. Diagnostic utility of contrast echocardiography and lung perfusion scan in patients with hepatopulmonary syndrome. *Gastroenterology* 1995;**109**:1283–1288.

26. Yonemura T, Yoshibayashi M, Uemoto S, *et al.* Intrapulmonary shunting in biliary atresia before and after living-related liver transplantation. *Br J Surg* 1999;**86**:1139–1143.

27. Barbe T, Losay J, Grimon G, *et al.* Pulmonary arteriovenous shunting in children with liver disease. *J Pediatr* 1995;**126**:571–579.

28. Condino AA, Ivy DD, O'Connor JA, *et al.* Portopulmonary hypertension in pediatric patients. *J Pediatr* 2005;**147**:20–26.

29. Laving A, Khanna A, Rubin L, Ing F, Dohil R, Lavine JE. Successful liver transplantation in a child with severe portopulmonary hypertension treated with epoprostenol. *J Pediatr Gastroenterol Nutr* 2005;**41**:466–468.

30. Yousef N, Habes D, Ackermann O, *et al.* Hepatorenal syndrome: diagnosis and effect of terlipressin therapy in 4 pediatric patients. *J Pediatr Gastroenterol Nutr* 2010;**51**:100–102.

31. Superina R, Shneider B, Emre S, Sarin SK, de Ville de Goyet J. Surgical guidelines for the management of extra-hepatic portal vein obstruction. *Pediatric Transplant* 2006;**10**:908–913.

32. Utterson EC, Shepherd RW, Sokol RJ, *et al.* Biliary atresia: clinical profiles, risk factors, and outcomes of 755 patients listed for liver transplantation. *J Pediatr* 2005;**147**:180–185.

33. Kasai M, Okamoto A, Ohi R, Yabe K, Matsumura Y. Changes of portal vein pressure and intrahepatic blood vessels after surgery for biliary atresia. *J Pediatr Surg* 1981;**16**:152–159.

34. Ohi R, Mochizuki I, Komatsu K, Kasai M. Portal hypertension after successful hepatic portoenterostomy in biliary atresia. *J Pediatr Surg* 1986;**21**:271–274.

35. van Heurn LW, Saing H, Tam PK. Portoenterostomy for biliary atresia: Long-term survival and prognosis after esophageal variceal bleeding. *J Pediatr Surg* 2004;**39**:6–9.

36. Miraglia R, Caruso S, Maruzzelli L, *et al.* MDCT, MR and interventional radiology in biliary atresia candidates for liver transplantation. *World J Radiol* 2011;**3**:215–223.

37. Sokal EM, Van Hoorebeeck N, Van Obbergh L, Otte JB, Buts JP. Upper gastro-intestinal tract bleeding in cirrhotic children candidates for liver transplantation. *Eur J Pediatr* 1992;**151**:326–328.

38. Bosch J, Abraldes JG, Berzigotti A, Garcia-Pagan JC. The clinical use of HVPG measurements in chronic liver disease. *Nat Rev Gastroenterol Hepatol* 2009;**6**:573–582.

39. D'Amico G, Pagliaro L, Pietrosi G, Tarantino I. Emergency sclerotherapy versus vasoactive drugs for bleeding oesophageal varices in cirrhotic patients. *Cochrane Database Syst Rev* 2010;(3):CD002233.

40. de Franchis R. Revising consensus in portal hypertension: report of the Baveno V consensus workshop on methodology of diagnosis and therapy in portal hypertension. *J Hepatol* 2010;**53**:762–768.

41. D'Amico G, Pagliaro L, Bosch J. The treatment of portal hypertension: a meta-analytic review. *Hepatology* 1995;**22**:332–354.

42. Ling SC, Walters T, McKiernan PJ, *et al.* Primary prophylaxis of variceal hemorrhage in children with portal hypertension: a framework for future research. *J Pediatr Gastroenterol Nutr* 2011;**52**:254–261.

43. Goncalves ME, Cardoso SR, Maksoud JG. Prophylactic sclerotherapy in children with esophageal varices: long-term results of a controlled prospective randomized trial. *J Pediatr Surg* 2000;**35**:401–405.

44. Zargar SA, Javid G, Khan BA, *et al.* Endoscopic ligation compared with sclerotherapy for bleeding esophageal varices in children with extrahepatic portal venous obstruction. *Hepatology* 2002;**36**:666–672.

45. Shashidhar H, Langhans N, Grand RJ. Propranolol in prevention of portal hypertensive hemorrhage in children: a pilot study. *J Pediatr Gastroenterol Nutr* 1999;**29**:12–17.

46. Ozsoylu S, Kocak N, Demir H, *et al.* Propranolol for primary and secondary prophylaxis of variceal bleeding in children with cirrhosis. *Turk J Pediatr* 2000;**42**:31–33.

47. Chalasani N, Boyer TD. Primary prophylaxis against variceal bleeding: beta-blockers, endoscopic ligation, or both? *Am J Gastroenterol* 2005;**100**:805–807.

48. Tripodi A, Mannucci PM. The coagulopathy of chronic liver disease. *N Engl J Med* 2011;**365**:147–156.

49. Hill ID, Bowie MD. Endoscopic sclerotherapy for control of bleeding varices in children. *Am J Gastroenterol* 1991;**86**:472–476.

50. Eroglu Y, Emerick KM, Whitingon PF, Alonso EM. Octreotide therapy for control of acute gastrointestinal bleeding in children. *J Pediatr Gastroenterol Nutr* 2004;**38**:41–47.

51. Stiegmann GV. Endoscopic ligation of esophageal varices. *Am J Surg* 1988;**156**:9B–12B.

52. Zemel G, Katzen BT, Becker GJ. Percutaneous transjugular portosystemic shunt. *JAMA* 1991;**266**:390–393.

53. Gooding I, Dondos V, Gyi KM, Hodson M, Westaby D. Variceal hemorrhage and cystic fibrosis: outcomes and implications for liver transplantation. *Liver Transplant* 2005;**11**:1522–1526.

54. Srinath A, Shneider BL. Congenital hepatic fibrosis and autosomal recessive polycystic kidney disease: an analytic review of the literature. *J Pediatr Gastroenterol Nutr* 2011.

55. Hall RJ, Lilly JR, Stiegmann GV. Endoscopic esophageal varix ligation: technique and preliminary results in children. *J Pediatr Surg* 1988;**23**:1222–1223.

56. McKiernan PJ, Beath SV, Davison SM. A prospective study of endoscopic esophageal variceal ligation using a multiband ligator. *J Pediatr Gastroenterol Nutr* 2002;**34**:207–211.

57. Infante-Rivard C, Esnaola S, Villeneuve JP. Role of endoscopic variceal sclerotherapy in the long-termmanagement of variceal bleeding: a meta-analysis. *Gastroenterology* 1989;**96**:1087–1092.

58. Brems J, Hiatt JR, Klein AS. Effect of a prior portasystemic shunt on subsequent liver transplantation. *Ann Surg* 1989;**209**:51–56.

59. Fonkalsrud EW. Surgical management of portal hypertension in childhood: long-term results. *Arch Surg* 1980;**115**:1042–1045.

60. Emre S, Dugan C, Frankenberg T, *et al.* Surgical porto-systemic shunts and the Rex by-pass in children: A single center experience. *HBP* 2009;**11**:252–257.

61. de Ville de Goyet J, Alberti D, Clapuyt P, *et al.* Direct bypassing of the extrahepatic portal venous obstruction in children: A new technique for combined hepatic portal revascularization and treatment of extrahepatic portal hypertension. *J Pediatr Surg* 1998;**33**:597–601.

62. Iwatsuki S, Starzl TE, Todo S, *et al.* Liver transplantation in the treatment of bleeding esophageal varices. *Surgery* 1988;**104**:697–705.

63. Heyman MB, LaBerge JM, Somberg KA, *et al.* Transjugular intrahepatic portosystemic shunts (TIPS) in children. *J Pediatr* 1997;**131**:914–919.

64. Lorenz JM. Placement of transjugular intrahepatic portosystemic shunts in children. *Tech Vasc Interv Radiol* 2008;**11**:235–240.

Laboratory assessment of liver function and injury in children

Vicky Lee Ng

The liver is a multifunctional organ that is involved in a number of critical excretory, synthetic, and metabolic functions. Biochemical assessment of these functions in children involves a number of tests performed in clinical laboratories. Many of the most commonly utilized serum chemistry tests, such as the aminotransferase and alkaline phosphatase (AP) levels, are often referred to as liver function tests, which is a misnomer as these do not actually measure or indicate liver function. Rather, these tests should be referred to as liver enzyme tests, with the term liver function tests reserved for true measures of hepatocyte synthetic function such as serum albumin levels and the prothrombin time (PT) or international normalized ratio. Any single biochemical test provides limited information that must be placed in the context of the entire clinical and historical picture. Currently available laboratory evaluative tests of the liver are used to: (1) screen for and document liver injury; (2) identify the type or pattern of liver disorder and the site of injury; (3) make a prognosis and follow-up children with chronic liver disease; and (4) serially monitor the course of liver disease, evaluate the response to treatment, and adjust a treatment regimen, when appropriate.

The widespread availability and frequent use of serum chemistry tests in children have resulted in an increase in the number of both normal and abnormal liver chemistry test values that must be evaluated by physicians. However, some limitations of liver biochemical tests must be recognized. First, screening laboratory tests may lack sensitivity. That is, if a liver chemistry test is normal, it does not ensure that the patient is free of liver disease. Children with chronic liver disease can have normal serum aminotransferase levels. Second, these tests are not specific for liver dysfunction. For example, serum aminotransferases may be elevated in patients with a non-hepatic disorder such as a musculoskeletal condition or cardiomyopathy. Finally, liver chemistry tests rarely provide a specific diagnosis; rather, they suggest a general category of liver disorder. For example, abnormal liver biochemical tests do not distinguish viral hepatitis from autoimmune hepatitis, or delineate intrahepatic from extrahepatic etiologies of cholestasis.

The sensitivity and specificity of screening laboratory tests in the detection of liver disease may be increased when utilized as a battery [1]. When more than one test within a battery is serially abnormal, then the probability of liver disease is higher. When all test results within the battery are normal, the probability of missing occult liver disease is lower. Ultimately, the clinical significance of any liver chemistry test abnormality in a child must be interpreted in the context of the clinical setting.

Tests to evaluate liver disease can be divided into five categories (Table 7.1).

1. *Tests that detect liver injury* are based on measurement of the serum level of endogenous substances released from damaged hepatocytes including alanine aminotransferase (ALT), aspartate aminotransferase (AST), and lactic acid dehydrogenase (LDH).

2. *Tests that detect impaired bile flow or cholestasis* are based on measurement of the serum level of endogenous substances released from damaged tissue such as alkaline phosphatase (AP), gamma-glutamyltransferase (GGT), and 5′-nucleotidase (5′NT).

3. *Tests of liver synthetic capacity* include the serum levels of albumin, PT and PTT, and individual clotting factors (such as factor VII and factor V). Triglyceride, cholesterol, lipid and lipoprotein synthesis also occur in the liver.

4. *Tests of hepatic excretory function* are based on measurements of serum concentrations of substances metabolized and transported by the liver, including endogenously produced compounds such as bilirubin and bile acids, as well as the determination of the rate of clearance of exogenously administered compounds, such as caffeine, lidocaine or para-aminobenzoic acid (PABA).

5. *Tests of hepatic metabolic function* reflect the central role of the liver in metabolic and regulatory pathways, including the detoxification and clearance of endogenous metabolites such as ammonia. Multiple metabolic abnormalities caused by specific inherited deficiencies of enzymes that reside almost exclusively in the liver, such as the urea cycle defects, can have a primary or secondary effect on the liver.

Table 7.1 Tests of liver function and injury

Test basis	Test
Endogenous substances *released* from damaged hepatocytes	Alanine aminotransferase Aspartate aminotransferase Lactic dehydrogenase
Endogenous substances reflecting impaired bile flow (cholestasis)	Gamma-glutamyltransferase Alkaline phosphatase 5'-Nucleotidase Leucine aminopeptidase Urobilinogen
Tests based on substances *synthesized* by the liver	Albumin Coagulation factors Serum lipids and lipoproteins Triglycerides Cholesterol
Tests based on substances *metabolized* and *transported* by the liver	Endogenous substances (serum bilirubin, serum bile acids) Exogenous substances (lidocaine, caffeine, aminopyrine, para-aminobenzoic acid)
Tests based on substances *detoxified and cleared* by the liver	Endogenous substances (ammonia)
Miscellaneous specific serum tests	Serum immunoglobulins Autoantibodies Plasma and urine amino acids

In this chapter, those tests most frequently used in assessing liver function and injury in children are discussed.

Tests based on substances released from injured liver

Aminotransferases

Assay of the serum aminotransferases (formerly known as transaminases), AST and ALT, are the liver chemistry tests most commonly used to assess injury to hepatocytes and to identify patients with liver disease.

The reversible transfer of the amino group from aspartic acid to the α-keto group of α-ketoglutaric acid to form oxaloacetic acid plus glutamic acid is catalyzed by AST (hence the former name of serum glutamic oxaloacetate transaminase). Similarly, ALT is the enzyme that catalyzes the reversible α-amino group transfer from the amino acid alanine to the α-keto group of α-ketoglutaric acid to yield pyruvic acid plus glutamic acid (hence its former name of serum glutamic pyruvic transaminase).

AST is present as both cytosolic and mitochondrial isoenzymes and is found in high concentrations in many tissues other than the liver, including heart muscle, skeletal muscle, kidney, brain, pancreas, lung, leukocytes, and red cells. ALT is a cytosolic enzyme that is present in highest concentrations in the liver. Elevation of enzyme activities in serum results from damage to or destruction of tissues rich in the aminotransferases, or to a change in cell membrane permeability allowing AST and/or ALT to leak from damaged cells into serum. However, because of the wide tissue distribution of AST, the hepatic origin of an isolated serum AST elevation should be confirmed by obtaining a serum ALT value. Differentiation of tissue sources by isoenzyme analysis is not routinely clinically available and typically not needed. A disproportionately isolated increase in serum AST should prompt a search for evidence of hemolysis (including difficult venipuncture attempts), acute rhabdomyolysis (such as seen during a systemic viral illness), a myopathic process, myocardial disease (including undiagnosed cardiomyopathy), or recent vigorous physical activity (such as long-distance running or weight lifting). Results of specific biochemical tests (such as serum haptoglobin, LDH, creatine phosphokinase, or aldolase) may verify hemolysis or myopathy/muscle disease as the underlying etiology of a disproportionately elevated serum AST. Spuriously high serum levels of AST can be caused by the presence of a macro-AST, formed by the enzyme complexing with an immunoglobulin, usually IgG, leading to decreased clearance, similar to the confusion that can occur in the case of macroamylasemia in the assessment of pancreatic diseases.

Concentrations of liver enzymes in plasma are widely used as indicators of liver disease. Screening for chronic liver disease is most commonly done using serum ALT activity; elevated ALT is widely considered to be an indicator of liver injury without providing a specific etiology. A study of over 5000 twin pairs from the TwinsUK Registry showed that variations in liver enzyme concentrations in plasma are highly heritable, suggesting an important role for genetic factors [2]. In adults, the clinically relevant upper limit of normal (ULN) for ALT is lower than frequently used [3]. The SAFETY (Screening ALT for Elevation in Today's Youth) study recently demonstrated the wide variability in the ULN of ALT used in acute care children's hospitals in the USA [4]. The authors concluded that ALT cut-off values are set too high for reliable detection of chronic liver disease in children and proposed consideration of lowering the ULN threshold to ALT >25 IU/L for boys and ALT >22 IU/L for girls [4]. Investigations of asymptomatic elevation of serum aminotransferases at a tertiary care hospital led to the findings of an underlying genetic disease in 12% of patients, including diagnoses of Wilson disease, α_1-antitrypsin deficiency, Alagille syndrome, hereditary fructose intolerance, glycogen storage disease, and ornithine transcarbamylase deficiency [5]. The presence of increased serum aminotransferases may be the only manifestation of celiac disease [6]. Non-alcoholic fatty liver disease is becoming increasingly common in children [7]; this can present as an isolated increase in serum ALT [8]. The differential diagnosis of elevated serum aminotransferase in a patient with a transplanted allograft mandates consideration of the time from transplantation surgery and prompt attention to the possibilities of rejection (hyperacute, acute cellular, or chronic), de novo autoimmune hepatitis, infection (hepatitis or intercurrent systemic), or biliary/vascular complications [9]. After blunt abdominal trauma, parallel elevations in aminotransferase levels may provide an early clue to liver injury [10]. In chronic liver diseases or in biliary obstruction (both intrahepatic and extrahepatic), AST and ALT elevations are usually less marked. A differential rise or fall in serum AST and ALT may, however, provide useful information, with a greater rise in ALT compared with AST seen with acute hepatitis, whereas a predominant rise in AST levels have been reported in fulminant echovirus infection and some metabolic diseases.

Some of the highest AST and ALT values (elevations >15 times normal) are seen following an acute episode of hypoxia or hypoperfusion (shock liver), and during the course of acute viral hepatitis, medication- or toxin-induced hepatotoxicity, and autoimmune hepatitis. Ischemic and hypoxic acute liver damage is more likely in patients with concomitant clinical conditions such as sepsis or low-flow hemodynamic states. However, there is a poor correlation between serum elevations of aminotransferases and the extent of liver cell necrosis seen on liver biopsy. Accordingly, serum AST and ALT elevations alone have limited prognostic value. Nevertheless, a rapid decline in aminotransferase levels, reflecting massive destruction and loss of viable hepatocytes, in association with increasing bilirubin levels and a coagulopathy portends a poor prognosis in the child with acute liver failure.

Serial measurements of aminotransferases are one of the important means of following the clinical activity of acute viral or autoimmune hepatitis in children, evaluating the response to immunosuppression therapy in chronic hepatitis or acute cellular rejection after liver transplantation, detecting drug-induced hepatotoxicity, and monitoring for progression or regression to liver injury [11]. Further understanding of the susceptibility to drug-induced liver injury requires an understanding of relevant mechanisms, the genetic and environmental factors influencing such mechanisms, and advances in toxicogenomics and proteomics.

The value of an increased AST:ALT ratio in adults as a non-invasive indicator of cirrhosis in chronic hepatitis C infection or to recognize undisclosed alcoholic liver disease has been debated [12]. Alcoholic patients, often deficient in pyridoxal 5′-phosphate, the coenzyme needed for ALT synthesis, have increased serum AST:ALT ratios, reflecting altered synthesis ratios in the liver [13]. Physiologically, impairment of functional hepatic blood flow leads to a resultant decrease in hepatic sinusoidal uptake of AST in patients with cirrhosis [12]. Pediatric experience with AST:ALT ratios is very limited; a retrospective review of 73 infants with chronic liver disease at one center demonstrated an increase in AST:ALT ratio over a 13-month period of follow-up in those with a worse clinical outcome [14]. An AST:ALT ratio

>4 in the appropriate clinical setting is highly suggestive of fulminant Wilson disease [15].

Lactate dehydrogenase

Lactate dehydrogenase is a cytoplasmic enzyme present in many tissues. There are five isoenzymes of LDH present in the serum and these can be separated using electrophoretic techniques. The slowest migrating band predominates in the liver. The differential diagnosis of elevated serum LDH levels includes skeletal or cardiac muscle injury, hemolysis, stroke, renal infarction, and acute and chronic liver disease. Because of limited specificity, serum LDH measurements rarely add information to that obtained from the aminotransferases alone. Uncommon clinical situations in which serum LDH may be diagnostically useful include the massive and transient elevation characteristic of ischemic hepatitis and the sustained elevation accompanying elevated serum AP, suggesting malignant infiltration of the liver.

Enzymes that detect impaired bile flow or cholestasis

Alkaline phosphatase

The APs are a group of isoenzymes originating in different tissues in the body that hydrolyze organic phosphate esters at alkaline pH, generating inorganic phosphate and an organic radical; the APs are true isoenzymes because they all catalyze this reaction. There are differences in their physicochemical properties. They are found in several tissues, including the canalicular membrane of hepatocytes, bone osteoblasts, the brush border of enterocytes in the small intestine, proximal convoluted tubules of the kidney, the placenta, and white blood cells. While the bone AP isoenzyme appears to be involved with calcification, the precise function of the liver AP isoenzyme is not known, although some postulate that it may participate in transport processes [16].

Activity of AP is normally demonstrable in serum, with the most likely sources being liver and bone. The serum level of AP varies considerably with age. Mean serum AP activity is higher in males aged 15–50 years of age; levels in females over 60 years equal or exceed those of age-matched males. The reasons for these differences are not known. Normal growing children and rapidly growing adolescents, in particular, have elevations of serum AP of bone origin, with good correlation with the rate of bone growth, which causes influx of enzymes from osteoid tissues. Therefore, an isolated increase in AP may not indicate hepatic or biliary disease if other liver biochemical tests are normal. Initial management may involve repeating the test, or confirming the hepatic origin with another liver chemistry test such as GGT or 5′NT (discussed in the next section).

Hepatobiliary disease leads to elevated serum AP through increased de novo synthesis of AP (induced and mediated by the action of bile acids) in the liver and leakage into the systemic circulation occurring through disruption of organelles and solubilization of phosphates bound to plasma membranes [17]. The extent of the abnormal elevation does not differentiate or discriminate intrahepatic from extrahepatic causes, nor do values differ significantly among various extrahepatic obstructive disorders such as choledochal cyst, bile duct stenosis, or sclerosing cholangitis. Similarly, values do not discriminate among various intrahepatic causes such as primary biliary cirrhosis, drug-induced hepatitis, and liver transplant rejection. Markedly increased AP levels are seen predominantly with infiltrative liver disorders (such as primary or metastatic tumor) or biliary obstruction. Conversely, serum AP levels can be normal despite extensive hepatic metastasis, or despite documented large duct obstruction.

A low serum AP level is seen in zinc deficiency and Wilson disease. Since zinc is a cofactor for AP, the measured activity of serum AP will be low in zinc deficiency states accompanying intestinal disorders such as acrodermatitis enteropathica and Crohn disease. Serum AP activity can be low in the fulminant presentation of Wilson disease.

The differential diagnosis of increased serum AP in the absence of liver disease includes pregnancy, familial inheritance, chronic renal failure and blood group types B or O, and transient hyperphosphatemia of infancy. During pregnancy, serum AP levels may double owing to increased activity from the placental isoenzyme. Unexplained elevation of AP activity was found to be familial, occurring in several healthy members of one family in an autosomal dominant inheritance pattern in the absence of bone or hepatic diseases [18]. Patients with blood groups O and B, who are ABH secretors and Lewis antigen-positive, may have increased amounts of serum intestinal AP activity, particularly after a fatty meal [19]. Measurement of AP in the fasting patient eliminates or reduces this elevated activity. Macro-APs, formed by the complexing of AP from liver or bone with immunoglobulin, are demonstrated as slow-moving forms on electrophoresis, but their significance is uncertain. Transient hyperphosphatemia of infancy is an apparently benign condition characterized by a marked transient and disproportional increase in serum AP lasting several weeks in the absence of any clinical, radiologic, or biochemical evidence of bone or liver pathology. The rise in AP is dramatic, often exceeding $10 \times$ ULN for the laboratory, with return to normal levels within 8 to 12 weeks. Awareness of this condition will curtail unnecessary extensive investigations for hepatobiliary disease [20,21].

In summary, because normal growing children have significant elevations of serum AP activity originating from influx into serum of the bone isoenzyme, this determination is of less value in the assessment of cholestasis in children, particularly in rapidly growing adolescents. The tissue origin of elevated AP activity can be determined by polyacrylamide gel electrophoresis, but this is not routinely available in most clinical laboratories. Heat denaturation of the enzyme in serum takes advantage of the fact that the liver isoenzyme is more resistant to denaturation than the bone form, but this method is

Table 7.2 Reference normal values for serum gamma-glutamyltransferase by patient age

Patient age	Sex	Normal serum level (U/L)
<1 month	M/F	<385
1 to 2 months	M/F	<225
2 to 4 months	M/F	<135
4 to 7 months	M/F	<75
7 months to 15 years	M/F	<45
>15 years	M	<75
>15 years	F	<55

Source: Hospital for Sick Children, Toronto, Canada, 1993 [24], with permission.

unreliable [22]. The most practical method most clinicians use to determine if an elevation of total serum AP activity signifies hepatic disease is to measure another enzyme that increases in cholestatic conditions and which is more specific to the liver, such as GGT or 5′NT.

Gamma-Glutamyltransferase

The microsomal enzyme GGT catalyzes the transfer of gamma-glutamyl groups from peptides such as glutathione to other amino acids. The enzyme is present in the cell membranes of multiple organs, including the kidney, pancreas, liver, spleen, brain, breast, and small intestine. Since it is found in so many tissues, including the biliary epithelium and hepatocyte, the usefulness of an elevated serum GGT is limited by its lack of specificity [23]. However, GGT *does not* increase in serum of patients with bone disease or children with active bone growth. Consequently, GGT is helpful in confirming the hepatic origin of elevated serum AP.

The newborn may have very high levels of GGT, up to five to $8 \times$ ULN for adults [23]. In premature infants in the first few days of life, the values of GGT may be even higher than in the full-term infant. Serum values then decline rapidly in both the full-term and premature infant and reach adult normal levels by 6 to 9 months of age [23]. Table 7.2 shows normal values of GGT by age used at the Hospital for Sick Children in Toronto, Canada, using the Eastman Kodak Ektachem 700 analyzer, a spectrophotometric method in common use in pediatric laboratory facilities because of the microliter quantities of serum required for analysis [24].

As with other microsomal enzymes, GGT activity is inducible by certain drugs. Hence elevated GGT levels are often found in children taking anticonvulsants such as phenobarbital and phenytoin. Valproic acid may not induce an increase in serum GGT, except in cases of true hepatotoxicity, making this biochemical test a good candidate for monitoring for liver injury during therapy with this anticonvulsant [25].

In up to 90% of cases of primary liver disease, elevated serum GGT is found, and hence it is not of great value in differential diagnosis. The highest levels are found in biliary obstruction, but extremely high levels are also found in intrahepatic cholestatic disorders such as Alagille syndrome. Serum GGT was most elevated in all children with biliary atresia, sclerosing cholangitis, paucity of intrahepatic bile ducts (Alagille syndrome), and cholestatic patients with α_1-antitrypsin deficiency [26]. The presence of increased serum GGT in both intrahepatic and extrahepatic cholestasis is variable and cannot be used to differentiate between them.

Normal or decreased serum GGT in the clinical setting of persistent jaundice is utilized as a test to distinguish between the different subtypes of genetic cholestatic syndromes [27]. Progressive familial intrahepatic cholestasis (PFIC) is a general term encompassing a group of illnesses characterized by persistent and profound cholestasis without extrahepatic pathology, typically presenting in the neonatal or infancy period, and with a progressive clinical course to cirrhosis. While not typically correlated with genotype data, elevated serum GGT is thought to distinguish PFIC type 3 (also known as multidrug resistance associated protein 3 (MDR3) disease) from the normal to low serum GGT levels more typical of PFIC type 1 (Byler disease) and type 2 (also known as bile salt export pump (BSEP) disease). A normal or low GGT with preserved normal liver structure also occurs in infants with benign recurrent intrahepatic cholestasis with a good long-term prognosis. Recent scientific advances have helped to clarify the molecular basis of many of these disorders [26–28]. As discussed in detail in Chapter 13, benign recurrent intrahepatic cholestasis type 1 is an autosomal recessive liver disease characterized by intermittent attacks of cholestasis; it starts at any age, lasts for several weeks to months, and shares a locus (chromosome 18q21) with PFIC type 1.

Elevations in GGT have been described in adults with a wide range of clinical conditions, including chronic alcoholism, exocrine pancreatic diseases, myocardial infarction, renal failure, chronic obstructive pulmonary disease, and diabetes. While measurement of serum GGT provide a sensitive indicator of the presence or absence of hepatobiliary disease, the usefulness of this assay is limited by its lack of specificity. Measurement of serum GGT levels is probably best used in combination to evaluate the meaning of elevations in other serum liver biochemical tests.

5′-Nucleotidase

The hydrolysis of nucleotides such as adenosine 5′-phosphate or inosine 5′-phosphate is catalyzed by 5′NT; these nucleotides are unique in having the phosphate group attached to the 5′ position of a pentose sugar moiety. The enzyme is found in the liver, intestine, brain, heart, blood vessels, and endocrine pancreas. Despite this widespread tissue distribution, marked serum elevations of 5′NT are found almost exclusively in the setting of liver disease. In the liver, 5′NT is located in both sinusoidal and canalicular membranes, but its precise physiologic purpose is not known. Serum 5′NT is substantially lower

in children than in adults, increases gradually with adolescence, and reaches a plateau after 50 years of age [29].

Serum 5′NT is elevated in hepatobiliary disease such as biliary obstruction, cholestasis of various etiologies, and hepatic infiltration. The spectrum of abnormal 5′NT values may parallel that of serum AP, probably because both enzymes have similar locations within the hepatocyte. However, unlike AP, serum 5′NT typically does not increase in the presence of bone disease. Elevated serum 5′NT in the presence of high ALT and AST suggest both hepatic and biliary tree involvement, as in patients with sickle cell disease [30]. The main value of 5′NT is its specificity for hepatobiliary disease when it is elevated in the non-pregnant patient, particularly with a concomitantly increased serum AP. Pregnancy also causes an increased value. Occasionally, 5′NT may be normal while the AP is elevated, yet the AP may still be of hepatic origin [29].

Leucine aminopeptidase

Leucine aminopeptidase catalyzes the hydrolysis of amino acids from the N-terminus of peptides and proteins, but its physiologic function is not known. The name derives from the fact that it reacts most readily with peptides containing leucine. Leucine aminopeptidase is found widely in human tissues, but activity is high in liver, particularly in biliary epithelium. Activity is increased in both pregnancy and hepatobiliary diseases, but not in bone disease. Values are the same in children and adults. Leucine aminopeptidase appears to be as sensitive in detecting obstructive biliary disease as 5′NT and AP, but also cannot differentiate among intrahepatic and extrahepatic causes of cholestasis [31]. Because of the common availability of AP, 5′NT, and GGT assays, leucine aminopeptidase has not found its way into common clinical use.

Tests of liver synthetic function
Albumin

Albumin, the principal serum protein, is synthesized only in the liver. The serum albumin level at any point in time reflects the rate of synthesis, rate of degradation, and volume of distribution. Albumin is synthesized in the rough endoplasmic reticulum of hepatocytes at a daily rate of 150 mg/kg in an adult and has a half-life in the serum of approximately 20 days. Albumin synthesis is regulated by changes in nutritional status, osmotic pressure, systemic inflammation, and hormone levels. The major functions of albumin are to maintain intravascular colloid osmotic pressure and to bind and serve as a carrier for a variety of compounds in serum, including bilirubin, inorganic ions such as calcium, as well as many drugs [32].

As serum albumin has a long half-life, low serum albumin levels are often taken as a sign of chronic liver disease rather than acute injury. However, a patient with compensated chronic liver disease may demonstrate an abrupt decrease in serum albumin concentration during an acute illness, such as sepsis or even a flu-like minor illness. This is caused partly by an acute decrease in synthesis below that already present owing to the parenchymal liver disease, possibly regulated by cytokines such as tumor necrosis factor and interleukin-1. Hypoalbuminemia is not specific for liver disease because it also occurs in the setting of protein-losing enteropathy, chronic infection, and nephrotic syndrome. In the absence of other non-hepatic etiologies, serum albumin can be useful in assaying hepatic synthetic function. Chronic inflammation, chronic liver disease, and protein malnutrition can inhibit albumin synthesis, whereas the presence of ascites causes an increased volume of distribution.

Tests of liver synthetic capacity

Coagulation disorders

Abnormal hemostasis is a common complication of liver disease [33]. The mechanisms resulting in these defects include (1) diminished hepatic synthesis of coagulation factors V, VII, IX, X, and XI, prothrombin and fibrinogen (reflected in prolongation of the PT); (2) dietary vitamin K deficiency from inadequate intake or malabsorption (based on intrahepatic or extrahepatic cholestasis and intestinal malabsorption); (3) dysfibrinogenemia; (4) enhanced fibrinolysis because of decreased synthesis of α_2-plasmin inhibitor; (5) disseminated intravascular coagulation; and (6) thrombocytopenia in hypersplenism. Due to the large functional reserve of the liver, failure of hemostasis may not be a complication of every liver disease and may not arise as a complication except in severe or chronic liver diseases. Therefore, testing for a coagulation defect is not a screening procedure; rather, it serves as a means of following the progress of the liver disease or for assessing the risk of bleeding before an invasive and traumatic diagnostic procedure is undertaken [34]. As storage capacity of vitamin K in the liver is limited, depletion occurs quickly when absorption is impaired, and the PT increases above normal ranges.

The PT is a measure of the time it takes for prothrombin (factor II) to be converted into thrombin in the presence of tissue extract (thromboplastin), calcium ions, and activated clotting factors V, VII, and X. Subsequently, there is a secondary reaction involving the polymerization of fibrinogen (factor I) to fibrin by thrombin. The result of the initial reaction that produced thrombin is expressed in seconds or as a ratio of the plasma PT to a control PT. This reaction evaluates the extrinsic pathway of coagulation and is prolonged if any of the involved factors (I, II, V, VII, and X) are deficient, either individually or in combination.

A prolonged PT is not specific for liver disease because it is seen in various congenital deficiencies of coagulation factors and in acquired conditions such as consumption of clotting factors (as in disseminated intravascular coagulation) and ingestion of drugs that affect the PT complex. Factor VIII, being made in non-hepatic tissues, is helpful in differentiating the depression of clotting factor activity and prolongation of hemostasis caused by severe liver disease alone (normal factor VIII) from that caused by accompanying disseminated intravascular coagulation (depressed factor VIII activity from consumption). Disseminated intravascular coagulation is more common in children with end-stage liver failure because of the increased risk of infection from general debilitation and synthetic deficiencies of plasma proteins such as complement and opsonins normally made by the liver.

In the presence of normal factor VIII activity, prolongation of the PT indicates plasma clotting factor deficiency from impaired hepatic synthesis or secondary to vitamin K deficiency. Recent intake of antibiotics that alter the intestinal flora should be considered. Since the plasma half-life of several of the clotting factors is short (e.g. 3–5 hours for factor VII), the PT will rapidly reflect changes in hepatic synthetic function, such as may occur in acute liver failure, and thereby provides a good indicator of prognosis [33]. Most patients with extrahepatic obstruction respond promptly to parenterally administered vitamin K. In patients with jaundice, the type of response to vitamin K is, therefore, of value in differential diagnosis, particularly because it can be surmised that parenchymal function is good if the PT returns to normal within 24 hours after a single parenteral injection of vitamin K. In some inherited metabolic diseases in the newborn, such as tyrosinemia, there may be profound prolongations of both PT and the partial thromboplastin time (clotting test) that may appear out of proportion to other parameters of liver dysfunction [35].

The PT test is not a sensitive index of chronic liver disease because even in severe cirrhosis, levels can be normal or only slightly prolonged. It does, however, have high prognostic value, particularly for patients with acute hepatocellular disease. A persistently abnormal PT in a previously well child can be the single laboratory test that draws attention to the possibility of the development of acute liver failure [36]. However, not all patients with prolonged PTs will be shown to have evidence of acute liver failure. In children with chronic cholestatic liver disease, an abnormal PT level refractory to maximal vitamin K therapy and decreasing serum albumin should raise for consideration the merits of a referral to a liver transplantation center for assessment.

Specific assays of clotting factors and other proteins involved in the hemostatic process may supply additional information in assessing patients with liver disease. Although fibrinogen levels are usually normal in hepatic disease because it is made both in the liver and in extrahepatic sites, increased catabolism of fibrinogen has been noted in patients with acute and chronic liver disease. Low levels of fibrinogen are seen in liver disease accompanied by disseminated intravascular coagulation when there is consumption of fibrinogen and other clotting factors. Conversely, high levels of fibrinogen can be seen in patients with hepatic diseases because fibrinogen is an acute phase reactant or from elevations specifically in cholestatic disease. Finally, some patients with liver disease develop a dysfibrinogenemia with accumulation of an abnormal fibrin monomer aggregate, which is manifested by a normal measured fibrinogen level in serum together with prolonged PT.

Table 7.3 Reference values for prothrombin time and activated partial thromboplastin time in the healthy premature (30 to 36 weeks of gestation) infant during the first 6 months of life

Postnatal age	Prothrombin time (s)[a]	Activated partial thromboplastin time (s)[a]
Day 1	13.0 (10.6–16.2)	53.6 (27.5–79.4)
Day 5	12.5 (10.0–15.3)	50.5 (26.9–74.1)
Day 30	11.8 (10.0–13.6)	44.7 (26.9–62.5)
Day 90	12.3 (10.0–14.6)	39.5 (28.3–50.7)
Day 180	12.5 (10.0–15.0)	37.5 (21.7–53.3)
Adult	12.4 (10.8–13.9)	33.5 (26.6–40.3)

[a] Values in parentheses are normal ranges.

Nearly all of the above data are derived from studies in adults because of the considerable lag in knowledge of the unique aspects of the hemostatic system in full-term and preterm infants and the young child. Some of the distinctions that have been recognized include differences in the concentration of clotting factors, differences in the ability to generate thrombin (i.e. the very process measured by the PT), and the ability to inhibit the activity of thrombin once it is formed [37]. Many of the clotting factors, including the vitamin K-dependent factors II, VII, IX, and X, are less than 70% of adult levels in both full-term and preterm newborns. It is now clear that the hemostatic system of the neonate is dynamic and evolving toward that of the normal adult. Therefore, in assessing liver dysfunction in young infants based on prolongation of the PT, normal values specific to the gestational age at term and the postnatal age need to be considered [38,39] (Table 7.3). Despite these prolongations in PT and activated partial thromboplastin time, clinical evidence indicates that the healthy infant is not at an increased risk of bleeding. By contrast, in the sick infant, further reductions in clotting factors will decrease the production of prothrombin, which may then result in bleeding observed in sick newborns with liver disease.

Lipids and lipoproteins

The liver plays a central role in production and degradation of lipoproteins [40]. Lipoprotein abnormalities are common in chronic cholestatic disorders of either intrahepatic or extrahepatic etiology [41]. Marked elevations in the plasma levels of cholesterol and phospholipids occur through the regurgitation into plasma of biliary phospholipids, which have secondary effects leading to an increase in plasma cholesterol due to enhanced hepatic synthesis of cholesterol. The cholesterol is transported in the blood in lipoprotein X, an unusual vesicular form of lipoprotein specific to cholestasis [41]. However, in non-cholestatic liver diseases, declining lipoprotein cholesterol may also reflect deteriorating liver function and is an indicator of prognosis.

In acute hepatocellular injury, levels of hepatic enzymes such as lecithin-cholesterol acyltransferase and triglyceride lipase are decreased. Patients with acute liver disease have increased levels of plasma triglycerides, a decreased percentage of cholesterol esters, and abnormal electrophoretic lipoprotein patterns. Mild hypertriglyceridemia is characteristic of acute hepatocellular injury, with accumulation of triglyceride-rich low density lipoprotein (LDL). Deficiency of hepatic triglyceride lipase may account for the increased LDL triglyceride levels seen in acute hepatitis [42]. However, attempts to correlate blood lipid and apolipoprotein levels with specific causes of liver dysfunction have been unsuccessful [42]. Some investigators advocate analyses of multiple apolipoproteins and subclasses, particularly apolipoprotein-AII, as a more sensitive index of liver dysfunction [43].

Tests based on substances metabolized and transported by the liver

Bilirubin

A more detailed discussion of the biochemistry and physiology of bilirubin metabolism is found in Chapter 12.

Bilirubin is a yellow tetrapyrrole pigment produced from the breakdown of ferroprotoporphyrin IX (heme), an integral part of heme-containing proteins. Approximately 75% of total bilirubin produced comes from the heme moiety of hemoglobin released from senescent erythrocytes destroyed in the reticuloendothelial cells of the liver, spleen, and bone marrow. The remaining bilirubin is produced from the premature destruction of red blood cell precursors in the bone marrow (i.e. ineffective erythropoiesis) and from the turnover and catabolism of other heme-containing proteins such as myoglobin, cytochromes, and peroxidases.

Unconjugated bilirubin must be taken up into the hepatocyte and conjugated into the glucuronide form by the endoplasmic reticulum enzyme bilirubin UDP-glucuronyltransferase; the water-soluble bilirubin mono- and diglucuronides are then excreted across the canalicular membrane into bile [44]. The molecular mechanisms of these processes have been delineated and reviewed [28].

When hepatic excretion of bilirubin glucuronides is impaired, serum levels of bilirubin glucuronides increase. Bilirubin glucuronides covalently bound to serum albumin form a fourth form of bilirubin, known as δ-bilirubin; δ-bilirubin is identified in the fourth fraction (the first three forms of bilirubin being α, β, and γ, corresponding to unconjugated, monoconjugated, and diconjugated species, respectively) to elute when bilirubin is fractionated by high-pressure liquid chromatography [45,46]. In both children and adults, the appearance of δ-bilirubin is associated with elevations of conjugated bilirubin and not with those disorders producing unconjugated bilirubin. Albumin-bound δ-bilirubin has a prolonged half-life of approximately 14 days, compared with the 4 hour half-life of bilirubin. The prolonged half-life of albumin-bound δ-bilirubin explains why some children with reversible hepatobiliary diseases have serum bilirubin levels that decline slower than one might expect during an otherwise satisfactory clinical recovery. The increase in δ-bilirubin accompanying the decrease in total serum bilirubin levels during recovery from an obstructive hepatobiliary disorder likely reflects decreased clearance of δ-bilirubin because of its protein-bound nature and larger size. The percentage of δ-bilirubin in jaundiced neonates is low compared with icteric adults. This may reflect delayed maturation of the enzymatic processes that produce protein-bound bilirubin from elevated conjugated bilirubin in serum.

Some clinical laboratories still use spectrophotometry to measure serum bilirubin as direct-reacting or indirect-reacting fractions. In this method, some bilirubin in the serum of jaundiced patients reacts directly with Ehrlich's diazo reagent (direct bilirubin), whereas some bilirubin requires alcohol as an accelerator for the reaction to proceed to a color product (indirect bilirubin). The value of indirect bilirubin is then calculated as the difference between the total value measured with the accelerator minus the direct value obtained without the accelerator (direct fraction). In this method, protein-bound δ-bilirubin is not detected as a separate species and is present in the direct fraction. Hence, direct bilirubin and conjugated bilirubin levels are not interchangeable [47]. Many clinical laboratories now measure and report separate true values for conjugated, unconjugated, and total bilirubin. The δ-bilirubin value can then be calculated as the difference between total bilirubin and the sum of the conjugated and unconjugated fractions. Use of high-pressure liquid chromatography can precisely quantify separate fractions of conjugated, unconjugated, and protein-bound or δ-bilirubin, but the method is not generally available for routine clinical use.

Unconjugated hyperbilirubinemia may result from hemolysis or from genetic diseases such as Crigler–Najjar syndrome, a rare genetic disease with deficiency of bilirubin UDP-glucuronyltransferase. It presents shortly after birth and is characterized by a severe or total impairment of bilirubin conjugation by the liver. Diminished expression of this enzyme is also the defect causing Gilbert syndrome, a benign, unconjugated hyperbilirubinemia occurring in up to 5% of the normal population. The term "physiologic jaundice" is used to describe the frequently observed jaundice in otherwise completely normal neonates, which is the result of a number of factors involving increased bilirubin production and decreased excretion. These entities are discussed in further detail in Chapter 12.

Conjugated hyperbilirubinemia (>15% of the total serum bilirubin) indicates hepatobiliary disease and is always pathologic. It is usually accompanied by bilirubin in the urine, the presence of which can be tested quickly and cheaply using a urine dipstick. The presence of bilirubin in the urine confirms the presence of conjugated hyperbilirubinemia because unconjugated bilirubin is not excreted in urine. Bilirubinuria can appear before overt clinical jaundice. Further diagnostic evaluations in this setting should never be delayed, with an approach focused on the age-specific onset of diseases affecting the developing liver. The merits of quickly diagnosing causes amenable to specific medical therapies (e.g. sepsis, hypopituitarism, and galactosemia) or to early surgical interventions (e.g. biliary atresia or choledochal cyst) prior to the development of comorbid complications must be emphasized. Various infectious, metabolic, toxic, genetic, and anatomic causes for a mechanical obstruction to bile flow or a functional impairment of any of the many processes involved in hepatic excretory function and bile secretion must be meticulously sought [48,49] as discussed in Chapter 8.

Although serum bilirubin levels increase in cholestatic disorders, the magnitude of the increase does not help to differentiate between intrahepatic and extrahepatic biliary disorders. Both conjugated and unconjugated bilirubins are retained in these disorders, and a wide range of elevated serum concentrations of each form of bilirubin may be observed. Cholestasis is associated with complex transcriptional and post-transcriptional alterations of hepatobiliary transporters and enzymes participating in bile formation. Extensive studies on genotype–phenotype correlations in monogenic diseases, such as PFIC and benign recurrent intrahepatic cholestasis, facilitate diagnostics and improve the risk assessment of hepatobiliary transporter gene variants in bile transport pathophysiology [27,28,50,51]. Genome-wide association scans are the next step in gathering information about contributors toward polygenic (multifunctional) cholestatic diseases [45,52].

Urobilinogen

Urobilinogen refers to a group of three colorless tetrapyrroles formed when unconjugated bilirubin (formed after the bilirubin glucuronides secreted into the upper small intestine are hydrolyzed to the unconjugated pigment) is reduced by the anaerobic intestinal microbial flora. Up to 20% of the urobilinogens produced daily are then reabsorbed from the intestine and undergo enterohepatic recirculation. The majority of the reabsorbed urobilinogen is taken up by the liver and then re-excreted into bile. A small amount is also excreted in the urine. In the lower intestinal tract, the urobilinogen tetrapyrroles spontaneously oxidize to produce the major color pigments of stool.

The formation of urobilinogen is decreased in all conditions in which biliary excretion of bilirubin is impaired. In the presence of hepatic dysfunction, more urobilinogen escapes hepatic uptake and biliary–enteric excretion and, thus, appears in the urine. As biliary obstruction becomes more complete, delivery of bilirubin to the intestinal tract is limited, and urine as well as stool urobilinogen excretion decrease to very low concentrations.

Some confounding factors must be considered in the measurement and interpretation of urinary urobilinogen. Excretion has some diurnal variation, with peak urinary output between 12:00 and 16:00 hours. Urinary excretion of urobilinogen depends strongly on urinary pH; tubular reabsorption increases and urobilinogen stability decreases as pH decreases.

Urobilinogen production and hence urinary excretion decrease with antibiotic treatment and diarrhea. These changes in urobilinogen unrelated to altered hepatobiliary function need to be considered when interpreting urinary urobilinogen values.

Bile acid tests

Bile acids are a class of endogenous organic anions synthesized from cholesterol exclusively in the hepatocytes; they are then conjugated to glycine or taurine and excreted into bile (reviewed in Chapter 33). Alterations in hepatic bile acid synthesis, intracellular metabolism, excretion, intestinal absorption, and plasma extraction are reflected in derangements in bile acid metabolism [53]. Bile acids are also able to activate a range of dedicated nuclear receptors that play a key role in the transcriptional control of critical steps of a wide range of hepatic functions ranging from bile acid homeostasis and bile formation, phase I/II metabolism of endo- and xenobiotics (such as bile acids and drugs, respectively), to hepatic lipids and glucose metabolism [54]. Nuclear receptors activated by bile acids are key for understanding the pathogenesis of several liver diseases and represent attractive drug targets in the treatment of cholestatic liver disease. The abnormal serum bile acid levels in cirrhosis of any cause is a consequence of decreased liver cell mass, decreased bile excretion, and the portosystemic shunting usually present in chronic liver disease.

Several methods to measure serum concentrations of bile acids are available, including enzymatic assays, in which the bacterial enzyme 3α-hydroxysteroid dehydrogenase is coupled to either fluorimetric or bioluminescence techniques; gas–liquid chromatography; radioimmunoassay; or a highly specific assay that combines gas–liquid chromatography and mass spectrometry [55,56]. The development of the technique of fast atom bombardment mass spectrometry in a handful of specialized laboratories has allowed the rapid screening of urine samples from infants and older children with suspected bile acid synthetic disorders using microliter amounts of sample directly, without requiring time-consuming sample preparation (see Chapter 33). Mass spectra are generated and indicate whether bile acid conjugates are present in an abnormal profile [53,55,56]. Such techniques of precise bile acid analysis have contributed heavily to our current knowledge of several inborn metabolic defects of bile acid synthesis.

Common causes of mildly elevated serum bile acid levels include portosystemic shunting and the postprandial state. Fasting serum bile acid levels are disproportionately elevated in certain cholestatic disease, such as primary sclerosing cholangitis and PFIC syndromes (all subtypes) in children, and primary biliary cirrhosis and pregnancy in adults. Serum bile acid levels are elevated in patients with liver biopsy-proven acute and chronic liver disease, even when serum bilirubin levels are normal. However, levels of serum bile acids do not provide specific information on the type of liver disease. Measuring serum bile acids may be less useful in children because of the presence of a relative "physiologic cholestasis" in neonates, which results in baseline elevations of serum levels even in healthy babies. These baseline elevations decrease within the first year of life, indicating a maturation of the bile acid transport processes. Using serum bile acid measurements to differentiate biliary atresia from other, non-obstructive causes of neonatal cholestasis, or to assess prognosis in children with α_1-antitrypsin deficiency, have been unsuccessful [57,58].

Exogenous substances used in tests to assess quantitative liver function

The tests for quantitative liver function, or true dynamic liver function tests, are based on uptake, metabolism, and excretion of a determinate substance. The ideal test would be inexpensive, easy to perform and analyze, safe, have a single pharmacokinetic profile with minimal drug interactions, have a high predictive value, and provide quick results [59]. No single test has yet met these ideal performance characteristics. Quantitative liver function tests are not suitable for use in screening for liver disease. They are more complex to perform and more expensive than conventional biochemical tests, but superior in monitoring the degree of liver dysfunction.

Two approaches have generally been used in the assessment of liver function: one is to measure the products of liver synthesis, whereas the other is to monitor hepatic clearance function. Dynamic function tests can be classified in two categories: those using elimination of a substrate for testing (e.g. indocyanine green clearance, caffeine clearance, and galactose elimination) and studies which detect metabolites of the substance administered (e.g. aminopyrine breath test, monoethylglycinexylidide test, and the PABA test).

Exogenously administered lidocaine is metabolized by oxidative de-ethylation (within the hepatic cytochrome P450 system) to monoethylglycinexylidide, which can be analyzed by common laboratory instrumentation thus making rapid evaluation of liver function possible. However, because the rate of monoethylglycinexylidide production declines significantly with age, results of this test must be interpreted for age [60]. This test may have the most clinical utility in evaluating liver function to determine the suitability of the donor liver for transplant and to measure graft function post-transplantation [61].

The use of PABA as a probe drug to quantify hepatic function has been reported to be a promising prognostic test for children with chronic liver disease and with fulminant liver failure [62,63]. PABA is a non-toxic, inexpensive, and orally administered probe drug that is readily absorbed from the gastrointestinal tract and undergoes biotransformation to three metabolites independent of phase I cytochrome P450 biotransformation reactions. Through phase II conjugation reactions, PABA combines with glycine (to form para-aminohippuric acid), with acetyl-CoA (to form para-acetamidobenzoic acid), or with both glycine and acetyl CoA (to form para-acetamidohippuric acid) [63]. With extensive hepatocellular damage, glycine conjugation and hepatic acetylation of PABA is rapidly lost. The measurement by high-pressure liquid chromatography of serum para-aminohippuric acid concentration at 30 minutes after oral administration was the most reliable early prognostic marker of outcome in 24 children with acute liver failure or acute severe hepatitis, with a sensitivity of 92%, and negative predictive value of 92%; this can be compared with a sensitivity of 54% and a negative predictive value of 63% with King's College criteria [62]. Further confirmatory multicenter studies are needed.

Tests based on substances cleared from plasma by the liver

Ammonia

The concentration of ammonia in blood is regulated by the balance of its production and clearance. Production is mainly in the large intestine by the action of bacterial urease on dietary protein and amino acids. Clearance of ammonia under normal circumstances occurs mainly by the liver through transformation of ammonia into urea via the urea cycle and into glutamine by transamination of α-ketoglutarate to glutamate and then to glutamine. The liver ordinarily removes 80% of the portal venous ammonia in a single pass.

In chronic liver diseases, disturbed urea cycle function caused by parenchymal liver cell destruction and portosystemic shunting permits large amounts of ammonia (and other putative toxins) to bypass the liver and exert their effects on the central nervous system [63]. Some ammonia is also made by the kidney and small intestine, a fact that becomes important when a patient is taking certain drugs such as the anticonvulsant valproic acid, which can cause an increase in serum ammonia independent of any hepatotoxicity because of the drug-induced ammonia production by the kidney.

Advanced liver disease is the most commonly encountered acquired cause of hyperammonemia. Any cause of severe liver failure can lead to a significant impairment of normal ammonia metabolism. Hepatic encephalopathy, which develops in patients with cirrhosis, can be precipitated by an episode of gastrointestinal bleeding, which enhances ammonia production by bacterial metabolism of the blood proteins in the colon. However, in children, levels of encephalopathy and serum ammonia have a poor correlation.

Patients with advanced cirrhosis can have normal fasting levels of ammonia. Conversely, non-fasting values of ammonia may be elevated even in a patient with mild liver disease. Therefore, fasting serum levels should be determined to reflect accurately the clearance of ammonia in blood. Serial measurements are useful because an increasing trend of fasting ammonia values has more value in assessing the development of advancing liver disease and hepatic encephalopathy than a single measurement in time.

Other causes of elevated blood ammonia include portosystemic shunts (either those created surgically or those of congenital origin), inherited defects of the urea cycle enzymes such as ornithine carbamoyltransferase deficiency, defects in mitochondrial fatty acid beta-oxidation, and Reye syndrome. When cirrhosis is accompanied by impaired venous drainage from the intestinal tract into the liver via the portal vein, venous anastomoses develop. These collateral vessels shunt ammonia of intestinal origin away from the liver and into the general systemic circulation and cause increases in blood ammonia. Impaired renal function also often accompanies severe liver disease, with decreasing urinary output leading to increasing blood urea concentration and increased excretion of urea into the intestine, where it is converted to ammonia. Finally, the patient with compensated liver disease and normal or near normal ammonia levels may develop the sudden onset of encephalopathy and increased serum ammonia if presented with a large protein load. This may occur during the setting of a large blood loss into the gastrointestinal tract, with or without the catabolic stress of sepsis, both of which are common events in patients with chronic liver disease [63].

Other laboratory tests to assess for liver disease in children

Serum globulins

Serum globulins can be quickly determined by subtracting the albumin concentration from the total protein level. Serum globulins can be further separated by using serum protein electrophoresis into α_1, α_2, β, and γ fractions. Within each of these fractions is a heterogeneous collection of different serum proteins. The α_1 fraction is composed principally of α_1-antitrypsin, ceruloplasmin, and orosomucoid (an α_1-acid glycoprotein), all of which are acute phase reactants and increase in response to liver disease and many inflammatory disorders. Haptoglobin makes up a large part of the α_2 fraction and is also an acute-phase reactant. Transferrin and β-lipoprotein make up a major portion of the β fraction. The principal constituents of the γ fraction are the immunoglobulins, particularly IgG, IgA, and IgM. Abnormalities may occur in the serum protein electrophoresis profile in various liver diseases, such as hypergammaglobulinemia seen in autoimmune hepatitis and low α_1 fraction peak in α_1-antitrypsin deficiency. Few of these abnormalities are a specific diagnostic aid. Serum immunoglobulins are produced by stimulated B-lymphocytes. Therefore, measurement of these substances is not a direct test of liver function or hepatocyte injury.

Plasma and urine amino acids

Measures of amino acids in the blood and urine may provide specific information critical to or supportive of the diagnosis of an inborn error of intermediary metabolism, such as hereditary tyrosinemia, methylmalonic acidemia, and defects of ureagenesis. These are discussed in further detail in Chapters 31, 34, and 38.

Genome-wide association studies

A recent genome-wide association study identified 42 loci associated with concentrations of liver enzymes in plasma and provided new insight into the genetic variation and pathways influencing liver biochemical tests such as ALT, AP, and GGT, as well as biological mechanisms involved in liver injury [65]. The 69 candidate genes identified include those involved in biliary transport; glucose, carbohydrate, and lipid metabolism; glycoprotein biosynthesis and cell surface glycobiology; inflammation and immunity; and glutathione metabolism [63]. Genome-wide association and complex mapping studies in inbred animals may in the future be tools to identify previously unsuspected modifier loci and eventually genes predisposing to cholestasis. A genome-wide association study in large patient cohorts with gallstones, fatty liver disease, viral hepatitis, chronic cholestatic liver diseases, and drug-induced liver injury have provided new insights into illness pathophysiology and suggest the contribution of previously unsuspected pathogenic pathways [49]. The ultimate goal is to define subgroups of patients at risk of developing liver diseases who would benefit from preventive measures and/or personalized

therapy. Comprehensive strategies for integrating genomic data and counseling of patients remain to be developed [49].

Conclusions

The initial evaluation of a serum liver chemistry value in a child must be assessed in the context of the findings of a detailed history and physical examination. A reliable literature to make unequivocal recommendations for the diagnostic evaluation of children with abnormal liver chemistry tests is lacking. In the individual patient care setting, additional serologic, radiologic, and histopathologic results may well be warranted. Advances in laboratory medicine have made possible increasingly sophisticated analysis of compounds in body fluids related to the liver function in both health and diseased states. Results from genome-wide association studies suggest potential hereditary contributions to tests of liver function. These analyses provide the clinician with valuable diagnostic as well as, on occasion, prognostic information. Some tests still are not widely available for routine clinical use. Others continue to lack the diagnostic sensitivity and specificity clinicians seek for the ideal liver injury and function tests. Further advances in our knowledge of the physiology and biochemistry of the normal and diseased liver will contribute to the fulfilment of this goal.

References

1. Adams PC, Arthur MJ, Boyer TD, *et al.* Screening in liver disease: report of an AASLD clinical workshop. *Hepatology* 2004;**39**:1204–1212.

2. Rahmioglu N, Andrew T, Cherkas L, *et al.* Epidemiology and genetic epidemiology of the liver function test proteins. *PLOS One* 2009;**4**:e4435.

3. Prati D, Taioli E, Zanella A, *et al.* Updated definitions of healthy ranges for serum alanine aminotransferase levels. *Ann Intern Med* 2002;**137**:1–10.

4. Schwimmer JB, Dunn W, Norman GJ, *et al.* SAFETY study: alanine aminotransferase cutoff values are set too high for reliable detection of pediatric chronic liver disease. *Gastroenterology* 2010;**138**:1357–1364.

5. Iorio R, Sepe A, Giannattasio A, Cirillo F, Vegnente A. Hypertransaminasemia in childhood as a marker of genetic liver disorders. *J Gastroenterol* 2005;**40**:820–826.

6. Farre C, Esteve M, Curcoy A, *et al.* Hypertransaminasemia in pediatric celiac disease patients and its prevalence as a diagnostic clue. *Am J Gastroenterol* 2002;**97**:3176–3181.

7. Cohen JC, Horton JD, Hobbs HH. Human fatty liver disease: old questions and new insights. *Science* 2011;**332** (6037):1519–1523.

8. Mencin AA, Lavine JE. Nonalcoholic fatty liver disease in children. *Curr Opin Clin Nutr Metab Care* 2011;**14**:151–157.

9. Kamath BM, Olthoff KM. Liver transplantation in children: update 2010. *Pediatr Clin North Am* 2010;**57**:401–414.

10. Keller MS, Coln CE, Trimble JA, Green MC, Weber TR. The utility of routine trauma laboratories in pediatric trauma resuscitations. *Am J Surg* 2004;**188**:671–678.

11. Kaplowitz N. Drug-induced liver injury. *Clin Infect Dis* 2004;**38**(Suppl 2): S44–S48.

12. Giannini E, Risso D, Botta F, *et al.* Validity and clinical utility of the aspartate aminotransferase-alanine aminotransferase ratio in assessing disease severity and prognosis in patients with hepatitis C virus-related chronic liver disease. *Arch Intern Med* 2003;**163**:218–224.

13. Diehl AM, Potter J, Boitnott J, *et al.* Relationship between pyridoxal 5′-phosphate deficiency and

aminotransferase levels in alcoholic hepatitis. *Gastroenterology* 1984;**86**:632–636.

14. Rosenthal P, Haight M. Aminotransferase as a prognostic index in infants with liver disease. *Clin Chem* 1990;**36**:346–348.

15. Berman DH, Leventhal RI, Gavaler JS, Cadoff EM, Van Thiel DH. Clinical differentiation of fulminant Wilsonian hepatitis from other causes of hepatic failure. *Gastroenterology* 1991;**100**:1129–1134.

16. Kaplan MM. Alkaline phosphatase. *Gastroenterology* 1972;**62**:452–468.

17. Seetharam S, Sussman NL, Komoda T, Alpers DH. The mechanism of elevated alkaline phosphatase activity after bile duct ligation in the rat. *Hepatology* 1986;**6**:374–380.

18. McEvoy M, Skrabanek P, Wright E, Powell D, McDonagh B. Family with raised serum alkaline phosphatase activity in the absence of disease. *BMJ (Clin Res Ed)* 1981; **282**(6272):1272.

19. Bamford KF, Harris H, Luffman JE, Robson EB, Cleghorn TE. Serum-alkaline-phosphatase and the ABO blood-groups. *Lancet* 1965; i:530–531.

20. Eymann A, Cacchiarelli N, Alonso G, Llera J. Benign transient hyperphosphatasemia of infancy. A common benign scenario, a big concern for a pediatrician. *J Pediatr Endocrinol Metab* 2010;**23**:927–930.

21. Teitelbaum JE, Laskowski A, Barrows FP. Benign transient hyperphosphatasemia in infants and children: a prospective cohort. *J Pediatr Endocrinol Metab* 2011;**24** (5–6):351–353.

22. Chopra S, Griffin PH. Laboratory tests and diagnostic procedures in evaluation of liver disease. *Am J Med* 1985;**79**:221–230.

23. Cabrera-Abreu JC, Green A. Gamma-glutamyltransferase: value of its measurement in paediatrics. *Ann Clin Biochem* 2002;**39**:22–25.

24. Hospital for Sick Children Toronto, Canada. *Reference Values and SI Unit Information*. Toronto: Hospital for Sick Children, 1993.

25. Deutsch J, Fritsch G, Golles J, Semmelrock HJ. Effects of anticonvulsive drugs on the activity of gammaglutamyltransferase and aminotransferases in serum. *J Pediatr Gastroenterol Nutr* 1986;**5**:542–548.

26. Maggiore G, Bernard O, Hadchouel M, Lemonnier A, Alagille D. Diagnostic value of serum gamma-glutamyl transpeptidase activity in liver diseases in children. *J Pediatr Gastroenterol Nutr* 1991;**12**:21–26.

27. van der Woerd WL, van Mil SW, Stapelbroek JM, *et al.* Familial cholestasis: progressive familial intrahepatic cholestasis, benign recurrent intrahepatic cholestasis and intrahepatic cholestasis of pregnancy. *Best Pract Res Clin Gastroenterol* 2010;**24**:541–553.

28. Wagner M, Zollner G, Trauner M. New molecular insights into the mechanisms of cholestasis. *J Hepatol* 2009;**51**:565–580.

29. Hill PG, Sammons HG. An assessment of 5′-nucleotidase as a liver-function test. *Q J Med* 1967;**36**(144):457–468.

30. Ahn H, Li CS, Wang W. Sickle cell hepatopathy: clinical presentation, treatment, and outcome in pediatric and adult patients. *Pediatr Blood Cancer* 2005;**45**:184–190.

31. Banks BM, Pineda EP, Goldbarg JA, Rutenburg AM. Clinical value of serum leucine aminopeptidase determinations. *N Engl J Med* 1960;**263**:1277–1281.

32. Doumas BT, Peters T, Jr. Serum and urine albumin: a progress report on their measurement and clinical significance. *Clin Chim Acta* 1997;**258**:3–20.

33. Tripodi A, Mannucci PM. The coagulopathy of chronic liver disease. *N Engl J Med* 2011;**365**:147–156.

34. Lisman T, Porte RJ. Rebalanced hemostasis in patients with liver disease: evidence and clinical consequences. *Blood* 2010;**116**: 878–885.

35. Croffie J, Gupta SK, Chong SK, Fitzgerald JF. Tyrosinemia type 1 should be suspected in infants with severe coagulopathy even in the absence of other signs of liver failure. *Pediatrics* 1999;**103**:675–678.

36. Squires RH, Jr., Shneider BL, Bucuvalas J, *et al.* Acute liver failure in children: the first 348 patients in the pediatric acute liver failure study group. *J Pediatr* 2006;**148**:652–658.

37. Andrew M, Paes B, Johnston M. Development of the hemostatic system in the neonate and young infant. *Am J Pediatr Hematol Oncol* 1990;**12**:95–104.

38. Andrew M, Paes B, Milner R, *et al.* Development of the human coagulation system in the full-term infant. *Blood* 1987;**70**:165–172.

39. Andrew M, Paes B, Milner R, *et al.* Development of the human coagulation system in the healthy premature infant. *Blood* 1988;**72**:1651–1657.

40. Dixon JL, Ginsberg HN. Hepatic synthesis of lipoproteins and apolipoproteins. *Semin Liver Dis* 1992;**12**:364–372.

41. Miller JP. Dyslipoproteinaemia of liver disease. *Baillieres Clin Endocrinol Metab* 1990;**4**:807–832.

42. Seidel D. Lipoproteins in liver disease. *J Clin Chem Clin Biochem* 1987;**25**:541–551.

43. Lontie JF, Dubois DY, Malmendier CL, *et al.* Plasma lipids and apolipoproteins in end-stage liver disease. *Clin Chim Acta* 1990;**195**(1–2):93–96.

44. Tukey RH, Strassburg CP. Human UDP-glucuronosyltransferases: metabolism, expression, and disease. *Annu Rev Pharmacol Toxicol* 2000;**40**:581–616.

45. Mullenbach R, Lammert F. An update on genetic analysis of cholestatic liver diseases: digging deeper. *Dig Dis* 2011;**29**:72–77.

46. Weiss JS, Gautam A, Lauff JJ, *et al.* The clinical importance of a protein-bound fraction of serum bilirubin in patients with hyperbilirubinemia. *N Engl J Med* 1983;**309**:147–150.

47. Davis AR, Rosenthal P, Escobar GJ, Newman TB. Interpreting conjugated bilirubin levels in newborns. *J Pediatr* 2011;**158**:562–565.

48. Hirschfield GM, Heathcote EJ, Gershwin ME. Pathogenesis of cholestatic liver disease and therapeutic approaches. *Gastroenterology* 2010;**139**:1481–1496.

49. Benchimol EI, Walsh CM, Ling SC. Early diagnosis of neonatal cholestatic jaundice: test at 2 weeks. *Can Fam Physician* 2009;**55**:1184–1192.

50. Davit-Spraul A, Fabre M, Branchereau S, *et al.* ATP8B1 and ABCB11 analysis in 62 children with normal gamma-glutamyl transferase progressive familial intrahepatic cholestasis (PFIC): phenotypic differences between PFIC1 and PFIC2 and natural history. *Hepatology* 2010;**51**:1645–1655.

51. Pawlikowska L, Strautnieks S, Jankowska I, *et al.* Differences in presentation and progression between severe FIC1 and BSEP deficiencies. *J Hepatol* 2010;**53**:170–178.

52. Krawczyk M, Mullenbach R, Weber SN, Zimmer V, Lammert F. Genome-wide association studies and genetic risk assessment of liver diseases. *Nat Rev Gastroenterol Hepatol* 2010;**7**: 669–681.

53. Clayton PT. Disorders of bile acid synthesis. *J Inherit Metab Dis* 2011;**34**:593–604.

54. Wagner M, Zollner G, Trauner M. Nuclear receptors in liver disease. *Hepatology* 2011;**53**:1023–1034.

55. Setchell KD, O'Connell NC. Bile acid synthesis and metabolism. In Walker W, Goulet O, Kleiman R, *et al.* (eds.) *Pediatric Gastrointestinal Disease: Pathophysiology, Diagnosis, Management*. Philadelphia, PA: Decker, 2004, pp. 1308–1343.

56. Setchell KD, Heubi JE. Defects in bile acid biosynthesis-diagnosis and treatment. *J Pediatr Gastroenterol Nutr* 2006;**43**(Suppl 1):S17–S22.

57. Javitt NB, Keating JP, Grand RJ, Harris RC. Serum bile acid patterns in neonatal hepatitis and extrahepatic biliary atresia. *J Pediatr* 1977;**90**:736–739.

58. Nemeth A, Samuelson K, Strandvik B. Serum bile acids as markers of juvenile liver disease in alpha 1-antitrypsin deficiency. *J Pediatr Gastroenterol Nutr* 1982;**1**:479–483.

59. Burra P, Masier A. Dynamic tests to study liver function. *Eur Rev Med Pharmacol Sci* 2004;**8**:19–21.

60. Orlando R, Palatini P. The effect of age on plasma MEGX concentrations. *Br J Clin Pharmacol* 1997;**44**:206–208.

61. Tanaka E, Inomata S, Yasuhara H. The clinical importance of conventional and quantitative liver function tests in liver transplantation. *J Clin Pharm Ther* 2000;**25**:411–419.

62. Lebel S, Nakamachi Y, Hemming A, *et al*. Glycine conjugation of para-aminobenzoic acid (PABA): a pilot study of a novel prognostic test in acute liver failure in children. *J Pediatr Gastroenterol Nutr* 2003;**36**:62–71.

63. Bachmann C. Mechanisms of hyperammonemia. *Clin Chem Lab Med* 2002;**40**:653–662.

64. Furuya KN, Durie PR, Roberts EA, *et al*. Glycine conjugation of para-aminobenzoic acid (PABA): a quantitative test of liver function. *Clin Biochem* 1995;**28**:531–540.

65. Chambers JC, Zhang W, Sehmi J, *et al*. Genome-wide association study identifies loci influencing concentrations of liver enzymes in plasma. *Nat Genet* 2011;**43**:1131–1138.

Chapter

8

Approach to the infant with cholestasis

Amy Feldman and Frederick J. Suchy

Jaundice sometimes appears at birth, indicated by the dark yellow color of the countenance and arising from obstructions of the liver. Cases are generally incurable.
Eli Ives of Yale University, America's first academic pediatrician, circa 1829 [1]

Introduction

Cholestasis may be defined physiologically as a measurable decrease in bile flow, pathologically as the histologic presence of bile pigment in hepatocytes and bile ducts and clinically as the accumulation in blood and extrahepatic tissues of substances normally excreted in bile (e.g. bilirubin, bile acids, and cholesterol). The process occurs as a result of impaired bile formation by the hepatocyte or from obstruction to the flow of bile through the intrahepatic and extrahepatic biliary tree [2,3]. In the neonate, the clinical and laboratory features of the many liver diseases presenting with cholestasis are quite similar. An important focus of the pediatric hepatologist is to differentiate intrahepatic from extrahepatic cholestasis and, if possible, establish a specific diagnosis [4]. Strategies for the treatment of metabolic or infectious liver disease and for the surgical management of biliary anomalies require early diagnosis. Even when treatment is not available or effective, infants with progressive liver disease usually benefit from optimal nutritional support and medical management of complications of cholestasis and possibly cirrhosis until liver transplantation is performed.

This chapter presents an overview of the approach to the infant with cholestatic liver disease. The diagnostic evaluation of these patients is emphasized. The incidence and scope of the problem are placed in perspective, and the differential diagnosis is reviewed, but the large numbers of specific disorders are not discussed here in detail. These disorders are covered comprehensively in subsequent chapters.

Incidence

The overall incidence of neonatal liver disease, most cases manifesting clinical or biochemical evidence of cholestasis, may be as high as 1 in 2500 live births. Of the many conditions that cause neonatal cholestasis, biliary atresia accounts for approximately 25%, genetic disorders for another 25%, metabolic disease for 20%, idiopathic neonatal hepatitis for 15%, α_1-antitrypsin deficiency for 10%, and viral illness for 5% [5]. So-called idiopathic neonatal hepatitis was the most common diagnosis in older series, with a reported incidence of 1 in 4800–9000 live births [6,7]. However, with the advent of new more accurate diagnostic methods that allow for diagnosis of disorders of bile acid synthesis, disorders of canalicular transport, storage diseases, mitochondrial diseases, and infectious diseases, the incidence of what was once called "idiopathic neonatal hepatitis" has decreased. The estimated incidence of biliary atresia ranges from 1 in 5000 to 1 in 21 000 live births, with cases occurring more frequently in Far Eastern than in Western countries [8]. In a prospective study conducted over 25 years in Atlanta, Georgia, the calculated incidence of biliary atresia was 0.73 cases per 10 000 live births, with a higher prevalence in African-American children than in white children [9]. Table 8.1 details the diagnoses of 1086 consecutive infants with conjugated hyperbilirubinemia referred over a 20-year period to King's College Hospital, a tertiary care center serving the majority of England [10]. The high percentage of patients with biliary atresia in this impressive series in part reflects the interest and expertise of these physicians in the diagnosis and surgical correction of biliary tract disorders. In another prospective study of 790 385 Australian infants by Danks *et al.* [7], 55 cases of biliary atresia (1 in 14 000 live births), 11 cases of intrahepatic biliary hypoplasia (1 in 70 000), and 99 cases of idiopathic neonatal hepatitis (1 in 8000) were observed. The time sequence of births for patients with neonatal hepatitis was fairly even in this study, but there was a suggestion of time–space clustering

Liver Disease in Children, Fourth Edition, ed. Frederick J. Suchy, Ronald J. Sokol, and William F. Balistreri. Published by Cambridge University Press. © Cambridge University Press 2014.

Table 8.1 Infants with conjugated hyperbilirubinemia referred to King's College Hospital between 1970 and 1990

Diagnosis	Number	Percentage
Biliary atresia	377	34.7
Idiopathic neonatal hepatitis	331	30.5
α_1-Antitrypsin deficiency	189	17.4
Other hepatitis	94	8.7
Alagille syndrome	61	5.6
Choledochal cyst	34	3.1

Modified from Mieli-Vergani et al. [10], with permission.

Table 8.2 Classification of cholestatic disorders[a]

Neonatal hepatitis
   Idiopathic
   Viral
      Cytomegalovirus
      Herpes (simplex, zoster, human type 6)
      Rubella
      Echovirus
      Reovirus type 3
      Adenovirus

      Coxsackievirus
      Enteroviruses
         Parvovirus B19
         Hepatitis B
         Human immunodeficiency virus
         Syncytial giant cell hepatitis with paramyxovirus-like inclusions

      Bacterial and parasitic
         Bacterial sepsis
         Urinary tract infection
         Syphilis
         Listeriosis
         Tuberculosis
         Toxoplasmosis
         Malaria

Bile duct obstruction
   Cholangiopathies
      Biliary atresia
      Choledochal cysts
      Non-syndromic paucity of interlobular bile duct
      Alagille syndrome
      Neonatal sclerosing cholangitis (with/without ichthyosis), **with Claudin 1 mutation**
      Spontaneous perforation of common bile duct
      Caroli disease
      Congenital hepatic fibrosis
      Bile duct stenosis

   Other
      Inspissated bile/mucous plug
      Cholelithiasis
      Tumors/masses (intrinsic and extrinsic)

Cholestatic syndromes
   PFIC caused by transport defects
      Type 1 (Byler's disease, defect in a P-type ATPase)
      Type 2 (defect in BSEP, a canalicular bile acid pump)
      Type 3 (defect in MDR3, a canalicular phospholipid transporter)

   Hereditary cholestasis with lymphedema (Aagenaes syndrome)
   Cholestasis of North American Indians
   Nielsen syndrome (Greenland Eskimos)
   Benign recurrent cholestasis (defect in same gene as PFIC type 1)

for some cases of biliary atresia. However, more recent studies have not supported this seasonal association [11]. In a study of 207 infants from Australia, the etiology of the cholestasis was idiopathic in 25%, metabolic/genetic in 23%, biliary obstruction in 20%, parenteral nutrition in 20%, infection in 9%, and bile duct hypoplasia in 3% [12].

Differential diagnosis of neonatal cholestasis

Liver dysfunction in the neonate, regardless of the etiology, is commonly associated with a failure of bile secretion and conjugated hyperbilirubinemia [13]. Jaundice is a frequent and early presenting feature of liver disease during early life rather than a late manifestation of advanced disease, as is seen in the older child or adult [13]. Owing to an immaturity of hepatic excretory function, a susceptibility to infection during the perinatal period, and the initial effects of congenital malformations and inborn errors of metabolism, the number of distinct disorders presenting with cholestasis is greater in the neonate than at any other time of life. A conceptually useful overview of the differential diagnosis of neonatal cholestasis is presented in Table 8.2. Although the origin or the predominating form of liver damage may be traced primarily to the level of the hepatocyte or to the biliary apparatus, there is considerable overlap between disorders in their clinical features as well as in the subsequent sites of injury. For example, injury to the biliary epithelium may be a prominent finding in neonatal infection with cytomegalovirus, α_1-antitrypsin deficiency, and some inborn errors of bile acid metabolism. Moreover, mechanical obstruction of the common bile duct invariably results in liver dysfunction and intrahepatic injury, which may include in the neonate significant giant cell transformation of hepatocytes. It is unclear in this setting whether giant cells, which appear to be a frequent, non-specific manifestation of neonatal liver injury, reflect the noxious effects of biliary obstruction or whether the hepatocytes as well as the biliary epithelium are damaged by a common insult such as a virus or toxin with tropism for both types of cells.

The term *neonatal hepatitis* refers to the histologic finding of extensive giant cell transformation of hepatocytes. The term is misleading because it implies an infectious process involving

Table 8.2 (cont.)

Neonatal Dubin–Johnson syndrome (MRP2
   deficiency)
Arthrogryposis, renal dysfunction, and cholestasis
   syndrome (VPS33B)
Metabolic disorders
   α₁-Antitrypsin deficiency
   Cystic fibrosis
   Neonatal iron storage disease
   Endocrinopathies
      Hypopituitarism (septo-optic dysplasia)
      Hypothyroidism/hyperthroidism
      McCune–Albright syndrome
      **HNF1β mutations with type 5 maturity-onset
         diabetes of the young**
      Donahue syndrome (leprechaunism)

   Amino acid disorders
      Tyrosinemia
      Hypermethionemia

   Storage disorders
      Niemann–Pick disease
      Gaucher disease
      Wolman disease
      Cholesterol ester storage disease
      Mucolipidosis type II (I cell disease)
      Mucopolysaccharidosis type VII
      Glycogen storage disease type IV
      Farber disease type IV

   Urea cycle disorders (arginase deficiency)
   Carbohydrate disorders
      Galactosemia
      Fructosemia
      Congenital disorders of glycosylation

   Mitochondrial disorders
      Respiratory chain defects
      **GRACILE syndrome (growth retardation,
         aminoaciduria, cholestasis, iron overload, lactic
         acidosis, early death)**
      Citrin deficiency

   Beta-oxidation defects
      Short-chain acyl-CoA dehydrogenase deficiency
      Long-chain acyl-CoA dehydrogenase deficiency

   Peroxisomal disorders
      Zellweger syndrome
      Infantile Refsum disease
      Other enzymopathies

   Bile acid synthetic defects
      **3β-Hydroxy Δ⁵C₂₇-steroid dehydrogenase
         isomerase**
      δ⁴-3-Oxosteroid 5β-reductase
      Oxysterol 7α-hydroxylase
      Sterol 27-hydroxylase
      **2-Methyl-CoA-racemase CoA/amino acid *N*-
         acyltransferase**

Table 8.2 (cont.)

   Defects in cholesterol biosynthesis
      **Smith–Lemli–Opitz syndrome (7-
         dehydrocholesterol reductase)**
      **Lathosterolosis (3β-hydroxysteroid-Δ⁵-
         desaturase)**
      Mevalonate kinase deficiency

Toxic
   Drugs
   Parenteral nutrition
   Aluminum
   Fetal alcohol syndrome
   Ceftriaxone lithiasis
   Prenatal methamphetamine exposure
Cardiovascular disorders
   Shock/hypoperfusion
   Congestive heart failure
   Perinatal asphyxia
   Veno-occlusive disease
   Extracorporeal membrane oxygenation
   Fetal arrhythmia
   Budd–Chiari syndrome
Chromosomal disorders
   Autosomal trisomies
   Turner syndrome

   Miscellaneous associations
      Neonatal leukemia, neuroblastoma, hepatoblastoma
      Histiocytosis X
      Neonatal lupus erythematosus
      Indian childhood cirrhosis
      Graft-versus-host disease
      Erythrophagocytic lymphohistiocytosis
      Erythroblastosis fetalis
      Fetal thrombotic vasculopathy
      Systemic juvenile xanthogranuloma
      Pseudo-TORCH syndrome
      **COACH syndrome (mutations in *MKS3*, *CC2D2A*, and
         RPGRIP1L)**
      Jeune syndrome
      Kabuki syndrome

ATPase, adenosine triphosphatase; BSEP, bile salt export pump; CoA,
coenzyme A; COACH, cerebellar vermis hypoplasia/aplasia, oligophrenia,
ataxia, coloboma, and hepatic fibrosis; HNF1β, hepatocyte nuclear factor-1β;
MDR3, multidrug resistance protein 3; MRP2, multidrug resistance-related
protein 2; PFIC, progressive familial intrahepatic cholestasis; TORCH,
toxoplasmosis, other, rubella, cytomegalovirus, and herpes (congenital
infections).
ᵃ The genetic defect has been identified and genetic testing is either feasible
   or available for disorders shown in bold.

the liver (such as the numerous forms of viral hepatitis), but it
has been used to describe virtually all forms of liver disease
after structural disorders of the biliary tree, such as biliary
atresia and choledochal cysts, have been excluded. Because of
improved imaging techniques, advances in virology, and the
application of sophisticated biochemical and molecular
methods to the diagnosis of inborn errors of metabolism, there

are fewer infants whose liver disease may be classified as idiopathic or cryptogenic. A disorder should now be designated as hepatitis only if an infectious agent can be documented or suspected on the basis of other clinical features associated with congenital infection. An increasing number of infections have been associated with neonatal hepatitis, including parvovirus B19, human herpesvirus 6, and HIV. The percentage of cases that can be classified as idiopathic will also be influenced by referral patterns, the prevalence of certain infections within a population, and the availability of specialized diagnostic techniques and biochemical assays.

Liver biopsies from 62 infants with neonatal giant cell hepatitis were recently studied [14]. The average age at liver biopsy was 2 months (73% male). Giant cell transformation affected an average of 36% of hepatocytes (range, 5–90%). Extramedullary hematopoiesis (both myelopoiesis and erythropoiesis) was found in 74% of the children. An actual "hepatitis" characterized by portal and lobular inflammation was mild to absent in 95%. Mild to moderate lobular cholestasis with a predominately canalicular distribution occurred in 84%. Bile ducts were hypoplastic in 32% but were not absent or reduced in number. Mild focal ductular proliferation was found in another 18% of biopsies. Portal or pericellular fibrosis was found in 30% and was advanced in 8%. A cause for cholestasis could not be established in 49% of patients. In the remaining patients, the specific diagnoses were hypopituitarism (16%), biliary atresia (8%), Alagille syndrome (6%), bile salt defects (6%), and several other disorders present at 5% or less. Histological features did not readily distinguish among the various etiologies; with the unexpected exception that bile duct hypoplasia was more common in hypopituitarism [14].

Spontaneously resolving forms of neonatal cholestasis may result from several factors including immaturity of bile secretion and perinatal disease leading to hepatic hypoxia or ischemia [15]. In one study of 70 infants with moderate portal and lobular fibrosis, multinucleated giant hepatocytes, and hematopoietic foci, 15 children had follow-up liver biopsies that were normal or improved [15]. The occurrence of so-called neonatal hepatitis in babies with other serious disorders, such as Down syndrome, hemolytic disease of the newborn, ischemic injury, or congenital heart disease, also suggests that systemic disease may either increase susceptibility to agents capable of causing hepatitis or further exacerbate an underlying immaturity of hepatic excretory function to the point of producing pathologic cholestasis.

Approximately 25% of cholestatic infants have evidence of an inherited molecular defect that leads to abnormalities in metabolism and substrate transport. Defects in bile acid transport, phospholipid transport, bile acid synthesis, and abnormal embryogenesis have been identified with variable presentations and prognoses [5]. The genes for several forms of progressive familial intrahepatic cholestasis (PFIC) have been identified and encode proteins critically important for bile formation [16,17]. Giant cell transformation of hepatocytes is the predominant histologic feature in type 2 PFIC because of mutations in the gene encoding the bile salt excretory pump [18].

Another feature often accompanying neonatal cholestasis is bile ductular paucity, a histologic finding implying a diminution in the number of interlobular bile ducts. The abnormality may be of primary importance in patients with so-called syndromic paucity of interlobular bile ducts (Alagille syndrome) but also may occasionally occur in other disorders including cytomegalovirus and rubella infections, α_1-antitrypsin deficiency, chromosomal monosomy and trisomy, cystic fibrosis, and bile acid synthesis defects [19]. The finding may not be present or may be difficult to recognize in the neonate; however, serial liver biopsies may demonstrate injury to bile ductular epithelial cells, a variable amount of associated inflammation, and a progressive decrease in the number of bile ductules per portal tract.

Manifestations of cholestatic liver disease in the neonate

Jaundice is the most overt physical sign of liver disease and occurs more commonly in the neonatal period than at any other time of life [20]. Unconjugated hyperbilirubinemia in the older patient is usually harmless, but in the neonate with an immature blood–brain barrier, it may be associated with deposition of free bilirubin in neuronal tissue and subsequent brain damage. In contrast, conjugated bilirubin is not toxic, but an elevated level is the most common presenting feature of liver disease in the neonate. Unconjugated jaundice is first appreciated in the head and progresses caudally to the palms and soles as the serum bilirubin increases. Jaundice becomes clinically apparent in the older child when the serum bilirubin concentration reaches 2–3 mg/dL, but the neonate may not appear icteric until the bilirubin level is >5 mg/dL. A serum conjugated (direct) bilirubin concentration of >1 mg/dL with a total bilirubin of <5 mg/dL, or over 20% of the total bilirubin concentration if the total is >5 mg/dL, is abnormal and requires evaluation [21]. Many clinical laboratories now employ the Ektachem method, which specifically measures direct bilirubin. A serum conjugated bilirubin concentration >1 mg/dL is abnormal using this assay.

The majority of infants with cholestatic liver disease present during the first month of life [13]. Differentiation of cholestatic jaundice from the common physiologic hyperbilirubinemia of the neonate or the prolonged jaundice occasionally associated with breast-feeding is essential. The initial goal of the physician must be to exclude rapidly life-threatening but potentially treatable disorders such as Gram-negative infection, endocrinopathies (such as panhypopituitarism), galactosemia, and inborn errors of bile acid metabolism. Prompt identification of cholestatic infants is also required to minimize the risk of hemorrhage from vitamin K deficiency. Because of early hospital discharges, some cholestatic infants may escape detection until the first well-baby examination at

6–8 weeks of age. The possibility of liver or biliary tract disease must be considered in any neonate jaundiced beyond 2 weeks of age. Between 2.4 and 15% of newborns will still be jaundiced at 2 weeks of age; the majority are breast-fed. These infants should be evaluated for cholestasis by measurement of total and conjugated serum bilirubin. However, with reliable follow-up, this testing may be deferred until 3 weeks of age in jaundiced breast-fed infants if stool color, urine color, and physical examination are normal. In one study, the incidence of jaundice in breast-fed babies at 4 weeks was 9%, but none had liver disease [22]. The utility of screening for neonatal liver disease remains unsettled. In a community-based study in which 27 654 neonates were tested for a serum conjugated bilirubin concentration $>18 \mu mol/L$ using the Ektachem method, a positive result requiring further testing was found in 107 babies. Gross hemolysis or insufficient sample size precluded analysis in 15.3% of the cases. Persistently elevated values on repeat testing was seen in 12 babies, 11 of whom had confirmed liver disease including neonatal hepatitis (six), biliary atresia (two), hypopituitarism (one), α_1-antitrypsin deficiency (one), and Alagille syndrome (one). The sensitivity and specificity of the test was 100% and 99.6%, respectively [23]. General application of this approach will likely require methods to measure conjugated bilirubin on dried blood spots. In Taiwan, a national screening program has been implemented through which an infant stool color card is placed into the child health booklet given to every neonate. This program has increased the national rate of the Kasai operation performed before 60 days of age from 49% to 66%, and it has increased the 3-month jaundice-free rate after the Kasai operation from 35% to 61% ($p < 0.001$). In addition, the 5-year jaundice-free survival rate with native liver increased from 27% to 64% ($p < 0.001$) and the 5-year overall survival rate increased from 56% to 89% ($p < 0.001$) [24].

The vast majority of infants with biliary atresia appear entirely well during the first 4–6 weeks of life apart from mild jaundice. However, the apparent well-nourished appearance of infants with biliary atresia may be a factor in a delay of diagnosis. Thorough anthropometric studies show that infants with biliary atresia have significantly decreased fat stores and lean body mass [25]. The added weight of an enlarged liver and spleen and the occasional finding of subclinical ascites may account for a relatively normal weight for age and weight for length on standardized growth curves [26].

Stools of a patient with biliary atresia are acholic, but early in the course of incomplete or evolving obstruction, stools may appear normally pigmented or only intermittently pigmented. Similarly, fluctuating levels of serum bilirubin do not eclude biliary atresia [27]. Liver disease also must be suspected in a jaundiced infant whose urine is dark yellow as opposed to colorless. Mieli-Vergani et al. [10] reported factors contributing to delayed referral of infants with biliary atresia. Lack of follow-up of neonatal jaundice, inadequate investigation of hemorrhagic disease, misdiagnosis of breast milk jaundice, and being misled by pigmented stools or a decrease in serum bilirubin were cited as reasons for late referral. Increased age at Kasai operation has been shown to be associated with worse survival, independent of other prognostic factors. In a recent study of 695 patients with biliary atresia who underwent the Kasai procedure in France, survival with native liver was best in children operated on in the first 30 days of life [28].

A stepwise discriminate analysis by Alagille [29] of many clinical and biochemical findings identified several variables that are useful in evaluating the cholestatic infant. In a series of 288 patients, the following features occurred more commonly in infants with intrahepatic cholestasis than in those with biliary atresia: male gender (66% versus 45%), low birth weight (2680 g versus 3230 g), later onset of jaundice (mean, 23 days versus 11 days), and later onset of acholic stools (mean, 30 days versus 16 days). An enlarged liver with a firm or hard consistency was present in 53% of those with intrahepatic cholestasis compared with 87% of those with extrahepatic cholestasis. The addition of another variable (progressive or irregular course of the jaundice) did not improve the results of the analysis. Therefore, this study indicates that, although clinical features are useful, there are no details in the history or physical examination that can identify all cases of biliary atresia [25].

The spectrum of illness is remarkably wide in infants with cholestatic jaundice [4]. Acholic stools are a cardinal feature of biliary obstruction but may also occur as a result of severe bile secretory failure at the level of the hepatocyte [25]. The affected infant may appear remarkably well, particularly during the evolution of biliary obstruction, or may manifest hepatic failure at birth. These infants also may be small for gestational age and fail to thrive. Congenital infection may be associated with low birth weight, microcephaly, purpura, and chorioretinitis. Dysmorphic facies may be observed in association with chromosomal aberrations and with syndromic paucity of interlobular bile duct [30]. Congenital malformations, including cardiac anomalies, polysplenia, intestinal malrotation, and situs inversus viscerum, may be found in almost a third of infants with biliary atresia [31]. Hepatomegaly is often a presenting feature of neonatal liver disease; if there is large duct obstruction, the liver is firm or even hard to palpation. In the polysplenia syndrome, a midline liver may be palpable in the hypogastrium. The spleen may be enlarged with infection or as a result of advanced prenatal liver disease and fibrosis, but it is usually of normal size early in the course of biliary tract disease. A mass in the right upper quadrant may be felt in approximately 50% of patients with a choledochal cyst. Pruritus and xanthomata, cutaneous manifestations of chronic cholestasis, are not observed in the neonate.

Irritability, poor feeding, vomiting, and lethargy are frequent symptoms in metabolic disorders such as galactosemia and tyrosinemia [32]. Ascites, edema, and coagulopathy may be present at birth or evolve rapidly during the first weeks of life after massive loss of hepatocytes through necrosis or apoptosis. A profound impairment of hepatic synthetic function, often in excess of that expected for the degree of cholestasis, may be an early indication of metabolic liver disease, such as neonatal iron storage disease or tyrosinemia. Neurologic abnormalities in the infant with liver disease may be primary symptoms, as found in mitochondrial disorders and Zellweger syndrome, or they may be secondary to hypoglycemia, hyperammonemia, or intracranial hemorrhage [33].

Evaluation of the cholestatic neonate

An algorithm for the investigation of the cholestatic infant is presented in Figure 8.1. The order in which this assessment proceeds may vary depending on the clinical findings that may strongly suggest a diagnosis. Box 8.1 lists the individual studies that are often used in this evaluation [34,35]. The optimal diagnostic strategy demands a cooperative medical and

surgical effort at a center prepared to investigate and manage potentially correctable abnormalities of the biliary tree as well as hepatocellular disorders [25]. The initial assessment should confirm rapidly that cholestasis is present, provide a baseline assessment of the severity of liver dysfunction, and exclude potentially treatable infectious, endocrine, and metabolic disorders. Next, in order to establish a specific diagnosis, a comprehensive plan for investigation is outlined, which should be guided by the initial history and physical examination. Because of the frequent lack of specific clinical features and overlap of many diagnostic studies, most cholestatic infants require a stepwise comprehensive evaluation. However, at any point during the process, a serologic test or imaging study may establish the probable cause of the liver disease. For example, ultrasonography may promptly demonstrate a choledochal

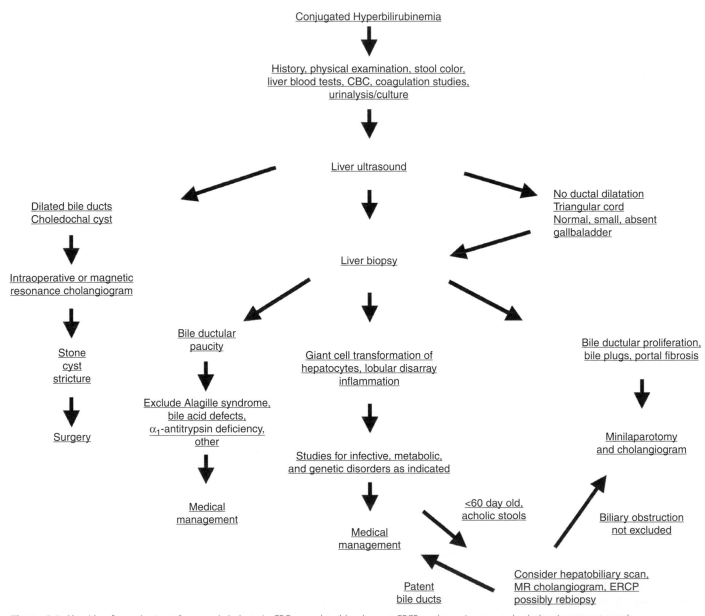

Figure 8.1 Algorithm for evaluation of neonatal cholestasis. CBC, complete blood count; ERCP, endoscopic retrograde cholangiopancreatography.

Box 8.1 Evaluation of the infant with cholestasis

Initial investigations

To establish the presence of cholestasis, define the severity of the liver disease, and detect readily treatable disorders:

- History, physical examination (including details of family history, pregnancy, early neonatal course, presence of extrahepatic anomalies, extrahepatic disease, stool color)
- Fractionated serum bilirubin analysis
- Serum tests for liver injury: alanine aminotransferase, aspartate aminotransferase, alkaline phosphatase, 5′-nucleotidase, gamma-glutamyltransferase
- Tests of liver function: prothrombin time, partial thromboplastin time, coagulation factors, serum albumin, serum ammonia, serum cholesterol, serum glucose
- Complete blood count, including platelet count
- Bacterial cultures of blood, urine, other as indicated
- Paracentesis if ascites: examine for bile and infection.

Investigations to establish a specific diagnosis

- Ultrasonography (MR cholangiography in selected cases)
- Serum α_1-antitrypsin level and phenotype
- Serologies for infectious disorders: hepatitis B surface antigen, TORCH (toxoplasmosis, other, rubella, cytomegalovirus, herpes), Epstein–Barr virus, parvovirus B19, human herpesvirus 6, HIV, other
- Sweat chloride analysis
- Metabolic screen: urine and serum amino acids, urine organic acids
- Serum thyroid hormone, thyroid-stimulating hormone (evaluation for hypopituitarism as indicated)
- Serum iron and ferritin
- Urine and serum analysis for bile acid and bile acid precursors
- Red blood cell galactose-1-phosphate uridyltransferase
- Viral cultures
- Genetic testing for Alagille syndrome, three types of progressive familial intrahepatic cholestasis, other
- Hepatobiliary scintigraphy
- Radiographs of skull and long bones for congenital infection and bone dysplasia and of the chest for lung and heart disease
- Bone marrow examination and skin fibroblast culture for suspected storage disease
- Percutaneous or endoscopic retrograde cholangiography (rarely indicated)
- Percutaneous liver biopsy: routine histology, immunohistochemistry, electron microscopy, viral culture, and enzymology as required
- Exploratory laparotomy and intraoperative cholangiogram.

Adapted with permission from Suchy and Shneider, 1992 [35].

---

cyst in a jaundiced infant, obviating the need to search for an infectious or metabolic basis for the liver disease. Increasing numbers of infants will be identified as a result of neonatal screening programs. Some US states are using mass spectroscopy in tandem with other methods to detect as many as 40 inherited disorders, some of which may present as cholestasis in the neonate, including hypothyroidism, cystic fibrosis, and galactosemia [36].

Numerous biochemical and imaging studies have been used in an effort to distinguish between infants with intrahepatic versus obstructive cholestasis and thus avoid unnecessary surgical exploration [37]. Standard liver biochemical tests show non-specific and variable elevation of serum direct bilirubin, aminotransferases, alkaline phosphatase, 5′-nucleotidase, and lipids [37,38]. Poor hepatic function at birth, including hypoglycemia and coagulopathy unresponsive to vitamin K, may reflect the prenatal effects of an inborn error of metabolism or an intrauterine infection. Because loss of hepatocyte mass in some metabolic disorders occurs by apoptosis rather than cell necrosis, serum aminotransferase values may be normal or only modestly elevated. Low or normal serum gamma-glutamyltransferase activity is found in the serum of patients with PFIC types 1 and 2, some inborn errors of bile acid metabolism, hypopituitarism, and benign recurrent cholestasis [17,39]. However, no single biochemical test or imaging study, or even combination of non-invasive tests, has proven to be of sufficient discriminatory value in excluding extrahepatic obstruction because approximately 10% of infants with intrahepatic cholestasis have clinical and laboratory studies that overlap with results from patients with biliary atresia. The presence of bile pigment in stools is sometimes cited as evidence against complete biliary obstruction, but the physician may be misled by historical information about stool color, by feces colored by bile-stained secretions and shed epithelial cells, and by the gradual evolution of bile duct obstruction. Aspiration and visual inspection of duodenal secretions for bile pigment or measurement of radioactivity in duodenal fluid after scintigraphy have been used by some workers to distinguish intrahepatic from extrahepatic cholestasis [40].

A variety of newer diagnostic tests are becoming part of the armamentarium of the hepatologist. Any infant with intrahepatic cholestasis of obscure etiology should be evaluated for a possible inborn error of bile acid metabolism by analysis of a urine sample for abnormal bile acid metabolites using fast atom bombardment mass spectroscopy. Identification of these infants is critical because some of these disorders are treatable by oral bile acid replacement. The genes for three distinct forms of PFIC and for Alagille syndrome have been cloned and are now commercially available.

Ultrasonography is often the most useful initial imaging modality for providing information about liver structure, size, and composition. A high-frequency, real-time examination can assess gallbladder size, detect gallstones and sludge in the bile ducts and gallbladder, demonstrate ascites, and define cystic or obstructive dilatation of the biliary tree. Extrahepatic anomalies also may be detected. Common bile duct dilatation >4 mm is associated with congenital choledochal malformations and inspissated bile requiring intervention. It is not a feature of biliary atresia [41]. Ultrasound findings associated with biliary atresia include absent, small (<1.5 cm), or empty gallbladder, a hypertrophied hepatic artery, or increased hepatic subcapsular flow on Doppler ultrasound [42]. However, these findings cannot be reliably used to diagnose biliary atresia. The sensitivity and specificity of a small or absent gallbladder in detecting biliary atresia varies from 73% to 100% and 67% to 100%, respectively, when data are compiled from several studies [21]. A triangular or tubular echogenic density or triangular cord representing a fibrous cone of tissue at the porta hepatis on a transverse or longitudinal scan has been proposed as a specific ultrasonographic finding for biliary atresia [43]. Recent literature suggests that this sign has a sensitivity of 62–93%, and a specificity of 96–100% [42].

While CT provides information similar to that obtained by ultrasonography, it is usually less useful in infants because of a paucity of intra-abdominal fat for contrast and the need for heavy sedation or general anesthesia.

Magnetic resonance (MR) cholangiography, performed with T_2-weighted turbo spin-echo sequences, is being widely used to assess the biliary tract in all age groups, with visualization previously possible only with transhepatic or endoscopic retrograde cholangiography (ERCP). In several pilot studies, MR cholangiography reliably demonstrated the common bile duct and gallbladder in normal neonates. Non-visualization of the common bile duct and demonstration of a small gallbladder characterized the findings in a small number of patients with biliary atresia. For example, in one study, MR cholangiography accuracy was 82% (19 of 23), sensitivity 90% (9 of 10), and specificity 77% (10 of 13) for the detection of extrahepatic biliary atresia, with a positive predictive value of 75% (9 of 12) and a negative predictive value of 91% (10 of 11) [44]. Further advances will be required before the reliability of MR cholangiography in evaluating the cholestatic infant can be established.

Hepatobiliary scintigraphy, using technetium-99m iminodiacetic acid derivatives, has been used to help to differentiate biliary atresia from other causes of neonatal cholestasis. Premedication with phenobarbital for 5 days before imaging can increase accuracy. In biliary atresia, there is usually a rapid hepatic extraction of tracer, but no subsequent excretion of tracer into the gastrointestinal tract. Unfortunately, some children with other forms of neonatal hepatitis also have decreased excretion of tracer, significantly lowering the specificity of this diagnostic modality. One study showed that 50% of patients with interlobular bile duct paucity but no extrahepatic obstruction failed to show biliary excretion of radionuclide, and 25% of patients with idiopathic neonatal hepatitis also demonstrated no biliary excretion [45]. However, the modality remains useful for assessing cystic duct patency in a patient with a hydropic gallbladder or with cholelithiasis.

Percutaneous transhepatic cholangiography or cholecystocholangiography may be required to visualize the biliary tract in selected patients. However, these techniques are more difficult to perform in infants because of the small size of the intrahepatic bile ducts and because most of the disorders in this age group do not result in dilatation of the intrahepatic bile ducts. Recently, laparoscopic cholecystocholangiography

has been used as a less invasive method for evaluating the biliary tract. In one study, 144 patients with suspected biliary atresia underwent laparoscopic cholangiography. In 21 (14.6%) where the gallbladder was atretic, laparoscopic cholangiogram was unable to be performed and biliary atresia was confirmed by subsequent laparotomy. Of the other 123 patients, 88 (71.5%) were successfully diagnosed with biliary atresia, 14 (11.4%) with biliary hypoplasia, and 21 (17.1%) with cholestasis [46].

Endoscopic retrograde cholangiography may be useful in the evaluation of selected infants with obstructive cholestasis [47]. In a recent study, ERCP was performed successfully under general anesthesia in 45 of 48 infants younger than 100 days of age (94%) with prolonged cholestasis. All three infants in whom ERCP failed had biliary atresia diagnosed by intraoperative cholangiography at laparotomy. Of the 45 successful ERCPs, 25 (52%) had findings suggestive of biliary atresia; and 22 of these patients (85%) were confirmed to have biliary atresia at laparotomy. The remaining three infants had cytomegalovirus hepatitis, total parenteral nutrition-related cholestasis, and non-syndromic biliary hypoplasia. In this study, ERCP had a positive predictive value of 88%, a negative predictive value of 100%, a sensitivity of 100%, and a specificity of 87% [48]. This approach also provides detailed information on anomalous arrangement of the pancreaticobiliary junction in patients with choledochal cysts. Considerable technical expertise is necessary for a successful examination in infants. Most require general anesthesia for a satisfactory examination. The greater availability of specially designed pediatric duodenoscopes will facilitate the use of ERCP in infants with obstructive cholestasis.

Percutaneous liver biopsy remains one of the important diagnostic steps in evaluating the cholestatic infant and may be performed in even the smallest infants using only local anesthesia and sedation. In several studies, a diagnosis of biliary atresia was possible after liver biopsy in 90–95% of patients, with one study finding that liver biopsy was 100% sensitive and 76% specific in detecting biliary atresia [49]. The characteristic features of large duct obstruction include bile duct proliferation, bile plugs in small bile ducts, and portal tract edema and fibrosis [50]. The basic lobular architecture is usually intact. However, these findings require time to develop and may not all be present in biopsy samples taken in the first weeks of life. Therefore, serial assessment and possibly a repeat liver biopsy, may be required until a specific diagnosis is established or extrahepatic obstruction is clearly excluded. In patients with intrahepatic disease, diffuse cellular swelling and giant cell transformation of hepatocytes, variable inflammation, and focal hepatocellular necrosis are commonly observed. Fibrosis, bile ductular injury, and even bile duct paucity may be present. Pseudoacinar arrangement of hepatocytes and steatosis suggest a metabolic liver disease. Periodic acid–Schiff-positive granules can suggest α_1-antitrypsin deficiency. Abnormal storage of material in hepatocytes or Kupffer cells and viral inclusions also may be found. Electron microscopy and immunohistochemical methods may aid in the identification and localization of these abnormalities. Liver tissue also may be frozen for later biochemical or molecular analysis.

Lai et al. [51] have studied the diagnostic efficacy of many of the approaches that have been covered individually in this chapter and used them in a 3-day prospective evaluation of 126 infants, including 84 with neonatal hepatitis (age 65.1 ± 24.1 days) and 42 with biliary atresia (age 60.3 ± 31.1 days). The diagnostic accuracy of various methods was as follows: liver histology, 96.8%; color of duodenal juice, 91.6%; peak radioisotope count in duodenal juice, 84.2%; ultrasonographic examination of the hepatobiliary system, 80.2%; and persistence of clay-colored stool, 80.2%. After stepwise logistic regression, the diagnostic methods of significance were liver biopsy, color of duodenal juice, abdominal ultrasonography, and stool color. However, stool color and the onset of jaundice could not differentiate severe neonatal hepatitis from biliary atresia. The diagnostic methods of significance then were liver biopsy and duodenal juice color. With this 3-day protocol, an overall diagnostic accuracy of 96.8% was attained. No cases of biliary atresia were missed, although four cases of neonatal hepatitis were misdiagnosed, resulting in unnecessary laparotomy.

In patients with features consistent with a diagnosis of biliary atresia, or in the small number in which doubt persists about the diagnosis after review of the imaging studies and liver biopsy, the patency of the biliary tree should be directly examined at the time of a minilaparotomy and intraoperative cholangiogram [25]. The adverse effects of a diagnostic laparotomy are minimal. High-risk patients with features of liver failure including uncorrectable coagulopathy, hepatic encephalopathy, and ascites do not have biliary atresia and do not require surgical exploration. The surgeon should avoid transecting a biliary tree that is patent but small in diameter because of biliary hypoplasia or a low rate of bile flow associated with severe intrahepatic cholestasis. Moreover, the dynamic nature of the neonatal obstructive cholangiopathies is exemplified by rare cases in which the patency of the extrahepatic bile ducts was initially proven on cholangiopathy but evolution to biliary atresia was later documented at autopsy or laparotomy.

References

1. Pearson HA. Lectures on the diseases of children by Eli Ives, MD, of Yale and New Haven: America's first academic pediatrician. *Pediatrics* 1986;**77**:680–686.

2. Trauner M, Meier PJ, Boyer JL. Molecular pathogenesis of cholestasis. *N Engl J Med* 1998;**339**:1217–1227.

3. Koopen NR, Muller M, Vonk RJ, Zimniak P, Kuipers F. Molecular mechanisms of cholestasis: causes and consequences of impaired bile formation. *Biochim Biophys Acta* 1998;**1408**:1–17.

4. Suchy FJ. Neonatal cholestasis. *Pediatr Rev* 2004;**25**:388–396.

5. Balistreri WF, Bezerra JA. Whatever happened to "neonatal hepatitis"? *Clin Liver Dis* 2006;**10**:27–53, v.

6. Dick MC, Mowat AP. Hepatitis syndrome in infancy: an epidemiological survey with 10 year follow up. *Arch Dis Child* 1985;**60**:512–516.

7. Danks DM, Campbell PE, Jack I, Rogers J, Smith AL. Studies of the aetiology of neonatal hepatitis and biliary atresia. *Arch Dis Child* 1977;**52**:360–367.

8. Hartley JL, Davenport M, Kelly DA. Biliary atresia. *Lancet* 2009;**374**:1704–1713.

9. Yoon PW, Bresee JS, Olney RS, James LM, Khoury MJ. Epidemiology of biliary atresia: a population-based study. *Pediatrics* 1997;**99**:376–382.

10. Mieli-Vergani G, Howard ER, Portman B, Mowat AP. Late referral for biliary atresia: missed opportunities for effective surgery. *Lancet* 1989;**i**:421–423.

11. Wada H, Muraji T, Yokoi A, *et al.* Insignificant seasonal and geographical variation in incidence of biliary atresia in Japan: a regional survey of over 20 years. *J Pediatr Surg* 2007;**42**:2090–2092.

12. Stormon MO, Dorney SF, Kamath KR, O'Loughlin EV, Gaskin KJ. The changing pattern of diagnosis of infantile cholestasis. *J Paediatr Child Health* 2001;**37**:47–50.

13. Bezerra JA, Balistreri WF. Cholestatic syndromes of infancy and childhood. *Semin Gastrointest Dis* 2001;**12**:54–65.

14. Torbenson M, Hart J, Westerhoff M, *et al.* Neonatal giant cell hepatitis: histological and etiological findings. *Am J Surg Pathol* 2010;**34**:1498–1503.

15. Jacquemin E, Lykavieris P, Chaoui N, Hadchouel M, Bernard O. Transient neonatal cholestasis: origin and outcome. *J Pediatr* 1998;**133**:563–567.

16. Emerick KM, Whitington PF. Molecular basis of neonatal cholestasis. *Pediatr Clin North Am* 2002;**49**:221–235.

17. Carlton VE, Pawlikowska L, Bull LN. Molecular basis of intrahepatic cholestasis. *Ann Med* 2004;**36**:606–617.

18. Thompson R, Strautnieks S. BSEP: function and role in progressive familial intrahepatic cholestasis. *Semin Liver Dis* 2001;**21**:545–550.

19. Yehezkely-Schildkraut V, Munichor M, Mandel H, *et al.* Nonsyndromic paucity of interlobular bile ducts: report of 10 patients. *J Pediatr Gastroenterol Nutr* 2003;**37**:546–549.

20. Balistreri WF. Intrahepatic cholestasis. *J Pediatr Gastroenterol Nutr* 2002;**35** (Suppl 1):S17–S23.

21. Moyer V, Freese DK, Whitington PF, *et al.* Guideline for the evaluation of cholestatic jaundice in infants: recommendations of the North American Society for Pediatric Gastroenterology, Hepatology and Nutrition. *J Pediatr Gastroenterol Nutr* 2004;**39**:115–128.

22. Crofts DJ, Michel VJ, Rigby AS, *et al.* Assessment of stool colour in community management of prolonged jaundice in infancy. *Acta Paediatr* 1999;**88**:969–974.

23. Powell JE, Keffler S, Kelly DA, Green A. Population screening for neonatal liver disease: potential for a community-based programme. *J Med Screen* 2003;**10**:112–116.

24. Lien TH, Chang MH, Wu JF, *et al.* Effects of the infant stool color card screening program on 5-year outcome of biliary atresia in Taiwan. *Hepatology* 201;**53**:202–208.

25. Sokol RJ, Mack C, Narkewicz MR, Karrer FM. Pathogenesis and outcome of biliary atresia: current concepts. *J Pediatr Gastroenterol Nutr* 2003;**37**:4–21.

26. Sokol RJ, Stall C. Anthropometric evaluation of children with chronic liver disease. *Am J Clin Nutr* 1990;**52**:203–208.

27. Davenport M. Biliary atresia. *Semin Pediatr Surg* 2005;**14**:42–48.

28. Serinet MO, Wildhaber BE, Broue P, *et al.* Impact of age at Kasai operation on its results in late childhood and adolescence: a rational basis for biliary atresia screening. *Pediatrics* 2009;**123**:1280–1286.

29. Alagille D. Cholestasis in the first three months of life. *Prog Liver Dis* 1979;**6**:471–485.

30. Kamath BM, Piccoli DA. Heritable disorders of the bile ducts. *Gastroenterol Clin North Am* 2003;**32**:857–875.

31. Sokol RJ, Mack C. Etiopathogenesis of biliary atresia. *Semin Liver Dis* 2001;**21**:517–524.

32. Kelly DA, McKiernan PJ. Metabolic liver disease in the pediatric patient. *Clin Liver Dis* 1998;**2**:1–30.

33. Goncalves I, Hermans D, Chretien D, *et al.* Mitochondrial respiratory chain defect: a new etiology for neonatal cholestasis and early liver insufficiency. *J Hepatol* 1995;**23**:290–294.

34. Suchy FJ. Clinical problems with developmental anomalies of the biliary tract. *Semin Gastrointest Dis* 2003;**14**:156–164.

35. Suchy FJ, Shneider BI. Neonatal jaundice and cholestasis. In Kaplowitz N (ed.) *Liver and Biliary Diseases.* Baltimore, MD: Williams & Wilkins, 1992, p. 446.

36. Rinaldo P, Tortorelli S, Matern D. Recent developments and new applications of tandem mass spectrometry in newborn screening. *Curr Opin Pediatr* 2004;**16**:427–433.

37. Balistreri WF, A-Kader HH, Setchell KD, *et al.* New methods for assessing liver function in infants and children. *Ann Clin Lab Sci* 1992;**22**:162–174.

38. Rosenthal P. Assessing liver function and hyperbilirubinemia in the newborn. National Academy of Clinical Biochemistry. *Clin Chem* 1997;**43**:228–234.

39. Maggiore G, Bernard O, Hadchouel M, Lemonnier A, Alagille D. Diagnostic value of serum gamma-glutamyl transpeptidase activity in liver diseases in children. *J Pediatr Gastroenterol Nutr* 1991;**12**:21–26.

40. Rosenthal P, Miller JH, Sinatra FR. Hepatobiliary scintigraphy and the string test in the evaluation of neonatal cholestasis. *J Pediatr Gastroenterol Nutr* 1989;**8**:292–296.

41. Fitzpatrick E, Jardine R, Farrant P, *et al.* Predictive value of bile duct dimensions measured by ultrasound in neonates presenting with cholestasis. *J Pediatr Gastroenterol Nutr* 2010;**51**:55–60.

42. Nievelstein RA, Robben SG, Blickman JG. Hepatobiliary and pancreatic imaging in children: techniques and an overview of non-neoplastic disease entities. *Pediatr Radiol* 2011;**41**:55–75.

43. Kanegawa K, Akasaka Y, Kitamura E, *et al.* Sonographic diagnosis of biliary atresia in pediatric patients using the "triangular cord" sign versus gallbladder length and contraction. *AJR Am J Roentgenol* 2003;**181**:1387–1390.

44. Norton KI, Glass RB, Kogan D, *et al.* MR cholangiography in the evaluation of neonatal cholestasis: initial results. *Radiology* 2002;**222**:687–691.

45. Gilmour SM, Hershkop M, Reifen R, Gilday D, Roberts EA. Outcome of hepatobiliary scanning in neonatal hepatitis syndrome. *J Nucl Med* 1997;**38**:1279–1282.

46. Huang L, Wang W, Liu G, *et al.* Laparoscopic cholecystocholangiography for diagnosis of prolonged jaundice in infants, experience of 144 cases. *Pediatr Surg Int* 2010;**26**:711–715.

47. Iinuma Y, Narisawa R, Iwafuchi M, *et al.* The role of endoscopic retrograde cholangiopancreatography in infants with cholestasis. *J Pediatr Surg* 2000;**35**:545–549.

48. Shanmugam NP, Harrison PM, Devlin J, *et al.* Selective use of endoscopic retrograde cholangiopancreatography in the diagnosis of biliary atresia in infants younger than 100 days. *J Pediatr Gastroenterol Nutr* 2009;**49**:435–441.

49. Zerbini MC, Gallucci SD, Maezono R, *et al.* Liver biopsy in neonatal cholestasis: a review on statistical grounds. *Mod Pathol* 1997;**10**:793–799.

50. Finegold MJ. Common diagnostic problems in pediatric liver pathology. *Clin Liver Dis* 2002;**6**:421–454.

51. Lai MW, Chang MH, Hsu SC, *et al.* Differential diagnosis of extrahepatic biliary atresia from neonatal hepatitis: a prospective study. *J Pediatr Gastroenterol Nutr* 1994;**18**:121–127.

Chapter

9

Medical and nutritional management of cholestasis in infants and children

Andrew P. Feranchak, Frederick J. Suchy, and Ronald J. Sokol

Introduction

When first encountering an infant or child with cholestatic liver disease, it is essential that diagnostic evaluation be conducted promptly in order to (1) recognize disorders amenable either to specific medical therapy (e.g. galactosemia, tyrosinemia, hypothyroidism, urinary tract infection) or to early surgical intervention (e.g. biliary atresia, choledochal cyst); (2) institute treatment directed toward enhancing bile flow; and (3) prevent and treat the varied medical, nutritional, and emotional consequences of chronic liver disease. Because many of the treatable causes require early diagnosis and prompt institution of therapy, the evaluation of the cholestatic infant should never be delayed. Although "physiologic cholestasis" (hypercholemia or elevated bile acids) may be present in the infant, there is no state of "physiologic conjugated hyperbilirubinemia". For the jaundiced infant, historical and clinical information such as color of the stools, birth weight, and presence of hepatomegaly may provide important clues as to the etiology of cholestasis. Consanguinity or liver disease in siblings suggests the possibility of metabolic, familial, or genetic disease. Review of the prenatal and postnatal course may reveal intrauterine infection, occurrence of hypoglycemia or seizures, and exposure to toxins/drugs (i.e. total parenteral nutrition (TPN)). Careful physical examination may reveal features of typical disorders or syndromes. For the older child and adolescent, a history of exposure to drugs/toxins (e.g. acetaminophen), the presence of vascular insufficiency, and the presence of underlying disease (e.g. inflammatory bowel disease) provide helpful clues. The diagnostic evaluation of the infant with cholestasis is detailed in Chapter 8.

Once the diagnosis is made, a limited number of disorders are amenable to specific treatments. Although less than 10% of infants with neonatal cholestasis are found to have treatable medical disorders, the individual patient will derive important benefits from early diagnosis and treatment. Those infants found to require surgical correction of anatomic causes of cholestasis likewise require early identification and therapy for optimal outcome. A classification scheme relating the availability of specific therapy to the individual causes of prolonged neonatal cholestasis is given in Table 9.1 [1].

In the majority of cases where there is no "curable" etiology or when surgical correction of biliary atresia is unsuccessful, medical management is largely supportive, directed at inducing choleresis, optimizing growth and nutrition, minimizing discomfort and disability, and aiding the child and the family in coping with the stress, social, and emotional effects of chronic liver disease. The success of therapeutic intervention, however, is limited by the residual functional capacity of the liver and by the rate of progression of the underlying liver disease. Since orthotopic liver transplantation in children has become standard therapy for end-stage liver disease, it is increasingly important to optimize the care, growth, and development of children with chronic liver disease in order to enhance their chances for successful liver transplant.

The ultimate prognosis for an affected child is related to the severity of the complications resulting from chronic cholestasis. These complications are attributable directly or indirectly to diminished bile flow plus (1) retention of substances normally excreted in bile (bile acids, bilirubin, cholesterol, and trace elements) with resultant hepatocyte apoptosis and necrosis and induction of portal fibrosis progressing to portal hypertension, cirrhosis, and liver failure; (2) transfer of constituents of bile into the systemic circulation, leading to pruritus, fatigue, hypercholesterolemia, and xanthoma formation; and (3) reduced delivery of bile to the small bowel, with decreased intraluminal bile acid concentrations leading to malabsorption of fat and fat-soluble vitamins. These departures from normal physiology lead to discomfort, failure to thrive, specific nutrient deficiencies, and psychological/behavioral problems in the developing child. A summary of medical treatment options for cholestasis, including medications, doses, and toxicity is given in Table 9.2 [2,3].

Retention of bile constituents

Hepatocellular injury: pathogenesis of cholestatic injury

The retention of endogenous bile acids in the hepatocyte during cholestasis is believed to be involved in the pathogenesis of progressive liver injury and may lead to perpetuation of

Liver Disease in Children, Fourth Edition, ed. Frederick J. Suchy, Ronald J. Sokol, and William F. Balistreri. Published by Cambridge University Press. © Cambridge University Press 2014.

Table 9.1 Treatable causes of neonatal cholestasis

Disease	Liver involvement	Treatment
Congenital infectious hepatitis		
Herpes simplex virus	Coagulative necrosis	Acyclovir IV
Syphilis	Hepatitis, periportal, and interlobular fibrosis	Penicillin G IV (50 000 U/kg daily for 10–14 days)
Listeria monocytogenes infection	Granulomatous hepatitis	Ampicillin IV (neonatal doses)
Tuberculosis	Granulomatous hepatitis	Consult neonatal infectious disease expert
Toxoplasmosis	Cholestasis	Pyrimethamine (1 mg/kg every 2–4 days) and sulfadiazine (50–100 mg/kg daily) for 21 days
HIV	Cholestasis	Consult neonatal infectious disease expert
Metabolic diseases		
Galactosemia	Cholestasis, steatosis, fibrosis, cirrhosis	Galactose-free diet
Hereditary tyrosinemia	Steatosis, fibrosis, cirrhosis	Low tyrosine/phenylalanine diet, nitisinone
Hereditary fructose intolerance	Steatosis, fibrosis	Fructose/sucrose-free diet
Hypothyroidism/hypopituitarism	Cholestasis	Thyroid, adrenal, growth hormone replacement
Cystic fibrosis	Biliary mucus plugging, cholestasis, focal biliary cirrhosis, multilobular cirrhosis, cholelithiasis	Oral pancreatic enzyme replacement, pulmonary therapy, fat-soluble vitamin supplements, UDCA
Bile acid synthesis defects		
Δ4-3-Oxosteroid-5β-reductase deficiency	Cholestasis, giant cell hepatitis	Cholic acid
3β-Hydroxysteroid dehydrogenase/isomerase deficiency	Cholestasis, giant cell hepatitis	Cholic acid
Neonatal iron storage disease	Cholestasis, fibrosis, cirrhosis	Antioxidant therapy,[a] liver transplantation, exchange transfusion, IV immunoglobulin
Drugs and toxins		
Drugs	Variable	Discontinue drug
Bacterial endotoxin (sepsis, urinary tract infections, etc.)	Cholestasis, hepatocyte necrosis	Appropriate IV antibiotic therapy
TPN-associated	Cholestasis, steatosis, bile duct proliferation, portal fibrosis, cirrhosis	Institute early enteral feedings, avoid excessive (IV) calories and protein, use neonatal amino acid solutions, UDCA (?), lipid modification
Anatomic lesions		
Extrahepatic biliary atresia	Cholestasis, bile duct proliferation, fibrosis, cirrhosis	Hepatoportoenterostomy
Choledochal cyst	Cholestasis, fibrosis, cirrhosis	Choledochoenterostomy
Spontaneous perforation of common bile duct	Peritonitis, ascites, cholestasis	Surgical drainage
Inspissated bile/calculi in common bile duct	Cholestasis, bile duct proliferation, fibrosis, cirrhosis	Biliary tract irrigation

IV, Intravenous; nitisinone, 2-(2-nitro-4-trifluoromethylbenzoyl)-1,3-cyclohexanedione; TPGS, tocopherol polyethylene glycol-1000 succinate; TPN, total parenteral nutrition; UDCA, ursodeoxycholic acid.

[a] Vitamin E (TPGS) 25 IU/kg per day oral; desferrioxamine 15 mg/h per kg body weight IV continuous infusion until ferritin <500 μg/L; selenium 2–3 μg/kg per day IV (in TPN); *N*-acetylcysteine 70 mg/kg dose every 4 hours via nasogastric tube or IV for 20 doses.

Source: from Sokol, 1990 [1], with permission.

Table 9.2 Medical treatment options for cholestasis

Treatment	Indications	Dosage	Toxicity
Bile acid-binding agents: cholestyramine, colestipol, aluminum hydroxide antacids, sucralfate (?)	Hypercholesterolemia, xanthoma, pruritus, hypercholemia(?)	250–500 mg/kg daily (cholestyramine and colestipol)	Constipation, hyperchloremic acidosis, binding of drugs, increased steatorrhea, intestinal obstruction
Naltrexone	Pruritus	50 mg/day (adults)	Nausea, headache, hepatotoxicity (?), opioid withdrawal reactions
Phenobarbital	Hypercholesterolemia, pruritus, hypercholemia(?)	3–10 mg/kg per day	Drowsiness, behavior changes, interference with vitamin d metabolism, risk for suicide and suicidal behavior
Rifampicin	Pruritus	10 mg/kg per day	Hepatotoxicity, drug interactions, hemolytic anemia, renal failure
Ursodeoxycholic acid	Pruritus, hypercholesterolemia, cholestasis, cystic fibrosis liver disease	10–30 mg/kg per day	Diarrhea, increased pruritus, hepatotoxicity(?)
Antihistamines	Pruritus	Diphenhydramine, 5–10 mg/kg daily or hydroxyzine, 2–5 mg/kg daily	Drowsiness
Ultraviolet B light	Pruritus		Skin burn
Carbamazepine	Pruritus	20–40 mg/kg/d	Hepatotoxicity, bone marrow suppression, fluid retention, behavioral changes

Source: from Sokol, 1990 [1], with permission.

cholestasis. Hydrophobic bile acids (i.e. monohydroxy and dihydroxy bile acids) are more hepatotoxic than the hydrophilic bile acids (trihydroxy bile acids and ursodeoxycholic acid ($3\alpha,7\beta$-dihydroxy-5β-cholan-24oic acid; UDCA)). These differences in hepatotoxicity may be related to effects on membrane properties, inhibition of microsomal enzymes, generation of free radicals, stimulation of cellular death receptors on the plasma membrane, activation of protein kinase signaling pathways and induction of pathologic mitochondrial permeability. In the pathogenesis of cholestatic liver injury, it appears that hydrophobic bile acids play an important role in activation of death receptors, induction of the mitochondrial permeability transition and various intracellular pathways of apoptosis and cellular necrosis.

To counteract the effects of retained toxic bile acids, several agents have been proposed to improve choleresis. Choleretic agents such as UDCA, tauroursodeoxycholic acid (TUDCA), and phenobarbital may potentially minimize the toxic effects of bile acids by enhancing hepatocyte excretion of bile acids into bile, improving bile acid-independent bile flow, stabilizing hepatocyte membranes, and protecting hepatocyte mitochondria from the permeability transition. In addition, UDCA and TUDCA may be hepatoprotective by displacing toxic bile acids in the bile acid pool and by producing a bicarbonate-rich hypercholeresis [4].

Treatment with choleretic agents: ursodeoxycholic acid

Ursodeoxycholic acid is the major bile acid of the black bear and has been used for centuries in traditional Chinese and Japanese medicine for the treatment of gallbladder and liver disease. It normally occurs in only small quantities (<3%) in human bile and is formed by 7β-epimerization of the primary bile salt, chenodeoxycholic acid, through the action of colonic bacteria. The difference in the position of the hydroxyl group (β instead of α) confers the marked hydrophilicity of UDCA compared with chenodeoxycholic acid.

Several mechanisms have been proposed to explain the potential beneficial effects of UDCA in the treatment of cholestatic liver diseases [5]. Since intracellular retention of hydrophobic bile acids is thought to lead to liver cell injury, replacement of these compounds with a non-toxic hydrophilic bile acid such as UDCA should theoretically reduce injury. It may be hepatoprotective by displacing toxic bile acids from both the bile acid pool and hepatocellular membranes. In vitro studies have demonstrated that UDCA has a direct hepatoprotective effect on cultured hepatocytes exposed to toxic, hyrophobic bile acids. In addition, UDCA has been shown to improve mitochondrial oxidative phosphorylation and prevent the mitochondrial membrane permeability transition, a key signaling pathway in both apoptotic and necrotic cell death. In vivo studies in the rat have also shown that administration of UDCA (either enterally or parenterally) ameliorates the effects of hydrophobic bile acid-induced cholestasis. While this cytoprotective effect may result from direct stabilization of the hepatocyte membrane, UDCA may also work by altering the bile salt pool with a decrease in hydrophobic bile salts. UDCA is poor at micelle formation and solubilization and is poorly absorbed from the proximal intestine [4]. Therefore, a large amount of orally administered UDCA reaches the terminal ileum where it interferes with the absorption of endogenous, more hydrophobic and toxic bile acids. Studies have demonstrated a significant increase in serum UDCA concentration (from 2% to 40%) during UDCA therapy, with a corresponding decrease in serum chenodeoxycholic and cholic acid levels. In addition to its effects on the bile salt pool composition, UDCA has a direct hypercholeretic effect. In rats, unconjugated UDCA secreted by the liver becomes protonated in the biliary ductule. The protonated UDCA is very lipophilic and is rapidly reabsorbed by biliary epithelial cells prior to reaching the small intestine, transported back to the liver, and secreted again [3]. This "cholehepatic shunt" mechanism leads to a significant hypercholeresis [4]. Identification of bile acid transporters on both the cholangiocyte apical (luminal) and basoletral membranes provides a more mechanistic understanding of this process. In addition to the effect on bile salt-dependent bile flow, UDCA also increases bile salt-independent flow through a direct effect on cholangiocyte calcium-activated chloride secretion, resulting in bicarbonate-rich choloresis. Lastly, UDCA may have an important immunomodulatory role, reducing immunologic injury associated with some cholestatic liver diseases. While normal hepatocytes do not express HLA class I or II antigens, cholestasis may induce abnormal HLA class I expression in these cells, resulting in cytotoxic T-cell-mediated lysis and further liver injury. In vivo studies in the mouse and in patients with primary biliary cirrhosis (PBC) have shown that UDCA therapy leads to a reduction in the expression of abnormal HLA class I proteins on hepatocytes.

The observation that some patients with chronic active hepatitis demonstrated improvement in biochemical markers of liver injury when treated for gallstones with UDCA led to trials of UDCA for a wide variety of cholestatic liver diseases. The evidence supporting use of UDCA for the treatment of specific cholestatic liver diseases will be reviewed below.

Primary biliary cirrhosis

The therapeutic efficacy of UDCA has been best demonstrated in the treatment of the cholestatic adult disease, PBC, an autoimmune fibrosing cholangiopathy. UDCA treatment markedly improves serum liver tests and histologic features of liver injury and fibrosis when administered at a daily dose of 13–15 mg/kg [6]. However, despite adequate dosing, approximately one-third of patients do not respond to therapy. The most significant therapeutic effect has been demonstrated in those patients with cirrhosis or higher serum bilirubin levels;

transplant-free survival may increase as much as 25% with UDCA treatment versus placebo. The cost-effectiveness of UDCA in the treatment of PBC has also been established. Therefore, UDCA is safe, efficacious, and cost-effective in the treatment of adults with PBC, although it does not prevent progressive disease in all patients. Unfortunately, the data establishing the effectiveness of UDCA in other adult and childhood cholestatic disorders have not been as definitive.

Primary sclerosing cholangitis

While the use of UDCA in primary sclerosing cholangitis (PSC) initially appeared promising, long-term controlled trials have not demonstrated any improvement in disease progression. In fact, high-dose UDCA (28–30 mg/kg daily) has been shown to increase the risk of adverse outcomes and increase the risk of colorectal neoplasia in patients with ulcerative colitis and PSC [7]. Additionally, UDCA has had little success in improving pruritus or fatigue associated with PSC. Long-term pediatric trials to determine a potential benefit of UDCA in childhood PSC are lacking and, given the poor results in adults, unlikely to occur.

Cystic fibrosis

The best data demonstrating a therapeutic effect of UDCA in pediatric cholestatic disorders are in the treatment of cystic fibrosis (CF). Clinically significant liver disease develops in 10–20% of patients with CF and 5–10% develop cirrhosis by adolescence [8]. The pathogenesis of CF-associated liver disease remains speculative. One model suggests that liver injury is the result of the retention of hepatotoxic bile salts secondary to obstruction of bile ducts by inspissated secretions and viscid mucus [8]. This provides a logical rationale for the use of UDCA as a potential cytoprotective agent and stimulator of bicarbonate-rich bile flow. Prospective clinical trials of UDCA in children with CF liver disease at daily doses of 10–20 mg/kg for 6–12 months have shown significant improvement in alanine aminotransferase, alkaline phosphatase, and gamma-glutamyltransferase (GGT) [8]. A double-blind, multicenter trial demonstrated improved biochemical and clinical parameters (as measured by the Shwachman score) after 1 year of treatment with UDCA (15 mg/kg daily). Several studies have reported a dose–response effect for UDCA in CF liver disease with maximal effect at a daily dosage of 20 mg/kg, suggesting that higher doses of UDCA may be necessary in CF than in other forms of cholestasis. In addition to improvement of liver blood tests, UDCA improved hepatobiliary excretory function (as measured by radionuclide hepatobiliary scintigraphy), liver histology, and nutritional status of patients with CF-related liver disease. Despite the improved biochemical, biliary excretory, and perhaps histologic data, it remains to be seen whether UDCA alters the natural course of liver disease in patients with CF. While there is a need for long-term pediatric studies, it appears prudent to use UDCA in patients with CF and evidence of liver disease, as recommended by the Cystic Fibrosis Foundation Hepatobiliary Disease Consensus Group [8].

However, given the recent results of UDCA in PSC, this recommendation may need to be revisited. For a more detailed discussion of the use of UDCA in cystic fibrosis please see Chapter 26.

Alagille syndrome

Balistreri *et al.* [9] in a study of 31 patients with Alagille syndrome, demonstrated a decrease in serum alanine aminotransferase and cholesterol levels, and a marked improvement in pruritus during UDCA therapy: 15 of the 31 patients had an initial clinical response with a decrease in pruritus after 1 month of therapy (15–30 mg/kg daily). In addition, 11 of the 16 initial non-responders showed improvement with an increase in the dose of UDCA (45 mg/kg daily). Several case studies have also reported an improvement in pruritus, serum liver enzymes, cholesterol, triglyceride, phospholipid levels, and xanthomas. While further studies are desirable, these preliminary reports suggest that the use of UDCA in Alagille syndrome is warranted. However, there are no data available as to alteration of the natural history of Alagille syndrome by UDCA therapy.

Progressive familial intrahepatic cholestasis

Progressive familial intrahepatic cholestasis (PFIC) is a group of childhood cholestatic diseases with at least three different subtypes: type 1 (Byler disease) is caused by mutations in *ATP8B1* and is associated with normal serum GGT levels; type 2 results from a defect in the canalicular bile salt export pump BSEP (*ABCB11*) and is associated with normal GGT levels; and type 3 is caused by a deficiency in the multidrug resistance-associated protein 3 (MDR-3, encoded by *ABCB4*) and associated with elevated GGT levels. Jacquemin *et al.* used UDCA (20–30 mg/kg daily) in 39 patients divided into two groups, based on serum GGT levels (group 1 normal GGT and group 2 elevated GGT) [10]. After 2–4 years of therapy, liver tests normalized in 32%, improved in 20%, and worsened in 48% in group 1. In group 2, liver tests normalized in 50%, improved in 29%, and worsened in 21%. Children with PFIC type 3 and missense mutations had less severe disease and more often a beneficial response to UDCA therapy [11]. While long-term data are lacking, empiric therapy with UDCA appears worthwhile in some patients with PFIC, but low GGT familial intrahepatic cholestasis is generally refractory to medical treatment and UDCA has not been effective in patients with benign recurrent intrahepatic cholestasis.

Bile acid synthesis defects

Several distinct abnormalities in primary bile salt synthesis have been described including Δ^4-3-oxosteroid-5β-reductase deficiency and 3β-hydroxysteroid dehydrogenase/isomerase deficiency. In these inherited defects, primary bile acid synthesis is absent or markedly impaired. Δ^4-3-Oxosteroid-5β-reductase deficiency results in increased synthesis of abnormal oxo-bile acids and neonatal liver failure. Patients with this defect have demonstrated a dramatic response to combined cholic acid therapy, with suppression of oxo-bile synthesis, normalization of liver blood tests, marked improvement in liver histology, and with long-term survival of a presumably fatal disorder. 3β-Hydroxysteroid dehydrogenase/isomerase deficiency is clinically similar to PFIC, with low GGT; however, patients do not have pruritus. The failure of normal bile acid synthesis and the accumulation of atypical bile acids in this disorder presumably account for the progressive liver injury [12]. Cholic acid and not UDCA leads to suppression of bile acid synthesis at the level of 7α-hydroxylase and decreased production of toxis bile acid intermediates.

Biliary atresia

Although UCDA is frequently used after portoenterostomy for treatment of biliary atresia, there is no evidence that it improves outcome or decreases complications such as recurrent cholangitis. Further studies are needed to determine whether subgroups of patients with biliary atresia (e.g. those with recurrent cholangitis after the establishment of bile flow) will benefit from UDCA therapy. Clearly, when portoenterostomy is unsuccessful or has not been performed, UDCA is of no benefit in biliary atresia.

Cholestasis associated with total parenteral nutrition

UDCA may improve liver tests in patients on long-term therapy with TPN, but there is little evidence that it alters the course of the disease. One limitation to the use of UDCA in patients at risk for the development of TPN-associated cholestasis is poor intestinal absorption of UDCA in patients with short gut. However, UDCA may bind bacterial endotoxin in the gut lumen and prevent its absorption, thereby reducing activation of Kupffer cells, inhibiting TNF generation, and reducing liver injury. This mechanism could explain a beneficial effect of UDCA therapy in children with short gut syndrome and bacterial overgrowth of the small bowel. As an alternative, TUDCA has not been of value in improving the liver disease in infants with short bowel syndrome and cholestasis.

Hepatic veno-occlusive disease and graft-versus-host disease

UDCA has been used both prophylactically and in the treatment of hepatic complications related to bone marrow transplantation. Compared with a historical control group, prophylactic treatment with UDCA decreased serum bilirubin levels, reduced the incidence of veno-occlusive disease, and improved survival after bone marrow transplantation. While improvement of serum liver tests was observed in patients with graft-versus-host disease of the liver, biochemical abnormalities returned after discontinuation of UDCA. Although further data are desirable, UDCA may be considered for the treatment of liver graft-versus-host disease and in the prevention of veno-occlusive disease following bone marrow transplantation, particularly in patients at high risk because of the type of chemotherapy used.

Summary of ursodeoxycholic acid treatment

The use of UDCA has proven long-term benefit in adult PBC. While further studies are needed, it appears prudent to use UDCA in the treatment of CF-associated liver disease, Alagille syndrome, PFIC, graft-versus-host disease, and veno-occlusive disease. There has been no proven benefit of its use in PSC, TPN-associated cholestasis, biliary atresia, chronic hepatitis, or orthotopic liver transplantation. It must be pointed out that, at present, no UDCA trials in children with cholestasis have shown that this therapy has altered the ultimate course of the underlying liver disease or survival [13]. However, most experience shows that it is safe to use in infants and children who do not have fixed obstruction to bile flow.

Treatment with choleretic agents: tauroursodeoxycholic acid

Concerns regarding the long-term use of UDCA have included its poor enteral absorption during cholestasis, poor biliary enrichment of the unconjugated form, and increased biotransformation to more hydrophobic bile acids such as lithocholic acid. Several recent studies have, therefore, focused on other hydrophilic bile acids TUDCA, the taurine conjugate of UDCA, which has been shown in vitro and in vivo to have greater cytoprotective effects than UDCA [14]. Possible mechanisms of its hepatoprotective action include membrane enrichment and stability, enhanced Kupffer cell phagocytosis, and calcium homeostasis and hepatocyte exocytosis. Data from animal studies and from preliminary trials in patients with PBC suggest that TUDCA is better absorbed, induces more favorable changes in the composition of the bile salt pool, and undergoes less biotransformation to hydrophobic species when compared with UDCA. Preliminary, short-term studies in adults with PBC have demonstrated that TUDCA was equally as beneficial as UDCA, with comparable doses (500 mg/day), in lowering serum liver enzyme levels. However, higher TUDCA doses (1000 and 1500 mg/day) resulted in greater bile pool enrichment with hydrophilic bile acids, both UDCA and TUDCA, and a significant decrease in both total and HDL cholesterol [14]. These preliminary studies are encouraging and further long-term adult trials and investigational trials in pediatric cholestatic disorders appear warranted. As noted above, TUDCA does not appear to be effective in treating TPN-related cholestasis in the infant with short bowel syndrome.

Other treatments

Other bile acid molecules

nor-Ursodeoxycholate, the C-23 analogue of ursodeoxycholate, is a potent choleretic agent that appears to be a promising treatment of PSC animal models and is currently under investigation in humans [15].

Phenobarbital

Phenobarbital therapy has been used for years as a choleretic and antipruritic agent for many cholestatic liver diseases. By increasing the bile acid independent fraction of bile flow, enhancing bile acid synthesis, inducing hepatic microsomal enzymes, and increasing hepatic Na^+-K^+-ATPase activity, it has been used in cholestasis to decrease serum bilirubin, lower circulating serum bile acids, and, by its hepatic microsomal stimulation and excretory enhancement, possibly help in the elimination of a pruritogenic substance. The usual daily dosage of phenobarbital is 3–10 mg/kg, aiming to achieve a serum level of approximately 10–20 μg/mL. High-dose phenobarbital therapy can be associated with sedation, and alterations in the metabolism of a wide variety of drugs including vitamin D may occur. Chronic phenobarbital therapy in children with seizure disorders has been associated with poor self-esteem, labile moods, neurotic symptoms, frank depression, and an increased risk for suicide and suicidal behavior. Although detailed study has not been conducted on the effects of phenobarbital on cognitive and behavior functions in children with chronic cholestasis, with the availability of other medications that reduce pruritus and stimulate bile flow, phenobarbital treatment is now used rarely for the treatment of cholestasis.

Glucocorticoids

While steroids have not been used as long-term choleretic agents, high-dose "bursts" of intravenous methylprednisolone have been shown to be effective in stimulating bile flow during episodes of refractory cholangitis after hepatic portoenterostomy treatment for extrahepatic biliary atresia. Short-term intravenous corticosteroid therapy is frequently used routinely in Asia following portoenterostomy for biliary atresia. One US study demonstrated an improvement in conjugated bilirubin levels and transplant-free survival in a group of patients with biliary atresia following portoenterostomy when treated with high-dose steroids in conjunction with antibiotics and UDCA compared with those who did not receive steroid treatment [16]. However, the lack of randomization confounds the interpretation of this and other reports of steroid use following portoenterostomy. Several controlled randomized studies are now in progress. There have not been any studies to suggest a beneficial effect of long-term steroid administration in cholestatic disorders; in view of the many complications of chronic steroid therapy, its use for chronic cholestasis is not warranted.

Cholecystokinin

Cholecystokinin, a peptide hormone secreted by the intestine in response to a meal, stimulates gallbladder contraction and relaxation of the sphincter of Oddi, and increases intestinal motility. A synthetic cholecystokinin-octapeptide (sincalide) has been developed and was believed to be of potential benefit in treating cholestasis associated with abnormal gallbladder function, such as TPN-cholestasis where lack of enteral nutrition is associated with a decrease in endogenous cholecystokinin secretion. While administration of sincalide may cause a decline in serum conjugated bilirubin levels, no significant improvement in serum aminotransferases or in the course of liver disease has been observed. A large multicentered randomized controlled trial of sincalide in infants at risk for TPN cholestasis found that it did not affect conjugated bilirubin levels, sepsis incidence, time to achieve 50% and 100% energy intake enterally, mortality rate, incidence of cholelithiasis, and number of days in intensive care and in hospital. Based on these results, sincalide should not be recommended for prevention of TPN cholestasis in infants at risk.

Nuclear receptor agonists

The identification of the proteins involved in hepatic bile acid uptake, transport, and excretion has provided a more mechanistic model of liver transport functions in both health and disease. Identification of these transport proteins has provided insight into the pathogenesis of many cholestatic liver disorders, while also advancing our basic knowledge of normal liver transport functions. One exciting area has been the identification of the regulatory pathways involved in the transcription and expression of these transport proteins, which involve the binding of ligands to specific nuclear receptors that regulate transcription [17]. Several nuclear receptors have been identified that regulate bile acid transport proteins and enzymes involved in bile acid synthesis, including the farnesoid X receptor (FXR), the constitutive androstane receptor (CAR), and the pregnane X receptor (PXR). Identification of these nuclear receptors suggests a new category of agents to treat cholestasis, namely specific receptor activators that will alter the expression of bile acid transporters directly.

The farnesoid X receptor is highly expressed in the liver and activated by bile acids, such as the hydrophobic bile acid chenodeoxycholic acid [17]. Binding of bile acids to FXR upregulates transcription of genes coding for BSEP, MDR-3 and multidrug resistance-associated protein 2, proteins responsible for the export of bile acids from the hepatocyte. Activation by FXR also inhibits the transcription of *CYP7A* and *CYP8B*, both involved in bile acid synthesis, and hence provides feedback inhibition of bile acid synthesis. Another membrane receptor for bile acids, TGR5, has expression and function that is distinct from FXR. These two bile acid receptors complement each other in maintaining bile acid homeostasis and mediating bile acid signaling. Presence of TGR5 may be important for preserving the bile acid pool and for preventing bile acid-induced toxicity. There has been considerable interest in developing agonists for these receptors in order to harness their potential hepatoprotective effects. Selective and dual agonists for these receptors have been developed (INT-747 for FXR, INT-777 for TGR5, and INT-767 for FXR/TGR5) [4] that reduce liver injury and promote biliary bicarbonate output in a mouse cholangiopathy model [18]. Human studies with the agents are forthcoming.

Another nuclear receptor found in liver, CAR, plays an important role in the detoxification of bile acids as well as mediating the response to xenobiotics such as phenobarbital. It appears to abrogate the hepatotoxicity associated with lithocholic acid. Agonists for CAR, including the herbal medicine Yin Shi Huang and phenobarbital, have been shown to reduce bile acid levels in adults with PBC as well as bilirubin levels in neonates. Another nuclear receptor, PXR, is closely related to CAR and regulates genes in the pathways affecting hepatic oxidation, conjugation, and transport. Interestingly, rifampicin is a ligand for PXR, and, therefore, the antipruritic effects of this drug may be by direct modulation of bile acid synthesis and transport activity [14].

Clearly the area of transcriptional regulation of the enzymes and proteins involved in bile acid synthesis and transport warrant further study. In the future, the use of nuclear receptor agonists may provide another useful therapeutic strategy in the treatment of cholestasis.

Progressive fibrosis and cirrhosis
Pathogenesis of liver fibrosis

The liver, with its unique regenerative capacity, has a remarkable ability to resorb scar after the underlying liver disease resolves spontaneously or is successfully treated. The long-term survival of children with chronic cholestatic liver disease will ultimately depend on the residual functional capacity of the liver and the rate of progression of the underlying disorder. Chronic cholestatic liver disease is, with rare exception, associated with hepatic fibrosis, a complex process that involves changes in the amounts of extracellular matrix components, activation of cells capable of producing matrix materials (e.g. hepatic stellate cells, fibroblasts), cytokine release, and tissue remodeling [19]. One result of the matrix protein accumulation is an imbalance in the relationship between the hepatic parenchymal cells and their blood supply, ultimately leading to increased intrahepatic vascular resistance, microcirculatory ischemia, and consequent portal hypertension, which are the hallmarks of hepatic cirrhosis. Although recent research has led to a greater understanding of the biological importance of the major macromolecules of the extracellular matrix in the pathogenesis of excessive collagen deposition and disturbances in hepatocyte growth, regeneration, and repair during progressive hepatic fibrosis, there is no established therapy to attenuate hepatic fibrogenesis. Current antifibrotic therapy is directed toward modulation of inflammatory mediators that stimulate hepatic stellate cells to proliferate and increase collagen production and stimulation of collagenase and other proteinases.

Treatment

Several potential antifibrotics have been evaluated in clinical trials, but none has proved effective [20]. Colchicine is an antifibrogenic drug that suppresses collagen biosynthesis directly by inhibiting polymerization of microtubules and blocking transcellular movement of procollagen. In addition, it has inhibitory effects on anti-inflammatory cells, reducing their ability to stimulate production of extracellular matrix components and accelerating breakdown of collagen by stimulating collagenase activity. Clinical trials of colchicine in adults with various types of cirrhosis have variably shown improvement in biochemical liver tests but have failed to demonstrate a decrease in mortality. More recent long-term studies in adults report no influence of colchicine therapy on progression of disease in patients with PBC and no improvement in hepatic histology in patients who have been treated for 8 years. One large placebo-controlled double-blinded trial of colchicine for 2–6 years in adults with alcohol-induced cirrhosis found no effect of colchicine on mortality, complications of portal hypertension, or liver fibrosis. Therefore, this drug cannot be recommended for adults with cirrhosis until there is evidence supporting its use.

Two other antifibrogenic agents that have been studied in adults with liver disease are D-penicillamine and glucocorticoids. The use of D-penicillamine in conditions of hepatic fibrogenesis was suggested by its inhibition of intra- and intermolecular collagen cross-linking. Prospective trials of D-penicillamine in patients with PBC, however, failed to show any significant clinical or histologic benefit or improvement in survival. Significant toxicity (bone marrow suppression, rash, dysgeusia) was observed relatively frequently in these trials and D-penicillamine is not used as an antifibrogenic agent in adults. In addition to their anti-inflammatory effects, glucocorticoids are believed to decrease collagen synthesis by different mechanisms. However, the unacceptable systemic effects of long-term glucocorticoid therapy (including osteoporosis) preclude its aggressive use to treat hepatic fibrogenesis. Antioxidants (e.g. vitamin E) have been shown to reduce fibrogenesis in animal models of cirrhosis induced by chemical agents, possibly by the reduction of lipid peroxide products that can stimulate collagen synthesis in hepatic stellate cells. Studies in adults with hepatitis C viral infection suggest a reduction in stellate cell activation and the extracellular matrix during vitamin E therapy. Further evaluation of the potential use of antioxidants in cholestatic liver disease is in progress.

Understanding the role of the hepatic stellate cell in the progressive fibrosis associated with many cholestatic disorders may lead to new treatment strategies to prevent ongoing cellular injury and interrupt fibrogenesis. While a number of antifibrogenic agents that target stellate cells are in the development phase and may prove to be beneficial in the future, the role of antifibrotic agents in the treatment of cholestatic disorders requires further study. The development of new agents to reduce fibrogenesis based on the molecular mechanisms of fibrogenesis will hopefully lead to more effective medical therapy to prevent progression to cirrhosis.

Transfer of bile constituents into systemic circulation

Defective hepatocyte canilicular transport results in hepatocyte retention of components of bile, with leakage or transport of these substances into the hepatic sinusoid, raising serum levels of bile acids, bilirubin, and triglycerides. Additionally, transfer of biliary phospholipids into plasma may lead to increased circulating levels of cholesterol and triglycerides. Other mechanisms contributing to elevated systemic concentrations of bile acids, cholesterol, and triglycerides include decreased uptake of bile acids by the hepatocyte, downregulation of basolateral bile acid transporters, and alterations in cholesterol synthesis and metabolism. Evidence suggests that, during cholestasis, hepatocytes demonstrate decreased uptake of bile acids owing to downregulation of the Na^+-taurocholate cotransporting polypeptide on the basolateral membrane. While this altered uptake may play a hepatoprotective role by preventing further accumulation of toxic bile acids in the hepatocyte, it further contributes to the systemic elevation of bile acids. The mechanisms underlying elevated serum levels of bile acids, cholesterol, and triglyceride may be complex, but the end result leads to significant and debilitating complications, including pruritus, fatigue, hyperlipidemia, and cutaneous xanthomas.

Pruritus

Pruritus is a distressing manifestation of both intrahepatic and extrahepatic cholestasis. Its severity can vary from mild with no interference of normal activities, to moderate with disturbance of sleep, to severe and intractable [21]. Because of incessant scratching, the resulting open skin lesions may predispose to secondary bacterial skin infections (particularly staphylococcal and streptococcal) and disfiguring scars. Interference with sleep at night and the inability to concentrate and be attentive at school may impair normal development and school performance. In adults, severe pruritus has driven some patients with PBC to contemplate suicide. Unremitting severe pruritus may, in itself, be an indication for liver transplantation. Usually, the pruritus is generalized, with the palms and soles, extensor surfaces of the extremities, face and ears, and upper trunk most severely affected. Children with paucity of interlobular bile duct disorders, PFIC, unsuccessful or failing portoenterostomy for treatment of biliary atresia, PSC, cholestatic forms of autoimmune chronic hepatitis, and benign recurrent intrahepatic cholestasis appear to be most severely affected with pruritus. Patients with bile acid synthesis and metabolism defects generally do not experience pruritus.

Pathogenesis

The pathogenesis of the pruritus of cholestasis is poorly understood [21]. Penicillate intraepidermal nerve endings, which arise from unmyelinated subepidermal free nerve endings, have been implicated as the sensor that mediates general pruritus; however, the mediators that stimulate these nerve endings during cholestasis are still unknown. Earlier studies had suggested that elevated serum and skin concentration of bile acids were responsible, but a direct causal relationship between itching and bile acid levels in skin and/or serum has not been confirmed. Other evidence refuting the role of bile acids in pruritus is the reduction of pruritus in patients with uremia and polycythemia vera by cholestyramine treatment, disease states not associated with bile acid retention. However, the absence of pruritus in children with bile acid synthesis defects and those with low serum concentrations of bile acids, despite significant cholestasis, argues for a role of circulating bile acids.

There is a significant component of the pruritus that may be of central neurogenic origin, possibly involving the opiate receptor system. This is based on the observation that pruritus is a recognized side effect of morphine and other opiate receptor agonists. Indeed, physicians who use meperidine for sedation prior to procedures are familiar with the "itching of the nose" behavior associated with the administration of this medication. This opioid-associated pruritus is reversed by opiate receptor antagonists (naloxone) but not by antihistamines. The central effect of opiates is mediated via opiate receptors in the brain. Bergasa *et al.* [17] injected serum from patients with PBC into the medullary dorsal horn of monkeys and induced itching, which was blocked by the opioid-receptor antagonist, naloxone. In a rat model of cholestasis, binding of a selective μ-opioid receptor ligand to μ-opioid receptors is altered in cholestasis. These μ-opioid receptors are downregulated, suggesting that cholestasis may be associated with chronically elevated levels of endogenous opioids. In chronic cholestatic liver disease, nalmefene, a specific oral opiate receptor antagonist, produces symptoms strikingly similar to the "withdrawal reaction" of opiate addiction. This observation suggests that patients with cirrhosis and impaired hepatocellular function are chronically exposed to increased levels of endogenous opiate receptor agonists, and it is further supported by the finding of elevated levels of the endogenous opiate ligands met-enkephalins and leu-enkephalins, in these patients. Furthermore, other evidence suggests that these elevated plasma levels of pentapeptide enkephalins allow them to cross the blood–brain barrier. Preliminary reports on the beneficial effects of opiate receptor antagonists (naloxone and nalmefene) in the pruritus of cholestasis likewise support the concept that increased availability of endogenous opiate ligands at central opiate receptors may stimulate the pruritus of cholestasis.

Experimental evidence has implicated the lysophospholipase autotaxin and its product, lysophosphatidic acid, as potential mediators of cholestatic pruritus [22]. In a recent study increased serum autotaxin was specific for pruritus of cholestasis but not for other pruritus-associated disorders such as uremia or Hodgkin disease. Rifampin treatment significantly reduced itch intensity and autotaxin activity in cholestatic patients with pruritus. In vitro studies showed that this effect required the expression of PXR. Other effective treatments for severe, refractory pruritus using the molecular adsorbents recirculation system or nasobiliary drainage improved itch intensity and was correlated with the reduction of autotaxin levels.

Findings advancing roles for lysophosphatidic acid and opioids in the pathogenesis of pruritus in cholestasis may not be mutually exclusive. Both mediators may be involved.

Treatment

The therapeutic agents most commonly used for pruritus in cholestasis are oral bile acid-binding resins (cholestyramine or colestipol), phenobarbital, rifampicin, UDCA, and carbamazepine [23]. Cool baths, moisturizers, topical steroid creams, topical anesthetics, antihistamines, and sedatives have offered little long-term relief, although they may be of temporary benefit in individual patients. In small children, fingernails should be trimmed, long-sleeve nightshirts worn, and occasionally the hands covered securely with stockings at night to minimize the effects of scratching. Plasmapharesis and ultraviolet light treatment have improved pruritus in adults with PBC. The possible use of opioid antagonists is being explored. Finally, partial biliary diversion, ileal exclusion, and liver transplantation are considered when all other therapeutic options have been exhausted.

Non-absorbable ion exchange resins

Cholestyramine, colestipol, and colesevelam hydrochloride are non-absorbable anion exchange resins that bind bile acids, cholesterol, many drugs, and presumably other toxic agents in the intestinal lumen, thereby increasing fecal excretion of these substances [23]. These bile acid-binding agents interrupt the enterohepatic circulation of bile acids, decreasing the negative feedback to the liver, enhancing conversion of cholesterol to bile acids, and possibly stimulating a choleresis. Because of the possible long-term benefit of reducing hepatic accumulation of potentially toxic bile acids, these agents are recommended for long-term management of intrahepatic cholestatic disorders. Because cholestyramine relieves pruritus without causing a change in serum bile acids, it is possible that it also removes other anionic molecules that may be contributing to pruritus.

Cholestyramine and colestipol are usually administered mixed with juice or water at a daily dose of 0.25–0.50 g/kg, given either before and after breakfast when bile flow is maximal or, less commonly, divided among two or three daily meals. Colestipol appears to be better tolerated than cholestyramine; however, cholestyramine bars are now available and are more palatable. No other medications or vitamins should be given orally for the 2 hours preceding or following administration of these resins because of the risk of binding to the resin and impaired absorption. Several other factors limit the use of cholestyramine and colestipol: the unpalatable nature of the compounds (which may lead to poor compliance); increased steatorrhea and fat-soluble vitamin deficiency because of further reduction in the already low concentrations of free bile acids in the intestinal lumen; constipation; intestinal obstruction from inspissation of the drug; and hyperchloremic metabolic acidosis. In a double-blind, randomized, placebo-controlled trial, the potent bile acid sequestrant colesevelam was not effective in treating cholestatic pruritus [24]. These compounds are generally contraindicated in the infant with biliary atresia and a Roux-en-Y portoenterostomy because of the risk that the compound may accumulate in and obstruct the reconstructed biliary intestinal conduit, leading to ascending cholangitis.

Rifampicin

Studies suggest that rifampicin, an antibiotic for tuberculosis, is an effective treatment for severe pruritus in PBC and in children with chronic cholestatic liver disease. In a comparison of rifampicin with phenobarbital for treatment of pruritus in biliary cirrhosis, 19 out of 21 patients who completed a 2-week course of rifampicin (10 mg/kg daily) had significant relief from pruritus compared with only 8 of 18 who took phenobarbital (3 mg/kg daily) [25]. For both drugs, relief of pruritus occurred after the first week of administration and both had similar effects in lowering serum aminotransferase levels and in inducing hepatic microsomal function. Rifampicin, however, reduced alkaline phosphatase, GGT, and serum bile acid levels, which did not respond to phenobarbital. Yerushalmi et al. [26] treated 24 children with cholestasis with rifampin (10 mg/kg daily, in two divided doses). After an average of 18 months of therapy, 10 patients had a complete response and 12 patients had a partial response as assessed by a clinical scoring system. Treatment was associated with a reduction in GGT and no clinical or biochemical toxicity of rifampin was observed. Complete response was more common in children with extrahepatic cholestasis (e.g. biliary atresia) than intrahepatic cholestasis (64% versus 10%).

Rifampicin is a ligand for PXR, which activates many pathways for biotransformation [22,23]. Proposed mechanisms for the effect of rifampicin on pruritus include enhancement of multidrug-resistance protein 2 production, activation of enzymes (UDP-glucuronosyltransferase-1A and cytochrome P4503A4), and stimulation of 6α-hydroxylation of bile acids, thereby promoting urinary excretion of dihydroxy and monohydroxy bile acids. The capacity to reduce lysophosphatidic acid levels may be more important than its effects on bile acid metabolism. Despite the apparent amelioration of pruritus with rifampicin, its propensity for toxic hepatitis requires careful monitoring. The other potential adverse effects associated with its use are drug interactions, hemolytic anemia, and renal failure. We have been very pleased with the response of children with a variety of cholestatic disorders to rifampicin treatment.

Opioid antagonists

Given the theory that cholestasis-associated pruritus may be caused by centrally mediated increased opioid tone, the use of several opioid antagonists have been investigated, including naloxone, nalmefene, and naltrexone. A small cross-over study in eight patients with PBC and a larger double-blind, controlled, cross-over trial in 29 patients with liver diseases of various causes demonstrated marked improvement in pruritus during intravenous, 24-hour naloxone infusions compared with placebo [17]. Mild neuropsychiatric disturbances, described as "ill-defined anxiety", were reported in four

patients in the larger study and no patients in the pilot study. This complication may be explained by a mild opiate withdrawal effect in the presence of the chronic increased opioid tone postulated to exist in patients with cholestasis. Because of the opioid receptor specificity of naloxone, these findings support the hypothesis that a mechanism underlying the pruritus of cholestasis is modulated by endogenous opioids. Although effective, naloxone has several limitations for long-term use, including a short half-life and large first-pass metabolism, which necessitate intravenous administration.

Nalmefene, another opioid antagonist, has a longer duration of action compared with naloxone and can be given orally, however, at the present time it is only available in the USA as a parenteral product. In an initial report of 11 patients with cirrhosis, nalmefene therapy (starting at a dose of 5 mg/day and gradually increasing to a maximum of 20–40 mg three times daily) resulted in a significant reduction in patient's pruritus scores and sense of fatigue. Distressingly, all 11 patients experienced withdrawal reactions consisting of nausea, abdominal pain, diaphoresis, tremor, and occasional hallucinations. Larger doses of nalmefene (up to 300 mg) given to healthy subjects have not produced withdrawal reactions, once again supporting the theory of increased opioid tone in patients with cholestasis-associated pruritus. A recent open-label trial of oral nalmefene also demonstrated a beneficial effect in relieving pruritus, but with fewer side adverse reactions reported [17]. In this study of 14 adults with cholestasis, the initial starting dose was 2 mg twice a day and was gradually increased, over 2–4 weeks, until a satisfactory clinical response was achieved (average maintenance dose was 60 mg/day, with a range of 20–240 mg/day) and continued for 2 to 26 months. Only five patients experienced withdrawal-like reactions, which did not preclude continuation of therapy. A significant decrease in visual analogue scores was noted in 13 patients and a decrease in scratching activity was noted in 12. Possible tolerance occurred in three patients and three patients experienced a marked exacerbation of pruritus after therapy was suddenly discontinued. This uncontrolled study suggests that orally administered nalmefene is of benefit to patients with cholestasis-associated pruritus and is associated with fewer withdrawal reactions with the lower starting dose.

The opioid antagonists investigated to date have severe limitations. Naloxone has a short half-life and can only be administered parenterally, while nalmefene treatment is associated with a severe opiate withdrawal reaction and is not currently licensed for clinical use. These limitations have prompted investigation of other opioid antagonists. Naltrexone is an opiate receptor antagonist with a bioavailability and half-life that lies between that of naloxone and nalmefene, and it can be administered orally. It is a structural analogue of naloxone and nalmefene that undergoes extensive first pass metabolism; however, the main metabolite, 6β-naltrexol, reaches a higher plasma levels than the parent drug and exerts long-lasting opiate antagonist activity. A large, double-blind, placebo-controlled study demonstrated significant decreases in both daytime and night-time itching (as recorded by the patient using the visual analogue scale) [27]. In this study, 16 adults with cholestasis were randomized with eight receiving oral naltrexone (50 mg/day for 4 weeks) and eight receiving placebo. Compared with the placebo group, the naltrexone-treated group had significantly decreased pruritus scores at the end of treatment, with associated improvement in sleep satisfaction and less fatigue compared with baseline scores prior to treatment. Withdrawal reactions were noted in four patients in the treatment group but were generally transient, with the exception of one patient who required discontinuation of treatment. Naltrexone may be an effective alternative therapy for patients with cholestasis-associated pruritus unresponsive to other antipruritics; however, larger, long-term studies are needed. The initial concerns over possible hepatotoxicity of naltrexone in studies of alcoholism were not validated in a review of adults. Nausea (9%) and headaches (6%) were the most common side effects of naltrexone.

The use of opioid antagonists may provide an effective alternative treatment for patients with severe pruritus unresponsive to other therapies; however, the significant side effects and withdrawal reactions may severely limit the general use of these medications. Further placebo-controlled trials are needed to determine safety, proper dosage, and long-term efficacy in children with cholestatic liver disease. Concerns regarding the effects of chronic opioid antagonism in the developing brain will also need to be addressed.

Phenobarbital

In addition to its choleretic effects, phenobarbital therapy has been beneficial in improving cholestasis-associated pruritus [23]. The mechanism of action in ameliorating pruritus is not entirely clear. The antipruritic action of phenobarbital has been demonstrated without corresponding decreases in circulating levels of bile acids, suggesting that the effect of phenobarbital may not be entirely explained by a decrease in bile acid levels. However, through microsomal enzyme stimulation and excretory enhancement, phenobarbital may eliminate another, as of yet unidentified, pruritogenic substance. The beneficial effect of phenobarbital in relieving cholestasis-associated pruritus has been demonstrated in a number of cholestatic disorders including adults with PBC and children with intrahepatic cholestasis. However, studies comparing the efficacy of phenobarbital with other antipruritics have not been as favorable. Rifampin appeared to improve cholestasis-associated pruritus to a greater degree and with fewer side effects than phenobarbital. As mentioned above, the sedative effects, irritability, and altered performance associated with phenobarbital therapy are undesirable and limit its chronic use in children.

Ursodeoxycholic acid

As discussed above, UDCA is a potent choleretic and has been shown to improve biochemical parameters associated with several cholestatic disorders [13]. Preliminary data in children

with chronic intrahepatic cholestasis suggest that UDCA administration may similarly result in significant improvement in refractory pruritus. However, in infants with biliary atresia and poor bile drainage following portoenterostomy, administration of UDCA may worsen pruritus and possibly lead to a significant worsening of liver dysfunction. The other side effect reported in children has been occasional diarrhea.

Partial biliary diversion and ileal exclusion

Partial external diversion of bile is being used as a treatment for refractory pruritus in children with severe intrahepatic cholestasis [28,29]. This surgical procedure consists of the construction of a 10–15 cm jejunal conduit from the dome of the gallbladder to the abdominal wall. The gallbladder is anastomosed end to side to the blind proximal portion of a jejunal conduit with the distal end of the conduit brought out to the skin as a permanent cutaneous stoma. Others have described using the appendix as a conduit between the gallbladder and skin. The bile collected in the stoma appliance is discarded. Of six patients with refractory pruritus who had this diversion, four with progressive intrahepatic cholestasis had complete clinical remission from pruritus within 48 hours of surgery and had no recurrence of itching in the 3–8 years of follow-up. There was also significant reversal of biochemical markers of cholestasis in these four children. The two patients with Alagille syndrome, in contrast, showed partial clinical improvement after 1–2 weeks and had mild, persistent itching after surgery [28]. Partial external biliary diversion has been combined with UDCA therapy in two children with Alagille syndrome and one with idiopathic intrahepatic cholestasis and has provided relief after failure of UDCA therapy alone. In a small study, partial biliary diversion led to resolution of pruritus, serum markers of cholestasis, and decreased progression of hepatic fibrosis in children with PFIC type 1 after a follow-up of 1–13 years [29]. Our own experience in five patients with PFIC has also been very favorable, with resolution of pruritus, normalization of liver blood tests, reversal of portal fibrosis, and improved growth following partial biliary diversion. Surprisingly, the characteristic granular inclusions ("Byler's bile") in caniliculi disappeared in electron micrographs of liver biopsies following the operation.

The mechanism by which this procedure produces these results is poorly understood. It is not known if a toxin in bile is discarded, if hepatic bile acid metabolism is altered, or if another process is taking place. Recently, it has been shown that the ileal bile acid transporter is upregulated in FIC1 disease, providing an explanation for the significant cholestasis and elevated bile acids in this disorder as well as providing a rationale for the use of biliary diversion. Partial external biliary diversion or ileal exclusion is an option that should be considered in planning the management of children with progressive intrahepatic cholestasis, particularly in those with intractable pruritus uncontrolled by medical therapy.

Ileal exclusion is a surgical internal ileal–colonic bypass of the distal ileum, which results in an interruption of the enterohepatic circulation of bile acids by the failure of bile acids to be actively transported in the terminal ileum. In patients who have undergone cholecystectomy, ileal exclusion has been suggested as an alternative for increasing fecal excretion of bile acids and reducing pruritus. Others have now used this surgery as primary therapy. Initial studies suggest that ileal exclusion may be as effective as partial biliary diversion (and cosmetically more acceptable to the child and family); however, its benefits may diminish over time. Further experience comparing these two procedures will be needed in order to develop solid recommendations.

Recently, nasobiliary drainage has been employed to effectively reduce pruritus in patients with exacerbations of benign recurrent intrahepatic cholestasis, a milder form of FIC1 and BSEP diseases. Ultraviolet light and the molecular adsorbent recirculating system have also been used with variable success [23].

Fatigue

It has long been appreciated that significant fatigue is associated with chronic cholestatic liver disease, particularly in adults, often out of proportion to that explained by chronic illness alone. Indeed, fatigue is the most common symptom reported by patients with PBC (in up to 80%). In addition, fatigue has been shown to adversely impact on job performance and family life and has been significantly associated with depression in PBC. The mechanism underlying fatigue in chronic cholestasis is unknown. Altered behavioral state has been linked to hepatic function as demonstrated by hepatic encephalopathy, where altered neurotransmission may play a role. The recent evidence that increased central opioid tone may play a role in cholestasis-associated pruritus suggests that altered central neurotransmission may play a role in other behavioral manifestations of cholestasis, such as fatigue. Studies by Swain and Maric suggest that this may in fact be the case [30]. The authors showed an abnormal pattern of behavior and altered function of the hypothalamic–pituitary–adrenal axis coexist in rats with cholestasis secondary to bile duct ligation, and they postulated that this might be implicated in the mediation of fatigue. It is interesting to note that an alteration of hypothalamic function has also been postulated to contribute to the hyperpigmentation in patients with PBC. The authors demonstrated that cholestatic rats, as compared with sham-operated controls, were more easily fatigued and spent a significantly longer time floating (as opposed to active swimming) when placed in a swim tank [30]. The administration of LY293284, a 5-hydroxytryptamine-1A receptor agonist [30], did not affect floating times in controls but corrected the prolonged floating times in cholestatic rats. This finding was interpreted as suggesting that the abnormal behavior state was attributable to altered transmission in serotonin neural pathways on which this receptor is located, and that it could be corrected by enhancing neurotransmission in these pathways. The preliminary studies regarding serotonin

neurotransmission are novel and will require further investigation. Other factors that may be involved in the fatigue associated with cholestatic liver disease include altered sleep patterns caused by pruritus, chronic disease, depression, chronic anemia, or poor nutritional status. The clinical manifestations of fatigue are more difficult to delineate in children with cholestasis; however, following liver transplant, parents frequently report that their child is more energetic, participates in new activities, and demonstrates improved school performance.

Hyperlipidemia/xanthomas

Hyperlipidemia and xanthomas are common consequences of severe intrahepatic cholestasis (e.g. Alagille syndrome) but are less severe in biliary atresia. With increasing impairment of bile flow during cholestasis, the plasma concentration of circulating lipidoproteins and individual lipids increase. The primary event is the regurgitation into plasma of biliary phospholipids, which produce secondary effects leading to an increase in plasma cholesterol perhaps through enhanced hepatic synthesis of cholesterol [31]. The cholesterol is transported in the blood in lipoprotein X, an unusual vesicular form of lipoprotein specific to cholestasis. Lecithin–cholesterol acyltransferase activity is also diminished during cholestasis, further altering lipoprotein metabolism. These pertubations can cause severe hypercholesterolemia (serum cholesterol 1000–2000 mg/dL) leading to cholesterol deposition in skin, mucous membranes, and arteries. The disfiguring effect of xanthomas on fine motor function of affected fingers and on self-image (Figure 9.1) should not be underestimated in young, developing children. The risk for atherosclerosis in children with chronic cholestasis is not known; however, severe hypercholesterolemia in Alagille syndrome has been associated with renal lipidoses, causing renal failure, and with atheromatous plaque deposition in the aorta within the first few years of life [31]. Atherosclerosis has been reported in adults with hypercholesterolemia caused by cholestasis but there does not appear to be an increased risk of atherosclerosis in women with PBC compared with healthy women. With longer survival in children with chronic cholestasis and hyperlipidemia associated with immunosuppressive drugs after liver transplantation, more attention may need to be focused on measures to reduce serum cholesterol levels in children with cholestatic disorders.

Treatment

Treatment is directed at increasing conversion of cholesterol to bile acids, reducing biliary regurgitation into the systemic circulation, and enhancing the elimination of bile acids and cholesterol. In general, the efficacy of therapeutic agents depends on generating increased bile flow and, therefore, requires a patent biliary tract. In some conditions, such as Alagille syndrome, spontaneous improvement in bile flow after age 2–3 years may lead to reduction of serum lipids.

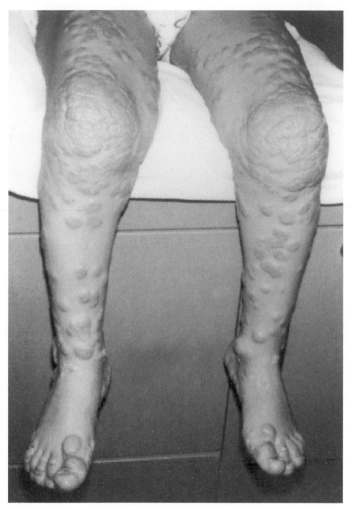

Figure 9.1 Extensive cutaneous xanthomas in a 4-year-old child with Alagille syndrome whose serum cholesterol levels were between 1000 and 2000 mg/dL.

Partial external diversion of bile has been effective in some children with xanthomas associated with intrahepatic cholestasis [3].

Non-absorbable ion exchange resins

Cholestyramine, colestipol, and colesevelam hydrochloride interrupt the enterohepatic circulation of bile acids by binding to intraluminal bile acids and increasing fecal excretion, thus decreasing negative feedback to the liver mediated through FXR and enhancing conversion of cholesterol to bile acids. The up-regulation of low density lipoprotein (LDL) receptors may also increase clearance of circulating LDL. Although these bile acid-binding resins effectively lower serum bile acid concentrations in most patients, a similar effect on serum cholesterol is not noted as frequently. The dose used and side effects are the same as for the treatment of pruritus mentioned previously.

Ursodeoxycholic acid

Cholesterol and lipoprotein metabolism are affected by UDCA in several ways. It directly stimulates receptor-dependent LDL uptake in the liver, decreases hydroxymethylglutaryl-CoA

(HMG-CoA) reductase activity, and indirectly decreases cholesterol absorption from the intestine by causing a marked reduction in the secretion of cholesterol into the bile. Encouraging results have been seen in some children with idiopathic intrahepatic cholestasis and with Alagille syndrome with resolution of xanthomas. These data suggest that UDCA therapy may significantly reduce hypercholesterolemia in children with chronic intrahepatic cholestasis. However, the resulting serum cholesterol levels are still higher than those in the normal population.

Cholesterol synthesis-blocking agents

Cholesterol synthesis-blocking agents (lovastatin, simvastatin) are effective in lowering serum cholesterol in familial heterozygous and non-familial hypercholesterolemia. The mechanism of action of these drugs centers on inhibition of HMG-CoA reductase, the rate-limiting enzyme in cholesterol synthesis. Studies have demonstrated that these statins have a synergistic effect with UDCA in reducing biliary cholesterol output and binary cholesterol saturation index, but they do not effect bile acid metabolism. Because these agents do little to the underlying pathophysiology in cholestasis and because of potential hepatotoxicity, they currently play little role in treating hypercholesterolemia in pediatric cholestasis.

Diet and other agents

Low cholesterol and saturated fat diets have been ineffective in reducing serum cholesterol in cholestatic patients unresponsive to bile acid-binding resins and phenobarbital. Moreover, restriction of fat in the diet will make the diet less palatable and lower dietary caloric content, thereby exacerbating the malnutrition common in cholestatic children. Other cholesterol-lowering agents (e.g. L-thyroxine, clofibrate) have likewise been unsuccessful in our experience. The serum lipid-lowering effect of phenobarbital appears to be modest; therefore its use must be counterbalanced by its effects of sedation, irritability, and drug interaction. Future studies may determine whether plasmapheresis or partial ileal bypass, therapies that have successfully lowered serum cholesterol in adults with familial and non-familial hypercholesterolemia, will be effective in cholestasis and whether these therapies are practical in selected cases. Partial biliary diversion and ileal exclusion have successfully reduced serum lipids in selected patients with Alagille syndrome (those patients without bridging fibrosis or cirrhosis on liver biopsy) [32]. Lastly, liver transplantation has been succesful in relieving hypercholesterolemia and reversing xanthomas in refractory cases.

Reduced delivery of bile to the intestine causing malabsorption

Steatorrhea, malnutrition, and growth failure

Malnutrition is a frequent complication in cholestatic children. Because of defects in the intraluminal phase of fat digestion, steatorrhea is invariably present in children with severe

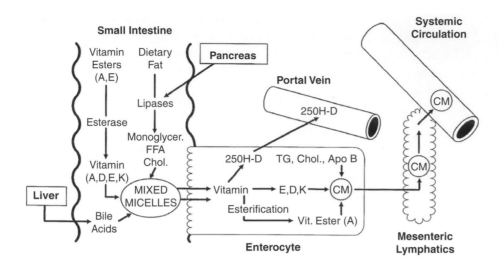

Figure 9.2 Pathways of absorption of dietary fat and the fat-soluble vitamins. FFA, free fatty acids; monoglycer., monoglycerides; TG, triglycerides; Apo B, apolipoprotein B; chol., cholesterol; CM, chylomicrons.

cholestasis and is one important cause of malnutrition. In addition, other factors that contribute to the malnutrition of chronic cholestasis include abnormalities in amino acid and glucose metabolism, increased resting energy expenditure, recurrent infections, anorexia and early satiety, gastroesophageal reflux, or vomiting secondary to compression of abdominal viscera by the enlarged liver, spleen, or ascites.

Bile acids are important amphipathic molecules that aid in the solubilization of dietary fat, allowing the interaction between pancreatic lipase and colipase that is essential for hydrolysis of dietary lipids. The monoglycerides and free fatty acids produced are then incorporated into mixed micelles, formed in the presence of bile acids and transported across the aqueous luminal environment into the intestinal epithelium (Figure 9.2). The decreased delivery of bile acids to the duodenum during cholestasis may lead to intraluminal bile acid concentrations that are inadequate for the formation of micelles, resulting in the malabsorption of dietary lipids and the fat-soluble vitamins.

Recent evidence suggests that children with liver disease have alterations in the growth hormone axis. The liver is an important endocrine organ producing factors such as insulin-like growth factor-1 (IGF-1) and IGF-binding proteins 1, 2, and 3 in response to stimulation by growth hormone. The majority of circulating IGF-1 is derived from liver and appears to mediate the anabolic actions of growth hormone. The production of normal levels of IGF-1 depends on normal liver function. In children with end-stage liver disease, IGF-1 levels fall to undetectable levels and serum growth hormone is increased [33]. Additionally, IGF-binding proteins 1 and 2 are elevated, while IGF-binding protein 3 is low. The low levels of IGF-1 and IGF-binding protein 3 despite high growth hormone levels suggests that resistance to growth hormone is present in chronic liver failure. Additionally, treatment of children with end-stage liver disease awaiting transplant and taking recombinant human growth hormone did not appear to improve body composition or growth.

Aside from the debilitation attributed to generalized and specific nutrient deficiencies, malnutrition has been associated with decreased brain growth, impairment of mental development, and decreased immunocompetence, with increased susceptibility of infection. For example, the severity of malnutrition and poor growth in children with biliary atresia before liver transplant is predictive of cognitive performance years after transplantation. Therefore, to improve neurocognitive outcomes, an aggressive approach to nutritional support is essential in the care of the pediatric patient with chronic liver disease. A summary of nutritional assessment, therapies, and potential side effects of the therapies are listed in Table 9.3.

Nutritional assessment

Nutritional assessment should be initiated at the first visit of the cholestatic child and used to monitor effects of nutritional rehabilitation [34]. Although helpful in following growth and development of normal children, serial weight for age, height for age, and weight-for-height measurements are less reliable for children with chronic liver disease [35]. Weight gain may result from hepatosplenomegaly and ascites and from excessive tissue sequestration of water because of poor intravascular colloid osmotic status, renal retention of salt and water, and hyperaldosteronism. Therefore, weight-for-age and weight-for-height measurements may incorrectly indicate better nutritional status than is present. The utility of serial height-for-age plots is likewise reduced in some infants and children with chronic cholestasis if the underlying disease (e.g. Alagille syndrome, familial cholestasis) influences growth independent of nutritional status. Instead, serial estimates of body fat using triceps and subcapsular skinfold thickness, and of body protein using midarm muscle circumference, compared with age-matched and height-matched normal values are a better estimation of nutritional status during chronic liver disease [35]. Other means of assessing body composition (e.g. dual

Table 9.3 Guidelines for nutritional management in chronic cholestasis

Nutritional factor	Index of assessment	Treatment options	Toxicity
Energy	Anthropometrics, triceps and subscapular skinfold thickness, serial measurements of weight/height, indirect calorimetry, fat malabsorption	Caloric goal: 125% of RDA based on weight for height at 50th percentile Glucose polymers (Polycose powder or solution) to ↑ to 24–27 cal/oz formula Supplemental night-time nasogastric drip feedings MCT infant formulae (Pregestimil, Alimentum) MCT oil supplements: 1–2 mL/kg daily in 2–4 doses	Financial burden, essential fatty acid deficiency Aspiration pneumonia
Essential fatty acids	Deficiency: triene:tetraene ratio >0.3, ↓ linoleic acid	Corn oil or oral lipid emulsions IV lipid emulsions	
Protein	Mid-arm muscle circumference, serum albumin, prealbumin, RBP, transferrin	Infants: protein intake 2–3 g/kg per day Hepatic encephalopathy: protein intake 0.5–1.0 g/kg per day Branched-chain amino acid supplements	Unknown
Fat-soluble vitamins			
Vitamin A	Deficiency: retinol:RBP molar ratio <0.8 or serum retinol < 20 mg/dL; relative dose response; conjunctival impression cytology; xerosis, Bitot spots, etc.	5000–25 000 U/day orally of water-miscible preparation of vit. A	Hepatotoxicity, pseudotumor cerebri, bone lesions, hypercalcemia
Vitamin D	Deficiency: calcifidiol <14 ng/mL	Vit. D (Drisdol), 3–10× RDA for age Rickets: calcifidiol (Calderol), 3–5 mg/kg per day Osteomalacia: calcitriol (Rocaltrol), 0.05–0.2 mg/kg per day	Hypercalcemia Hypercalcemia, nephrocalcinosis
Vitamin E	Deficiency: vit. E:total lipid ratio <0.6 mg/g (age <1 year), <0.8 mg/g (age >1 year)	α-Tocopherol (acetate) 25–200 IU/kg per day TPGS (Liqui E), 15–25 IU/kg per day	Potentiation of vit. K deficiency coagulopathy, diarrhea, hyperosmolality (TPGS)
Vitamin K	Deficiency: prolonged prothrombin time, Elevated PIVKA-II	Mephyton, 2.5 mg twice/wk to 5.0 mg/d AquaMEPHYTON (IM) 2–5 mg every 4 wk	
Water-soluble vitamins		Prevent deficiency of water-soluble vitamins dose: 1–2× RDA	Fat-soluble vitamin toxicity
Minerals and trace elements			
Calcium	Deficiency in steatorrhea despite corrected vit. D status	25–100 mg/kg per day up to 800–1200 mg/day	Hypercalcemia, hypercalciuria
Phosphorus	Low serum phosphorus despite corrected vit. D and calcium status	25–50 mg/kg per day up to 500 mg/day	Gastrointestinal intolerance
Magnesium	Deficiency: serum Mg <1.4 mEq/L	Magnesium oxide, 1–2 mEq/kg daily orally or 50% solution of magnesium sulfate, 0.3–0.5 mEq/kg IV over 3 hours (max. 3–6 mEq)	Respiratory depression, lethargy, coma
Zinc	Deficiency: plasma zinc <60 μg/dL	Zinc sulfate solution (10 mg/mL elemental zinc) 1 mg/kg/d orally for 2–3 mo	↓ Intestinal absorption of copper and iron
Selenium	Deficiency: plasma Se <40 μg/L	1–2 μg/kg per day oral sodium selenite or 1–2 μg/kg per day Se in TPN	Dermatologic changes (skin eruptions, pathologic nails, hair loss), dyspepsia, diarrhea, anorexia
Iron	Deficiency: ↓ serum iron, ↑ total iron-binding capacity, iron saturation index <16%	5–6 mg/kg per day elemental iron	Teeth staining, hemorrhagic gastroenteritis, metabolic acidosis, coma, liver failure

↑, increased; ↓, decreased; IM, intramuscularly; IV, intravenous; MCT, medium-chain triglyceride; PIVKA-II, protein induced in vitamin K absence; RBP, retinol-binding protein; RDA, recommended daily allowance; TPGS, tocopherol polyethylene glycol-1000 succinate; TPN, total parenteral nutrition.

electron X-ray absorptiometry) may provide additional information but are most useful in a research setting. Measurement of visceral protein status (serum albumin, prealbumin, retinol-binding protein, and transferrin) may also be helpful; however, liver synthetic failure and vitamin A deficiency may confound interpretation of these tests. Retinol-binding protein and pre-albumin, with half-lives of 12 hours and 2 days, respectively, respond rapidly and are useful parameters to follow during nutritional repletion. Indirect calorimetry may be utilized to estimate oxygen consumption and caloric requirements if weight gain is poor despite seemingly adequate caloric intake.

Hepatic osteodystrophy

Metabolic bone disease associated with chronic liver disease is frequently referred to as hepatic osteodystrophy [36,37]. It is characterized by reduced formation and increased resorption of bone; chronic cholestasis and advanced cirrhosis are major risk factors. In children the term encompasses not only low bone mineral density and fractures but also rickets (vitamin D deficiency of growing bone), spine abnormalities, and growth failure. The process depletes existing bone mass and also damages growth plates, leading to short stature. Fractures occur in 10–28% of children prior to orthotopic liver transplantation and in 12–38% after the transplant. Pathogenetic mechanisms in the cholestatic child are multifactorial and only partially understood. They include genetic factors, abnormalities of calcium, vitamin D, vitamin K and bilirubin metabolism, IGF-1 deficiency, hypogonadism, drugs harmful to bone, lifestyle factors (such as immobility), malnutrition, and low body mass index.

Bone mineral density generally improves after liver transplantation in long-term follow-up studies. However, bone loss after transplantation may continue owing to the adverse effects of immunosuppressive drugs (glucocorticoids and calcineurin inhibitors) on bone remodeling.

Nutritional therapy

Malnutrition is common in children with end-stage liver disease and so nutritional support assumes an important role in children awaiting orthotopic liver transplantation. Indeed, one component of pediatric end-stage liver disease is growth failure (weight and height <2 standard deviations below the mean). In a prospective study of 100 infants with biliary atresia, growth failure after portoenterostomy was associated with transplantation or death by 24 months of age [38]. Most patients (82%) in the "good outcome" group were receiving nutritional supplementation at the time of portoenterostomy versus only 36% of the patients in the "poor outcome" group [39,40].

Energy

In the presence of steatorrhea and increased energy expenditure, the goal for caloric intake should be approximately 125% of the recommended dietary allowance based on ideal body weight (50th percentile of weight for height). Additional calories may be needed to provide for catch-up growth if a significant deficit in weight is present. The infant formula can be mixed with less water to provide 24 or 27 kcal/ounce. Alternatively, glucose polymers (8 cal/5 mL; Polycose powder, Ross Laboratories, Columbus, OH, USA) or medium-chain triglycerides (MCT) oil (7.7 cal/mL; Mead Johnson, Evansville, IN, USA) can be added to the standard 20 cal/ounce dilution of the formula. Whenever possible, oral feeding is preferred, but with increasing anorexia and debilitation secondary to progressive liver disease, supplemental nocturnal nasogastric infusions may be required in order to meet caloric and fluid requirements and prevent or reverse inadequate weight gain, particularly in those children awaiting liver transplantation. The use of narrow-bore, soft, weighted silastic or polyurethane feeding tubes is generally well tolerated, with minimal risk of aspiration or upper gastrointestinal hemorrhage. Compared with bolus gavage feeding techniques, continuous formula infusion leads to better energy balance and reduces the hazard of significant regurgitation [41]. Nocturnal nasogastric feedings can be safely administered in the home. Because of portal hypertensive gastropathy and the development of gastric varices, gastrostomy tubes are not used in this setting. Occasionally, parenteral nutrition through an indwelling central venous catheter is required to assure adequate weight gain while a child is bridged to liver transplantation [40].

Fat

In general, infant formulae containing significant quantities of MCT, C_8–C_{12} fatty acids, will provide better energy balance during cholestasis. Unlike long-chain triglycerides, which require bile acid micelles for solubilization, MCT are relatively water soluble and directly absorbed into the portal circulation. For this reason, MCT oil-containing diets have been used successfully to reduce steatorrhea, improve energy balance, and promote growth in children with chronic cholestasis. Pregestimil (Mead Johnson) and Alimentum (Ross Laboratories, Columbus, OH, USA) are MCT oil-predominant formulae frequently used in cholestasis, containing approximately 60% and 50% of fat calories as MCT oil, respectively. Breast-fed infants with chronic cholestasis should be supplemented with these formulae if growth is not adequate. It is not unusual, however, that unremitting steatorrhea in the breast-fed cholestatic infant requires weaning to an MCT oil-containing formula as the only means of attaining adequate weight gain and growth if total fluid intake is limited by the child's appetite or because of ascites or organomegaly.

Protein

It is essential that adequate protein intake be preserved (2.0–3.0 g/kg daily in small infants) while delivering optimal energy intake. Plasma aminograms of patients with chronic cholestasis and cirrhosis are often abnormal; with low levels of branched-chain amino acids (BCAAs) and an elevated ratio of aromatic amino acids to BCAAs. These abnormalities reflect disturbed amino acid kinetics and relate to increased BCAA utilization in muscle, where, under the influence of hyperinsulinemia, they provide an alternative substrate source for gluconeogenesis, and to impaired hepatic enzymatic processing of aromatic amino acids. There is some evidence to suggest that diets relatively rich in BCAA may confer significant advantages in nutritional therapy for chronic liver disease. In an animal model of cholestasis, oral supplementation with BCAA improved nitrogen retention, body composition, and growth. Additionally, a randomized study in children with end-stage liver disease demonstrated improved nutritional status and body composition in those who were fed the BCAA-enriched formula. However, MCT-containing complete BCAA formulae are rather expensive and not readily available. If hepatic encephalopathy occurs, dogma is that daily protein intake may need to be limited to 0.5–1.0 g/kg. However, it has been recently shown that nutritional rehabilitation using enteral drip feedings (140% of recommended caloric intake, 4 g/kg per day protein) in children with severe chronic liver disease awaiting liver transplant led to improved nutritional status without hyperammonemia or adverse clinical and biochemical effects. This relatively large amount of protein was well tolerated although it did contain 31% of protein calories as BCAA. However, stable levels of plasma ammonia were not accompanied by any significant change in amino acid profiles during therapy. Our own clinical experience indicates that similar protein intakes of MCT oil-containing formulae are well tolerated without hyperammonemia or signs of hepatic encephalopathy unless liver failure is advanced.

Essential fatty acids

The combination of malabsorption of long-chain triglycerides and inadequate intake of energy can lead to essential fatty acid (EFA) deficiency [32,42]. The EFAs are those fatty acids that cannot be generated in mammalian organisms by desaturation and elongation of shorter fatty acids. Linoleic acid (18:2 omega-6) and linolenic acid (18:3 omega-3) are the two main EFAs. Arachidonic acid (20:4 omega-6), derived from linoleic acid, should also be considered an EFA. Deficiency of essential fatty acids may produce growth impairment, a dry scaly rash, thrombocytopenia, impair immune function, and inhibit eicosanoid pathways. These long-chain fatty acids are poorly absorbed if bile flow is diminished, as in chronic cholestasis. Since infants have small linoleic acid stores, fat malabsorption in cholestasis places them at a higher risk of developing EFA deficiency. In addition, ingested linoleic and linolenic acids may be preferentially oxidized for energy if caloric intake/absorption is inadequate. Importantly, Pregestimil (Mead Johnson Nutrition) and Alimentum (Abbott Nutrition) contain only 7–14% of calories, respectively, as linoleic acid. It is generally accepted that the minimum amount of linoleic acid necessary to prevent EFA deficiency is 3–4% of dietary calories. If 30–40% of dietary fat is malabsorbed during cholestasis, the absorbed amount of linoleic acid may be only borderline adequate using these infant formulae. Several reports document biochemical evidence (low linoleic acid levels, triene:tetraene ratio >0.3) [43] of EFA deficiency in infants with cholestasis receiving these types of formula. Clearly, other formulae containing 85% of fat calories as MCT oil and under 3% of calories as EFAs (e.g. Portagen; Mead Johnson) may induce EFA deficiency and should not be used in chronic cholestasis. Corn oil or safflower oil (linoleic acid 5.4 and 7.2 g/mL, respectively) can be added to foods, and lipid emulsions (e.g. Microlipid, 0.40 g linoleic acid/mL) can be added to formula to provide additional linoleic acid if needed. Linoleic acid levels and the plasma triene:tetraene ratio should be measured in the cholestatic child with poor growth to evaluate for the possibility of EFA deficiency and the need for EFA supplementation.

Fat-soluble vitamins

The intestinal absorption of vitamins A, D, E, and K is strongly dependent on adequate hepatic secretion of bile acids into the intestinal lumen (Figure 9.2) [35]. When intraluminal bile acid concentrations are below the critical micellar concentration of 1.5–2.0 mmol/L, malabsorption of fat-soluble vitamins is common. The use of bile acid-binding agents (e.g. cholestyramine) as treatment for cholestasis may further impair absorption. In addition, vitamin A and vitamin E esters require hydrolysis by an intestinal esterase that is bile acid-dependent prior to intestinal absorption. When cholestasis begins in infancy, depletion of meager body stores present at birth occurs rapidly, resulting in biochemical and clinical features of fat-soluble vitamin deficiency as early as age 4–12 months if supplementation is not initiated. The frequency of biochemical evidence of fat-soluble vitamin deficiency despite "routine" vitamin supplementation is approximately 35–50% for vitamin A, 66% for vitamin D, 50–75% for vitamin E, and 25% for vitamin K [35,41]. Evaluation of vitamin status, supplemental doses, and monitoring differ for each vitamin and will be considered separately [44]. In a recent prospective study, biochemical fat-soluble vitamin deficiency was commonly observed in infants with biliary atresia and persistent cholestasis despite administration of a liquid containing d-α-tocopheryl polyethylene glycol succinate (TPGS) with multiple fat-soluble vitamins [41].

Vitamin A

Vitamin A comprises retinol and its derivatives that have the same β-ionone ring and qualitatively similar biologic activities [44]. The principal vitamin A compounds – retinol, retinal (retinaldehyde), retinoic acid, and retinyl esters – differ in the terminal C-15 group at the end of the side-chain. Vitamin A is present in the diet as retinyl esters derived almost exclusively from animal sources (liver and fish liver oils, dairy products, kidney, and eggs) and provitamin A carotenoids (mainly beta-carotene), which are distributed widely in green and yellow vegetables. The Recommended Daily Allowance (RDA) is 375 μg retinol equivalents for 0–1 years of age, 400 μg for 1–3 years, 500 μg for 4–6 years, and 700–1000 μg for older children and adults (1 μg retinol equivalent = 3.3 IU vitamin A).

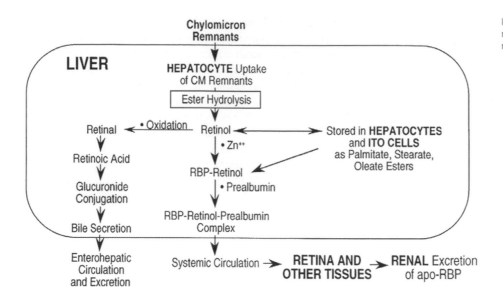

Figure 9.3 Processes involved in hepatic metabolism of vitamin A. CM, chylomicrons; RBP, retinol-binding protein.

The functions of vitamin A are maintenance of proper vision, epithelial cell integrity, and regulation of glycoprotein synthesis and cell differentiation [35].

Following micellar solubilization and hydrolysis by pancreatic esterase in the intestinal lumen, retinol is absorbed into the enterocyte, undergoes re-esterification with palmitate, stearate, or oleate, and is then incorporated into newly synthesized chylomicrons or very low density lipoproteins (VLDL) for transport into the mesenteric lymphatics (Figure 9.2). Upon reaching the bloodstream, the triglyceride content of the chylomicra is hydrolyzed, and the retinyl ester-rich chylomicron remnants are taken up by the liver. In the hepatocyte (Figure 9.3), retinyl esters may be hydrolyzed, releasing the free retinol, which can be transported into the sinusoids bound in a 1:1 molar ratio with retinol-binding protein (RBP) in a ternary complex with prealbumin (transthyretin). Circulating RBP-bound retinol is the transport form that delivers retinol to target tissues such as the retina. Alternatively, retinyl esters may be stored in the hepatocyte or transported as RBP-bound retinol from the hepatocyte to hepatic stellate cells (lipocytes, Ito cells), the storage site of over 80% of hepatic vitamin A under normal conditions.

Several alterations in hepatic metabolism of vitamin A occur in chronic cholestasis, and deficiency of vitamin A has been observed in 35–69% of children with chronic cholestatic liver disease [35]. Intraluminal solubilization of vitamin A and other carotenoids is compromised by lack of bile flow, resulting in malabsorption of vitamin A. If protein malnutrition, zinc deficiency, or depressed hepatic synthetic function are present, hepatic synthesis and secretion of RBP is diminished, leading to low plasma levels of retinol and impaired delivery of retinol to target tissues.

The evaluation of vitamin A status in cholestasis is confounded by a reportedly poor correlation between serum and hepatic vitamin A concentrations. In patients without liver disease, serum retinol levels <20 µg/dL generally correlate with deficient hepatic stores of vitamin A. However, in children with cholestatic liver disease, serum retinol may not correlate with hepatic stores of vitamin A.

Because of these inaccuracies in using serum retinol alone to define vitamin A status, other potential indices have been proposed for the evaluation of vitamin A status during cholestasis, including the relative dose–response (RDR), retinol:RBP ratio, and ocular measures including conjunctival impression cytology, ophthalmologic slit-lamp examination, and the rapid darkfield adaptation test.

The RDR, considered the best non-invasive test of vitamin A status, is based on the observation that when hepatic stores of vitamin A are normal, plasma retinol concentration does not change significantly following administration of a small oral loading dose of exogenous vitamin A. However, when hepatic vitamin A reserves are low, the plasma retinol concentration increases markedly after the administration of an exogenous vitamin A dose, reaching a peak several hours after the dose. This paradoxical effect observed during vitamin A deficiency is most likely the result of rapid mobilization of hepatic RBP bound to incoming retinol in an attempt to redistribute the absorbed vitamin A to peripheral tissues. The standardized RDR is expressed as the percentage increase in plasma retinol 5 hours after an oral loading dose of vitamin A. However, use of the oral RDR test in cholestasis is potentially problematic because of poor absorption of the oral dose of vitamin A. The RDR test can be performed utilizing an intramuscular injection of vitamin A (Aquasol A; ASTRA Pharmaceutical, Westboro, MA, USA) [43]. In a study of 23 patients with cholestatic liver disease and 10 patients with non-cholestatic liver disease (controls), vitamin A deficiency was identified in 10 of the cholestatic patients and none of the control patients utilizing the intramuscular RDR (Figure 9.4). Comparing other tests with the intramuscular RDR revealed that serum retinol alone was a good screening measure with a sensitivity of 90% and a specificity of 78% to detect vitamin A deficiency [45] (Table 9.4).

Table 9.4 Comparison of indices of vitamin A status in cholestasis

	Sensitivity (%)[a]	Specificity (%)[a]
Retinol	90	78
Retinol-binding protein	40	91
Retinol:retinol-binding protein ratio	60	74
Oral relative dose response	80	100
Conjunctival impression cytology	44	48
Slit lamp	20	66

[a] For the detection of vitamin A deficiency.
Source: modified from Feranchak *et al.*, 2005 [43].

It has been proposed that the molar ratio of serum retinol:RBP may reflect hepatic stores more accurately. However, in a larger controlled study the ratio did not improve the detection of vitamin A deficiency over serum retinol level alone [43].

Another measure used in assessing vitamin A status is conjunctival impression cytology. In this test, a small piece of filter paper is applied to the bulbar conjunctiva after local anesthesia, patted gently, and peeled off slowly. After fixation and staining, the morphology of adherent epithelial cells is evaluated histologically for abnormalities in epithelial cell morphology, decreased number of goblet cells, and mucin spots covering <25% of the sample, all of which are consistent with vitamin A deficiency. One small study showed that conjunctival impression cytology correctly identified the vitamin A status of children with chronic cholestasis. However, the test

(a)

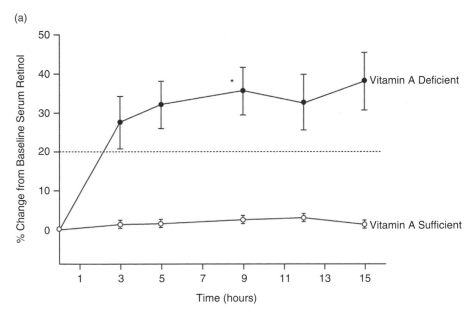

(b)

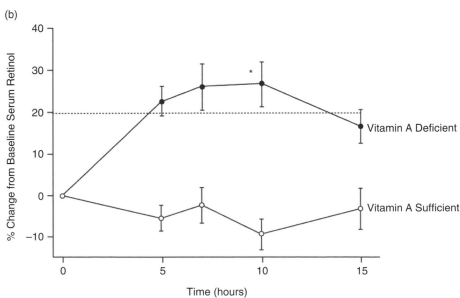

Figure 9.4 Relative dose–response (RDR) tests for the detection of vitamin A deficiency. (a) Modified intramuscular RDR. Percentage rise in serum retinol level from baseline following intramuscular injection of vitamin A. Mean values ± SEM are shown at each time point. A rise of >20% at 9 hours is considered abnormal and indicative of vitamin A deficiency. All patients with vitamin A deficiency had a >20% rise in serum retinol by 9 hours. Conversely, all patients with vitamin A sufficiency had no significant rise in serum retinol following the injection (normal response). (b) Modified oral RDR. Percentage rise in serum retinol level from baseline following an oral dose of vitamin A (1500 IU) given concurrently with vitamin E (25 IU/kg tocopherol polyethylene glycol succinate). A rise of >20% at 10 hours is considered abnormal. Mean values ± SEM are shown at each time point. (Reproduced with permission from Feranchek *et al.* [43].)

may have a lower specificity particularly in Western or developed nations. In fact, conjunctival impression cytology had a sensitivity of only 44% and a specificity of 48% to detect vitamin A deficiency in this study [43]. Likewise, ophthalmologic examination was also a poor discriminator of vitamin A deficiency in this population. Direct measures of visual acuity and darkfield adaptation have been used to assess vitamin A deficiency but may not be feasible in younger children.

A modified version of the RDR was subsequently developed using oral administration of TPGS vitamin E plus retinyl palmitate, with the TPGS promoting solubilization and absorption of oral vitamin A and, thus, mitigating against the need for parenteral RDR to assess vitamin A status. In fact, the oral RDR had a sensitivity of 80% and a specificity of 100% to detect vitamin A deficiency in this group of patients with chronic cholestasis (Figure 9.4) [43]. Based on these findings, serum retinol level as an initial screen followed by confirmation with a modified oral RDR test may be the most effective means of identifying vitamin A deficiency in these patients.

It is important to detect vitamin A deficiency in children with chronic cholestatic liver disease as deficiency may lead to xerophthalmia, keratomalacia, and irreversible damage to the cornea, as well as night blindness and pigmentary retinopathy. Although these ocular findings are rare in children with chronic cholestasis, the potential for impairment of vision exists. Vitamin A deficiency may also potentially put patients at risk for infection and abnormalities in biliary epithelialization of Roux-en-Y conduits following hepatic portoenterostomy. The effect of vitamin A deficiency on immune function during cholestasis has not been evaluated.

The recommended oral supplements of vitamin A range from 5000 to 25 000 IU/day of water-miscible preparations of vitamin A (Aquasol A; ASTRA Pharmaceutical, Westboro, MA, USA) [44]. The water-soluble form of vitamin E, TPGS, has been shown to solubilize and improve intestinal absorption of other lipid-soluble molecules, such as cyclosporine and vitamin D, during cholestasis. Therefore oral coadministration of vitamin A supplements with TPGS may improve absorption of vitamin A during cholestasis and would most likely result in the need for smaller doses of vitamin A (e.g. 5000 to 10 000 IU/day).

Because of the known hepatotoxicity of vitamin A, careful monitoring during vitamin A repletion and supplementation is mandatory. In adults, chronic administration of 25 000 IU vitamin A for 6 years may lead to cirrhosis. Vitamin A toxicity is also manifested by increased intracranial pressure in children, painful bone lesions, precocious bone growth, and desquamative dermatitis. To monitor for vitamin A toxicity during high-dose vitamin A therapy, serum retinyl esters, normally not present, should be monitored. Elevated retinyl esters are associated with hepatotoxicity. Plasma levels of retinol and RBP are not reliable means of detecting vitamin A toxicity. Whether other indices of vitamin A status, such as the molar ratio of serum retinol:RBP, will be useful in assessing toxicity in children with chronic cholestasis is currently not known.

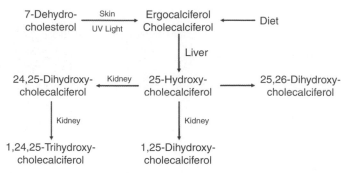

Figure 9.5 Vitamin D metabolism.

Vitamin D

Vitamin D (calciferol) refers to two secosteroids, vitamin D_2 (ergocalciferol) and vitamin D_3 (cholecalciferol) [44]. They differ in their side-chains; vitamin D_2 has a methyl group at C-24 and a double bond at C-22 to C-23. Vitamin D_2 is derived from plants and fungi and is added to vitamin D-supplemented cow's milk. The RDA is 400 IU (10 μg vitamin D_3) in infants (<6 months) and 600 IU (15 μg vitamin D_3) in older children and adults [35]. The absorption of vitamin D_2 is dependent on micellar solubilization; therefore, vitamin D_2 malabsorption has been observed in cholestasis (Figure 9.2). Vitamin D_3 is synthesized in the skin from 7-dehydrocholesterol upon exposure to sunlight. Dietary vitamin D is absorbed in the jejunum and ileum and is then either transported into the lymphatics in chylomicrons (vitamin D_2 and D_3) or absorbed directly into the portal system (calcifidiol (25-hydroxyvitamin D)). In the blood, vitamin D is transported primarily bound to a vitamin D-binding protein synthesized in the liver. Vitamins D_2 and D_3 subsequently undergo 25-hydroxylation in the liver to form calcifidiol, which is the major circulating form of vitamin D (Figure 9.5). From the liver, calcifidiol bound to vitamin D-binding protein is transported to the kidney for 1α-hydroxylation to form 1,25-dihydroxyvitamin D (calcitriol). Calcitriol is the biologically active form of vitamin D that stimulates intestinal absorption of calcium and phosphorus, renal reabsorption of filtered calcium, and the mobilization of calcium and phosphorous from bone. In the presence of low serum calcium, increased levels of parathormone activate 1α-hydroxylase in the kidney, increasing circulating levels of calcitriol and thus stimulating calcium absorption. A 24-hydroxylation step in the kidney may result in the synthesis of 24,25-dihydroxyvitamin D, which appears necessary for adequate bone mineralization.

The primary manifestations of vitamin D deficiency are related to the effects of calcitriol on calcium metabolism [37]. Hypocalcemia, hypophosphatemia, tetany, osteomalacia, and rickets are the most common clinical features [46]. During cholestasis, several factors predispose to vitamin D deficiency. Absorption of ingested vitamin D_2 is impaired although 25-hydroxylation in the liver is intact. Hepatic secretion of vitamin D-binding protein may be reduced in liver disease, leading to lower levels of bound calcifidiol. Consequently, the

(a)

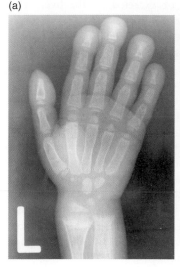

(b)

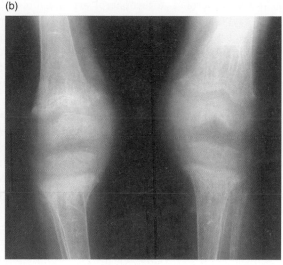

Figure 9.6 Extensive rickets caused by prolonged vitamin D deficiency in a 6-year-old child with biliary atresia and a non-functioning portoenterostomy who did not receive vitamin D supplements. (a) Radiograph of the wrist shows that the provisional zones of calcification at the distal ends of the radius and ulna are extensively frayed, cupped, and irregularly mineralized. The carpal and metacarpal bones and the distal shafts of the radius and ulna are diffusely osteopenic and coarse in texture (osteomalacia). This patient also had a markedly delayed bone age. Note the pronounced flattening and rounding of the soft tissues surrounding the terminal phalanges consistent with severe digital clubbing. (b) Bone films of the same patient's legs demonstrate marked osteopenia in the shafts. The metaphyses of the distal femur and proximal tibia and fibula are poorly calcified, widened, and frayed, denoting advanced rickets.

photosynthesized vitamin D_3 becomes a more important source of vitamin D. However, because of chronic debilitation, many children with chronic cholestatic liver disease are not exposed to adequate sunlight, thus decreasing the cutaneous synthesis of vitamin D_3. Phenobarbital therapy during cholestasis has also been shown to alter vitamin D metabolism, resulting in rickets. Before the development of newer vitamin D analogues, approximately 29% of children with cholestasis had radiographic evidence of rickets (Figure 9.6), while up to 80% had decreased bone mineral density based on iodine-131 photonabsorptiometry. Although patients with chronic cholestasis may normalize vitamin D status with therapy, they may continue to show evidence of metabolic bone disease. This suggests that factors other than calcium malabsorption and decreased serum calcifidiol levels contribute to the osteopenia commonly observed in children with chronic cholestasis. The clinical evaluation of vitamin D status in cholestatic children is performed initially by measuring serum calcifidiol. Serum calcium, magnesium, phosphorus, alkaline phosphatase, and parathormone levels, as well as bone X-rays or bone densitometry can be used to identify osteomalacia, osteopenia, or rickets. A serum calcifidiol <14–$15\,\mu g/L$ is indicative of vitamin D deficiency. The serum level of calcitriol is more indicative of calcium than vitamin D status, with a high level indicative of calcium deficiency, and it is not essential for routine monitoring for vitamin D deficiency.

It is currently recommended that children with chronic cholestasis have periodic monitoring of serum calcifidiol levels and normal intake of calcium and phosphorus in the diet [35]. If vitamin D deficiency is present, oral vitamin D_3 (Drisdol; Winthrop-Breon Laboratories, New York, USA) can be administered in a daily dose of 3–10 times the RDA for age; however, close monitoring of serum calcifidiol levels is required. If vitamin D is provided in a multiple vitamin supplement, it should be accounted for in the daily vitamin D dose. Intestinal absorption of these supplements may be improved by the coadministration of oral TPGS–vitamin E as a solubilizing agent. If patients fail to respond, have significant bony changes, or have severe cholestasis, supplementation with calcitriol (Rocaltrol; Roche Laboratories, Nutley, NJ, USA) at a daily dose of 0.05–$0.2\,\mu g/kg$ should be administered. This requires monitoring (including calcitriol levels) because there is no physiologic regulation of this compound. Rocaltrol is expensive and is available in North America only in capsule form; therefore, the contents should be aspirated into a syringe to allow for proper dosing (given with meals) in small children. Serum concentrations of calcifidiol (or calcitriol if Rocaltrol is used) should be rechecked in 1–2 months until normalization and then every 3–6 months thereafter. Monitoring for vitamin D toxicity should include urine calcium:creatinine ratio, serum calcium and phosphorus, and serum calcifidiol (or calcitriol). The principal manifestations of vitamin D intoxication are hypercalcemia, leading to depression of the central nervous system and ectopic calcification, and hypercalciuria, leading to nephrocalcinosis and nephrolithiasis. While bisphosphonate drugs have been used to prevent and treat osteoporosis associated with PBC in adults, the use of these agents in cholestatic children requires further study.

Vitamin E

The term vitamin E refers to a group of eight compounds called the tocopherols and the tocotrienols, which consist of substituted hydroxylated chromanol ring systems linked to an isoprenoid side-chain [44]. The four major forms of vitamin E (alpha, beta, delta, and gamma) differ by the number and position of the methyl group substitutions on the chromanol ring, and in their bioactivity. Alpha-tocopherol has the highest biologic activity and is the predominant form in foodstuffs with the exception of soy and other vegetable oils, which contain high levels of γ-tocopherol. The common dietary sources of vitamin E are the oil-containing grains, plants, and vegetables. The RDA is 15 mg/day *d*-α-tocopherol ((*RRR*)-α-tocopherol) in adults and less (4–11 mg/day) in children [49] (1 mg *d*-α-tocopherol = 1 tocopherol equivalent; 1 mg *dl*-α-tocopheryl acetate (*all-rac*-α-tocopherol) = 1 IU).

The ingested vitamin E requires solubilization by bile acids into mixed micelles and hydrolysis by pancreatic or intestinal esterases (bile acid dependent) prior to traversing the unstirred water layer in the intestinal lumen into the enterocyte [35] (Figure 9.2). Absorption occurs by a non-saturable, non-carrier-mediated passive diffusion process. Absorbed α- and γ-tocopherol are then incorporated in the enterocyte into chylomicrons and VLDL and are secreted into the mesenteric lymphatics, finally reaching the systemic circulation. Upon reaching the blood, vitamin E is transported predominantly in LDL and high density lipoprotein (HDL). The α- and γ-tocopherol remaining in chylomicrons is taken up by the hepatocyte. Alpha-tocopherol (particularly *d*-α-tocopherol) is preferentially resecreted as a component of hepatic-derived VLDL and perhaps HDL (Figure 9.7). Both γ- and δ-tocopherols as well as non-natural stereoisomers of

α-tocopherol are metabolized or excreted by the liver. The hepatic tocopherol-transfer protein appears to play a role in the hepatic discrimination process by which *d*-α-tocopherol is incorporated into lipoproteins and other forms of vitamin E are not [50]. The delivery of vitamin E to peripheral tissues involves lipoprotein lipase hydrolysis of chylomicrons and LDL binding to cell receptors.

The impaired secretion of bile acids during cholestasis results in malabsorption of vitamin E. Vitamin E is the most hydrophobic of the fat-soluble vitamins and, therefore, has the greatest requirement for intraluminal bile acids for absorption. Vitamin E absorption, measured by the oral vitamin E tolerance test, is profoundly depressed in cholestatic children who are vitamin E deficient [49]. Coadministration of bile acids enhances the absorption of vitamin E [50]. The frequency of vitamin E deficiency in children with chronic cholestasis is 49–77% despite the administration of "routine" oral supplements [49].

The physiologic role of vitamin E in the maintenance of structure and function of the human nervous system and skeletal muscle was recognized by the discovery of a progressive degenerative neuromuscular disorder associated with vitamin E deficiency during cholestasis and other states of fat malabsorption. Involved regions include the spinocerebellar tracts; cranial nerve nuclei III and IV; large-caliber myelinated axons in peripheral nerves, the posterior columns of the spinal cord, and gracillus and cuneatus nuclei in the brainstem; skeletal muscle; and the ocular retina (Figure 9.8). Clinical manifestations of vitamin E deficiency appear as hyporeflexia at approximately 18–24 months of age in children with prolonged neonatal cholestatic disorders, and this may be accompanied by sural nerve lesions even before 1 year of age. Uncorrected vitamin E deficiency during childhood leads to sequential development of neurologic symptoms including truncal and limb ataxia, depressed vibratory and position sensation, impairment in balance and coordination, peripheral neuropathy, proximal muscle weakness, ophthalmoplegia, and

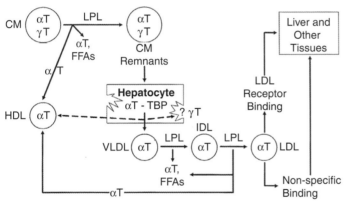

Figure 9.7 Proposed lipoprotein transport and delivery of vitamin E to the liver and peripheral tissues. CM, chylomicron; TBP, tocopherol-binding protein; LPL, lipoprotein lipase; *α*T, α-tocopherol; *γ*T, γ-tocopherol; FFAs, free fatty acids.

Figure 9.8 Sites of neuromuscular involvement of vitamin E deficiency and corresponding clinical manifestations.

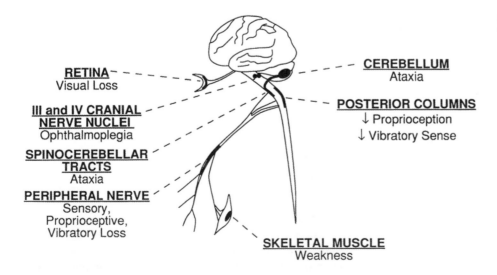

RETINA
Visual Loss

III and IV CRANIAL NERVE NUCLEI
Ophthalmoplegia

SPINOCEREBELLAR TRACTS
Ataxia

PERIPHERAL NERVE
Sensory, Proprioceptive, Vibratory Loss

CEREBELLUM
Ataxia

POSTERIOR COLUMNS
↓ Proprioception
↓ Vibratory Sense

SKELETAL MUSCLE
Weakness

retinal dysfunction. Significant cognitive and behavioral abnormalities have also been described in association with prolonged vitamin E deficiency. The neurologic lesions may be irreversible to a substantial degree if vitamin E deficiency remains untreated. Studies have demonstrated reversal or prevention of neurologic degeneration if vitamin E deficiency is corrected before age 3–4 years, whereas older children with more severe neurologic symptoms show a more limited response to therapy; this mandates aggressive evaluation and normalization of vitamin E status early in the course of chronic cholestasis in children. Deficiency of vitamin E has also been associated with hemolytic anemia in premature infants fed a diet high in polyunsaturated fatty acids but this has not been reported in cholestasis.

The major function of vitamin E is its role as an antioxidant, protecting cell membrane polyunsaturated fatty acids and thiol-rich proteins from oxidant damage initiated by free radical reactions. Vitamin E has also recently been shown to be an agonist for the PXR nuclear receptor. The possibility that vitamin E deficiency may worsen cholestatic liver injury has been proposed based on the observation that lipid peroxidation increases in the cholestatic rat liver, and that vitamin E deficiency combined with a diet containing over 30% of calories as fat may exacerbate cholestatic hepatic injury in the rat. In addition, pro-oxidants, such as copper and manganese, which accumulate during cholestasis, increase free-radical generation and the requirement for vitamin E and other antioxidants.

The assessment of vitamin E status during cholestasis should utilize the ratio of the serum vitamin E concentration to total serum lipid concentrations (E:lipid) [51]. Elevated circulating lipid levels during cholestasis cause vitamin E to partition into the plasma lipoproteins and may increase the serum vitamin E concentration into the normal range (5–20 μg/mL) in a vitamin E-deficient patient. Calculation of the ratio of E:lipid compensates for this phenomenon [51]. Vitamin E deficiency is indicated by a ratio <0.6 mg/g in children under 1 year of age, and <0.8 mg/g for older children [35,49]. For vitamin E repletion of deficient patients, we aim to achieve an E:lipid ratio of 0.8–1.0 mg/g. Measurement of vitamin E in adipose tissue assesses vitamin E stores; however, it requires adipose biopsies and few laboratories perform this analysis.

To prevent the development of vitamin E deficiency, routine supplementation with vitamin E is indicated in all infants and young children with chronic cholestasis. In older children and adults, vitamin E stores will maintain adequacy of vitamin E status for at least 6–12 months. Newly diagnosed infants with cholestatic disorders are treated with 25 IU/kg daily of vitamin E (α-tocopherol, α-tocopheryl acetate, α-tocopheryl succinate, or α-tocopheryl nicotinate) or 15–25 IU/kg daily of a liquid preparation of the water-soluble TPGS (Liqui-E; 26.6 IU/mL, Twin Laboratories, Ronkonkoma, NY, USA; or Aqua-E; 20 IU/mL, Yasoo Health, Johnson City, TN, USA). Vitamin E is given as a single morning dose with breakfast (when bile flow is maximal) or at least 2 hours apart

from medications that can interfere with its absorption (e.g. cholestyramine, iron). Alternatively, capsules of vitamin E (100–400 IU) can be slit open and the oil carefully squeezed into the infant or child's mouth followed by formula or breast-feeding, or into solid food in order to deliver these large doses in an inexpensive manner. If TPGS is used, 25 IU/kg daily is almost always effective in normalizing vitamin E status. If other forms of vitamin E are used, doses are increased by 25–50 IU/kg daily up to a 100–200 IU/kg daily maximum if there is no response in serum E:lipid ratio in 3–4 weeks. If vitamin E status fails to normalize (reaching E:lipid ratio >0.8 mg/g) after several months of therapy with 100 IU/kg daily of the standard vitamin E preparations, either TPGS or intramuscular injections of vitamin E (Ephynal, 50 mg/mL; Hoffman LaRoche, Basel, Switzerland) will need to be instituted. The effective dose for this parenteral form of vitamin E is 0.5–1.0 IU/kg daily given as 0.5–1.0 mL intramuscular injections every 3–10 days to provide the calculated dose [52]. In a US multicenter trial, all 60 vitamin E-deficient children with cholestasis who failed to respond to large doses of standard vitamin E responded to 15–30 IU/kg daily of TPGS without detectable side effects [45]. Therefore, intramuscular vitamin E is only used in the rare instances of TPGS failure.

Vitamin E therapy is monitored by obtaining trough E:lipid ratios every 2–3 months and by performing serial neurologic examinations. Attempts are made to keep serum vitamin E levels <25–30 μg/mL; however, to achieve an E:lipid ratio >0.8 mg/g, it is occasionally necessary to allow serum vitamin E to exceed this range in the severely hyperlipidemic child. Once normalization of the serum E-lipid ratio has been achieved, these checks are repeated every 6 months during continued vitamin E supplementation unless there is a major change in the severity of cholestasis. If profound neurologic deficits are present, serial visual evoked response or somatosensory evoked response measurements may be helpful in documenting neurologic improvement. Vitamin E toxicity is rare. Normal adults appear to tolerate oral doses of 100–800 mg daily without clinical signs or biochemical evidence of toxicity. Because up to 3–4% of the polyethylene glycol contained in TPGS may be absorbed, there is a small risk of inducing a hyperosmolar state if glomerular filtration rate is decreased through renal failure or dehydration. Therefore, TPGS should be administered cautiously in these circumstances. One additional concern is the potential exacerbation of vitamin K-deficient coagulopathy. Adults without liver disease who received very large doses of vitamin E (>1000–1500 IU/day) in conjunction with warfarin therapy had significantly prolonged prothrombin time beyond that expected from the warfarin alone. Presumably the excess vitamin E inhibited the gamma-carboxylation reaction of vitamin K. Therefore, to prevent this occurrence in cholestatic children receiving large doses of vitamin E, vitamin K status should be corrected, prothrombin time monitored, and excessively high serum vitamin E levels should be avoided. In addition, large parenteral doses of vitamin E that achieved extremely high serum vitamin E levels (>40–$50\,\mu g/mL$) in preterm infants (without significant liver disease) have been associated with an increased incidence of bacterial and fungal sepsis, presumably through inhibition of neutrophil function (generation of free radicals). Proper monitoring of serum vitamin E levels in cholestatic patients should prevent this possible complication. Finally, intravenous use of an untested form of α-tocopheryl acetate solubilized in polysorbate (Eferol) led to fatal liver injury in a number of preterm infants. It was most likely the polysorbate and not the vitamin E that was toxic. This product was promptly removed from the market when this toxicity was recognized.

Vitamin K

Vitamin K belongs to the family of 2-methyl-1,4 naphthoquinones and exists in three forms. Phylloquinone (vitamin K_1) is obtained from leafy vegetables, soybean oil, fruits, seeds, and cow's milk. Menaquinone (vitamin K_2), which has 60% of the activity of vitamin K_1, is synthesized by intestinal bacteria. Menadione (vitamin K_3) is not a natural form but is synthesized chemically and has better water solubility than the two natural forms. The RDA for infants is $5\,\mu g$ phylloquinone or menaquinone for the first 6 months, $10\,\mu g$ during the second 6 months, and $1\,\mu g/kg$ body weight for older children [35].

The absorption of vitamin K requires bile and pancreatic secretions and is, therefore, impaired during cholestasis. Small intestinal absorption of vitamin K_1 is by a saturable process requiring metabolic energy, while K_2 absorption occurs by passive diffusion. The absorbed vitamin K is incorporated in the enterocyte into chylomicrons and is transported to the blood via the lymph (Figure 9.2). In the liver, vitamin K is taken up in chylomicron remnants and incorporated into VLDL and ultimately into LDL for transport to tissues. Little vitamin K is stored in the liver.

Vitamin K is necessary for the post-translational gamma-carboxylation of glutamic acid residues of the vitamin K-dependent coagulation proteins (factors II, VII, IX, and X, protein C, and protein S). Carboxylation allows these proteins to bind calcium, thus leading to activation of the clotting factors. In addition, there is a family of other vitamin K-dependent proteins ("gla proteins") found in all tissues, the function of which are largely unknown. Osteocalcin is one such gla protein involved in bone mineralization. Vitamin K status may impact bone mineralization. Vitamin K deficiency causes a coagulopathy that can present in infancy with intracranial bleeding. Malabsorption of vitamin K, as well as frequent antibiotic suppression of intestinal floral production of vitamin K, predisposes to deficiency during cholestasis [47]. In one study, 10 of 43 patients (23%) with biliary atresia who had undergone portoenterostomy were found to be vitamin K deficient [48].

Vitamin K status is clinically evaluated by measuring the prothrombin time/international normalized ratio (INR), which is dependent on the vitamin K-dependent clotting factors [35]. If the prothrombin time/INR is prolonged in comparison with the partial thromboplastin time, then this most likely represents vitamin K deficiency. Response of prothrombin time to intramuscular injection of vitamin K is the most accurate means of diagnosing deficiency. A more sensitive measure of vitamin K status is analysis of plasma levels of protein-induced in vitamin K absence (PIVKA-II). Factor II, VII, IX, and X assays offer no real advantage over the prothrombin time and are not only costly but also unavailable in many laboratories. Serum vitamin K levels can be measured but do not represent vitamin K stores, are only available in research laboratories, and may not correlate with prothrombin time/INR measurements.

Since children with chronic liver disease have other risk factors for bleeding (e.g. development of esophageal varices, portal hypertensive gastropathy, platelet dysfunction, thrombocytopenia, and diminished hepatic synthesis of other coagulation factors), vitamin K deficiency should be routinely prevented. Oral forms of vitamin K supplements of 2.5 to 5.0 mg two to seven times a week should be given to all children with chronic cholestasis [39]. Vitamin K_1 (Mephyton; Aton Pharma, Lawrenceville, PA, USA) is preferred because it lacks toxicity if given in excess. Coadministration of Mephyton with TPGS may also theoretically enhance its absorption. Vitamin K_3 (Synkavite; Roche Laboratories), more water soluble and therefore better absorbed, may be needed if there is no response to vitamin K_1. However, large doses of vitamin K_3 have the potential for hepatotoxicity if completely absorbed, and massive hemolysis in infants with glucose-6-phosphate dehydrogenase deficiency has been reported. Synkayvite is currently not available in North America. If oral vitamin K supplementation is unsuccessful, intramuscular or intravenous injection of vitamin K (AquaMEPHYTON) every 3–4 weeks at a dose of 2–5 mg prevents and reverses vitamin K deficiency-induced coagulopathy [35].

Water-soluble vitamins

Little is known about the nutritional status of water-soluble vitamins during chronic childhood cholestasis. In adults with chronic liver disease, however, deficiency of vitamins B_1, B_6, C, and folic acid have been described [50]. Therefore, it seems prudent to supplement the vitamins normally present in the diet with an additional one to two times the RDA of water-soluble vitamins contained in standard pediatric multivitamin supplements. Since these supplements also contain additional amounts of the fat-soluble vitamins, these should be taken into account when calculating supplemental doses for each vitamin, particularly for vitamins A and D.

Calcium and phosphate

Appropriate intake of the bone minerals calcium and phosphate should be ensured. Phosphate supplementation may be particularly important in treating and preventing rickets. Fat malabsorption during cholestasis decreases the intestinal absorption of calcium and phosphate through formation of insoluble soaps. Mineral deficiency may develop and potentially contribute to bone disease unresponsive to normalization of vitamin D status [3]. In addition to encouraging high calcium and phosphate foods, enteral daily supplements of 25–100 mg/kg elemental calcium and of 25–50 mg/kg phosphorus may be necessary to reverse bone abnormalities. Calcium may be administered as inexpensive chewable calcium carbonate antacid tablets (e.g. Tums, Rolaids). Serum calcium and phosphorus concentrations, urine calcium:creatinine ratio, and the fractional excretion of phosphate should be used to monitor supplementation with these minerals.

Magnesium

Hypomagnesemia has been described in both adults and children with cirrhosis. The mechanism for the low plasma magnesium is believed to be related to malabsorption, hyperaldosteronism leading to increased renal excretion of magnesium, hepatic fibrosis, decreased albumin/gammaglobulin ratio, and chronic malnutrition. Like serum zinc, serum magnesium may be normal in the presence of depleted total body stores or be low with normal stores. Isolated magnesium deficiency is actually rare because of very effective control of magnesium homeostasis by the kidney. But if magnesium depletion is present, it may lead to hypocalcemia as a result of decreased synthesis and secretion of parathormone.

It has been postulated that negative magnesium balance may be a contributing factor to the metabolic bone disease of chronic liver disease. In a small group of children with cholestasis, all were found to be magnesium depleted with significantly reduced serum parathormone levels [51]. Furthermore, reduced bone mineral density in children with chronic cholestasis was associated with reduced urinary excretion of an intravenous loading dose of magnesium, indicating magnesium deficiency [53]. Supplementation with magnesium oxide for at least 12 months led to improvement in bone mineral density in these children. These data need to be corroborated to delineate the role of magnesium in cholestatic metabolic bone disease. Magnesium deficiency is treated with 1–2 mEq/kg daily of oral magnesium oxide. Acute states of magnesium depletion may be treated with a 0.3–0.5 mEq/kg dose (3–6 mEq maximum) of a 50% solution of magnesium sulfate given intravenously over 3 hours and repeated over the remainder of the 24-hour period. Magnesium excess may cause respiratory depression, lethargy, and coma.

Zinc

Zinc is an essential trace metal present in over 100 zinc metalloenzymes and a range of transcription proteins. The RDA for infants and children is 5–10 mg/day. Deficiency of zinc leads to poor linear growth, hypogeusia, anorexia, impaired immune function, and an erythematous vesicular eruption on the face and distal extremities. Delayed recovery from infectious diarrheal states has also been reported. Low plasma zinc is common in infants with chronic cholestasis [51]. In a series of 27 children awaiting liver transplantation, 42% were reported to have low plasma zinc concentrations [54]. The reduced zinc concentrations may be related to poor intake of zinc-containing foods, malabsorption of zinc, reduced levels of serum albumin available for binding and transport of zinc, compartmentation of zinc into the liver as part of the acute phase response, or increased zinc excretion in urine. Inappropriately elevated urinary zinc excretion rapidly reverses after liver transplant. Unfortunately, plasma zinc concentrations do not correlate well with total body zinc status. In children with cirrhosis, normal plasma zinc levels have been observed in the presence of diminished hepatic zinc concentrations. Therefore, identifying infants and children with chronic zinc deficiency may be difficult. If infants are growing poorly with inadequate oral intake or if plasma zinc concentration is low (<60 µg/dL), we recommend supplementation with 1 mg/kg daily of elemental zinc as a zinc sulfate solution (zinc 10 mg/mL) for 2 to 3 months as a therapeutic trial. Further study of zinc balance and the effects of zinc deficiency in cholestasis are needed.

Selenium

As part of the enzyme glutathione peroxidase, selenium functions as an antioxidant catalyzing the reduction of lipid hydroperoxides and of hydrogen peroxide to water. Other selenoproteins have also been discovered recently. The RDA for selenium is 10 µg/day in infants and 15–50 µg/day in children and adolescents. The plasma selenium concentration of the majority of healthy infants and children falls within the range 50–150 µg/L, with the mean around 100 µg/L. Selenium deficiency may cause a cardiomyopathy and a skeletal myopathy manifested by weakness and muscle pain. Keshan disease is an endemic form of cardiomyopathy caused by selenium deficiency and found in China. Milder selenium deficiency is associated with macrocytosis of erythrocytes and loss of hair pigment. Plasma selenium <40 µg/L (0.5 mmol/L) indicate mild and <10 µg/L (0.12 mmol/L) severe selenium deficiency. While biochemical deficiency of selenium may occur in 13–33% of children with chronic cholestasis, with plasma selenium levels <20 µg/L, clinical manifestations of selenium deficiency is extremely rare [54]. Whether selenium deficiency potentiates the skeletal myopathy of vitamin E-deficient children is not known. Although definite recommendations cannot be made, it seems prudent to monitor plasma selenium levels periodically in children with severe cholestasis, particularly those with poor growth. Consumption of selenium-rich foods such as cereals, meat, eggs, and dairy products should be encouraged. If serum selenium levels are low, oral supplementation with 1–2 µg/kg sodium selenite daily should be considered. For infants and children on parenteral nutrition, an intravenous dose of 2 µg/kg daily is recommended for repletion therapy followed by 1 µg/kg daily for long-term TPN maintenance. Plasma selenium levels should be monitored during and after supplementation with a goal of 50–150 µg/L.

Iron

Iron deficiency results from a combination of decreased intake and chronic blood loss from esophageal varices, portal hypertensive gastropathy, and prolonged bleeding from other sites because of coagulopathy and thrombocytopenia. A 32% incidence of iron deficiency anemia has been reported in children with end-stage liver disease [55]. Low serum iron, increased total iron-binding capacity and a saturation index <16% suggest a diagnosis of iron deficiency. Treatment is elemental iron at a daily dose of 5–6 mg/kg during deficiency, and 1–2 mg/kg daily to compensate for ongoing blood loss. Correction of vitamin E deficiency, if present, should be performed concomitantly with iron therapy to prevent precipitation of hemolysis. The role of iron deficiency in the developmental delays, psychological, and emotional problems encountered during chronic cholestasis has not been investigated.

Copper, manganese, and aluminum

Copper accumulates in the liver during all forms of cholestasis because its major excretory pathway is through the biliary route. To compensate for this impaired excretion of copper, liver synthesis and secretion of ceruloplasmin is increased, leading to elevated serum concentrations of ceruloplasmin and copper during cholestasis. Extraordinarily elevated hepatic copper concentrations, sometimes well within the range found in patients with Wilson disease, have been observed in children with various forms of cholestasis. Although there has been no convincing demonstration of toxicity of copper during childhood cholestasis, the possible interaction between copper, a pro-oxidant capable of stimulating the generation of free radicals, particularly in the face of depletion of antioxidants (such as vitamin E, selenium, and glutathione), in an already injured liver deserves further attention. Two small, uncontrolled trials of the copper chelator D-penicillamine in children with chronic cholestasis failed to demonstrate any improvement in liver function or histology, although copper chelation was achieved. However, all children had advanced liver disease at the time of chelation therapy and no attempts were made to correct antioxidant deficiencies. Currently, copper chelation is not recommended for childhood cholestatic disorders that are not inborn errors of copper metabolism. Low copper diets and removing or lowering copper supplements from parenteral nutrition infusates administered to cholestatic children are recommended but have not been thoroughly investigated.

Manganese is another trace element that is excreted primarily in bile and accumulates in the liver in infants with biliary atresia. The major toxicity of manganese appears to be related to the central nervous system, where it may accumulate in the globus pallidus and subthalamic nuclei during cholestasis, causing basal ganglia injury. Increasing evidence suggests that manganese deposition is responsible for the T_1-weighted MRI signal hyperintensity observed in the globus pallidus of cirrhotic patients and correlates with elevated blood manganese levels. Both chronic liver disease and the presence of portal-systemic shunting have been significantly associated with brain manganese accumulation. In a study of autopsy specimens, globus pallidal manganese concentrations were significantly higher in patients with a history of chronic liver disease who died of hepatic coma compared with controls. The association of extrapyramidal symptoms in patients with cirrhosis and hyperintense pallidal signaling on MRI suggests a role for manganese in hepatic encephalopathy. In a report of a child with Alagille syndrome, dystonia and tremor, whole blood manganese levels were associated with symmetric hyperintense globus pallidi on T_1-weighted MRI. Following liver transplantation, neurologic function improved, blood manganese levels normalized, and the MRI signal abnormality completely resolved.

Additionally, rats injected with high doses of manganese simultaneously with bilirubin developed cholestatic liver disease, raising concern for possible hepatotoxicity of manganese during cholestasis. Pending further investigation, it is recommended that manganese supplements be withheld from parenteral nutrition solutions administered to infants and children with cholestasis. Furthermore, since intravenous nutrition solutions are contaminated with variable amounts of manganese, plasma manganese levels should be monitored in cholestatic patients receiving TPN. As intestinal absorption of both iron and manganese are increased during iron deficiency, iron deficiency may increase the susceptibility to manganese toxicity. Patients with chronic liver disease should avoid manganese supplements without concurrent iron supplementation.

Aluminum is commonly found in aluminum hydroxide antacids and sucralfate, and as a contaminant in many TPN constituents and other common intravenous products (e.g. calcium gluconate, albumin, potassium phosphate). This metal appears to have hepatotoxic effects in large doses. Because biliary excretion is an important route of elimination of orally absorbed aluminum, it is possible that cholestasis may lead to accumulation of aluminum in the liver. Consequently, the use of aluminum-containing medications should be discouraged in cholestasis unless absolutely necessary until more is known about hepatic metabolism and potential hepatotoxicity of aluminum.

General pediatric care

The long-term management of the child with chronic liver disease is directed not only toward the medical treatment of the varied complications of the underlying liver disease but also to optimizing growth and development, alleviating psychological/emotional problems in the developing child, and helping the family cope with the emotional and financial stresses resulting from raising a child with chronic disease.

Growth and development

Deficits in both growth and mental development observed in children with chronic liver disease are believed to arise from a combination of the following factors: prolonged illness, repeated hospitalizations, and malnutrition and nutrient deficiencies associated with the underlying liver disease [34,53]. Children with early-onset liver disease (younger than 1 year of age) score significantly lower on verbal, performance, and full-scale IQ testing. Furthermore, in contrast to children with a later onset of liver disease (over 1 year of age), those with early onset are more compromised in linear growth and head circumference, and have lower serum vitamin E levels, consistent with the results of earlier studies. Although it is generally difficult to predict cognitive outcomes accurately based on testing in the first 2 years of life, developmental testing (McCarthy Scales of Children's abilities) 4–7 years after portoenterostomy demonstrated slight mental delay and learning disabilities. Although the number of children studied has been small, this once again emphasizes the importance of aggressive nutritional management and correction of malnutrition and micronutrient deficiencies (e.g. vitamin E) particularly in children who develop chronic cholestatic liver disease within the first year of life. It has also been suggested that delaying transplantation in children with biliary atresia and poor growth may compromise their eventual intellectual development. Periodic testing of cognitive and motor development will help to identify those children at risk for developmental delay and learning disabilities so that appropriate intervention can be initiated early.

For the adolescent, chronic liver disease has many frustrating complications including primary or secondary amenorrhea and delayed puberty. Adolescent females with severe liver disease often have amenorrhea that resolves as the liver disease abates. However, the use of spironolactone, frequently used as a diuretic in the treatment of patients with ascites, has been associated with primary or secondary amenorrhea in adolescents with chronic liver disease. The mechanism of action is believed to be suppression of estrogen or androgen synthesis by spironolactone or binding at estrogen or androgen receptors, resulting in negative feedback regulation of gonadotropins. In the reported cases, regular menses began shortly after discontinuation of spironolactone. It is, therefore, recommended that if amenorrhea develops during spironolactone therapy alternative treatments, such as triamterene, should be considered.

Immunizations

In general, children with chronic liver disease should receive routine childhood immunizations, with the exception of patients who had recently undergone portoenterostomy for biliary atresia, and those who have had a liver transplantation. For patients who have recently undergone a hepatoportoenterostomy, the DPT combination vaccination (diphtheria and pertussis (whooping cough) and tetanus) may be delayed temporarily following surgery. The occurrence of fever and irritability that is common following DPT immunization is difficult to differentiate clinically from cholangitis and would necessitate admission into the hospital for treatment of presumed cholangitis. In addition, dehydration and decreased bile flow secondary to poor intake and fever following DPT vaccination may predispose to bile stasis and cholangitis. Vaccines with live viruses are generally contraindicated in children who have undergone liver transplantation. Therefore, it is recommended that children who are scheduled to have a liver transplant and who are older than 12 months should be given the measles, mumps, and rubella vaccine, and varicella vaccine, preferably at least 1 month before transplantation. Only inactivated polio vaccine (Salk) should be given to transplant recipients and their household contacts because the attenuated virus in oral polio vaccine can spread from person to person in a household. Immunization with influenza and pneumococcal vaccines should be encouraged as well in the absence of contraindications. Passive immunization with immunoglobulin should be employed for prophylaxis after exposure to other infections (e.g. varicella-zoster immunoglobulin for varicella). Hepatitis A and B vaccines should be routinely administered at the earliest recommended ages.

Dental hygiene

Discoloration of teeth and dental caries are common in children with chronic liver disease. The yellow–green staining of primary teeth in infants with chronic cholestasis is attributed to exposure of the developing dentin and enamel to hemosiderin, biliverdin, and bilirubin. The degree of pigment deposition may be proportionate to the serum concentration of bilirubin. Unless the child continues to have severe cholestasis through 8 years of age when formation of permanent teeth is completed, permanent teeth are unlikely to be affected. However, surface discoloration of teeth may occur in all ages and may result from oral bacteria causing black or green stains as a result of poor oral hygiene, use of sweetened acidic iron preparations leaving black iron sulfide deposits, dental caries, and ingested food products. The numerous oral medications taken by children with chronic liver disease usually contain sweeteners and have a syrupy consistency, increasing the risk for development of dental caries. The poor absorption of calcium, phosphorus, and vitamin D in chronic cholestasis may likewise lead to decreased integrity of dental structures and increased susceptibility to development of dental caries. Restriction of sugar-containing medications, stressing good oral hygiene, and frequent dental examinations and surveillance will aid in the prevention of dental caries, gingivitis, or abscesses, which may develop into severe infections in this group of relatively immunocompromised patients. Lastly, cosmetic treatment of discolored teeth may become necessary for self-esteem as the child grows older.

Family support

Chronic liver disease presents an enormous stress not only on the affected child but also on the family. Stresses identified by families caring for a child with chronic liver disease include parental fear that the child might die; guilt over having "caused" the liver disease in some way; parenting inadequacy to fulfill the child's "special needs;" pain from seeing their child frequently experience discomfort and physical pain (e.g. medical procedures); financial concerns; uncertainty and fear of the future; lack of control and taking control; and strained relationships among family members. In addition, because many children with chronic liver disease are hospitalized frequently, families are often separated for long and indefinite periods of time, disrupting normal routines. Early identification of these stresses and attention to these aspects of the child's care should help to improve the quality of life for the child and the family. Establishing friendships and communication between patients, parents, and the medical team, as well as patient and family education, offers invaluable support in dealing with the emotional stress and turmoil associated with living with chronic liver disease. Organizing family and patient support groups locally is recommended. National foundations and patient advocacy groups can also supply families with useful information, contacts with other families, and "chat rooms" on the Internet.

Conclusions

Cholestatic liver disease in infancy and childhood is heterogeneous in etiology and natural history. Because specific medical/surgical therapy is available for many cholestatic disorders, prompt diagnosis is imperative before irreversible liver damage occurs. Anticipation and recognition of the varied medical, nutritional, emotional, and psychological consequences of chronic cholestasis will optimize growth and development, and minimize discomfort and disability. For those children who will eventually require orthotopic liver transplantation, supportive medical care, including aggressive nutritional therapy, may enhance their chances for a successful operation as well as normal growth and development following transplantation. An improved understanding of the molecular and cellular mechanisms causing liver injury and fibrosis in cholestasis is needed. It is hoped that new biotechonology and translational approaches will lead to the development of newer treatment strategies designed to prevent, reverse, and treat these disorders.

References

1. Sokol RJ. Medical management of neonatal cholestasis. In Balistreri WF, Stocker JT (eds.) *Pediatric Hepatology*. Philadelphia, PA: Hemisphere, 1990, p. 43.

2. Suchy FJ. Neonatal cholestasis. *Pediatr Rev* 2004;**25**:388–396.

3. Ng VL, Balistreri WF. Treatment options for chronic cholestasis in infancy and childhood. *Curr Treat Option Gastrol* 2005;**8**:419–430.

4. Maillette de Buy Wenniger LJ, Oude Elferink RP, Beuers U. Molecular targets for the treatment of fibrosing cholangiopathies. *Clin Pharmacol Ther* 2012;**92**:381–387.

5. Roma MG, Toledo FD, Boaglio AC, *et al.* Ursodeoxycholic acid in cholestasis: linking action mechanisms to therapeutic applications. *Clin Sci* 2011;**121**:523–544.

6. Beuers U, Lindor KD. A major step towards effective treatment evaluation in primary biliary cirrhosis. *J Hepatol* 2011;**55**:1178–1180.

7. Mendes F, Lindor KD. Primary sclerosing cholangitis: overview and update. *Nat Rev Gastroenterol Hepatol* 2010;**7**:611–619.

8. Sokol RJ, Durie PR. Recommendations for management of liver and biliary tract disease in cystic fibrosis. Cystic Fibrosis Foundation Hepatobiliary Disease Consensus Group. *J Pediatr Gastroenterol Nutr* 1999;**28**(Suppl 1): S1–s13.

9. Balistreri WF. Bile acid therapy in pediatric hepatobiliary disease: the role of ursodeoxycholic acid. *J Pediatr Gastroenterol Nutr* 1997;**24**:573–589.

10. Jacquemin E, Hermans D, Myara A, *et al.* Ursodeoxycholic acid therapy in pediatric patients with progressive familial intrahepatic cholestasis. *Hepatology* 1997;**25**:519–523.

11. Jacquemin E, De Vree JM, Cresteil D, *et al.* The wide spectrum of multidrug resistance 3 deficiency: from neonatal cholestasis to cirrhosis of adulthood. *Gastroenterology* 2001;**120**:1448–1458.

12. Sundaram SS, Bove KE, Lovell MA, Sokol RJ. Mechanisms of disease: Inborn errors of bile acid synthesis. Nature clinical practice. *Gastroenterol Hepatol* 2008;**5**:456–468.

13. Narkewicz MR, Smith D, Gregory C, *et al.* Effect of ursodeoxycholic acid therapy on hepatic function in children with intrahepatic cholestatic liver disease. *J Pediatr Gastroenterol Nutr* 1998;**26**:49–55.

14. Xu C, Li CY, Kong AN. Induction of phase I, II and III drug metabolism/ transport by xenobiotics. *Arch Pharmacal Res* 2005;**28**:249–268.

15. Ponsioen CY. Novel developments in IBD-related sclerosing cholangitis. Best practice & research. *Clin Gastroenterol* 2011;**25**(Suppl 1):S15–S18.

16. Meyers RL, Book LS, O'Gorman MA, *et al.* High-dose steroids, ursodeoxycholic acid, and chronic intravenous antibiotics improve bile flow after Kasai procedure in infants with biliary atresia. *J Pediatr Surg* 2003;**38**:406–411.

17. Bergasa NV. The itch of liver disease. *Semin Cutaneous Med Surg* 2011;**30**:93–98.

18. Baghdasaryan A, Claudel T, Gumhold J, *et al.* Dual farnesoid X receptor/TGR5 agonist INT-767 reduces liver injury in the Mdr2$^{-/-}$ (Abcb4$^{-/-}$) mouse cholangiopathy model by promoting biliary HCO(−)(3) output. *Hepatology* 2011;**54**:1303–1312.

19. Hernandez-Gea V, Friedman SL. Pathogenesis of liver fibrosis. *Ann Rev Pathol* 2011;**6**:425–456.

20. Cohen-Naftaly M, Friedman SL. Current status of novel antifibrotic therapies in patients with chronic liver disease. *Ther Adv Gastroenterol* 2011;**4**:391–417.

21. Bunchorntavakul C, Reddy KR. Pruritus in chronic cholestatic liver disease. *Clin Liver Dis* 2012;**16**: 331–346.

22. Kremer AE, van Dijk R, Leckie P, *et al.* Serum autotaxin is increased in pruritus of cholestasis, but not of other origin, and responds to therapeutic interventions. *Hepatology* 2012;**56**: 1391–1400.

23. Imam MH, Gossard AA, Sinakos E, Lindor KD. Pathogenesis and management of pruritus in cholestatic liver disease. *J Gastroenterol Hepatol* 2012;**27**:1150–1158.

24. Kuiper EM, van Erpecum KJ, Beuers U, *et al*. The potent bile acid sequestrant colesevelam is not effective in cholestatic pruritus: results of a double-blind, randomized, placebo-controlled trial. *Hepatology* 2010;**52**:1334–1340.

25. Bachs L, Pares A, Elena M, Piera C, Rodes J. Comparison of rifampicin with phenobarbitone for treatment of pruritus in biliary cirrhosis. *Lancet* 1989;**i**:574–576.

26. Yerushalmi B, Sokol RJ, Narkewicz MR, Smith D, Karrer FM. Use of rifampin for severe pruritus in children with chronic cholestasis. *J Pediatr Gastroenterol Nutr* 1999;**29**:442–447.

27. Wolfhagen FH, Sternieri E, Hop WC, *et al*. Oral naltrexone treatment for cholestatic pruritus: a double-blind, placebo-controlled study. *Gastroenterology* 1997;**113**:1264–1269.

28. Whitington PF, Whitington GL. Partial external diversion of bile for the treatment of intractable pruritus associated with intrahepatic cholestasis. *Gastroenterology* 1988;**95**:130–136.

29. Ng VL, Ryckman FC, Porta G, *et al*. Long-term outcome after partial external biliary diversion for intractable pruritus in patients with intrahepatic cholestasis. *J Pediatr Gastroenterol Nutr* 2000;**30**:152–156.

30. Swain MG, Maric M. Improvement in cholestasis-associated fatigue with a serotonin receptor agonist using a novel rat model of fatigue assessment. *Hepatology* 1997;**25**:291–294.

31. Longo M, Crosignani A, Podda M. Hyperlipidemia in chronic cholestatic liver disease. *Curr Treat Options Gastroenterol* 2001;**4**:111–114.

32. Simopoulos AP. Essential fatty acids in health and chronic disease. *Am J Clin Nutr* 1999;**70**(3 Suppl):560S–569S.

33. Bucuvalas JC, Cutfield W, Horn J, *et al*. Resistance to the growth-promoting and metabolic effects of growth hormone in children with chronic liver disease. *J Pediatr* 1990;**117**:397–402.

34. Sokol RJ, Stall C. Anthropometric evaluation of children with chronic liver disease. *Am J Clin Nutr* 1990;**52**:203–208.

35. Sokol RJ. Fat-soluble vitamins and their importance in patients with cholestatic liver diseases. *Gastroenterology Clin North Am* 1994;**23**:673–705.

36. Hogler W, Baumann U, Kelly D. Growth and bone health in chronic liver disease and following liver transplantation in children. *Pediatr Endocrinol Rev* 2010;**7**:266–274.

37. Hogler W, Baumann U, Kelly D. Endocrine and bone metabolic complications in chronic liver disease and after liver transplantation in children. *J Pediatr Gastroenterol Nutr* 2012;**54**:313–321.

38. DeRusso PA, Ye W, Shepherd R, *et al*. Growth failure and outcomes in infants with biliary atresia: a report from the Biliary Atresia Research Consortium. *Hepatology* 2007;**46**:1632–1638.

39. Chin SE, Shepherd RW, Thomas BJ, *et al*. Nutritional support in children with end-stage liver disease: a randomized crossover trial of a branched-chain amino acid supplement. *Am J Clin Nutr* 1992;**56**:158–163.

40. Sullivan JS, Sundaram SS, Pan Z, Sokol RJ. Parenteral nutrition supplementation in biliary atresia patients listed for liver transplantation. *Liver Transplant* 2012;**18**:120–128.

41. Shneider BL, Magee JC, Bezerra JA, *et al*. Efficacy of fat-soluble vitamin supplementation in infants with biliary atresia. *Pediatrics* 2012;**130**:e607–e614.

42. Simopoulos AP, Leaf A, Salem N, Jr. Essentiality of and recommended dietary intakes for omega-6 and omega-3 fatty acids. *Ann Nutr Metab* 1999;**43**:127–130.

43. Feranchak AP, Gralla J, King R, *et al*. Comparison of indices of vitamin A status in children with chronic liver disease. *Hepatology* 2005; **42**:782–792.

44. Sathe MN, Patel AS. Update in pediatrics: focus on fat-soluble vitamins. *Nutr Clin Pract* 2010;**25**:340–346.

45. Sokol RJ, Butler-Simon N, Conner C, *et al*. Multicenter trial of d-alpha-tocopheryl polyethylene glycol 1000 succinate for treatment of vitamin E deficiency in children with chronic cholestasis. *Gastroenterology* 1993;**104**:1727–1735.

46. de Albuquerque Taveira AT, Fernandes MI, Galvao LC, *et al*. Impairment of bone mass development in children with chronic cholestatic liver disease. *Clin Endocrinol* 2007;**66**:518–523.

47. Strople J, Lovell G, Heubi J. Prevalence of subclinical vitamin K deficiency in cholestatic liver disease. *J Pediatr Gastroenterol Nutr* 2009;**49**:78–84.

48. Yanofsky RA, Jackson VG, Lilly JR, *et al*. The multiple coagulopathies of biliary atresia. *Am J Hematol*. 1984;**16**:171–180.

49. Sokol RJ. Assessing vitamin E status in childhood cholestasis. *J Pediatr Gastroenterol Nutr* 1987;**6**:10–13.

50. Said HM. Intestinal absorption of water-soluble vitamins in health and disease. *Biochem J* 2011;**437**:357–372.

51. Heubi JE, Higgins JV, Argao EA, Sierra RI, Specker BL. The role of magnesium in the pathogenesis of bone disease in childhood cholestatic liver disease: a preliminary report. *J Pediatr Gastroenterol Nutr* 1997;**25**:301–306.

52. Umusig-Quitain P, Gregorio GV. High incidence of zinc deficiency among Filipino children with compensated and decompensated liver disease. *J Gastroenterol Hepatol* 2010;**25**:387–390.

53. Kaller T, Boeck A, Sander K, *et al*. Cognitive abilities, behaviour and quality of life in children after liver transplantation. *Pediatric Transplant* 2010;**14**:496–503.

54. Chin SE, Shepherd RW, Thomas BJ, *et al*. The nature of malnutrition in children with end-stage liver disease awaiting orthotopic liver transplantation. *Am J Clin Nutr* 1992;**56**:164–168.

55. Mattar RH, Azevedo RA, Speridiao PG, *et al*. [Nutritional status and intestinal iron absorption in children with chronic hepatic disease with and without cholestasis.]. *J Pediatr* 2005;**81**:317–324.

Chapter

10

Neonatal hepatitis and congenital infections

Philip Rosenthal

Introduction

Neonatal hepatitis refers to a heterogeneous group of disorders that result in a somewhat similar morphologic change in the liver of an infant younger than 3 months of age in response to various insults. The term *neonatal hepatitis* has been used at times to include all causes of cholestasis in infancy in which extrahepatic biliary obstruction is excluded. Although in the majority of cases an etiology cannot be found, specific infectious and metabolic causes have been identified that may present as neonatal hepatitis. At final diagnosis, neonatal hepatitis is responsible for approximately 40% of the cases of infants with cholestasis and is the most frequently encountered liver disorder of early infancy. Males usually predominate over females (2:1). Additionally, some familial cases have been reported, suggesting either a maternal environmental factor or autosomal recessive inheritance.

Histologically, there is a loss of the lobular architecture with preservation of the zonal distribution of portal tracts and central veins. There is ballooning degeneration of hepatocytes with fusion of hepatocyte membranes and nuclear transformation into multinucleated giant cells. These multinucleated giant cells are believed to be the response of immature hepatocytes to most forms of injury and are a non-specific finding in neonatal liver biopsy samples. There may be abundant extramedullary hematopoiesis and variable inflammation (Figure 10.1). Cholestasis may be marked because the newborn already is in a relative state of physiologic cholestasis. Finding cytoplasmic inclusions, steatosis, or storage material, or elucidating a positive family history, may aid in distinguishing metabolic, viral, and familial causes of neonatal hepatitis.

This chapter reviews known causes of neonatal hepatitis with intrahepatic cholestasis, concentrating in particular on associated congenital infections. It has become increasingly clear that the term neonatal hepatitis is too vague and is no longer clinically or therapeutically appropriate. Hepatitis in a neonate caused by a known etiologic agent that may be amenable to therapy needs to be differentiated from idiopathic neonatal hepatitis, in which etiologic agents are unknown and probably multiple. This becomes increasingly important as new therapeutic regimens are developed.

Routes of infection

The newborn may acquire infection transplacentally in utero, during delivery, or after birth. The study of transplacental infection has been hampered by the latency of many viruses. It has been well established that transplacental passage may result in congenital syphilis, toxoplasmosis, rubella, and cytomegalovirus (CMV) infections. The secondary liver abnormalities at birth may be inactive because of remote in utero infection, with the consequent scarred cirrhotic liver, or relatively new, with an acute hepatitis. An essential factor in the transmission of the infection from the mother to the fetus is the time of maternal infection during the pregnancy. In general, infectious agents cross the placenta best during the third trimester. This is particularly true for syphilis, toxoplasmosis, and hepatitis B virus (HBV).

Perinatal acquisition of infection may be the result of the upward spread of bacterial agents from vaginitis, endometritis, or placentitis. Inhalation or swallowing of infected amniotic fluid may transmit the infection to the fetus. During labor and delivery, direct contact with pathogens in vaginal or uterine secretions or contaminated blood may result in neonatal infection. *Listeria*, herpes simplex, and CMV may be transmitted by this route and can cause neonatal hepatitis.

Postnatal infection less frequently results in neonatal hepatitis. Close contact with maternal infecting secretions (oral, nasal, breast milk) is possible. Blood or blood product transfusions may contain agents that could result in a neonatal hepatitis.

Etiologic agents
Bacterial infections

The reticuloendothelial system in the liver and spleen is responsible for effectively clearing bacteria from the bloodstream. However, in the neonate, the reticuloendothelial system is often immature and there may be diminished

Liver Disease in Children, Fourth Edition, ed. Frederick J. Suchy, Ronald J. Sokol, and William F. Balistreri. Published by Cambridge University Press. © Cambridge University Press 2014.

(a)

(b)

(c)

(d)

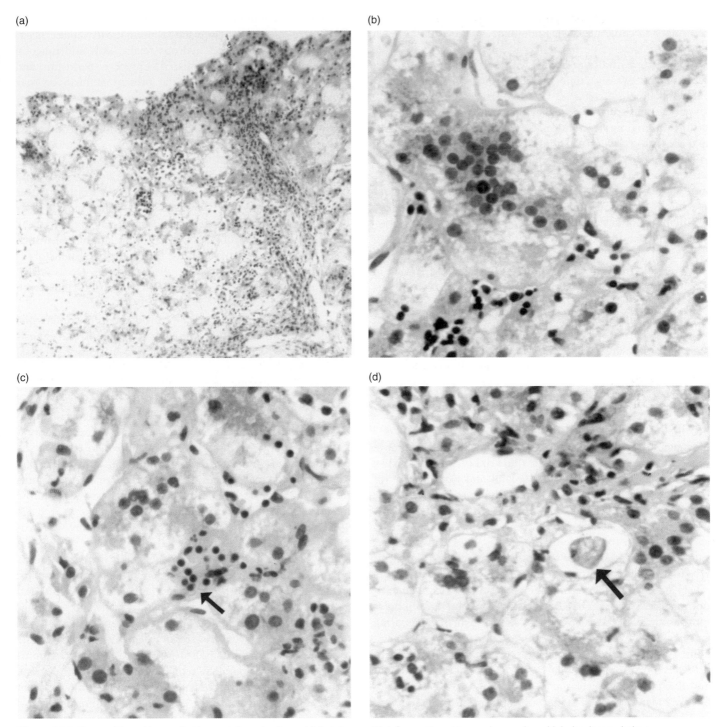

Figure 10.1 Neonatal hepatitis; needle biopsy at 6 weeks of age. (a) Portal area with inflammation at top and parenchymal lobular disarray below (original magnification 40×). (b) Ballooned hepatocytes and multinucleated giant cell (original magnification 450×). (c) Extramedullary hematopoiesis (arrow) (original magnification 450×). (d) Necrotic hepatocyte (Councilman body, arrow) (original magnification 450×). (Hematoxylin & eosin stain.)

amounts of complement and opsonins, which impair the neonate's ability to handle bacterial infections adequately. Hepatic injury from systemic bacterial infections may result from direct invasion of hepatocytes and Kupffer cells, from circulating toxins, or as a result of fever or hypoxia.

Hepatomegaly and jaundice may be clinical signs of neonatal sepsis with hepatic involvement [1]. Both Gram-positive and Gram-negative organisms have been implicated, with Gram-negative bacteria being the most frequent etiologic agents reported [2]. Hepatotoxicity is believed to be secondary to circulating endotoxin from the bacterial cell walls and secondary to cholestasis [3]. Endotoxin is known to diminish bile flow in isolated perfused liver preparations [4].

Laboratory studies in infants with bacterial infection often reveal a leukocytosis, conjugated hyperbilirubinemia, and elevated alkaline phosphatase levels. Serum aminotransferase levels are only slightly to moderately elevated. A prolonged prothrombin time and abnormal clotting factors may be related to a coexisting disseminated intravascular coagulopathy.

Percutaneous liver biopsies are rarely performed in infants with sepsis because of the accompanying abnormal coagulation parameters and because the findings are often non-specific [5]. There may be bile stasis, focal hepatocyte necrosis, a polymorphonuclear portal infiltrate, giant cell transformation, and Kupffer cell hyperplasia. Occasionally, culture of the hepatic tissue may be positive.

The most frequent bacterial organism isolated resulting in a neonatal hepatitis is *Escherichia coli*. *Streptococcus* group B is rarely implicated. *Listeria monocytogenes* infection invariably results in hepatic manifestations.

Liver abscesses, the result of hepatic injury from umbilical catheterization, are uncommonly observed [6]. When present, *E. coli* and *Staphylococcus aureus* are the most common pathogens isolated and are presumed secondary to colonization of the umbilical stump.

Urinary tract infection

Neonatal bacterial infections associated with jaundice have frequently been associated with the urinary tract [7]. They commonly present between the second and eighth weeks of postnatal life. These infections are rarely associated with fever or urinary symptoms. There may be a history of lethargy, irritability, poor feeding, and, occasionally, vomiting or diarrhea. Males are more frequently affected than females. Anatomic abnormalities of the genitourinary tract are infrequent. Hepatomegaly is frequently apparent. Laboratory studies reveal a conjugated hyperbilirubinemia, mildly increased aminotransferase levels, and leukocytosis with an increase in polymorphonuclear cells. Urinalysis shows pyuria, and urine culture usually reveals *E. coli*. Blood cultures may be transiently positive. Hepatic pathology is relatively benign, with non-specific findings of bile stasis, periportal inflammation, and Kupffer cell hyperplasia.

Treatment consists of appropriate antibiotic therapy to avoid significant morbidity and mortality. Resolution of the jaundice may be delayed despite successful bacterial eradication because of the formation of bilirubin–protein conjugates in the serum. An underlying metabolic disease (e.g. galactosemia) must be considered in all infants with cholestasis and Gram-negative bacterial infections.

Congenital syphilis

Despite penicillin and routine maternal screening, congenital syphilis remains a problematic perinatal infection. In utero, transplacental transmission of *Treponema pallidum* spirochetes

to the fetus may result in a mild to severe range of symptoms [8]. Severe infections may result in prematurity, apnea, hepatosplenomegaly, jaundice, hydrops fetalis, skin and mucosal lesions, rhinitis, osteochondritis, osteomyelitis, periostitis, and pseudoparalysis. Findings may be present at birth or may develop over days to weeks. Milder infections may present with anicteric hepatitis, poor weight gain, or purulent nasal discharge. Laboratory abnormalities include a conjugated hyperbilirubinemia and elevated serum aminotransferase levels.

Liver histology classically reveals an intralobular dissecting fibrosis with centrilobular mononuclear infiltration. Silver stains may demonstrate spirochetes. In milder infections or in late presentation, the histologic features may not be typical. There may be portal fibrosis and portal inflammation, which are non-specific signs of hepatitis. Unless the clinical history is obtained, the diagnosis could easily be missed. Occasionally, congenital syphilis may lead to fulminant hepatic failure with subsequent liver calcifications [9].

Congenital syphilis should be considered in the differential diagnosis of any neonate with hepatitis. A definitive diagnosis can be made if spirochetes are identified in skin or mucosal lesions. Serologic testing of serum and cerebrospinal fluid analysis using specific treponemal antibody tests (e.g. microhemagglutination test for *T. pallidum*, fluorescent treponemal antibody absorption) and non-specific non-treponemal reagin and flocculation tests (e.g. Venereal Disease Research Laboratory test, rapid plasma reagin, automated reagin test) may be required to distinguish syphilis from other spirochetal diseases. Serology may be positive in normal unaffected infants for up to 3 months after birth because of passively acquired maternal antibodies confounding the diagnosis.

Treatment includes parenteral penicillin therapy. Erythromycin and ceftriaxone are reserved for penicillin allergy, but efficacy has not been proved and penicillin desensitization is preferable. Tetracycline or doxycycline, although useful in adults, should not be used in pregnant mothers or infants because of effects on developing teeth and bones. If penicillin G cannot be administered, alternative treatment recommendations can be found at the Centers for Disease Control and Prevention website (http://www.cdc.gov/nchstp/dstd/penicillinG.htm). After appropriate therapy, serology may remain positive for up to 2 years. Serum aminotransferase levels may remain elevated after onset of therapy for a prolonged period. Prognosis may ultimately depend on the extent of hepatic damage before the institution of therapy. Chronic liver disease has not been reported in infants appropriately treated for congenital syphilis.

Tuberculous hepatitis

Neonatal infection of the liver with tuberculosis is exceedingly rare. Infection may occur by way of placental spread from miliary tuberculosis in the mother, by inhalation with pulmonary involvement, or by aspiration of contaminated amniotic fluid. Usually, respiratory symptoms predominate. Hepatic lesions have caseating necrosis with surrounding giant cells and epithelioid cells with tubercle bacilli [10]. The clinical course is usually rapidly fatal. If a newborn is suspected of having congenital tuberculosis, a Mantoux skin test (5 tuberculin units of purified protein derivative), chest radiographs, lumbar puncture, and cultures should be obtained rapidly. Regardless of the skin test results, which are frequently negative in congenital tuberculosis, treatment should be initiated promptly with isoniazid, pyrazinamide, rifampin, and streptomycin or kanamycin.

Toxoplasmosis

Maternal infection with the intracellular protozoan parasite is usually acquired by contact with the oocytes excreted in cat feces or ingestion of inadequately cooked meat (lamb, beef, or pork). Maternal infection may be asymptomatic or mild but is a prerequisite for the development of congenital toxoplasmosis during gestation [11]. The majority of infected newborns may be asymptomatic [12]. Hepatitis may be the only indicator of infection. Serious disease is primarily related to hepatic and central nervous system involvement [13]. Manifestations of congenital infection with *Toxoplasma gondii* may include purpura, microcephaly, chorioretinitis, intracranial calcification, meningoencephalitis, and psychomotor retardation. Most infants with congenital toxoplasmosis have hepatosplenomegaly, but jaundice may be variable.

Liver biopsy may show a generalized hepatitis with areas of necrosis. Intracellular bile stasis and periportal infiltration with histiocytes, lymphocytes, granulocytes, and eosinophils may accompany hepatocyte necrosis. *Toxoplasma* organisms may be seen in the liver using fluorescent antibody staining. Plain abdominal roentgenograms may show hepatic microcalcifications, the result of calcification of necrotic lesions.

Diagnosis may be made prenatally by detection of the parasite in fetal blood or amniotic fluid or from the placenta, cord, or infant's peripheral blood using mouse inoculation or polymerase chain reaction (PCR) of its genomic material. Serologic diagnosis can be made by immunoglobulin (Ig) M or IgA or persistent (over 12 months); IgG anti-*Toxoplasma* antibody tests are determined in the infant's blood. A case of congenital toxoplasmosis diagnosed by the use of exfoliative cytology of neonatal ascites has been reported [14]. Mothers known to be infected during pregnancy may be treated with sulfadiazine and pyrimethamine or spiramycin (an investigational drug in the USA) in an attempt to prevent congenital infection. Infants with documented infection may be treated with pyrimethamine and sulfadiazine, with folinic acid added to prevent hematologic toxicity of therapy. Although further cellular invasion may be prevented, pre-existing damage and intracellular organisms may not be influenced by this regimen.

Viral infections

Cytomegalovirus

Cytomegalovirus may be acquired transplacentally, at delivery, or postnatally from infected secretions (saliva or breast milk) or from transfusion of blood products [15]. Significant

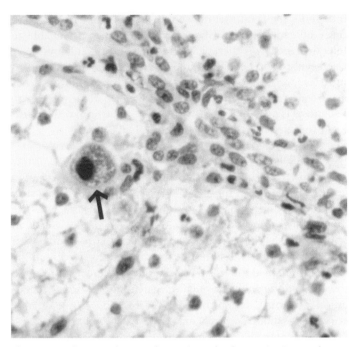

Figure 10.2 Cytomegalovirus infection. Large hard-appearing intranuclear inclusion (arrow). Adjacent portal tract has acute and chronic inflammatory infiltrate. (Hematoxylin & eosin, original magnification 450×.)

congenital CMV disease has been reported in the offspring of liver transplant recipients [16]. Most congenitally infected infants remain asymptomatic. The minority (5–10%) develop clinically apparent infection, but, unfortunately, these may include low birth weight, microcephaly, periventricular cerebral calcifications, chorioretinitis, thrombocytopenia, purpura, deafness, and psychomotor retardation. Hepatosplenomegaly and conjugated hyperbilirubinemia are often seen in neonatal CMV infection [17,18]. The hepatosplenomegaly may be secondary to significant extramedullary hematopoiesis.

Liver biopsy may reveal significant giant cell transformation. The presence of large intranuclear inclusion bodies in bile duct epithelium and occasionally in hepatocytes or Kupffer cells, and intracytoplasmic inclusion bodies in hepatocytes, confirms the diagnosis (Figure 10.2) [17]. Bile stasis, inflammation, fibrosis, and bile duct proliferation are also featured.

Diagnosis of CMV infection includes culture of the nasopharynx, saliva, and urine. Culture of the liver may yield positive results, but the yield is usually not as good as from the urine [19]. The detection of CMV in hepatic tissue can be improved with the use of electron microscopy, viral DNA by PCR, and monoclonal antibody techniques [20,21]. Serologic tests are also useful for CMV diagnosis and IgM CMV-specific antibodies can be monitored.

Long-term follow-up of congenital CMV-infected patients may show resolution of hepatomegaly but development of portal hypertension despite the absence of cirrhosis [22,23]. Treatment for congenital CMV infection includes use of the antiviral drug ganciclovir and CMV immunoglobulin intravenously. Foscarnet may be used as an alternative drug in cases of ganciclovir-resistant virus or in patients unable to tolerate ganciclovir therapy. Valganciclovir and cidofovir have also been used in neonates with CMV infection, but side effects must be weighed before use. Liver transplantation also has been used rarely for infants with severe hepatic involvement. Prognosis is poor for infants with severe infection, with neurologic sequelae frequently occurring.

Herpes hepatitis

Hepatitis from herpes simplex may present as part of a generalized disease in the newborn [24]. Symptoms may not appear until 4–8 days of age, which coincides with the incubation period for herpes. Congenital herpes infection may present with microcephaly and necrotic, ulcerative, vesicular, or purpuric lesions on the mucosal surfaces or the skin. Although the liver may be mildly affected, more often there is jaundice, hepatosplenomegaly, and abnormal coagulation factors. Gastrointestinal bleeding, coagulopathy, encephalitis, and seizures may be present in severe cases. Diagnosis may be confirmed by typical cutaneous lesions, by identification of the virus in skin lesions using direct fluorescent antibody staining or enzyme immunoassay detection of herpes antigens, cell culture, and PCR of herpes simplex viral DNA [25]. Acute and convalescent sera may be tested for increases in herpes simplex antibody titers to confirm acute infection, but serologic diagnosis is less helpful than viral isolation, which has become the more rapid diagnostic procedure of choice.

An asymptomatic maternal genital lesion is often the cause of the neonatal infection, with herpes simplex type 2 accounting for the majority of congenital herpes infections. Fetal scalp monitoring, prolonged rupture of membranes, prematurity, and low birth weight may contribute to the risk of infection. Infection in the newborn can be avoided by cesarean section delivery. Other less common sources of neonatal infection include transmission from a parent from a non-genital infection (e.g. from the hands or mouth) or postnatal infection from another infected infant in the nursery, probably from the hands of personnel caring for the infants.

Liver histology reveals necrosis (either multifocal or generalized) with characteristic intranuclear acidophilic inclusions in hepatocytes. Multinucleated giant cells also may be present (Figure 10.3). Culture of liver tissue may confirm the diagnosis but may take up to a week to be positive. Morphologic demonstration of herpesvirus is usually faster. Immunohistochemical staining using commercially available antisera can demonstrate herpesvirus in tissue [26]. The closely related varicella–zoster virus, which can produce an identical histologic appearance in the liver, can be distinguished by the difference in cutaneous rash. The CMV intranuclear inclusions are much larger than those of herpesvirus intranuclear inclusions, and there may be bile duct cell involvement in CMV infection, aiding in the diagnosis [27]. Herpes simplex viral DNA may be detected by PCR.

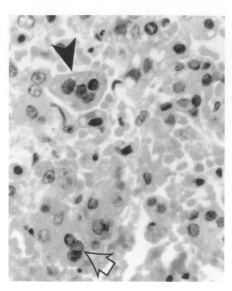

Figure 10.3
Herpesvirus infection. Viable hepatocytes adjacent to areas of necrosis. A multinucleated giant cell (solid arrow) and pale intranuclear inclusions with rim of chromatin (open arrow) are noted. (Hematoxylin & eosin, original magnification 450×.)

Without treatment, the outcome invariably is death. The use of antiviral therapy (acyclovir) in conjunction when necessary with liver transplantation has significantly improved the outlook for herpes-infected neonates with severe disease limited to the liver [25,28]. Acyclovir has become the drug of choice because of its ease of administration and lower toxicity. Prophylactic use of acyclovir in exposed newborns is not recommended because of potential drug toxicity and the low risk of disease to most newborns.

Rubella

The incidence of congenital rubella has diminished because of the widespread use of rubella vaccine [29]. Hepatic involvement in congenital rubella is common [30,31]. Hepatomegaly is always found, and splenomegaly, jaundice, and cholestasis with a conjugated hyperbilirubinemia and elevated serum alkaline phosphatase and aminotransferases may also feature. Congenital rubella is associated with ophthalmologic (cataracts, microphthalmia, glaucoma, chorioretinitis), cardiac (patent ductus arteriosus, peripheral pulmonic stenosis, atrial or ventricular septal defects), auditory (sensorineural deafness), and neurologic (microcephaly, meningoencephalitis, retardation) anomalies. Growth retardation, thrombocytopenia, and purpuric skin lesions (blueberry muffin) may be observed.

Humans are the sole source of rubella infection. Postnatal rubella is transmitted by direct or droplet contact with nasopharyngeal secretions. Congenitally infected infants may shed rubella virus in nasopharyngeal secretions and urine for up to 1 year and transmit infection to contacts.

Liver histology reveals mononuclear infiltrates of the portal zones with intralobular fibrosis and extramedullary hematopoiesis (Figure 10.4). There may be giant cell transformation, focal areas of necrosis, cholestasis, and evidence of bile duct proliferation. An increased incidence of biliary atresia has been reported in these infants [18].

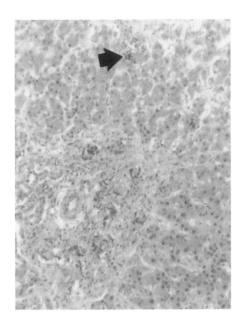

Figure 10.4 Congenital rubella infection. Portal and periportal fibrosis and extramedullary hematopoiesis (arrow). (Hematoxylin & eosin, original magnification 100×.)

Diagnosis may be made by isolation of virus from the nose by inoculation of appropriate tissue culture. Throat swabs, urine, blood, and cerebrospinal fluid may yield positive cultures, particularly in congenitally infected infants. Serologic testing is also useful in confirming the diagnosis. Specific rubella IgM antibody is indicative of recent postnatal or congenital infection. The use of PCR for prenatal and postnatal diagnosis of congenital rubella is also being utilized.

Treatment is supportive. Control of rubella has been attempted by the routine immunization of all infants and the testing of all women for evidence of protective antibody to rubella before marriage. Infants with congenital rubella usually recover from the hepatitis without the development of hepatic failure. However, significant morbidity and mortality in these infants usually are the result of the cardiac lesions or hemorrhage.

Hepatitis A

Although hepatitis A virus (HAV) is a frequent cause of hepatitis in childhood, it is not a frequent cause of hepatitis in the newborn [32]. Acquisition of HAV by blood transfusions has been reported in the neonatal period [33]. Most of these neonates developed serologic evidence of acute HAV infection but were clinically and biochemically asymptomatic. Although rare, neonatal cholestasis resulting from vertical transmission of HAV has been reported [34,35].

In general, HAV is spread by the orofecal route. Infection occurs at a younger age in lower socioeconomic groups and is endemic in developing countries. Children usually are anicteric and have a milder course than do adults. No HAV carrier state exists, and chronic HAV infection does not occur.

Serologic testing for IgM- and IgG-specific anti-HAV antibodies is commercially available. Recent infection is denoted by an elevated titer of IgM anti-HAV.

Treatment is supportive. Enteric precautions should be observed. If the mother is not jaundiced, no special care of the infant is recommended. Breast-feeding may occur as long as proper hygiene is practiced. If the mother is jaundiced, immunoglobulin is recommended, although its efficacy in this situation is not proven. Limited data exist on the use of the HAV vaccine in infants; the currently available vaccines in the USA are approved for children over 1 year of age.

Hepatitis B

Overall in the USA, HBV is an uncommon cause of neonatal hepatitis. However, in certain regions of the USA and in parts of the world, it is common for perinatal transmission of HBV to occur from a chronic HBV carrier mother or the mother with acute HBV infection during the third trimester of pregnancy [36]. Perinatal transmission of HBV is also more likely if the mother is positive for the HBV antigen (HBeAg) and thus has HBV DNA circulating in the bloodstream. If the infant does not acquire HBV infection at birth, close contact with other family members places the infant at high risk for acquisition of the virus, making pre-exposure HBV immunization imperative.

The majority of infants who develop hepatitis B through vertical transmission show evidence of HBV surface antigen (HBsAg) positivity between 4 and 16 weeks of age and become asymptomatic carriers. However, some infants develop a chronic active form of hepatitis B, and others, with time, develop cirrhosis and hepatocellular carcinoma. A coinfection or superinfection with delta hepatitis virus (hepatitis D (HDV)) is also possible. It is rare for perinatally acquired HBV to result in an acute icteric hepatitis [37]. These infants may have a benign course, with the development of anti-HBsAg and loss of HBsAg, or uncommonly may progress to a rapidly fulminant and fatal hepatitis.

All mothers with the potential for HBV infection should be screened for HBsAg. In many US states, the law requires that all pregnant women have their HBV status investigated during their pregnancy. For infants whose mothers are found to be HBsAg positive, immunoprophylaxis should be instituted at birth. Neonates born to mothers who are HBsAg positive should be bathed carefully soon after birth to remove potentially infected maternal blood or secretions. Hepatitis B immunoglobulin (HBIG) should be administered intramuscularly (0.5 mL) as soon as possible after birth and preferably within 12 hours. Efficacy of HBIG after 12 hours and before 48 hours is presumed but unproved. At another distant injection site, HBV vaccine (0.5 mL) should be administered intramuscularly using a different syringe at the same time as HBIG. The second and third doses of vaccine are given at 1–2 and 6 months after the first. For preterm infants who weigh <2 kg at birth born to HBsAg-positive mothers, the initial vaccine dose should not be counted in the required three doses to complete the immunization series, so these preterm infants receive a total of four doses. The need for booster doses of HBV vaccine for children and adults with a normal immune system is not recommended as immune memory remains intact for 15 years or more. The Infectious Disease Advisory Committee of the American Academy of Pediatrics recommends routine immunization with HBV vaccine of all infants regardless of risk factors or maternal HBV status. Although the cost–benefits of this approach will not be immediate, it is anticipated that, within 10–20 years of this practice, HBV infection could be effectively controlled and potentially eliminated as a significant cause of liver disease within the USA.

Diagnosis of HBV uses commercially available serologic tests for HBV antigens (HBsAg and HBeAg) and antibodies to HBsAg, HBV core antigen (HBcAg), and HBeAg. In acute infection, HBsAg positivity detects the great majority of cases. However, because HBsAg is also positive in chronic infection, IgM anti-HBcAg presence can be used to establish acute or recent HBV infection. Quantitative tests of serum HBV DNA by PCR or branched-chain DNA methods are commercially available and useful in the selection and monitoring of patients for therapy.

Liver biopsy is seldom necessary for the diagnosis of acute HBV infection. Focal or single-cell necrosis with clear cells, balloon cells, and acidophilic bodies is usually evident. There may be centrilobular necrosis with surrounding mononuclear infiltrate as well as bile stasis and Kupffer cell enlargement.

There is no specific treatment for acute HBV infection. For chronic hepatitis B in childhood, interferon-alfa2b therapy and lamivudine have been approved for use in children with evidence of viral replication (HBV DNA or HBeAg positivity) and increased serum aminotransferase levels [38]. Interferon therapy requires an injection three times a week for 24 weeks. Lamivudine requires 52 weeks of daily oral administration. With interferon, 26% of children became HBeAg negative and 10% lost HBsAg. With lamivudine, 23% had HBeAg seroconversion and only 2% lost HBsAg. Adefovir dipivoxil is approved by the US Food and Drug Administration (FDA) for use in children over 12 years of age. Currently, trials are under way using the orally administered drugs entecavir for children under 16 years of age and tenofovir disoproxil fumarate in adolescents 12–17 years of age with chronic hepatitis B.

Hepatitis C

The signs and symptoms of hepatitis C are similar to those of hepatitis A and B. Acute disease is associated with jaundice in only 25% of patients, and abnormalities in serum liver function tests occur less frequently than with hepatitis B infection. Most infections are asymptomatic. Transmission of hepatitis C virus (HCV) can occur by way of parenteral administration of blood or blood products, but the majority of cases in the USA are not associated with blood transfusion. High-risk groups for HCV infection include parenteral drug users, people transfused with blood or blood products, healthcare workers who are frequently exposed to blood, and people with household or sexual contact with an infected person. Perinatal transmission of HCV has been demonstrated [39].

Seroprevalence among pregnant women in the USA is estimated at 1–2%, with maternal–fetal transmission at about 5%. Maternal coinfection with HIV has been associated with an increased risk of perinatal transmission of HCV. Vertical transmission of HCV may depend on the HCV genotype and the serum titer of maternal viral RNA. Serum HCV antibody and HCV RNA have been detected in breast milk, but HCV transmission to infants by breast-feeding has not been demonstrated [40]. The rate of vertical transmission of HCV is identical in breast-fed and bottle-fed infants. A key feature of HCV hepatitis is its propensity to progress to chronic hepatitis and more severe hepatic dysfunction. About 60–80% of children with hepatitis C progress to chronicity, and cirrhosis develops in at least 20% of these [41,42]. Hepatitis C has been associated with the development of hepatocellular carcinoma [43].

The two major tests currently available for the laboratory diagnosis of HCV infections are antibody assays for HCV and those for detecting and quantitating HCV RNA. The antibody test involves a sensitive enzyme-linked immunosorbent assay. If positive, confirmation in the past was made by a recombinant immunoblot assay. Both assays detect IgG antibodies; no IgM assays are available. Highly sensitive PCR assays for detection and quantification of HCV RNA and a nucleic acid-based amplification test are commercially available and have largely replaced the recombinant immunoblot assay for confirmation. These tests are costly, but they may be useful for monitoring patients undergoing therapy and for identifying infection early in infants because maternal antibody can cross the placenta and interfere with the ability to detect antibody produced by the infant.

Interferon, pegylated interferon, and pegylated interferon in combination with ribavirin have been found to be safe and efficacious in the treatment of chronic hepatitis C in adults and children [44–48]. Combination therapy (interferon with ribavirin) was shown to result in higher rates of sustained virologic, biochemical, and histologic response then interferon alone. Combination pegylated interferon and ribavirin are FDA approved for use in children with chronic HCV infection. The use of immunoglobulin for postexposure prophylaxis against HCV infection is not recommended based on the lack of clinical efficacy in humans and animal laboratory studies. Furthermore, immunoglobulin is manufactured from plasma documented to be negative for anti-HCV antibodies.

Delta hepatitis (hepatitis D)

Delta hepatitis virus requires infection with HBV because the outer coat of the complete HDV is HBsAg. If HDV infection occurs at the same time as HBV infection, this is referred to as a coinfection. If HDV infection occurs in a person who is already chronically infected with HBV, this is referred to as a superinfection. Transmission of HDV can be by parenteral, percutaneous, or mucous membrane inoculation. It may also be transmitted by blood or blood products, intravenous drug use, or sexual contact if HBsAg is present in the person's blood. Transmission of HDV from mother to newborn infant is unusual. Spread of HDV may also occur among families with HBsAg carriers. Infection with HDV is most commonly found in southern Italy, eastern Europe, South America, Africa, and the Middle East. Although there is a high prevalence of HBV infection in the Far East, HDV is uncommon there. In the USA, HDV is found most frequently in intravenous drug abusers, hemophiliacs, and immigrants from endemic areas.

Diagnosis of HDV infection can be made using commercially available anti-HDV antibody test, IgM-specific anti-HDV, and delta antigen tests. Differentiation of HDV coinfection from superinfection can be established by use of IgM anti-HBcAg, which is present only with acute HBV infection.

Treatment of HDV infection is supportive. Use of interferon therapy in limited trials has been disappointing [49]. Because HDV cannot be transmitted in the absence of HBV, care in avoiding HDV should be taken by HBV-positive individuals. Successful immunization with HBV vaccine affords protection from HDV infection.

Hepatitis E (enterically transmitted non-A, non-B hepatitis)

Transmission of hepatitis E virus is by the orofecal route. The disease is more common in adults than children and is associated with a significantly high incidence of mortality in pregnant women. Cases have been reported in epidemics and have usually been traced to contaminated water. Endemic enterically transmitted non-A, non-B hepatitis has been reported in the USA, but most reported cases have occurred among travelers to endemic regions.

Diagnosis is established by exclusion of other known causes of acute hepatitis (i.e. HAV, HBV, HCV, and HDV). Serologic tests that detect antibody (IgM) to the hepatitis E virus and hepatitis E viral RNA detection by PCR of stool or serum are available in commercial and research laboratories to confirm the diagnosis. Treatment is supportive. Passive immunoprophylaxis with immunoglobulin prepared in the USA has not been effective.

GB virus C (hepatitis G)

Two viruses belonging to the Flaviviridae family, GB virus C and hepatitis G virus (HGV), are variants of the same viral species and distantly related to HCV. Although there is considerable evidence demonstrating persistent viral infection, this virus has not been demonstrated to cause disease in humans or other primates. An association with post-transfusion hepatitis has been reported, but most infected children remain asymptomatic. Mother-to-infant transmission of HGV has been documented, resulting in a high viral persistence rate and lack of immune response to the virus [50,51]. In mothers coinfected with either HIV or HCV and HGV, HGV transmission is more frequent and occurs at a higher rate than that for HCV. Transmission of HGV can be through blood or blood products, injection drug use, or sexual contact.

No serologic test is commercially available. An indirect immunoassay, which uses the E2 (envelope) protein as an antigenic target, is available for research purposes. GB virus C RNA can be detected in serum samples using a reverse transcriptase PCR method.

Because the virus has not been demonstrated to cause either persistent hepatitis or symptomatic disease, treatment is supportive. Although HGV has been demonstrated to be sensitive to treatment with interferon therapy, the infection frequently recurs once therapy is terminated [52].

Transfusion-transmitted virus

Transfusion-transmitted virus (TTV) is an unenveloped, single-stranded DNA virus that has been implicated as a cause of post-transfusion hepatitis [53]. The virus has been found to contaminate blood and blood product transfusions and has been found in the feces [54]. No data have been published on maternal–neonatal transmission of this virus. Coinfection with HCV has been noted. Like HGV, TTV does not seem to be linked to biochemical signs of liver disease.

No serologic test is currently available. The viral DNA has been detected by use of PCR using semi-nested primers [55]. In preliminary studies in adults coinfected with HCV and TTV, interferon therapy seemed useful in TTV eradication.

Enteroviral hepatitis

Although many viruses may produce disease in the newborn, only a few viruses are frequently encountered. Among the less frequent viruses, which may on occasion result in nursery epidemics of significant clinical illness, are viruses within the enterovirus classification. These generally include non-polio enteroviruses, including coxsackieviruses, echoviruses, and enteroviruses. Transmission may have occurred during the prenatal, intrapartum, or perinatal period. A maternal history of a viral syndrome or fever just before delivery may be elicited. Initially the infant may appear healthy and vigorous. However, poor feeding, fever, lethargy, diarrhea, jaundice, and skin rash signal clinical infection. These non-specific signs, however, do not help to distinguish these viruses from other bacterial or viral etiologies. In the majority of cases, these infections are benign and self-limited. However, there are reports of death resulting from enteroviral infections in neonates [56,57]. Fatal and massive hepatic necrosis with failure has been reported with infections of coxsackievirus group B and echovirus groups 6, 9, 11, 14, and 19. These patients demonstrated jaundice, markedly elevated serum aminotransferases, disseminated intravascular coagulation, and progressive hepatic failure.

Diagnosis is made by viral isolation from the throat, rectum, or other sites of clinical involvement, or using biopsy material. Tissue culture techniques may not be adequate for viral isolation, and suckling mouse inoculation may be required to isolate the offending virus. Sera for antibody testing during the acute and convalescent periods should be collected and stored because an increase in titer for an isolated virus suggests a causal role. Because no common enterovirus antigen is available, serologic screening without viral isolation is generally not performed. Use of PCR to test for the presence of enteroviral RNA in cerebrospinal fluid is available in several research laboratories.

There is no specific approved therapy for enteroviral infections. Good supportive care, attention to bleeding problems, and treatment of secondary bacterial infections are important considerations. Intravenous immunoglobulin has been used in life-threatening neonatal enteroviral infections in hope of the presence of a high antibody titer to the infecting virus. Pleconaril is an investigational drug that inhibits viral attachment to host cell receptors and uncoating of viral nucleic acid. It has potent anti-enterovirus activity and has shown promise in treatment of neonatal echovirus and coxsackievirus B infections, including severe hepatitis [58].

Parvovirus hepatitis

Parvovirus B19 is most often associated with erythema infectiosum (fifth disease) and is usually manifested by mild systemic symptoms, fever, and the distinctive "slapped cheek" rash. However, it has been reported to cause liver disease ranging from an acute hepatitis to fulminant hepatitis with an associated aplastic anemia [59,60].

Laboratory diagnosis can be made by testing for parvovirus B19 IgM antibody. Presence of IgG serum antibody indicates prior infection and immunity. Commercial, research, and state health department laboratories provide assays using the PCR or nucleic acid hybridization techniques that are useful for detecting chronic infection.

Treatment with monoclonal anti-CD52 antibodies has been successful in a few cases [60]. In immunodeficient patients with chronic infection, intravenous immunoglobulin therapy should be considered.

Human herpesvirus 6 infection

Human herpesvirus 6 (HHV-6) infection has been identified as the etiologic agent for roseola infantum (exanthema subitum, sixth disease). Young children usually present with an acute febrile illness for several days, with rapid defervescence followed by an erythematous maculopapular rash lasting 1–2 days. Acute liver failure and chronic hepatitis in an infant associated with HHV-6 has been reported [61]. The presence of HHV-6 DNA in liver tissue was confirmed by both in situ hybridization and PCR.

Reovirus 3 infection

The concept of infantile obstructive cholangiopathy postulated by Landing [62] suggests a common etiologic agent for several neonatal liver diseases, including biliary atresia and neonatal hepatitis. Reovirus 3 has been proposed as a candidate virus serving as an etiologic agent for biliary atresia and neonatal hepatitis. Infection of weanling mice results in hepatic lesions similar to those observed in neonates with neonatal hepatitis. Several early studies suggested elevated reovirus type 3

antibody titers in the sera of infants with biliary atresia and neonatal hepatitis. Reovirus 3 was also detected in the porta hepatis of an infant with biliary atresia and in a monkey infected with reovirus that developed biliary atresia. However, this association has not been confirmed. Studies using molecular techniques have yielded mixed results [63,64]. If reovirus 3 infection results in biliary atresia or neonatal hepatitis in human newborns, only some of the cases may be attributed to its presence.

Paramyxovirus infection

Ten patients with an unusual form of giant cell hepatitis associated with a severe clinical course have been reported [65]. Two of the patients were infants 5 months and 7 months of age. Both infants had features of autoimmune chronic active hepatitis, and one infant also had evidence of autoimmune hemolytic anemia. Histopathologic and electron microscopic evaluation of the liver biopsy samples from these infants showed the presence of syncytial multinucleated giant cells replacing hepatocyte cords most prominently in the centrilobular region, as well as severe acute and chronic hepatitis with bridging necrosis of hepatocytes, ballooning, and dropout of hepatocytes, cholestasis, and small round cell inflammation within the lobule. Ultrastructural studies revealed the presence of virus-like structures within the giant cells resembling the nucleocapsids of paramyxoviruses. Inoculation from one of the patients into two chimpanzees failed to induce biochemical or histologic evidence of hepatitis. However, in one animal, an increase in titer of antibodies to measles virus and parainfluenza 4 was found. The giant cells in these infants were larger and of different morphology to the giant cells usually encountered in neonatal hepatitis and biliary atresia. Paramyxoviruses should be considered in patients with severe sporadic hepatitis.

Human immunodeficiency virus infection

Infection with HIV in children is associated with a broad spectrum of disease and a varied clinical course. Acquired immunodeficiency syndrome (AIDS) represents the most severe form. The great majority of cases of AIDS in children are the result of vertical transmission from an infected mother. Other infections (e.g. HBV, HCV) may be transmitted to the newborn more efficiently when the mother is coinfected with HIV. Other routes of HIV transmission include sexual contact with an infected individual and exposure to infected blood or blood products. Clinical manifestations of HIV infection often involve the gastrointestinal tract and the liver and include generalized lymphadenopathy, hepatomegaly, splenomegaly, failure to thrive, oral candidiasis, recurrent diarrhea, parotitis, cardiomyopathy, hepatitis, nephropathy, central nervous system disease, lymphoid interstitial pneumonia, recurrent invasive bacterial infections, opportunistic infections, and malignancies.

Although liver involvement is frequently observed in HIV infection, whether the liver lesions are primary or secondary to opportunistic infection in an immunosuppressed host is difficult to determine. Children with HIV infection have demonstrated hepatosplenomegaly and elevated serum aminotransferases. Histology has revealed both lobular and portal changes with lymphocytic infiltration, piecemeal necrosis, hepatocellular and bile duct damage, sinusoidal cell hyperplasia, and endothelialitis [66]. In adults with HIV infection with abnormal liver test abnormalities, fever for longer than 2 weeks, or hepatomegaly who undergo liver biopsy, the most common biopsy-derived diagnosis has been *Mycobacterium avium* complex [67]. Other frequently diagnosed infections have included *Mycobacterium tuberculosis*, other *Mycobacterium* species, and other opportunistic infections. Biliary tract abnormalities, including papillary stenosis and sclerosing cholangitis, have been observed. The most common neoplasm has been lymphoma. The efficacy of liver biopsy in HIV-infected people is still unknown. Liver biopsy may be a helpful diagnostic tool in HIV-positive patients with fever, hepatomegaly, or liver test abnormalities.

Diagnosis of HIV infection is made by serum antibody tests (enzyme immunoassays), except in children under 18 months of age because of passive maternal antibody acquisition across the placenta. Western blot or immunofluorescent antibody tests should be used for confirmation of positive results. In young children (18 months), the preferred tests are HIV culture and detection of HIV genomic sequences by PCR.

Antiretroviral therapy is the standard of care for HIV-infected children. Therapeutic strategies are rapidly changing in this field, so consultation with an expert or enrollment of an HIV-infected child into an available clinical trial is recommended.

Neonatal lupus erythematosus

Hepatic involvement expressed as neonatal cholestasis has been associated with neonatal lupus erythematosus [68,69]. Hepatomegaly and splenomegaly have been noted in 20–40% of reported cases. Several infants with neonatal lupus erythematosus have been reported with liver histology demonstrating giant cell transformation, ductal obstruction, and extramedullary hematopoiesis. It is postulated that maternal autoantibodies passing by way of a transplacental mechanism result in an immune response in the infant that results in hepatic injury. This is an extension of the theory that maternal autoantibodies to Sjögren syndrome antigen A and Sjögren syndrome antigen B cause congenital heart block in infants with neonatal lupus erythematosus whose initial pathologic lesion is myocardial inflammation. Clearly, a prospective study investigating maternal autoantibodies and the incidence of liver involvement in neonatal lupus erythematosus is required before this hypothesis can be proved.

Chromosomal disorders

Both neonatal hepatitis and biliary atresia have been associated with trisomy 17–18 syndrome (trisomy E) and trisomy 21 (Down syndrome) [70,71]. Intrahepatic cholestasis and variable combinations of hepatocellular and portal tract involvement have been observed. Giant cell transformation and focal obliteration of bile ducts have been seen. Diffuse lobular fibrosis surrounding proliferating ductular elements and residual hepatocytes, which proved fatal, was observed in a group of infants with Down syndrome. The possibility of a viral etiology for the hepatic lesions observed was not sufficiently excluded. Whether the chromosomal defects directly contribute to the hepatic dysfunction observed in these infants is unknown.

Familial intrahepatic cholestatic syndromes

The familial intrahepatic cholestatic syndromes are discussed in detail in Chapters 13 and 14. Affected children often present in infancy or early childhood because of their propensity to develop cholestasis, and so have often been classified under the umbrella of neonatal hepatitis. These children may have disease limited to the liver or have abnormalities, often striking, in other organs. Laboratory findings vary widely depending on the condition. Typical obstructive cholestasis with jaundice, pruritus, and hypercholesterolemia may dominate the picture, although certain syndromes are atypical, with normal serum cholesterol levels, normal gamma-glutamyltransferase levels, and cholestasis.

Among these syndromes are conditions that are fatal in childhood, whereas others are essentially benign. Investigation of many of the conditions in this group has led to clear identification and characterization within the past few years [72–75].

Pseudo-TORCH syndrome (Baraitser–Reardon syndrome)

Intracranial calcifications may be observed in neonates with environmental or metabolic disturbances. The predominant environmental factors associated with intracranial calcifications are congenital infections with toxoplasmosis, rubella, CMV, herpes, and others (TORCH). Yet, there are infants in whom all confirmatory tests for congenital infection are negative. Reports of more than one affected child within a sibship have led to the recognition of an autosomal recessive congenital infection-like syndrome called pseudo-TORCH syndrome [76–78]. In addition to the intracranial calcifications, microcephaly, seizures, neurologic delay, hepatomegaly, splenomegaly, raised serum aminotransferases (aspartate aminotransferase, alanine aminotransferase) and thrombocytopenia have been observed [79]. A liver biopsy performed at 2 months of age in a child with this syndrome showed preserved liver architecture without any sign of inflammation or focal necrosis. Abundant iron pigmentary accumulations were observed within many hepatocytes in association with features of cholestasis. Aicardi–Goutière syndrome shares many of the features of pseudo-TORCH syndrome but differs by the presence of cerebrospinal fluid lymphocytosis with raised levels of interferon-α. Two boys of consanguineous parents demonstrating the phenotypic overlap of Aicardi-Goutière and pseudo-TORCH syndromes have been reported.

Coombs-positive giant cell hepatitis

Although giant cell hepatitis is a frequent pattern of injury in the neonate, it is unusual after infancy. Coombs-positive giant cell hepatitis is a rare disease of early childhood with unknown etiology and a variable response to immunosuppressive therapy [80]. An immune dysregulation mechanism is postulated. Liver histology reveals severe giant cell transformation with cholestasis, marked inflammation, clusters of neutrophils, spotty hepatocyte necrosis, and fibrosis. Many reports in the literature suggest this disorder is distinct and has an aggressive course. Liver transplantation for giant cell hepatitis with autoimmune Coombs-positive hemolytic anemia has had inconsistent success, with reports of recurrence of disease in the graft [81].

Differential diagnosis

A diverse group of disorders may present in the neonate as cholestasis with a conjugated hyperbilirubinemia. A logical, well-organized, and rapid evaluation of the infant with conjugated hyperbilirubinemia is mandatory. Although the differential list is long and may be intimidating, the work-up is relatively straightforward. The initial evaluation should determine the severity of the hepatic dysfunction. It should identify specific metabolic, infectious, endocrinologic, toxic, or surgically correctable disorders amenable to therapy. The initial evaluation should identify recognizable genetic or congenital disorders and determine the need for further investigation. Statistically, approximately 75% of all cases of neonatal cholestasis are the result of biliary atresia or neonatal hepatitis. Neonatal hepatitis is the most common diagnosis of infants with neonatal cholestasis. Epidemiologic data suggest two categories of neonatal hepatitis: a sporadic form and a familial form. The increased incidence of neonatal hepatitis within some families suggests that a metabolic or genetic cause is responsible. Unfortunately, no etiologic factor has been identified in these cases. Some of these familial cases may have forms of progressive familial intrahepatic cholestasis.

Discriminating among the several forms of familial intrahepatic cholestasis may be aided by a comparison of several factors. These include birth weight; age of onset of cholestasis; associated anomalies of the heart, eyes, bones, or kidneys; pattern of cholestasis (episodic or continuous); laboratory parameters; biopsy findings; outcome; and presumed inheritance pattern.

Clinical presentation

Differentiating extrahepatic from intrahepatic cholestasis remains the challenge for the clinician because early recognition of extrahepatic obstruction may be amenable to surgical intervention. Furthermore, avoiding unnecessary and potentially harmful surgery is always warranted. Unfortunately, there is no pathognomonic symptom to distinguish biliary atresia from neonatal hepatitis. Infants in both groups present with jaundice and acholic stools. Observation of the stools by an experienced individual is an inexpensive and highly useful procedure. Verbal reports of stool pigment from the parents in my experience are notoriously inaccurate. Pruritus does not occur until later in the course. The liver is enlarged on physical examination. Clinical features may be useful in helping to discriminate between biliary atresia and neonatal hepatitis.

Biliary atresia is more common in girls with normal birth weight, whereas neonatal hepatitis is more common in boys [81,82]. Familial occurrence favors neonatal hepatitis. An associated polysplenia syndrome favors biliary atresia. Intermittent pigmentation of stools favors intrahepatic cholestasis, whereas consistently acholic stools favor a diagnosis of biliary atresia. Unfortunately, severe intrahepatic cholestasis also may result in acholic stools. With neonatal hepatitis, jaundice may persist after the first week of physiologic jaundice of the newborn, so jaundice may already be observed as abnormal during the second week of life. In contrast, a jaundice-free interval between the disappearance of physiologic jaundice and the onset of pathologic obstructive jaundice may be seen in patients with biliary atresia.

Pathologic jaundice requires biochemical confirmation with fractionation of the serum bilirubin. A conjugated hyperbilirubinemia with elevated serum aminotransferase levels, alkaline phosphatase, and gamma-glutamyltransferase is seen. Although many attempts have been made to discriminate intrahepatic from extrahepatic cholestasis based on biochemical profiles, overlap between groups has significantly hampered this approach.

Ultrasonographic examination of the liver, radionuclide hepatobiliary imaging, collection of duodenal fluid by a tube or string device, endoscopic retrograde cholangiopancreatography, percutaneous transhepatic cholangiography, and percutaneous liver biopsy all provide valuable information to aid in discrimination of intrahepatic and extrahepatic cholestasis. The combination of procedures performed depends on the results, skills, and expertise of the institution. However, there will still be patients for whom an intraoperative cholangiogram is necessary. Use of new therapeutic regimens (i.e. ursodeoxycholic acid) should not be instituted until a definitive diagnosis has been made. Early surgical intervention is the preferred treatment for biliary atresia.

Histopathology

In neonatal hepatitis, alterations in the parenchyma of the liver are more prominent than alterations in the portal zone [83–87] (Figure 10.5). Giant cells are usually more prominent than in biliary atresia and may be ballooned or may show degeneration [86,87]. Necrosis of giant cells in the parenchyma may result in neutrophil infiltration. Extramedullary hematopoiesis

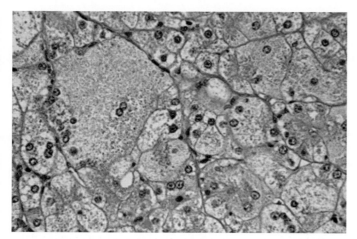

Figure 10.5 Neonatal hepatitis with giant cell transformation. Centrizonal region shows enlarged giant hepatocytes and scattered lobular sinusoidal mononuclear infiltrates. (Hematoxylin & eosin, original magnification 100×).

and hemosiderin deposition in parenchymal and Kupffer cells are generally more prominent in neonatal hepatitis than in biliary atresia. Intralobular inflammation and Kupffer cell hyperplasia are usually apparent in neonatal hepatitis, whereas portal and periportal inflammation is more apparent in biliary atresia. Cholestasis may be variable in neonatal hepatitis with pigment granules in parenchymal and Kupffer cells and intercellular bile plugs present. With severe cholestasis in neonatal hepatitis, bile plugs may be seen in portal ductules but usually not to the extent seen in biliary atresia. Bile ductular proliferation may occasionally be observed in neonatal hepatitis but is usually much more prominent in cases of biliary atresia.

By light and electron microscopic studies, the multinucleated giant cells in neonatal hepatitis appear to be of parenchymal origin. The number of nuclei in the giant cells may vary, as may their positions centrally or peripherally within the cytoplasm. By hematoxylin and eosin staining, the cytoplasm of multinucleated giant cells seen in neonatal hepatitis is pale. This may be the result of glycogen content or hydropic changes. Brownish pigment granules present in the giant cells may be a combination of bilirubin, hemosiderin, or lipofuscin deposition. Histochemical analysis of multinucleated giant cells in neonatal hepatitis reveals intense periodic acid–Schiff staining with diastase digestion, signifying glycogen presence [86]. Additionally, there is intense staining for glucose-6-phosphatase, succinic dehydrogenase, nicotinamide adenine dinucleotide, and nicotinamide adenine dinucleotide phosphate diaphorases. Inclusions that are acid phosphatase

positive are numerous, and there is increased alkaline phosphatase staining at the sinusoidal border.

Electron microscopic evaluation of multinucleated giant cells in neonatal hepatitis reveals well-preserved nuclei, mitochondria, endoplasmic reticulum, and plasma membranes [86,87]. Numerous intracytoplasmic vacuoles, bilirubin deposits, and nuclei are present. The formative mechanisms of giant cells have been debated, although fusion of several mononuclear hepatocytes to form a giant cell appears to be the most plausible explanation [86]. The mechanism whereby there is loss of giant cells spontaneously with time is also unknown. Giant cells appear to have a lifespan of several months, and their disappearance seems to parallel resolution of cholestasis. Their presence seems to be a non-specific response of the immature liver to injury [84]. Their biologic significance is unknown, and although they are more commonly seen in the newborn, they also may be seen on occasion in the livers of adults with various viral- or drug-induced hepatic disorders [65]. A girl with neonatal hepatitis progressing to cirrhosis and hepatocellular carcinoma by 28 months of age has been reported [88].

Prognosis

Prognosis of patients with neonatal hepatitis may be variable and depends on the extent of parenchymal injury and fibrosis [89–93]. In general, patients with neonatal hepatitis have a better prognosis than infants with biliary atresia or metabolic liver diseases, which are not amenable to diet therapy. Sporadic cases of neonatal hepatitis have a better prognosis than familial cases or cases with associated conditions such as α_1-antitrypsin deficiency. Quoted recovery rates from neonatal hepatitis are in the 60–80% range for sporadic forms, whereas for familial forms the recovery rate is in the 20–40% range. However, the impact of early recognition and intervention with diet therapy, vitamin supplementation, choleretic agents, and hepatic transplantation on the prognosis for neonatal hepatitis awaits further study.

Acknowledgements

I thank Samuel H. Pepkowitz of the Department of Pathology and Laboratory Medicine, Cedars-Sinai Medical Center, and Linda Ferrell of the Department of Pathology, University of California, San Francisco, for help with photographing the figures and creating the legends.

References

1. Hamilton JR, Sass-Kortsak A. Jaundice associated with severe bacterial infection in young infants. *J Pediatr* 1963;**63**:121–132.

2. Zimmerman HJ, Fang M, Utili R, *et al.* Jaundice due to bacterial infection. *Gastroenterology* 1979;**77**:362–374.

3. Andres JM, Walker WA. Effect of *Escherichia coli* endotoxin on the developing rat liver. I. Giant cell induction and disruption in protein metabolism. *Pediatr Res* 1979;**13**:1290–1293.

4. Bolder U, Ton-Nu HT, Schteingart CD, *et al.* Hepatocyte transport of bile acids and organic anions in endotoxemic rats: impaired uptake and secretion. *Gastroenterology* 1997;**112**:214–225.

5. Borges MAG, DeBrito T, Borges JMG. Hepatic manifestations in bacterial infections of infants and children. Clinical features, biochemical data and

morphologic hepatic changes. *Acta Hepatogastroenterol* 1972;**19**:328–344.

6. Lam HS, Li AM, Chu WCW, *et al*. Malpositioned umbilical venous catheter causing liver abscess in a preterm infant. *Biol Neonate* 2005;**88**:54–56.

7. Garcia FJ, Nager AL. Jaundice as an early diagnostic sign of urinary tract infection in infancy. *Pediatrics* 2002;**109**:846–851.

8. Hoarau C, Ranivoharimina V, Chavet-Queru MS, *et al*. Congenital syphilis: update and perspectives. *Sante* 1999;**9**:38–45.

9. Herman TE. Extensive hepatic calcification secondary to fulminant neonatal syphilitic hepatitis. *Pediatr Radiol* 1995;**25**:120–122.

10. Kumar R, Gupta N, Sabharwal A, Shalini. Congenital tuberculosis. *Indian J Pediatr* 2005;**72**:631–633.

11. Montoya JG, Rosso F. Diagnosis and management of toxoplasmosis. *Clin Perinatol* 2005;**32**:705–726.

12. Desmonts G, Couvreur J. Congenital toxoplasmosis. A prospective study of 378 pregnancies. *N Engl J Med* 1974;**290**:1110–1116.

13. Schmidt DR, Hogh B, Andersen O, *et al*. Treatment of infants with congenital toxoplasmosis: tolerability and plasma concentrations of sulfadiazine and pyrimethamine. *Eur J Pediatr* 2005;**165**:19–25.

14. Nicol KK, Geisinger KR. Congenital toxoplasmosis: diagnosis by exfoliative cytology. *Diagn Cytopathol* 1998;**18**:357–361.

15. Bellomo-Brandao MA, Andrade PD, Costa SC, *et al*. Cytomegalovirus frequency in neonatal intrahepatic cholestasis determined by serology, histology, immunohistochemistry and PCR. *World J Gastroenterol* 2009;**15**:3411–3416.

16. Laifer SA, Ehrlich GD, Huff DS, *et al*. Congenital cytomegalovirus infection in offspring of liver transplant recipients. *Clin Infect Dis* 1995;**20**:52–55.

17. Zuppan CW, Bui HD, Grill BG. Diffuse hepatic fibrosis in congenital cytomegalovirus infection. *J Pediatr Gastroenterol Nutr* 1986;**5**:489–491.

18. Watkins JB, Sunaryo FP, Berezin SH. Hepatic manifestations of congenital and perinatal disease. *Clin Perinatol* 1981;**8**:467–480.

19. Weller TH, Hanshaw JB. Virologic and clinical observations on cytomegalic inclusion disease. *N Engl J Med* 1962;**266**:1233–1244.

20. Snover DC, Horwitz CA. Liver disease in cytomegalovirus mononucleosis: a light microscopical and immunoperoxidase study of six cases. *Hepatology* 1984;**3**:408–412.

21. Greenfield C, Sinickas V, Harrison LC. Detection of cytomegalovirus by the polymerase chain reaction. A simple, rapid and sensitive non-radioactive method. *Med J Aust* 1991;**154**:383–385.

22. Berenberg W, Nankervis G. Long-term followup of cytomegalic inclusion disease of infancy. *Pediatrics* 1970;**46**:403–410.

23. Dressler S, Linder D. Noncirrhotic portal fibrosis following neonatal cytomegalic inclusion disease. *J Pediatr* 1978;**93**:887–888.

24. Thompson C, Whitley R. Neonatal herpes simplex virus infections: where are we now? *World J Gastroenterol* 2009;**15**:3411–3416.

25. Twagira M, Hadzic N, Smith M, *et al*. Disseminated neonatal herpes simplex virus (HSV) type 2 infection diagnosed by HSV DNA detection in blood and successfully managed by liver transplantation. *Eur J Pediatr* 2004;**163**:166–169.

26. Nakamura Y, Yamamoto S, Tanaka S, *et al*. Herpes simplex viral infection in human neonates: an immunohistochemical and electron microscopic study. *Human Pathol* 1985;**16**:1091–1097.

27. Raga J, Chrystal V, Coovadia HM. Usefulness of clinical features and liver biopsy in diagnosis of disseminated herpes simplex infection. *Arch Dis Child* 1984;**59**:820–824.

28. Egawa H, Inomata Y, Nakayama S, *et al*. Fulminant hepatic failure secondary to herpes simplex virus infection in a neonate: a case report of successful treatment with liver transplantation and perioperative acyclovir. *Liver Transplant Surg* 1998;**4**:513–515.

29. Schluter WW, Reef SE, Redd SC, *et al*. Changing epidemiology of congenital rubella syndrome in the United States. *J Infect Dis* 1998;**178**:636–641.

30. Monif GRG, Asofsky R, Sever JL. Hepatic dysfunction in the congenital rubella syndrome. *BMJ* 1966;**1**:1086–1088.

31. Strauss L, Bernstein J. Neonatal hepatitis in congenital rubella. *Arch Pathol* 1968;**86**:317–327.

32. Duff P. Hepatitis in pregnancy. *Semin Perinatol* 1998;**22**:277–283.

33. Noble RC, Kane MA, Reeves SA, *et al*. Posttransfusion hepatitis A in a neonatal intensive care unit. *JAMA* 1984;**252**:2711–2715.

34. Renge RL, Dani VS, Chitambar SD, Arankalle VA. Vertical transmission of hepatitis A. *Indian J Pediatr* 2002;**69**:535–536.

35. Leikin E, Lysikiewicz A, Garry D, Tejani N. Intrauterine transmission of hepatitis A virus. *Obstet Gynecol* 1996;**88**:690–691.

36. Poland GA, Jacobson RM. Prevention of hepatitis B with the hepatitis B vaccine. *N Eng J Med* 2004;**351**:2832–2838.

37. Tang JR, Hsu HY, Lin HH, *et al*. Hepatitis B surface antigenemia at birth: a long-term follow-up study. *J Pediatr* 1998;**133**:374–377.

38. Suskind DL, Rosenthal P. Chronic viral hepatitis. *Adolesc Med Clin* 2004;**15**:145–158.

39. Granovsky MO, Minkoff HL, Tess BH, *et al*. Hepatitis C virus infection in the mothers and infants cohort study. *Pediatrics* 1998;**102**:355–359.

40. Kumar RM, Shahul S. Role of breast-feeding in transmission of hepatitis C virus to infants of HCV-infected mothers. *J Hepatol* 1998;**29**:191–197.

41. Chang MH. Chronic hepatitis virus infection in children. *J Gastroenterol Hepatol* 1998;**13**:541–548.

42. Realdi G, Alberti A, Rugge M, *et al*. Long-term follow-up of acute and chronic non-A, non-B post-transfusion hepatitis: evidence of progression to liver cirrhosis. *Gut* 1982;**23**:270–275.

43. Hasan F, Jeffers LJ, De Medina M, *et al*. Hepatitis-C associated hepatocellular carcinoma. *Hepatology* 1990;**12**:589–591.

44. McHutchison JG, Gordon SC, Schiff ER, *et al*. Interferon alfa-2b alone or in combination with ribavirin as initial treatment for chronic hepatitis C. Hepatitis Interventional Therapy Group. *N Engl J Med* 1998;**339**:1485–1492.

45. Fried MW, Shiffman ML, Reddy KR, *et al*. Peginterferon alfa-2a plus ribavirin for chronic hepatitis C virus

infection. *N Engl J Med*
2002;**347**:975–982.

46. Gonzalez-Peralta RP. Treatment of chronic hepatitis C in children. *Pediatr Transplant* 2004;**8**:639–643.

47. Bortolotti F, Iorio R, Nebbia G, *et al.* Interferon treatment in children with chronic hepatitis C: long-lasting remission in responders, and risk for disease progression in non-responders. *Dig Liver Dis* 2005;**37**:336–341.

48. Schwarz KB, Gonzalez-Peralta RP, Murray KF, *et al.* The combination of ribavirin and peginterferon is superior to peginterferon and placebo for children and adolescents with chronic hepatitis C. *Gastroenterology* 2011;**140**:450–458.

49. Dalekos GN, Galanakis E, Zervou E, *et al.* Interferon-alpha treatment of children with chronic hepatitis D virus infection: the Greek experience. *Hepatogastroenterology* 2000;**47**:1072–1076.

50. Chen HL, Chang MH, Lin HH, *et al.* Antibodies to E2 protein of hepatitis G virus in children: different responses according to age at infection. *J Pediatr* 1998;**133**:382–385.

51. Zanetti AR, Tanzi E, Romano L, *et al.* Multicenter trial on mother-to-infant transmission of GBV-C virus. The Lombardy Study Group on Vertical/Perinatal Hepatitis Viruses Transmission. *J Med Virol* 1998;**54**:107–112.

52. Woelfle J, Berg T, Keller KM, *et al.* Persistent hepatitis G virus infection after neonatal transfusion. *J Pediatr Gastroenterol Nutr* 1998;**26**:402–407.

53. Naoumov NV, Petrova EP, Thomas MG, *et al.* Presence of a newly described human DNA virus (TTV) in patients with liver disease. *Lancet* 1998;**352**:195–197.

54. Okamoto H, Akahane Y, Ukita M, *et al.* Fecal excretion of a nonenveloped DNA virus (TTV) associated with posttransfusion non-A-G hepatitis. *J Med Virol* 1998;**56**:128–132.

55. Koidl C, Michael B, Berg J, *et al.* Detection of transfusion transmitted virus DNA by real-time PCR. *J Clin Virol* 2004;**29**:277–281.

56. Abzug MJ. Prognosis for neonates with enterovirus hepatitis and coagulopathy. *Pediatr Infect Dis J* 2001;**20**:758–763.

57. Kawashima H, Ryou S, Nishimata S, *et al.* Enteroviral hepatitis in children. *Pediatr Int* 2004;**46**:130–134.

58. Abzug MJ. Presentation, diagnosis, and management of enterovirus infections in neonates. *Paediatr Drugs* 2004;**6**:1–10.

59. Pardi DS, Romero Y, Mertz LE, *et al.* Hepatitis-associated aplastic anemia and acute parvovirus B19 infection: a report of two cases and a review of the literature. *Am J Gastroenterol* 1998;**93**:468–470.

60. Granot E, Miskin H, Aker M. Monoclonal anti-CD52 antibodies: a potential mode of therapy for parvovirus B19 hepatitis. *Transplant Proc* 2001;**33**:2151–2153.

61. Tajiri H, Tanaka-Taya K, Ozaki Y, *et al.* Chronic hepatitis in an infant, in association with human herpesvirus-6 infection. *J Pediatr* 1997;**131**:473–475.

62. Landing BH. Considerations of the pathogenesis of neonatal hepatitis, biliary atresia and choledochal cyst: the concept of infantile obstructive cholangiopathy. *Prog Pediatr Surg* 1974;**4**:113–139.

63. Steele MI, Marshall CM, Lloyd RE, *et al.* Reovirus 3 not detected by reverse transcriptase-mediated polymerase chain reaction analysis of preserved tissue from infants with cholestatic liver disease. *Hepatology* 1995;**21**:697–702.

64. Tyler KL, Sokol RJ, Oberhaus SM, *et al.* Detection of reovirus RNA in hepatobiliary tissues from patients with extrahepatic biliary atresia and choledochal cysts. *Hepatology* 1998;**27**:1475–1482.

65. Phillips MJ, Blendis LM, Poucell S, *et al.* Syncytial giant-cell hepatitis: sporadic hepatitis with distinctive pathological features, a severe clinical course, and paramyxoviral features. *N Engl J Med* 1991;**324**:455–460.

66. Kahn E, Greco MA, Daum F, *et al.* Hepatic pathology in pediatric acquired immunodeficiency syndrome. *Human Pathol* 1991;**22**:1111–1119.

67. Poles MA, Dieterich DT, Schwarz ED, *et al.* Liver biopsy findings in 501 patients infected with human immunodeficiency virus (HIV). *J AIDS Hum Retrovirol* 1996;**11**:170–177.

68. Laxer RM, Roberts EA, Gross KR, *et al.* Liver disease in neonatal lupus

erythematosus. *J Pediatr* 1990;**116**:238–242.

69. Lee LA, Sokol RJ, Buyon JP. Hepatobiliary disease in neonatal lupus: prevalence and clinical characteristics in cases enrolled in a national registry. *Pediatrics* 2002;**109**:E11.

70. Alpert LI, Strauss L, Hirschhorn K. Neonatal hepatitis and biliary atresia associated with trisomy 17–18 syndrome. *N Engl J Med* 1969;**280**:16–20.

71. Schwab M, Niemeyer C, Schwarzer U. Down syndrome, transient myeloproliferative disorder, and infantile liver fibrosis. *Med Pediatr Oncol* 1998;**31**:159–165.

72. Pratt DS. Cholestasis and cholestatic syndromes. *Curr Opin Gastroenterol* 2005;**21**:270–274.

73. van Mil SW, Houwen RH, Klomp LW. Genetics of familial intrahepatic cholestasis syndromes. *J Med Genet* 2005;**42**:449–463.

74. Krantz ID, Piccoli DA, Spinner NB. Alagille syndrome. *J Med Genet* 1997;**34**:152–157.

75. Bull LN, van Eijk MJ, Pawlikowska L, *et al.* A gene encoding a P-type ATPase mutated in two forms of hereditary cholestasis. *Nat Genet* 1998;**18**:219–224.

76. Vivarelli R, Grosso S, Cioni M, *et al.* Pseudo-TORCH syndrome or Baraitser–Reardon syndrome: diagnostic criteria. *Brain Dev* 2001;**23**:18–23.

77. Sanchis A, Cervero L, Bataller A, *et al.* Genetic syndromes mimic congenital infections. *J Pediatr* 2005;**146**:701–705.

78. Knoblauch H, Tyennstedt C, Brueck W, *et al.* Two brothers with findings resembling congenital intrauterine infection-like syndrome (pseudo-TORCH syndrome). *Am J Med Genet A* 2003;**120**:261–265.

79. Hadzic N, Portmann B, Lewis I, Mieli-Vergani G. Coombs positive giant cell hepatitis: a new feature of Evans' syndrome. *Arch Dis Child* 1998;**78**:397–398.

80. Akylidiz M, Karasu Z, Arikan C, *et al.* Successful liver transplantation for giant cell hepatitis and Coombs-positive haemolytic anemia: a case report. *Pediatr Transplant* 2005;**9**:630–633.

81. Balistreri WF, Grand R, Hoofnagle JH, *et al.* Biliary atresia: current concepts and research directions. Summary of a

symposium. *Hepatology* 1996;**23**:1682–1692.

82. Bates MD, Bucuvalas JC, Alonso MH, *et al.* Biliary atresia: pathogenesis and treatment. *Semin Liver Dis* 1998;**18**:281–293.

83. Tazawa Y, Abukawa D, Maisawa S, *et al.* Idiopathic neonatal hepatitis presenting as neonatal hepatic siderosis and steatosis. *Dig Dis Sci* 1998;**43**:392–396.

84. Shet TM, Kandalkar BM, Vora IM. Neonatal hepatitis: an autopsy study of 14 cases. *Indian J Pathol Microbiol* 1998;**41**:77–84.

85. Nishinomiya F, Abukawa D, Takada G, *et al.* Relationships between clinical and histological profiles of non-familial idiopathic neonatal hepatitis. *Acta Paediatr Jpn* 1996;**38**:242–247.

86. Ruebner B, Thaler MM. Giant-cell transformation in infantile liver disease. In Javitt NB (ed.) *Neonatal Hepatitis and Biliary Atresia.* [DHEW publication 79-1296.] Bethesda, MD: US Department of Health, Education and Welfare, 1979, pp. 299–314.

87. Park WH, Kim SP, Park KK, *et al.* Electron microscopic study of the liver with biliary atresia and neonatal hepatitis. *J Pediatr Surg* 1996;**31**:367–374.

88. Moore L, Bourne AJ, Moore DJ, *et al.* Hepatocellular carcinoma following neonatal hepatitis. *Pediatr Pathol Lab Med* 1997;**17**:601–610.

89. Suita S, Arima T, Ishii K, *et al.* Fate of infants with neonatal hepatitis: pediatric surgeons' dilemma. *J Pediatr Surg* 1992;**27**:696–699.

90. Dick MC, Mowat AP. Hepatitis syndrome in infancy: an epidemiological survey with 10 year follow-up. *Arch Dis Child* 1985;**60**:512–516.

91. Lee PI, Chang MH, Chen DS, *et al.* Prognostic implications of serum alpha-fetoprotein levels in neonatal hepatitis. *J Pediatr Gastroenterol Nutr* 1990;**11**:27–31.

92. Chang MH, Hsu HC, Lee CY, *et al.* Neonatal hepatitis: a follow-up study. *J Pediatr Gastroenterol Nutr* 1987;**6**:203–207.

93. Deutsch J, Smith AL, Danks DM, *et al.* Long-term prognosis for babies with neonatal liver disease. *Arch Dis Child* 1985;**60**:447–451.

Biliary atresia and other disorders of the extrahepatic bile ducts

William F. Balistreri, Jorge A. Bezerra, and Frederick C. Ryckman

Introduction

Biliary atresia and related disorders of the biliary tract, such as choledochal cysts, must be considered in the differential diagnosis of prolonged conjugated hyperbilirubinemia in the newborn (neonatal cholestasis).

Neonatal hepatobiliary diseases, including biliary atresia, choledochal cysts, and "idiopathic" neonatal hepatitis, have historically been viewed as a continuum – a gradation of manifestations of a basic underlying disease process in which giant cell transformation of hepatocytes is strongly associated with inflammation at any level of the hepatobiliary tract. These disease entities may be polar end-points of a common initial insult, as originally stated in the unifying hypothesis of Landing [1]. The end result represents the sequelae of the inflammatory process at the primary site of injury. Landing suggested that this inflammatory process may injure bile duct epithelial cells, leading to either duct obliteration (biliary atresia) or weakening of the bile duct wall with subsequent dilatation (choledochal cyst). The lesions may be dependent on the stage of fetal or early postnatal development when the injury occurs and the site within the developing hepatobiliary tree at which the injury occurs [1,2]. The recent observation that extrahepatic bile ducts develop cystic dilatations following rotavirus infection in newborn mice genetically primed to have a prominent T helper lymphocyte type 2 response suggests that the lesions may also be dependent on the type of immune response to the viral insult [3]. A relationship between the pathogenesis of these obstructive cholangiopathies of infancy and the process of development (embryogenesis) is suggested by the association with disorders of situs determination such as the polysplenia syndrome and the observation of the so-called ductal plate malformation within the liver of a few patients with biliary atresia. The ductal plate malformation is postulated to represent either a primary developmental anomaly or disruption of a developmental sequence early in fetal life, resulting in incomplete regression of the immature bile ducts [2]. In contrast, most patients with biliary atresia have the late-onset type, which probably occurs after the anatomic formation of intra- and extrahepatic bile ducts; this represents injury

(destruction) of fully formed structures [1]. The dynamic nature of the underlying process has been further suggested by an apparent postnatal evolution of patent to atretic ducts: patients initially shown to have "neonatal hepatitis" with a patent biliary system were subsequently found to have acquired biliary atresia. The overlap concept is additionally supported by the frequent documentation of intrahepatic ductal injury in patients with extrahepatic biliary atresia. Depletion of intrahepatic bile ducts is observed regularly at autopsy in children with biliary atresia who were never subjected to a biliary drainage procedure [4].

In biliary atresia, the initial insult remains undefined. For example, although viral infection is a postulated initial insult, no specific viral agent has been reproducibly detected in tissue from affected infants, and there is no conclusive serologic evidence of their presence [5]. Other theories (discussed below) include defective embryogenesis or an innate or development-specific dysregulation of the immune response to injury [6]. Greater understanding of how the neonatal immune system responds to a perinatal viral insult will provide insight into early mechanisms that disrupt the mucosal integrity of the bile ducts, obstruct the lumen, and sustain the activation of cells that produce the ongoing liver injury [5,6]. Further studies are warranted; biliary atresia and related disorders continue to offer clinicians and scientists stimulating challenges.

This chapter reviews the current status of diagnosis and management of these disorders, as well as advances in the intriguing quest for an understanding of their pathogenesis.

Biliary atresia

Biliary atresia is the end result of a destructive, idiopathic, inflammatory process that affects intra- and extrahepatic bile ducts, leading to fibrosis and obliteration of the biliary tract, and eventual development of biliary cirrhosis [5]. This disorder should be of interest to all individuals involved in basic and clinical studies of diseases of the liver; the rapidly progressive fibro-obliterative process may represent a paradigm for other forms of hepatobiliary injury, perhaps reflecting an

Liver Disease in Children, Fourth Edition, ed. Frederick J. Suchy, Ronald J. Sokol, and William F. Balistreri. Published by Cambridge University Press. © Cambridge University Press 2014.

inter-relationship between genetic predisposition and environmental exposure [5].

Biliary atresia is the most common cause of chronic cholestasis in infants and children, and because of the high frequency of progression to end-stage liver disease, it is the most frequent indication for liver transplantation in the pediatric age group. There is general agreement that the older theory that biliary atresia was caused by failure of recanalization of embryonic bile ducts should be abandoned. The lesion, in most patients, is not a true congenital malformation but seems to be acquired in late gestation or after birth. Studies of liver samples obtained from patients with biliary atresia at the time of diagnosis revealed unique proinflammatory features [7,8]; how the inflammatory process produces complete or partial sclerosis of the extrahepatic (and intrahepatic) biliary ducts is now the subject of ongoing studies [5–8]. This idiopathic process leads to obliteration or discontinuity of the hepatic or common bile ducts at any point from the porta hepatis to the duodenum. In most patients, cordlike remnants of the extrahepatic ducts are encountered at surgery.

Incidence

Biliary atresia occurs worldwide, affecting an estimated 1 in 8000–15 000 live births. There is a slight female predominance in most series. One population-based birth defects surveillance system for infants with biliary atresia in metropolitan Atlanta calculated an incidence rate of 0.73 per 10 000 live births [9]. There was significant seasonal clustering of the disease, with rates three times higher in infants born between December and March. Rates were significantly higher among non-white infants. The demonstration of significant seasonal clustering in this and other studies supports the theory that biliary atresia may be caused by environmental exposure (consistent with a viral cause) during the perinatal period [5].

Clinical forms

Two different forms of biliary atresia are recognized, with disparate pathogenesis: a fetal or embryonic form, and a peri- or postnatal form. In patients with the less common fetal form (10–35% of all patients), cholestasis is present from birth, with no jaundice-free interval. Bile duct remnants may not be detectable in the hepatic hilum, and there is a high frequency (10–20%) of associated malformations such as the "polysplenia syndrome," which may be associated with cardiovascular defects, asplenia or abdominal situs inversus, intestinal malrotation, and positional anomalies of the portal vein and hepatic artery. Extrahepatic anomalies reported in patients with biliary atresia are outlined in Table 11.1.

The fetal form of biliary atresia probably has the greatest contribution from genetic factors in its pathogenesis, in the form of defective embryogenesis. In contrast, the postnatal form may be the result of an acquired obliteration. These two forms have not been distinguished on the basis of histology of

Table 11.1 Extrahepatic anomalies reported in patients with biliary atresia

System	Anomalies
Splenic anomalies	Polysplenia, double spleen, asplenia
Portal vein anomalies	Preduodenal position, absence, cavernomatous transformation
Abdominal abnormalities	Situs inversus, intestinal malrotation, annular pancreas, duodenal atresia, esophageal atresia, jejunal atresia
Cardiac anomalies	Dextrocardia, atrial situs ambiguus, ventricular inversion
Immotile cilia syndrome (Kartagener syndrome)	
Renal anomalies	Polycystic kidney, renal agenesis, hypoplastic kidneys
Cleft palate	

porta hepatis specimens; both forms may have inflamed and obliterated bile duct segments in this resected tissue mass.

In the series of Davenport et al. [10] of 308 patients with biliary atresia, 23 (7.5%) had polysplenia, 2 had double spleens, and 2 had asplenia. All 27 had anomalies that may occur in the polysplenia syndrome; the investigators used the term "biliary atresia splenic malformation syndrome" to describe all such infants. Infants with this syndrome had a lower birth weight and a higher incidence of maternal diabetes compared with non-syndromic cases. The extrahepatic anatomy of the biliary tract also reportedly was different, including instances of what they termed biliary agenesis. These findings suggest that either the timing or the nature of the lesion of this "fetal" subgroup may differ from that of the more common "postnatal" disorder. We believe that the postnatal form of biliary atresia may be the result of the sporadic occurrence of a virus-induced or virus-initiated progressive obliteration of the bile ducts, with some degree of intrahepatic bile duct injury [5,11]. Biliary atresia in both subtypes appears to involve an ongoing inflammatory process that produces complete sclerosis of extrahepatic bile ducts and progression to cirrhosis; whether the lesion noted in the intrahepatic bile ducts results from an extension of the extrahepatic lesion or is a consequence of cholestasis is not defined. It is believed that ductal plate malformation and segmental agenesis of bile ducts in porta hepatis specimens are identified more commonly in the fetal form, but an analysis of several portal tracts from eight infants with the perinatal form of biliary atresia and six infants with biliary atresia splenic malformation syndrome identified no association between ductal plate malformation and either clinical form of disease [12].

There is no proven difference in histological features of the liver between infants with and without congenital anomalies. A third form or clinical variant is defined by the presence of cystic dilatation of extrahepatic bile ducts, in addition to the fibrosing obstruction of duct segments. Some of the infants with biliary cysts are detected prenatally during routine ultrasound examination of the fetus; jaundice and acholic stools may present soon after birth or after a variable period of time. In a review of a large cohort with biliary atresia, biliary cysts occurred in approximately 8% of patients [13]. Infants with this cystic variant were younger at presentation, but a delay in performing a portoenterostomy beyond 70 days of age was associated with poor long-term survival with the native liver. The anatomical details of this variant, the earlier age at presentation, and the differences in outcome raise the possibility that it differs in pathogenic mechanisms of disease.

Clinical features

Despite the postulated variant cause and multifactorial pathogenesis, there is consistency in the clinical features of biliary atresia: affected infants present with jaundice (conjugated hyperbilirubinemia) and acholic stools. The presence of hepatomegaly, failure to thrive, pruritus, and coagulopathy depends on the level of progression of disease. Affected infants usually are born at term, are of normal birth weight, and weight gain is appropriate early in the course. Patients with biliary atresia occasionally present with bleeding as a result of vitamin K deficiency. Examination may reveal hepatomegaly and splenomegaly. Ascites and wasting may be seen as late manifestations if biliary cirrhosis has supervened. Increased awareness to ensure early diagnosis and development of methods to prevent progressive hepatic fibrosis are currently needed. Early recognition of babies who have biliary atresia is particularly critical for optimal intervention; ideally, biliary atresia should be identified by the time of the first well-baby visit after discharge from the hospital. The importance of a prompt and precise diagnosis must be stressed to all pediatric healthcare providers. In the UK, an educational effort (the Yellow Alert campaign) was established to indicate the significance of jaundice persisting after 14 days of age. Population screening also has been considered, including the use of stool color cards to identify at-risk infants. In Taiwan, population screening with these cards resulted in an increase in the national rate of portoenterostomy before 60 days of age from 60% to 74.3% [14]. The ultimate goals are to define the pathogenesis of biliary atresia and establish preventive strategies.

Cause and pathogenesis

Although our understanding of the cause of biliary atresia has remained unchanged for several decades, there is now greater knowledge regarding the pathogenesis of the disease from patient-based studies and the use of experimental models of bile duct injury [5,6]. Theoretic considerations of the cause of biliary atresia have been based on epidemiologic and clinical features. Two critical clinical features offer potential clues about chief biologic processes. The first is that the onset of disease is restricted to the perinatal or immediate postnatal period (<4 months). The second is the presence of inflammation and fibrosis of the extrahepatic bile ducts. In the "typical" patient, the structural changes present in the hepatobiliary tract suggest a progression of the lesion from acute cholangitis to fibrotic obliteration of the ducts (Figure 11.1). The dynamic nature of the obliterative process is illustrated by the fact that atresia has been found at autopsy or re-exploration in infants previously shown to have patent extrahepatic ducts or "neonatal hepatitis."

Multiple studies have focused on normal and altered bile duct morphogenesis and the role of various factors (infectious or toxic agents and metabolic insults) in isolation or in combination with a genetic or immunologic susceptibility to biliary atresia [5]. Biliary atresia is not thought to be inherited in the majority of patients. The absence of documented recurrence in siblings of infants with biliary atresia and reports of dizygotic and monozygotic twins discordant for biliary atresia appears to exclude simple Mendelian inheritance in the vast majority of patients [5]. The concept that an acquired obliterative process underlies biliary atresia is attractive and suggests that a virus-related inflammation may initiate the sequence that leads to fibrosis and luminal obstruction. In support of this concept, giant multinucleate hepatocytes have been noted in up to 40% of liver biopsy samples obtained early in life from patients with biliary atresia.

Viral infection

A favored theory implicates occult viral infection as the inciting mechanism. The demonstration of significant seasonal clustering provides support for the theory that biliary atresia may be caused by environmental exposure (consistent with a viral cause) during the perinatal period. Multiple potential etiopathogenic viruses have been ruled out as "suspects." Hepatitis A, B, and C virus infections are not related to biliary atresia [5], and there was no apparent increase in the incidence of biliary atresia during rubella epidemics. Cytomegalovirus (CMV), which characteristically infects the biliary epithelium, has been suggested as a cause of biliary atresia. For example, a Swedish study showed a higher prevalence of CMV antibodies in mothers of infants with biliary atresia, and CMV DNA was present in livers from 9 of 18 infants with biliary atresia [15]. A role for CMV in the pathogenesis of biliary atresia, however, was not supported by studies examining porta hepatis specimens by in situ hybridization and polymerase chain reaction using CMV DNA probes [16]. Exposure to CMV remains a potential causative factor because of the viral tropism to the bile duct epithelium, but future studies will need to employ new approaches that detect virus-specific epitopes in memory lymphocytes. A high prevalence of human papillomavirus has been detected in liver tissue and in cervical swabs from mothers of patients with biliary atresia. There is no animal model, however, demonstrating the consequences of human papillomavirus infection in an immature liver, nor have these findings been confirmed. Mason et al. [17] detected retroviral antibody reactivity in patients with biliary atresia attributable either to an autoimmune response to antigenically related cellular proteins or to an immune response to uncharacterized viral proteins that share antigenic determinants with these retroviruses. Further studies are needed.

The viral agents most frequently implicated in the pathogenesis of biliary atresia include reovirus and rotavirus. Serologic reactivity to reovirus type 3 and reovirus particles in the porta hepatis have been found in children with biliary atresia [5]. It had been known for some time that this virus could cause an obliterative cholangiopathy in weanling mice; a similarity exists between the hepatitis with biliary tract inflammation induced by reovirus type 3 infection in the weanling mouse model and the progressive postnatal fibrotic obliteration of the extrahepatic bile ducts and liver cell injury noted in biliary atresia [5]. Reovirus type 3 infection, therefore, has been implicated as the initial insult in the sequence of events resulting in the observed lesions. Murine reovirus infection may lead to necrosis of bile duct epithelium and hepatocytes, inflammatory infiltration, and possibly identifiable viral inclusions in bile duct epithelial cells. Pathologic changes in reovirus-infected mice, including distal stenosis of the common bile duct and dilation of the proximal bile duct, remain after infectious virus or viral antigens can no longer be detected [18]. Infection of newborn mice with reovirus in the first days of life, however, did not produce obstruction of extrahepatic bile ducts [19]. Previous attempts to show an association between reoviruses and human hepatobiliary disease have yielded conflicting results.

Reoviruses have not been isolated from human hepatobiliary tissue, but reovirus antigen was detected in the bile duct remnant resected from an infant with biliary atresia, and reovirus-like virion particles were seen in this tissue by electron microscopy [18]. Using reverse transcriptase polymerase chain reaction, reovirus was found in hepatobiliary samples of 55% of patients with biliary atresia and 78% with choledochal cyst, whereas the virus was present in tissues of only 8–21% of appropriately matched controls [20]. More work is needed to establish causative relationship between reovirus and biliary atresia.

Riepenhoff-Talty et al. [21] reported the development of extrahepatic biliary obstruction in newborn mice orally inoculated with group A rotavirus. These investigators also presented evidence for polymerase chain reaction amplification of group C rotavirus sequences from livers of patients with biliary atresia, for immunoreactivity to group C rotavirus in serum of patients with biliary atresia, and for group C rotavirus particles in the stool of patients with biliary atresia [22]. Additional studies in newborn mice have clearly shown the lesion to reside in the biliary epithelium. This model of rotavirus-induced biliary injury has proved valuable in studying the mechanisms of biliary atresia because it recapitulates two consistent clinical features of the disease in humans: the onset of disease in the immediate neonatal period and the progressive cholangiopathy [5,6].

Additional studies are needed to further investigate a relationship between reovirus, rotavirus, or any other virus in the pathogenesis of biliary atresia. Investigation into the contribution of virus-initiated immune or autoimmune mechanisms of hepatobiliary injury in these disorders may yield information essential for development of treatment or prevention strategies. One example is the observation that the incidence of biliary atresia appeared to decrease in Taiwan after the introduction of rotavirus vaccine [23]. It is unlikely, however, that antiviral therapy alone would alter the natural history of biliary atresia if the pathologic process is an immunologic reaction to a preceding viral injury, without ongoing viral replication.

Defect in morphogenesis

The hypothesis that a defect in morphogenesis of the biliary tract is a mechanism for the pathogenesis of biliary atresia is appealing, particularly considering the coexistence of other anomalies, particularly anomalies of visceral organ symmetry (Table 11.1) that occur in 10–20% of infants with biliary atresia. Tan et al. [24] compared the developing biliary system of normal human embryos and fetuses with the resected extrahepatic biliary remnants from 205 patients with biliary atresia. At the porta hepatis level, the primary biliary ductal plate underwent a specific sequence of remodeling between 11 and 13 weeks after fertilization, resulting in the formation of large tubular bile ducts surrounded by thick mesenchyme. Luminal continuity with the extrahepatic biliary tree was maintained throughout gestation. Contrary to previous speculation, no "solid phase" was documented during the development of the extrahepatic bile duct. Examination of the biliary remnants in biliary atresia showed that the porta hepatis was encased in fibrous tissue, with a variable pattern of obliteration of the common hepatic and common bile ducts. There were similarities on anti-cytokeratin immunostaining between the abnormal ductules within the porta hepatis in biliary atresia and the normal developing bile ducts during the first trimester. The investigators proposed that biliary atresia may be caused by failure of the remodeling process at the hepatic hilum, with persistence of fetal bile ducts poorly supported by mesenchyme. They further postulated that, as bile flow increases perinatally, bile leakage from these abnormal ducts may trigger an intense inflammatory reaction, with subsequent obliteration of the biliary tree. It remains to be demonstrated whether these processes are causative or whether the histological features result from the activation of cellular circuits in response to poorly defined insults. Among these are infectious or immune insults that can interfere with the normal remodeling process at the hepatic hilum and with ductal plates within the liver.

Several genes have been implicated in the abnormal development of the biliary system and potentially in the pathogenesis of biliary atresia [5,6,25]. Anomalies of visceral organ symmetry, including complete abdominal situs inversus, severe jaundice, and death within the first week of life, have been reported in transgenic mice that have a recessive

(a)

(b)

(c)

(d)

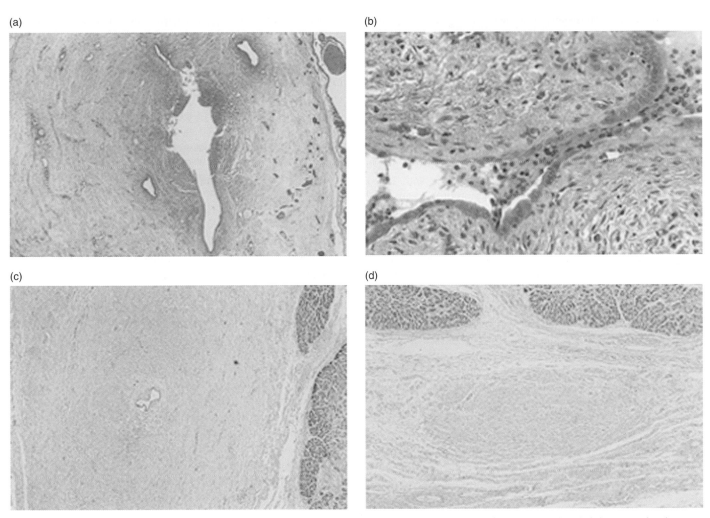

Figure 11.1 Stages of biliary atresia. (a) Patent bile duct in a specimen from porta hepatis exhibits periductal inflammation and epithelial erosion; elsewhere in this patient, the duct was obliterated by reactive tissue (magnification 37×). (b) Detail of eroded bile duct shows regressive epithelial change, periductal edema, and mild inflammation (magnification 250×). (c) At the autopsy of a patient with biliary atresia, a minute remnant of common bile duct has intact epithelium (magnification 100×). (d) Minute fibrous cord represents the final stage of biliary atresia (magnification 100×). In many patients, the atretic duct is not visible to the naked eye. (Hematoxylin & eosin staining.)

insertional mutation in the proximal region of mouse chromosome 4 and deletion of the inversin (*inv*) gene [26]. Presumably, the gene mutated in this *inv* mouse ordinarily directs a critical phase in the morphogenetic program for establishing visceral symmetry and for early development of the extrahepatic biliary tree, with duct obstruction and failure to excrete solute from the liver into the small intestine. These results suggest that the *inv* plays an essential role in the morphogenesis of the hepatobiliary system in mice, but the role in pathogenesis of biliary atresia remains undefined in view of the inability to detect abnormalities of *INV* in children with laterality defects and biliary atresia [27].

An interesting series of observations clarified the morphogenesis and differentiation of the intrahepatic bile ducts [2,28]. In a study of human liver samples from different stages of fetal development and immunostaining with anti-cytokeratin antibodies specific for bile duct epithelial cells, investigators showed that bile ducts arise within the mesenchyme

surrounding portal vein radicals. Presumed primitive hepatic precursor cells differentiate into a single layer of cytokeratin-staining cells and then form a double layer. At focal points, these cells then scatter and remodel as a single layer around a lumen. In livers from some infants with biliary atresia, there was evidence for an arrest in remodeling such that lumens are not formed (ductal plate malformation) [2,28]. The c-*MET* oncogene was suggested to play a potential role in mediating differentiation of mesenchymal tissue into epithelial cells, scattering and remodeling these epithelial cells in a manner that results in formation of a lumen [5]. However, no biliary abnormality was reported in mice with targeted inactivation of the receptor. In contrast, histological and functional abnormalities in the biliary tract have been reported in mice with genetic mutations in *Jagged, Notch, Hes1, Hnf6, Hnf1b, Foxm1b, Foxf1, Foxa1/Foxa2, Sox17,* and *Lgr4*, which raises questions about the potential role of these genes as susceptibility factors or modifiers of disease in humans [5,6,25].

Proinflammatory mechanisms of disease

Several lines of evidence point to a proinflammatory response that targets the bile ducts in patients with biliary atresia. One theory holds that a viral or toxic insult to the biliary epithelium leads to newly expressed antigens on the surface of bile duct epithelia, which in the proper genetically determined immunologic milieu (e.g. the presence of major histocompatibility molecules) are recognized by T-lymphocytes that elicit a cellular immune injury. In support of this notion, Silveira *et al.* [29] reported an association of the human leukocyte antigen (HLA)-B12 allele and haplotypes HLA-A9B5 and HLA-A28B35 with biliary atresia. Other haplotypes of potential involvement include HLA-Cw4/7, HLA-A33, HLA-B44, and HLA-DR6 and a higher prevalence of polymorphisms in *CD14*, *MIF* (encoding migratory inhibitory factor) and SNP rs17095355 on 10q24 [6]. This field will benefit from future validation studies in a large patient population.

Histological and immunostaining analyses of the liver and extrahepatic remnants suggest that lymphocytes, dendritic cells, and Kupffer cells may play key roles in the regulation of inflammation and destruction of bile ducts in infants with biliary atresia. Both CD4 T-cells and natural killer cells increase in livers at diagnosis and are associated with epithelial cell pyknoses within intrahepatic portal tracts, porta hepatis, and common bile duct remnants [6,30]. Not surprisingly, the liver expresses high levels of cytokines and receptors, such as tumor necrosis factor-α, interleukin-2 and its receptor, the transferring receptor CD71, and interferon-γ. More direct evidence for an effector role of T-lymphocytes emerged from a report that liver and bile duct remnants of patients with biliary atresia have oligoclonal expansion of CD4 and CD8 T-cells [31]. These technically challenging experiments add functional relevance to this group of antigen-specific T-cells, and set the stage for future studies investigating their relationship to molecular epitopes in cholangiocytes. One example is the detection of elevated levels of anti-enolase antibodies in about 35% of infants with biliary atresia [32].

The prevailing hypothesis that proinflammatory cytokines are important to the pathogenesis of biliary atresia has been tested in the rotavirus-mouse model. In this model, blocking of signals regulated by interferon-γ, α$_2$-integrin and interleukin-15 prevented bile duct obstruction and the phenotype of biliary atresia [6,33]. Searching for the cellular basis of cytokine production and biliary obstruction, individual mononuclear cells were depleted in newborn mice to examine their contribution to the atresia phenotype. While the loss of CD4 cells had no obvious influence on the biliary injury, individual depletion of CD8 lymphocytes, NK lymphocytes, dendritic cells, or macrophages decreased the epithelial injury and/or prevented the obstruction of extrahepatic bile ducts, with improved growth and long-term survival in experimental mice [3,6,34]. The similarities between the phenotypes produced by the loss of these cell types and cytokines suggest that they work in concert to promote duct obstruction, and may constitute therapeutic targets to block progression of liver disease.

One feature that deserves special note is the restriction of onset of disease to the first few months of life in infants and the first few days of life in mice, suggesting that the mechanisms of disease are substantially influenced by developmental factors. One likely factor is the influence of genes regulating embryogenesis, such as *CFC1*, SNP rs17095355, and others (see above). However, the lack of congenital malformations in the majority of patients opens the possibility for a greater influence of other biological processes. Among them is an inflammatory response triggered by the presence of rare maternal cells in the liver of affected infants (maternal chimerism). Evidence for this process is largely circumstantial at this time. Another relates to the paucity of regulatory T-lymphocytes in the liver and other peripheral tissues in the first 3 days of life in mice. These regulatory cells have an important immunomodulatory function; their absence leads to an array of autoimmune phenotypes. The regulatory T-cells were reported to be nearly absent in mouse livers following rotavirus challenge in the first 3 days of life [35]. In contrast, when rotavirus was injected at 7 days of age, a time when the liver was populated by regulatory T-cells, mice were resistant to the biliary atresia phenotype. How these results apply to susceptibility of biliary injury in humans, however, is unknown at this time.

The combined genetic and cell depletion studies in mice uncover a continuum of biological events that produce obstruction of extrahepatic bile ducts in a fashion that recapitulates some features of the disease in humans. The events begin with a viral infection (e.g. rotavirus) that targets the bile duct epithelium and primes macrophages and dendritic cells ("initiating" phase). This is followed by activation of NK cells that injure cholangiocytes and disrupt mucosal continuity (phase of epithelial injury). An amplification of the adaptive immune response by CD4 and CD8 T-cells and by the release of proinflammatory cytokines form a cellular plug at the site of epithelial injury (phase of obstruction), followed by the evolution to collagen deposition to produce the atresia phenotype (Figure 11.2).

Environmental toxic exposure

To date, the only supportive patient-based evidence for a role of a toxic insult as a causative factor of biliary atresia is the time–space clustering of cases. In animals, unusual outbreaks of hepatobiliary injury in lambs and calves in New South Wales, Australia, occurred in 1964 and 1988, with pathologic specimens displaying features akin to the pathology seen in humans with biliary atresia. Despite the localized geographic distribution of the outbreaks, an extensive investigation for causative phytotoxins or mycotoxins was unrevealing [36].

Vascular abnormalities

Developmental abnormalities in the position of the portal vein and in hepatic artery anatomy at the porta hepatis are common in patients with biliary atresia. There are no consistent experimental data, however, to confirm the hypothesis

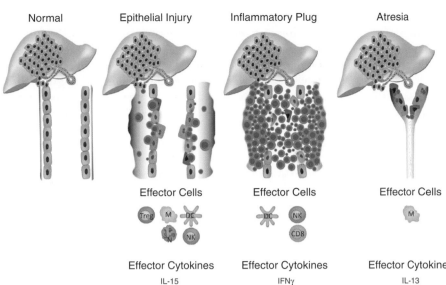

Normal   Epithelial Injury   Inflammatory Plug   Atresia

Effector Cells   Effector Cells   Effector Cells

Effector Cytokines   Effector Cytokines   Effector Cytokines

IL-15   IFNγ   IL-13
NKG2D   IL-12   TGFβ
RAE-1   TNFα   CTGF
MIP-2   Osteopontin
Integrin

Figure 11.2 Proposed model of pathogenesis of biliary atresia identifies a continuum of disease, in which an initial insult targets the bile duct epithelium and activates an immune response that obstructs the duct lumen (inflammatory plug) and rapidly progresses to fibrosis and atresia. At the stage of epithelial injury, macrophages (M), neutrophils (N), dendritic cells (DC) and natural killer (NK) cells work collaboratively to injure cholangiocytes and use several effector cytokines. Regulatory T (Treg) lymphocytes are proposed to suppress the response of dendritic cells and lymphocytes. At the stage of inflammatory plug, the adaptive immune system makes use of DC, NK, and CD8 T-cells and cytokines to amplify the inflammatory response. In the later stages of atresia, alternatively activated macrophages and fibrosis-related cytokines promote tissue fibrosis. IFNγ, interferon-γ; IL, interleukin; TNFα, tumor necrosis factor-α; NKG2D, activating receptor on NK cells; RAE-1, mRNA export factor; MIP-2, macrophage inflammatory protein 2; TGFβ, transforming growth factor-β; CTGF, connective tissue growth factor.

that a vascular basis, such as ischemia, is a cause of the progressive duct injury seen in biliary atresia [37]. In utero devascularization or ligation of the extrahepatic bile duct has been attempted in some animal models, and lesions similar to the less common "correctable" variants of biliary atresia have been produced; however, other studies have been inconclusive.

Diagnosis of biliary atresia

Various laboratory tests, imaging methods, and biopsy samples have been utilized in attempts to establish the diagnosis of biliary atresia, particularly in differentiating it from various forms of intrahepatic cholestasis (idiopathic neonatal hepatitis). In our experience, the most reliable information is obtained by review of hepatic histopathology followed by direct visualization of obliterated extrahepatic bile ducts (intraoperative cholangiography). Percutaneous liver biopsy has a diagnostic accuracy of 95% if a sample of adequate size, containing five to seven portal spaces, is obtained and carefully interpreted.

Evaluation

Our approach to the work-up of an infant with cholestasis is shown in Box 11.1. We recommend the following sequential approach:

1. Prompt recognition of cholestasis is essential. Jaundice in an infant must not be attributed erroneously to physiologic hyperbilirubinemia or to breast-feeding; fractionation of the serum bilirubin usually separates out these later conditions, which cause a predominant elevation (>80%) of unconjugated bilirubin levels.

Box 11.1   Evaluation of infants with cholestasis

General evaluation

1. Clinical evaluation (family and gestational history, feeding history, physical examination, assessment of stool color)
2. Index of hepatic synthetic function (prothrombin time) INR
3. Cultures (blood, urine, spinal fluid) as indicated
4. Determination of serum bile acid levels (followed by *qualitative analysis* of urinary bile acid profile if abnormal)
5. Gamma-glutamyltransferase
6. Serum electrolytes (to exclude acidosis)

Specific evaluation (to exclude or confirm a specific diagnosis)

- α-1-antitrypsin phenotype
- Thyroxine and thyroid-stimulating hormone
- Sweat chloride-mutational analysis (to exclude cystic fibrosis)
- Ferritin–transferrin concentration and saturation
- Metabolic screen (urine-reducing substances, urine/serum amino acids, organic acids, succinyl acetone)
- Hepatitis B surface antigen, anti-HIV, and Venereal Disease Research Laboratory titers for syphilis (in selected, high-risk patients)
- Abdominal ultrasonography
- Liver biopsy

2. The evaluation should be expeditiously performed to rule out potentially devastating illnesses such as sepsis, endocrine disorders, and nutritional hepatotoxicity attributable to metabolic disease (e.g. galactosemia). Definitive detection is usually straightforward, and

institution of appropriate treatment for these conditions may prevent further liver injury. Early recognition of specific, treatable primary causes of neonatal cholestasis then is attempted. Early in the evaluation of any infant with cholestasis, other clinical issues need to be addressed. Hypoprothrombinemia may be present regardless of the cause of cholestasis; administration of vitamin K may prevent spontaneous, life-threatening bleeding, such as intracranial hemorrhage.

3. "Idiopathic" neonatal intrahepatic cholestasis must be differentiated from biliary atresia because the prognosis and management differ significantly. In infants with biliary atresia, progressive fibrosis rapidly occurs; therefore, significant delay in diagnosis or treatment must be avoided.

No single test is entirely satisfactory in discriminating intrahepatic cholestasis from biliary atresia; however, historical and clinical features may aid in the differential diagnosis. Neonatal hepatitis is reported to have a familial incidence of 15–20%; the intrafamilial recurrence risk is negligible for biliary atresia. Infants with biliary atresia may look well, become clinically jaundiced at 3–6 weeks of age, and have slowly progressive elevation of serum bilirubin levels but seldom have pruritus or skin xanthoma. The liver is enlarged and firm; splenomegaly occurs as cirrhosis develops. Stools of patients with biliary atresia are acholic at presentation, but early in the course, during the evolving process of bile duct obliteration, they may contain some bile pigment. Acholic stools are either intermittent or delayed in onset in a quarter of patients with biliary atresia and are present in some patients with neonatal hepatitis. The consistent presence of pigmented stools excludes biliary atresia.

Duodenal fluid may be obtained to assess the bilirubin content; if bile-stained fluid is collected, biliary atresia is excluded. Hepatobiliary scintigraphy using iminodiacetic acid analogues has been used to provide discriminatory data. In biliary atresia, hepatocyte function is intact early in the disease; therefore, uptake of the imaging agent is unimpaired but excretion into the intestine is absent. Conversely, in intrahepatic cholestasis, tracer uptake is sluggish or impaired but excretion into the bile and intestine eventually occurs. Oral administration of phenobarbital, 5 mg/kg daily for 5 days before the study, is required to enhance biliary excretion of the isotope and, therefore, the sensitivity of the procedure. However, in our experience, this may delay the evaluation process and is rarely definitive. Techniques that are used extensively in evaluation of adults with cholestatic disease, such as percutaneous transhepatic and endoscopic retrograde cholangiography, are not of proven value in children. The role of magnetic resonance cholangiography is undefined. Ultrasonography may detect dilation of the biliary tract, the presence of a choledochal cyst, or, in patients with biliary atresia, absence of the gallbladder.

Ultrasound can also identify a sonographic finding known as a *triangular cord*, a fibrous cone of tissue at the bifurcation of the portal vein that has been highly associated with biliary atresia [38].

Numerous diagnostic algorithms incorporating these features have been proposed in an attempt to select those infants who are surgical candidates and to avoid unnecessary surgery. Discriminatory analysis of clinical, biochemical, and histological data obtained from 288 infants younger than 3 months presenting with neonatal cholestasis allowed for an accurate differentiation in 85% of the patients studied [39]. In infants with intrahepatic disease, the following features occurred significantly more frequently than in infants with biliary atresia: male gender, low birth weight, later onset of jaundice (mean of 23 versus 11 days of age), later onset of acholic stools (mean of 30 versus 16 days), and pigmented stools within 10 days after admission (79% versus 26%). Patients with biliary atresia more frequently had hepatomegaly, and the liver usually had a firm or hard consistency. Despite the use of scoring systems such as this, about 10% of infants with intrahepatic cholestasis cannot be distinguished from those with biliary atresia. Unnecessary explorations are, of course, to be avoided; however, delay in establishing a diagnosis also is unwarranted because the data suggest that the success rate for surgical management of patients with biliary atresia rapidly declines with age.

Role of liver biopsy

In our experience, clinical examination, careful and repeated examination of the stool, and needle biopsy of the liver correctly identify the majority of patients with biliary atresia. In most patients, biopsy can be performed safely using the Menghini technique of percutaneous aspiration with sedation and local anesthesia. An accurate, biopsy-based diagnosis is possible in up to 95% of patients and avoids unnecessary surgery in patients with intrahepatic disease. Early in the progression of biliary atresia, the liver shows preservation of the basic hepatic architecture, with bile ductular proliferation, canalicular and cellular bile stasis, and portal or perilobular edema and fibrosis (Figure 11.3). Bile plugs in the portal ducts are relatively specific but are found in only 40% of biopsy specimens. Portal fibrosis with wide swaths of connective tissue extending into the liver substance develops in older infants but may be established as early as 3 months after birth. Approximately 25–40% of infants have portal inflammatory infiltration and hepatocyte giant cell transformation indistinguishable from neonatal hepatitis. These portal tract findings contrast with those of neonatal hepatitis, in which variable, often severe, intralobular cholestasis may be accompanied by focal hepatocellular necrosis (Figure 11.4). Bile ducts show little or no alteration in idiopathic intrahepatic cholestasis. Portal inflammatory infiltrates are present in both conditions and tend to be more prominent in idiopathic intrahepatic cholestasis. Portal area stroma is more likely to show edema in patients with biliary atresia. Giant cell transformation and extramedullary

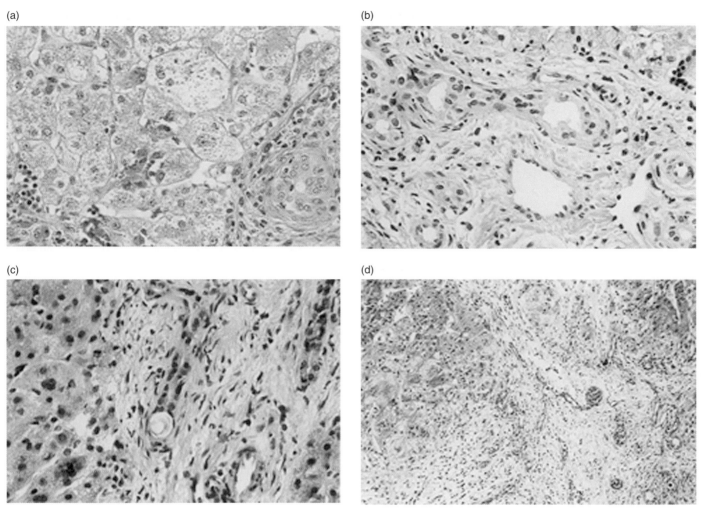

Figure 11.3 Intrahepatic changes in biliary atresia. (a) Giant cell transformation of hepatocytes, sinusoidal erythropoiesis, and slight bile duct proliferation may overlap with neonatal hepatitis (magnification 250×). (b,c) Histologic changes that are diagnostic of biliary obstruction include unequivocal proliferation of interlobular bile ducts, portal stromal edema, and bile concretions in ducts (magnification 250×). (d) Advanced changes in this liver biopsy specimen suggest transition to biliary cirrhosis, which is unusual before 3 months after birth (magnification 100×). (Hematoxylin & eosin stain.)

hematopoiesis, particularly sinusoidal erythropoiesis, are found in a large percentage of infants with either condition and have no diagnostic specificity. In very young infants, the initial biopsy may be inconclusive; rebiopsy after 7–14 days may be more definitive.

The scoring systems discussed above have been evaluated in the differential diagnosis between obstructive and non-obstructive forms of neonatal cholestasis [40,41]. The accuracy, sensitivity, and specificity rates reported by Zerbini *et al.* [41] were all 94%; the model then was applied to a new sample of 74 needle liver biopsy specimens. The accuracy, sensitivity, and specificity rates were 91%, 100%, and 76%, respectively. In a multicenter study, analysis of 97 liver biopsy samples was carried out by a group of pediatric pathologists; the histological features that best predicted biliary atresia on the basis of logistic regression were bile duct proliferation, portal fibrosis, and absence of sinusoidal fibrosis, with a positive predictive value of 90.7% [40]. This suggests that if extrahepatic obstruction cannot be ruled out, limited exploration with

cholangiography and repeat needle or wedge biopsy of the liver should be performed; if atresia is apparent, the biliary tract can be explored further.

Role of surgical exploration

When the suspicion of biliary obstruction is high, operative exploration should be performed to document the presence and the site of obstruction and to direct attempts at surgical drainage. Cholangiography and meticulous exploration of the entire biliary tree should be carried out. The decision made at the operating table may be aided by observations of features usually associated with biliary atresia, such as consistency (coarse, fibrotic) and color (green) of the liver, and the presence of subcapsular telangiectasia (early vascular obstruction secondary to fibrosis). The presence of biliary epithelium and the size of residual ducts can be evaluated in frozen sections of the transected porta hepatis.

The approach outlined here is not without pitfalls; caution should be exercised in interpretation of certain studies,

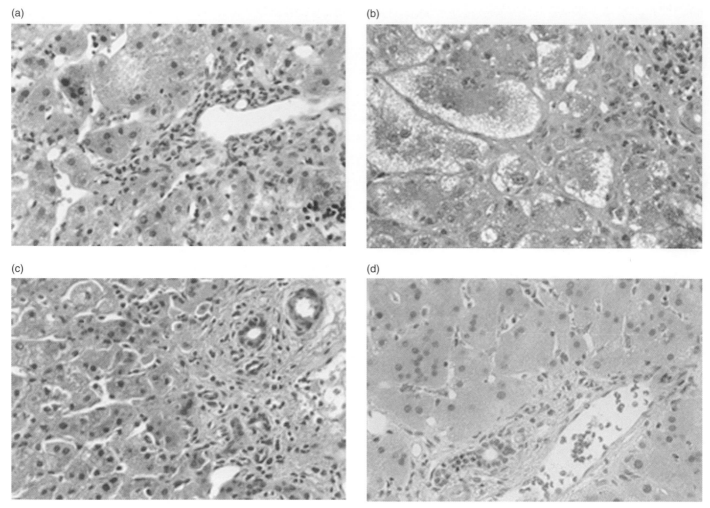

Figure 11.4 Neonatal hepatitis. Inflammation is typically mild. Giant cell transformation is variable in severity and extent in these four examples. Interlobular bile ducts may be inconspicuous (a), slightly proliferative (b), or normal (c,d). Pseudotubular metaplasia of zone 1 hepatocytes may occur along fibrotic portal zone margins (c). Mild cholestasis and giant cell transformation of hepatocytes (d) may linger for months, as in this 3-month-old infant, who eventually recovered. (Hematoxylin & eosin staining, magnification 250×.)

particularly in very young infants. In four patients reported by Markowitz *et al.* [42], scintigraphic evidence of biliary atresia was present, and intraoperative cholangiography failed to demonstrate any proximal intrahepatic biliary radicals; therefore, hepatoportoenterostomy was performed. There was inadequate postoperative drainage with cholangitis, development of cirrhosis in two, and death from hepatic failure in one infant. Subsequently, a histological and clinical diagnosis of intrahepatic cholestasis (Alagille syndrome) was made in each of the four patients. The progression of the hepatic disease in these patients demonstrated that portoenterostomy had severely and adversely altered the course of their disease. During cholangiography, an absence of retrograde flow into the proximal intrahepatic ducts does not exclude the presence of a patent, albeit hypoplastic, extrahepatic biliary duct system in a patient with intrahepatic disease. The liver disease in intrahepatic cholestasis syndromes (e.g. Alagille syndrome) is not amenable to surgical correction, and portal dissection should not be attempted.

Management of biliary atresia

At present, there is no specific medical therapy for patients with biliary atresia. The first breakthrough in the surgical therapy of patients with biliary atresia occurred in the late 1950s when Dr. Morio Kasai and associates described microscopic bile ducts within the fibrous remnant of the atretic biliary tree at the porta hepatis [43]. This led to the critical observation that if the extrahepatic bile ducts were removed at a time at which there was continuity between the microscopic ducts in the ductal plate at the porta hepatis and the intrahepatic biliary system, the progression of biliary atresia could be arrested. This operation, the *Kasai hepatoportoenterostomy*, has become the current standard surgical approach [43–47]. As experience has grown, there have been minor though significant technical improvements in the hepatoportoenterostomy. For example, extension of the dissection beyond the portal vein bifurcation, which incorporates a larger amount of biliary remnants and improves bile flow.

The principles of contemporary surgical management for biliary atresia are based, in part, on the conclusions of the 1983 National Institutes of Health Consensus Conference on Liver Transplantation: (1) hepatoportoenterostomy should be the primary surgical therapy for biliary atresia; (2) transplantation is appropriate therapy for patients with biliary atresia who fail primary hepatoportoenterostomy; (3) liver transplantation should be delayed as long as possible to permit maximum growth; (4) transplantation should be deferred until progressive cholestasis, hepatocellular decompensation, or severe portal hypertension supervenes; and (5) multiple attempts to revise an unsuccessful Kasai procedure are not warranted because they can make liver transplantation more difficult and dangerous [5,44,48].

Surgical management

Sequential surgical therapy for biliary atresia is divided into two steps: the establishment of a secure diagnosis, then the construction of the portoenterostomy. The importance of establishing an unequivocal diagnosis before proceeding to hepatoportoenterostomy cannot be overstated. The initial step in the exploration should both confirm the diagnosis of biliary atresia and exclude other diagnoses not improved by operative intervention, such as various forms of intrahepatic cholestasis. This can be done through direct observation and definition of the distal biliary ductal anatomy using cholecystocholangiography. The liver in patients with biliary atresia is firm and shows a cholestatic brown–green discoloration often accompanied by multiple subcapsular telangiectasias. The gallbladder remnant is usually fibrotic but may contain a small amount of clear mucoid secretions. Early in the course of the disease, the hilar structures and the biliary ductal remnant may show a considerable amount of edema. In older children, these structures are fibrotic and more difficult or impossible to identify. If these findings are accompanied by a fibrotic gallbladder, cholangiography is not necessary and biliary atresia is confirmed. If the gallbladder is not obliterated, gentle cholecystocholangiography is undertaken to further define the operative course. Because of the small gallbladder volume and minimal ductal size in infants, the cholangiogram should be visualized from its onset using fluoroscopy to avoid overdistension and extravasation, which preclude successful visualization of ductal structures. If the ductal system is normal or the bile ducts are small but patent, a generous wedge and needle biopsy is obtained; however, biliary reconstruction should be specifically avoided. If flow into the distal biliary tract is seen but no proximal flow is documented, a light spring-loaded vascular occlusion clamp should be placed on the supraduodenal biliary structures before additional attempts to visualize the proximal ductal system. The Kasai hepatoportoenterostomy should be undertaken if no proximal patency is documented.

Anatomic variants of biliary atresia

The anatomy of the abnormal extrahepatic bile ducts in patients with biliary atresia is variable. The currently accepted classification of anatomic variants of biliary atresia is based on that proposed by the Japanese Society of Pediatric Surgeons, which divides the abnormal anatomy into three principal types: type 1, atresia of the common bile duct; type 2, atresia of the common hepatic duct; and type 3, atresia of the right and left hepatic ducts. Further subdivisions include the variable morphology of the gallbladder and the distal common bile duct. Absence of the proximal biliary tree has been termed biliary agenesis. "Correctable" lesions – distal common bile duct atresia with a patent portion of the extrahepatic duct up to the porta hepatis and joining the intrahepatic ducts – allow direct drainage into a Roux-en-Y anastomosis. The most commonly encountered lesion (seen in 75–85%), however, is obliteration of all of the ducts throughout the porta hepatis (type 3), presenting an apparently "non-correctable" type of atresia. Minute bile duct remnants or residual channels may be present in the fibrous tissue within the porta hepatis. These channels are often in continuity with the intrahepatic ductal system and, therefore, should provide drainage. If flow is not established rapidly in these ducts, progressive obliteration ensues. Biliary drainage is attempted by excision of the obliterated extrahepatic ducts and apposition of the resected surface of the transected porta hepatis to the bowel mucosa in the Roux-en-Y loop hepatoportoenterostomy – the Kasai procedure. The unusual patient with "agenesis" in porta hepatis specimens does not respond to Kasai drainage procedures.

Hepatoportoenterostomy

When the diagnosis of biliary atresia is secure, the second phase of the operative procedure, the Kasai hepatoportoenterostomy, is begun. The traditional dissection of the portal fibrous mass begins by transecting the distal duct remnant above the duodenal margin, mobilizing the gallbladder remnant from its hepatic bed, and dissecting this fibrous remnant from the anterior portal vein wall. It is important to emphasize that in biliary atresia, the bile ducts are not absent but rather replaced by fibrous tissue. The anatomic course of the ductal remnants follows the normal biliary position within the portal triad to reach the liver hilum. The fibrous remnant then proceeds posteriorly and passes superior to but within the bifurcation of the portal vein to reach the capsular surface of the liver [44,47]. Individual small portal vein branches passing directly into the fibrous mass must be divided. This allows downward displacement of the portal vein bifurcation, which facilitates full dissection of the fibrous triangular mass before its transection at the level of the liver capsule (Figure 11.5).

In the original Kasai hepatoportoenterostomy, the fibrous triangle was dissected and divided between the right and left branches of the portal vein at the level of the posterior surface of the portal vein. Further revision of this technique has shown that meticulous dissection of the lateral fibrous triangle tissues allows more of the segmental biliary structures to be included in the divided hilar tissue. On the right, the dissection is carried to the dorsal aspect of the anterior portal branch and over the bifurcation of the anterior and posterior portal vein branches. The left portal vein is also dissected to the umbilical

(a)

(b)

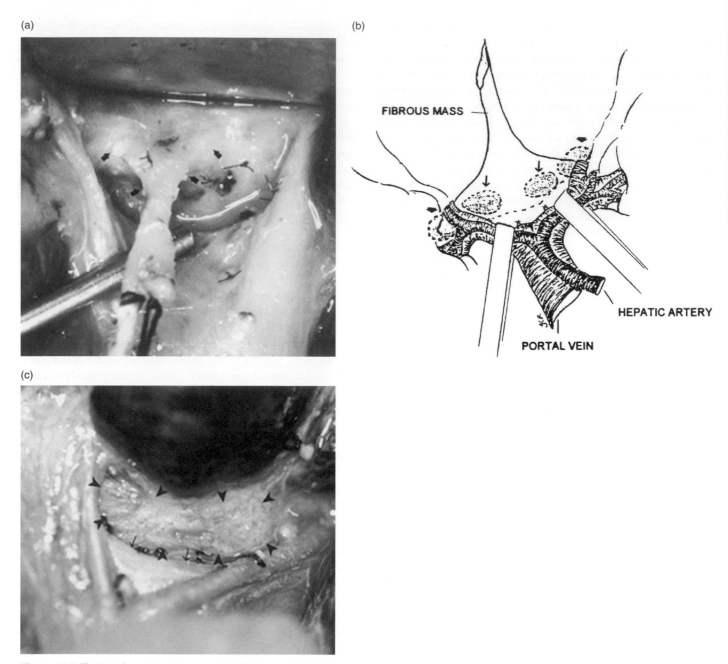

FIBROUS MASS

HEPATIC ARTERY

PORTAL VEIN

(c)

Figure 11.5 The Kasai hepatoportoenterostomy. (a) Division site. Fibrous triangle (arrows) dissected superior to the bifurcation of the portal vein before division. The portal vein must be retracted inferiorly to visualize the posterior surface of the fibrous mass and the liver capsule. (b) Kasai procedure. Schematic representation of fibrous triangular mass before its division and the location (stippled areas) of the primary biliary remnants within the classic dissection limits (small arrows) and within the extended dissection areas (broad arrows). (c) Completed hilar dissection. The fibrous mass is divided parallel and at the level of the liver capsule within the bifurcation of the portal vein (small arrows). Divided fibrous mass margins outlined with arrowheads.

point, which often requires division of the parenchymal bridge surrounding the round ligament between segments 3 and 4 of the liver [45,46]. The fibrous remnant tissue is divided sharply along a plane parallel to and at the level of the hepatic capsule. Deeper dissections into the hepatic parenchyma have not led to improved results. Hemostasis at the transected remnant is achieved by warm irrigation and direct pressure. Suture ligation and electrocautery are discouraged because they may damage the small ductal remnants critical for success.

Roux-en-Y drainage using a 35–40 cm isoperistaltic retrocolic jejunal limb is preferred because this limb may be used later for transplantation if necessary. This limb should be fashioned from the most proximal portion of the jejunum, allowing bile to return to the proximal intestine, improving nutrient and medication absorption. The Roux-en-Y hilar anastomosis should be undertaken using absorbable monofilament suture material to avoid the presence of a nidus for later infection. This suture margin is placed just outside of the divided hilar tissue margin to avoid transfixing any ductal remnants. The anastomotic suture line should surround or invaginate the vascular branches, incorporating all the fibrous tissue within the lumen. This technique excludes the portal vein wall from the cut surface and inhibits its attachment to and scarring of the potential ductal drainage area. Anti-reflux valves are not recommended, but the anastomosis is fashioned to inhibit enteric flow into the drainage limb.

In patients in whom cholangiography indicates distal patency of the common bile duct with good luminal caliber and proximal biliary ductal atresia, a hepatic portocholecystostomy (gallbladder Kasai) procedure is an alternative to conventional hepatoportoenterostomy. In this procedure, the gallbladder is mobilized from its hepatic fossa, protecting the cystic arterial supply. The distal gallbladder is transected, and an opening is sutured to the biliary hilum, replacing the Roux-en-Y drainage limb. In these patients, drainage through the distal biliary structure and intact sphincter of Oddi virtually eliminates ascending cholangitis in the postoperative period, as long as the distal biliary structures are large enough to accommodate normal bile flow.

Prognosis after surgery

A proportion of patients with biliary atresia will derive long-term benefit from hepatoportoenterostomy. In most patients, however, variable degrees of hepatic dysfunction persist, often because of severe intrahepatic cholangiopathy. The long-term prognosis is related directly to the establishment of successful bile flow and the disappearance of jaundice, with increased long-term survival with the native liver in children with serum bilirubin <1 mg/dL within 3 months of hepatoportoenterostomy; in these children the 10-year survival ranges from 73% to 92% [5,25]. In those patients in whom jaundice remains and bile flow is inadequate, the 3-year survival rate decreases to 20%. Even in patients with transient bile flow whose jaundice does not resolve, some benefit, namely growth to a size sufficient to receive a transplant, is often achievable.

The variable prognosis after hepatoportoenterostomy is related to several factors; one of these factors is age at operation. With the Kasai procedure, the timing of the surgery correlates with outcome. In some series, it has been reported that bile flow has been re-established in more than 80% of infants who were referred for surgery within 60 days after birth [5,25,43,48,49]. The success rate drops dramatically, to under 20%, in those older than 90 days at the time of operation. Consequently, performance of the Kasai procedure after 3 months of age may be justified, but only in selected cases. A second factor is size of the ducts visualized in tissue from the porta hepatis. Microscopic ductal patency of more than 150 μm should determine successful postoperative bile flow, although this concept is not universally recognized. For those patients with smaller or no identifiable epithelial-lined structures in fibrous tissue, the success rate is low [50,51]. Prognosis after portoenterostomy procedures may also be correlated with the degree or proliferation of the periductular glands; the hilar

biliary plexus may act as a drainage route for bile in these patients. A third determinant is the experience and operative technique of the surgeon.

The rate of progression of the liver disease may be the overall limiting factor; a nearly universal finding is the presence of a persistent intrahepatic inflammatory process, which may partially account for the poor results and the development of portal hypertension. The continuing nature of the disease process may be caused by an immunologically mediated injury or the toxicity of bile acids. Examining histological markers at diagnosis may be predictive of clinical outcome and prognosis. For example, quantification of the extent of portal fibrosis by applying a computerized system or detecting the presence of extensive bile duct proliferation may be associated with a poor outcome. Other strategies include the presence of molecular signature for inflammation or fibrosis at the time of hepatoportoenterostomy, with markers of fibrosis having decreased survival with the native liver [6].

Another factor affecting prognosis is prevention of secondary postoperative complications, namely bacterial cholangitis, which is a constant threat and may lead to reobstruction [50,52–55]. Patients who previously had good bile excretion may have repeated episodes of fever, increased jaundice, acholic stools, leukocytosis, and evidence of bacteremia (contamination with intestinal flora). Intrahepatic portal vein thrombosis can aggravate pre-existing presinusoidal resistance caused by progressive parenchymal fibrosis, which is the end result of intrahepatic inflammation or recurrent bouts of ascending cholangitis. Intrahepatic biliary cysts have been noted in about 20% of patients with biliary atresia; episodes of cholangitis may precede discovery of the cysts. Hepatic artery resistance index has been measured by Doppler ultrasonography and has been found to predict rapid deterioration and death in children with biliary atresia [5].

Role of reoperation following hepatoportoenterostomy

Several series have emphasized the potential value of reoperation in patients with cessation of bile flow after initial success or in patients with refractory cholangitis. In many patients, debridement or revision of the scarred area may result in the re-establishment of bile flow. If a patient had poor bile flow initially, reoperation is usually unsuccessful in establishing flow. Reoperation should be limited to infants in whom active bile drainage is achieved after the initial operative procedure, leading to an anicteric state followed by abrupt cessation of bile excretion. Evaluation for reoperation is usually considered after appropriate treatment of the infant with antibiotics for the possibility of ascending cholangitis. These infants should have had favorable hepatic histology and biliary ductal remnants at their initial operation. Reconstitution of suitable bile flow following debridement or revision of the scarred hilar area is successful in more than half the patients undergoing reoperation using these highly selective criteria [47,53]. Subsequent tertiary re-exploration should be limited to patients with established bile drainage with suspected mechanical obstruction originating in the intestinal conduit. The increased intraperitoneal and perihepatic adhesions that complicate subsequent liver transplantation are most often the consequence of repetitive but misdirected attempts to reoperate on poorly selected candidates with a poor prognosis for improvement or recurrent episodes of bacterial peritonitis.

Medical treatment following hepatoportoenterostomy

The goals of postoperative management of infants with biliary atresia are three-fold: (1) prevention of cholangitis, (2) stimulation of choleresis, and (3) nutritional support. Infants typically receive parenteral broad-spectrum antibiotics perioperatively and for 2 to 5 days after surgery, followed by oral prophylaxis with trimethoprim-sulfamethoxazole (5 mg/kg trimethoprim daily) or another antibiotic for 3–12 months. Ursodeoxycholic acid (10 mg/kg per day), a more hydrophilic bile acid, has been used by many centers to improve choleresis. Although a few studies have documented the efficacy of ursodeoxycholic acid in promoting choleresis, weight gain, decreased pruritus, and improved liver enzymes, it has no obvious impact on long-term survival or the need for transplant between treated and non-treated patients [56]. Corticosteroids are used postoperatively in some centers; dosing regimens, duration of treatment, and outcomes are variable among published reports [57,58]. Future multicenter randomized controlled clinical trials are required to determine objectively the role of corticosteroids in the treatment of infants following portoenterostomy.

Infants should receive approximately 125% of the Recommended Dietary Calorie Allowance based on weight for height at the 50th percentile, with additional calories often needed if biliary drainage is marginal. If cholestasis is present, infants require supplementation and close monitoring to prevent the consequences of vitamin deficiencies: vitamin A 5000–25 000 IU/day, vitamin D 1200–4000 IU/day, vitamin E 25 IU/kg per day (in a miscible form: d-α-tocopheryl polyethylene glycol 1000 succinate (TPGS)), and vitamin K 2.5 mg three times per week. Doses must be adjusted based on serum levels of specific vitamins and prothrombin time/international normalized ratio (for vitamin K). Unfortunately, malnutrition frequently develops with persistent cholestasis; liver disease progresses despite adequate nutritional support, and coagulopathy not responsive to vitamin K supplementation develops late in the course of the liver disease.

Outcome

Progressive biliary cirrhosis and hepatic failure may occur despite apparent success in achieving bile drainage. Factors that contribute to failure include stenosis of the anastomosis, ascending cholangitis, and progressive loss of intrahepatic bile ducts that may have been injured before the drainage procedure. Liver transplantation is necessary in infants with a failed hepatoportoenterostomy, manifest by progressive

hepatocellular decompensation, jaundice, refractory growth failure with hepatic synthetic dysfunction and the development of a coagulopathy, or intractable portal hypertension with recurrent gastrointestinal hemorrhage or hypersplenism. The risk of death or need for liver transplantation has been estimated at 50% at 6 years after the initial episode of esophageal variceal hemorrhage. Patients with a serum bilirubin ≤4 mg/dL at the first episode of esophageal variceal hemorrhage had a transplant-free survival rate of more than 80% for 4 years after this episode; those with serum bilirubin of 4–10 mg/dL had 50% survival at 1 year, and those with serum bilirubin >10 mg/dL had 50% survival at 4 months [59]. Therefore, compared with the risk for an age-matched child who did not have esophageal variceal hemorrhage, the risk of death or transplant for a child with esophageal variceal hemorrhage was 12-fold greater when the total serum bilirubin was >10 mg/dL, seven-fold when it was 4–10 mg/dL, and 0.6-fold when it was ≤4 mg/dL or less.

A late complication of biliary atresia-associated portal hypertension is the hepatopulmonary syndrome, defined as intrapulmonary vascular dilatation with shunting and arterial desaturation. This syndrome is associated with decreased exercise tolerance and digital clubbing and seems to correlate with the presence of cutaneous spider telangiectasia. Hepatopulmonary syndrome may be reversed by liver transplantation; however, patients with hepatopulmonary syndrome are more susceptible to postoperative complications. Portopulmonary hypertension, another of the pulmonary vascular disorders complicating chronic liver disease, is defined as pulmonary arterial hypertension associated with severe liver disease or portal hypertension. Portopulmonary hypertension, when left untreated, is fatal; mean survival in adults is 15 months. The criteria for portopulmonary hypertension include an elevated mean pulmonary arterial pressure (>25 mmHg at rest), increased pulmonary vascular resistance, and normal pulmonary capillary wedge pressure in the presence of portal hypertension. Clinical symptoms are subtle and may be overlooked. Children with portal hypertension who develop a new heart murmur, dyspnea, or syncope, or who are being evaluated for liver transplantation, require evaluation for portopulmonary hypertension. Electrocardiography and chest radiography are insensitive screening tests; hence an echocardiogram and cardiology evaluation may be needed to confirm the diagnosis.

Although the success rate for biliary enteric anastomosis in patients with biliary atresia cannot be predicted, it remains the most reasonable initial approach. A retrospective study was carried out to define the long-term outcome of children who have undergone surgery for biliary atresia [60]. Of 122 children, 38% were alive after 10 years; however, firm hepato- and splenomegaly were present in about 75%. Normal liver enzymes and an absence of portal hypertension were observed in only 9% of the children. These results suggest that although hepatoportoenterostomy may be helpful, about 80% of such children eventually require liver transplantation.

Liver transplantation

Biliary atresia remains the primary indication for liver transplantation in the pediatric age group, constituting about 50% of children undergoing transplantation. Liver transplantation should be delayed as long as possible to permit maximal growth. Repeated attempts at revision of the hepatoportoenterostomy or portosystemic shunting, however, may be ineffective and render eventual transplantation more difficult.

Children undergoing liver replacement today can expect survival rates approaching 90% as a result of improved techniques of preoperative management, resolution of major intraoperative technical problems associated with microvascular reconstruction of the hepatic vasculature, and precise postoperative immunosuppression and management of infectious diseases [61]. The remaining factor that limits widespread application and prevents access by all pediatric candidates to transplantation is the *scarcity* of adequate donor organs. The surgical techniques necessary to allow all variations of whole, split liver, and living donor transplantation were developed in an attempt to meet this desperate need, yet increasing numbers of potential recipients overwhelm these resources. The disparity in size-matched pediatric donors is compounded by the preponderance of children with biliary atresia among the candidates for liver transplantation in the pediatric population; 55% of deaths in children from liver diseases occur before 2 years of age. In these patients, liver replacement is necessary at a very young age and small size, in view of the rapid progression of the hepatic disease and poor nutritional status. This creates an "epidemiologic disparity" because most pediatric donors are of school age or older. The use of reduced-size liver transplantation as an initial strategy is successful in both improving patient survival and decreasing the waiting-list mortality rate [62]. Since the institution of segmental transplantation at Cincinnati Children's Hospital Medical Center, the number of deaths while awaiting donor organ availability and the incidence of hepatic artery thrombosis has been substantially reduced. Before the introduction of reduced-size liver transplantation at our center, 29% of children listed for transplantation died because of the lack of donor organ availability. After the implementation of reduced-size liver transplant techniques, the waiting-list mortality rate has been reduced to 2% in our center, with similar reductions in other centers. Although 45% of children still undergo transplantation with a status of high medical urgency, the wider range of donors available using reduced-size allografts has allowed the selection of donors with improved hemodynamic stability and liver function. These procedures established the successful techniques needed to advance both living donor and split liver transplantation, both of which increase the donor pool rather than redistributing the resources. However, these procedures encompass increased perioperative risks to the recipient (and living donor) [63]. Reduced-size liver transplantation is not the ideal solution; however, expansion of the donor pool may be possible through extension of the surgical techniques used to prepare reduced-size allografts. The need for orthotopic liver transplantation in small children stimulated the development of other innovative operative procedures based on the concept of reduced-size allografts; these include split liver transplantation and the use of living, related organ donors. Liver transplantation survival rates for living donor, split, and reduced-size transplantation are similar to those with whole-organ graft transplantation in children older than 2 years.

Despite the high overall success rate of liver transplantation in children, multiple challenges remain, including improvement of methods of preoperative management to address the problems of malnutrition, improvement of methods of immune suppression to prevent graft loss and avoid lymphoproliferative disease and other infectious complications, and development of protocols to avoid growth suppression. Children are particularly sensitive to the consequences of both under-immunosuppression (linked to rejection) and over-immunosuppression (linked to post-transplantation lymphoproliferative disease, renal insufficiency, infection). The latter is complicated by the fact that children appear to be more immunoresponsive than adults.

Liver transplantation as primary therapy for biliary atresia

Those who propose primary transplantation as the procedure of choice for children with biliary atresia cite several potential advantages, including the lack of adhesions in a previously undisturbed abdomen leading to a decreased need for blood products. In the past, survival of children younger than 1 year of age was compromised; however, experienced transplant centers now report 1-year survival of more than 85%, even in these critical infants [63]. However, the most compelling argument against primary transplantation centers on inadequate donor resources. Mortality awaiting transplantation is highest in those over 1 year of age, and an influx of biliary atresia infants would further increase the disparity and mortality. Selection of candidates for primary transplantation is not well accepted, except possibly in patients in whom liver disease is so advanced (advanced age and cirrhosis) that bile flow cannot be restored. Conservative decision making should be practiced in this regard, knowing that even partial return of bile flow may delay transplantation to an age at which prognosis is more favorable and a donor organ more readily available.

The limitations and potential pitfalls of primary liver transplantation have led to adaptation of a *sequential approach* in the management of biliary atresia (Figure 11.6). Hepatoportoenterostomy would obviate the need for transplantation for patients in whom the procedure was a long-term success and delay transplantation in another significant proportion. In our opinion, therefore, sequential surgical therapy for biliary atresia should begin with creation of an hepatoportoenterostomy. Infants with poor response will undergo transplantation within the first 2 years. Children with initially "successful" drainage but with progressive liver disease with portal hypertension, hypersplenism, variceal hemorrhage, and malnutrition will need orthotopic liver

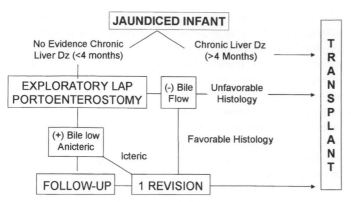

Figure 11.6 Flow chart for patients with biliary atresia. Management strategy after sequential Kasai hepatoportoenterostomy procedure followed, when needed, by liver transplantation. Dz, disease.

transplantation at a later date. Occasionally, long-term survivors may not require transplantation.

Chardot *et al.* [64] reviewed all patients with biliary atresia living in France and born between the years 1986 and 1996. A total of 472 patients were identified; the 10-year overall survival rate was 68%. Independent prognostic factors for overall survival were the performance of the Kasai operation, age at operation, anatomic pattern of extrahepatic bile ducts, polysplenia syndrome, and experience of the managing center. Survival with native liver depended on the same independent prognostic factors. These data support the concepts that the Kasai operation should remain the first-line treatment of biliary atresia and that early performance of this operation and treatment in an experienced center should reduce the need for liver transplantation in infancy and childhood and provide children with the best chance of survival. High survival rates for patients with biliary atresia can be achieved through the complementary and sequential utilization of early primary therapy with the Kasai portoenterostomy followed by liver transplantation if necessary. This series also emphasized the value of "center experience" in achieving these high success rates [64]. The Kasai procedure is technically difficult, and success in achieving bile flow is related to the skill with which this procedure is performed. The need for primary transplantation is not well accepted, except possibly in those patients in whom liver disease is so advanced that bile flow cannot be restored. Studies such as this argue for conservative decision making in this regard. Optimizing the outcome of the hepatoportoenterostomy can be obtained by addressing the controllable factors involved in the prognosis: early diagnosis and referral to a center experienced in the care of children with this disorder.

Outcome of orthotopic liver transplantation in children

The most important factor determining post-transplant survival at our center is the severity of the patient's illness at the time of transplantation. Survival in infants has improved with increasing experience. Infants younger than 1 year now have 1-year survival rates >85%. This increase in survival results from technical operative improvements and experienced care management. A major challenge is the high frequency of virus-related disease in children, particularly Epstein–Barr virus related. As the survival rates following orthotopic liver transplantation in children have increased, healthcare providers have begun to measure the overall health status of liver transplant recipients (functional outcome) as a complement to traditional measures of medical outcomes. The overriding objective of hepatic transplantation in children is complete rehabilitation with improved quality of life, as discussed in Chapters 43 and 44. Factors contributing to the attainment of this goal include improved nutritional status with appropriate growth and development as well as enhanced motor and cognitive skills, allowing social reintegration.

Future

The ultimate goal is to prevent biliary atresia. To accomplish that objective, a multicenter, multifaceted effort is necessary. The US National Institutes of Health have established a consortium – The Childhood Liver Disease Research and Education Network – consisting of 15 pediatric clinical research centers in the USA (http://www.childrennetwork.org). The individual centers and a data-coordinating center will accelerate advances in the understanding, diagnosis, and clinical management of biliary atresia and related pediatric liver diseases. Their goals are to (1) determine the etiology of the disorder, (2) develop rapid and sensitive means for diagnosis, (3) define the natural history of biliary atresia, (4) determine the optimal medical and surgical treatment strategies, and (5) identify risk factors for progression of the disease.

The consortium has developed a prospective clinical database and a repository of tissue, serum, and plasma samples and has recently reported an analysis of the outcomes of infants with biliary atresia. This database will be a valuable resource in the quest to achieve the goals outlined here and thus clearly represents an important first step in our fight against this disease.

Choledochal cyst

Choledochal cysts are considered to be congenital anomalies of the biliary tract characterized by varying degrees of cystic dilatation at various segments of the biliary tract (extrahepatic or intrahepatic). The frequency of choledochal cysts is about 1 in 15 000 live births in Western countries and as high as 1 in 1000 live births in Japan. There is a marked female predominance (4:1) regardless of the racial origin. A choledochal cyst (or congenital bile duct cyst) may be detected at any age and in any portion of the bile duct. Choledochal cysts can be classified into five subtypes (Figure 11.7, Table 11.2). Although cysts uncommonly present in the neonatal period, this consideration must be included in the differential diagnosis of neonatal cholestasis; antenatal diagnosis has been described. Cysts are present in up to 2% of infants with obstructive jaundice. Infants present in a manner simulating biliary atresia and, if unrecognized, may have progressive disease. Prolonged obstruction results in biliary cirrhosis, portal hypertension resulting from cirrhosis, and pressure on the portal vein by the distended cyst. Recurrent pancreatitis is an unusual complication of the malformation.

Clinical features

The classic triad of intermittent abdominal pain, jaundice, and right epigastric mass varies in incidence; this triad is usually not present in infants and is uncommon in older children, occurring in about 20%. Jaundice (conjugated hyperbilirubinemia) is the common manifestation. Abdominal pain may be a presenting symptom, often with elevated serum amylase

Table 11.2 Classification of bile duct cysts

Type	Features
I	Cystic dilatation of the common bile duct
Ia	Large saccular cystic dilatation
Ib	Small localized segmental dilatation
Ic	Diffuse (cylindric) fusiform dilatation
II	Diverticulum of the common bile duct and/or the gallbladder
III	Choledochocele
IV	Multiple cysts
IVa	Intrahepatic and extrahepatic (most common form)
IVb	Extrahepatic only
V	Fusiform intrahepatic dilatations (relation to Caroli disease?)

levels. The lesion may be detected at any age, with 18% appearing before 1 year of age. Older children may have mild chronic liver disease, which may reflect variable degrees of common bile duct obstruction. In certain patients, the lesion appears to be a true congenital malformation and is associated with other anomalies of the biliary tree, such as double common duct, double gallbladder, and accessory hepatic ducts, as well as polycystic and hypoplastic kidneys. Complete distal biliary obstruction may also be seen in infants, with no detectable biliary remnant at the site of the distal common bile duct. In these infants, the histological changes in the liver are indistinguishable from biliary atresia or constitute a distinct clinical subgroup [65]. Adults with choledochal cyst disease commonly have acute biliary tract or pancreatic symptoms. It is possible that the variability in age and clinical course represents two distinct entities: congenital disease (in infants) versus acquired disease (in older children).

Spontaneous perforation of a choledochal cyst in infancy may occur. Of 187 patients with infantile choledochal cyst treated at one hospital, 13 cases of spontaneous perforation were encountered; 8 patients were found to have biliary peritonitis, and 5 had sealed perforation [66]. The cause of the perforation is postulated to be biliary epithelial irritation as a result of reflux of pancreatic juice caused by pancreaticobiliary malunion associated with mural immaturity, rather than an abnormal rise in ductal pressure or congenital mural weakness at a certain point.

Pathogenesis

The pathogenesis of choledochal cysts is undetermined; there are several theories. Cysts may represent (1) anomalous union of the common bile duct and the pancreatic duct proximal

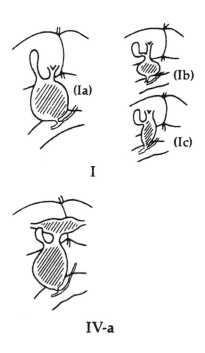
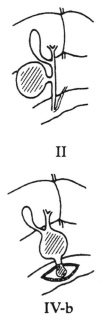
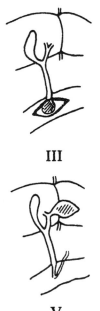

Figure 11.7 Classification of congenital bile duct cysts; see Table 11.2 for descriptions of each type.

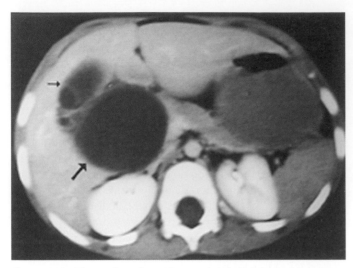

Figure 11.8 CT scan of an infant with a type I choledochal cyst. A large arrow indicates the cyst, a small arrow the gallbladder.

to the sphincter of Oddi, which may permit reflux of pancreatic enzymes into the common bile duct with resultant inflammation, localized weakness, and dilatation; (2) congenital segmental weakness of the common bile duct wall; or (3) obstruction of the distal common bile duct leading to dilatation. Interestingly, a recent study in a mouse model of rotavirus-induced biliary atresia showed a high incidence of dilatation of extrahepatic bile ducts in mice with overexpression of T helper lymphocyte type 2 cytokines, suggesting that the formation of cysts may depend, at least in part, on the type of tissue response following an injury [3]. Further research is needed.

Diagnosis

In most infants, the diagnosis is suggested if non-invasive imaging studies are undertaken for vague right upper quadrant symptoms (Figure 11.8). Ultrasonography should be the initial procedure in the evaluation of suspected choledochal cyst. Radiographs of the upper gastrointestinal tract may outline the mass as it displaces the first and second portion of the duodenum but are unnecessary.

Ultrasonography may be helpful in the preoperative differential diagnosis of choledochal cysts in neonates and infants. Cysts are larger, intrahepatic ducts are dilated, and gallbladders are not atretic in patients with choledochal cysts compared with patients with biliary atresia.

The accuracy of antenatal ultrasonography in the diagnosis of choledochal cysts is not known. We detected choledochal cysts in five patients through antenatal ultrasonography (at 17–35 weeks of gestational age). All had cystic dilatation of the common bile duct (type I cysts). All those with distal obstruction by operative cholangiography had varying degrees of fibrosis. Each improved following surgical excision and porto- or choledochoenterostomy. Redkar *et al.* [67] studied

13 patients with proven biliary disease who had abnormal antenatal scans at a mean of 20 weeks. Two infants had type I cystic biliary atresia, and one had a non-communicating segmental dilatation of the bile duct in a type III biliary atresia. The remainder had choledochal cysts and included two patients with intrahepatic cysts. The correct diagnosis was made antenatally in only two patients (15%). Of the remaining patients, seven were diagnosed with intra-abdominal cysts of unknown cause, three with duodenal atresia, and one with an ovarian cyst. Antenatal diagnosis offers the possibility of early definitive surgery for uncomplicated choledochal dilatation and the chance for improved outcome for surgically treated biliary atresia.

Treatment

The goal is complete surgical excision of the cyst mucosa, with a Roux-en-Y choledochojejunostomy proximal to the most distal lesion. This allows direct bile duct mucosa-to-bowel mucosa anastomosis, with the lowest risk of stenosis or stricture. This strategy has evolved from historic attempts at aspiration and external drainage, internal decompression and drainage into the duodenum (cyst duodenostomy), or direct anastomosis of the cyst to a jejunal Roux-en-Y loop. Each of these drainage techniques retained the wall of the cyst with its abnormal mucosa. Poor drainage leading to stasis and persistent cyst inflammation resulted in stricture formation, biliary lithiasis, and an increased risk of malignant evolution within the cyst wall. The recommended treatment currently includes elimination of the entire cyst mucosal wall by complete excision of the extrahepatic cyst and of the extrahepatic biliary tree and the creation of a retrocolic, isoperistaltic jejunal Roux-en-Y loop of 35–45 cm. Internal or external biliary transanastomotic stents rarely are needed because of the large size of the anastomosis (Figure 11.9).

In patients in whom prolonged or recurrent inflammation within and surrounding the cyst has complicated identification of the portal vasculature, the cyst can be transected along its anterolateral wall, allowing complete excision of the mucosa while retaining the fibrous cyst wall overlying the hepatic artery and portal vein. This protects the critical portal vascular structures and allows excision of all of the abnormal lining of the cyst.

The distal remnant of the common bile duct should be closed through the open base of the choledochal cyst, taking great care not to injure the often ectopically located pancreatic duct junction. Failure to remove this distal, often retroduodenal, portion of the cyst may lead to recurrence.

It is important to define the extent of any intrahepatic cystic disease at the time of choledochal cyst excision. This is best undertaken with an intraoperative cholangiogram or through preoperative percutaneous transhepatic or endoscopic retrograde cholangiography. If the cystic disease is in continuity with the primary bile duct cyst and no

(a)

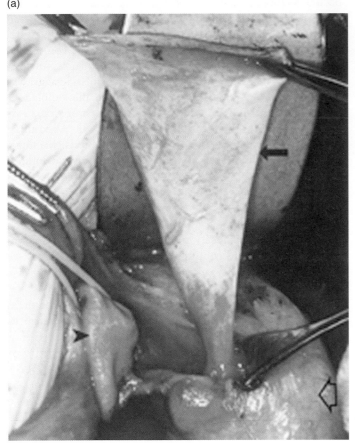

(b)

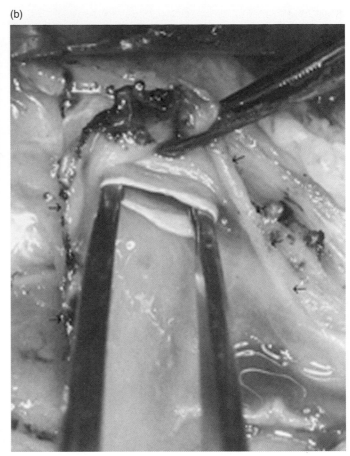

Figure 11.9 Surgical management of choledochal cyst. (a) Operative photograph of the "Lilly" dissection showing the inflammatory wall of the proximal choledochal cyst separated from the internal lining "mucosa" (arrow). The distal cyst wall is identified by the arrowhead. (b) Transection of the mucosal dissection just proximal to the proper hepatic duct bifurcation and prepared for reconstruction as an end-to-side choledochojejunostomy using an isoperistaltic jejunal Roux-en-Y loop. Arrows outline the retained outer wall of the choledochal cyst.

intervening strictures leading to stasis are present, reconstruction at the hepatic hilum is appropriate therapy. If intrahepatic cystic disease with interposed areas of stenosis (Caroli disease) is present, such decompressive methods are not applicable. Segmental multifocal cystic disease isolated to a single hepatic lobe can be treated successfully by cyst excision and hepatic lobectomy. If the intrahepatic disease is diffuse and involves all hepatic lobes, liver transplantation may be necessary if complete and successful decompressive drainage is not possible.

Complications and outcome

Cholangitis may occur in up to 15% of patients following surgery, even with the Roux-en-Y procedure, but is much less common than with direct anastomosis to the duodenum; the latter procedure is not advisable. The high rate of stricture (73%) after cyst enterostomy is also preventable by total cyst excision and Roux-en-Y reconstruction. Pancreatitis is uncommon but may occur secondary to proximal pancreatic duct or sphincter stenosis or stones.

Malignancy in choledochal cysts

Carcinoma has been reported in residual cystic tissue in up to 26% of patients, an incidence that is 20 times greater than that in the general population. The typical malignancy is adenocarcinoma of the bile duct or gallbladder; less commonly squamous cell carcinoma and cholangiocarcinoma have been described. The risk of developing malignancy increases with age, making complete excision of the cyst and proximal bile duct mucosa an essential component of the operation in older patients. Malignant change also may occur in areas of the biliary tree remote from the cyst. The increased risk of malignant degeneration and the dismal prognosis once cancer has developed warrant complete cyst excision, even in asymptomatic patients, including those with prior cyst enterostomies.

Spontaneous perforation of the common bile duct

Spontaneous perforation of the common bile duct is a rare curiosity. The typical onset of symptoms (mild jaundice, ascites, acholic stools, poor weight gain, and vomiting)

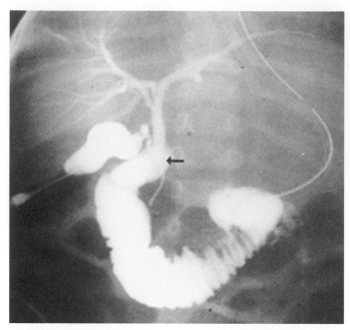

Figure 11.10 An infant with a bile duct stricture at the junction of the cystic duct with the proper hepatic duct (arrow). The hypoplastic distal common bile duct is seen. The patient was treated with a choledochojejunostomy into an isoperistaltic jejunal Roux-en-Y loop.

occurs before 3 months of age. Progressive abdominal distension occurs, with bile staining of umbilical and inguinal hernias and of the abdominal wall. The diagnosis is suggested by the relatively modest degree of conjugated hyperbilirubinemia with minimal elevation of aminotransferase levels in association with acholic stools. Sonography may reveal ascites or loculated fluid around the gallbladder [68], and hepatobiliary scintigraphy may demonstrate evidence of activity outside the biliary tract [69]. Abdominal paracentesis yields clear, bile-stained ascitic fluid. Histologically, the liver manifests cholestasis with a normal lobular pattern. Operative cholangiography usually demonstrates the presence of the perforation, frequently in association with obstruction at the distal end of the common bile duct, secondary to stenosis, segmental atresia, or inspissated bile. The rather constant location of the perforation at the junction of the cystic and common bile ducts is highly suggestive of a developmental weakness at this site (Figure 11.10). Drainage with suture closure of the perforation may be a satisfactory treatment. Internal diversion through a Roux-en-Y loop of jejunum may be used for drainage in some infants.

References

1. Landing BH. Considerations of the pathogenesis of neonatal hepatitis, biliary atresia and choledochal cyst: the concept of infantile obstructive cholangiopathy. *Prog Pediatr Surg* 1974;**6**:113–139.

2. Desmet VJ. Congenital diseases of intrahepatic bile ducts: variations on the theme "ductal plate malformation". *Hepatology* 1992;**16**:1069–1083.

3. Li J, Bessho K, Shivakumar P, *et al.* Th2 signals induce epithelial injury in mice and are compatible with the biliary atresia phenotype. *J Clin Invest* 2011;**121**:4244–4256.

4. Landing BH, Wells TR, Ramicone E. Time course of the intrahepatic lesion of extrahepatic biliary atresia: a morphometric study. *Pediatr Pathol* 1985;**4**:309–319.

5. Balistreri WF, Grand R, Hoofnagle JH, *et al.* Biliary atresia: current concepts and research directions. Summary of a symposium. *Hepatology* 1996;**23**:1682–1692.

6. Bessho K, Bezerra JA. Biliary atresia: will blocking inflammation tame the disease? *Annu Rev Med* 2011;**62**:171–185.

7. Bezerra JA, Tiao G, Ryckman FC, *et al.* Genetic induction of proinflammatory immunity in children with biliary atresia. *Lancet* 2002;**360**:1563–1659.

8. Mack CL, Tucker RM, Sokol RJ, *et al.* Biliary atresia is associated with CD4+ Th1 cell-mediated portal tract inflammation. *Pediatr Res* 2004;**56**:79–87.

9. Yoon PW, Bresee JS, Olney RS, James LM, Khoury MJ. Epidemiology of biliary atresia: a population-based study. *Pediatrics* 1997;**99**:376–382.

10. Davenport M, Savage M, Mowat AP, Howard ER. Biliary atresia splenic malformation syndrome: an etiologic and prognostic subgroup. *Surgery* 1993;**113**:662–668.

11. Balistreri WF. Neonatal cholestasis. *J Pediatr* 1985;**106**:171–184.

12. Pacheco MC, Campbell KM, Bove KE. Ductal plate malformation-like arrays in early explants after a Kasai procedure are independent of splenic malformation complex (heterotaxy). *Pediatr Dev Pathol* 2009;**12**:355–360.

13. Davenport M, Caponcelli E, Livesey E, Hadzic N, Howard E. Surgical outcome in biliary atresia: etiology affects the influence of age at surgery. *Ann Surg* 2008;**247**:694–698.

14. Hsiao CH, Chang MH, Chen HL, *et al.* Universal screening for biliary atresia using an infant stool color card in Taiwan. *Hepatology* 2008;**47**:1233–1240.

15. Fischler B, Ehrnst A, Forsgren M, Orvell C, Nemeth A. The viral association of neonatal cholestasis in Sweden: a possible link between cytomegalovirus infection and extrahepatic biliary atresia. *J Pediatr Gastroenterol Nutr* 1998;**27**:57–64.

16. Jevon GP, Dimmick JE. Biliary atresia and cytomegalovirus infection: a DNA study. *Pediatr Dev Pathol* 1999;**2**:11–14.

17. Mason AL, Xu L, Guo L, *et al.* Detection of retroviral antibodies in primary biliary cirrhosis and other idiopathic biliary disorders. *Lancet* 1998;**351**:1620–1624 [erratum *Lancet* 1998;**352**:152].

18. Mack CL. The pathogenesis of biliary atresia: evidence for a virus-induced autoimmune disease. *Semin Liver Dis* 2007;**27**:233–242.

19. Szavay PO, Leonhardt J, Czech-Schmidt G, Petersen, C. The role of reovirus type 3 infection in an established murine model for biliary atresia. *Eur J Pediatr Surg* 2002;**12**:248–250.

20. Tyler KL, Sokol RJ, Oberhaus SM, *et al.* Detection of reovirus RNA in hepatobiliary tissues from patients with

extrahepatic biliary atresia and choledochal cysts. *Hepatology* 1998;**27**:1475–1482.

21. Riepenhoff-Talty M, Schaekel K, Clark HF, *et al.* Group A rotaviruses produce extrahepatic biliary obstruction in orally inoculated newborn mice. *Pediatr Res* 1993;**33**:394–399.

22. Riepenhoff-Talty M, Gouvea V, Evans MJ, *et al.* Detection of group C rotavirus in infants with extrahepatic biliary atresia. *J Infect Dis* 1996;**174**:8–15.

23. Lin YC, Chang MH, Liao SF, *et al.* Decreasing rate of biliary atresia in Taiwan: a survey, 2004–2009. *Pediatrics* 2011;**128**:e530-e536.

24. Tan CE, Davenport M, Driver M, Howard ER. Does the morphology of the extrahepatic biliary remnants in biliary atresia influence survival? A review of 205 cases. *J Pediatr Surg* 1994;**29**:1459–1464.

25. Sokol RJ, Shepherd RW, Superina R, *et al.* Screening and outcomes in biliary atresia: summary of a National Institutes of Health workshop. *Hepatology* 2007;**46**:566–581.

26. Yokoyama T, Copeland NG, Jenkins NA, *et al.* Reversal of left-right asymmetry: a situs inversus mutation. *Science* 1993;**260**:679–682.

27. Schon P, Tsuchiya K, Lenoir D, *et al.* Identification, genomic organization, chromosomal mapping and mutation analysis of the human *INV* gene, the ortholog of a murine gene implicated in left-right axis development and biliary atresia. *Hum Genet* 2002;**110**:157–165.

28. Desmet VJ. Intrahepatic bile ducts under the lens. *J Hepatol* 1985;**1**:545–559.

29. Silveira TR, Salzano FM, Donaldson PT, *et al.* Association between HLA and extrahepatic biliary atresia. *J Pediatr Gastroenterol Nutr* 1993;**16**:114–117.

30. Moyer K, Kaimal V, Pacheco C, *et al.* Staging of biliary atresia at diagnosis by molecular profiling of the liver. *Genome Med* 2010;**2**:33.

31. Mack CL, Falta MT, Sullivan AK, *et al.* Oligoclonal expansions of CD4+ and CD8+ T-cells in the target organ of patients with biliary atresia. *Gastroenterology* 2007;**133**:278–287.

32. Lu BR, Brindley SM, Tucker RM, Lambert CL, Mack CL. Alpha-enolase autoantibodies cross-reactive to viral

proteins in a mouse model of biliary atresia. *Gastroenterology* 2010;**139**:1753–1761.

33. Jafri M, Donnelly B, Allen S, *et al.* Cholangiocyte expression of alpha2beta1-integrin confers susceptibility to rotavirus-induced experimental biliary atresia. *Am J Physiol Gastrointest Liver Physiol* 2008;**295**:G16–G26.

34. Saxena V, Shivakumar P, Sabla G, *et al.* Dendritic cells regulate natural killer cell activation and epithelial injury in experimental biliary atresia. *Sci Transl Med* 2011;**3**:102ra194.

35. Miethke AG, Saxena V, Shivakumar P, *et al.* Post-natal paucity of regulatory T cells and control of NK cell activation in experimental biliary atresia. *J Hepatol* 2010;**52**:718–726.

36. Harper P, Plant JW, Unger DB. Congenital biliary atresia and jaundice in lambs and calves. *Aust Vet J* 1990;**67**:18–22 [erratum p. 167].

37. Klippel CH. A new theory of biliary atresia. *J Pediatr Surg* 1972;**7**:651–654.

38. Choi SO, Park WH, Lee HJ, Woo SK. "Triangular cord": a sonographic finding applicable in the diagnosis of biliary atresia. *J Pediatr Surg* 1996;**31**:363–366.

39. Alagille D. *Cholestasis in the First Three Months of Life.* New York: Grune & Stratton, 1979, pp. 471–485.

40. Russo P, Magee JC, Boitnott J, *et al.* Design and validation of the biliary atresia research consortium histologic assessment system for cholestasis in infancy. *Clin Gastroenterol Hepatol* 2011;**9**:357–362.

41. Zerbini MC, Gallucci SD, Maezono R, *et al.* Liver biopsy in neonatal cholestasis: a review on statistical grounds. *Mod Pathol* 1997;**10**:793–799.

42. Markowitz J, Daum F, Kahn EI, *et al.* Arteriohepatic dysplasia. I. Pitfalls in diagnosis and management. *Hepatology* 1983;**3**:74–76.

43. Kasai M, Watanabe I, Ohi, R. Follow-up studies of long term survivors after hepatic portoenterostomy for "noncorrectible" biliary atresia. *J Pediatr Surg* 1975;**10**:173–182.

44. Ryckman FC, Alonso MH, Bucuvalas JC, Balistreri WF. Biliary atresia: surgical management and treatment options as they relate to outcome. *Liver Transplant Surg* 1998;**4**:S24–33.

45. Endo M, Katsumata K, Yokoyama J, *et al.* Extended dissection of the portahepatis and creation of an intussuscepted ileocolic conduit for biliary atresia. *J Pediatr Surg* 1983;**18**:784–793.

46. Hashimoto T, Otobe Y, Shimizu Y, *et al.* A modification of hepatic portoenterostomy (Kasai operation) for biliary atresia. *J Am Coll Surg* 1997;**185**:548–553.

47. Ohi R, Ibrahim M. Biliary atresia. *Sem Pediatr Surg* 1992;**1**:115–124.

48. Ryckman F, Fisher R, Pedersen S, *et al.* Improved survival in biliary atresia patients in the present era of liver transplantation. *J Pediatr Surg* 1993;**28**:382–386.

49. Lally KP, Kanegaye J, Matsumura M, *et al.* Perioperative factors affecting the outcome following repair of biliary atresia. *Pediatrics* 1989;**83**:723–726.

50. Chandra RS, Altman RP. Ductal remnants in extrahepatic biliary atresia: a histopathologic study with clinical correlation. *J Pediatr* 1978;**93**:196–200.

51. Ohya T, Miyano T, Kimura K. Indication for portoenterostomy based on 103 patients with Suruga II modification. *J Pediatr Surg* 1990;**25**:801–804.

52. Davenport M, De Ville de Goyet J, Stringer MD, *et al.* Seamless management of biliary atresia in England and Wales (1999–2002). *Lancet* 2004;**363**:1354–1357.

53. Ohi R, Hanamatsu M, Mochizuki I, Ohkohchi N, Kasai M. Reoperation in patients with biliary atresia. *J Pediatr Surg* 1985;**20**:256–259.

54. Gottrand F, Bernard O, Hadchouel M, *et al.* Late cholangitis after successful surgical repair of biliary atresia. *Am J Dis Child* 1991;**145**:213–215.

55. Lunzmann K, Schweizer P. The influence of cholangitis on the prognosis of extrahepatic biliary atresia. *Eur J Pediatr Surg* 1999;**9**:19–23.

56. Balistreri WF. Bile acid therapy in pediatric hepatobiliary disease: the role of ursodeoxycholic acid. *J Pediatr Gastroenterol Nutr* 1997;**24**:573–589.

57. Davenport M, Stringer MD, Tizzard SA, *et al.* Randomized, double-blind, placebo-controlled trial of cortico-steroids after Kasai portoenterostomy for biliary atresia. *Hepatology* 2007;**46**:1821–1827.

58. Petersen C, Harder D, Melter M, *et al.* Postoperative high-dose steroids do not improve mid-term survival with native liver in biliary atresia. *Am J Gastroenterol* 2008;**103**: 712–719.

59. Miga D, Sokol RJ, Mackenzie T, *et al.* Survival after first esophageal variceal hemorrhage in patients with biliary atresia. *J Pediatr* 2001;**139**:291–296.

60. Laurent J, Gauthier F, Bernard O, *et al.* Long-term outcome after surgery for biliary atresia. Study of 40 patients surviving for more than 10 years. *Gastroenterology* 1990;**99**:1793–1797.

61. Ryckman FC, Fisher RA, Pedersen SH, Balistreri WF. Liver transplantation in children. *Sem Pediatr Surg* 1992;**1**:162–172.

62. Ryckman FC, Flake AW, Fisher RA, *et al.* Segmental orthotopic hepatic transplantation as a means to improve patient survival and diminish waiting-list mortality. *J Pediatr Surg* 1991;**26**:422–427; discussion 427–428.

63. Tiao GM, Alonso M, Bezerra J, *et al.* Liver transplantation in children younger than 1 year: the Cincinnati experience. *J Pediatr Surg* 2005;**40**:268–273.

64. Chardot C, Carton M, Spire-Bendelac N, *et al.* Prognosis of biliary atresia in the era of liver transplantation: French national study from 1986 to 1996. *Hepatology* 1999;**30**:606–611.

65. De Matos V, Erlichman J, Russo PA, Haber BA. 2005. Does "cystic" biliary atresia represent a distinct clinical and etiological subgroup? A series of three cases. *Pediatr Dev Pathol* 2005;**8**:725–731.

66. Ando K, Miyano T, Kohno S, Takamizawa S, Lane G. Spontaneous perforation of choledochal cyst: a study of 13 cases. *Eur J Pediatr Surg* 1998;**8**:23–25.

67. Redkar R, Davenport M, Howard ER. Antenatal diagnosis of congenital anomalies of the biliary tract. *J Pediatr Surg* 1998;**33**:700–704.

68. Haller JO, Condon VR, Berdon WE, *et al.* Spontaneous perforation of the common bile duct in children. *Radiology* 1989;**172**:621–624.

69. So SK, Lindahl JA, Sharp HL, Cook AM, Leonard AS. Bile ascites during infancy: diagnosis using Disofenin Tc 99m sequential scintiphotography. *Pediatrics* 1983;**71**:402–405.

Neonatal jaundice and disorders of bilirubin metabolism

Mark Bartlett and Glenn R. Gourley

Introduction

Elevation of the serum bilirubin level is a common finding during the first week of life. This can be a transient phenomenon that will resolve spontaneously or it can signify a serious or even potentially life-threatening condition. There are many causes of hyperbilirubinemia and each has its own therapeutic and prognostic implications. Independent of the cause, elevated serum bilirubin levels can be potentially toxic to the newborn infant. This chapter will review perinatal bilirubin metabolism and address assessment, etiology, toxicity, and therapy for neonatal jaundice. Finally, the diseases in which there is a primary disorder in the metabolism of bilirubin will be reviewed regarding their clinical presentation, pathophysiology, diagnosis, and treatment. For more extensive referencing, see this chapter in the third edition of this textbook [1].

Bilirubin metabolism

Production and circulation

Bilirubin (from Latin, *bilis*, bile; *rube*, red) is formed from the degradation of heme-containing compounds (Figure 12.1). The largest source for the production of bilirubin is hemoglobin. However, other heme-containing proteins are also degraded to bilirubin, including the cytochromes, catalases, tryptophane pyrrolase, and muscle myoglobin.

The formation of bilirubin is initiated by cleaving the tetrapyrrole ring of protoheme (protoporphyrin IX), which results in a linear tetrapyrrole (biliverdin). The first enzyme system involved in the formation of bilirubin is microsomal heme oxygenase. Heme oxygenase reduces the porphyrin iron (FeIII to FeII) and hydroxylates the α-methine ($=C-$) carbon. This carbon is then oxidatively excised from the tetrapyrrole ring, yielding carbon monoxide and opening the ring structure; this is associated with oxygenation of the two carbons adjacent to the site of cleavage. The cleaved α-carbon is excreted as carbon monoxide, which also functions as a neurotransmitter. The iron released by heme oxygenase can be reutilized by the body. The resultant linear tetrapyrrole is

biliverdin IXα The stereospecificity of the enzyme produces cleavage almost exclusively at the α-carbon of the tetrapyrrole.

In utero, bilirubin IXβ (cleavage between the two β-carbons, Figure 12.1) is the first bile pigment seen and can be found in bile or meconium by 15 weeks of gestation. Small amounts of bilirubin IXβ are also found in adult human bile. The central (C-10) carbon on biliverdin IXα is then reduced from a methine to a methylene group ($-CH_2-$) forming bilirubin IXα. This is accomplished by the cytosolic enzyme biliverdin reductase. The proximity of this enzyme results in very little biliverdin ever being present in the circulation. The daily production rate of bilirubin is 6 to 8 mg/kg in healthy term infants and 3 to 4 mg/kg in healthy adults. In mammals, approximately 80% of bilirubin produced daily originates from hemoglobin. Degradation of hepatic and renal heme appears to account for most of the remaining 20%, reflecting the very rapid turnover of certain of these heme proteins. Catabolism of hemoglobin occurs very largely from the sequestration of erythrocytes at the end of their lifespan (120 days is adult humans, 90 days in newborns.). A small fraction of newly synthesized hemoglobin is degraded in the bone marrow. This process, termed "ineffective erythropoiesis," normally represents <3% of daily bilirubin production but may be substantially increased in people with hemoglobinopathies, vitamin deficiencies, and heavy metal intoxication. Infants produce more bilirubin per unit body weight because red blood cell mass is greater and red blood cell lifespan is shorter in infants. Additionally, hepatic heme proteins represent a larger fraction of total body weight in infants. Although bilirubin has long been thought of solely as a waste product of heme catabolism, there are data to suggest that some mild degree of hyperbilirubinemia may be helpful because of the antioxidant capacity of bilirubin and its potential role as a free-radical scavenger and cytoprotectant.

Bilirubin is poorly soluble in aqueous solvents and requires biotransformation to more water-soluble derivatives for excretion from the body. This poor solubility is related to the structure of bilirubin. Rather than being linear (structure 5, Figure 12.1), bilirubin undergoes extensive internal hydrogen

Liver Disease in Children, Fourth Edition, ed. Frederick J. Suchy, Ronald J. Sokol, and William F. Balistreri. Published by Cambridge University Press. © Cambridge University Press 2014.

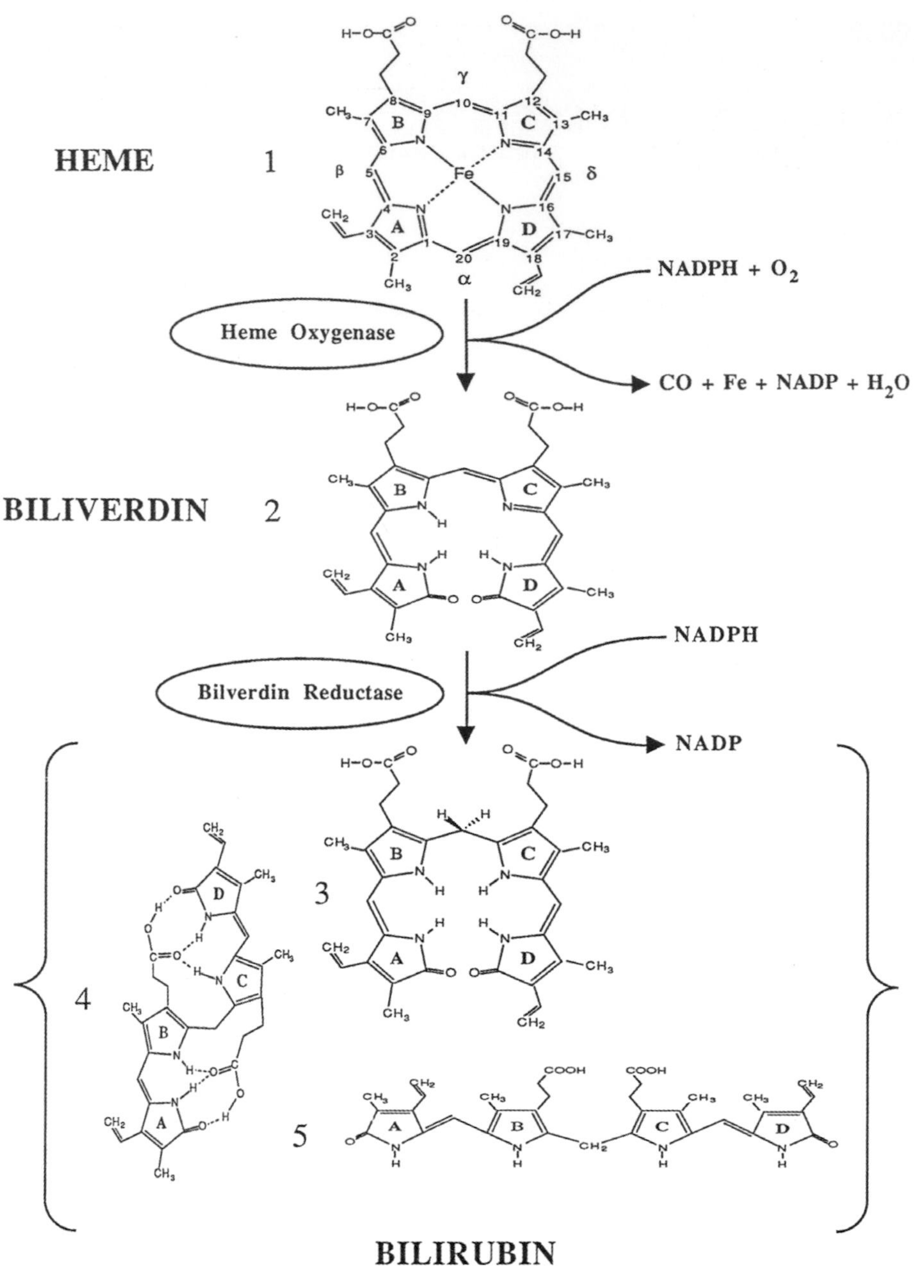

Figure 12.1 Chemical structures depicting the conversion of heme to bilirubin. Bilirubin is frequently represented by any of the three structures (2–4) shown at the bottom.

bonding (structure 4, Figure 12.1). This shields the polar propionic acid side-chains and makes bilirubin very non-polar and lipophilic. The carbon–carbon double bonds at positions 4–5 and 15–16 can assume two different configurations (similar to *cis* and *trans*) depending on whether the higher priority atoms or groups (based on atomic number) are on the same (*Z, zusammen*, German: "together") or opposite (*E, entgegen*, "opposite") sides of the double bond. The naturally occurring form of bilirubin, (4Z,15Z)-bilirubin IXα, can be represented by any of the three structures [2–4] depicted at the bottom of Figure 12.1. Knowledge of this stereochemistry is important in understanding phototherapy.

The poor aqueous solubility makes a carrier molecule, albumin, necessary for bilirubin transport from its sites of production in the reticuloendothelial system to the liver for excretion (Figure 12.2). Each albumin molecule possesses a single high-affinity binding site for one molecule of bilirubin. A binding affinity of this magnitude implies that, at normal serum bilirubin levels, all bilirubin will be transported to the liver bound to albumin, with negligible amounts free to diffuse into other tissues.

Hepatocyte uptake

The structure of the liver is well suited for the uptake of bilirubin by individual hepatocytes. Cords of hepatocytes are arranged radially so that adjacent sinusoids border all hepatocytes. The flow of blood through the sinusoids is slower than

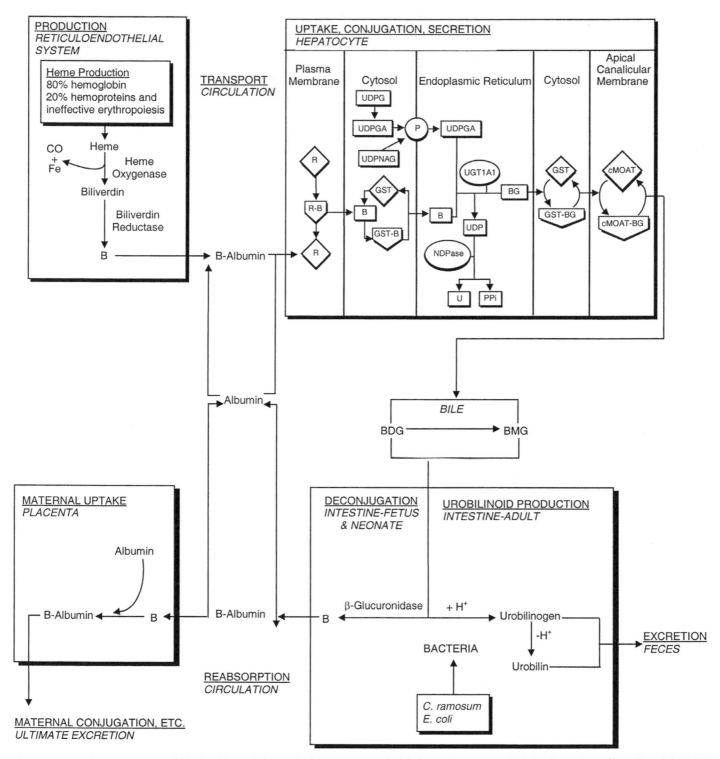

Figure 12.2 A schematic overview of bilirubin (B) metabolism in the fetus, neonate, and adult. R, membrane carrier; GST, glutathione *S*-transferase (ligandin); UDPG, uridine diphosphate glucose; UDPGA, uridine diphosphate glucuronic acid; UDPNAG, uridine diphosphate *N*-acetyl glucosamine; P, permease; UGT1A1, bilirubin UDP-glucuronosyltransferase; NDPase, nucleoside diphosphatase; PPi, inorganic pyrophosphate; BDG/BMG, bilirubin di- or mono-glucuronide; cMOAT, canalicular multispecific organic anion transporter (also known as multidrug resistance-associated protein 2 (MRP2) and encoded by *ABCC2*); BG, bilirubin glucuronide.

that of other capillary beds because it is generated by portal venous pressure rather than arterial pressure. Albumin-bound bilirubin passes from the plasma into the tissue fluid space (space of Disse) between the endothelium and the hepatocyte since the sinusoidal endothelium of the liver lacks the basal laminae that are found in other organ capillary systems. The pores of the endothelium allow direct contact with the plasma membrane of the hepatocyte.

A hepatocyte with a schematic illustration of bilirubin metabolism is shown in Figure 12.2. In the first step, bilirubin dissociates from its albumin carrier and enters the hepatocyte either via a membrane receptor carrier or by passive diffusion. The carrier in the basolateral plasma membrane, known as organic anion transporting polypeptide 2 (human OATP2 recently named OATP1B1 under new nomenclature; transporter symbol SLC21A6) also transports other bilirubin glucuronides and bromsulfopthalein. This carrier protein is competitively inhibited by simultaneous exposure to bromsulfophthalein and indocyanine green

Once within the aqueous environment of the hepatocyte, bilirubin is again bound by a protein carrier, glutathione S-transferase, traditionally referred to as ligandin. This is a family of cytosolic proteins that have enzymatic activity and also bind non-substrate ligands. Although the affinity of purified glutathione S-transferase for bilirubin is less than that of albumin, this compound is thought to prevent bilirubin and its conjugates from refluxing back into the circulation.

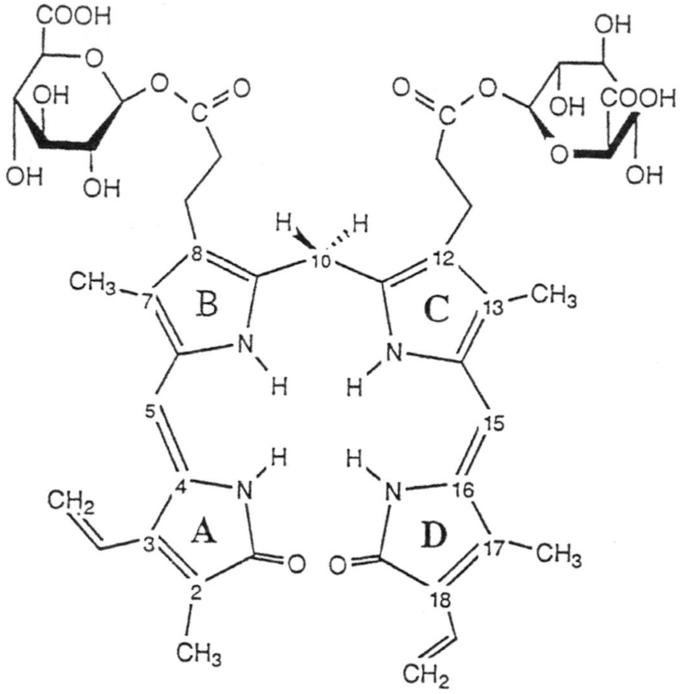

Conjugation

Inside the endoplasmic reticulum (microsomes) of the hepatocyte, bilirubin is conjugated with glucuronic acid. The glucuronic acid donor is uridine diphosphate glucuronic acid. The conjugation results in an ester linkage formed with either or both of the propionic acid side-chains on the B and C pyrrole rings of bilirubin (Figure 12.3). The enzyme responsible for this esterification is bilirubin UDP-glucuronosyltransferase (OMIM (Online Mendelian Inheritance in Man) database *191740; http://www.ncbi.nlm.nih.gov/sites/entrez?db=omim).

The specific isoform responsible for bilirubin conjugation is UGT1A1. This is part of the UDP glycosyltransferase superfamily of enzymes encoded by *UGT1* gene complex on chromosome 2 that is involved with metabolism of many xenobiotic and endogenous substances. *UGT1* encodes several isoforms and has a complex structure consisting of four common exons [5] and 13 variable exons encoding different isoforms (Figure 12.4). Numerous *UGT1* mutant alleles have been described which cause Gilbert syndrome (GS) and Crigler–Najjar (CN) syndrome types I and II. The isoform UGT1A1 catalyzes the formation of bilirubin mono- and diglucuronides. In normal adult humans, the majority of bilirubin conjugates are excreted in the bile as bilirubin diglucuronides (~80%) (Figure 12.5, middle panel). Lesser amounts of bilirubin monoglucuronides (~15%) are also excreted along with very small amounts of unconjugated bilirubin other bilirubin conjugates (e.g. glucose, xylose, and mixed diesters). In infants, since there is lower UGT1A1 activity, bile contains less bilirubin diglucuronide and more bilirubin monoglucuronide than the adult (Figure 12.6, middle panel).

Excretion of bilirubin conjugates

Following conjugation, bilirubin conjugates are excreted against a concentration gradient from the hepatocyte through the canalicular membrane into the bile. Data suggests that bilirubin glucuronides are transported across the canalicular membrane by both ATP-dependent and membrane potential-dependent transport systems. The ATP-dependent transporter responsible for bilirubin glucuronide passage from the hepatocyte through the canalicular membrane is canalicular multi-specific organic anion transporter (cMOAT; OMIM *601107). cMOAT is a member of the ATP-binding cassette (ABC)

Figure 12.3 Bilirubin diglucuronide. In bilirubin monoglucuronide, only one propionic acid side-chain (C-8 or C-12) is glucuronidated.

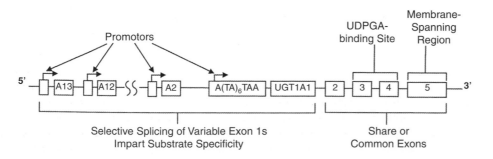

Promotors

Selective Splicing of Variable Exon 1s
Impart Substrate Specificity

UDPGA-binding Site

Membrane-Spanning Region

Share or Common Exons

Figure 12.4 The human gene for UDP-glucuronosyltransferase-1 (*UGT1*). UDPGA, uridine diphosphate glucuronic acid.

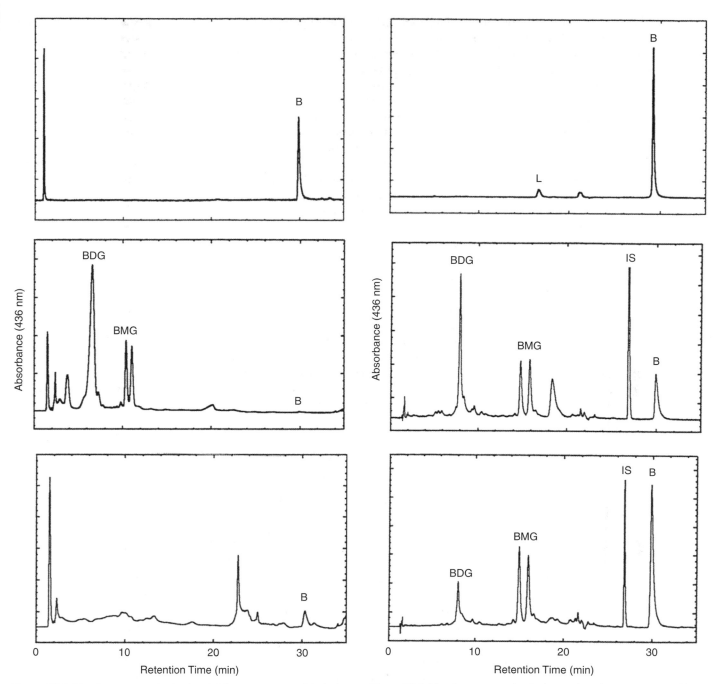

Figure 12.5 Bile pigment excretion in the adult human as assessed by high performance liquid chromatography. Chromatograms represent analysis of serum (20 μl, top), duodenal bile (20 μl, middle), and stool extract (equivalent to 50 mg of wet stool, bottom) from a normal man. Scale of *y* axes varies. Serum bile pigments are almost all bilirubin (B). The bilirubin diglucuronides (BDG) and monoglucuronides (BMG) that predominate in adult bile are not present in adult feces because of metabolism by intestinal bacteria.

Figure 12.6 Bile pigment excretion in the newborn human as assessed by high performance liquid chromatography. Chromatograms represent analysis of serum (20 μl, top) of an infant receiving phototherapy in the first week of life, and duodenal bile (20 μl, middle) and stool extract (equivalent to 50 mg of wet stool, bottom) from a normal full-term, formula-fed female infant on day 3 of life. Serum bile pigments include lumirubin (L). Scale of *y* axes varies. Neonates lack an intestinal bacterial flora and, hence, large quantities of bilirubin diglucuronides (BDG), and monoglucuronides (BMG) and bilirubin (B) are present in feces. IS, internal standard.

transporter superfamily and is homologous to the multidrug resistance-associated protein (MRP2); it is also known as ABCC2 since it is encoded by *ABCC2*. This transporter is involved with ATP-dependent transport across the apical canalicular membrane of a variety of endogenous compounds and xenobiotics including bilirubin mono- and diglucuronide. Genetic mutations which alter these ABC transporters cause diseases which include cystic fibrosis, hyperinsulinemia, progressive familial intrahepatic cholestasis types 2 and 3, adrenoleukodystrophy, multidrug resistance, and Dubin–Johnson syndrome (DJS). This mechanism can be saturated with increasing amounts of bilirubin or bilirubin conjugates.

Under normal conditions, there is evidence that bilirubin conjugates equilibrate across the sinusoidal membrane of hepatocytes. This results in small amounts of bilirubin conjugates being present in the systemic circulation. If there is diminished hepatic glucuronidation of bilirubin (e.g. in the neonate), there will be a decreased amount of bilirubin conjugates present in the serum. In full-term newborns, there is an increase in the serum level of bilirubin diconjugates ($0.55 \pm 0.25\%$ on days 2–4 and $1.62 \pm 0.99\%$ on days 9–13) that is consistent with the maturation of bilirubin glucuronidation. In contrast, in premature infants younger than 33 weeks of gestation, bilirubin diconjugates were very low and remained so, suggesting a more severe immaturity of the glucuronidation process.

In many pathologic circumstances, bilirubin mono- and diglucuronides are not excreted from the hepatocyte fast enough to prevent significant reflux back into the circulation. The resulting elevation of serum bilirubin conjugate levels results in the transesterification of bilirubin glucuronide with an amino group on albumin, producing a covalent bond between albumin and bilirubin [2]. This product is formed spontaneously and is known as δ-bilirubin. δ-Bilirubin is not formed in hyperbilirubinemic conditions unless there is elevation of the conjugated bilirubin fraction. Both δ-bilirubin and bilirubin conjugates are direct reacting in the van den Bergh test, which explains how direct bilirubin may continue to be elevated in patients who otherwise are recovering from an hepatic insult; δ-bilirubin lingers because of the long half-life (~20 day) of albumin.

Enterohepatic circulation

When bilirubin conjugates enter the intestinal lumen (Figure 12.2), several possibilities for further metabolism arise. In adults, the normal bacterial flora hydrogenate various carbon double bonds in bilirubin to produce assorted urobilinogens (Figure 12.7). Subsequent oxidation of the middle (C-10) carbon produces the related urobilins. Since there are a large number of unsaturated bonds in bilirubin, there are many compounds formed by reduction and oxidation of these bonds. This large family of related reduction–oxidation products of bilirubin is known as the urobilinoids [3] and is excreted in the feces. The conversion of bilirubin conjugates to urobilinoids is important because it blocks the intestinal absorption of bilirubin, known as the enterohepatic circulation [4]. Neonates lack an intestinal bacterial flora and are more likely to absorb bilirubin from the intestine. This difference in bile pigment excretion between adults and neonates is demonstrated by comparing Figures 12.5 and 12.6 (lower panels).

Bilirubin conjugates in the intestine can also act as substrate for either bacterial or endogenous tissue β-glucuronidase, which hydrolyses glucuronic acid from bilirubin glucuronides. The unconjugated bilirubin produced is more rapidly absorbed from the intestine [6]. In the fetus, tissue β-glucuronidase is detectable by 12 weeks of gestation and facilitates intestinal bilirubin absorption, which enables bilirubin to be cleared via the placenta. Following birth, increased intestinal β-glucuronidase can increase the neonate's likelihood of experiencing higher serum bilirubin levels [7]. Breast-milk can contain high levels of β-glucuronidase and this is one factor related to the higher jaundice levels seen in breast-fed infants [8]. Feeding specific nutritional ingredients, such as L-aspartic acid, that inhibit β-glucuronidase has been shown to result in increased fecal bilirubin excretion and lower levels of jaundice [9].

Jaundice assessment

Jaundice (French *jaune*, yellow) and icterus (Greek *ikteros*, jaundice) both refer to the yellow discoloration of the tissues (skin, sclerae, etc.) caused by deposition of bilirubin. Jaundice is a sign that hyperbilirubinemia exists (i.e. total serum bilirubin is approximately >1.4 mg/dL (23.8 µmol/L) after 6 months of age). The degree of yellow is directly related to the level of serum bilirubin and the related amount of bilirubin deposition into the extravascular tissues. Hypercarotenemia can impart a yellow hue to the skin but the sclerae remain white. There are many conditions associated with neonatal jaundice. Some of these states are so commonly recognized as to be termed "physiologic." Alternatively, jaundice can be a sign of severe hemolysis, infection, or liver failure.

Measurement of the total serum bilirubin concentration allows quantification of jaundice. In 2009, an expert panel of the American Academy of Pediatrics recommended that universal predischarge bilirubin screening, using total serum bilirubin or transcutaneous bilirubin measurements, would help to reduce risk of subsequent severe hyperbilirubinemia [10]. Two components of total serum bilirubin can be routinely measured in the clinical laboratory: conjugated bilirubin ("direct" reacting because in the van den Bergh test color development takes place directly without adding methanol), and unconjugated bilirubin ("indirect" fraction). Although the terms "direct" and "indirect" are used equivalently with conjugated and unconjugated bilirubin, it is now known that this is not quantitatively correct since the direct fraction includes both conjugated bilirubin and δ-bilirubin. Elevation of either of these fractions can result in jaundice. There is a long history of undesirable variability in the measurement of serum bilirubin fractions. The Jendrassik–Grof procedure is the method of choice for total bilirubin measurement, although this method also has problems. When the total serum bilirubin level is high, factitious elevation of the direct fraction has been reported.

Newer methods, high performance liquid chromatography (HPLC) and multilayered slide technology, have been developed that can more accurately determine the various bilirubin fractions (unconjugated, monoconjugated, diconjugated, and albumin bound). High performance liquid

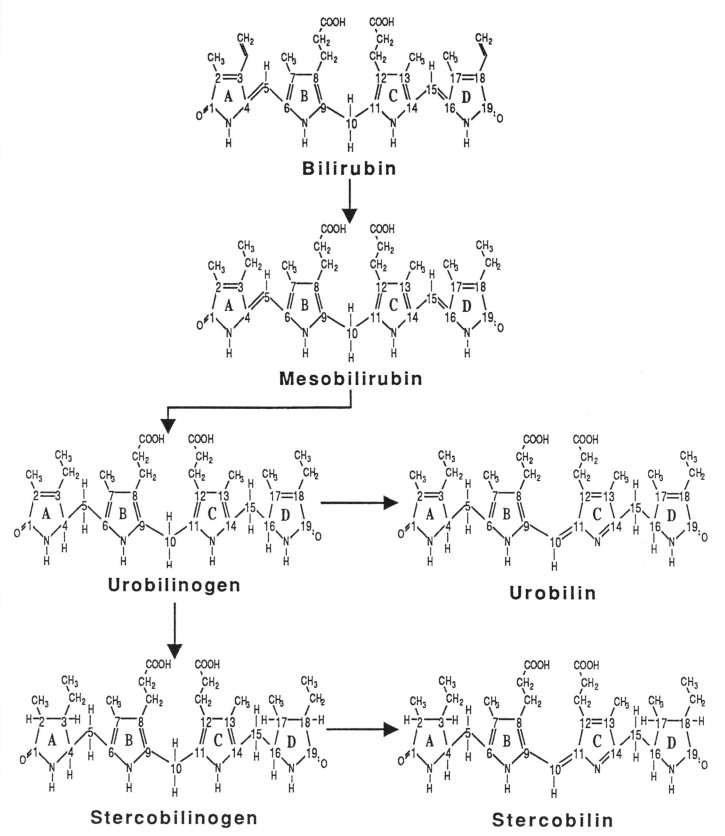

Figure 12.7 The reduction and oxidation of bilirubin to a family of related compounds known collectively as urobilinoids. Only several examples are given of this much larger family.

chromatography is superior but too expensive and time consuming for the clinical laboratory. Analysis with automated multilayered slide technology is in use in many clinical laboratories. This allows measurement of specific conjugated and unconjugated bilirubin fractions without inclusion of δ-bilirubin. The conjugated bilirubin measurement is an earlier indicator of relief from biliary cholestasis than is direct bilirubin because of the long half-life of δ-bilirubin.

Non-invasive methods to measure jaundice levels also exist and have been shown to be particularly useful in neonates. Current commercially methods available include the BiliCheck (Respironics, Pittsburgh, PA, USA) and the Minolta/Hill-Rom Air-Shields Transcutaneous Jaundice Meter 103 (Air-Shields, Hatboro, PA, USA). The device is touched to the skin in a painless manner with the immediate resulting point-of-care measurement of transcutaneous bilirubin that correlates highly with transcutaneous serum bilirubin.

Neonatal jaundice

In general, infants are not jaundiced at the moment of birth. This is because of the impressive ability of the placenta to clear bilirubin from the fetal circulation. However, within the next few days most infants develop elevated serum bilirubin levels (>1.4 mg/dL). As the serum bilirubin rises the skin becomes more jaundiced in a cephalocaudal manner. Icterus is first observed in the head and progresses caudally to the palms and soles. Kramer found the following serum indirect bilirubin levels as jaundice progressed: head and neck, 4–8 mg/dL; upper trunk, 5–12 mg/dL; lower trunk and thighs, 8–16 mg/dL; arms and lower legs, 11–18 mg/dL; palms and soles >15 mg/dL [11]. Hence, when the bilirubin was >15 mg/dL, the entire body was icteric. However, darker skin tones can make jaundice difficult to estimate visually. Jaundice is best observed by blanching the skin with gentle digital pressure under well-illuminated (white light) conditions. At least one-third of infants develop visible jaundice. A combined analysis of several large studies involving thousands of infants during the first week of life showed that moderate jaundice (bilirubin >12 mg/dL) occurs in at least 12% of breast-fed infants and 4% of formula-fed infants, while severe jaundice (>15 mg/dL) occurs in 2% and 0.3% of these feeding groups, respectively [12].

In recent decades, changes in perinatal care have made severe neonatal jaundice a larger problem and there was a re-emergence of kernicterus. This prompted guidelines from the American Academy of Pediatrics aimed at assessing the risk of severe hyperbilirubinemia, evaluating the causes and optimizing therapy for neonatal jaundice. The American Academy of Pediatrics updated their 1994 guidelines [13] for the management of hyperbilirubinemia in newborn infants in 2004 [14] and an expert panel further clarified these recommendations in 2009 [10].

Jaundice can be caused by increased bilirubin production, decreased bilirubin excretion or a combination of these mechanisms:

- increased production of bilirubin
  - fetal–maternal blood group incompatibilities
  - extravascular blood in body tissues
  - polycythemia
  - red blood cell abnormalities (hemoglobinopathies, membrane and enzyme defects)
  - induction of labor
  - decreased excretion of bilirubin
- increased enterohepatic circulation of bilirubin
  - breast-feeding
  - inborn errors of metabolism
  - hormones and drugs
  - prematurity
  - hepatic hypoperfusion
  - cholestatic syndromes
  - obstruction of the biliary tree
- combined increased production and decreased excretion of bilirubin
  - sepsis
  - intrauterine infection
  - congenital cirrhosis.

Figure 12.8 presents a clinical approach to assess these diagnoses.

The term "physiologic jaundice" has been used to describe the frequently observed jaundice in otherwise completely normal neonates. Physiologic jaundice is the result of a number of factors involving increased bilirubin production and decreased excretion. Jaundice should always be considered as a sign of a possible disease and not assumed to be physiologic. Specific characteristics of neonatal jaundice to be considered abnormal until proven otherwise include (1) development before 36 hours of age, (2) persistence beyond 10 days of age, (3) serum bilirubin >12 mg/dL at any time, and (4) elevation of the direct reacting fraction of bilirubin (>2 mg/dL or 30% of the total serum bilirubin) at any time.

There are a number of epidemiologic risk factors related to neonatal jaundice. Some of the factors associated with increased neonatal bilirubin levels are male sex, low birth weight, prematurity, certain races (Asian, American Indian, Greek), maternal medications (e.g. oxytocin, promethazine hydrochloride), premature rupture of the membranes, increased weight loss after birth, delayed meconium passage, breast-feeding, and neonatal infection. Delivery with the vacuum extractor increases the risk of cephalohematoma and neonatal jaundice. Data suggest pancuronium is associated with an increased risk of hyperbilirubinemia. There is a close correlation between umbilical cord serum bilirubin level and subsequent hyperbilirubinemia. Maternal serum bilirubin level at the time of delivery, and transplacental bilirubin gradient, also correlate positively with neonatal serum bilirubin concentrations. Other factors are associated with decreased neonatal bilirubin levels including black race, exclusive formula feeding, gestational age 41 weeks, maternal smoking and certain drugs given to the mother (e.g. phenobarbital).

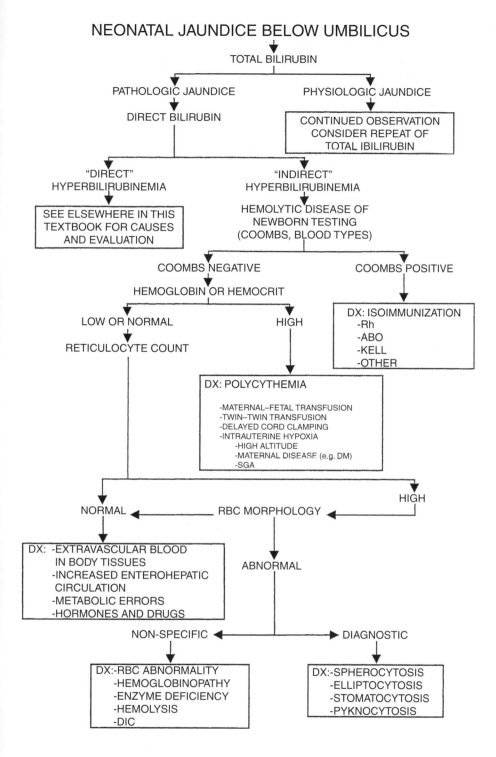

Figure 12.8 One possible approach to the clinical evaluation of neonatal jaundice. Dx, diagnosis; DIC, disseminated intravascular coagulation; DM, diabetes mellitus; Rh, rhesus.

Neonatal jaundice caused by increased production of bilirubin

Isoimmunization

The most common cause of severe early jaundice is fetal–maternal blood group incompatibility, with resulting isoimmunization. Maternal immunization develops when erythrocytes leak from fetal to maternal circulation. Fetal erythrocytes carrying different antigens are recognized as foreign by the maternal immune system, which then forms antibodies against them (maternal sensitization). These antibodies (immunoglobulin (Ig) G) cross the placental barrier into the fetal circulation and bind to fetal erythrocytes. In rhesus incompatibility, sequestration and destruction of the antibody-coated erythrocytes takes place in the reticuloendothelial system of the fetus. In ABO incompatibility, hemolysis is intravascular, complement mediated, and usually not as severe as in rhesus disease. Significant hemolysis can also result from incompatibilities between minor blood group antigens (e.g. Kell). Although hemolysis is predominantly associated with elevation of unconjugated bilirubin, the conjugated fraction can also be elevated.

Rhesus incompatibility problems do not usually develop until the second pregnancy. Therefore, prenatal blood typing and serial testing of rhesus-negative mothers for the development of rhesus antibodies provide important information to guide possible intrauterine care. If maternal rhesus antibodies develop during pregnancy, potentially helpful measures include serial amniocentesis (with bilirubin measurement), ultrasound assessment of the fetus, intrauterine transfusion, and premature delivery. The prophylactic administration of anti-D gammaglobulin has been most helpful in preventing rhesus sensitization. The newborn infant with rhesus incompatibility presents with pallor, hepatosplenomegaly, and a rapidly developing jaundice in the first hours of life. If the problem is severe, the infant may be born with generalized edema (fetal hydrops). Laboratory findings in the neonate's blood include reticulocytosis, anemia, a positive direct Coombs test, and a rapidly rising serum bilirubin level. Exchange transfusion continues to be an important therapy for seriously affected infants. Intravenous gammaglobulin has been shown to reduce the need for exchange transfusions in both rhesus and ABO hemolytic disease.

Clinically, ABO incompatibility usually presents with the first pregnancy. Development of ABO hemolytic disease is largely limited to blood group A or B infants born to group O mothers. Development of jaundice is not as rapid as with rhesus disease and a serum bilirubin >12 mg/dL on day 3 of life is typical. Laboratory abnormalities include reticulocytosis (>10%), increased spherocytes, and a weakly positive direct Coombs test, although this is sometimes negative. Anti-A or anti-B antibodies may be seen in the serum of the newborn if examined within the first few days of life before they rapidly disappear.

Extravascular blood

Extravascular blood within the body (e.g. cephalohematoma, ecchymoses, petechiae, and hemorrhage) can be rapidly metabolized to bilirubin by tissue macrophages. Although the diagnosis can often be made on physical examination, occult intracranial, intestinal, or pulmonary hemorrhage can also produce hyperbilirubinemia. Similarly, swallowed blood can be converted to bilirubin by the heme oxygenase of intestinal epithelium. The Apt test can be used to distinguish blood of maternal or infant origin because of differences in alkali resistance between fetal and adult hemoglobin.

Polycythemia

Polycythemia can cause hyperbilirubinemia because the absolute increase in red cell mass results in elevated bilirubin production through normal rates of erythrocyte breakdown.

A number of mechanisms may result in neonatal polycythemia (usually defined by venipuncture hematocrits >65%). During placental separation at the time of birth, bleeding may occur from the maternal circulation into the fetus (maternal–fetal transfusion) or because of a delay in cord clamping. Twin–twin transfusions can also result in polycythemia. Similarly intrauterine hypoxia and maternal diseases such as diabetes mellitus can result in neonatal polycythemia. Therapy for symptomatic polycythemia is partial exchange transfusion, although therapy for asymptomatic polycythemia remains controversial.

Red blood cell abnormalities

A number of specific abnormalities related to the red blood cell can result in neonatal jaundice, including hemoglobinopathies, and red blood cell membrane and enzyme defects. Hereditary spherocytosis is not usually a neonatal problem but hemolytic crises can occur and present with a rising bilirubin level and a falling hematocrit. A family history of spherocytosis, anemia, or early gallstone disease (before age 40) is helpful in suggesting this diagnosis. The characteristic spherocytes seen in the peripheral blood smear may be impossible to distinguish from those seen with ABO hemolytic disease. Other hemolytic anemias associated with neonatal jaundice include drug-induced hemolysis, deficiencies of the erythrocyte enzymes (glucose-6-phosphate dehydrogenase (G6PD), pyruvate kinase, and others), and hemolysis induced by vitamin K or bacteria. Alpha-thalassemia can result in severe hemolysis and lethal hydrops fetalis. Gamma-beta thalassemia may also present with hemolysis and severe neonatal hyperbilirubinemia. There are a wide variety of clinical findings associated with the thalassemias, extending from profound intrauterine hydrops and death to mild neonatal jaundice and anemia, to no jaundice or anemia. Southeast Asian ovalocytosis has been associated with severe hyperbilirubinemia. These red blood cell abnormalities are more likely to result in hyperbilirubinemia in the presence of GS as described later in this chapter. Drugs or other substances responsible for hemolysis can be passed to the fetus across the placenta or to the neonate via the breast milk.

Induction of labor with oxytocin

Induction of labor with oxytocin has been shown to be associated with neonatal jaundice. There is a significant association between hyponatremia and jaundice in infants of mothers who received oxytocin to induce labor. The vasopressin-like action of oxytocin prompts electrolyte and water transport such that the erythrocyte swells and increased osmotic fragility and hyperbilirubinemia can result.

Neonatal jaundice caused by decreased excretion of bilirubin

Increased enterohepatic circulation of bilirubin

Increased enterohepatic circulation of bilirubin is believed to be an important factor in neonatal jaundice. Neonates are at risk for the intestinal absorption of bilirubin because (1) their bile contains increased levels of bilirubin monoglucuronide, which allows easier conversion to bilirubin; (2) they have significant amounts of β-glucuronidase within the intestinal lumen, which hydrolyses bilirubin conjugates to bilirubin that is more easily absorbed from the intestine; (3) they lack an intestinal flora to convert bilirubin conjugates to urobilinoids; and (4) meconium contains significant amounts of bilirubin. Conditions which prolong meconium passage (e.g. Hirschsprung disease, meconium ileus, meconium plug syndrome) are associated with hyperbilirubinemia. The enterohepatic circulation of bilirubin can be blocked by the enteral administration of compounds that bind bilirubin such as agar, charcoal, and cholestyramine.

Breast-feeding

Breast-feeding has been clearly identified as a factor related to neonatal jaundice. Breast-fed infants have significantly higher serum bilirubin levels than formula-fed infants on each of the first 5 days of life, and this unconjugated hyperbilirubinemia can persist for weeks to months. Jaundice during the first week of life is sometimes described as "breast-feeding jaundice" in order to differentiate it from "breast-milk jaundice syndrome," which occurs after the first week of life. The former is frequently associated with inadequate breast milk intake, whereas the latter generally occurs in otherwise thriving infants. There is probably overlap between these conditions and physiologic jaundice. There are conflicting data regarding efforts to attribute this jaundice to increased lipase activity in the breast milk, resulting in elevated levels of free fatty acids, which could inhibit hepatic UGT1A1. It has been suggested that the enterohepatic circulation of bilirubin can be facilitated by the presence of β-glucuronidase or some other substance in human milk. In a mouse model in which mouse *Ugt1a1* was replaced with the human gene, human breast milk but not formula feeding appeared to suppress intestinal IκB kinase α and β, resulting in inactivation of nuclear factor-κB and loss of production of intestinal UGT1A1, thereby exacerbating hyperbilirubinemia [12]. Activation of the intestinal xenobiotic nuclear receptors PXR and CAR contribute to the induction of *UGT1A1*. Other factors possibly related to jaundice in breast-fed infants include caloric intake, fluid intake, weight loss, delayed meconium passage, intestinal bacterial flora, and inhibition of UGT1A1 by an unidentified factor in the milk. It has been suggested that a healthy breast-fed infant with unconjugated hyperbilirubinemia but with normal hemoglobin concentration, reticulocyte count, and blood smear, plus no blood group incompatibility and no other abnormalities on physical examination, may be presumed to have early breast-feeding jaundice. Since there is no specific laboratory test to confirm a diagnosis of breast-milk jaundice, it is important to rule out treatable causes of jaundice before ascribing the hyperbilirubinemia to breast-milk. Some infants with presumed breast milk jaundice exhibit elevated serum bile acid levels, suggesting mild hepatic dysfunction or cholestasis, although in general this is not the case. Waiting until the serum bilirubin level reaches 15 mg/dL before evaluating an otherwise well-appearing breast-fed infant is an approach [10]. Breast-fed infants who are fed specific nutritional ingredients, such as L-aspartic acid, that inhibit β-glucuronidase [15] excrete more fecal bilirubin and have lower levels of jaundice [9] than breast-fed infants who receive no supplements. No commercial preparations of these specific ingredients are presently available.

Hormones

Various hormones may cause development of neonatal unconjugated hyperbilirubinemia. Congenital hypothyroidism can present with serum bilirubin >12 mg/dL prior to the development of other clinical findings. Prolonged jaundice is seen in one-third of infants with congenital hypothyroidism. Similarly, hypopituitarism and anencephaly may be associated with jaundice caused by inadequate thyroxine, which is necessary for hepatic clearance of bilirubin.

Drugs

Certain drugs may affect the metabolism of bilirubin and result in hyperbilirubinemia or displacement of bilirubin from albumin. Such displacement increases the risk of kernicterus and can be caused by sulfonamides [16], moxalactam, and ceftriaxone (independent of its sludge-producing effect). The popular Chinese herb Chuen-Lin, given to 28–51% of Chinese newborn infants, has been shown to have a significant effect in displacing bilirubin from albumin. Pancuronium bromide and chloral hydrate have been suggested as causes of neonatal hyperbilirubinemia.

Maternal diabetes

Infants of diabetic mothers have higher peak bilirubin levels and a greater frequency of hyperbilirubinemia than normal neonates. While polycythemia is one possible mechanism, other potential reasons for this hyperbilirubinemia include prematurity, substrate deficiency for glucuronidation (secondary to hypoglycemia), and poor hepatic perfusion (secondary to respiratory distress, persistent fetal circulation, or cardiomyopathy).

Lucey–Driscoll syndrome

The Lucey–Driscoll syndrome consists of neonatal hyperbilirubinemia within families in whom there is in vitro inhibition of UGT1A1 by both maternal and infant serum. It is presumed that this is caused by gestational hormones.

Prematurity

Prematurity is frequently associated with unconjugated hyperbilirubinemia in the neonatal period. Hepatic UGT1A1 activity is markedly decreased in premature infants and rises steadily from 30 weeks of gestation until reaching adult levels 14 weeks after birth [17]. In addition there may be deficiencies for both uptake and secretion. Bilirubin clearance improves rapidly following birth.

Hepatic hypoperfusion and liver disease

Hepatic hypoperfusion can result in neonatal jaundice. Inadequate perfusion of the hepatic sinusoids may not allow sufficient hepatocyte uptake and metabolism of bilirubin. Causes include patent ductus venosus (e.g. with respiratory distress syndrome), congestive heart failure, and portal vein thrombosis. Other specific liver diseases described elsewhere in this text can result in neonatal jaundice.

Neonatal jaundice from both increased production and decreased excretion of bilirubin

In neonatal diseases with jaundice caused by increased production of bilirubin and decreased excretion, both conjugated and unconjugated bilirubin fractions can be elevated. Bacterial sepsis increases bilirubin production by bacterial hemolysin release, which promotes erythrocyte hemolysis. Endotoxins released by bacteria can also decrease canalicular bile formation.

Toxicity of neonatal jaundice

Kernicterus (German: *kern*) is the neuropathologic finding associated with severe unconjugated hyperbilirubinemia and is named for the yellow staining of certain regions of the brain, particularly the basal ganglia, hippocampus, cerebellum, and nuclei of the floor of the fourth ventricle. Clinical findings associated with kernicterus, termed bilirubin encephalopathy, include sluggish Moro reflex, opisthotonos, hypotonia, vomiting, high-pitched cry, hyperpyrexia, seizures, paresis of gaze ("setting sun sign"), oculogyric crisis, and death. Long-term findings include spasticity, choreoathetosis, and sensorineural hearing loss. Milder forms of bilirubin encephalopathy include cognitive dysfunction and learning disabilities. Although the neonatal period is the most common time for bilirubin-related brain damage, the neurotoxicity of bilirubin has also been documented in older children and adults with CN syndrome type I [18].

The absolute level of serum bilirubin has not been a good predictor of the risk of severe neonatal jaundice. However, it has long been known that kernicterus is likely with serum unconjugated bilirubin levels >30 mg/dL and unlikely with values <20 mg/dL. In one study, 90% of the patients who had serum bilirubin >35 mg/dL either died or had cerebral palsy or physical retardation. Alternatively, no developmental retardation was found in 129 infants with serum bilirubin <20 mg/dL. Albumin concentration is an important variable because of the high affinity binding with bilirubin, and the ratio of bilirubin to albumin is a risk factor which has been included in the most recent American Academy of Pediatrics guidelines [14]. Drugs and organic anions also bind to albumin and can displace bilirubin [19], thereby increasing the free bilirubin that can diffuse into cells and causing toxicity at lower bilirubin levels, for example when sulfafurazole (sulfisoxazole) was given to premature infants. There is considerable debate at present regarding the risk of bilirubin encephalopathy in otherwise healthy full-term infants, with the suggestion that such infants are not at risk until the serum bilirubin rises to >20 mg/dL. While it has been acknowledged that total serum bilirubin may not be the most important factor related to risk, there are, at present, no other generally accepted tests (e.g. albumin saturation, reserve bilirubin-binding capacity, or free bilirubin) that are more helpful in identifying infants at risk for bilirubin encephalopathy.

Another approach aimed at measuring early changes in the central nervous system caused by bilirubin uses brainstem auditory evoked potentials. Abnormalities have been demonstrated in jaundiced infants and shown to improve after exchange transfusion. Data have shown that even moderate hyperbilirubinemia (mean 14.3 mg/dL (SD, 2.8)) affects brainstem auditory evoked potentials, specific components of the Brazelton Neonatal Behavioral Assessment Scale, and cry characteristics. Somatosensory evoked potentials, which have their pathway through the region of the basal ganglia, also show abnormalities with jaundice and have been suggested as another method of monitoring the central nervous system effects of bilirubin. At present neither brainstem auditory evoked potentials nor somatosensory evoked potentials are measured routinely.

Management of neonatal jaundice

Hyperbilirubinemia is the most frequent reason that infants are readmitted to the hospital in the first weeks of life. The most important step in treatment of jaundice is determination of the primary etiology. However, independent of the etiology of the jaundice, elevation of the serum unconjugated bilirubin fraction prompts concern about possible kernicterus. When the unconjugated bilirubin fraction is elevated, care must be given to avoid administration of agents that bind to albumin and displace bilirubin, thus promoting kernicterus. Although historically, sulfonamides are the most well-known bilirubin-displacing agents, drugs such as ceftriaxone and ibuprofen are also strong bilirubin displacers with a potential for inducing bilirubin encephalopathy. Therapeutic options to lower unconjugated bilirubin levels include phototherapy, exchange transfusion, interruption of the enterohepatic circulation, enzyme induction, and alteration of breast-feeding.

Phototherapy consists of irradiation of the jaundiced infant with light. Photon energy derived from light changes the structure of the bilirubin molecule in two ways (Figure 12.9) allowing bilirubin to be excreted into bile or urine without the usual requirement for hepatic glucuronidation. One change involves a 180 degree rotation around the double bonds between either the A and B or the C and D rings, converting the normal Z configuration to the E configuration. (4Z,15E)-Bilirubin is preferentially formed and can spontaneously reisomerize to native bilirubin. More importantly a new seven-membered ring structure can be formed between rings A and B, resulting in "lumirubin" [20] or "cyclobilirubin."

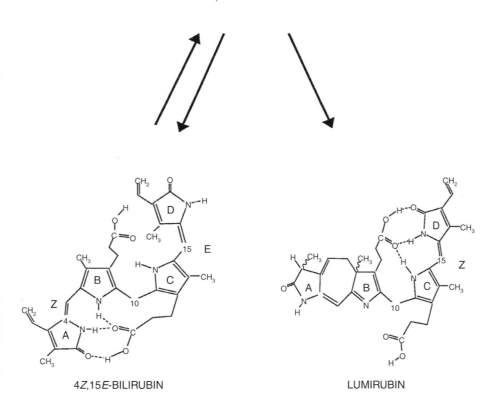

Figure 12.9 The major products of phototherapy. Light induces an isomerization of (4Z,15Z)-bilirubin to produce the configurational isomer (4Z,15E)-bilirubin and the structural isomer lumirubin. Both isomers interrupt the internal hydrogen bonding and expose the propionic acid side-chains, thus increasing the polarity of the compound and allowing excretion in bile without hepatic glucuronidation.

Both changes interfere with the internal hydrogen bonding of native bilirubin and by exposing the propionic acid groups result in a more polar compound. Therefore, the lumirubin and *E* isomers can be excreted directly into bile. Lumirubin appears to be the major route by which bilirubin is eliminated with phototherapy. There are conflicting data about the best choice of light for phototherapy. Phototherapy devices utilizing woven fiberoptic pads are currently available, effective, safe, eliminate the need for eye patches and permit greater time for maternal–infant bonding. In general, phototherapy is used to prevent serum bilirubin concentrations from reaching levels necessitating exchange transfusion. Phototherapy is now frequently carried out at home, a practice accepted and recommended by the American Academy of Pediatrics [21]. Phototherapy is generally safe. In extremely premature infants (<800 g birth weight), prolonged phototherapy and low peak serum bilirubin levels (<9.4 mg/dL) have been shown to be independently associated with blindness. This could possibly be related to direct effects of light on the unshielded immature eye or decreased antioxidant protection by low serum bilirubin levels. Phototherapy should not be employed without prior diagnostic evaluation of the cause of the jaundice. In term, healthy newborns, phototherapy may be stopped when the serum bilirubin level falls below 14 to 15 mg/dL, and hospital discharge need not be delayed to observe for a rebound in the bilirubin level.

Exchange transfusion is the most rapid method to acutely lower the serum bilirubin concentration. Indications for exchange transfusion vary and can be related to either anemia or elevated serum bilirubin level. In neonatal hemolytic disease, suggested indications for transfusion include (1) anemia (hematocrit <45%), positive direct Coombs test, and bilirubin >4 mg/dL in the cord blood; (2) postnatal rise in serum bilirubin concentration that exceeds 1 mg/dL per hour for more than 6 hours; (3) progressive anemia and rate of increase in serum bilirubin of >0.5 mg/dL per hour; and (4) continuing progression of anemia despite control of hyperbilirubinemia. Sometimes exchange transfusion for hemolytic disease can be avoided through the use of high-dose intravenous immunoglobulin therapy [22]. Suggested indications for exchange transfusion because of hyperbilirubinemia alone in term infants include either a bilirubin concentration >15 mg/dL for more than 48 hours or a ratio of total serum bilirubin (mg/dL) divided by serum albumin (g/dL) >8 [14]. Although there are many well-described risks with exchange transfusion, mortality is low (<0.6%) if it is performed properly.

There are a number of pharmacologic approaches to the prevention and treatment of neonatal hyperbilirubinemia [23]. The enterohepatic circulation can be interrupted by enteral administration of agents that bind bilirubin in the intestine and prevent reabsorption. Such agents include agar, cholestyramine, activated charcoal, and calcium phosphate. Increased intestinal peristalsis would be expected to allow less time for bilirubin absorption. Frequent feedings and rectal stimulation are associated with lower serum bilirubin levels.

Since neonatal hepatic UGT1A1 activity is low in neonates [17], it is not surprising that induction of this hepatic enzyme results in lower serum bilirubin levels. Such induction in the neonate can be accomplished with prenatal maternal use of phenobarbital or diphenylhydantoin. Even low-birth-weight infants (<2000 g) have been shown to respond to in utero phenobarbital therapy with significantly increased serum levels of conjugated bilirubin and decreased need for phototherapy. In the postnatal period, use of phenobarbital by the neonate has the same bilirubin-lowering effect.

Optimization of breast-feeding in the perinatal period is important. If the bilirubin level is rising, recommendations support encouraging mothers to breast-feed more frequently, with an average interval between feeds of 2 hours and no feeding supplements or at least 8–10 feedings per 24 hours [14]. A strong dose–response relationship has been shown between feeding frequency and a decreased incidence of hyperbilirubinemia. More frequent nursing may not increase intake but may increase peristalsis and stool frequency, thus promoting bilirubin excretion. Frequency of breast-feeding during the first 24 hours of life has been shown to be correlated significantly with the frequency of meconium passage.

The serum bilirubin level at which breast-feeding should be discontinued, because of breast milk jaundice syndrome, is controversial and recommendations vary from 14 to 20 mg/dL. When breast-feeding is interrupted, formula feeding may be initiated for 24 to 48 hours, or breast- and formula-feeding can be alternated [13]. No studies have addressed the cost-effectiveness of various formulae in their jaundice-lowering effects, although two independent studies have shown that infants exclusively fed Nutramigen (a casein hydrolysate formula, Mead Johnson) have lower jaundice levels than infants fed routine formula [24]. Supplementing breast-fed infants with small volumes of specific nutritional ingredients has been shown to result in increased fecal bilirubin excretion and lower transcutaneous bilirubin levels, although no commercial preparations of these ingredients are currently available. A fall in the serum bilirubin of 2 to 5 mg/dL is consistent with a diagnosis of breast-milk jaundice. Breast-feeding may then be resumed with the acknowledgement that serum bilirubin levels may rise for several days but will gradually level off and decline. If breast-feeding is to be resumed following the interruption, it is important to preserve lactation with the use of a breast pump. In one study, interruption of breast-feeding for approximately 50 hours (during which time a formula was given) was shown to have the same bilirubin-lowering effect as a similar duration of phototherapy. Interruptions of breast-feeding for 24 to 48 hours have been shown to be successful at lowering serum bilirubin levels and avoiding the need for phototherapy in 81 of 87 jaundiced infants. Formula feedings to Asian neonates receiving phototherapy resulted in greater decrease of serum bilirubin levels than in infants who were exclusively breast-fed. Careful counseling and support can prevent the interruption of breast-feeding from becoming a permanent discontinuance of nursing. Alternative approaches to treat neonatal hyperbilirubinemia have included metalloporphyrins to block the production of bilirubin, and hemoperfusion, although neither is commonly used.

Disorders of bilirubin metabolism

The disorders described in this section, summarized in Tables 12.1 and 12.2, are those in which there is a primary abnormality in bilirubin metabolism without other liver disease. The disorders can best be understood in the context of the normal pathway in which bilirubin is cleared from the circulation (Figure 12.2). Defects in these metabolic steps are responsible for the disorders to be described in the final section of this chapter.

Gilbert syndrome
Clinical presentation

Gilbert syndrome (OMIM 143 500) was first described in 1901 by Gilbert and Lereboullet [25]. It is characterized by a hereditary chronic or recurrent, mild unconjugated hyperbilirubinemia with otherwise normal liver function tests. The serum unconjugated bilirubin elevation is variable and usually ranges from 1 to 4 mg/dL (17–68 μmol/L). Frequently, patients are first identified when elevated serum bilirubin is found on screening blood chemistry or mild jaundice (perhaps only

Table 12.1 Comparison of disorders of unconjugated hyperbilirubinemia

	Gilbert syndrome	Crigler–Najjar type I	Crigler–Najjar type II
Prevalence	3%	Rare	Rare
Inheritance	Autosomal dominant or recessive	Autosomal recessive	Autosomal recessive, rarely dominant
Genetic defect	*UGT1A1*	*UGT1A1*	*UGT1A1*
Hepatocyte defect site	Microsomes ± plasma membrane	Microsomes	Microsomes
Deficient hepatocyte function	Glucuronidation ± uptake	Glucuronidation	Glucuronidation
Bilirubin UDP-glucuronosyltransferase activity	5–53% of controls	Severely decreased	2–23% of controls
Hepatocyte uptake	Decreased in 20–30%	Normal	Normal
Serum total bilirubin (mg/dL)	0.8–4.3	15–45	8–25
Serum bilirubin decrease with phenobarbital (%)	70	0	77
Serum bilirubin composition (%)[a]			
Unconjugated (normal 92.6%)	98.8	~100	99.1
Diglucuronide (normal 6.2%)	1.1	0	0.6
Monoglucuronide (normal 0.5%)	0	0	0
Bile bilirubin conjugates			
Diglucuronide (normal ~80%)	60	0 to trace	5–10
Monoglucuronide (normal ~1.5%)	30	Predominant if measurable	90–95
Other routine liver function tests	Normal	Normal	Normal
Prognosis	Benign	Kernicterus common	Occasional kernicterus

[a] By high performance liquid chromatography.

scleral icterus) is noted during a period of fasting associated with a non-specific viral illness or religious activities. There are generally no negative implications for health or longevity associated with GS and it may be inherited in either an autosomal dominanat or recessive fashion [26].

Although GS is a congenital disorder, it rarely becomes clinically apparent until after puberty. The reasons for this are not known but have been suggested to be related to the hormonal changes of puberty. Steroid hormones can suppress hepatic bilirubin clearance. Odell speculated that some infants with non-hemolytic neonatal jaundice are manifesting GS [27]. Use of genetic markers (see below) has allowed investigation of the role GS plays in neonatal jaundice. Individuals carrying such markers have been shown to have a more rapid rise in their jaundice levels during the first 2 days of life [28], a predisposition to prolonged or severe neonatal hyperbilirubinemia, variably increased jaundice when the GS polymorphism occurs with pyloric stenosis or is coinherited with hematological abnormalities such as G6PD deficiency, beta-thalassemia or hereditary spherocytosis. Studies from several different parts of the world indicate that GS, as

detected by *UGT1A1* analysis, does play some role in neonatal jaundice. Kaplan *et al.* [29] noted that neither G6PD deficiency nor the GS type *UDPGT1* promoter polymorphism (also known as UGT1A1*28) alone increased the incidence of hyperbilirubinemia in their study, but both in combination did (Figure 12.10). They speculated that this gene interaction may serve as a paradigm of the interaction of benign genetic polymorphisms in the causation of disease; that is, it may take two genetic abnormalities to produce disease symptoms.

Pathophysiology

Gilbert syndrome is a heterogeneous group of disorders all of which share at least a 50% decrease in hepatic UGT1A1 activity. Some individuals with GS have delayed uptake of bilirubin into the hepatocyte; others have delayed biotransformation, and others demonstrate both abnormalities. Immunohistochemical staining for UGT1A1 shows a clear reduction throughout the hepatic lobule in specimens from individuals with GS, when compared with normal controls [30].

Table 12.2 Comparison of disorders of conjugated hyperbilirubinemia

	Rotor syndrome	Dubin–Johnson syndrome
Prevalence	Rare	Rare
Inheritance	Autosomal recessive	Autosomal recessive
Genetic defect	*SLCOIB1, SLCOIB3*	*ABCC2*
Hepatocyte defect site	(?) Glutathione *S*-transferase and plasma membrane	Apical canalicular membrane
Deficient hepatocyte function	Organic anion transport	Cannalicular secretion of bilirubin conjugates
Brown–black liver	No	Yes
Serum total bilirubin (mg/dL)	2–7	1.5–6.0
Serum conjugated bilirubin (%)	>50	>50
Other routine liver function tests	Normal	Normal
Oral cholecystogram	Usually visualizes	Usually does not visualize
Technetium-99m hepatobiliary iminodiacetic acid cholescintigraphy		
Liver	Poor to no visualization	Intense, prolonged visualization
Gallbladder	Poor to no visualization	Delayed or non-visualization
Clearance tests		
Sulfobromophthalein	Serum levels elevated (delayed clearance)	Serum levels normal at 45 min but elevated at 90–120 min
Indocyanine green	Delayed clearance	Normal
Response to estrogens or pregnancy	No change	Increased jaundice
Total urinary coproporphyrin excretion (isomers I + III)	2.5 to 5.0 times increased	Normal
Urinary coproporphyrin isomer I composition (%) (normal 25%)	Usually <80% of total	>80% of total
Prognosis	Benign (asymptomatic)	Benign (occasional abdominal complaints, probably incidental)

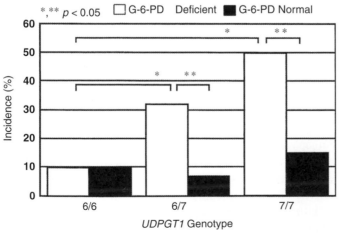

Figure 12.10 Incidence (percentage) of hyperbilirubinemia (serum total bilirubin ≥257 μmol/L) in glucose-6-phosphate dehydrogenase (G-6-PD)-deficient neonates and normal controls, stratified for the three genotypes of the UGT1A1 promoter. (Reprinted from Kaplan *et al.*, 1997 [29] © 1997, with permission from the National Academy of Sciences, USA.)

The elucidation of the structure of *UGT1*, which encodes a number of UDP-glucuronosyltransferase isozymes, led to the discovery of *UGT1A1* mutations or polymorphisms associated with GS. In white populations, the homozygous finding of an additional TA repeat in the promoter region or so-called TATA box (i.e. (TA)$_7$TAA, rather than (TA)$_6$TAA) of *UGT1A1* has been shown to be a necessary, although not sufficient, condition for GS. Individuals who are heterozygous for (TA)$_7$ have significantly higher serum bilirubin levels than the homozygous wild type (TA)$_6$ [31]. In Asian populations, the (TA)$_7$ mutation is relatively rare but several different *UGT1A1* mutations have been associated with GS. These Asian mutations involve exon 1 of *UGT1A1* rather than the TATA promoter region. One of the most common mutations in Asians, a mutation in exon 1 causing Gly71Arg change (also known as UGT1A1*6), has also linked GS and severe neonatal hyperbilirubinemia [32]. It has been reported that, although with white subjects the promoter TA repeat number and bilirubin level are strongly positively correlated, in other ethnic groups such as Africans, in whom two other variants $(TA)_5$ and $(TA)_8$ have been identified, there is a negative correlation. Rarely the $(TA)_8$ variant has been reported in white patients; consequently, the ethnic implications of these genetic polymorphisms of *UGT1A1* require further analysis.

Diagnosis and treatment

Generally, GS can be diagnosed when there is a mild, fluctuating unconjugated hyperbilirubinemia, the rest of the liver function tests are normal, and there is no hemolysis. Hemolysis can add confusion because it can result in similar findings and it is not unusual in GS. Hence other tests are sometimes used to aid in diagnosis.

One diagnostic test involves the intravenous administration of niotinic acid (niacin) with assessment of the subsequent rise in serum bilirubin concentration. Nicotinic acid is usually administered to adults in a dose of 50 mg over 30 seconds. Non-conjugated serum bilirubin is then measured every 30 to 60 minutes for the next 4 to 5 hours. In individuals with GS, the bilirubin rise is higher and clearance is delayed longer than in normals. Nicotinic acid causes increased osmotic fragility and hemolysis of red blood cells, with sequestration in the spleen. Splenic heme oxygenase is also induced, with rapid conversion of heme to bilirubin. Hence, the prolonged serum bilirubin levels are related to delayed hepatic clearance of bilirubin. Nicotinic acid infusion has been suggested to be a better method to diagnose GS than a 400 kcal fast because delayed bilirubin clearance was seen after nicotinic acid in GS subjects who otherwise had normal serum bilirubin levels. The nicotinic acid test is not useful in differentiating GS from chronic liver disease as both groups showed positive tests.

Rifampin, given to fasting or non-fasting adults in one oral dose of 900 mg, increases total serum bilirubin levels in normal controls and those with GS, although there is an exaggerated increase in GS (fasting: >1.9 mg/dL increase in bilirubin concentration 2–6 hours after rifampin; non-fasting: >1.5 mg/dL increase 4–6 hours after rifampin). This exagerated rise in serum bilirubin enabled differentiation of 10 healthy control patients and 15 patients with GS with high sensitivity and specificity.

Fractionation of the total serum bilirubin using alkaline methanolysis and thin-layer chromatography can also aid in diagnosing GS. This allows precise measurement of the conjugated and unconjugated bilirubin levels and has shown that in GS approximately 6% of the total serum bilirubin is conjugated, compared with approximately 17% in normals and those with chronic hemolysis. Individuals with chronic persistent hepatitis had 28% of their total bilirubin present as conjugates. Fasting did not change the percentage of conjugates in GS, despite the rise in total serum bilirubin concentration. An overlap of only three individuals was seen among 77 with GS and 60 normal subjects. Other studies support these findings. In patients with GS, fractionation of the total serum bilirubin by HPLC showed significantly decreased bilirubin monoglucuronides (1.1% versus 6.2%

in normals) and increased unconjugated bilirubin (98.8 versus 92.6 in normals).

Genetic testing can be useful in the investigation of prolonged neonatal jaundice. The *UGT1A1* TA repeat can be determined for non-Asian subjects and the Gly71Arg mutation for Asian subjects. This test is performed by many genetic laboratories around the world (see http://genetests.org).

There are no significant negative implications regarding morbidity or mortality with GS. In general, drug metabolism studies have revealed no major dangers, although there appears to be an increased incidence of slow acetylators and lorazepam clearance is decreased 20–40%. Concurrent genetic deficiencies in other xenobiotic pathways may put individuals with GS at increased risk of drug toxicity to such compounds as acetaminophen, cancer chemotherapeutic agents CPT-11 (irinotecan) or TAS-103, or the viral protease inhibitor indinavir. Therefore, some suggest that screening for GS is of clinical importance. No specific treatment is necessary for GS, although phenobarbital has been shown to lower serum bilirubin levels in these patients. Higher rates of gallstones have been reported in patients with thalassemia major who have GS. If the well-documented antioxidant effect of bilirubin provides a biological advantage, then the mild hyperbilirubinemia of GS might actually be a significant benefit in such things as vascular disease in which free radicals are involved in pathogenesis. The Framingham Heart Study concluded that homozygous *UGT1A1*28* allele carriers with higher serum bilirubin concentrations exhibit a strong association with lower risk of cardiovascular disease. One Taiwanese study demonstrated GS related to the Gly71Arg mutation may be protective against non-alcoholic fatty liver disease.

Crigler–Najjar syndrome

Clinical presentation

In 1952, Crigler and Najjar described seven infants with congenital familial non-hemolytic jaundice who developed severe unconjugated hyperbilirubinemia shortly after birth and died from kernicterus within months [33]. These infants were from three related families. The serum bilirubin concentration reached 25–35 mg/dL despite a lack of hemolytic disease. Other liver function tests were normal. Liver histology was normal except for the deposition of bile pigments. Subsequent reports document that bilirubin levels varied from 15 to 45 mg/dL and the main risk for patients with CN syndrome is kernicterus [34]. An excellent review of the neurologic perspectives of CN syndrome has been published [35]. Although some patients survive into the second decade with normal development, the possibility of developing late kernicterus is always a concern, even in adulthood. Of the four studies of long-term outcomes, one does suggest that normal development can be attained with proper management [36].

In 1969, Arias *et al.* [37] described a second, more frequent, type of severe non-hemolytic hyperbilirubinemia. The previous syndrome was termed type I (OMIM 218 800), while the new findings were termed CN syndrome type II or Arias syndrome (OMIM 606 785). Hyperbilirubinemia is less severe in patients with type II and varies from approximately 8 to 25 mg/dL. Hence, these individuals have a much lower incidence of kernicterus, although such damage occurs.

Pathophysiology

Both type I and type II CN syndrome are generally inherited in an autosomal recessive manner. Both result from mutations in the *UGT* complex [38]. Patients with one normal allele demonstrate normal metabolism of bilirubin. The genetic details determine the severity of clinical disease. In CN syndrome type I, there is a complete absence of functional UGT1A1, while in type II UGT1A1 activity is markedly reduced. In type I, 18 of 23 described mutations of *UGT1* are found in the common exons 2 to 5 (Figure 12.4) and thus affect many UGT1 isozymes [38,39]. Intronic mutations causing CN syndrome type I have also been reported. However, in type II, four out of nine known mutations are found in exon 1A1. In both types, assays of liver tissue from affected patients demonstrate negligible or very low UGT1A1 activity. Hence, patients with these disorders experience a profound block in bilirubin excretion because they lack the ability to conjugate bilirubin with UDP glucuronic acid. Liver biopsy is not helpful in differentiating types I and II. Study of the resected livers from four patients with CN syndrome type I undergoing liver transplantation showed that there was heterogeneous glucuronidation of various substrates other than bilirubin. In family studies of patients with CN syndrome type I, partial deficiencies have been found in the glucuronidation of salicylate and menthol among siblings, parents, and grandparents.

The major differentiating characteristic between the types is the response to drugs that stimulate hyperplasia of the endoplasmic reticulum. When patients with type II received phenobarbital or diphenylhydantoin, there is a significant decline in the serum bilirubin level, increased hepatic clearance of radiolabeled bilirubin, and increased biliary levels of bilirubin diglucuronides (Figure 12.11). In a study of five patients with CN syndrome type II, the magnitude of the phenobarbital-induced decrease in serum bilirubin ranged from 2.1 to 12.1 mg/dL (27 to 72%) with pre- and post-phenobarbital serum bilirubin levels ranging from 7.8 to 16.9 and 4.7 to 10.1 mg/dL, respectively [40]. Summarizing data from seven earlier studies regarding the response of patients with type II to oral phenobarbital treatment, revealed the following: 11 females and 13 males had a total mean serum bilirubin of 15.7 mg/dL (SD, 13.8) prior to phenobarbital. After doses ranging from 90 to 390 mg/day, or 4 mg/kg daily, the serum bilirubin decreased to 12.0 mg/dL (SD, 4.0) (77% (SD, 13)). The lowest total serum bilirubin following phenobarbital therapy was 5.9 mg/dL. In contrast, patients with CN syndrome type I show neither decrease in serum bilirubin nor significantly increased biliary bilirubin conjugates in response to drugs (Figure 12.11). The response to phenobarbital is the criterion used to differentiate between these two

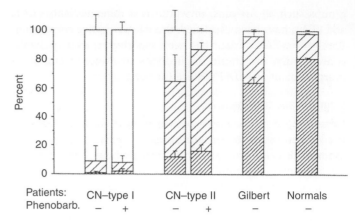

Figure 12.11 Bile pigment composition in bile from 8 normal individuals, 3 with Crigler–Najjar (CN) syndrome type I, 3 with type II, and 16 with Gilbert syndrome receiving (+) or not receiving (–) phenobarbital (phenobarb.). Relative bile pigment composition is indicated in the vertical columns as percentage of total ± SD. White, unconjugated bilirubin; intermediate hatching, bilirubin monoconjugate; dark hatching, bilirubin diconjugate. (From Sinaasappel and Jansen, 1991 [40] © 1991, with permission from the American Gastroenterological Association.)

disorders [41]. Bile analysis has also been suggested as another method to differentiate types I and II. In type I, bile contains insignificant bilirubin conjugates (<10%) and unconjugated bilirubin predominates. In type II, bile contains small amounts of bilirubin conjugates and those present are predominantly bilirubin monoglucuronides (>60%).

Diagnosis and treatment

Although CN syndrome can be diagnosed during the prenatal period, evaluation of infants with CN syndrome more typically begins during the first days of life when serum bilirubin exceed 20 mg/dL. The conjugated fraction will not be elevated except possibly for the factitious elevation sometimes seen when the total serum bilirubin level is very high. Infants should be evaluated for hemolysis, hypothyroidism, infection, and other more common causes of jaundice. Formula feedings will help to identify those infants with jaundice related to human milk. During this period of testing, the magnitude of the serum bilirubin elevation should prompt use of phototherapy to avoid kernicterus. Exchange transfusion may be necessary. Despite these efforts, patients with CN syndrome will have persistent jaundice. There is currently no widely available simple clinical test to confirm the diagnosis, but it can be excluded by finding significant amounts of bilirubin conjugates in neonatal stools if collected prior to establishment of sufficient intestinal bacteria to convert bilirubin conjugates to urobilinoids. Analysis of duodenal bile with HPLC will show negligible bilirubin mono- or diglucuronides in type I, whereas in type II these conjugates are present but in low concentration. The ratio of serum bilirubin conjugates (as determined by alkaline methanolysis with thin-layer chromatography) to total bilirubin, although abnormally low, does not allow differentiation of patients with CN syndrome from those with GS.

Similar overlap occurs with HPLC fractionation of serum bilirubin conjugates. Analysis of DNA can be very helpful in establishing the correct diagnosis. Currently, sequencing of the coding region for known CN mutations can be performed at selected laboratories (see http://genetests.org].

A world registry of patients with CN syndrome type I aimed at developing management guidelines has been published [42]. Phenobarbital (4 mg/kg daily in infants) should be used when there is concern about deficiency of UGT1A1. Within 48 hours patients with type II can demonstrate a significant decrease in serum bilirubin levels (as detailed above) and an increased biliary excretion of bilirubin mono- and diglucuronides, while the patients with type I will show no significant response. Occasionally, patients with type II do not respond to the first trial of phenobarbital therapy, but subsequent trials months later will demonstrate the significant decrease in serum bilirubin level [41]. However, despite the decrease in serum bilirubin in response to phenobarbital, patients with type II will usually continue to manifest a significant hyperbilirubinemia (approximately 5–15 mg/dL). Phototherapy for 8 to 12 hours daily has been the primary modality to keep serum bilirubin levels <20 mg/dL during the first several months of life, since patients with CN syndrome type I can excrete all bilirubin photoisomers. These patients will require lifelong treatment with phototherapy until more definitive therapy such as liver transplant. Phototherapy has been found to be least intrusive when given at night and improvements have been made in effectiveness and comfort. Although phototherapy is very helpful in infancy, in adolescence social inconvenience and compliance problems can bring increased risk of kernicterus.

A long-term study of patients with CN syndrome in the Amish and Mennonite communities demonstrated significant treatment success. By focusing on effective phototherapy, including higher dosing of light, percentage skin exposed, use of white sheets and mirrors, and attention to light power calculation, brain damage and mortality could be eliminated.

Other therapeutic considerations involve the oral administration of binding agents such as agar or cholestyramine, or calcium phosphate. These agents bind to bilirubin in the intestinal lumen after phototherapy or through direct intestinal permeation. They prevent the enterohepatic circulation of bilirubin. Problems associated with the use of cholestyramine include cost, taste, and concern about bile salt depletion and fat malabsorption. Problems regarding agar include significant variation in bilirubin binding affinity among various preparations and batches. During acute episodes of severe hyperbilirubinemia after the first year of life, one center has had success with continuous phototherapy, albumin infusions to bind bilirubin, ursodiol to optimize bile salt-dependent bile flow, and dextrose to maintain euglycemia [36]. Plasmapheresis has been shown to rapidly decrease serum bilirubin levels. Drugs that bind to albumin should be avoided at all times. Tin-mesoporphyrin (stannsoporfin; 2 to 4 μmol/kg) [43] is suggested to offer a promising, although still experimental, additional therapy for controlling episodes of acute, severe jaundice.

Because patients with CN syndrome have good hepatic function other than conjugating bilirubin, they are ideal candidates for auxiliary liver transplantation. This option has recently become clinically available. More commonly, orthotopic liver transplantation has been performed. Ideally the timing of transplantation would precede irreversible neurologic injury. Successful cloning of UGT1A1 offers the hope of future gene therapy to correct this deficiency; however, currently, clinicians must focus on optimizing care of these patients with effective phototherapy and the use of emergency protocols during exacerbations.

Rotor syndrome

Clinical presentation

Rotor syndrome (OMIM 237 450), first described in 1948, is a familial disorder that involves chronic elevation of both the conjugated and unconjugated serum bilirubin fractions. Half or more of the total serum bilirubin is conjugated and total bilirubin levels usually range from 2 to 7 mg/dL, but occasionally may reach 20 mg/dL. Liver functions tests are otherwise normal and there is no evidence of hemolysis. Liver histology is normal when examined with both light and electron microscopy. Oral cholecystograms reveal normal gallbladder opacification. This disorder can present in early childhood or possibly the first months of life, if coinherited with G6PD deficiency or heterozygous β thalassemia, and manifests no gender predisposition. Family studies suggest an autosomal recessive mode of inheritance.

Pathophysiology

In a recent analysis of eight affected families, Rotor syndrome was linked to mutations predicted to cause complete and simultaneous deficiencies of the organic anion transporting polypeptides OATP1B1 and OATP1B3, thereby disrupting hepatic reuptake of bilirubin glucuronide [44]. Patients with Rotor syndrome also demonstrate a delayed plasma clearance of both sulfobromophthalein and indocyanine green, and heterozygotes show delayed sulfobromophthalein clearance with values intermediate between normals and those with homozygous Rotor syndrome. Glutathione S-transferase serves as an intracellular carrier protein for certain organic molecules, acting as an intracellular equivalent to albumin in blood plasma. A patient with Rotor syndrome has been shown to have a deficiency of hepatic glutathione S-transferase, and this would be consistent with observations regarding the pathogenesis of this disorder. Deficiency of glutathione S-transferase would result in impaired uptake of bilirubin within the cytosol. In addition, since bilirubin conjugates are bound to glutathione S-transferase while awaiting excretion from the hepatocyte via the canalicular membrane, deficient intracellular storage would result in leakage of bilirubin conjugates back into the circulation. Serum elevations of both conjugated and non-conjugated bilirubin result.

Another important observation in Rotor syndrome relates to the urinary excretion of coproporphyrin. In normal healthy individuals, only the I and III isomers of coproporphyrin are excreted in the urine. In Rotor syndrome, there is a marked increase in urinary coproporphyrin excretion and, usually, less than 80% of the total (I + III) is isomer I. Heterozygotes demonstrate urinary coproporphyrin values that are intermediate between normals and homozygotes. Urinary excretion of coproporphyrin is believed to be increased because biliary excretion is impaired, similar to findings in other liver diseases.

Diagnosis and treatment

A diagnosis of Rotor syndrome should be considered in all individuals having elevation of both conjugated and non-conjugated serum bilirubin fractions along with otherwise normal liver function tests. The diagnosis can be confirmed by measuring urinary coproporphyrin levels, which are 2.5 to 5 times higher than normal levels [45]. Of the total urinary coproporphyrin isomers I plus III, isomer I constitutes <80% of the total in Rotor syndrome [46]. Use of technetium-99m hepatobiliary iminodiacetic acid cholescintigraphy has also been shown to be useful to diagnose Rotor syndrome and demonstrates poor to no visualization of the liver.

Patients with Rotor syndrome require no specific therapy and are asymptomatic. Although jaundice is a lifelong finding, it is associated with no morbidity or mortality.

Dubin–Johnson syndrome

Clinical presentation

Dubin–Johnson syndrome (OMIM 237 500), first described in 1954 [47], involves elevation of both the conjugated and unconjugated serum bilirubin fractions. More than half of the total serum bilirubin is conjugated, and total bilirubin levels usually range from 1.5 to 6 mg/dL, although they have been reported as high as 25 mg/dL during intercurrent illness. Patients with DJS sometimes report vague abdominal complaints although this is not believed to reflect serious pathology. Although hepatomegaly is sometimes seen, liver functions tests are otherwise normal, including bile acids, and there is no evidence of hemolysis. Although this syndrome occurs in both sexes, males predominate and present at an earlier age. It occurs in all races; however, Iranian and Moroccan Jews have an increased incidence. It is usually diagnosed after puberty, although cases have also been reported in neonates, at which time cholestasis can be significant. It is inherited as an autosomal recessive trait with heterozygotes manifesting normal serum bilirubin levels. This syndrome is far more common than Rotor syndrome and jaundice can be worsened by pregnancy and oral contraceptives. Often patients with DJS have non-visualizing gallbladders when undergoing oral cholecystogram.

A striking characteristic of DJS is the brown to black discoloration of the liver. There is still debate about the identity of this pigment, which is located in the lysosomes. Although originally thought to be lipofuscin, more recent data provide conflicting evidence for a relationship to melanin or polymerized epinephrine or other metabolites that accumulate in the lysosomes. It is hypothesized that these pigments accumulate in the liver because of impaired secretion of various metabolites from the hepatocyte into the bile. This pigment disappears from the liver during acute viral hepatitis, with subsequent reappearance. Other than this striking pigmentation, the liver is histologically normal.

Pathophysiology

The primary defect in DJS is deficient hepatic excretion of non-bile salt organic anions at the apical canalicular membrane, by MRP2, a member of the ABC transport system (see above) [48]. MRP2 is encoded by a single copy gene, *ABCC2*, located on chromosome 10q24. Mutations of this gene have been shown to produce a highly defective MRP2 that is associated with DJS. Although hepatic sulfobromophthalein clearance tests are no longer performed, they nicely demonstrate the effect of deficient transport via the canalicular membrane, characteristic of DJS. Data suggest that sulfobromophthalein hepatic storage is normal but there is a 90% decrease in its excretory transport maximum. Hence, in DJS, deficient excretion of bilirubin glucuronides at the canalicular membrane, in the presence of otherwise normal intrahepatic metabolism, results in reflux of conjugated bilirubin back into the circulation.

Patients with this disorder have an increase in the urinary excretion of coproporphyrin I, with a concomitant decrease in the excretion of coproporphyrin III. This results in a total coproporphyrin excretion (I + III) that is normal or only slightly increased, but which consists of >80% coproporphyrin I (normal 25%) [49]. In heterozygotes, the coproporphyrin I:III ratio is intermediate between normals and homozygotes, although there is some overlap between heterozygotes and normals.

Diagnosis and treatment

A diagnosis of DJS should be considered in all individuals having elevation of conjugated bilirubin in the serum along with otherwise normal liver function tests. The diagnosis can be confirmed by measuring urinary coproporphyrin levels of isomers I and III. While the total coproporphyrin level will be approximately normal, more than 80% will be isomer I. This finding is pathognomonic for DJS when congenital erythropoietic porphyria or arsenic poisoning have been excluded. Although oral cholecystogram may fail to visualize the gallbladder, ultrasound examination will show a normal biliary tree. Cholescintigraphy demonstrates prolonged intense visualization of the liver with delayed appearance of the gallbladder and only faint or non-visualization of the biliary ducts.

Patients with DJS require no specific therapy. Avoidance of the oral contraceptive has been recommended since this can increase jaundice. Anticipatory guidance regarding jaundice increasing during pregnancy is also appropriate. Although jaundice is a lifelong finding, it is associated with no morbidity or mortality, as demonstrated in a 30 year follow-up of 10 Japanese individuals [50].

References

1. Gourley GR. Neonatal jaundice and disorders of bilirubin metabolism. In Suchy FJ, Sokol RJ, Balistreri WF (eds.) *Liver Disease in Children*, 3rd edn. New York: Cambridge University Press, 2007, pp. 270–309.

2. Weiss JS, Guatam A, Lauff JJ, *et al.* The clinical importance of a protein-bound fraction of serum bilirubin in patients with hyperbilirubinemia. *N Engl J Med* 1983;**309**:147–150.

3. Billing BH. Intestinal and renal metabolism of bilirubin including enterohepatic circulation. In Ostrow JD (ed.) *Bile Pigments and Jaundice*. New York: Marcel Dekker, 1986, pp. 255–269.

4. Poland RL, Odell GB. Physiologic jaundice: the enterohepatic circulation of bilirubin. *N Engl J Med* 1971;**284**:1–6.

5. Mackenzie PI, Owens IS, Burchell B, *et al.* The UDP glycosyltransferase gene superfamily: recommmended nomenclature update based on evolutionary divergence. *Pharmacogenetics* 1997;**7**:255–269.

6. Lester R, Schmid R. Intestinal absorption of bile pigments. I. The enterohepatic circulation of bilirubin in the cat. *J Clin Invest* 1963;**42**:736–746.

7. Gourley GR, Arend RA. β-Glucuronidase and hyperbilirubinemia in breast-fed and formula-fed babies. *Lancet* 1986;**i**:644–646.

8. Gourley GR. Pathophysiology of breast-milk jaundice. In Polin RA, Fox WW (eds.) *Fetal and Neonatal Physiology*, 2nd edn. Philadelphia, PA: Saunders, 1998, pp. 1499–1505.

9. Gourley GR, Li Z, Kreamer BL, Kosorok MR. A Controlled, randomized, double-blind trial of prophylaxis against jaundice among breastfed newborns. *Pediatrics* 2005;**116**:385–391.

10. Maisels MJ, Bhutani VK, Boggs T, *et al.* Hyperbilirubinemia in the newborn infant ≥35 weeks' gestation: an update with clarification. *Pediatrics* 2009;**124**:1193–1198.

11. Kramer LI. Advancement of dermal icterus in the jaundiced newborn. *Am J Dis Child* 1969;**118**:454–458.

12. Fujiwara R, Chen S, Karin M, *et al.* Reduced expression of *UGT1A1* in intestines of humanized UGT1 mice via inactivation of NF-κB leads to hyperbilirubinemia. *Gastroenterology* 2012;**142**:109–118.

13. American Academy of Pediatrics. Practice parameter: management of hyperbilirubinemia in the healthy term newborn. *Pediatrics* 1994;**94**:558–565.

14. American Academy of Pediatrics Subcommittee on Hyperbilirubinemia. Management of hyperbilirubinemia in the newborn infant 35 or more weeks of gestation. *Pediatrics* 2004;**114**:297–316.

15. Kreamer BL, Siegel FL, Gourley GR. A novel inhibitor of β-glucuronidase: L-aspartic acid. *Pediatric Res* 2001;**50**:460–466.

16. Odell GB. Studies in kernicterus. I. Protein binding of bilirubin. *J Clin Invest* 1959;**38**:823.

17. Kawade N, Onishi S. The prenatal and postnatal development of UDP-glucuronyltransferase activity towards bilirubin and the effect of premature birth on this activity in the human liver. *Biochem J* 1981;**196**:257–260.

18. Rubboli G, Ronchi F, Cecchi P, *et al.* A neurophysiological study in children and adolescents with Crigler–Najjar syndrome type I. *Neuropediatrics* 1997;**28**:281–286.

19. Odell GB. The dissociation of bilirubin from albumin and its clinical implications. *J Pediatr* 1959;**55**:268–279.

20. McDonagh AF, Palma LA, Lightner DA. Phototherapy for neonatal jaundice: stereospecific and regioselective photoisomerization of bilirubin bound to human serum albumin and NMR characterization of intramolecular cyclized photoproducts. *J Am Chem Soc* 1982;**104**:6867–6869.

21. Greenwald JL. Hyperbilirubinemia in otherwise healthy infants. *Am Fam Physician* 1988;**38**:151–158.

22. Alpay F, Sarici SU, Okutan V, *et al.* High-dose intravenous immunoglobulin therapy in neonatal immune haemolytic jaundice. *Acta Paediatr* 1999;**88**:216–219.

23. Valaes TN, Harvey-Wilkes K. Pharmacologic approaches to the prevention and treatment of neonatal hyperbilirubinemia. *Clin Perinatol* 1990;**17**:245–273.

24. Gourley GR, Kreamer B, Cohen M, Kosorok MR. Neonatal jaundice and diet. *Arch Pediatr Adolesc Med* 1999;**153**:184–188.

25. Gilbert A, Lereboullet P. La cholemie simple familiale. *Sem Med* 1901;**21**:241–243.

26. Bosma P, Chowdhury JR, Jansen PH. Genetic inheritance of Gilbert's syndrome. *Lancet* 1995;**346**:314–315.

27. Odell GB. *The Estrogenation of the Newborn. Neonatal Hyperbilirubinemia*. New York: Grune & Stratton, 1980, pp. 39–41.

28. Bancroft JD, Kreamer B, Gourley GR. Gilbert syndrome accelerates development of neonatal jaundice. *J Pediatr* 1998;**132**:656–660.

29. Kaplan M, Renbaum P, Levy-Lahad E, *et al.* Gilbert syndrome and glucose-6-phosphate dehydrogenase deficiency: a dose-dependent genetic interaction crucial to neonatal hyperbilirubinemia. *Proc Natl Acad Sci USA* 1997;**94**:12128–12132.

30. Debinski HS, Lee CS, Dhillon AP, *et al.* UDP-Glucuronosyltransferase in Gilbert's syndrome. *Pathology* 1996;**28**:238–241.

31. Bosma PJ, Chowdhury JR, Bakker C, *et al.* The genetic basis of the reduced expression of bilirubin UDP-glucuronosyltransferase 1 in Gilbert's syndrome. *N Engl J Med* 1995;**333**:1171–1175.

32. Akaba K, Kimura T, Sasaki A, *et al.* Neonatal hyperbilirubinemia and a common mutation of the bilirubin uridine diphosphate-glucuronosyltransferase gene in Japanese. *J Hum Genet* 1999;**44**:22–25.

33. Crigler JF, Najjar VA. Congenital familial nonhemolytic jaundice with kernicterus. *Pediatrics* 1952;**10**:169–180.

34. Gourley GR. Bilirubin metabolism and kernicterus. *Adv Pediatr* 1997;**44**:173–229.

35. Shevell MI, Majnemer A, Schiff D. Neurologic perspectives of Crigler–Najjar syndrome type I. *J Child Neurol* 1998;**13**:265–269.

36. Strauss KA, Robinson DL, Vreman HJ, *et al.* Management of hyperbilirubinemia and prevention of kernicterus in 20 patients with Crigler–Najjar disease. *Eur J Pediatr* 2006;**165**:306–319.

37. Arias IM, Gartner LM, Cohen M, Ezzer JB, Levi AJ. Chronic nonhemolytic

unconjugated hyperbilirubinemia with glucuronyl transferase deficiency. *Am J Med* 1969;**47**:395–409.

38. Clarke DJ, Moghrabi N, Monaghan G, *et al.* Genetic defects of the UDP-glucuronosyltransferase-1 (*UGT1*) gene that cause familial non-haemolytic unconjugated hyperbilirubinaemias. *Clin Chim Acta* 1997;**266**:63–74.

39. Labrune P, Myara A, Hadchouel M, *et al.* Genetic heterogeneity of Crigler–Najjar syndrome type I: a study of 14 cases. *Hum Genet* 1994;**94**:693–697.

40. Sinaasappel M, Jansen PL. The differential diagnosis of Crigler–Najjar Disease, types 1 and 2, by bile pigment analysis. *Gastroenterology* 1991;**100**:783–789.

41. Rubaltelli FF, Novello A, Zancan L, Vilei MT, Muraca M. Serum and bile bilirubin pigments in the differential diagnosis of Crigler–Najjar disease. *Pediatrics* 1994;**94**:553–556.

42. van der Veere CN, Sinaasappel M, McDonagh AF, *et al.* Current therapy for Crigler–Najjar syndrome type 1: report of a world registry. *Hepatology* 1996;**24**:311–315.

43. Rubaltelli FF. Current drug treatment options in neonatal hyperbilirubinaemia and the prevention of kernicterus. *Drugs* 1998;**56**:23–30.

44. van de Steeg E, Stránecký V, Hartmannová H, *et al.* Complete OATP1B1 and OATP1B3 deficiency causes human Rotor syndrome by interrupting conjugated bilirubin reuptake into the liver. *J Clin Invest* 2012;**122**:519–528.

45. Wolkoff AW, Wolpert E, Pascasio FN, Arias IM. Rotor's syndrome. a distinct inheritable pathophysiologic entity. *Am J Med* 1976;**60**:173–179.

46. Shimizu Y, Naruto H, Ida S, Kohakura M. Urinary coproporphyrin isomers in Rotor's syndrome: a study in eight families. *Hepatology* 1981;**1**:173–178.

47. Dubin IN, Johnson FB. Chronic idiopathic jaundice with unidentified pigment in liver cells: a new clincopathologic entity with a report of 12 cases. *Medicine* 1954;**33**:155–197.

48. Toh S, Wada M, Uchiumi T, *et al.* Genomic structure of the canalicular multispecific organic anion-transporter gene (*MRP2/CMOAT*) and mutations in the ATP-binding-cassette region in Dubin–Johnson syndrome. *Am J Hum Genet* 1999;**64**:739–746.

49. Frank M, Doss M, de Carvalho DG. Diagnostic and pathogenetic implications of urinary coproporphyrin excretion in the Dubin–Johnson syndrome. *Hepatogastroenterology* 1990;**37**:147–151.

50. Machida I, Wakusawa S, Sanae F, *et al.* Mutational analysis of the *MRP2* gene and long-term follow-up of Dubin–Johnson syndrome in Japan. *J Gastroenterol* 2005;**40**:366–370.

Familial hepatocellular cholestasis

Frederick J. Suchy, Shikha S. Sundaram, and Benjamin L. Shneider

Introduction

Inherited cholestasis of hepatocellular origin has long been described in the neonate or during the first year of life [1]. Many of these infants were categorized as having idiopathic neonatal hepatitis after biliary atresia, metabolic diseases, and congenital infections were excluded [2,3]. The prognosis in familial cholestasis was poor compared with sporadic cholestasis that sometimes had an identifiable etiology. As the clinical and genotypic heterogeneity of these inherited disorders has become apparent, it is now recognized that patients may present initially and progress to end-stage liver disease at ages ranging from infancy to adulthood [4]. There may be significant overlap in clinical features such as intense pruritus and a low serum concentration of gamma-glutamyltransferase (GGT). The histopathology, immunohistochemical staining, and hepatic ultrastructure may provide additional diagnostic clues as to the underlying defect. However, the identification of the genes responsible for several of these disorders now allows a specific diagnosis in many cases, may suggest therapy with varying success based on the genotype of the patient, and has advanced our understanding of molecular mechanisms of bile secretion and acquired cholestasis. It is not surprising that, so far, mutations in three genes encoding ATP-dependent transport proteins localized to the canalicular membrane that result in progressive cholestasis and liver injury have been discovered. The features of these disorders are compared in Table 13.1. Other genes encoding proteins involved in membrane transport, vesicular trafficking, and integrity of the cell junction may also be mutated in some patients. Owing to an immaturity of hepatic excretory function, cholestasis may occasionally occur in inherited diseases because of systemic illness rather than a primary defect in the liver (see Table 9.1). These disorders will not be considered in this review.

Progressive familial intrahepatic cholestasis type 1

Byler disease and benign recurrent intrahepatic cholestasis (BRIC), diseases that are now known to be caused by defects in the gene *ATP8B1* (once known as *FIC1*), were some of the first clinically well-described forms of familial intrahepatic cholestasis (FIC) [1,2]. A large part of the published literature regarding these disorders predates the molecular genetics of these diseases, so completely accurate genotype–phenotype correlation is not possible. In 1959, BRIC was first described as an intermittent form of intrahepatic cholestasis characterized by variable periods of intense pruritus often associated with jaundice [2]. The age of onset is variable, but it typically occurs during childhood or adolescence. The severity and duration of attacks also vary, and triggering features are not well known. The benign designation of BRIC refers to the general lack of progressive liver disease, although the pruritus is far from benign during an intense episode.

Byler disease was initially described in direct descendents of Jacob Byler [1,3]. Unlike BRIC and despite an intermittent nature of the disease at its onset, the pruritus and liver disease in Byler disease are eventually persistent and progressive.

Classically, FIC1 disease was considered to be two different disorders: Byler diease or progressive familial intrahepatic cholestasis type 1 (PFIC1) and BRIC. However, we now view these two disorders as two ends of a continuum and so this historical nomenclature of Byler disease and BRIC may be outdated [4]. Many clinicians now refer to all these diseases in a general sense as FIC1 disease.

Clinical features

Progressive familial intrahepatic cholestasis type 1 is an autosomal recessive liver disease characterized by unremitting cholestasis with pruritus and jaundice that usually starts before the age of 1 year and progresses to cirrhosis and liver failure [5–7]. Serum GGT activity is normal and aminotransferase levels are only minimally elevated. The latter may distinguish the presentation of FIC1 from bile salt export pump (BSEP) disease (PFIC type 2) [6]. The average age at onset is 2 months, but some patients are affected as neonates and rarely cholestasis may not be manifest until adolescence. Diarrhea, malabsorption, and failure to thrive are common in the first months of life. Fat-soluble vitamin malabsorption can lead to a potentially fatal bleeding diathesis from vitamin K deficiency, rickets

Liver Disease in Children, Fourth Edition, ed. Frederick J. Suchy, Ronald J. Sokol, and William F. Balistreri. Published by Cambridge University Press. © Cambridge University Press 2014.

Table 13.1 Progressive familial intrahepatic cholestasis

	Type 1	Type 2	Type 3
Transmission	Autosomal recessive	Autosomal recessive	Autosomal recessive
Chromosome	18q21-22	2q24	7q21
Gene	*ATP8B1/FIC1*	*ABCB11/BSEP*	*ABCB4/MDR3*
Protein	Familial intrahepatic cholestasis 1 (FIC1)	Bile salt export pump (BSEP)	Multidrug resistance-associated protein 3 (MDR3)
Location	Wide tissue distribution including almost all epithelial cells: on apical membranes	Hepatocyte canalicular membrane	Hepatocyte canalicular membrane
Function	ATP-dependent aminophospholipid flippase; may influence farsenoid X receptor-mediated signaling; may alter function and stability of membrane proteins	ATP-dependent bile acid transport	ATP-dependent PC translocation
Phenotype	Progressive cholestasis with severe pruritus, diarrhea, steatorrhea, growth failure, sensorineural hearing loss, pancreatitis, respiratory disease	Rapidly progressive cholestatic giant cell hepatitis, growth failure, pruritus, hepatocellular carcinoma	Later-onset cholestasis, portal hypertension, minimal pruritus, intraductal and gallbladder lithiasis
Histology	Initial bland cholestasis; coarse, granular canalicular bile on EM	Neonatal giant cell hepatitis, amorphous canalicular bile on EM	Bile ductular proliferation, periportal fibrosis, eventually biliary cirrhosis
Biochemical features	Normal serum GGT; minimal to modest serum aminotransferase elevation, high serum bile acid levels, low biliary bile acid secretion	Normal serum GGT; high serum, low biliary bile acid concentrations	Elevated serum GGT; low to absent biliary PC; absent serum lipoprotein X; normal biliary bile acid concentrations
Treatment	Biliary diversion, ileal exclusion, liver transplantation – but post-orthotopic liver transplantation diarrhea, pancreatitis, steatorrhea, fatty liver with possible progression to cirrhosis	Biliary diversion, liver transplantation (possible recurrent disease after transplantation)	Ursodeoxycholic acid if residual PC secretion; liver transplantation

EM, electron microscopy; PC, phosphatidylcholine.

from vitamin D deficiency, and neuromuscular dysfunction from vitamin E deficiency. The disorder typically does not progress to end-stage liver disease during early childhood but gradually evolves to cirrhosis in the second decade of life. As such, hepatosplenomegaly eventually develops as a manifestation of progressive liver disease. Few patients with early onset of cholestasis have survived into the third decade without treatment. Several patients have also been described with recurrent attacks of cholestasis beginning in infancy and that eventually became permanent as adults.

Pruritus is the dominant feature of cholestasis in the majority of patients and is often out of proportion to the level of jaundice. It may initially vary in intensity and may be exacerbated during intercurrent illness. Pruritus may not be noticed until 6 months of age because the neural pathways necessary for concerted scratching are not fully developed. However, affected infants often are irritable and fretful and sleep poorly with onset of cholestasis. Scratching is usually evident first as digging at the ears and eyes, which are the first areas to show evidence of excoriation. By 1 year of age, patients may show generalized mutilation of skin, usually most severe on the extensor surfaces of the arms and legs and on the flanks of the back. The pruritus is very disabling and often responds poorly to pharmacologic therapies. In contrast to other cholestatic disorders, these patients do not develop xanthomas.

Growth failure is another major feature of PFIC1. Most patients have short stature (less than the fifth percentile), although their weight for height is often normal, giving a stocky appearance. Delayed onset of puberty and sexual development is characteristic of patients surviving until adolescence without treatment. Patients receiving effective treatment experience normal sexual development, and several have borne normal children. Intellectual development and school performance are generally normal in patients receiving effective treatment but often are delayed before treatment, probably as a result of constant pruritus and associated problems with sleep and inattention.

There is an association of FIC1 disease with a variety of extrahepatic manifestations, which we now understand may be the result of the wide tissue distribution of *ATP8B1* expression. The more commonly described extrahepatic manifestations include recurrent pancreatitis, diarrhea that is independent of cholestasis, sensorineural hearing loss, chronic cough/wheezing, and somatic short stature., Many of these problems persist and may even worsen after liver transplantation, supporting the notion that they are the result of *ATP8B1* expression in organs other than the liver. Severe diarrhea and progressive steatohepatitis are particularly problematic after liver transplantation. Steatosis is only seen after liver transplantation and can be progressive leading to cirrhosis in less than ten years [8].

A form of benign recurrent intrahepatic cholestasis (BRIC1) is characterized by attacks of jaundice and pruritus separated by symptom-free intervals [9]. Patients may also experience fatigue, anorexia, steatorrhea, dark-colored urine, and weight loss. Progression to cirrhosis and long-term complications of chronic liver disease do not occur or occur later in the course compared with individuals with more severe FIC1 disease. The disorder is caused by mutations in *ATP8B1* and is inherited as an autosomal recessive trait.

The age of presentation of the first attack of jaundice ranges from 1–50 years, but jaundice usually occurs before the age of 20 years. Attacks usually are preceded by a minor illness and consist of a preicteric phase of 2–4 weeks (characterized by malaise, anorexia, and pruritus) and an icteric phase that may last from 1 to 18 months. In some patients, hormonal factors such as the use of oral contraceptives or pregnancy have been associated with precipitation of an attack. Patients may have severe coughing during episodes, as is seen sometimes in patients with PFIC1.

During the icteric phase, the concentrations of serum bile acid, bilirubin, and alkaline phosphatase are increased. Serum GGT concentration, however, remains low. Liver biopsy results are very benign, often showing no pathologic change even during an episode. Some specimens show hepatocellular cholestasis and cholate injury, mostly centrilobular. During the asymptomatic period, all parameters are normal: clinical, laboratory, and liver histology.

Laboratory findings

The laboratory findings in PFIC1 and BRIC1 are remarkable for the presence of low serum GGT and normal or near normal serum cholesterol levels, even in the presence of severe cholestasis [10]. Patients may have serum GGT >100 IU/L while receiving microsomal inducers such as phenobarbital. Serum concentrations of alkaline phosphatase, bilirubin, and bile salts do not differ from those seen in several other cholestatic disorders and may be normal or near normal early in the course of the disease. Serum aminotransferase levels are usually no higher than twice normal values. Patients with PFIC1 or a prolonged episode of BRIC1 frequently develop complications of cholestasis, including fat-soluble vitamin deficiency. Sweat chloride and sodium levels may be elevated. With progressive liver injury, features of hepatic failure and portal hypertension develop that are similar to those of any other end-stage liver disease.

A low serum GGT level is highly unusual in the presence of cholestasis. It should suggest the possibility of one of the forms of PFIC or BRIC. However, the differential diagnosis should include inborn errors of bile acid synthesis. In PFIC and BRIC, serum concentrations of primary bile acids are markedly elevated, whereas in bile synthetic defects, the serum contains abnormal bile acid precursors but no primary bile acids. Pruritus is an uncommon manifestation in bile acid synthetic defects.

The mechanism for the low serum concentration of GGT in PFIC and BRIC is not clear. This enzyme is normally bound to the canalicular membrane by a glycosyl phosphatidylinositol (GPI) anchor. In obstructive cholestasis, when excessive amounts of bile salts accumulate in the canalicular lumen under increased pressure, GGT is released from the membrane by detergent action and refluxes back into serum, possibly via leaky intercellular junctions. However, in PFIC and BRIC, alterations in lipid bilayer characteristics may lead to release of canalicular enzymes into bile. Immunohistochemical studies indicate that some canalicular proteins, including GGT and carcinoembryonic antigen, are poorly expressed at the caniculus in PFIC1 [11].

Consistent with severe cholestasis, total serum bile acid concentrations are markedly elevated (usually >200 μmol/L; normal, <10 μmol/L) with an elevated ratio of chenodeoxycholic acid to cholic acid conjugates, usually >10:1. The total biliary bile acid concentrations are generally low (0.1–0.3 μmol/L; normal, >20 μmol/L), with a predominance of cholic acid conjugates. These findings have suggested a defect in biliary excretion, particularly of chenodeoxycholic acid conjugates.

Histopathology

A bland hepatocellular and canalicular cholestasis with some pseudo-acinar transformation are the most uniform histologic findings early in the course of the disease (Figure 13.1) [10,11]. Minimal giant cell formation and ballooning of hepatocytes also may be found. Giant cells are present more often during infancy and may regress with age. Bile duct damage is minimal in infants but may be more prominent later, leading to ductal paucity. The degenerating biliary epithelium shows apoptotic changes consisting of small hyperchromatic nuclei, attenuated cytoplasm, and loss of duct lumina, but inflammation is absent. The typical progression of fibrosis starts early, with 76% of patients having some fibrosis by 2 years of age, and fibrosis may appear initially either as pericentral sclerosis or portal fibrosis, or sometimes both. Portal to central bridging then develops in association with lacy lobular fibrosis and eventually leads to cirrhosis. Proliferating bile ductules are observed at the edge of the portal tracts in patients with significant fibrosis. The rate of progression of the fibrosis is highly variable but correlates loosely with the severity of the clinical disease. The natural history of the disease is rarely observed in the current era as clinical interventions alter the

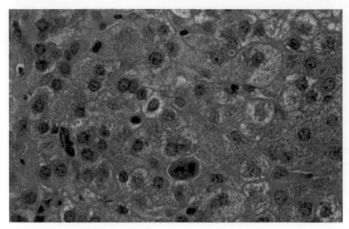

Figure 13.1 Histopathology in progressive familial intrahepatic cholestasis type 1. Liver biopsy from a 2-year-old patient showing swelling of hepatocytes, a bland hepatocellular, and canalicular cholestasis, and occasional necrotic hepatocytes (Courtesy of Dr. Kevin Bove.)

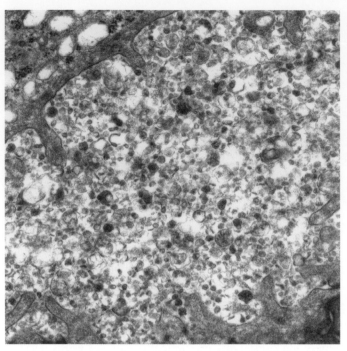

Figure 13.2 Ultrastructural pathology of progressive familial intrahepatic cholestasis type 1. Electron microscopy of liver from a patient shows distended bile canaliculi with microvilli that are reduced in number and length. Bile canaliculi contain unusually coarse and granular bile (so-called Byler's bile). (Courtesy of Dr. Alex Knisely.)

course of disease. Mallory hyaline and hepatocellular carcinoma may be seen with very advanced disease.

Unfortunately, well-characterized and clinically useful antibodies against the FIC1 protein do not exist, so routine direct histochemical analysis cannot be performed to diagnose FIC1 disease. Indirect analysis of GGT staining may suggest a diagnosis of FIC1 disease [11].

Electron microscopy on liver samples from patients who are not receiving ursodeoxycholic acid (UDCA) shows distended bile canaliculi with microvilli that are reduced in number and length (Figure 13.2). Bile canaliculi contain unusually coarse and granular bile (so-called Byler's bile). In some confirmed cases of PFIC1, aggregated vesicles of membranous material rather than coarse granular bile are observed. Bile is retained in hepatocytes and Kupffer cells and is predominantly periportal in localization. The pericanalicular ectoplasm is often thickened. These ultrastructural abnormalities are highly suggestive of, but not absolutely specific for, PFIC1 [10,11].

Genetics

Gene linkage analysis of BRIC and Byler disease indicated that the same gene is involved in both of these diseases, and is mapped to chromosome 18q21. Refined linkage analysis and gene sequencing of patients with well-characterized disease ultimately led to the discovery that defects in the P-type ATPase (FIC1 or ATP8B1) are responsible for FIC1 disease [12]. *ATP8B1* contains 28 exons, spans at least 77 kb, and yields no alternatively spliced transcripts [5]. The FIC1 protein consists of 1251 amino acid residues and has the 10 predicted membrane-spanning domains typical of P-type ATPases. Mutational analyses in 180 families with PFIC1 and 50 families with BRIC1 identified 54 distinct disease mutations, including 10 mutations predicted to disrupt splicing, 6 nonsense mutations, 11 small insertion or deletion

mutations predicted to induce frameshifts, 1 large genomic deletion, 2 small in-frame deletions, and 24 missense mutations [5]. Mutations of *ATP8B1* were detected in 30% and 41%, respectively, of the PFIC and BRIC families screened. Most mutations were rare, occurring in one to three families, or were limited to specific populations. Compound heterozygotes were commonly observed (9 in 39 with PFIC1 and 12 in 20 with BRIC1). There was also a correlation with the type of mutation and clinical severity. Based on sequence analysis and the predicted effects of specific mutations, it is hypothesized that BRIC-like disease is the result of functionally less severe mutations in *ATP8B1*. Missense mutations were more common in BRIC1 (58% versus 38% in PFIC1), whereas nonsense, frameshifting, and large deletion mutations were more common in PFIC1 (41% versus 16% in BRIC1) [5]. In one study, 14 of 16 patients with BRIC1 were either homozygous or compound heterozygous for the I661T mutation, which was frequently found in European patients [5]. Nonsense mutations at the 5′ end of the *ATP8B1* coding region are typically associated with severe disease, whereas mutations at the 3′ end are associated with milder and intermittent disease. A functional assay examining signaling by the nuclear receptor farsenoid X receptor (FXR) suggests that disease severity correlates with FIC1 function [13]. Those with BRIC type mutant FIC1 may have reduced plasma membrane targeting that can be partially corrected by chemical chaperones [14].

Pathophysiology

Occurrence of FIC1 appears to be the result of abnormalities in the enterohepatic circulation of bile acids. In vivo clearance of radiolabeled bile acids in patients with Byler disease and careful examination of biliary bile acids suggest that there is reduced hepatic canalicular excretion of bile salts. Clinical response to partial biliary diversion or ileal exclusion indicates that enhanced intestinal reabsorption of bile acids may also be involved in the disease process. Animal models of Byler disease have not yielded a simple explanation of the molecular events involved in FIC1 [15–17]. The genetic mutation initially described in the Byler's kindred, causing G308V, was introduced into mice. Adult *Atp8b1G308V/G308V* mice expressed mRNA for FIC1 but not protein. The mice were normal appearing, although serum aspartate aminotransferase and bile salts were elevated compared with wild-type littermate controls. Paradoxically, bile flow and hepatic excretion of bile salts were enhanced in the Byler mice. Cholate feeding of the *Atp8b1G308V/G308V* mice exacerbated the pathology and suggested that abnormal regulation of bile acid homeostasis is operative in the pathogenesis of FIC1.

The Byler mouse has been a clearer model of some aspects of extrahepatic disease. Hearing deficits, as assessed by auditory brainstem responses, develop in Byler mice as they age [18]. The protein FIC1 is produced in the hair cells of the organ of Corti and the organ of Corti degenerates as the Byler mice age. Bacteria-induced lung injury is worsened in Byler mice and correlates with the cardiolipin clearance from lung fluid [19].

At present, the exact molecular pathophysiology of FIC1 is uncertain. This is in contrast to defects in BSEP and multidrug resistance protein (MDR) 3, in which the presumed pathophysiology follows directly from protein function. Based on sequence and homology analysis, it has been presumed that FIC1 is a P-type ATPase that functions as an aminophospholipid flippase, transferring aminophospholipids from the outer to inner hemi-leaflet of cell membranes. Aminophospholipid translocase activity has been demonstrated in rat liver canalicular membrane vesicles that contained FIC1. Transfection of a mutagenized Chinese hamster ovary cell line that lacks FIC1 cells with *ATP8B1* cDNA resulted in the production of FIC1 in membrane preparations and energy-dependent translocation of a fluorescent analogue of phosphatidylserine [20]. Coexpression of an accessory protein CDC50A or CDC50B enhances and may be essential for the phospholipid flippase activity of FIC1 [21]. These data suggest that FIC1 is an aminophospholipid transporter that helps to maintain the appropriate asymmetric distribution of aminophospholipids between the inner and outer leaflets of the plasma membrane. Lipid bilayer composition may influence the activity of integral membrane proteins and more importantly may increase the susceptibility of the membrane to the detergent effects of bile. Cholesterol depletion is found in FIC1-deficient canalicular membranes and this depletion is associated with diminished BSEP function [22]. Byler mice have diminished resistance of

the bile canalicular membrane to hydrophobic bile acids. As such, canalicular ectoenzymes are sloughed into bile and there is a marked reduction in the cholesterol content of the bile canalicular membrane, which would be expected to diminish BSEP activity and lead to cholestasis. The relevance of lipid asymmetry at the canalicular membrane is highlighted by the counteracting effects of aminophospholipid flipping and phosphatidylcholine flopping demonstrated in the *Atp8b1* and *Abcb4* double knockout mice [23]. In this model, the deleterious effects of *Abcb4* loss of function are partially rescued by the superimposition of *Atp8b1* dysfunction.

Alterations in FIC1 may alter apical membrane protein production independent of flippase activity [24]. Asymmetry of aminophospholipids in lipid bilayers may also play a role in regulating important lipid-dependent signaling pathways.

The protein FIC1 is produced at the canalicular membrane of the hepatocyte and at the apical membrane of bile duct epithelial cells and enterocytes [20,25]. It is abundant along the entire length of the gastrointestinal tract from the stomach to the colon and is also found in the pancreas. There does not appear to be a direct linkage between FIC1 and bile acid transport proteins.

An alternative hypothesis for the pathogenesis of Byler disease is based upon the supposition that *ATP8B1* expression may influence post-translational modification of FXR, leading to enhancement of its nuclear localization and transcriptional activity [13,26,27]. The FXR is a nuclear protein that is integral to the bile acid responsiveness of a variety of genes involved in bile acid biosynthesis and transport. It positively regulates the expression of BSEP and negatively regulates the expression of the ileal apical sodium-dependent bile acid transporter. In FIC1 deficiency, it is proposed that there is diminished FXR

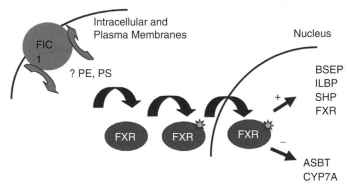

Figure 13.3 Hypothetical model of the effect of familial intrahepatic cholestasis 1 (FIC1). This is a membrane protein that alters membrane aminophospholipid asymmetry and transduces an unknown signaling pathway (curved arrows). This leads to a post-translational modification of the farsenoid X receptor (FXR), possibly through some type of phospholipid-dependent signaling pathway (indicated by the attached star). The post-translational modification is necessary for nuclear translocation of FXR. FXR in the nucleus then activates itself (FXR), the ileal lipid-binding protein (ILBP), the inhibitory transcription factor, the short heterodimer partner (SHP), and the bile salt export pump (BSEP). FXR, via the effect of SHP, inhibits the expression of the apical sodium-dependent bile acid transporter (ASBT) and cholesterol 7α-hydroxylase (CYP7A). PE, phosphatidylethanolamine; PS, phosphatidylserine. (Modified from Chen *et al.*, 2004 [26].)

activity, leading to reduced production of the canalicular BSEP and increased production of the ileal apical sodium-dependent bile acid transporter. The net effect of these changes would be enhanced reabsorption of intestinal bile acids coupled with diminished hepatic excretion of bile acids, yielding marked hypercholanemia and diminished hepatic bile acid secretion (Figure 13.3). Analysis of ileum from individuals with FIC1 disease reveals evidence of diminished FXR signaling and increased expression of the ileal apical sodium-dependent bile acid transporter [26]. These findings have not been observed in the Byler mice [16]. Assessment of FXR signaling and BSEP expression in human liver from individuals with Byler disease has yielded conflicting results and is limited by small numbers of samples and inadequate controls. Silencing FIC1 in primary human hepatocytes is associated with diminished FXR signaling and reduced endogenous BSEP production [27].

Progressive familial intrahepatic cholestasis type 2

Following the identification of the gene underlying PFIC1 and better delineation of its clinical features, it became clear that there was genetic and clinical heterogeneity in patients with PFIC and low serum GGT. A second locus for PFIC was then mapped to 2q24 by homozygosity mapping and linkage analysis in six consanguineous families of Middle Eastern origin [7]. Mutations were defined later in a liver-specific gene of unknown function, initially called the *sister of P-glycoprotein*, which was found within this region. Further studies revealed that this gene's protein, a member of the ATP-binding cassette family of transporters, was located exclusively on the canalicular membrane of hepatocytes and functioned as an ATP-dependent BSEP. Numerous mutations in *ABCB11* (was *BSEP*) have been defined in patients with the form of PFIC linked to 2q24 (now named PFIC2) [28]. The phenotype of these patients is consistent with defective bile salt excretion at the hepatocyte canalicular membrane. Mutations of *ABCB11* have also been detected in some patients with BRIC. Variants of *ABCB11* have also been associated with drug-induced cholestasis and some cases of intrahepatic cholestasis of pregnancy [29].

The protein BSEP consists of 1321 amino acid residues (molecular mass ~160 kDa) and, in keeping with other members of the ABC superfamily, has a predicted topology of 12 membrane-spanning domains [29]. It has a tandemly duplicated structure with each half of the molecule composed of six predicted transmembrane domains and a large cytoplasmic nucleotide-binding domain. The protein transports monovalent monovalent bile acids with high affinity. Expression of *ABCB11* is regulated by FXR, which is activated by bile acids.

Clinical features

Patients with PFIC2 usually present in the neonatal period with progressive cholestasis [7,30]. In general, these patients lack the relapsing course seen in the early stages of PFIC1 and

instead have a more rapid progression to cirrhosis without therapy [7]. Irritability and bleeding related to vitamin K deficiency are commonly seen. Rickets is another complication caused by vitamin D deficiency. Patients may clinically manifest vitamin deficiencies even in the absence of jaundice. Failure to thrive occurs, related to fat malabsorption and poor intake. The majority of patients have hepatomegaly; significant splenomegaly implies portal hypertension related to advanced fibrosis or cirrhosis [28]. Cholelithiasis has been observed in at least 30% of patients, owing to impaired bile acid secretory function and supersaturation of bile with cholesterol. Similar to patients with PFIC1, these patients do not have xanthomas. Extrahepatic features may help to distinguish PFIC1 and PFIC2. Watery diarrhea, pancreatitis, and impaired hearing occur in PFIC1 but not in PFIC2 [7].

Pruritus is the dominant feature of the disorder in the majority of patients before complications of cirrhosis develop [6,31]. Pruritus is often out of proportion to the level of jaundice and is not clinically evident in the first months of life.

Patients with PFIC2 are at risk for developing hepatocellular carcinoma and cholangiocarcinoma [28]. Malignancy may occur as early as 10 months of age and in patients with normalized liver tests following biliary diversion [29].

Patients fitting the phenotype of BRIC have recently been described with mutations in *ABCB11* [29]. These patients had at least two recurrent episodes of cholestasis and were clinically healthy and biochemically normal between attacks. The age of onset and total number of recurrent episodes were highly variable. Cholelithiasis occurred in 7 of 11 patients with BRIC2. Several patients had a relatively early onset of the disease and developed permanent cholestasis as adults after initial periods of recurrent attacks.

There has been a recent association of single-nucleotide polymorphisms of *ABCB11* with intrahepatic cholestasis of pregnancy [29]. A patient with transient neonatal cholestasis has also been reported with a small heterozygous deletion in the long arm of chromosome 2 [31].

Laboratory findings

Patients with PFIC2 have low serum GGT and normal or near normal serum cholesterol levels [28,32]. The serum GGT concentration may increase to >100 IU/L in patients receiving microsomal inducers such as phenobarbital and rifampicin. Serum concentrations of alkaline phosphatase, bilirubin, and bile salts do not differ from those seen in many other cholestatic disorders. In contrast to patients with PFIC1, serum aminotransferase levels are usually elevated to at least five times normal values. Patients frequently develop complications of cholestasis, including fat-soluble vitamin malabsorption and steatorrhea [32].

Histopathology

Liver morphology in PFIC2 shows a neonatal hepatitis with giant cell transformation of hepatocytes and lobular cholestasis that may persist beyond infancy [10]. Canalicular cholestasis is

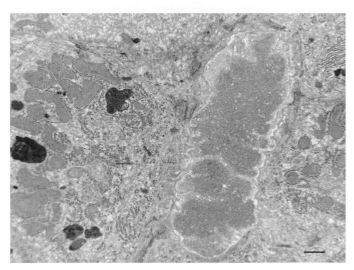

Figure 13.4 Ultrastructural pathology in progressive familial intrahepatic cholestasis type 2. Amorphous bile is observed in the canaliculus of this 2-year-old patient with absent hepatic immunostaining for bile salt export pump and low gamma-glutamyltransferase cholestasis. Bile canaliculi are distended, and microvilli are reduced in number and length (magnification 8000×, bar = 1.25 μm). (Image courtesy of Ronald Gordon, Mount Sinai School of Medicine.)

prominent, particularly in zone 3. Balloon cholestasis of hepatocytes and isolated hepatocyte necrosis may be found. Injury to hepatocytes results in perivenular, pericellular, and periportal fibrosis with progression to cirrhosis. There is mild ductular proliferation and scattered polymorphonuclear leukocytes in portal tracts. The interlobular bile ducts are normal.

Electron microscopy (Figure 13.4) demonstrates effaced microvilli and dilated bile canaliculi that contain finely granular or filamentous bile.

Genetics

Progressive familial intrahepatic cholestasis type 2 is inherited as an autosomal recessive trait. *ABCB11* is located on chromosome 2q24 and consists of 28 exons. Well over 100 different mutations in *ABCB11* have been discovered, including missense, nonsense, deletions and insertions, and slice site mutations [28]. These variants lead to inherited cholestasis of varying severity and predispose to acquired cholestasis, such as drug-induced cholestasis and intrahepatic cholestasis of pregnancy. The most common defects are missense mutations, and these were present in at least one allele in 79% of 109 families. There is some correlation of mutations with ethnicity with mutations found on at least one allele leading to E297G and D482G in 58% European families. In PFIC2, about half the mutations resulted in an early stop codon or a frameshift in the encoded protein [33]. The other PFIC2 mutations and all BRIC2 mutations were non-synonymous. Heterogeneity in clinical phenotype from a particular single gene mutation suggests contributions from additional genetic and/or environmental modifiers to the severity of the disease [29].

In a 2001 report describing the genetic analysis of 194 patients with low-GGT PFIC, 103 mutant *ABCB11* alleles were found in 63 families [34]. In this group, there were 5 different nonsense mutations, 19 different missense mutations, 8 different 1 or 2 base pair insertions or deletions, 2 major gene rearrangements, and 1 complete gene deletion. In 22 of these families, the affected patients were homozygotes; in 41 families, the affected individuals were compound heterozygotes. In a more recent study of 109 families, 82 different mutations (52 novel) were identified (9 nonsense mutations, 10 small insertions and deletions, 15 splice-site changes, 3 whole-gene deletions, 45 missense changes) [28]. Two protein-truncating mutations conferred particular risk of hepatocellular carcinoma, with 8/21 patients (38%) carrying them developing malignancy versus 11/107 patients (10%) with potentially less severe genotypes. In BRIC2, "milder" missense mutations are found more commonly than those leading to an absence of protein on the canalicular membrane and these mutations may occur in less conserved regions of the gene than in the critical Walker A/B motifs [31].

The more severe mutations result in a marked reduction or complete loss of BSEP expression on the canalicular membrane [28,30]. Of a group of patients with *ABCB11* mutations, 10 of 11 showed no BSEP on the canalicular membrane by immunohistochemical staining [30]. These patients had a variety of abnormalities in *ABCB11*, including missense, nonsense, and deletional mutations. No *ABCB11* mutations were found in any of the eight patients with positive canalicular BSEP staining. This suggests that in the majority of patients with PFIC2, the gene defect is severe enough to produce no product or a protein that cannot be inserted into the canalicular membrane. Immunolocalization may provide a means of diagnosing PFIC2 in the clinical setting [10]. Howvever, detectable BSEP does not exclude the possibility of a functional BSEP defect.

The majority of known *ABCB11* missense mutations and single-nucleotide polymorphisms have been analyzed and frequently result in impaired BSEP processing in the endoplasmic reticulum or aberrant pre-mRNA splicing. Primary defects at either the protein or the mRNA level (or both) contribute significantly to BSEP deficiency. Specific therapies may be feasible using agents to correct abnormal protein processing with BSEP cell surface expression or to modulate splicing defects [35].

Pathophysiology

The clinical implications of defective canalicular BSEP are quite clear; there will be markedly diminished bile salt secretion and progressive cholestasis [31]. In patients studied by Jansen *et al.* [30], biliary bile salt concentrations were 0.2 ± 0.2 mmol/L (<1% of normal) in patients with PFIC2 versus 18.1 ± 9.9 mmol/L (~40% of normal) in patients with other forms of PFIC. Both biliary cholesterol and phospholipid secretion were also markedly reduced. A bile salt kinetic study in one BSEP-deficient patient showed a dramatic decrease in bile salt secretion, with most of the bile salt pool confined to a "central compartment" consisting of liver, blood, and the extracellular space. Owing to bile secretory failure, bile salts and other biliary constituents are retained in the hepatocyte and lead to progressive liver damage. Seven patients studied by Jansen *et al.* [30] were treated with UDCA but were able to excrete very low amounts of UDCA into bile. These findings indicate that in addition to secretion of the primary bile salts, cholic acid, and chenodeoxycholic acid, BSEP is largely responsible for canalicular transport of UDCA.

Targeted inactivation of *Bsep* (homologue of *Abcb11*) in mice has yielded some surprising results [29]. The *Bsep*$^{-/-}$ mice were growth retarded but exhibited no signs of overt cholestasis or abnormalities in serum liver biochemical tests. As expected, the secretion of cholic acid in mutant mice was greatly reduced (6% of wild type), but total bile salt output in mutant mice was about 30% of wild type. Production of the Mdr1 P-glycoprotein was enhanced in these mice and provided an alternative but incomplete mechanism for bile salt secretion [29]. Secretion of a large amount of tetrahydroxylated bile acids occurred in mutant but not wild-type mice. These results suggest that hydroxylation and an alternative canalicular transport mechanism for bile acids compensate for the absence of Bsep function and protected the mutant mice from severe cholestatic damage. However, feeding the mutant mice with a more hydrophobic bile salt, cholic acid, led to severe cholestasis characterized by jaundice, weight loss, elevated plasma bile acid concentrations, elevated serum aminotransferases, cholangiopathy (with proliferation of bile ductules and cholangitis), liver necrosis, and high mortality [29].

A number of missense mutations in *ABCB11* that have been associated with PFIC2 have been studies in vitro [29]. Five mutants, G238V, E297G, G982R, R1153C, and R1268Q, prevented the protein from trafficking to the apical membrane, and E297G, G982R, R1153C, and R1268Q also abolished taurocholate transport activity, possibly by causing BSEP to misfold. Mutant C336S may not be disease causing as it had no effect on transport activity or apical trafficking of BSEP; D482G did not affect the apical expression but partially decreased the transport activity of BSEP. Mutant G238V was rapidly degraded in both MDCK and Sf9 cells, and a proteasome inhibitor resulted in intracellular accumulation of this and other mutants, suggesting proteasome-mediated degradation is involved in processing of mutant BSEP. These studies provide useful information on amino acid residues that are critical for BSEP function.

The consequences of mutant E297G and D482G have also been studied [29]. Both arise from missense mutations affecting the second intracellular loop and the first ATP-binding domain, respectively. Introduction of these residue changes into the human BSEP resulted in a significantly reduced BSEP production in kidney cell lines. Most of the D482G and some of the E297G BSEP was retained intracellularly, probably in the endoplasmic reticulum in an immature,

core-glycosylated form. However, the transport function of the BSEP mutants assessed in membrane vesicles isolated from transfected HEK293 cells was normal. These studies indicate that impaired membrane trafficking is the abnormality produced by the E297G and D482G mutants. As a strategy to treat certain forms of PFIC2, it may be feasible to develop agents that can induce trafficking of BSEP mutants that retain transport activity to the canalicular membrane.

Treatment of progressive familial and benign recurrent intrahepatic cholestasis

The treatment of PFIC includes standard measures related to the management of chronic cholestasis and specific approaches to these forms of intrahepatic cholestasis. Fat-soluble vitamin supplementation and monitoring are necessary for all forms of chronic cholestasis. Coagulopathy in the newborn period has resulted in intracranial hemorrhage and death in children with PFIC, particularly when vitamin K is not administered in the newborn period. Nutritional supplementation with medium-chain triglycerides may be necessary for adequate caloric assimilation. The most difficult therapeutic issue in PFIC relates to management of pruritus. Conventional therapies with antihistamines and UDCA are of limited efficacy in this patient population. Opioid antagonists are problematic to administer and not terribly efficacious. Variable and typically temporary response may be observed with rifampicin. Therefore, most common medical approaches to the intractable pruritus associated with cholestasis are often ineffective in PFIC1 and PFIC2.

Interruption of the enterohepatic circulation has yielded excellent clinical, biochemical, and histological responses in a number of children with progressive intrahepatic cholestasis. The exact mechanism(s) by which this intervention works is unclear, although it is likely that there is a significant change in the composition of the bile acid pool [36]. At present, it is unclear if these approaches are optimal for specific genetic forms of PFIC. It is possible that these interventions may be best for severe FIC1 (PFIC1) and milder phenotypic variants of PFIC2. There are two major surgical techniques to permanently interrupt the enterohepatic circulation, namely cutaneous external biliary diversion and internal partial ileal exclusion. In the first procedure, one end of a jejunal conduit is anastamosed to the dome of the gallbladder and the other is used to form a cutaneous ostomy. Bile in the gallbladder then flows either out of the ostomy or into the intestine. Typically 30–70% of bile drains out of the ostomy and is discarded. This procedure, first described by Whitington and Whitington [37], yields excellent clinical responses in a significant percentage of patients with low-GGT intrahepatic cholestasis (presumed FIC1 disease in many cases). The response often includes complete amelioration of pruritus and importantly biochemical and histological stabilization and possible improvement [36]. The response may be transiently diminished in females near the time of puberty. In addition, some children develop episodes that resemble BRIC after successful biliary diversion.

Modifications of this procedure including internal diversion to the colon and use of a "button" have been described as means to obviate the need for a chronic ostomy bag.

An alternative, although less commonly used, surgical approach to interrupting the enterohepatic circulation of bile acid involves internal partial ileal exclusion [31,32]. The vast majority of intestinal bile salts are reabsorbed in the distal ileum, that is, the distal 20–25% of the small intestine. Therefore, exclusion of this segment of intestine may lead to bile acid wasting, as has been extensively demonstrated in the surgical treatment of hypercholesterolemia. The small intestine is transected at a point that demarcates the distal 15% of the small intestine, and a blind loop is formed with the distal ileal segment. The proximal loop of the intestine is sewn end to side to the cecum, completing the internal bypass of the distal ileum. There is limited experience with this surgical approach in PFIC, although some success has been reported. Avoidance of an ostomy is attractive for many patients and their families. Accurate assessment of the appropriate amount of ileum for bypass is likely to be critical; too little is unlikely to be therapeutic and too much is likely to yield bile acid-induced diarrhea. At present, it is not clear if there will be compensatory responses in the intestine that will ultimately diminish the long-term effectiveness of ileal exclusion in PFIC.

The evidence base for the efficacy of surgical treatments of PFIC is inadequate. A review of published studies reveals a relatively small number of non-cirrhotic patients (<100) with low-GGT PFIC who were treated with one of several different procedures, including partial external biliary diversion, ileal exclusion, and cholecystoappendicostomy. Patients were usually referred for intractable pruritus. Approximately 75% of patients in these studies were reported to have improved, but the end-points were highly variable and included improved pruritus, liver tests, and growth. In some cases, progression of liver disease decreased and there was even regression of fibrosis and ultrastructural abnormalities. Genotyping was carried out in only a few patients, so it was often not possible to know whether PFIC1, PFIC2, or some other disorder was being treated. Further studies are needed to correlate the outcome of surgical therapy with the genotype of the patient. Mutational analysis may be used eventually to predict which patients are most likely to benefit from surgery.

Pharmacologic interruption of the enterohepatic circulation using bile acid transport inhibitors or potent bile acid sequestrants is a theoretical alternative to these surgical approaches [32]. Extreme caution should be considered with the latter approach as low intraluminal bile acid levels can predispose to severe fat-soluble vitamin deficiency with potentially life-threatening coagulopathy. Temporary endoscopic nasobiliary drainage was used to induce long-standing remissions in three adults with BRIC1 who had been refractory to medical therapies [38]. Pruritus disappeared within 24 hours, with normalization of serum bile acid concentrations. This approach might be useful in selected cases to help to determine whether a permanent surgical approach will be efficacious.

Ursodeoxycholic acid is frequently given to patients with PFIC1 and PFIC2 in a daily dosage of 10–20 mg/kg. Liver tests may improve, but the drug has little benefit in patients with severe pruritus [31]. Moreover, there is no evidence that UDCA alters the natural history of these disorders, including the need for biliary diversion or liver transplantation, or shortens the duration or frequency of episodes of BRIC.

Liver transplantation remains an option for the management of end-stage liver disease in PFIC and as an alternative approach in patients with refractory and severe pruritus [39]. In BSEP and MDR3 disease, in which the disease is hepatocyte specific, liver transplantation is usually a definitive approach. In contrast, in FIC1 disease, liver transplantation is potentially fraught with a number of potential complications related to the extrahepatic expression of *ATP8B1*. The most prominent post-transplantation problems include intractable diarrhea, hepatic steatosis, poor growth, and recurrent pancreatitis. The steatosis can be progressive, leading to cirrhosis in less than 10 years [8]. Interestingly, post-transplant steatosis and diarrhea was responsive to biliary diversion. Therefore, in FIC1 disease, non-transplantation surgical approaches should be considered the preferred first-line of therapy.

Ten children with PFIC2 have been reported who developed recurrent normal GGT cholestasis mimicking primary BSEP deficiency after liver transplantation [40]. Time to onset of biochemical low GGT, cholestasis, and histologic evidence of cholestasis without rejection ranged from 9 months to 17 years after liver transplantation [41]. As in their original disease, there is extensive giant cell transformation of hepatocytes on liver biopsy. When assay was possible, anti-BSEP antibodies were found in these patients that were not found in the serum of patients who had undergone transplantation for BSEP disease and who did not develop recurrence. Genotyping showed genetic defects in *ABCB11* that were predicted to lead to a congenital absence of BSEP protein. Therefore, pretransplant tolerance to native human BSEP by B-cells and/or T-cells was less likely to occur after its introduction in the allograft. Intensification of immunosuppression regimens were variably and typically only temporarily successful in treating recurrent cholestasis, and recurrent disease with circulating high-titer antibodies against BSEP usually occurred after retransplantation. In those cases where a second transplant was performed for "recurrent" disease, recurrence always ensued with progressive disease leading to death. Therefore, clinical decision making in children with BSEP disease manifest by absent BSEP protein is problematic. One must balance the ongoing risk of development of hepatocellular carcinoma in the native liver with the risk of recurrent disease in a new transplanted liver.

Progressive familial intrahepatic cholestasis type 3

Progressive familial intrahepatic cholestasis type 3 is an autosomal recessive disease with some clinical features that overlap with PFIC1 and PFIC2, particularly with presentation in early life, but it can be distinguished from these disorders by an elevation in serum GGT and by histologic findings of bile ductular proliferation, portal fibrosis, and inflammation with patency of the intra- and extrahepatic bile ducts [42–44]. These patients have a defect in biliary phospholipid secretion related to mutations in *ABCB4* (once known as *MDR3* and encoding the class III multidrug resistance P-glycoprotein MDR3). The spectrum of disease associated with this genetic defect has expanded to include distinct presentations in older children and adults.

Clinical features

Patients may present in infancy with jaundice, hepatomegaly, splenomegaly, and acholic stools. In contrast to PFIC1 and PFIC2, the age of symptom onset is extremely broad, ranging from 1 month to 20.5 years (mean, ~3.5 years). Patients with truncated proteins secondary to homozygous nonsense mutations present early, while homozygous or heterozygous missense mutations present later. In a series of 31 patients reported by Jacquemin *et al.* [45], clinical signs of cholestasis were uncommon in the neonate but were manifest by 1 year of age in one-third of patients. Pruritus occurs less frequently than in the other types of PFIC and is usually mild. Height and weight may be below normal as the disease progresses. Liver disease tends to evolve slowly to biliary cirrhosis with or without overt cholestatic jaundice. Splenomegaly is common, detected in 27 of 31 children at a mean age of 5.5 years (range, 8 months to 20.5 years). Esophageal varices were found in 19 patients at a mean age of 9 years (range, 5–20.5), leading to variceal hemorrhage in 9 children at a mean age of 11.5 years (range, 5–20.5). In 18 patients, liver transplantation was required at a mean of 7.5 years (range, 2–12.5) because of complications of portal hypertension, liver failure, or severe cholestasis [45]. Asymptomatic disease leading to cirrhosis, portal hypertension, and variceal bleeding in adolescent and young adults has also been reported. Cholangiography performed in a limited number of cases has been normal [45].

A single patient with PFIC3 has been described who developed hepatocellular carcinoma, but cholangiocarcinoma has not been reported. Regular screening in patients with PFIC3 for hepatic carcinoma is recommended.

Mutations in *ABCB4* may also cause low phospholipid associated cholelithiasis syndrome. Affected patients suffer from symptomatic cholesterol cholelithiasis, usually before age 40 years, along with intrahepatic sludge and microlithiasis [46]. These patients experience symptom recurrence, even after cholecystectomy, because of intrahepatic cholesterol deposits and bile duct inflammation. Affected patients often report a family history of cholesterol gallstones. Recurrence can be prevented by treatment with ursodeoxycholate [47]. Consistent with a defect in MDR3, bile analysis show cholesterol supersaturation together with low phospholipid concentration, resulting in a high cholesterol saturation index, which promotes cholesterol crystallization and stone formation.

A predisposition to develop gallstones in these patients is not surprising as phospholipids are the main carrier and solvent of cholesterol in hepatic bile [46]. In addition, patients with intrahepatic brown stones distinct from cholesterol stones have also been described with *ABCB4* mutations.

Approximately one-third of cases of intrahepatic cholestasis of pregnancy has been associated with heterozygous mutations in *ABCB4* [47–49]. Affected women appear to have adequate levels of *ABCB4* under normal conditions but become symptomatic under the physiologic stress of pregnancy. They develop generalized pruritus, rarely accompanied by jaundice, which is exacerbated late in gestation. These women may have subclinical or symptomatic steatorrhea, with weight loss and fat-soluble vitamin deficiencies. Serum alanine aminotransferase and bile acid concentrations are increased, while bilirubin is typically normal. The serum GGT level may be normal or increased. Pruritus may cause severe discomfort for the mother. Most concerning, however, is the significant risk intrahepatic cholestasis of pregnancy carries for the fetus, with high rates of prematurity and risk of fetal distress or stillbirth, often after 35 weeks of gestation [44]. Cholestasis recurs in 60–70% of subsequent pregnancies and may also occur during administration of oral contraceptives [48]. Fluctuation in both estrogen and progesterone may contribute to the symptomatic presentation, as evidenced by symptom development late in gestation, when hormone levels are high, resolving after delivery when hormone levels return to baseline, and being more frequent in twin pregnancies, in which higher hormone levels are present [44]. Prenatal mutation analysis in kinships known to be affected by intrahepatic cholestasis of pregnancy is available.

It has also been suggested that some cases of transient neonatal cholestasis may be related to heterozygous defects in canalicular ATP-dependent transport systems involved in bile formation, such as MDR3. Defects in MDR3 have also been reported in young adults with biliary fibrosis and cirrhosis [47,50].

Laboratory studies

The serum concentration of GGT is elevated in PFIC3, often more than 13 times the normal value, in contrast to PFIC1 and PFIC2. This distinguishes the disorder from the other forms of PFIC but not from other inherited and acquired cholestatic liver diseases in which the serum GGT is usually elevated. Other commonly used liver tests are variably elevated, including serum aminotransferases (5 times normal), conjugated bilirubin (2 times normal), and alkaline phosphatase (2 times normal). Serum cholesterol concentration is usually normal. The total serum bile acid concentration is elevated to as high as 25 times the normal value, but biliary bile acid concentrations are normal [42,44].

The cardinal feature of PFIC3 is a markedly reduced concentration of biliary phospholipid. In nine carefully studied patients with PFIC3, the mean biliary phospholipid

(a)

(b)

(c)

(d)

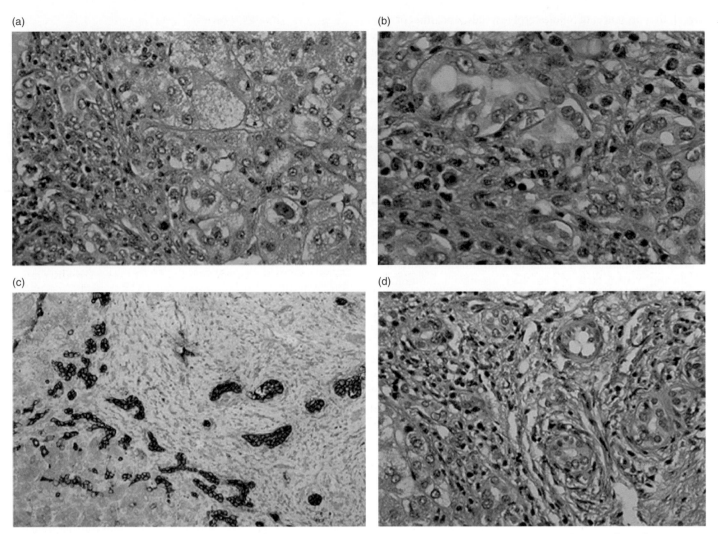

Figure 13.5 Histopathology of liver in a child with progressive familial intrahepatic cholestasis type 3. (a) Cholestatic hepatitis with giant cell transformation and isolated eosinophilic necrotic hepatocyte. Portal zone at the left shows bile ductular proliferation and mild mixed inflammatory infiltrate. (b) Bile ducts are increased in number, tortuous, and lined by swollen reactive epithelium. Inflammatory cells include lymphocytes, plasma cells, and occasional polymorphonuclear leukocytes. Bile stasis in ducts is absent. (c) A cytokeratin immunostain shows increased numbers of periportal ductules and interlobular bile ducts. (d) In type 3, progressive bile duct injury is associated with periductal fibroblast proliferation, as shown here, and eventually fibrosis. (Courtesy of Drs. Kevin Bove and James Heubi.)

concentration was 1.4 mmol/L, compared with 29.1 mmol/L in a group of control cholestatic children [45]. Ratios of biliary bile acid to phospholipid and cholesterol to phospholipid were approximately five-fold higher than in control samples.

Because measurement of biliary phospholipids is impractical in the evaluation of most patients, measurement of serum lipoprotein X may serve as a surrogate marker for PFIC3 and is available through several commercial clinical laboratories. Serum lipoprotein X is absent from the serum of patients with homozygous *ABCB4* mutations. Lipoprotein X is the predominant lipoprotein in the plasma of cholestatic patients. Lipoprotein X is probably composed of biliary vesicles that are formed at the subapical compartment of the hepatocyte, transcytosed to sinusoidal membrane, and released into plasma. This process is absolutely dependent on MDR3, but the precise mechanism has not been defined.

Molecular analysis of *ABCB4* may be used to confirm the diagnosis of PFIC3, low phospholipid associated cholelithiasis or intrahepatic cholestasis of pregnancy [42].

Histopathology

The morphology of PFIC3 is distinct from that of PFIC1 and PFIC2. Significant bile ductular proliferation and mixed inflammatory infiltrates (Figure 13.5) are observed in the early stages despite patency of intra- and extrahepatic bile ducts [43,45]. Cytokeratin immunostaining confirms marked bile ductular proliferation. Cholestasis with giant cell transformation and isolated eosinophilic necrotic hepatocytes may also be present. Periductal sclerosis affecting the interlobular bile ducts eventually occurs. Extensive portal fibrosis evolves into biliary cirrhosis in older children. Electron microscopy may reveal the presence of cholesterol crystals and loss of bile canalicular microvilli [43]. Bile canalicular immunostaining for MDR3 protein is variable and depends on the type of *ABCB4* mutation. Mutations leading to synthesis of a truncated protein show a complete absence of canalicular immunostaining for MDR3 protein [43] but missense mutations may demonstrate faint or normal MDR3 staining. Consequently, normal canalicular staining does not exclude the possibility of PFIC [43,44].

Genetics

ABCB4 is located on chromosome 7q21. In the largest reported series, 17 different *ABCB4* mutations were found in 22 of 31 patients with the PFIC3 phenotype [45]. Eleven missense mutations and six mutations predicted to yield a truncated protein were identified. Patients with homozygous mutations producing a truncated protein had negative immunohistochemical canalicular staining for MDR3 protein and no biliary phospholipid excretion. The lack of MDR3 protein may be the result of rapid breakdown of a truncated protein or a premature stop codon that causes instability and decay of *ABCB4* mRNA, as evidenced by minimal to undetectable *ABCB4* mRNA in the livers of some affected patients. However, MDR3 protein could be demonstrated in some patients with missense mutations and was associated with low but detectable amounts of biliary phospholipids. Most of these missense mutations were found in the highly conserved Walker A and Walker B motifs, essential for ATP binding, such that ATPase activity and membrane transport would be disrupted. Other missense mutations, located in transmembrane domains, might have effects on substrate binding, transport activity, and intracellular trafficking of MDR3 [33]. Residual MDR3 function in patients with missense mutations results in milder disease with later onset and slower progression.

Pathophysiology

The function of MDR3 was suggested by studies in mice with homozygous disruption of *Mdr2* (homologue of human *ABCB4*) [42,51]. The *Mdr2*$^{-/-}$ mice developed a cholangiopathy characterized histologically by bile ductular proliferation, portal inflammation, and progressive fibrosis. Hepatocellular carcinoma developed in mice surviving over 1 year. These mice had low to absent concentrations of biliary phosphatidylcholine but maintained normal bile salt secretion. Both human MDR3 and mouse Mdr2 (Figure 13.6) are members of the ATP-binding cassette family of transporters that serve as phospholipid flippases essential for biliary phospholipid secretion [42]. These transporters are located exclusively on the canalicular membrane of the hepatocyte and work in conjunction with the BSEP. The bile salt export pump moves bile salts from the hepatocyte into the canalicular lumen. Phosphatidylcholine is flipped from the cytoplasmic leaflet to the luminal side of the canalicular membrane by MDR3. Bile salts incorporate phosphatidylcholine that has

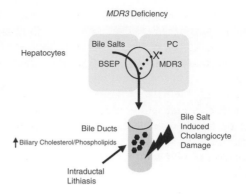

Figure 13.6 Pathophysiology of biliary tract disease in progressive familial intrahepatic cholestasis type 3 (multidrug resistance-associated protein 3 (MDR3) deficiency). Phosphatidylcholine (PC) in bile normally protects cholangiocytes from bile salt (BS) toxicity by forming mixed micelles. However, a mutation of the gene *ABCB4* encoding MDR3 results in decreased biliary PC secretion (dotted line) and high BS-to-PC ratio, leading to bile duct injury (cholangitis and ductular proliferation). A mutation of *ABCB4* also results in a decreased biliary PC concentration and high cholesterol (Chol)-to-PC ratio. The high biliary cholesterol saturation index promotes crystallization of cholesterol and the lithogenicity of bile.

been flipped to the outer leaflet either directly in contact with MDR3 or from projections of phosphatidylcholine from the luminal leaflet into small mixed phosphatidylcholine–bile salt micelles [52]. These micelles interact with the two cholesterol half-transporters of the ABC family (encoded by *ABCG5* and *ABCG8*, respectively), which transfers cholesterol partly into the aqueous phase so it can be captured by the micelles. Mixed bile salt/phosphatidylcholine/cholesterol micelles move down the biliary tract into the gallbladder and duodenum. These mixed micelles are thought to protect the canalicular and cholangiocyte membranes from bile acid-induced cell injury.

Fickert *et al.* provided direct evidence for cholangiocyte injury leading to an obliterative cholangitis in *Mdr2*$^{-/-}$ mice [53]. To visualize leakage of bile from the biliary tree, fluorescent-labeled UDCA was injected intravenously. There was disruption of tight junctions and basement membranes, with bile acid leakage into portal tracts of *Mdr2*$^{-/-}$ but not wild-type mice. The bile acid-induced injury led to the induction of a portal inflammatory (CD11b, CD4) infiltrate and activation of proinflammatory (tumor necrosis factor-α, interleukin-1β) and profibrogenic cytokines (transforming growth factor-β1) [53]. These mediators resulted in activation of periductal myofibroblasts, producing periductal fibrosis, the separation of the peribiliary plexus from cholangiocytes, and eventually atrophy and death of the cholangiocytes. Although non-micellar toxic bile acids may directly produce chemical/detergent damage to bile ducts, these studies indicate that the peribiliary vascular plexus may be displaced from the biliary epithelium by the expanding fibrotic bands, leading to ischemic ductal injury.

Whereas biliary bile salt concentrations are normal in patients with PFIC3, serum bile salt levels are elevated. Downregulation of transporters involved in bile acid uptake, including the sodium-cotransporting peptide (NTCP) and several members of the organic anion-transporting polypeptide family, explains in part the elevated serum bile acid levels in this disorder. In contrast, the multi-drug resistance protein 4 (MRP4) is strongly upregulated at the mRNA and protein level, mediating bile salt efflux into serum. It is not known how and why bile salts are directed to MRP4 rather than to the canalicular BSEP, which is expressed normally in PFIC3.

In addition, expression of *Abcb4* in rodents can be induced through the regulation of FXR. The homologous human gene *ABCB4* also has a functional FXR response element [44]. In rodents, fibrates also induce *Abcb4*, mediated by peroxisome proliferator activated receptor-α [44].

Treatment

Patients with PFIC3 should receive nutritional support including supplements of fat-soluble vitamins. Pruritus is usually mild in this condition and may not require specific therapy. Oral administration of UDCA appears to be of value, with normalization of liver tests in approximately 60% of patients [42,44]. The rationale underlying this therapy is that enrichment of bile with this hydrophilic bile acid reduces cytotoxic injury to hepatocytes and bile ducts and stimulates bile flow. In the $Mdr2^{-/-}$ mouse model, feeding of UDCA led to significant improvement in liver disease. Jacquemin *et al.* [45] found that UDCA was effective in some patients with *ABCB4* missense mutations who maintained residual biliary phospholipid secretion. There was no improvement, however, in patients with nonsense mutations, who have a complete lack of biliary phospholipids. These patients progress to biliary cirrhosis and liver failure at a variable rate and ultimately require liver transplantation [42,44]. In addition to cadaveric transplant, living related donor transplant from *ABCB4* heterozygotes can be performed without adverse outcomes in transplant recipients.

Hepatocyte transplantation has also shown promise in *Mdr2* (homologue of *ABCB4*) knockout mice, although it has not been studied in humans. Transgenic *MDR3*-expressing hepatocytes as well as normal $Mdr2^{+/+}$ hepatocytes have been transplanted in $Mdr2^{-/-}$ mice. Transplanted hepatocytes partially repopulated the liver, restored phospholipid secretion, and diminished liver pathology. A similar approach may be considered for treatment of patients with PFIC3. Partial external biliary diversion, widely used in PFIC1 and PFIC2, is not recommended for PFIC3.

Intrahepatic cholestasis of pregnancy is best treated by delivery, after which symptoms resolve within 2 weeks [44]. Delivery of affected pregnancies by 36–38 weeks, depending on severity of disease, has been recommended. Prior to this, UDCA may provide symptomatic relief [44]. Studies using *S*-adenosylmethionine, involved in phosphatidylcholine synthesis, either alone or in combination with UDCA remain inconclusive [54].

Patients with low phospholipid associated cholelithiasis syndrome may also respond to treatment with long-term UDCA [42,44]. In addition, animal models suggest that drugs that increase MDR3 expression via FXR (such as 6α-hydroxylated bile salts), cholesterol biosynthesis inhibitors (such as hydroxymethylglutaryl-CoA reductase inhibitors) and drugs such as fibrates that upregulate transcription of *ABCB4* via peroxisome proliferator activated receptor-α may be of benefit in the treatment of low phospholipid associated cholelithiasis syndrome, but require careful human studies [44]. Finally, the approach of inducing other canalicular proteins that would functionally complement MDR3 has also been suggested.

Hereditary cholestasis with lymphedema

Patients of Norwegian decent with intrahepatic cholestasis and lymphedema have been described. The disease is not limited to Norwegians and has been reported in Italian, Japanese, and English children. The cause of this syndrome and the relation between peripheral lymphatic obstruction and cholestatic liver disease remain unknown. It has been suggested that deficiency of intrahepatic lymphatics contributes to the cholestasis [55]. Study of reported cases supports an autosomal recessive mode of inheritance. There is one report, however, of a mother and child with the disease, suggesting autosomal dominant inheritance. The locus (LS1) for the disorder, at least in Norwegian patients, has been mapped to a 6.6 centimorgan interval on chromosome 15q. All Norwegian patients are likely homozygous for the same disease mutation, inherited from a shared ancestor. A second locus has been proposed based on a report of a Serbian–Romanian patient with features atypical of the Norwegian form of the disease. The patient had low serum cholesterol and GGT concentrations and progressed rapidly to end-stage liver disease. The disorder did not map to the *LCS1*, *ATP8B1*, and *ABCB11* loci.

The clinical course in the first months of life is dominated by cholestasis with malabsorption. Jaundice appears in most patients within 2–4 weeks of life and always before 2 months. The stools are usually acholic. Growth and weight gain may be poor during infancy. Lymphedema is rarely present at birth or at the time patients initially are found to be cholestatic. Lymphedema is observed in the lower extremities, usually in early childhood, and has been attributed to lymphatic vessel hypoplasia.

The cholestatic liver disease tends to improve with age, with most patients having a normal serum bilirubin concentration by 3 or 4 years of age [56]. Serum bile acid concentrations may remain elevated even after jaundice improves. Serum aminotransferase levels may be high during the first year of life but gradually return to the normal range before school age. Serum GGT is increased only modestly in this syndrome, about twice the upper normal value [55]. These patients, however, may have an exaggerated increase in GGT after treatment with phenobarbital. Cholestasis occurs episodically in older children, with cholestatic periods lasting 2–6 months. Puberty and pregnancy seem to be important initiators of cholestatic episodes later in life. The liver disease tends to be mild in most patients, but several older children and adults have progressed to cirrhosis [56]. Two siblings with particularly marked cholestasis, including severe pruritus and hepatic fibrosis, responded well to partial cutaneous biliary diversion (PF Whitington, unpublished observations). Neither has had progression of liver disease in more than 16 years of follow-up.

Liver histopathology in early childhood shows massive giant cell transformation of hepatocytes and intracellular retention of bile pigment. Patients in clinical remission may have liver morphology close to normal. Some patients may have bile plugs and a slight increase in portal fibrosis. Of 26 patients reported by Aagenaes [56], four have developed biopsy-proven cirrhosis. A 50-year-old woman with cirrhosis developed hepatocellular carcinoma.

Treatment is limited to avoiding complications of malabsorption during episodes of cholestasis, particularly fat-soluble vitamin deficiency. Lymphedema tends to become the dominant symptom of disease later in life and may be disabling in some patients. It may improve later in life and can be controlled in some patients by symptomatic treatment such as physiotherapy and wrapping of the lower extremities.

The ARC syndrome: arthrogryposis multiplex congenita, renal dysfunction, and cholestasis

Severe cholestasis may occur in association with arthrogryposis multiplex congenita and renal disease (ARC syndrome) [57]. The neurogenic muscular atrophy is related to rarefaction of the anterior horn cells of the spinal cord. Additional cerebral manifestations may be observed if the patient survives infancy, including severe developmental delay, hypotonia, nerve deafness, poor feeding, microcephaly, and defects of the corpus callosum. An increased risk of bleeding is caused by platelet dysfunction. The cholestatic liver disease is usually present at birth. An unexpected finding in these patients has been the normal serum concentration of GGT. Some patients have cholestasis and pigmentary change in the liver, similar to the Dubin–Johnson syndrome. Other patients have had paucity of intrahepatic bile ducts and giant cell transformation of hepatocytes as the predominant features. Bile duct paucity and lipofuscin disposition may be seen in a wide range of liver diseases and probably represent non-specific changes resulting from a common insult. Pigmentary change, bile duct paucity, and giant cell transformation may coexist in some patients. The varying liver histology probably represents a spectrum of injury found in the same disorder. With survival beyond infancy, progressive cholestasis and paucity of intrahepatic bile ducts may occur in this disorder, with progression to cirrhosis. Patients also may develop renal tubular cell degeneration with nephrocalcinosis.

The pattern of inheritance deduced from reported cases has been consistent with an autosomal recessive trait. The gene for the disorder was localized to chromosome 15q26.1. Fourteen affected kindreds were then used to identify germline mutations in the gene VPS33B, which is a homologue of the class C yeast vacuolar protein sorting gene Vps33, the product of which is involved in vacuolar biogenesis and the late stages of protein trafficking from the Golgi to the vacuole [58]. Consistent with the protean manifestations of the disorder, VPS33B is widely expressed in fetal and adult tissues. In liver biopsy specimens from patients with ARC syndrome, there was a marked disturbance in localization of plasma membrane proteins, including carcinoembryonic antigen, dipeptidyl peptidase and GGT, suggesting a defect in regulation of intracellular protein trafficking. There is a recent report of a patient with cholestasis, neurologic defects, ichthyosis, and aminoaciduria who was homozygous for a novel VPS33 mutation but did not have arthrogryposis.

North American Indian cholestasis

Thirty North American Indian children have been documented with a severe non-syndromic form of intrahepatic cholestasis [59]. The disorder is inherited as an autosomal recessive trait. Cholestatic jaundice was present in 21 (70%) within the neonatal period. Clinical jaundice disappeared in most patients during the first year of life, but the conjugated fraction of bilirubin was elevated in 75% by the age of 1 year. The serum concentration of GGT was also elevated. Other patients presented with no history of jaundice but initially were seen for gastrointestinal bleeding or for hepatomegaly later in childhood. Ongoing cholestasis was associated with chronic pruritus, persistent elevation of serum aminotransferase, serum alkaline phosphatase, and serum bile acid concentrations [59]. Normal or moderately increased serum cholesterol levels were found in most patients. Progression to periportal fibrosis and cirrhosis was typical in childhood and adolescence. Early onset of portal hypertension and variceal hemorrhage necessitated portosystemic shunts in 13 of the 30 children. Ten of fourteen deaths were related to chronic liver disease. Liver transplantation is the only effective therapy.

Giant cell hepatitis, bile stasis, and neoductular proliferation characterized histopathology early in the course of the disorder. Later, portal fibrosis became evident and was followed by rapid progression to biliary cirrhosis. The electron microscopic changes were initially thought to be distinctive. Bile canaliculi appeared slightly dilated, with preservation or partial loss of microvilli. There was marked widening of the pericanalicular ectoplasm with abundant pericanalicular microfilaments [59]. Immunofluorescence microscopy confirmed that the prominent pericanalicular filamentous web was composed of actin-containing microfilaments. Because these contractile proteins may be involved in canalicular motility and generation of bile flow, microfilament dysfunction was proposed as the cause of cholestasis in these children. These findings have been questioned and now are thought to be non-specific and secondary to cholestatic injury, perhaps a cholangiopathy. The hepatic ultrastructure cannot be reliably distinguished from other inherited forms of cholestasis [59].

The gene for the disorder was mapped to chromosome 16q22 and recently identified [60]. The product of this gene, called cirhin, is a protein of 686 amino acid residues with unknown function. Cirhin is preferentially synthesized in embryonic liver and has been localized to the nucleolus [60]. The disease-causing mutation, leading to a R565W change, is thought to change the predicted secondary structure of cirhin but has no effect on its nucleolar localization.

Familial hypercholanemia

Most patients with familial hypercholanemia are of Amish descent and present with pruritus, malabsorption, poor growth, and, in some cases, bleeding and rickets from deficiency of vitamins K and D, respectively [61]. The disorder is inherited as an autosomal recessive trait. Serum bile acids are elevated and may fluctuate significantly. Serum bilirubin, GGT, and cholesterol levels are usually normal. Serum aminotransferase levels are normal to slightly increased. Liver histology is available for only a few patients and may be normal or show a mild reactive hepatitis or canalicular cholestasis [61]. Symptoms usually respond to treatment with UDCA.

The phenotype in these patients initially suggested a possible defect in uptake of conjugated bile acids across the basolateral membrane of the hepatocyte. However, expression of mRNA and protein synthesis for NTCP was normal in liver biopsy specimens from two affected children and NTCP could also be detected on the basolateral membrane by indirect immunofluorescent microscopy. Moreover, no mutations were found on complete sequencing of the coding regions of SLC10A1, encoding NTCP, in both patients.

Recent studies of 17 Amish individuals from 12 families with familial hypercholanemia have identified mutations in genes encoding the tight junction protein 2 (TJP2) and the bile acid-CoA:amino acid N-acyltransferase (BAAT) [61].

Eleven patients were homozygous for a mutation in TJP2 and five were homozygous for a mutation in BAAT. Five individuals who were homozygous for a mutation in TJP2 also carried a BAAT mutation in one allele. One individual who was homozygous for a mutation in BAAT also carried a TJP2 mutation in one allele.

Tight junction protein 2 participates in the formation of intercellular barriers separating bile from blood and controlling paracellular solute diffusion. It is proposed that mutations in TJP2 increase paracellular permeability to bile acids and probably other small molecules. This "short circuiting" with leakage of bile acids into blood is likely to adversely affect bile flow and result in intestinal concentrations of bile acids inadequate for micelle formation and normal absorption of dietary fat and fat-soluble vitamins.

Bile acid-CoA:amino acid N-acyltransferase mediates conjugation of bile acids with glycine and taurine. Unconjugated bile acids are poor substrates for transport by NTCP and BSEP and for the nuclear receptor FXR that regulates bile acid homeostasis in the liver and intestine [61]. It is proposed that unconjugated bile acids diffuse back into blood and less so into bile, leading to high serum and low biliary bile acid concentrations.

Conclusions

The progress made in our understanding of inherited cholestatic liver diseases has been dramatic. New insights into hepatobiliary physiology and the behavior of liver transport proteins in acquired liver disease have also come from studies on PFIC. It is uncertain whether the heterozygous state or polymorphisms in the genes underlying these disorders can be associated with liver disease or affect the outcome of other forms of cholestasis, such as biliary atresia. Moreover, at least 30% of patients with low-GGT forms of PFIC and BRIC have no mutations in ATP8B1 and ABCB11. Additional work is required to discover the genetic basis and define the pathophysiology of these disorders [26].

References

1. Clayton RJ, Iber FL, Ruebner BH, McKusick VA. Byler disease. Fatal familial intrahepatic cholestasis in an Amish kindred. *J. Pediatr* 1965;**67**:1025–1028.

2. Summerskill WHJ, Walshe JM. Benign recurrent intrahepatic "obstructive" jaundice. *Lancet* 1959;**ii**:686–690.

3. Carlton VEH, Knisely AS, Freimer NB. Mapping of a locus for progressive familial intrahepatic cholestasis (Byler disease) to 18q21-q22, the benign recurrent intrahepatic cholestasis region. *Hum Mol Genet* 1995;**4**:1049–1053.

4. van Mil SW, Klomp LW, Bull LN, Houwen RH. FIC1 disease: a spectrum of intrahepatic cholestatic disorders. *Semin Liver Dis* 2001;**21**:535–544.

5. Klomp LW, Vargas JC, van Mil SW, et al. Characterization of mutations in ATP8B1 associated with hereditary cholestasis. *Hepatology* 2004;**40**:27–38.

6. Pawlikowska L, Strautnieks S, Jankowska I, et al. Differences in presentation and progression between severe FIC1 and BSEP deficiencies. *J Hepatol* 2010;**53**:170–178.

7. Davit-Spraul A, Fabre M, Branchereau S, et al. ATP8B1 and ABCB11 analysis in 62 children with normal gamma-glutamyl transferase progressive familial intrahepatic cholestasis (PFIC): phenotypic differences between PFIC1 and PFIC2 and natural history. *Hepatology* 2010;**51**:1645–1655.

8. Miyagawa-Hayashino A, Egawa H, Yorifuji T, et al. Allograft steatohepatitis in progressive familial intrahepatic cholestasis type 1 after living donor liver transplantation. *Liver Transpl* 2009;**15**:610–618.

9. Luketic VA, Shiffman ML. Benign recurrent intrahepatic cholestasis. *Clin Liver Dis* 2004;**8**:133–149, vii.

10. Morotti RA, Suchy FJ, Magid MS. Progressive familial intrahepatic

cholestasis (PFIC) type 1, 2, and 3: a review of the liver pathology findings. *Semin Liver Dis* 2011;**31**:3–10.

11. Knisely AS, Gissen P. Trafficking and transporter disorders in pediatric cholestasis. *Clin Liver Dis* 2010;**14**:619–633.

12. Bull LN, van Eijk MJT, Pawlikowska L, *et al*. Identification of a P-type ATPase mutated in two forms of hereditary cholestasis. *Nat Genet* 1998;**18**:219–224.

13. Frankenberg T, Miloh T, Chen FY, *et al*. The membrane protein ATPase class I type 8B member 1 signals through protein kinase C zeta to activate the farnesoid X receptor. *Hepatology* 2008;**48**:1896–1905.

14. van der Velden LM, Stapelbroek JM, Krieger E, *et al*. Folding defects in P-type ATP 8B1 associated with hereditary cholestasis are ameliorated by 4-phenylbutyrate. *Hepatology* 2010;**51**:286–296.

15. Pawlikowska L, Groen A, Eppens EF, *et al*. A mouse genetic model for familial cholestasis caused by ATP8B1 mutations reveals perturbed bile salt homeostasis but no impairment in bile secretion. *Hum Mol Genet* 2004;**13**:881–892.

16. Groen A, Kunne C, Paulusma CC, *et al*. Intestinal bile salt absorption in Atp8b1 deficient mice. *J Hepatol* 2007;**47**:114–122.

17. Paulusma CC, Groen A, Kunne C, *et al*. Atp8b1 deficiency in mice reduces resistance of the canalicular membrane to hydrophobic bile salts and impairs bile salt transport. *Hepatology* 2006;**44**:195–204.

18. Stapelbroek JM, Peters TA, van Beurden DH, *et al*. ATP8B1 is essential for maintaining normal hearing. *Proc Natl Acad Sci USA* 2009;**106**:9709–9714.

19. Ray NB, Durairaj L, Chen BB, *et al*. Dynamic regulation of cardiolipin by the lipid pump Atp8b1 determines the severity of lung injury in experimental pneumonia. *Nat Med* 2010;**16**:1120–1127.

20. Ujhazy P, Ortiz D, Misra S, *et al*. Familial intrahepatic cholestasis 1: studies of localization and function. *Hepatology* 2001;**34**:768–775.

21. Paulusma CC, Folmer DE, Ho-Mok KS, *et al*. ATP8B1 requires an accessory protein for endoplasmic reticulum exit and plasma membrane lipid flippase activity. *Hepatology* 2008;**47**:268–278.

22. Paulusma CC, de Waart DR, Kunne C, Mok KS, Elferink RP. Activity of the bile salt export pump (ABCB11) is critically dependent on canalicular membrane cholesterol content. *J Biol Chem* 2009;**284**:9947–9954.

23. Groen A, Romero MR, Kunne C, *et al*. Complementary functions of the flippase ATP8B1 and the floppase ABCB4 in maintaining canalicular membrane integrity. *Gastroenterology* 2011;**141**:1927–37 e1–4.

24. Verhulst PM, van der Velden LM, Oorschot V, *et al*. A flippase-independent function of ATP8B1, the protein affected in familial intrahepatic cholestasis type 1, is required for apical protein expression and microvillus formation in polarized epithelial cells. *Hepatology* 2010;**51**:2049–2060.

25. van Mil SW, van Oort MM, van den Berg IE, *et al*. Fic1 is expressed at apical membranes of different epithelial cells in the digestive tract and is induced in the small intestine during postnatal development of mice. *Pediatr Res* 2004;**56**:981–987.

26. Chen F, Ananthanarayanan M, Emre S, *et al*. Progressive familial intrahepatic cholestasis, type 1, is associated with decreased farnesoid X receptor activity. *Gastroenterology* 2004;**126**:756–764.

27. Chen F, Ellis E, Strom SC, Shneider BL. ATPase class I type 8B member 1 and protein kinase Czeta induce the expression of the canalicular bile salt export pump in human hepatocytes. *Pediatr Res* 2010;**67**:183–187.

28. Strautnieks SS, Byrne JA, Pawlikowska L, *et al*. Severe bile salt export pump deficiency: 82 different *ABCB11* mutations in 109 families. *Gastroenterology* 2008;**134**:1203–1214.

29. Lam P, Soroka CJ, Boyer JL. The bile salt export pump: clinical and experimental aspects of genetic and acquired cholestatic liver disease. *Semin Liver Dis* 2010;**30**:125–133.

30. Jansen PL, Strautnieks SS, Jacquemin E, *et al*. Hepatocanalicular bile salt export pump deficiency in patients with progressive familial intrahepatic cholestasis. *Gastroenterology* 1999;**117**:1370–1379.

31. Davit-Spraul A, Gonzales E, Baussan C, Jacquemin E. Progressive familial intrahepatic cholestasis. *Orphanet J Rare Dis* 2009;**4**:1.

32. Alissa FT, Jaffe R, Shneider BL. Update on progressive familial intrahepatic cholestasis. *J Pediatr Gastroenterol Nutr* 2008;**46**:241–252.

33. Dixon PH, Weerasekera N, Linton KJ, *et al*. Heterozygous *MDR3* missense mutation associated with intrahepatic cholestasis of pregnancy: evidence for a defect in protein trafficking. *Hum Mol Genet* 2000;**9**:1209–1217.

34. Thompson R, Strautnieks S. BSEP: function and role in progressive familial intrahepatic cholestasis. *Semin Liver Dis* 2001;**21**:545–550.

35. Byrne JA, Strautnieks SS, Ihrke G, *et al*. Missense mutations and single nucleotide polymorphisms in *ABCB11* impair bile salt export pump processing and function or disrupt pre-messenger RNA splicing. *Hepatology* 2009;**49**:553–567.

36. Kurbegov AC, Setchell KD, Haas JE, *et al*. Biliary diversion for progressive familial intrahepatic cholestasis: improved liver morphology and bile acid profile. *Gastroenterology* 2003;**125**:1227–1234.

37. Whitington PF, Whitington GL. Partial external diversion of bile for the treatment of intractable pruritus associated with intrahepatic cholestasis. *Gastroenterology* 1988;**95**:130–136.

38. Stapelbroek JM, van Erpecum KJ, Klomp LW, *et al*. Nasobiliary drainage induces long-lasting remission in benign recurrent intrahepatic cholestasis. *Hepatology* 2006;**43**:51–53.

39. Shneider BL. Liver transplantation for progressive familial intrahepatic cholestasis: the evolving role of genotyping. *Liver Transplant* 2009;**15**:565–566.

40. Jara P, Hierro L, Martinez-Fernandez P, *et al*. Recurrence of bile salt export pump deficiency after liver transplantation. *N Engl J Med* 2009;**361**:1359–1367.

41. Siebold L, Dick AA, Thompson R, *et al*. Recurrent low gamma-glutamyl transpeptidase cholestasis following liver transplantation for bile salt export pump (BSEP) disease (posttransplant recurrent BSEP disease). *Liver Transplant* 2010;**16**:856–863.

42. Davit-Spraul A, Gonzales E, Baussan C, Jacquemin E. The spectrum of liver diseases related to *ABCB4* gene

mutations: pathophysiology and clinical aspects. *Semin Liver Dis* 2010; **30**:134–146.

43. Morotti RA, Suchy FJ, Magid MS. Progressive familial intrahepatic cholestasis (PFIC) type 1, 2, and 3: a review of the liver pathology findings. *Semin Liver Dis* 2011; **31**:3–10.

44. Sundaram SS, Sokol RJ. The Multiple facets of ABCB4 (MDR3) deficiency. *Curr Treat Options Gastroenterol* 2007;**10**:495–503.

45. Jacquemin E, De Vree JM, Cresteil D, *et al.* The wide spectrum of multidrug resistance 3 deficiency: from neonatal cholestasis to cirrhosis of adulthood. *Gastroenterology* 2001;**120**:1448–1458.

46. Rosmorduc O, Hermelin B, Poupon R. *MDR3* gene defect in adults with symptomatic intrahepatic and gallbladder cholesterol cholelithiasis. *Gastroenterology* 2001;**120**:1459–1467.

47. Lucena JF, Herrero JI, Quiroga J, *et al.* A multidrug resistance 3 gene mutation causing cholelithiasis, cholestasis of pregnancy, and adulthood biliary cirrhosis. *Gastroenterology* 2003;**124**:1037–1042.

48. Jacquemin E, Cresteil D, Manouvrier S, Boute O, Hadchouel M. Heterozygous non-sense mutation of the *MDR3* gene in familial intrahepatic cholestasis of pregnancy. *Lancet* 1999;**353**:210–211.

49. Schneider G, Paus TC, Kullak-Ublick GA, *et al.* Linkage between a new splicing site mutation in the *MDR3* alias

ABCB4 gene and intrahepatic cholestasis of pregnancy. *Hepatology* 2007;**45**:150–158.

50. Ziol M, Barbu V, Rosmorduc O, *et al.* *ABCB4* heterozygous gene mutations associated with fibrosing cholestatic liver disease in adults. *Gastroenterology* 2008;**135**:131–141.

51. Smit JJ, Schinkel AH, Oude Elferink RP, *et al.* Homozygous disruption of the murine Mdr2 P-glycoprotein gene leads to a complete absence of phospholipid from bile and to liver disease. *Cell* 1993;**75**:451–462.

52. Small DM. Role of ABC transporters in secretion of cholesterol from liver into bile. *Proc Natl Acad Sci USA* 2003;**100**:4–6.

53. Fickert P, Fuchsbichler A, Wagner M, *et al.* Regurgitation of bile acids from leaky bile ducts causes sclerosing cholangitis in *Mdr2* (*Abcb4*) knockout mice. *Gastroenterology* 2004;**127**:261–274.

54. Binder T, Salaj P, Zima T, Vitek L. Randomized prospective comparative study of ursodeoxycholic acid and S-adenosyl-L-methionine in the treatment of intrahepatic cholestasis of pregnancy. *J Perinat Med* 2006;**34**:383–391.

55. Drivdal M, Trydal T, Hagve TA, Bergstad I, Aagenaes O. Prognosis, with evaluation of general biochemistry, of liver disease in lymphoedema cholestasis syndrome 1 (LCS1/Aagenaes

syndrome). *Scand J Gastroenterol* 2006;**41**:465–471.

56. Aagenaes O. Hereditary cholestasis with lymphoedema (Aagenaes syndrome, cholestasis-lymphoedema syndrome). New cases and follow-up from infancy to adult age. *Scand J Gastroenterol* 1998;**33**:335–345.

57. Nezelof C, Dupart MC, Jaubert F, Eliachar E. A lethal familial syndrome associating arthrogryposis multiplex congenita, renal dysfunction, and a cholestatic and pigmentary liver disease. *J Pediatr* 1979;**94**:258–260.

58. Gissen P, Johnson CA, Morgan NV, *et al.* Mutations in *VPS33B*, encoding a regulator of SNARE-dependent membrane fusion, cause arthrogryposis–renal dysfunction–cholestasis (ARC) syndrome. *Nat Genet* 2004;**36**:400–404.

59. Drouin E, Russo P, Tuchweber B, Mitchell G, Rasquin-Weber A. North American Indian cirrhosis in children: a review of 30 cases. *J Pediatr Gastroenterol Nutr* 2000;**31**:395–404.

60. Chagnon P, Michaud J, Mitchell G, *et al.* A missense mutation (R565W) in cirhin (*FLJ14728*) in North American Indian childhood cirrhosis. *Am J Hum Genet* 2002;**71**:1443–1449.

61. Carlton VE, Harris BZ, Puffenberger EG, *et al.* Complex inheritance of familial hypercholanemia with associated mutations in *TJP2* and *BAAT*. *Nat Genet* 2003;**34**:91–96.

Alagille syndrome

Binita M. Kamath, Nancy B. Spinner, and David A. Piccoli

Introduction

Alagille syndrome (ALGS) is an autosomal dominant, multi-system disorder which was first described in 1969 by Daniel Alagille as a constellation of clinical features in five different organ systems [1]. The diagnosis was based on the presence of intrahepatic bile duct paucity on liver biopsy in association with at least three of the major clinical features: chronic cholestasis, cardiac disease (most often peripheral pulmonary stenosis), skeletal abnormalities (typically butterfly vertebrae), ocular abnormalities (primarily posterior embryotoxon), and characteristic facial features. Advances in molecular diagnostics have enabled an appreciation of the broader disease phenotype with recognition of renal and vascular involvement [2,3]. There is significant variability in the extent to which each of these systems is affected in an individual, if at all [4,5]. It was originally estimated that ALGS had a frequency of 1 in 70 000 live births, although this was based on the presence of neonatal cholestasis. However, this is clearly an underestimate as molecular testing has demonstrated that many individuals with a disease-causing mutation do not have neonatal liver disease and the true frequency is likely closer to 1 in 30 000 [5].

Alagille syndrome is caused by mutations in *JAGGED1* (*JAG1*), encoding a ligand Jagged1 in the Notch signaling pathway [6,7]. Mutations in *JAG1* are identified in 94% of clinically defined probands [8]. Recently, mutations in *NOTCH2* have been identified in a few patients with ALGS who do not have *JAG1* mutations [9]. This exciting development has enhanced our understanding of the heterogeneity of this disorder, although much remains to be understood about the tremendous variability seen in affected individuals and the likely genetic modifiers involved.

Clinical features

A strikingly large number of abnormalities have been associated with ALGS. These problems are best organized into those features that are structural defects in the embryogenesis of the fetus or postnatal infant, functional defects resulting from abnormalities of embryogenesis, or complications of long-standing anatomic or biochemical abnormalities. The last are not truly features of the syndrome, but quite commonly are substantial problems. For example, the hepatic duct paucity is a result of a defect in organogenesis, but the coagulopathy is commonly a complication of fat malabsorption or end-stage liver disease. The severe limitations in height seen in many patients may be a feature of the skeletal development seen in ALGS or a complication of malnutrition, although clearly the two may coexist. Similarly, the marked increase in long-bone fractures may result from an intrinsic abnormality of bone structure and development in ALGS, or be a complication of vitamin D and nutrient malabsorption, or a combination of both issues.

There are several large series of patients with ALGS reported, and the characteristics of the disease are slightly divergent with respect to disease severity (Table 14.1) [2,10–14]. This likely reflects the differences in (1) dates of the reports, with treatment strategies changing over time; (2) evolving interpretation of the features and complications of the disorder; and (3) the characteristics of the reporting medical center. The tertiary nature of an institution and the availability of liver and cardiac transplantation at those centers influence the apparent severity of the disorder in each of these studies. These reports are weighted with the severely affected index cases in families and thus there is a high prevalence of clinical features, particularly hepatic disease (Table 14.1). Kamath *et al.* [5] studied the feature frequency and morbidity in mutation-positive relatives separately, thereby excluding the severely affected index cases. In mutation-positive relatives, the presence of significant cardiac and hepatic disease was less than in the probands. In the relatives, the frequency of liver disease was only 31%, compared with 97% in the probands, and 45% of the relatives had no clinical or biochemical hepatic involvement at all. Therefore, the clinical consequence of carrying a *JAG1* mutation is less severe than previously thought, and the disease certainly seems to have a better overall outcome [15]. This point is important for genetic counseling.

Liver Disease in Children, Fourth Edition, ed. Frederick J. Suchy, Ronald J. Sokol, and William F. Balistreri. Published by Cambridge University Press. © Cambridge University Press 2014.

Table 14.1 Clinical features of Alagille syndrome from reported series

	Alagille *et al.* (1987) [10]	Deprettere *et al.* (1987) [11]	Hoffenberg *et al.* (1995) [12]	Emerick *et al.* (1999) [2]	Quiros-Tejeira *et al.* (1999) [13]	Subramaniam *et al.* (2011) [14]
No. of patients	80	27	26	92	43	117
Bile duct paucity (%)	100	81	80	85	83	75
Cholestasis (%)	91	93	100	96	100	89
Murmur (%)	85	96	96	97	98	91
Vertebral anomalies (%)	87	33	48	51	38	37
Facies (%)	95	70	92	96	98	77
Ocular anomalies (%)	88	56	85	78	73	61
Renal involvement (%)	73	-	19	40	50	23
Intracranial bleeding (%)	-	-	12	14	12	-

Hepatic features

The majority of patients with ALGS who are symptomatic with liver disease present in the first year of life. The hepatic manifestations typically vary from mild to severe cholestasis. Hepatitis (elevated alanine and aspartate aminotransferases) is present in many infants but generally is less important than the cholestasis. Synthetic liver failure is extremely uncommon in the first year of life. Hepatomegaly is recognized in 93–100% of patients with ALGS and is common in infancy [2,10]. Splenomegaly is unusual early in the course of the disease but eventually is found in up to 70% of patients [2]. Jaundice is present in the majority of symptomatic patients and typically presents as a conjugated hyperbilirubinemia in the neonatal period. The magnitude of the hyperbilirubinemia is typically less than the degrees of cholestasis and pruritus. The pruritus seen is among the most severe of any chronic liver disease. It rarely is present before 3–5 months of age but is seen in most children by the third year of life, even in some who are anicteric.

The most striking laboratory abnormalities are in the measures of cholestasis and bile duct damage. Elevations of serum bilirubin up to 30 times normal and serum bile salt elevations of 100 times normal are not uncommon. Bile salt elevations are common, even if the bilirubin concentration is normal. Levels of markers of bile duct damage, including gamma-glutamyltransferase and alkaline phosphatase, are usually significantly elevated. The amounts of other substances typically excreted in bile are also increased in blood. Cholesterol levels may exceed 1000–2000 mg/dL. The aminotransferases are typically elevated three- to ten-fold but may be normal in some patients with cholestasis. Hepatic synthetic function is usually well preserved.

Multiple xanthomas are common sequelae of severe cholestasis (Figure 14.1). The timing for the formation of xanthomas relates to the severity of the cholestasis and correlates with a serum cholesterol >500 mg/dL. They typically form on the extensor surfaces of the fingers, the palmar creases, the nape of the neck, the ears, the popliteal fossa, the buttocks, and around the inguinal creases (Figure 14.1). These xanthomas increase in number over the first few years of life and may disappear subsequently as cholestasis improves.

The natural history of the liver disease in ALGS has a unique course. For those children with significant cholestasis in infancy, the hepatic involvement generally follows a more severe course in the first 5 years of life after which it appears to improve for most patients. This spontaneous improvement is poorly understood, but well documented. In approximately 10–20%, the cholestasis persists unabated or progresses to end-stage liver disease. For those children with mild cholestasis or hepatitis in early childhood, there is no progression of liver disease in later life. It is difficult to prognosticate early on which ALGS children with cholestasis in early childhood will eventually require liver transplantation and who will spontaneously improve. There are no known genotypic or radiologic predictors of liver disease progression in ALGS. A recent review of laboratory data of patients with ALGS recently showed that high bilirubin and cholesterol levels before the age of 5 years may aid in distinguishing high- from low-risk patients. More specifically, total bilirubin >6.5 mg/dL (111 μmol/L), conjugated bilirubin >4.5 mg/dL (77 μmol/L), and cholesterol >520 mg/dL (13.3 mmol/L) are strongly associated with severe liver disease in later life whereas levels lower than this are associated with a good hepatic outcome [16]. These data may assist the clinician in predicting which children

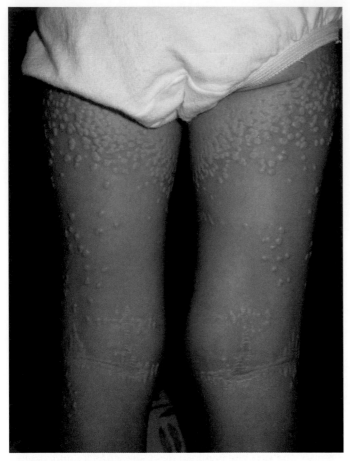

Figure 14.1 Xanthomas involving the extensor surfaces of the legs and thighs in Alagille syndrome.

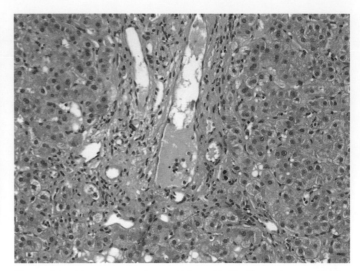

Figure 14.2 Liver specimen from an infant with Alagille syndrome with bile duct paucity. The portal tract is shown without any identifiable interlobular bile duct (hematoxylin & eosin, magnification 200×). (Courtesy of Pierre A. Russo MD.)

might go on to resolve their cholestasis and thereby avoid unnecessary liver transplantation in young children with ALGS.

Liver transplantation is eventually necessary in 21–31% of patients [17]. Several of these series are older and with current therapies this frequency is likely to be lower. Indications for transplantation include one or more problems including synthetic dysfunction, intractable portal hypertension, bone fractures, pruritus, and growth failure. Liver transplantation for ALGS is discussed in further detail under Management.

There have been numerous reports of hepatocellular carcinoma in patients with ALGS, including as young as 4 years of age. These have occurred in the presence and the absence of cirrhosis. Although there have been occasional reports of extrahepatic malignancies in ALGS, the overall incidence does not seem to be increased dramatically.

Histopathology

Bile duct paucity has been considered the most important and constant feature of ALGS. The normal bile duct:portal space ratio is between 0.9 and 1.8. Bile duct paucity is defined histologically in a full-term or older infant as a ratio of bile duct to portal tract that is <0.9 (Figure 14.2). It is important to note that bile ductules should not be included. The interlobular bile duct typically is located more centrally in the portal tract; the bile ductule is located peripherally. An adequate number of true portal tracts must be examined to arrive at an accurate ratio. It has been shown that a reasonably accurate estimation can be made with needle biopsy specimens containing as few as six portal tracts [18]. The bile duct:portal tract ratio in older infants with ALGS is usually less than 0.5–0.75 [19,20].

Bile duct paucity, however, is not present in infancy in many patients ultimately shown to have ALGS. Furthermore, a systematic study of the histopathology of adults with mild, non-cholestatic ALGS has not been performed. Paucity is present in about 89% of patients reported in large series [2,10–13]. The frequency of paucity in these series varies in large part with the criteria used to define ALGS. Older studies required paucity to consider the diagnosis of ALGS; newer studies focusing on the systemic manifestations or the presence of *JAG1* mutations identify paucity in only 80–85% of patients.

Several studies of serial liver biopsies have demonstrated that paucity is more common later in infancy and childhood [2,18,21]. Emerick *et al.* [2] found that paucity was present in 60% of 48 infants younger than 6 months of age but in 95% of 40 who underwent biopsy after 6 months. The progression to paucity typically accompanies a worsening of clinical hepatic disease in infancy over a period of months or years. Occasional reports have demonstrated, however, that the progression to paucity is not an absolute feature of ALGS. Hypotheses explaining this progression to paucity include a destruction of ducts postnatally and a differential maturation of portal tracts and their incumbent ducts. The factors that lead to a decrease in the number of ducts are not yet understood (see below under Notch signaling pathway and bile duct development).

Table 14.2 Frequent cardiovascular anomalies in a cohort of 200 patients with Alagille syndrome[a]

Primary cardiovascular anomaly	%
Cardiovascular anomalies seen on imaging	76
Right-sided anomalies:	55
Tetralogy of Fallot	12
Valvar pulmonary stenosis	8
Branch pulmonary artery stenosis	35
Left-sided anomalies: aortic stenosis, aortic coarctation, etc.	7
Other anomalies:	14
Ventricular septal defect	5
Atrial septal defect	5
Other	4
Normal or not imaged	25
Peripheral pulmonary stenosis murmur, without documented anomaly	19
No peripheral pulmonary stenosis murmur, with normal or no imaging	7

[a] Adapted from McElhinney et al., 2002 [23].

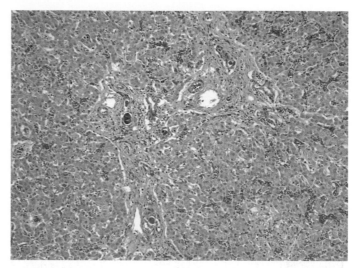

Figure 14.3 Liver specimen from a 1-month-old patient with Alagille syndrome demonstrating marked bile duct proliferation (hematoxylin & eosin, magnification 100×). (Courtesy of Pierre A. Russo MD)

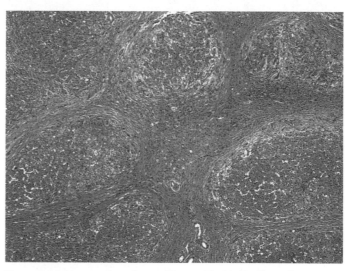

Figure 14.4 Liver specimen from a 16 year old with Alagille syndrome. There is established cirrhosis. Portal tracts are expanded and fibrotic. There is a complete absence of interlobular bile ducts (hematoxylin & eosin, magnification 100×). (Courtesy of Pierre A. Russo MD)

Ductular proliferation is present in a small number of infants with ALGS, leading to significant potential diagnostic confusion (Figure 14.3). This is seen most commonly in association with portal inflammation. As with any infantile cholestatic condition, giant cell hepatitis may be a predominant feature in the infant with ALGS. In part because of the variability in the early histopathology of the liver in ALGS, a number of patients have been misdiagnosed as having biliary atresia [2,12,13]. Histologic cholestasis is prominent early, but in many patients this tends to disappear unless there is progression to end-stage liver disease. An interesting characteristic of the hepatic histopathology of ALGS is the uncommon progression to cirrhosis (Figure 14.4). Typically, diseases with duct deficit and obstruction manifested by severe cholestasis progress to end-stage liver disease and cirrhosis. Not only does this not occur in most patients with ALGS, but the biochemical cholestasis and its clinical manifestations most commonly improve with time, despite the lack of reappearance of interlobular ducts.

Cardiac involvement

The early reports of ALGS by Watson and Miller [22] focused on the association of cholestatic liver disease, butterfly vertebrae, and particular facies in patients with familial dominant pulmonary arterial stenosis. In a comprehensive evaluation of 200 subjects with ALGS, cardiovascular involvement was present in 94% [23], with right-sided lesions being the most prevalent (Table 14.2). Pulmonary artery anomalies are the most common abnormality identified (76%) and may occur in isolation or in combination with structural intracardiac disease [23] (Figure 14.5). Pulmonary artery involvement may result in differential lung perfusion (Figure 14.6). Intracardiac lesions were present in 24% of 92 patients with ALGS [2]. The most common congenital defect is tetralogy of Fallot (TOF), which occurs in 7–12% [2,23]. It appears that severe forms of TOF (particularly TOF with pulmonary atresia) occur with greater frequency in the ALGS population than in the general population of individuals with TOF. Approximately 40% of patients with ALGS demonstrating TOF have pulmonary

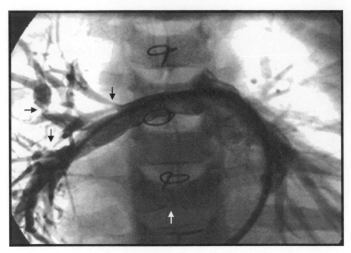

Figure 14.5 Right pulmonary arteriogram demonstrating multiple stenoses (black arrows) in a patient with prior surgery for tetralogy of Fallot, peripheral pulmonic stenoses, a butterfly vertebrae (white arrow), and a deletion of chromosome 20p12.

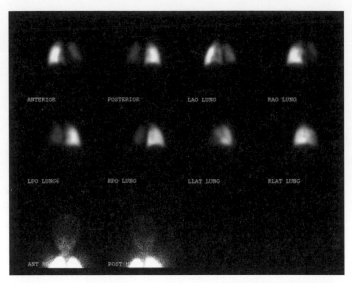

Figure 14.6 Lung perfusion scan from a patient with Alagille syndrome demonstrating differential blood flow within the pulmonary tree. The right lung receives more than 86% of pulmonary blood flow secondary to stenosis of the left pulmonary artery.

atresia. There is no correlation between the type or exonic location of the *JAG1* mutation and the nature of the cardiovascular involvement.

The exact incidence of severe neonatal cardiac disease is probably underestimated in all series of patients with ALGS because of the reliance on hepatic disease for ascertainment. Family members of ALGS probands with the full phenotype have been described with apparent isolated cardiac disease and the same familial *JAG1* mutation [5]. A small number of individuals with non-syndromic cardiac disease and *JAG1* mutations have been reported. Recently, 144 individuals with isolated right-sided cardiac defects were screened for *JAG1* mutations and 3% of those with TOF and 6% of those with pulmonary stenosis/peripheral pulmonary stenosis had *JAG1* mutations [24]. None of these children had identifiable liver disease, thus further expanding the phenotype of *JAG1*-associated ALGS.

In a large ALGS series, cardiac surgery was performed in infancy in 11% [2]. The mortality rates were 33% for those with TOF and 75% for those with TOF with pulmonary atresia. The survival of patients with ALGS with these lesions is markedly lower than for patients (with these lesions) without ALGS. This may be a result, in part, of the common presence of significant stenoses in the distal pulmonary artery, or of other systemic manifestations of the syndrome (Figure 14.5). Non-surgical invasive techniques have been used successfully for patients with ALGS, including valvuloplasty, balloon dilatation, and stent implantation. Heart–lung transplantation has been performed in combination with liver transplantation in a child with ALGS.

Cardiac disease accounts for nearly all of the early deaths in ALGS. Patients with intracardiac disease have approximately a 40% rate of survival to 6 years of life, compared with a 95% survival rate in patients with ALGS without intracardiac lesions [2]. Cardiovascular disease contributes significantly to the injury caused by the disorder and has been implicated in the increased post-transplantation mortality rate seen in some series.

Vascular involvement

Vascular anomalies have been noted in ALGS from some of the earliest descriptions of this syndrome. Pulmonary artery involvement is a hallmark feature of the condition and one of the most common manifestations. However, the literature documents multiple case reports of intracranial vessel abnormalities and other vascular anomalies in ALGS.

Unexplained intracranial bleeding is a recognized complication and cause of mortality in ALGS. Intracranial bleeds occur in approximately 15% of patients, and the hemorrhage is fatal in 30–50% of these events [2,12]. There does not seem to be any pattern to the location and/or severity of the intracranial bleeding, which ranges from massive fatal events to asymptomatic cerebral infarcts. Epidural, subdural, subarachnoid, and intraparenchymal bleeding have been reported. The majority of this bleeding has occurred in the absence of significant coagulopathy. Head trauma, typically of a minor degree, has been associated with the bleeding in a number of patients. The majority of cases of bleeding are spontaneous, however, with no clear risk factors. Lykavieris *et al.* [25] studied a cohort of 174 individuals with ALGS and identified 38 patients (22%) who had 49 bleeding episodes. All these hemorrhages occurred in the absence of liver failure, with normal median platelet counts and prothrombin times, suggesting that patients with ALGS may be at particular risk for bleeding.

Underlying vessel abnormalities in the central nervous system that could explain the occurrence of bleeding and

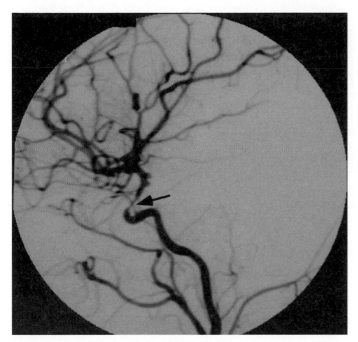

Figure 14.7 Moyamoya disease in Alagille syndrome. Cerebral angiogram demonstrating multiple areas of vascular stenoses (arrow).

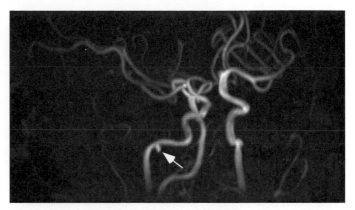

Figure 14.8 Aneurysm of the external carotid artery (arrow) in a 17 year old with Alagille syndrome without CNS symptoms found by routine screening.

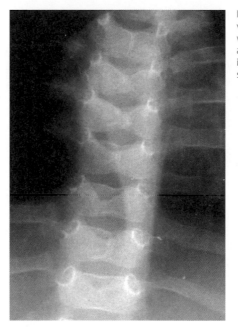

Figure 14.9 Butterfly vertebrae at T5 and T6, with vertebral anomalies at T4, T7, T8, and T9, in an infant with Alagille syndrome.

stroke in ALGS have been described in some of these patients [3,12,26]. Aneurysms of the basilar and middle cerebral arteries and various internal carotid artery anomalies have been described. Moyamoya disease (progressive intracranial arterial occlusive disease) also has been previously described in several children with ALGS (Figure 14.7). Emerick *et al.* [26] prospectively studied 26 patients with ALGS using MRI with angiography of the head. Cerebrovascular abnormalities were detected in 10 of 26 patients (38%). All the symptomatic patients had detected abnormalities, and 23% of screened, asymptomatic patients had detected anomalies. These results suggest that MRI with angiography is useful in detecting these lesions and may have a valuable role in screening for treatable lesions such as aneurysms (Figure 14.8). The current recommendation is for all asymptomatic patients with ALGS to have a screening MRI/MR angiography as a baseline and for physicians to have a low threshold for reimaging patients with ALGS in the event of any symptoms, head trauma, or suspicious neurologic signs.

Systemic vascular abnormalities have also been documented in ALGS. Aortic aneurysms and coarctations, renal artery, celiac artery, superior mesenteric artery, and subclavian artery anomalies have all been described. Kamath *et al.* [3] evaluated a large cohort of patients with ALGS and identified 9% (25 of 268) with non-cardiac vascular anomalies or events. In addition, vascular accidents accounted for 34% of the mortality in this cohort. These findings suggest that vascular abnormalities have been under-recognized as a potentially devastating complication of ALGS.

Skeletal involvement

Vertebral abnormalities are described in the initial reports of this syndrome. The most characteristic finding is the sagittal cleft or butterfly vertebrae, which is found in 33–87% of patients with ALGS [2,11–13] (Figures 14.9 and 14.10). This relatively uncommon anomaly may occur in normal individuals and is also seen in other multisystem abnormalities, such as 22q deletion syndrome and VATER (vertebral defects, anal atresia, tracheoesophageal fistula, radial and renal defect) syndrome. The affected vertebral bodies are split sagittally into paired hemivertebrae because of a failure of the fusion of the anterior arches of the vertebrae. Generally, these are asymptomatic and of no structural significance. The mildly affected vertebrae have a central lucency. A fully affected vertebra has a pair of separate

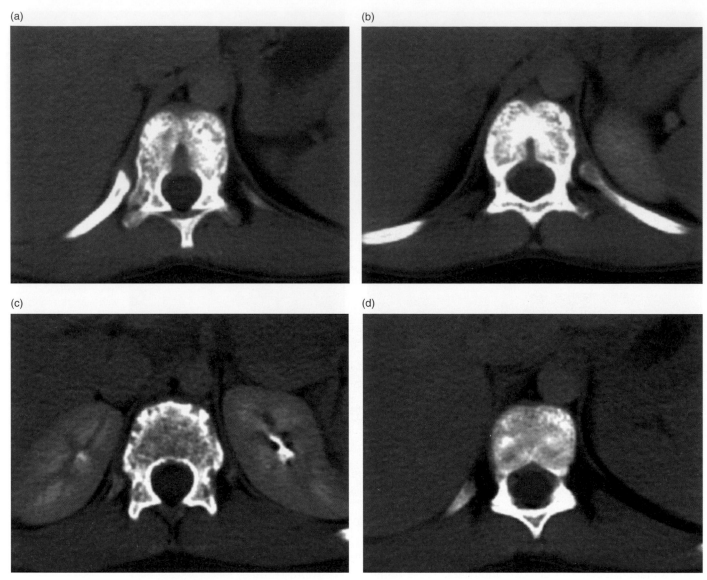

(a)

(b)

(c)

(d)

Figure 14.10 CT images of vertebral anomalies in Alagille syndrome. (a) A butterfly vertebral body. (b) A vertebral body with a posterior sagittal cleft. (c) A vertebral body with marked cortical irregularity. (d) A nearly normal vertebral body.

triangular hemivertebrae whose apices face each other like the wings of a butterfly. Other associated skeletal abnormalities include an abnormal narrowing of the adjusted interpedicular space in the lumbar spine, a pointed anterior process of C1, spina bifida occulta, fusion of the adjacent vertebrae, hemivertebrae, the absence of the 12th rib, and the presence of a bony connection between ribs. In addition, supernumerary digital flexion creases have been described in one-third of patients [27].

Severe metabolic bone disease with osteoporosis and pathologic fractures is common in patients with ALGS. Recurrent fractures, particularly of the femur, have been cited as a major indication for hepatic transplantation. Preliminary survey data suggest that there is a propensity toward pathologic lower extremity long bone fractures in ALGS [28].

A number of factors may contribute to osteopenia and fractures, including severe chronic malnutrition, vitamin D and vitamin K deficiency, chronic hepatic and renal disease, magnesium deficiency, and pancreatic insufficiency. It is not yet known whether there is an intrinsic defect in cortical or trabecular structure of the bones in patients with ALGS. Olsen *et al.* [29] evaluated bone status in prepubertal children with ALGS and identified significant deficits in bone size and bone mass that were related to fat absorption but not dietary intake.

Patients with ALGS are frequently found to have short stature; and this is likely multifactorial in origin, resulting from cholestasis and malabsorption, congenital heart disease and genetic predisposition. A validated growth curve for ALGS individuals is not yet available.

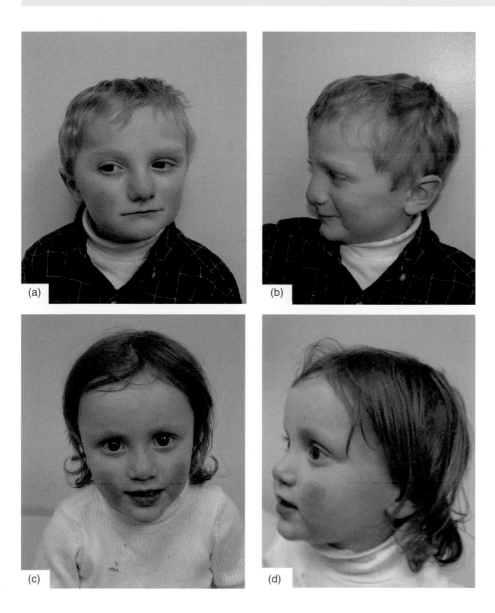

Figure 14.11 Characteristic facies of children with Alagille syndrome. (Courtesy of Ian D. Krantz MD.)

Facial features

A characteristic facial appearance is described in the original reports of ALGS and is probably one of the most penetrant features of the syndrome (for *JAG1*-associated disease). These features include a prominent forehead, deep-set eyes with moderate hypertelorism, a pointed chin, and a saddle or straight nose with a bulbous tip. The combination of these features gives the face a triangular appearance (Figure 14.11). The facies may be present early in infancy but in general becomes more dramatic with increasing age. The usefulness of the facies as a major diagnostic criterion has been challenged because of subjectivity and interobserver differences. In one study, photographs of patients with ALGS and patients with other known early-onset liver diseases were presented to dysmorphologists, who were able to correctly identify patients with *JAG1* mutations 79% of the time [30]. The facies in adults were least well identified in this study. They also reported that the facies change with age (Figure 14.12). In adults, the forehead is much less prominent and the protruding chin is more noticeable. The correct identification of these adults, who commonly have minimal signs and symptoms of ALGS, would help physicians in the evaluation of adults with apparently idiopathic cardiac, hepatic, or renal disease. It should be noted that, amongst the few patients reported to date, there appears to be a lower penetrance of characteristic facial features in patients with ALGS and *NOTCH2* mutations and it is, therefore, a less valuable diagnostic tool in this group.

Ocular involvement

The ocular abnormalities of patients with ALGS do not generally affect vision but are important as diagnostic tools. A large and varied number of ocular abnormalities have been

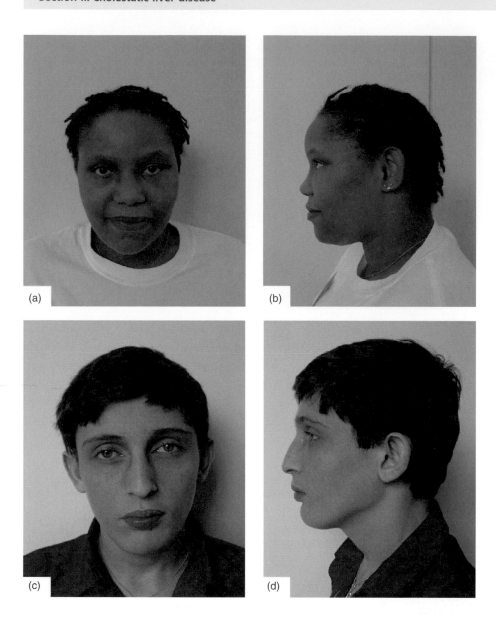

Figure 14.12 Characteristic facies of adults with Alagille syndrome. (Courtesy of Ian D. Krantz MD.)

described, although posterior embryotoxon is the most important diagnostically. Posterior embryotoxon is a prominent, centrally positioned Schwalbe's ring (or line) at the point at which the corneal endothelium and the uveal trabecular meshwork join (Figure 14.13). Posterior embryotoxon occurs in 56–88% of patients with ALGS (Table 14.1) and was also detected in 22% of children evaluated in a general ophthalmology clinic [31]. Posterior embryotoxon is seen in other multi-system disorders as well, such as chromosome 22q deletion. The Axenfeld anomaly, seen in 13% of patients with ALGS, is a prominent Schwalbe's ring with attached iris strands and is associated with glaucoma. In addition, Rieger anomaly, microcornea, keratoconus, congenital macular dystrophy, shallow anterior chambers, exotropia, ectopic pupil, band keratopathy, cataracts, strabismus, iris hypoplasia, choroidal folds, and anomalous optic disks have been reported in ALGS.

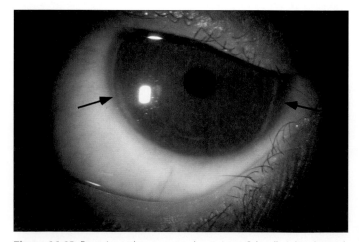

Figure 14.13 Posterior embryotoxon and prominent Schwalbe's line (arrows).

In a large series of patients with ALGS studied systematically, Hingorani *et al.* [32] identified posterior embryotoxon in 21 of 22 patients (95%), iris abnormalities in 10 (45%), diffuse fundic hypopigmentation in 13 (57%), speckling of the retinal pigment epithelium in 7 (33%), and optic disk abnormalities in 17 (76%). The frequency of these findings, higher than in other reported series, suggests that a formal ophthalmologic slit-lamp examination can provide one of the most crucial clues to the diagnosis of ALGS in infancy.

Nischal *et al.* [33] found ultrasound evidence of optic disk drusen using ocular ultrasonography in at least one eye in 95% and bilateral disk drusen in 80% of patients with ALGS but in none of the liver patients without ALGS whom they studied. This was substantiated in a recent study in which 91% of patients with ALGS had optic nerve drusen [34]. This is markedly higher than the incidence in the normal population (0.3–2%), suggesting that this newer ophthalmologic sign may be an extremely useful diagnostic tool.

Renal involvement

Renal involvement in ALGS has been widely reported on an individual case basis or as part of a larger report on general features of ALGS (Figure 14.14). The prevalence of renal involvement in larger series has ranged from 40 to 73% such

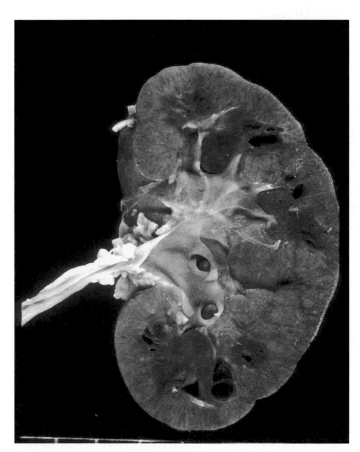

Figure 14.14 Diffuse renal cystic dysplasia in a patient with paucity of bile ducts. (Courtesy of Pierre A. Russo MD.)

that it has been proposed that renal anomalies now be considered a disease-defining criterion in ALGS (Table 14.1). In a large retrospective study, there was a prevalence of 39% of renal anomalies or disease and the most common renal involvement was renal dysplasia (58.9%), with renal tubular acidosis (9.5%), vesico-ureteric reflux (8.2%) and urinary obstruction (8.2%) following [35]. Renal insufficiency is relatively uncommon in ALGS but renal replacement therapy and even transplantation has been reported. Hypertension in patients with ALGS could be of cardiac, vascular, or renal etiology.

Functional and structural evaluation of the kidneys should be undertaken in all patients. The role of renal tubular acidosis in early growth failure is unclear, but administration of bicarbonate is necessary in some individuals. Renal function should be reassessed during the evaluation for hepatic transplantation.

Growth

Severe growth retardation is seen in 50–87% of patients [2,10,12,13]. Malnutrition resulting from malabsorption is a major factor in this failure to thrive, and chronic wasting as documented by height, weight, and anthropometry is severe in patients with ALGS [36,37]. Rovner *et al.* [37] assessed growth failure in 26 prepubertal children with ALGS and found that more than half the children were less than fifth percentile for weight and height and 20% had a diet poor in calories, fat, and other nutrients. There appear to be limitations to linear growth even if protein–calorie malnutrition is not evident. Patients with growth failure appear to be insensitive to exogenous growth hormone [38]. Many adults appear to have short stature, although a systematic study of adult height in ALGS has not been completed.

Diarrhea in a patient with ALGS may be a result of cholestasis and/or pancreatic insufficiency. Virtually all patients with ALGS had steatorrhea in one series [37]. Early data suggested that pancreatic insufficiency was an important problem in ALGS; however, more recent data suggest that this may not actually be the case [39].

Neurodevelopment and quality of life

Neurocognitive and developmental delay have been reported in 16–52% of patients with ALGS in general cohort studies [2,10,11,19]. Intellectual impairment was reported in the earliest description of ALGS in which 30% of the children had an IQ of 60–80 [19]. This is a significant proportion, as in a typically developing population, only 9% of individuals are expected to have an IQ below 80. Alagille *et al.* [10] went on to review 80 children and found that 16% had an IQ of less than 80, in the range that all of these children would qualify for special academic services. In another comprehensive cohort study of patients with ALGS, 16% (15/92) were found to have gross motor delay on routine pediatric screening [2]. Two in this cohort had defined psychiatric illnesses, namely major depressive disorder and oppositional defiant personality disorder and attention deficit/hyperactivity disorder. More recently, a questionnaire-based study noted that 49% of children with ALGS were in or had received special education, suggestive of a high prevalence of developmental delay or learning disabilities [40]. Interestingly, in this same study there was an increase in mental health diagnoses compared with the normative population (18% versus 5–10%), depression (10% versus 5%), and attention problems (32% versus 19%). It is certainly possible that some of these studies include children who did not receive adequate nutritional support in the earlier years, contributing to these findings, but the entire picture remains unclear without a prospective systematic study.

There has been one preliminary survey study of heath-related quality of life in ALGS [40]. The children with ALGS, aged 5–18 years, had a lower rating than a normal pediatric population and a group with juvenile rheumatoid arthritis. In this cohort, 18% of patients with ALGS were also diagnosed with a mental health problem. The ALGS-specific questionnaire in this same study revealed itching was a significant issue, with 75% of children having some form of scratching, and 32% with destruction of the skin [40]. Parents reported that xanthomas restricted physical activity and were upsetting to the children because of the effect on the physical appearance. These preliminary data suggest evidence of a significant clinical issue that warrants further investigation.

Survival outcomes

Cardiac, hepatic, and vascular disease account for the majority of deaths in ALGS, although the true frequency of death is variable, reflecting the heterogeneity of the disorder. The presence of complex intracardiac disease at diagnosis is the only predictor of an excessive early mortality rate, and cardiac disease accounts for the majority of deaths in early childhood. Overall, vascular events or defects account for most of the mortality in ALGS: 34% in a large series [3]. Quiros-Tejeira et al. [13] reported a 72% survival rate in 43 patients at a mean follow-up of 8.9 years in a population in which 20 (47%) received hepatic transplantation. Hoffenberg et al. [12] estimated the rate of survival to age 19 without transplantation to be approximately 50% in 26 patients who presented with cholestasis, but with transplantation (which in this series had a 100% survival rate), the 20-year survival rate was estimated at 87%. Emerick et al. [2] estimated the 20-year survival rate in 92 patients to be 75% overall, 80% for those not requiring hepatic transplantation and 60% for those requiring transplantation. For patients with structural intracardiac disease, however, the survival rate was only 40% at 7 years.

Diagnostic considerations

The majority of infants with ALGS are evaluated for conjugated hyperbilirubinemia in the first weeks or months of life. The differential diagnosis and general evaluation for conjugated hyperbilirubinemia are discussed in Chapter 8. Occasionally, ALGS is misdiagnosed as biliary atresia because of the overlap of biochemical, scintigraphic, histologic, and cholangiographic features. Serum bilirubin, bile acid, and gamma-glutamyltransferase typically are elevated in both of these disorders. Ultrasound should identify choledochal cysts and cholelithiasis accurately, but both patients with biliary atresia and those with ALGS may have small or apparently absent gallbladders. Excretion of nuclear tracer (technetium-99m–diisopropylacetanilidoiminodiacetic acid) into the duodenum eliminates biliary atresia from consideration, but non-excretion of tracer is also possible in ALGS. There was no excretion of scintiscan in 61% of 36 infants with ALGS [2]. Excretion was evident only after 24-hour follow-up in another 25% of these 36 patients.

If biliary atresia remains a diagnostic possibility after the initial non-invasive evaluation, a liver biopsy should follow, particularly if the studies suggest non-communication from the liver to the duodenum. Although a liver biopsy is not mandatory to diagnose ALGS, it remains an important step in differentiating between ALGS and biliary atresia. In biliary atresia, bile duct proliferation is the typical histologic lesion. In ALGS, paucity is evident in 60% of infants younger than 6 months but in 95% of older patients [2]. Unfortunately, there may be a normal number of ducts early in the course of biliary atresia and also in some patients with ALGS, and bile duct proliferation occasionally occurs in infants with ALGS. In very young infants in whom the percutaneous liver biopsy is not diagnostic, it may be helpful to delay exploration for 1 or 2 weeks and repeat the biopsy (recognizing that the success of therapy for biliary atresia is correlated with surgery before 60 days of age). Giant cell hepatitis is also seen in both disorders. Finally it should be noted that bile duct paucity, if present, is not diagnostic of ALGS and other diagnoses should be considered (Table 14.3).

A cholangiogram is indicated if there is scintigraphic and histologic evidence to support a diagnosis of biliary atresia.

Table 14.3 Causes of bile duct paucity

Type	Causes
Genetic disorders	Alagille syndrome Down syndrome Other chromosomal abnormalities
Metabolic disorders	α_1-Antitrypsin deficiency Cystic fibrosis Hypopituitarism
Infections	Congenital cytomegalovirus infection Congenital rubella infection Congenital syphilis
Immunologic disorders	Graft-versus-host disease Chronic hepatic allograft rejection Sclerosing cholangitis
Other disorders	Zellweger syndrome Ivemark syndrome Idiopathic disorders

Percutaneous cholangiography is technically difficult in this age group but possible in expert hands. An operative cholangiogram has been the gold standard procedure to evaluate the extrahepatic and intrahepatic biliary tree. Cholangiography of any type, however, is likely to be misleading if interpreted without attention to history, examination, biochemistry, and radiologic evaluation. The extra- and intrahepatic ducts are extremely small in patients with ALGS, and the cholangiogram commonly does not demonstrate communication proximally. In 37% of 19 cholangiograms in infants with ALGS, there was no opacification of the proximal extrahepatic ducts, and in another 37%, the proximal extrahepatic tree was abnormally small [2]. The intrahepatic ducts were normal in only 10% of 19 infants with ALGS, small or hypoplastic in 16%, and not visualized in 74%. Therefore, even the apparent gold standard test to differentiate ALGS and biliary atresia can be misleading. Unfortunately, it is very unlikely that mutational analysis can be performed within an appropriate window to meet the deadline for a timely Kasai procedure for biliary atresia and, therefore, clinical parameters remain the only available tool to distinguish the two diagnoses. It is important to do so as a Kasai procedure may be associated with a poorer outcome in ALGS (see Management).

Clinical features in extrahepatic organ systems may also help in the diagnostic evaluation. The list of abnormalities identified in the "major" organ systems and the list of other affected organs have grown appreciably. It should be noted that several of the defining features are present in normal individuals or in other conditions. Heart murmurs are present in 6% of all newborns and posterior embryotoxon appears in 22% of the general population. As mentioned above, butterfly vertebrae are seen in 11% of patients with 22q11 deletion. Furthermore, the facial features of patients with ALGS are subtle during the first months of life, making this an unreliable diagnostic tool in infancy.

With the advent of molecular testing for ALGS (see Genetics of Alagille syndrome) and the broader appreciation of the phenotypic variability, the diagnostic criteria for ALGS can be modified. To make a clinical diagnosis for the index case (proband) in the family, it seems reasonable to continue with a version of the original Alagille criteria, modified only in no longer requiring histology. Therefore, ALGS can be diagnosed clinically on the basis of cholestasis with at least three features from the list of characteristic Alagille facies, consistent cardiac disease, posterior embryotoxon, butterfly vertebrae, typical ALGS renal disease, and a structural vascular anomaly. In families with one definite clinically defined proband, other members with two features are likely to have a gene defect and should be considered as having ALGS. Others with typical ALGS manifestations but no mutation in *JAG1* or *NOTCH2* ultimately may be shown to have defects in other Notch or Jagged ligands, but may be considered to have ALGS based on clinical criteria. A revised list of diagnostic criteria is proposed in Table 14.4.

As molecular testing becomes more readily available and requested by cardiologists and nephrologists, it is likely that

Table 14.4 Diagnostic criteria for Alagille syndrome

Mutation in *JAG1* or *NOTCH2*[a]	Family history of Alagille syndrome	Number of clinical criteria required[b]
Identified	None (proband)	At least 1[c]
Identified	Present	Any or none
Not identified[d]	None (proband)	3 or more
Not identified	Present	2 or more

[a] The mutation identified must be likely to cause a functional change in the protein and predicted to be pathologic. It cannot be a non-disease-causing polymorphism.
[b] Clinical criteria for diagnosis include consistent hepatic (bile duct paucity and/or cholestasis); cardiac, renal, ocular, or skeletal involvement; a structural vascular anomaly; or characteristic facies.
[c] The exact terminology regarding an individual with a disease-causing mutation but no apparent clinical features of Alagille syndrome remains to be determined. This individual cannot be described as having a clinical syndrome but still carries disease risks of Alagille syndrome, such as stroke, and has a 50% chance of disease transmission to offspring. For the purposes of making the diagnosis of Alagille syndrome in a proband, at least one clinical feature is required in addition to a mutation.
[d] This table presumes that "not identified" mutations are mostly those which have not been sought (genotyping not done). Different screening laboratories and techniques have mutation detection rates ranging from 60 to 94% in clinically defined Alagille syndrome. If a mutation is exhaustively sought and found to be negative, the likelihood of true Alagille syndrome goes down significantly, particularly if the clinical manifestations are not cardinal features.

patients with isolated or limited manifestations will be diagnosed as having ALGS. Any individual with a clear mutation in *JAG1* or *NOTCH2* has the syndrome, although the exact terminology surrounding this diagnosis likely needs revision as Daniel Alagille clearly intended to describe a constellation of features associated with liver disease. Perhaps a molecular definition is warranted with the term ALGS being reserved for those individuals with liver disease and associated features. Regardless of the exact terminology used, it should be noted that all these individuals have a 50% chance of passing the mutation to their offspring, with no predictive ability about the phenotype in those children.

Management

The therapy for cholestasis and its associated abnormalities is discussed in detail in Chapter 9. Patients with ALGS present significant management challenges and these have been comprehensively reviewed elsewhere [16,41]. Cholestasis commonly is profound and the pruritus associated with ALGS cholestatic liver disease can be severe and may occur even without jaundice. Bile flow may be stimulated with the choleretic ursodeoxycholic acid, but in many patients, the pruritus continues unabated. Care should be taken to keep the skin hydrated with emollients, and fingernails should be trimmed to prevent further damage. Therapy with antihistamines may provide some temporary relief, but many patients require additional therapy with agents such as rifampin, cholestyramine, or naltrexone. Biliary diversion has been successful in a number of patients [42,43]. Emerick and Whitington [42] studied nine patients with ALGS and severe mutilating pruritus who underwent partial external biliary diversion. Mean pruritus scores were significantly lower 1 year after the procedure, and eight of the nine had only mild scratching when not distracted. Three of the nine also had complete resolution of extensive xanthomas. Therefore, biliary diversion may be offered as a viable therapy before transplantation, which was previously the only option for intractable pruritus.

Hepatoportoenterostomy is inappropriate in ALGS and may increase the amount of liver injury and progression to hepatic fibrosis. In a limited retrospective study comparing patients with ALGS with matched patients with biliary atresia after Kasai procedures, the ALGS cohort had a significantly higher rate of liver transplantation (47% versus 14%) and sustained higher mortality [44]. These data suggest that the Kasai procedure is not a marker for severe underlying liver disease but that the Kasai procedure itself has a detrimental effect on outcome.

Failure to thrive and malnutrition need to be addressed aggressively and early on in life. There is significant malabsorption of long-chain fat; therefore, formulae supplemented with medium-chain triglycerides have some nutritional advantage. Essential fatty acid deficiency in patients with ALGS has been reported, however, with acral lesions resembling porphyria that responded to parenteral supplementation of essential fatty acids. The increased caloric needs in ALGS result from malabsorption of fats and fat-soluble vitamins but do not appear to be related to markedly increased basal metabolism [45]. Many patients are unable to eat enough to provide the substantial quantities of energy required for growth and development, and nasogastric or gastrostomy tube feedings can provide necessary supplementation and aid greatly in administration of medication.

Fat-soluble vitamin deficiency is present to a variable degree in most patients with significant ALGS. Oral or parenteral supplementation is necessary for prevention of vitamin deficiencies and their sequelae. Multivitamin preparations may not provide the correct ratio of fat-soluble vitamins; vitamins are best administered as individual supplements tailored to the specific needs of the patient with consistent monitoring of blood levels to insure vitamin sufficiency.

Liver transplantation is required in 21–31% of patients with ALGS based on case series [46]. Indications for transplant are end-stage liver disease secondary to chronic cholestasis, severe complications of cholestasis such as failure to thrive, portal hypertension, and recurrent fractures. Hypercholesterolemia alone is not an indication for liver transplantation as it has been shown not to be atherogenic in other cholestatic conditions [47].

Liver transplantation in patients with ALGS is complicated by the associated comorbidities, particularly cardiac, renal, and vascular involvement. A detailed renal evaluation is warranted in any patient with ALGS prior to liver transplantation, including urinalysis, blood pressure, renal ultrasonography, glomerular filtration rate, serum cystatin C, and blood gas measurement. If renal impairment is documented, renal-sparing immunosuppressive protocols should be considered, including low target levels of calcineurin inhibitors and early introduction of mycophenolate mofetil or sirolimus. Vascular involvement should be assessed with CT or MR angiography of the head, neck, and abdomen. Cardiac pretransplant work-up is based on information acquired with echocardiography and electrocardiography. However, the peripheral branches of the pulmonary arteries and the degree of right ventricular hypertrophy are insufficiently appreciated using these modalities. Investigators at King's College London have suggested a pretransplant dynamic stress test with dobutamine to stimulate perioperative conditions with concomitant cardiac catheterization [48]. If the patient achieves >40% increase in the cardiac output, then the cardiac reserve is considered adequate for liver transplantation.

Living-related transplantation in ALGS requires careful consideration. In general, in North America, living-related transplantation has not been offered to donors with a known disease-causing mutation as the donor may suffer from subclinical liver disease. In Japan, the outcomes in 20 children have been reported and are good, with a 1-year survival rate of 80% [49]. They recommend comprehensive radiologic vascular assessment with CT or MR angiography and a liver biopsy, but not genetic testing. On a cautionary note, Gurkan *et al.* [50] reported two instances in which apparently unaffected parents underwent donor operations that were unsuccessful because of a paucity of duct structures discovered intraoperatively. Therefore, the recommendation in North America is for potential donors to undergo screening for the known mutation in the proband and for them generally not to be used as donors if positive for the mutation.

The survival rate of patients with ALGS undergoing liver transplantation has significantly improved in recent years with careful selection of transplant candidates and better management of concomitant cardiac disease. Combined case series show a 1-year post-transplantation patient survival rate of 79%. A recent report by Arnon *et al.* from the United Network for Organ Sharing dataset of 461 ALGS [51] who underwent liver transplantation from 1987 to 2008, revealed 1- and 5-year patient survival of 83% and 78%, respectively. Early death in the first 30 days was significantly higher in patients with ALGS compared with those with biliary atresia. Death from graft failure and neurologic and cardiac complications were also significantly higher in the ALGS cohort.

Genetics of Alagille syndrome

Alagille syndrome is inherited in an autosomal dominant manner, with highly variable expressivity. It is a genetically heterogeneous disorder and may be caused by either mutations in *JAG1* (seen in 94% of clinically defined probands) or

NOTCH2 (seen in 0.8%) [6,7,9]. Jagged1 is a cell surface protein that serves as a ligand for the four Notch receptors (Notch1–4), and together these proteins begin the cascade of events that turn on the Notch signaling pathway. The Notch signaling pathway is involved in the determination of cell fate and as such plays a crucial role in normal development.

Gene identification and mutation analysis

Alagille syndrome was recognized to have an autosomal dominant mode of inheritance in the first reports by Alagille and Watson and Miller. The site of the gene responsible for ALGS was first suggested more than 10 years later by the identification of visible gene deletions and translocations on the short arm of chromosome 20 [52]. Based on the clues provided by the cytogenetics, two groups identified mutations in JAG1 as the cause of ALGS in 1997 [6,7]. Jagged1 is a single-pass transmembrane protein with an extracellular and an intracellular domain. The genomic sequence is composed of 26 exons, and the standard strategy to screen for JAG1 mutations is to analyze the coding regions of each of the exons in addition to about 20 intronic bases surrounding each exon to identify potential splice site mutations. To date, more than 430 JAG1 mutations have been identified in patients with ALGS. The frequency of mutations was around 60–70% in older studies. However, more recently, a cohort of patients was exhaustively studied with sequencing of the genomic coding region and cDNA, in addition to analysis of full and partial gene deletions, and the mutation rate was found to be 94% [8]. The frequency of sporadic mutations (i.e. new in the proband) is approximately 56–70%.

The JAG1 mutations identified in patients with ALGS have been found distributed across the entire coding region, with no real hotspots [53]. The majority of the mutations are predicted to result in premature termination of the protein in the extracellular domain. Approximately 75% of patients with ALGS have protein-truncating (frameshift or nonsense or splice site) mutations [8,54,55]. Approximately 7% have gene deletions. Missense mutations are identified in 15%. Haploinsufficiency, a decrease in the amount of the normal protein, is hypothesized to be the mechanism causing ALGS. However, there is evidence to support the role of other potential mechanisms, such as the dominant negative effect of mutant transcripts [54].

The Notch2 protein is also a single-pass transmembrane protein. NOTCH2 is made up of 34 exons occupying 158 099 bp of genomic DNA, which codes for an 11 433 bp message. Screening of this gene for mutations in ALGS has been accomplished by sequencing of the genomic DNA. To date 10 patients with unique NOTCH2 mutations have been described [9,56].

In a small fraction (3–5%) of individuals with ALGS, there are deletions of chromosome 20p. Genome-wide single nucleotide polymorphism analysis of 25 patients with ALGS revealed 21 deletions ranging from 95 kb to 14.62 Mb [57]. Patients with deletions greater than a critical 5.4 MB region had additional phenotypic features not usually associated with ALGS, such as developmental delay and hearing loss. Interestingly deletions up to 5.4 MB did not confer additional clinical findings although there was haploinsufficiency for several genes other than JAG1.

Notch signaling pathway

JAG1 encodes for a ligand in the Notch signaling pathway, which is a highly evolutionarily conserved intercellular signaling mechanism. There are five ligands (Dll1, Dll3, Dll4, Jagged1 and Jagged2) and four Notch (1–4) receptors known to date in mammals. Jagged1 is a single pass type I membrane protein with an extracellular domain made of a N-terminal region, a delta/serrate/LAG2 (DSL) domain, 16 epidermal growth factor (EGF) tandem repeats, and a cysteine-rich, juxta-membrane region [58]. The DSL domain is required for binding with the Notch receptor and EGF1 and EGF2 are important for increasing the affinity with this receptor. The Notch receptor consists of an extracellular segment, formed by multiple EGF-like repeats, a transmembrane part, and an intracellular domain. Once the receptor–ligand interaction has occurred, the intracellular domain is cleaved from the inner surface of the membrane and translocates into the nucleus, where it regulates the transcription of different downstream genes, such as HES1/HEY2 [59].

The finding that mutations in JAG1 and NOTCH2 cause ALGS indicates that Notch signaling is important in the development of the organ systems affected, namely the liver, heart, skeleton, eye, face, and kidney. Studies of the pattern of expression of the various Notch receptors and ligands confirm that JAG1 is expressed in the locations and at the times expected for a gene that contributes to the normal development of the organs affected in ALGS (heart, liver, skeleton, kidney) [59]. While the Jag1 knockout heterozygous mouse did not phenocopy ALGS, a Jag1/Notch2 double heterozygote was found to have liver, cardiac, ocular, and renal manifestations similar to those seen in human ALGS [60].

Genotype–phenotype correlations

JAG1 mutations

Although the ALGS phenotype is highly variable, there is no apparent correlation with JAG1 genotype in the majority of patients. There is extreme variability of ALGS phenotype within families, suggesting other genetic or environmental factors contribute significantly to the clinical manifestations of the disease. A study of 53 JAG1 mutation-positive relatives of a cohort of ALGS probands demonstrated that only 53% met the clinical criteria for a diagnosis of ALGS, including 11 (21%) with clinical features that would have led to a diagnosis of ALGS and 17 (32%) who had mild features that would have only been apparent on targeted evaluation following the diagnosis of a proband in their family (i.e. discovery of elevation of liver enzymes or posterior embryotoxon in an asymptomatic individual) [5].

Missense mutations offer clues regarding the mechanism of disease that follows *JAG1* deletion. A well-described example is the mutation G274D that affects the second EGF repeat of the JAG1 protein and leads to impaired folding. This mutation has been associated with TOF in the absence of liver disease [61]. A mutation leading to a G274D change has been described as "leaky" in that some of the protein does appear on the cell surface but it can partially initiate Notch signaling. This mechanism was previously thought to account for the cardiac-only phenotype in these patients. However more recently a molecular study of 144 patients without ALGS with TOF or pulmonic stenosis revealed *JAG1* missense mutations in 2% and 4%, respectively [24]. Two of these mutations were clearly completely haploinsufficient, were not present at the cell surface, and could not initiate Notch signaling. However, these mutations were still not associated with the full manifestations of ALGS. Clearly changes in *JAG1* do not provide the full answer to disease phenotype in ALGS and these data are additional evidence of the presence of genetic modifiers.

NOTCH2 *mutations*

Data from the mouse had implicated *Notch2* in the etiology of clinical features associated with ALGS. To date 10 individuals with complete or partial features of classical ALGS have been found to have *NOTCH2* mutations [9,56]. Functional assays support the role of most of these as disease causing. From a phenotypic standpoint, individuals with *NOTCH2*-related ALGS appear to have less penetrance of the characteristic facial features and less skeletal involvement.

Notch signaling pathway and bile duct development

The exact mechanism whereby *JAG1* mutations lead to paucity of intrahepatic bile ducts and ALGS liver disease is not fully elucidated; however, there is substantial evidence that biliary development and tubular morphogenesis are mediated by NOTCH signaling. Normally during embryogenesis, bipotential hepatoblasts differentiate into hepatocytes or biliary epithelial cells. The hepatoblasts form a single and then a double layer in certain areas around the portal vein and its branches, forming the ductal plate. Ductal plate remodeling gives rise to tubular structures that eventually become bile ducts. Mutant mouse models have been particularly important in studying the role of the Notch signaling pathway in this process.

The doubly heterozygous *Jag1*^{null}/*Notch2* hypomorphic mouse has bile duct paucity and a few biliary cells adjacent to the portal vein. Similar findings are seen in mice homozygous for the *Notch2* hypomorphic allele. In the *Jag1/Notch2* doubly heterozygous mouse and the liver-specific *Notch2* conditional knockout, the ductal plate forms normally but the ductal plate remnants are present postnatally [62]. These and other data suggest *Notch2* is required for bile duct formation in the mouse. It appears that Notch signaling has a role in remodeling of the ductal plate into mature bile ducts late in gestation and in the early postnatal period.

Recent studies in mice have shown that Notch2 signaling in bipotential hepatoblasts not only drives cell differentiation into biliary epithelial cell but also is associated with increased biliary epithelial cell survival and tubulogenesis during embryonal bile duct development [63]. In addition, recombination signal-binding protein immunoglobulin kappa J (RBP-κJ)-knockout mice (RBP-κJ is a DNA-binding partner for NOTCH receptors) are found to have decreased number of biliary epithelial cells [64]. It appears that Notch signaling maintains biliary epithelial cells postnatally and can drive mature hepatocytes toward a biliary fate. Finally, Sparks *et al.* [65] recently showed that the three-dimensional biliary architecture in mice is also dependent upon the concentration of Notch signaling. In that study, impaired Notch signaling had a dose-dependent effect in decreasing the density of biliary branches. *NOTCH2* appears to have the principal role in biliary structure formation and tubulogenesis.

The role of *Jag1* in liver and bile duct development in mice models, perhaps surprisingly, does not support a major role for this gene in normal bile duct development in the embryonic period. Mice carrying a *Jag1* mutation targeted to hepatoblasts have no significant hepatic phenotype. In a recent interesting study, Hoffmann *et al.* [15] showed that Jag1 inactivation in the portal vein mesenchyme leads to bile duct paucity. It appears that Jag1-dependent signaling in the portal vein mesenchyme is essential for the morphogenesis of biliary epithelial cells and the organization of mature bile ducts in the mouse. These data clarify the role of Jag1 in bile duct formation and support the notion of ALGS having a primarily vascular etiology.

Notch signaling pathway and cardiovascular development

The importance of Notch signaling in cardiac development has been substantiated by the finding that *NOTCH1* mutations are associated with inherited aortic valve anomalies, such as bicuspid aortic valve [66]. In addition, the *Jag1/Notch2* mouse displays right-sided outflow tract anomalies, implicating this ligand-receptor pair in cardiac outflow tract development.

Embryogenesis of the heart is a complex process where mesoderm-derived cells become organized into the heart tube, which later rotates to create the normal heart, primarily composed of cardiomyocytes. These normally derive from undifferentiated cells within the heart tube. Impaired Notch signaling does not allow for normal cell fate specification and differentiation, interfering with normal cardiac embryogenesis. Notch signaling is also necessary for the formation of normal endocardiac cushions and valves. It appears that Notch signaling in the cardiac neural crest is pivotal in inducing cell-fate decisions, and Notch inhibition in this area leads to ALGS-like right-sided cardiac lesions [67].

Notch ligands and receptors are expressed in vascular endothelium or supporting cells, and, in particular, studies in mouse embryos show strong expression of *Jag1* in all major arteries [68]. Further evidence of the role of *JAG1* and NOTCH in vascular development is provided by the phenotype of targeted Notch pathway mutants. Mice homozygous for a mutation in *Jag1* die from hemorrhage during early embryogenesis because of defects in angiogenic vascular remodeling in the yolk sac and embryo. A human model also exists to support a role for the Notch pathway in vascular homeostasis. In adults, CADASIL (cerebral autosomal dominant arteriopathy with subcortical infarcts and leukoencephalopathy), a degenerative disorder characterized by late-onset strokes and dementia, is caused by mutations in the Notch3 receptor that result in alterations of vascular smooth muscle cells.

Genetic testing

Molecular sequencing is now widely commercially available for *JAG1* and for *NOTCH2* on a limited basis. Genotyping for both are also available as research tools. An evaluation by fluorescence in situ hybridization for deletions including *JAG1* will identify these deletions in less than 7% of patients. A molecular diagnosis can assist in an atypical ALGS and is also useful for genetic counseling and prenatal diagnosis. *JAG1* sequencing identifies mutations in individuals with clinically defined ALGS in the majority of cases (>90%). Individuals that have clinical features of ALGS but are not found to be carrying *JAG1* mutations should have sequence analysis of *NOTCH2* [9].

The most straightforward approach to screening is direct sequencing of the coding region of these genes, as data show that this approach identifies mutations in close to 95% of patients [8]. Once a *JAG1* mutation is identified in a proband, it is relatively simple to test parents and other relatives for the identified mutation. Mutations are inherited from an affected parent in 30–50% of patients, whereas the mutations appear de novo in 50–70% [53,54]. If a parental mutation is identified, there is a 50% risk for each future offspring to inherit the *JAG1* mutation. However, it should be emphasized that expressivity of the disorder is highly variable, and it is not currently possible to predict disease severity. If no parental mutation is identified, then the recurrence risk is limited to the chance of germline mosaicism, which for multiple different disorders is estimated at from 1 to 3%. There have also been cases of parental somatic mosaicism observed in apparently unaffected individuals. Prenatal testing may also be carried out in a family once the proband's mutation is identified. Testing can help to reassure parents of children with de novo mutations, who may be concerned about germline mosaicism. Testing has also aided in the diagnosis of ALGS in patients with minor or atypical manifestations and has expanded the spectrum of ALGS manifestations.

Prenatal genetic testing has been used to aid in the diagnosis of ALGS. This requires amniocentesis or chorionic villous sampling and assessment for a known *JAG1* mutation. Preimplantation genetic diagnosis has also been successfully performed in ALGS. It is imperative to counsel parents undergoing any type of prenatal testing carefully since there are no genotype–phenotype correlations in ALGS, so it is not possible to make predictions about a child's clinical course based on the type or presence of a mutation.

Conclusions

Alagille syndrome is a complex condition in which the molecular basis is well understood but the absence of identified genotype–phenotype correlations and the broad variability poses management challenges. Renal and vascular involvement should likely be included in the diagnostic criteria. The discovery of two disease-related genes and a broader phenotype that includes individuals with no liver disease suggests that a redefinition of this syndrome is warranted based on molecular defects, possibly reserving the term ALGS for those with liver disease and associated features.

References

1. Alagille D, Thomassin HE. L'atresie des voies biliaires intrahepatiques avec voies biliaires extrahepatiques permeables chez l'enfant. *J Par Pediatr* 1969:301–318.

2. Emerick KM, Rand EB, Goldmuntz E, *et al.* Features of Alagille syndrome in 92 patients: frequency and relation to prognosis. *Hepatology* 1999;**29**:822–829.

3. Kamath BM, Spinner NB, Emerick KM, *et al.* Vascular anomalies in Alagille syndrome: a significant cause of morbidity and mortality. *Circulation* 2004;**109**:1354–1358.

4. Crosnier C, Lykavieris P, Meunier-Rotival M, Hadchouel M. Alagille syndrome. The widening spectrum of arteriohepatic dysplasia. *Clin Liver Dis* 2000;4:765–778.

5. Kamath BM, Bason L, Piccoli DA, Krantz ID, Spinner NB. Consequences of *JAG1* mutations. *J Med Genet* 2003;**40**:891–895.

6. Li L, Krantz ID, Deng Y, *et al.* Alagille syndrome is caused by mutations in human *JAGGED1*, which encodes a ligand for Notch1. *Nat Genet* 1997;**16**:243–251.

7. Oda T, Elkahloun AG, Pike BL, *et al.* Mutations in the human *JAGGED1* gene are responsible for Alagille syndrome. *Nat Genet* 1997;**16**:235–242.

8. Warthen DM, Moore EC, Kamath BM, *et al. JAGGED1 (JAG1)* mutations in Alagille syndrome: increasing the mutation detection rate. *Hum Mutat* 2006;**27**:436–443.

9. McDaniell R, Warthen DM, Sanchez-Lara PA, *et al. NOTCH2* mutations cause Alagille syndrome, a heterogeneous disorder of the Notch signaling pathway. *Am J Hum Genet* 2006;**79**:169–173.

10. Alagille D, Estrada A, Hadchouel M, *et al.* Syndromic paucity of interlobular bile ducts (Alagille syndrome or arteriohepatic dysplasia): review of 80 cases. *J Pediatr* 1987;**110**:195–200.

11. Deprettere A, Portmann B, Mowat AP. Syndromic paucity of the intrahepatic bile ducts: diagnostic difficulty; severe morbidity throughout early childhood. *J Pediatr Gastroenterol Nutr* 1987;**6**:865–871.

12. Hoffenberg EJ, Narkewicz MR, Sondheimer JM, *et al.* Outcome of syndromic paucity of interlobular bile

ducts (Alagille syndrome) with onset of cholestasis in infancy. *J Pediatr* 1995;**127**:220–224.

13. Quiros-Tejeira RE, Ament ME, Heyman MB, *et al.* Variable morbidity in Alagille syndrome: a review of 43 cases. *J Pediatr Gastroenterol Nutr* 1999;**29**:431–437.

14. Subramaniam P, Knisely A, Portmann B, *et al.* Diagnosis of Alagille syndrome-25 years of experience at King's College Hospital. *J Pediatr Gastroenterol Nutr* 2011;**52**:84–89.

15. Hofmann JJ, Zovein AC, Koh H, *et al.* Jagged1 in the portal vein mesenchyme regulates intrahepatic bile duct development: insights into Alagille syndrome. *Development* 2010;**137**:4061–4072.

16. Kamath BM, Munoz PS, Bab N, *et al.* A longitudinal study to identify laboratory predictors of liver disease outcome in Alagille syndrome. *J Pediatr Gastroenterol Nutr* 2010;**50**:526–530.

17. Kamath BM, Schwarz KB, Hadzic N. Alagille syndrome and liver transplantation. *J Pediatr Gastroenterol Nutr* 2010;**50**:11–15.

18. Kahn E. Paucity of interlobular bile ducts. Arteriohepatic dysplasia and nonsyndromic duct paucity. *Perspect Pediatr Pathol* 1991;**14**:168–215.

19. Alagille D, Odievre M, Gautier M, Dommergues JP. Hepatic ductular hypoplasia associated with characteristic facies, vertebral malformations, retarded physical, mental, and sexual development, and cardiac murmur. *J Pediatr* 1975;**86**:63–71.

20. Treem WR, Krzymowski GA, Cartun RW, *et al.* Cytokeratin immunohistochemical examination of liver biopsies in infants with Alagille syndrome and biliary atresia. *J Pediatr Gastroenterol Nutr* 1992;**15**:73–80.

21. Dahms BB, Petrelli M, Wyllie R, *et al.* Arteriohepatic dysplasia in infancy and childhood: a longitudinal study of six patients. *Hepatology* 1982;**2**:350–358.

22. Watson GH, Miller V. Arteriohepatic dysplasia: familial pulmonary arterial stenosis with neonatal liver disease. *Arch Dis Child* 1973;**48**:459–466.

23. McElhinney DB, Krantz ID, Bason L, *et al.* Analysis of cardiovascular phenotype and genotype-phenotype correlation in individuals with a *JAG1*

mutation and/or Alagille syndrome. *Circulation* 2002;**106**:2567–2574.

24. Bauer RC, Laney AO, Smith R, *et al.* *JAGGED1* (*JAG1*) mutations in patients with tetralogy of Fallot or pulmonic stenosis. *Human Mutat* 2010;**31**:594–601.

25. Lykavieris P, Crosnier C, Trichet C, Meunier-Rotival M, Hadchouel M. Bleeding tendency in children with Alagille syndrome. *Pediatrics* 2003;**111**:167–170.

26. Emerick KM, Krantz ID, Kamath BM, *et al.* Intracranial vascular abnormalities in patients with Alagille syndrome. *J Pediatr Gastroenterol Nutr* 2005;**41**:99–107.

27. Kamath BM, Loomes KM, Oakey RJ, Krantz ID. Supernumerary digital flexion creases: an additional clinical manifestation of Alagille syndrome. *Am J Med Genet* 2002;**112**:171–175.

28. Bales CB, Kamath BM, Munoz PS, *et al.* Pathologic lower extremity fractures in children with Alagille syndrome. *J Pediatr Gastroenterol Nutr* 2010;**51**:66–70.

29. Olsen IE, Ittenbach RF, Rovner AJ, *et al.* Deficits in size-adjusted bone mass in children with Alagille syndrome. *J Pediatr Gastroenterol Nutr* 2005;**40**:76–82.

30. Kamath BM, Loomes KM, Oakey RJ, *et al.* Facial features in Alagille syndrome: specific or cholestasis facies? *Am J Med Genet* 2002;**112**:163–170.

31. Rennie CA, Chowdhury S, Khan J, *et al.* The prevalence and associated features of posterior embryotoxon in the general ophthalmic clinic. *Eye* 2005;**19**:396–399.

32. Hingorani M, Nischal KK, Davies A, *et al.* Ocular abnormalities in Alagille syndrome. *Ophthalmology* 1999;**106**:330–337.

33. Nischal KK, Hingorani M, Bentley CR, *et al.* Ocular ultrasound in Alagille syndrome: a new sign. *Ophthalmology* 1997;**104**:79–85.

34. Strachan D, Kamath B, Wengraf C. How we do it: use of a venous cannulation needle for endoscopic Teflon injection to the vocal folds. *J Laryngol Otol* 1995;**109**:1184–1185.

35. Kamath BM, Podkameni G, Hutchinson AL, *et al.* Renal anomalies in Alagille syndrome: a disease-defining feature. *Am J Med Genet* 2012;**158A**:85–89.

36. Arvay JL, Zemel BS, Gallagher PR, *et al.* Body composition of children aged 1 to 12 years with biliary atresia or Alagille syndrome. *J Pediatr Gastroenterol Nutr* 2005;**40**:146–150.

37. Rovner AJ, Schall JI, Jawad AF, *et al.* Rethinking growth failure in Alagille syndrome: the role of dietary intake and steatorrhea. *J Pediatr Gastroenterol Nutr* 2002;**35**:495–502.

38. Bucuvalas JC, Horn JA, Carlsson L, Balistreri WF, Chernausek SD. Growth hormone insensitivity associated with elevated circulating growth hormone-binding protein in children with Alagille syndrome and short stature. *J Clin Endocrinol Metab* 1993;**76**:1477–1482.

39. Kamath BM, Whitington PF, Piccoli DA, for the Childhood Liver Disease Research and Education Network (ChiLDREN). Pancreatic insufficiency is not a prevalent problem in Alagille syndrome. *J Pediatr Gastroenterol Nutr* 2012;**55**:612–614.

40. Elisofon SA, Emerick KM, Sinacore JM, Alonso EM. Health status of patients with Alagille syndrome. *J Pediatr Gastroenterol Nutr* 2010;**51**:759–765.

41. Kamath BM, Loomes KM, Piccoli DA. Medical management of Alagille syndrome. *J Pediatr Gastroenterol Nutr* 2010;**50**:580–586.

42. Emerick KM, Whitington PF. Partial external biliary diversion for intractable pruritus and xanthomas in Alagille syndrome. *Hepatology* 2002;**35**:1501–1506.

43. Yang H, Porte RJ, Verkade HJ, De Langen ZJ, Hulscher JB. Partial external biliary diversion in children with progressive familial intrahepatic cholestasis and Alagille disease. *J Pediatr Gastroenterol Nutr* 2009;**49**:216–221.

44. Kaye AJ, Rand EB, Munoz PS, *et al.* Effect of Kasai procedure on hepatic outcome in Alagille syndrome. *J Pediatr Gastroenterol Nutr* 2010;**51**:319–321.

45. Wasserman D, Zemel BS, Mulberg AE, *et al.* Growth, nutritional status, body composition, and energy expenditure in prepubertal children with Alagille syndrome. *J Pediatr* 1999;**134**:172–177.

46. Kamath BM, Schwarz KB, Hadzic N. Alagille syndrome and liver transplantation. *J Pediatr Gastroenterol Nutr* 2010;**50**:11–15.

47. Nagasaka H, Yorifuji T, Egawa H, *et al.* Evaluation of risk for atherosclerosis in Alagille syndrome and progressive familial intrahepatic cholestasis: two congenital cholestatic diseases with different lipoprotein metabolisms. *J Pediatr* 2005;**146**:329–335.

48. Razavi RS, Baker A, Qureshi SA, *et al.* Hemodynamic response to continuous infusion of dobutamine in Alagille's syndrome. *Transplantation* 2001;**72**:823–828.

49. Kasahara M, Kiuchi T, Inomata Y, *et al.* Living-related liver transplantation for Alagille syndrome. *Transplantation* 2003;**75**:2147–2150.

50. Gurkan A, Emre S, Fishbein TM, *et al.* Unsuspected bile duct paucity in donors for living-related liver transplantation: two case reports. *Transplantation* 1999;**67**:416–418.

51. Arnon R, Annunziato R, Miloh T, *et al.* Orthotopic liver transplantation for children with Alagille syndrome. *Pediatr Transplant* 2010;**14**:622–628.

52. Byrne JL, Harrod MJ, Friedman JM, Howard-Peebles PN. del(20p) with manifestations of arteriohepatic dysplasia. *Am J Med Genet* 1986;**24**:673–678.

53. Spinner NB, Colliton RP, Crosnier C, *et al.* JAGGED1 mutations in Alagille syndrome. *Hum Mutat* 2001;**17**:18–33.

54. Crosnier C, Driancourt C, Raynaud N, *et al.* Mutations in *JAGGED1* gene are predominantly sporadic in Alagille syndrome. *Gastroenterology* 1999;**116**:1141–1148.

55. Yerushalmi B, Sokol RJ, Narkewicz MR, Smith D, Karrer FM. Use of rifampin for severe pruritus in children with chronic cholestasis. *J Pediatr Gastroenterol Nutr* 1999;**29**:442–447.

56. Kamath BM, Bauer RC, Loomes KM, *et al.* NOTCH2 mutations in Alagille syndrome. *J Med Genet* 2012;**49**:138–144.

57. Kamath BM, Thiel BD, Gai X, *et al.* SNP array mapping of chromosome 20p deletions: genotypes, phenotypes, and copy number variation. *Hum Mutat* 2009;**30**:371–378.

58. Gridley T. Notch signaling in vascular development and physiology. *Development* 2007;**134**:2709–2718.

59. Crosnier C, Attie-Bitach T, Encha-Razavi F, *et al.* JAGGED1 gene expression during human embryogenesis elucidates the wide phenotypic spectrum of Alagille syndrome. *Hepatology* 2000;**32**:574–581.

60. McCright B, Lozier J, Gridley T. A mouse model of Alagille syndrome: Notch2 as a genetic modifier of Jag1 haploinsufficiency. *Development* 2002;**129**:1075–1082.

61. Eldadah ZA, Hamosh A, Biery NJ, *et al.* Familial tetralogy of Fallot caused by mutation in the *JAGGED1* gene. *Hum Mol Genet* 2001;**10**:163–169.

62. Lozier J, McCright B, Gridley T. Notch signaling regulates bile duct morphogenesis in mice. *PLoS ONE.* 2008;**3**:e1851.

63. Tchorz JS, Kinter J, Muller M, *et al.* Notch2 signaling promotes biliary epithelial cell fate specification and tubulogenesis during bile duct development in mice. *Hepatology* 2009;**50**:871–879.

64. Zong Y, Panikkar A, Xu J, *et al.* Notch signaling controls liver development by regulating biliary differentiation. *Development* 2009;**136**:1727–1739.

65. Sparks EE, Huppert KA, Brown MA, Washington MK, Huppert SS. Notch signaling regulates formation of the three-dimensional architecture of intrahepatic bile ducts in mice. *Hepatology* 2010;**51**:1391–1400.

66. Garg V, Muth AN, Ransom JF, *et al.* Mutations in *NOTCH1* cause aortic valve disease. *Nature* 2005;**437**:270–274.

67. High FA, Zhang M, Proweller A, *et al.* An essential role for Notch in neural crest during cardiovascular development and smooth muscle differentiation. *J Clin Invest* 2007;**117**:353–363.

68. Jones EA, Clement-Jones M, Wilson DI. *JAGGED1* expression in human embryos: correlation with the Alagille syndrome phenotype. *J Med Genet* 2000;**37**:663–668.

Intestinal failure-associated liver disease

Jason Soden and Ronald J. Sokol

Introduction

Intestinal failure (IF) is defined as the end result of any gastrointestinal disorder in which functional intestinal mass is insufficient to allow adequate growth, hydration, and electrolyte balance in children and adults. Inherent in this definition is the requirement for parental nutrition (PN), which is provided to maintain fluid, energy, protein, electrolyte, and micronutrient delivery in the absence of adequate intestinal function. In the pediatric population, IF may be the end result of various primary etiologies, although the most common is short bowel syndrome (SBS) following congenital or acquired disorders, including necrotizing enterocolitis (NEC), small intestinal atresia, volvulus, and gastroschisis. Table 15.1 summarizes the most common etiologies of pediatric IF.

Because patients with IF are, by definition, dependent on PN, they are at risk for numerous complications associated both with their underlying disease and with PN administration. Traditionally, the most important complication associated with long-term total PN (TPN) administration in infants and children has been the development of progressive liver disease. In 1975, Rager and Finegold first reported the development of cholestasis in 9 of 15 premature infants on PN, an observation that was reported less than 10 years after the initial use of PN for infants with SBS [1]. This entity, historically referred to as "PN-associated cholestasis" or "PN-associated liver disease," has been an important negative factor in predicting outcomes and survival in the pediatric population with IF. The terminology implies that PN itself is the predominant factor responsible for liver injury in IF. Over time, a better understanding of the various risk factors for liver disease in the individual patient with IF has led to the broader, yet synonomous, description of intestinal failure-associated liver disease (IFALD).

Clinical presentation and natural history

The clinical spectrum of IFALD ranges from mild elevation of hepatocellular enzymes to severe, cholestatic liver injury with fibrosis and end-stage liver disease. In infants, particularly

Table 15.1 Causes of intestinal failure in children

	Causes
Short bowel syndrome	
Neonatal/infants	Atresia Midgut volvulus Gastroschisis Necrotizing enterocolitis Long segment aganglionosis Congenital short bowel syndrome
Older children	Trauma Mesenteric infarction Radiation enteritis Inflammatory bowel disease (rare)
Motility disorders	
Primary (congenital)	Neuropathic, myopathic
Secondary (acquired)	Neuropathic, myopathic
Mucosal abnormalities	
Primary enteropathies	Microvillous inclusion disease Primary epithelial dysplasia (tufting enteropathy) Congenital disorders of glycosylation
Immune mediated	Primary immunodeficiency syndromes Autoimmune enteropathies

premature neonates, the classic presentation includes cholestatic jaundice. Historically, cholestasis (defined as elevation of conjugated bilirubin >2 mg/dL) was reported to be present in 40–60% of infants on long-term PN [2]. In a retrospective review of all neonates that underwent abdominal surgery between 2001 and 2006 and required PN, 24% had cholestasis, defined as two consecutive elevated conjugated bilirubin levels over at least 14 days [3]. Cholestasis may develop as early as 2–6 weeks after PN initiation [4,5]. Laboratory abnormalities associated with elevated conjugated bilirubin include elevations in serum alkaline phosphatase and gamma-

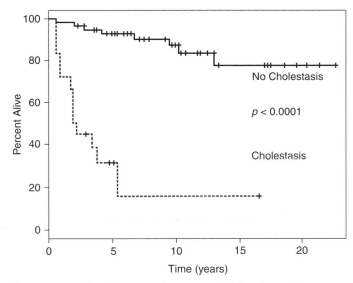

Figure 15.1 Kaplan–Meier curve illustrating probability of survival in a retrospective cohort of 78 patients with short bowel syndrome/intestinal failure with or without early persistent cholestatic jaundice. This study analyzed 25 years of retrospective data collected from 1975 to 2000. (With permission from Quiros-Tejeira *et al.*, 2004 [9].)

glutamyltransferase as well as aspartate aminotransferase (AST) and alanine aminotransferase (ALT). Elevation in alkaline phosphatase may be particularly challenging to interpret in the patient with IF because of micronutrient deficiencies such as zinc and vitamin D.

With ongoing PN administration, persistent biochemical cholestasis may evolve to the expected sequelae of progressive cholestatic liver injury, including fibrosis, portal hypertension, and liver synthetic dysfunction. In the patient with SBS, where enteral nutritional management is often optimized by use of a gastrostomy tube for feeding, portal hypertensive gastropathy may present with hemorrhage at the gastrostomy site. Histologically, intrahepatic cholestasis is predicted to progress to portal fibrosis within 8–12 weeks of continued PN exposure, and cirrhosis develops in >12 weeks [6]. The risk of developing end-stage liver disease has been reported to range from 15% to 90% of children with IF depending on the duration of PN [1,7]. Hepatocellular carcinoma has been reported as both a short- and long-term outcome in IFALD [8].

Importantly, the presence of IFALD is a major factor in predicting outcome of children with IF. Because the disease is progressive based on duration of PN exposure, evolving liver disease in a child that requires PN support has been a common and difficult complication to manage. In a retrospective analysis of 78 children with SBS over a 25 years at a single center, early, persistent cholestasis was identified as a key factor impacting survival in patients (Figure 15.1) [9].

In addition to the classic pediatric presentation of cholestatic liver injury, some patients, typically older children and adults, may develop elevation of liver enzymes alone, without the presence of cholestasis. In a retrospective analysis of 107 adults on long-term PN, nearly 40% developed abnormal liver chemistries (defined as any laboratory value >1.5 times normal range) [10]. Histologically, the adult-type PN-associated liver injury has been characterized by a steatohepatitis and portal fibrosis.

Occurrence of IFALD is considered to be reversible in that return to full enteral nutrition (along with discontinuation of PN), is associated with eventual biochemical and histological resolution in most patients. In those with advanced cirrhosis and portal hypertension, hepatic function may remain impaired even after PN has been discontinued.

Because the clinical management of patients with IF often requires prolonged periods of bowel rest, biliary stasis and subsequent biliary sludge or stone development is also relatively common. Cholelithiasis has been found in 40% of children requiring long-term PN, more common in patients with ileal resection and SBS [11]. Inspissated bile, biliary sludge, or gallstones may lead to frank biliary obstruction. Obstruction should be suspected in the patient with IF that develops acute worsening of conjugated bilirubin, acholic stools, or a Murphy's sign on physical examination. If cholelithiasis obstructing the bilary tree is encountered, the patient should be managed with routine surgical and endoscopic procedures. If no gallstones are encountered, diagnostic and therapeutic decision making may include endoscopic retrograde cholangiopancreatography, percutaneous transhepatic cholangiography, or intraoperative cholangiography.

Liver histology

Liver histology in IFALD demonstrates predominantly cholestasis or steatosis. Although these findings may be present in patients with IFALD of any age, there are features that track with age. In neonates and infants, liver histopathology is reflective of the predominant cholestatic injury observed clinically. In an autopsy study of neonates who had received TPN, the predominant findings included intracellular and canalicular cholestasis, bile duct proliferation, extramedullary hematopoiesis, periportal inflammation, portal tract bile duct plugging, and fibrosis [12]. In multiple studies, progression in liver fibrosis correlated with time of exposure to PN (Figure 15.2) [6,12]. It is relevant to point out that these histologic findings, as well as the progression to fibrosis, are characteristic of other neonatal cholestatic diseases, particularly biliary atresia. In fact, IFALD histology can be indistinguishable from biliary atresia. Steatosis is a common finding in older children and adults, often in combination with cholestasis, but rare in infants. In a recent retrospective study [13], the liver biopsies of 89 patients on PN were reviewed, and findings were segregated between patients who were <6 months and >12 months of age at the time of PN initiation: 91% of the younger cohort had cholestasis compared with 67% of the older cohort. Only 26% of the younger cohort had steatosis, compared with 58%

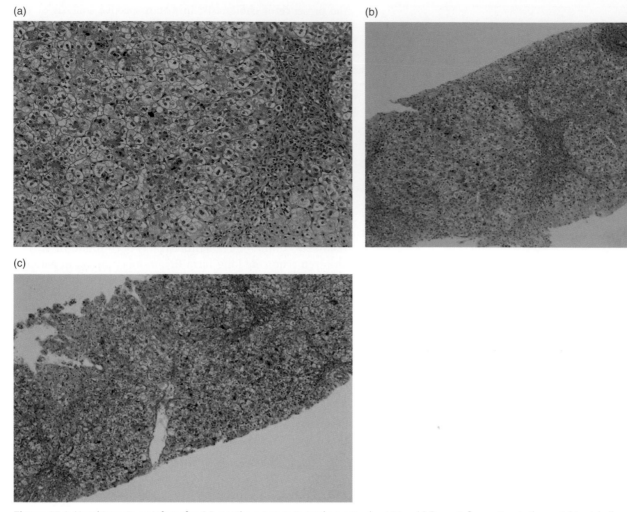

Figure 15.2 Liver biopsy in an infant after 3.5 months exposure to total parenteral nutrition. (a) Dense inflammation in the portal tract, ballooning hepatocytes, and canalicular bile plugging (hematoxylin & eosin, magnification ×20). (b,c) Fibrous expansion with bridging fibrosis (Ishak stage 3–4 out of 6) (b, hematoxylin & eosin, magnification ×10; c, trichrome staining magnification ×10).

of the older group (Table 15.2). The explanation for this age-related variation in histology may involve the immaturity of expression of bile acid and other canalicular transporters in infancy, promoting a propensity toward cholestasis upon injury.

An important issue in the clinical and histologic follow-up of IFALD is a discrepancy that potentially exists between biochemical cholestasis and histologic fibrosis. In a retrospective review of 83 liver biopsy specimens, serum direct bilirubin was normal (<2 mg/dL) in 55% of patients whose biopsies showed fibrosis [14]. Other recent studies have supported the lack of relationship between elevations of aminotransferases and the degree of hepatocellular fibrosis [13,15]. Therefore, risks for liver fibrosis and associated clinical sequelae, including portal hypertension and synthetic dysfunction, may persist independent of laboratory assessment. Liver biopsies should be obtained and followed when clinically indicated, and, if possible, at any surgical procedure where the surgeon may obtain a biopsy without imposing greater risk.

Risk factors and pathogenesis

The development and progression of IFALD is likely to be the result of a confluence of factors in the patient with IF. When reviewed in isolation, no single factor has been implicated as causative of liver injury in all patients on PN. Rather, there is a multifactorial pathogenesis leading to the end result of progressive cholestatic liver injury. Taking into account what is known about clinical risk factors for IFALD development, the most important categories include (1) underlying patient factors, including prematurity; (2) acute factors, including the occurrence of sepsis; (3) surgical factors, including anatomy, luminal or biliary stasis, and underlying disease; and (4) factors related to PN, including excess or deficiencies of macronutrients, micronutrients, or contaminants (Figure 15.3). Within this last category is the important subject of parenteral lipid composition. Historically, there have been multiple studies that have examined individual risk factors for IFALD, with data primarily

Table 15.2 Frequency of liver histopathologic findings in infants and children with intestinal failure-associated liver disease

	0–6 months at start (No. (%))	>1 year at start % (No. (%))
Total No.	53	36
Cholestasis	48 (91)	24 (67)
Steatosis*	14 (26)	21 (58)
Portal inflammation		
None	4 (84)	0
Mild	39 (73)	29 (80)
Moderate	10 (19)	7 (20)
Lobular inflammation		
None	2 (4)	0
Mild	42 (79)	33 (91)
Moderate	9 (17)	3 (8)
Ballooning and feathery changes		
None	5 (95)	5 (14)
Mild	16 (30)	18 (50)
Moderate	17 (32)	13 (36)
Severe*	15 (28)	0
Apoptosis		
Absent	5 (9)	9 (25)
Rare	37 (70)	3 (8)
Easily found*	11 (21)	1 (3)
Portal fibrosis	48 (91)	48 (91)
Stage 0	3 (6)	1 (3)
Stage 1	2 (4)	7 (19)
Stage 2	16 (30)	21 (58)
Stage 3	14 (26)	7 (19)
Stage 4*	18 (34)	0
Periventricular fibrosis		
None	9 (17)	11 (31)
Mild	15 (28)	17 (47)
Moderate	20 (38)	6 (17)
Severe	9 (17)	2 (6)
Ductopenia		
Present	12 (23)	9 (25)
Absent	28 (53)	21 (58)
Intermediate	13 (24)	6 (17)

* $p < 0.05$ for difference between two age groups.
Source: with permission from Zambrano *et al.*, 2004 [12].

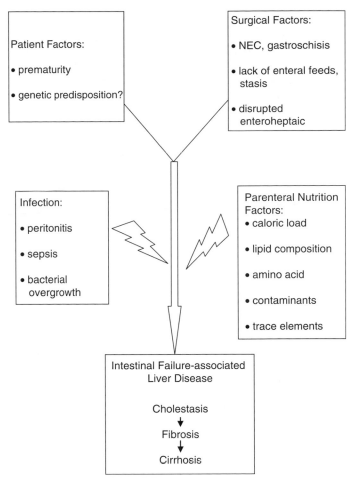

Figure 15.3 A confluence of factors contribute to the pathogenesis of intestinal failure-associated liver disease. Host factors, including prematurity, and surgical factors are important predisposing issues. Components of the parenteral nutrition itself, including parenteral lipids, share an important role in pathogenesis. Intercurrent infections, including catheter-associated sepsis and small bowel bacterial overgrowth, are common, and contribute to progression and severity of liver injury. NEC, necrotizing enterocolitis.

Patient (host) factors

Prematurity

One of the earliest factors identified as a risk for IFALD is prematurity. Using low birth weight as a correlate of gestational age, Beale *et al.* [16] reported a 50% incidence of PN-associated liver disease in infants born at <1000 g, a fivefold increase in risk compared with infants born at >1500 g. This finding has been supported in multiple studies [4,17]. In a retrospective, multicenter analysis of 1366 neonates who received ≥14 days of PN, the odds ratio of developing PN-associated liver disease was 30.7 in neonates with birth weight <500 g and 13.1 in those <750 g [4].

There are several potential factors to explain why the premature or low-birth-weight neonate may be at higher risk for IFALD development [1]. Immature enterohepatic circulation in the neonatal liver may predispose to cholestasis [18]. At a molecular level, this is likely related to developmentally

generated retrospectively. Challenges in interpreting these studies lie in the fact that the clinical subgroups often contain a diverse population of patients with heterogeneous gestational ages, underlying surgical diseases, and variability in treatment. Therefore, it has been difficult to draw definitive conclusions with regards to any single etiologic factor as causative of liver injury in the patient with IFALD. This chapter will highlight some of the more established clinical risk factors associated with IFALD, focusing on potential mechanisms of pathogenesis.

regulated expression of nuclear receptors (e.g. the farsenoid X receptor (FXR)) and their effect on expression of bile acid transporters [19]. Accumulation of toxic bile acids may precipitate secondary oxidant injury, to which the neonatal liver may be more predisposed because of antioxidant and other deficiencies (such as glutathione deficiency) [20].

Acute factors

Sepsis

Sepsis, typically related to venous catheter infections, is common in the pediatric IF population. A multicenter, retrospective analysis of 272 infants with IF found that 3.3/person-year new catheter-related bloodstream infections occurred in infants on PN [21]. The occurrence of infection has been well demonstrated as a key risk factor in the development of IFALD [17]. In a retrospective analysis of 42 postsurgical infants on PN $\geq$3 months, the majority of patients who developed cholestasis did so within 14 days of an episode of infection and patients who developed early infections (<6 weeks of life) were most likely to develop cholestasis [7]. This clinical correlation between age of first infection and severity of IFALD was further supported by a histological study that compared 16 infants with IFALD who had severe liver fibrosis with 14 with normal/mild fibrosis; the incidence of infection was significantly greater, and age at first infection was significantly lower, in the severe fibrosis subgroup[22].

The relationship between sepsis and cholestasis is well established, and there are several pathophysiologic mechanisms that support this clinical association. Within the liver, circulating endotoxin (lipopolysaccharide) activates Kupffer cells, stimulating the release of proinflammatory cytokines, which generate an inflammatory cascade. Kupffer cell activation likely occurs through endotoxin binding to membrane receptors causing induction of Toll-like receptor-dependent pathways [23]. At the hepatocellular level, endotoxinemia and subsequent release of cytokines lead to downregulation of bile acid transporters. On the basolateral hepatocyte aspect, decreased expression of the transporting proteins sodium taurocholate co transporting polypeptide and organic anion transporting polypeptide lead to decreased uptake of circulating bile acids. On the apical canalicular level, decreased expression of the bile salt export pump (BSEP) and multidrug resistance-associated protein 2 lead to accumulation of bile acids and other organic ions within the hepatocyte, stimulating further downstream hepatotoxic effects.

Surgical factors

Intestinal and biliary stasis

Several clinical factors precipitate alterations in normal gastrointestinal motility in patients with IF. There is often a requirement for prolonged avoidance of enteral feedings when there are congenital intestinal malformations or postsurgical issues. Feeding intolerance in malabsorptive diarrhea is common in the patient with SBS, and this may require interval periods of decreased or absent enteral feeding. As the foreshortened bowel undergoes adaptation, there is compensatory luminal dilatation to improve the absorptive surface area. When the bowel is overly distended, motility is altered, promoting stasis. Alterations in enteral feeding lead to decreased circulation of enteral hormones, including cholecystokinin, glucagon, gastrin, and enteroglucagon [1]. Decreased secretion of cholecystokinin and other regulatory gastrointestinal hormones predisposes to stasis within the biliary tree as well as in the intestinal lumen. Precipitation and sludge of bile, exaggerated when there are anatomic alterations in enterohepatic circulation (e.g. in the patient with ileal resection), also contribute to the propensity for cholelithiasis and IFALD development.

In addition to affecting gut motility, intestinal stasis and postsurgical anatomic alterations (absence of ileocecal valve, bowel dilation, anastomotic narrowing or dysfunction) predispose the patient with IF to small bowel bacterial overgrowth (SBBO). Bacterial overgrowth is an important factor in the clinical management of patients with IF. Because objective evaluation for SBBO is difficult to obtain and interpret, there are no conclusive studies that directly link SBBO as a causative factor in IFALD. Theoretically, however, the accumulation and overpopulation of enteric organisms, often Gram-negative bacteria, lead to enteritis, altered intestinal permeability to bacterial cell wall products (pathogen-associated molecular patterns), and bacterial translocation. Translocation, in turn, is likely to drive clinical episodes of Gram-negative sepsis (catheter-associated bloodstream infections) in the patient with IF. There may also be subclinical translocation of bacteria, without frank bacteremia, that further drives the activation of inflammatory cascades and the downregulation of bile acid transport pumps within the hepatocyte and liver.

Underlying disease

An understanding of the above pathogenic factors (prematurity, sepsis, intestinal stasis) offers support to the identification of surgical etiologies in IF that provide higher risk for IFALD development and progression. The most common etiology of SBS in the pediatric population is NEC. It occurs in premature infants, often presenting with acute, severe bowel necrosis and secondary peritonitis. The premature infant with compromised bowel and NEC may require emergency surgical management, bowel resection, and often prolonged periods of limited enteral feeding. In addition, the patient with SBS following NEC has a prolonged PN requirement starting at an early age, typically initiated in a setting of peritoneal contamination or systemic sepsis and continued in the setting of anatomically disrupted bowel integrity and impaired motility. It is no surprise, then, that the occurrence of severe NEC directly correlates with incidence of IFALD [24].

In addition to NEC, infants with gastroschisis and prolonged PN requirement have been implicated as having a higher risk for IFALD development and progression [4]. The patient with gastroschisis, particularly with concomitant intestinal atresia and SBS, may have a significantly dilated and often dysfunctional bowel, further predisposing to SBBO, altered intestinal permeability, PN requirement, and sepsis.

At present, there are no studies that conclusively link a defined postsurgical anatomy (e.g. jejunal resection, ileal resection) with occurrence of IFALD. However, the absence of the ileocecal valve has been well established as a risk factor for both SBBO and prolonged PN requirement in comparison with an intact ileocecal valve and colon after surgery or stoma takedown [25]. It can be extrapolated that this anatomic variation may also predispose to IFALD based at least on the risk of prolonged PN exposure.

Parenteral nutrition factors

The interplay between host factors and components of the administered PN itself likely fuel the liver injury in IFALD. It is clear that the histologic progression in IFALD correlates with duration of PN exposure, implying that PN administration is key to the development of cholestasis and liver injury. Because the prescription of PN entails multiple factors – fluids, electrolytes, micronutrients, macronutrients, administration rate, additives – isolation of specific variables has been challenging and has led to multiple hypotheses historically as to what parenteral components or deficiencies are most likely to contribute to IFALD.

Excessive energy and/or carbohydrate load

Excessive delivery of parenteral calories (>110–120 kcal/kg daily) or carbohydrate (>15–20 mg/kg per min) may lead to hyperglycemia, hyperinsulinemia, and hepatic steatosis. Steatosis is an important feature in the liver injury in adults with IFALD. In cholestatic injury associated with pediatric-type IFALD, steatosis is not generally present. In the present era, when attention to reduction of intravenous lipids has gained predominance in IF management, there is a compensatory increase in parenteral carbohydrate delivery to maintain adequate energy provision. Future studies will be relevant to re-examine the relationship between carbohydrate composition and liver injury.

Amino acid component

As a key macronutrient and energy source of PN, amino acid dosing and sources have been analyzed for their potential role in IFALD pathogenesis. There is reasonable evidence to suggest that a higher cumulative administered dose of parenteral amino acids is associated with higher risk of IFALD in infants. Steinbach et al. [26] found that the development of cholestasis in 122 patients on PN was more likely in neonates with a higher cumulative amino acid dose *and* longer duration of exposure to PN, factors that are essentially dependent on one another. Although the cumulative duration and dose of parenteral amino acid exposure is a relevant risk factor, there is no evidence that the initial dose of amino acid or rate of advancement is significant in IFALD development [17].

There is speculation that the formulation of parenteral amino acid solution may affect the development of IFALD. In comparing two standard amino acid formulations (Aminosyn PF and TrophAmine), Forchielli et al. [27] found no difference in development of cholestasis, whereas several years later, Wright et al. [28] suggested that Aminosyn PF was more likely to lead to cholestasis in a retrospective analysis of neonates on PN for ≥21 days. Therefore, there is inconclusive evidence regarding the formulation of amino acid solution in IFALD pathogenesis.

A deficiency in conditional amino acids in the neonate may also predispose to development of cholestasis. Premature neonates have decreased levels of cystathionase, which synthesizes taurine (and cysteine) from methionine [1]. Taurine is essential to the conjugation of bile acids and, therefore, taurine deficiency might lead to reduced bile acid secretion and subsequent accumulation of toxic bile acids. In an animal model of PN-associated cholestasis, supplementation with taurine improved bile acid secretion [29].

Carnitine depletion has been demonstrated in both animal models and human studies after PN administration [30]. Carnitine plays a key role in mitochondrial fatty acid oxidation and so its deficiency may impair energy utilization while increasing oxidative stress within the liver. Despite these findings, there has been no proven therapeutic benefit of carnitine supplementation on IFALD development [31].

Choline deficiency has been associated with the development of steatosis in patients on PN [32]. In children, choline deficiency has been associated with elevation of serum AST and ALT [33]. However, choline deficiency has not been shown to be associated with the development of cholestatic injury in children.

Lipid emulsions

Among the studies attempting to identify a single causative parenteral factor in the pathogenesis of IFALD, promising work has implicated lipid emulsions. At present, the fat component of PN in the USA is conventionally provided through a soybean-based intravenous lipid emulsion. Consensus guidelines have recommended that lipid emulsions account for 25–40% of non-protein calories administered in PN, making a daily dose of 2–3.5 g/kg [34]. Commonly used intravenous lipids are soybean- or plant-based lipid emulsions. Currently, the US Food and Drug Administration has approved two lipid solutions for parenteral use, soybean-based Intralipid (Fresenius Kabi, Stockholm, Sweden) and soybean and safflower-based Liposyn II (Hospira, Lake Forest, IL, USA). These plant-derived lipid oils are composed primarily of omega-6 polyunsaturated fatty acids. In general, long-chain polyunsaturated fatty acids can be categorized as omega-6 and omega-3. Omega-6 fatty acids, including linoleic acid, are precursors of arachidonic acid, which, in turn, forms the structural backbone of proinflammatory eicosanoids. In contrast, the omega-3 fatty acids (e.g. α-linoleic acid) are synthesized into

Table 15.3 Composition of lipid emulsion products

	Intralipid	Omegaven	SMOFlipid
Manufacturer	Baxter/ Fresenius Kabi	Fresenius Kabi	Fresenius Kabi
Oil source (g)			
Soy Ban	10	0	3
Safflower	0	0	0
Medium-chain triglycerides	0	0	3
Olive oil	0	0	2.5
Fish oil	0	10	1.5
Alpha-tocopherol (mg/L)	38	150–296	200
Phytosterol (mg/L)	348 ± 33	0	47.6
Fat composition (g)			
Linoleic acid	5.0	0.1–0.7	2.9
α-Linoleic acid	0.9	<0.2	0.3
Eicosapentanoic acid	0	1.28–2.82	0.3
Docosahexaenoic acid	0	1.44–3.09	0.05
Oleic acid	2.6	0.6–1.3	2.8
Palmitic acid	1.0	0.25–1.00	0.9
Stearic acid	0.35	0.05–0.20	0.3
Arachidonic acid	0	0.1–0.4	0.05

Source: adapted from Le *et al.*, 2010 [35].

anti-inflammmatory derivatives of EPA and docosahexaenoic acid. At present, several other lipid solutions are approved for use in Europe that contain a higher ratio of omega-3 to omega-6 fatty acids, including fish oil-based Omegaven (Fresenius Kabi) and SMOFlipid (Fresenius Kabi). Table 15.3 contains details of the components of currently available parenteral lipid emulsions [35].

In 2000, Colomb *et al.* [36] reported a series of 10 infants on PN that developed cholestasis in temporal correlation with increased dosage of soy-based lipid emulsion. More recently, Diamond *et al.* [37] reported that a key risk factor for development of advanced IFALD (serum conjugated bilirubin ≥5.9 mg/dL) was days of exposure to a daily parenteral lipid dose of ≥2.5 g/kg. Recently, some have recommended dose reduction or elimination of soy-based lipid emulsions and replacement with novel lipid solutions, including products derived from omega-3 fatty acids (fish oil) [38–40]. The pathophysiology of liver injury following soy lipid emulsion administration includes considerations of the biologic effects of fatty acids, as well as the potential role of plant-derived sterols (phytosterols).

In reviewing the role of intravenous lipids as the primary mediator of liver injury, supporting data have been obtained from animal models and human studies in which omega-6-based fatty acids are reduced or replaced with omega-3 based fatty acids. Studies of the effects of these therapeutic maneuvers in children will be reviewed in the "Treatment" section of this chapter. An initial report described two children with IF in whom cholestasis biochemically normalized after elimination of Intralipid and initiation of Omegaven [41]. This led to a re-examination of the role of lipid emulsions both clinically and in animal models of liver disease. A primary hypothesis supporting the potential benefit of omega-3- versus omega-6-based lipid solutions is the downstream anti-inflammatory properties of the omega-3 fatty acids compared with the potentially proinflammatory omega-6 forms. Several studies have clarified that this change in fatty acid profile may alter immunomodulatory pathways both within the liver and systemically [42,43]. As an example of direct anti-inflammatory effects within the liver, decreased markers of hepatitis (ALT and liver biopsy scores) and decreased proinflammatory cytokine expression (tumor necrosis factor-α, interferon-γ, interluekin-1β, and interleukin-6) were seen following supplementation with omega-3 fatty acids compared with controls in a mouse model of steatohepatitis [44].

In the clinical setting, the provision of proinflammatory omega-6 fatty acids has potential implications in the child with intestinal failure, where there are constant hurdles including peritonitis, catheter-associated bloodstream infections, and bacterial overgrowth and translocation. These infants and children are at risk for sepsis and increased intestinal permeability to macromolecules, and they may face subclinical events of bacteremia and endotoxinemia. Therefore, the administration of a potentially anti-inflammatory omega-3 fatty acid may help to blunt systemic inflammatory responses that mitigate end-organ pathways, including liver injury in IFALD.

Aside from alterations in proinflammatory/anti-inflammatory balance, omega-6 fatty acid administration may also favor the development of hepatic steatosis [45]. In contrast, murine models of steatosis have shown reduced histologic fat accumulation after administration of omega-3 fatty acid [46]. This effect of omega-3 fatty acid may be mediated through stimulation of fatty acid beta-oxidation or reduced hepatic lipogenesis, as shown in experimental models [45].

Another important component of intravenous lipid emulsions are the phytosterols, plant-based naturally occurring plant sterols that resemble cholesterol but have an alkylated side-chain. Elevated plasma phytosterol levels was reported in five children with cholestatic liver disease associated with PN [47]. In all patients, phytosterol levels and serum bilirubin improved following reduction in amount of lipid emulsion. The role of phytosterols in the pathogenesis of cholestasis may be through decreased bile acid synthesis or decreased bile acid secretion. For example, injection of phytosterols to neonatal piglets led to decreased bile flow and increased serum bilirubin [48]. Similarly, rat hepatocytes in culture exposed to phytosterols demonstrated decreased morphological cannalicular expression and decreased bile flow [48]. In another experimental model, neonatal piglets who received a fish oil-based intravenous lipid emulsion in PN had improved cholestasis and bile flow compared with those receiving soybean oil-derived lipid [49]. Although the latter study did not measure phytosterols specifically, these clinical and laboratory results suggest that the development of cholestasis in IFALD may be, in part, mediated by phytosterols in soybean-based lipid solutions. More recent studies demonstrate a correlation between phytosterol levels and the degree of both biochemical and histological injury in IFALD [50].

Molecular mechanisms to explain the apparent effect of TPN, lipid emulsion, and, more specifically, phytosterols on cholestasis development may involve alterations in expression of canalicular phospholipid and bile acid transporters. The effects of TPN administration on *Mdr2* RNA expression, which encodes for a canalicular phospholipid flippase, has been evaluated in mice [51]. The animals receiving TPN had significantly decreased expression of *Mdr2* correlating with elevated serum bile acid levels. In further experiments, there was no significant difference in *Mdr2* expression in mice that received PN with and without lipid emulsion, although serum bile acid levels were normal in mice that did not receive lipid [52]. Canalicular bile acid transport may occur through several proteins including BSEP, which is regulated by FXR. Administration of phytosterol (stigmasterol) led to decreased FXR in murine hepatocytes in primary culture, and further ameliorated BSEP expression, suggesting a direct role of phytosterols in the pathogenesis of cholestasis through FXR-mediated pathways that alter canalicular BSEP expression [53]. More recent investigations have demonstrated that both stigmasterol injection and soybean-based lipid administration led to similar changes in parameters of liver injury (elevated AST, ALT, bile acid, and bilirubin) and decreased FXR and BSEP expression in a murine model of PN liver injury; these effects were blunted when the animal received saline, PN without lipid, or PN with fish oil-based lipid [54]. Furthermore, addition of stigmasterol to fish oil-based lipid led to similar measures of liver injury and FXR/BSEP expression as in the soybean oil group [54]. These data support the pathogenic role of phytosterol in IFALD development, specifically cholestasis, through inhibition of FXR-mediated BSEP pathways or other canalicular biliary transporters. Alterations in human genotypes of bile acid transport expression may explain clinical phenotypes that are more susceptible to lipid-mediated IFALD.

Other contaminants or toxicities

Aluminum and chromium toxicities have been reported in PN-treated patients; however, neither of these parenteral contaminants have been linked to the pathogenesis of IFALD [2]. Photo-oxidation of both lipid emulsion and vitamin components in PN solutions leads to downstream oxidative stress, which theoretically may affect the liver; however, no direct cause-and-effect relationship between these factors has been seen in the development of IFALD [55].

Toxic serum levels of both manganese and copper have been reported in cholestatic patients on long-term PN [56,57]. Because these trace elements undergo hepatic clearance via bile excretion, the cholestatic patient is predisposed to retention and accumulation of these minerals. Manganese toxicity may further exacerbate cholestasis, with evidence of more severe IFALD in children with cholestasis and manganese toxicity compared with those with normal manganese levels. Typical recommendations are to eliminate manganese from trace element delivery in cholestatic patients with IF. Since copper deficiency states (from excess fecal losses in patients with SBS) have been reported in addition to copper toxicity in PN administration, copper may safely be administered, but serum levels should be monitored closely [58].

Treatment
Intestinal failure management

The primary treatment goal in the management of IFALD is to graduate a patient off PN. A progressive normalization in serum bilirubin was seen in 12 patients with IFALD after advancement to 100% enteral calories (and elimination of PN) (Figure 15.4) [3]. An organized, multispecialty approach to intestinal rehabilitation involving pediatric gastroenterology, pediatric surgery, nutrition, and pharmacy may improve time to weaning of PN. Nutritional management should be aimed at targeting appropriate enteral caloric sources, often with early initiation of trophic feedings and ongoing reliance upon continuous tube feeding, with careful monitoring and management of malabsorption and fluid and electrolyte status. Attention to fat-soluble vitamin and trace element status is important in the cholestatic infant with IF. Medical and pharmacologic management includes use of antisecretory agents, antimotility therapy, and surveillance for and treatment of SBBO. Surgical comanagement includes early stoma closure, and, when indicated, the use of bowel tapering and lengthening procedures, including serial transverse enteroplasty, to enhance absorptive surface, motility, and tolerance of enteral feedings.

Considering the important association between sepsis and IFALD development and progression, prevention of catheter-associated infections should be a central goal in the management of IF and, secondarily, IFALD prevention. Recently, ethanol locks have gained favor as a means of reducing the incidence of catheter-associated infections in children on PN [59]. More preliminary experience with antibiotic locks suggests this therapy may also have a role in preventing episodes of sepsis in IF.

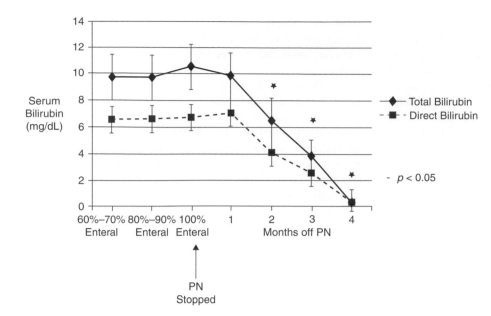

Figure 15.4 This retrospective review of 12 patients demonstrates the expected improvement in cholestasis once enteral autonomy is achieved. Once parenteral nutrition (PN) is discontinued, there is eventual normalization of serum bilirubin concentration. (With permission from Javid *et al.*, 2011 [5].)

Modification of non-lipid factors in parenteral nutrition

Careful attention to caloric requirements in the daily administration of PN should reduce hypercaloric administration, which could exacerbate steatosis and liver injury. In addition, cycling of PN (defined as non-continuous PN administration) has long been considered to be a favorable infusion option. From a patient-care perspective, cycling of PN allows the patient and family time off the infusion pump, which is associated with improved patient and caregiver quality of life [17]. Past studies have examined cycling of PN as a potentially hepatoprotective step in PN administration. A retrospective review showed decreased incidence of cholestasis in neonates with gastroschisis who received cycled PN compared with those receiving continuous PN [60]. In order to initiate non-continuous PN administration, the patient must be able to maintain adequate glycemic control during hours on and off infusion.

As discussed above, attention to trace elements in the cholestatic infant on PN should include avoidance of parenteral manganese, as well as reduction and surveillance of parenteral copper. There is insufficient evidence to support routine glutamine supplementation as a means to reduce the incidence of IFALD.

Modification of parenteral lipid

To date, no single therapy in the management of patients with IFALD has offered the therapeutic momentum present in the current era of IF management, much of which surrounds the approach to parenteral lipid modification. Following the publication of the small case series in 2006 [41] describing

resolution in IFALD in two patients following Omegaven (fish oil based), there has been a general change in clinical practice surrounding reduction or replacement of traditional soybean-based lipid emulsions. It should be emphasized that Omegaven is not approved by the US Food and Drug Administration and can only be used in the USA under Investigational New Drug status.

The initial clinical experience and publications surrounding fish oil-based lipid emulsions came from the Boston Children's Hospital [41,61]. A retrospective study compared a cohort of 18 infants with SBS/IF and cholestasis (direct bilirubin >2 mg/dL) who were treated by discontinuation of Intralipid (2–3 g/kg daily) and initiation of Omegaven (1 g/kg daily) with an historical cohort of 22 infants; the Omegaven group achieved reversal of cholestasis at a significantly shorter time interval (9.4 weeks versus 44.1 weeks) [62]. Similar results were seen in a larger, open label trial of 42 infants, in which 19 of 38 patients who received fish oil lipid emulsion achieved reversal of cholestasis compared with 2 of 36 patients in a soybean oil group (Figure 15.5) [40]. Several smaller, retrospective series have documented the effectiveness of Omegaven in reversing cholestasis and IFALD [15,62,63]. Although a randomized controlled trial has not been conducted, the data are compelling.

The above data have led investigators to consider whether it is the elimination of soybean lipid emulsions, the reduction in dose of lipid, or the addition of fish oil lipid emulsions that offers the therapeutic benefit. A prospective study examined parenteral lipid reduction in a soybean-based lipid emulsion from an historical control of 31 patients receiving 3 g/kg daily and a treatment group of 31 receiving 1 g/kg twice per week [38]. Bilirubin levels were significantly decreased in the lipid-reduction group compared with the controls, suggesting a

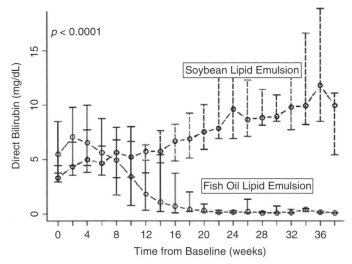

Figure 15.5 Time to reversal of cholestasis (as defined by serum bilirubin <2 mg/dL) in 42 infants with intestinal failure treated with fish oil-based lipid solution (Omegaven) compared to contemporary cohort of 49 infants who received soybean oil-based lipid (Intralipid). (With permission from Gura *et al.*, 2008 [62].)

lipid emulsion has been well tolerated. There is a single case report of an infant who developed reversible hemolytic anemia associated with fish oil lipid therapy [66].

Pharmacologic management

No single pharmacologic strategy has been proven to be effective in the prevention or management of IFALD. Choleritic agents (e.g. ursodeoxycholic acid) are widely used in this setting. Studies supporting the efficacy of ursodeoxycholic acid in IFALD have typically been small, retrospective, single-center reviews [17]. An open-label trial of tauroursodeoxycholic acid showed no benefit in treatment compared with control [67]. There are questions as to whether sufficient oral ursodeoxycholic acid can be absorbed in patients with IF to promote bile flow.

A large, multicenter, double-blind, randomized controlled trial was conducted to evaluate the effect of intravenous cholecystokinin-octapeptide (CCK-OP) for prevention of IFALD in 243 neonates. Treatment failed to reduce incidence of PN-associated liver injury and the frequency of cholelithiasis compared with a control group [68].

Reports of other therapeutic strategies in IFALD include the use of *N*-acetylcysteine (treatment) and high-dose oral erythromycin (prevention) to promote motility and sooner tolerance of enteral feedings [17]. Further studies into these and other pharmacologic modalities are necessary in order to better estimate their role in armamentarium of IFALD management.

Transplantation

Progressive liver disease in the setting of IF has historically been the predominant indication for multivisceral (combined liver and small intestine) transplantation in children. At present, 1-year survival following intestinal transplantation is 80%, and 5-year survival approaches 50% [69]. Considering these outcome statistics, current efforts to better characterize and treat IFALD offer potentially more favorable options than that of transplantation. In limited clinical situations, a patient with IF may show progressive tolerance to advancing enteral nutrition yet continue to manifest progressive end-stage liver disease. In these situations, in which the expectation is that the patient will achieve full enteral autonomy, isolated liver transplantation is a therapeutic option. With newer medical and surgical approaches to managing IF, the hope is that intestinal adaptation and reduction of IFALD will reduce the need for liver, intestinal, or multivisceral transplantation in children with IF.

lower dose of soybean-based lipid emulsion would be effective. However, eight patients in the lipid-reduction group were identified as having mild essential fatty acid deficiency, which corrected with more frequent administration of the low dose of lipid emulsion.

The potential risks of reducing or eliminating soybean-based (omega-6) fatty acids include that of deficiency of essential fatty acids. It is recommended protocol to survey biochemically for evidence of essential fatty acid deficiency in patients who undergo parenteral lipid modification. So far, conventional dosing of fish oil-based lipid emulsions (1 g/kg daily) has not resulted in documented essential fatty acid deficiency [64]. A retrospective review examined 12 children with advanced IFALD (conjugated bilirubin ≥5.9 mg/dL or ≥2.9 mg/dL with evidence of liver dysfunction) treated with 1 g/kg daily Omegaven in addition to 1 g/kg daily Intralipid [39]. Nine patients sustained normalization of serum bilirubin. This approach may theoretically provide a more balanced fatty acid and lipid profile. From that respect, a newer product containing soybean, medium-chain triglycerides, olive oil, and fish oil lipid emulsion (SMOFlipid, Fresenius Kabi) appears to be safe and well tolerated in infants with SBS, and in a randomized, double-blind study comparing SMOF with standard soybean lipid emulsion, the SMOF group showed lower serum bilirubin [65]. This product is not yet available in the USA. In general, the administration of fish oil-based

References

1. Carter BA, Shulman RJ. Mechanisms of disease: update on the molecular etiology and fundamentals of parenteral nutrition associated cholestasis. *Nat Clin Pract Gastroenterol Hepatol* 2007;**4**:277–287.

2. Kelly DA. Intestinal failure-associated liver disease: what do we know today? *Gastroenterology* 2006;**130**(Suppl 1): S70–S77.

3. Javid PJ, Collier S, Richardson D, *et al.* The role of enteral nutrition in the

reversal of parenteral nutrition-associated liver dysfunction in infants. *J Pediatr Surg* 2005;**40**:1015–1018.

4. Christensen RD, Henry E, Wiedmeier SE, Burnett J, Lambert DK. Identifying patients, on the first day of life, at high-risk of developing parenteral nutrition-associated liver disease. *J Perinatol* 2007;**27**:284–290.

5. Javid PJ, Malone FR, Dick AA, *et al.* A contemporary analysis of parenteral nutrition-associated liver disease in surgical infants. *J Pediatr Surg* 2011;**46**:1913–1917.

6. Mullick FG, Moran CA, Ishak KG. Total parenteral nutrition: a histopathologic analysis of the liver changes in 20 children. *Mod Pathol* 1994;**7**:190–194.

7. Sondheimer JM, Asturias EM. Infection and cholestasis in neonates with intestinal resection and long-term parenteral nutrition. *J Pediatr Gastroenterol Nutr* 1998;**27**:131–137.

8. Yeop I, Taylor C, Narula P, *et al.* Hepatocellular carcinoma in a child with intestinal failure associated liver disease. *J Pediatr Gastroenterol Nutr* 2012;**54**:695–697.

9. Quiros-Tejeira RE, Ament ME, Reyen L, *et al.* Long-term parenteral nutritional support and intestinal adaptation in children with short bowel syndrome: a 25-year experience. *J Pediatr* 2004;**145**:157–163.

10. Luman W, Shaffer JL. Prevalence, outcome and associated factors of deranged liver function tests in patients on home parenteral nutrition. *Clin Nutr* 2002;**21**:337–343.

11. Roslyn JJ, Berquist WE, Pitt HA, *et al.* Increased risk of gallstones in children receiving total parenteral nutrition. *Pediatrics* 1983;**71**:784–789.

12. Zambrano E, El-Hennawy M, Ehrenkranz RA, Zelterman D, Reyes-Mugica M. Total parenteral nutrition induced liver pathology: an autopsy series of 24 newborn cases. *Pediatr Dev Pathol* 2004;**7**:425–432.

13. Naini BV, Lassman CR. Total parenteral nutrition therapy and liver injury: a histopathologic study with clinical correlation. *Hum Pathol* 2012;**43**:826–833.

14. Fitzgibbons SC, Jones BA, Hull MA, *et al.* Relationship between biopsy-proven parenteral nutrition-associated liver fibrosis and biochemical cholestasis in children with short bowel syndrome. *J Pediatr Surg* 2010;**45**:95–99; discussion 99.

15. Soden JS, Lovell MA, Brown K, Partrick DA, Sokol RJ. Failure of resolution of portal fibrosis during omega-3 fatty acid lipid emulsion therapy in two patients with irreversible intestinal failure. *J Pediatr* 2010;**156**:327–331.

16. Beale EF, Nelson RM, Bucciarelli RL, Donnelly WH, Eitzman DV. Intrahepatic cholestasis associated with parenteral nutrition in premature infants. *Pediatrics* 1979;**64**:342–347.

17. Rangel SJ, Calkins CM, Cowles RA, *et al.* Parenteral nutrition-associated cholestasis: an American Pediatric Surgical Association Outcomes and Clinical Trials Committee systematic review. *J Pediatr Surg* 2012;**47**:225–240.

18. Balistreri WF, Heubi JE, Suchy FJ. Immaturity of the enterohepatic circulation in early life: factors predisposing to "physiologic" maldigestion and cholestasis. *J Pediatr Gastroenterol Nutr* 1983;**2**:346–354.

19. Karpen SJ. Nuclear receptor regulation of hepatic function. *J Hepatol* 2002;**36**:832–850.

20. Sokol RJ, Taylor SF, Devereaux MW, *et al.* Hepatic oxidant injury and glutathione depletion during total parenteral nutrition in weanling rats. *Am J Physiol* 1996;**270**:G691–G700.

21. Squires RH, Duggan C, Teitelbaum DH, *et al.* Natural history of pediatric intestinal failure: initial report from the Pediatric Intestinal Failure Consortium. *J Pediatr* 2012;**161**:723–728.

22. Hermans D, Talbotec C, Lacaille F, *et al.* Early central catheter infections may contribute to hepatic fibrosis in children receiving long-term parenteral nutrition. *J Pediatr Gastroenterol Nutr* 2007;**44**:459–463.

23. El Kasmi KC, Anderson AL, Devereaux MW, *et al.* Toll like receptor 4 dependent Kupffer cell activation and liver injury in a novel mouse model of parenteral nutrition. *Hepatology* 2012;**55**:1518–1528.

24. Duro D, Mitchell PD, Kalish LA, *et al.* Risk factors for parenteral nutrition-associated liver disease following surgical therapy for necrotizing enterocolitis: a Glaser Pediatric Research Network Study. *J Pediatr Gastroenterol Nutr* 2011;**52**:595–600.

25. Duro D, Kamin D, Duggan C. Overview of pediatric short bowel syndrome. *J Pediatr Gastroenterol Nutr* 2008;**47**(Suppl 1):S33–S36.

26. Steinbach M, Clark RH, Kelleher AS, *et al.* Demographic and nutritional factors associated with prolonged cholestatic jaundice in the premature infant. *J Perinatol* 2008;**28**:129–135.

27. Forchielli ML, Gura KM, Sandler R, Lo C. Aminosyn PF or trophamine: which provides more protection from cholestasis associated with total parenteral nutrition? *J Pediatr Gastroenterol Nutr* 1995;**21**:374–382.

28. Wright K, Ernst KD, Gaylord MS, Dawson JP, Burnette TM. Increased incidence of parenteral nutrition-associated cholestasis with aminosyn PF compared to trophamine. *J Perinatol* 2003;**23**:444–450.

29. Guertin F, Roy CC, Lepage G, *et al.* Effect of taurine on total parenteral nutrition-associated cholestasis. *J Parenter Enteral Nutr* 1991;**15**:247–251.

30. Tibboel D, Delemarre FM, Przyrembel H, *et al.* Carnitine deficiency in surgical neonates receiving total parenteral nutrition. *J Pediatr Surg* 1990;**25**:418–421.

31. Wales PW, Diamond IR. Intestinal failure-associated liver disease. In Duggan CP, Guru KM, Jaksic T (eds.) *Clinical Management of Intestinal Failure.* Boca Raton, FL: CRC Press, 2012, pp. 247–263.

32. Buchman AL, Dubin MD, Moukarzel AA, *et al.* Choline deficiency: a cause of hepatic steatosis during parenteral nutrition that can be reversed with intravenous choline supplementation. *Hepatology* 1995;**22**:1399–1403.

33. Misra S, Ahn C, Ament ME, *et al.* Plasma choline concentrations in children requiring long-term home parenteral nutrition: a case control study. *J Parenter Enteral Nutr* 1999;**23**:305–308.

34. Koletzko B, Goulet O, Hunt J, Krohn K, Shamir R. 1. Guidelines on paediatric parenteral nutrition of the European Society of Paediatric Gastroenterology, Hepatology and Nutrition (ESPGHAN) and the European Society for Clinical Nutrition and Metabolism (ESPEN), supported by the European Society of Paediatric Research (ESPR). *J Pediatr Gastroenterol Nutr* 2005;**41**(Suppl 2): S1–S87.

35. Le HD, Fallon EM, de Meijer VE, *et al.* Innovative parenteral and enteral nutrition therapy for intestinal failure. *Semin Pediatr Surg* 2010;**19**:27–34.

36. Colomb V, Jobert-Giraud A, Lacaille F, *et al.* Role of lipid emulsions in cholestasis associated with long-term parenteral nutrition in children. *J Parenter Enteral Nutr* 2000;**24**:345–350.

37. Diamond IR, de Silva NT, Tomlinson GA, *et al.* The role of parenteral lipids in the development of advanced intestinal failure-associated liver disease in infants: a multiple-variable analysis. *J Parenter Enteral Nutr* 2011;**35**:596–602.

38. Cober MP, Killu G, Brattain A, *et al.* Intravenous fat emulsions reduction for patients with parenteral nutrition-associated liver disease. *J Pediatr* 2012;**160**:421–427.

39. Diamond IR, Sterescu A, Pencharz PB, Kim JH, Wales PW. Changing the paradigm: omegaven for the treatment of liver failure in pediatric short bowel syndrome. *J Pediatr Gastroenterol Nutr* 2009;**48**:209–215.

40. Puder M, Valim C, Meisel JA, *et al.* Parenteral fish oil improves outcomes in patients with parenteral nutrition-associated liver injury. *Ann Surg* 2009;**250**:395–402.

41. Gura KM, Duggan CP, Collier SB, *et al.* Reversal of parenteral nutrition-associated liver disease in two infants with short bowel syndrome using parenteral fish oil: implications for future management. *Pediatrics* 2006;**118**:e197–e201.

42. Lee S, Gura KM, Kim S, *et al.* Current clinical applications of omega-6 and omega-3 fatty acids. *Nutr Clin Pract* 2006;**21**:323–341.

43. Wanten GJ, Calder PC. Immune modulation by parenteral lipid emulsions. *Am J Clin Nutr* 2007;**85**:1171–1184.

44. Schmocker C, Weylandt KH, Kahlke L, *et al.* Omega-3 fatty acids alleviate chemically induced acute hepatitis by suppression of cytokines. *Hepatology* 2007;**45**:864–869.

45. Diamond IR, Sterescu A, Pencharz PB, Wales PW. The rationale for the use of parenteral omega-3 lipids in children with short bowel syndrome and liver disease. *Pediatr Surg Int* 2008;**24**:773–778.

46. Alwayn IP, Gura K, Nose V, *et al.* Omega-3 fatty acid supplementation prevents hepatic steatosis in a murine model of nonalcoholic fatty liver disease. *Pediatr Res* 2005;**57**:445–452.

47. Clayton PT, Bowron A, Mills KA, *et al.* Phytosterolemia in children with parenteral nutrition-associated cholestatic liver disease. *Gastroenterology* 1993;**105**: 1806–1813.

48. Iyer KR, Spitz L, Clayton P. BAPS prize lecture: new insight into mechanisms of parenteral nutrition-associated cholestasis: role of plant sterols. British Association of Paediatric Surgeons. *J Pediatr Surg* 1998;**33**:1–6.

49. van Aerde JE, Duerksen DR, Gramlich L, *et al.* Intravenous fish oil emulsion attenuates total parenteral nutrition-induced cholestasis in newborn piglets. *Pediatr Res* 1999;**45**:202–208.

50. Kurvinen A, Nissinen MJ, Andersson S, *et al.* Parenteral plant sterols and intestinal failure associated liver disease in neonates: a prospective nationwide study. *J Pediatr Gastroenterol Nutr* 2012;**54**:803–811.

51. Tazuke Y, Kiristioglu I, Heidelberger KP, Eisenbraun MD, Teitelbaum DH. Hepatic P-glycoprotein changes with total parenteral nutrition administration. *J Parenter Enteral Nutr* 2004;**28**:1–6.

52. Tazuke Y, Teitelbaum DH. Alteration of canalicular transporters in a mouse model of total parenteral nutrition. *J Pediatr Gastroenterol Nutr* 2009;**48**:193–202.

53. Carter BA, Taylor OA, Prendergast DR, *et al.* Stigmasterol, a soy lipid-derived phytosterol, is an antagonist of the bile acid nuclear receptor FXR. *Pediatr Res* 2007;**62**:301–306.

54. El Kasmi K, Anderson A, Devereaux M, Noe M, Sokol R. Soy lipid-derived phytosterols are responsible for parenteral nutrition associated liver injury (PNALI) in a mouse model. *Hepatology* 2011;**54**:89A.

55. Lavoie JC, Chessex P, Gauthier C, *et al.* Reduced bile flow associated with parenteral nutrition is independent of oxidant load and parenteral multivitamins. *J Pediatr Gastroenterol Nutr* 2005;**41**:108–114.

56. Blaszyk H, Wild PJ, Oliveira A, Kelly DG, Burgart LJ. Hepatic copper in patients receiving long-term total parenteral nutrition. *J Clin Gastroenterol*, 2005;**39**:318–320.

57. Fell JM, Reynolds AP, Meadows N, *et al.* Manganese toxicity in children receiving long-term parenteral nutrition. *Lancet* 1996;**347**:1218–1221.

58. Frem J, Sarson Y, Sternberg T, Cole CR. Copper supplementation in parenteral nutrition of cholestatic infants. *J Pediatr Gastroenterol Nutr* 2010;**50**:650–654.

59. Oliveira C, Nasr A, Brindle M, Wales PW. Ethanol locks to prevent catheter-related bloodstream infections in parenteral nutrition: a meta-analysis. *Pediatrics* 2012;**129**:318–329.

60. Jensen AR, Goldin AB, Koopmeiners JS, *et al.* The association of cyclic parenteral nutrition and decreased incidence of cholestatic liver disease in patients with gastroschisis. *J Pediatr Surg* 2009;**44**:183–189.

61. Gura KM, Parsons SK, Bechard LJ, *et al.* Use of a fish oil-based lipid emulsion to treat essential fatty acid deficiency in a soy allergic patient receiving parenteral nutrition. *Clin Nutr* 2005;**24**:839–847.

62. Gura KM, Lee S, Valim C, *et al.* Safety and efficacy of a fish-oil-based fat emulsion in the treatment of parenteral nutrition-associated liver disease. *Pediatrics* 2008;**121**:e678–e686.

63. Cheung HM, Lam HS, Tam YH, Lee KH, Ng PC. Rescue treatment of infants with intestinal failure and parenteral nutrition-associated cholestasis (PNAC) using a parenteral fish-oil-based lipid. *Clin Nutr* 2009;**28**:209–212.

64. de Meijer VE, Le HD, Meisel JA, Gura KM, Puder M. Parenteral fish oil as monotherapy prevents essential fatty acid deficiency in parenteral nutrition-dependent patients. *J Pediatr Gastroenterol Nutr* 2010;**50**:212–218.

65. Goulet O, Antebi H, Wolf C, *et al.* A new intravenous fat emulsion containing soybean oil, medium-chain triglycerides, olive oil, and fish oil: a single-center, double-blind randomized study on efficacy and safety in pediatric patients receiving home parenteral nutrition. *J Parenter Enteral Nutr* 2010;**34**:485–495.

66. Mallah HS, Brown MR, Rossi TM, Block RC. Parenteral fish oil-associated burr cell anemia. *J Pediatr* 2010;**156**:324–326 e1.

67. Heubi JE, Wiechmann DA, Creutzinger V, *et al.* Tauroursodeoxycholic acid (TUDCA) in the prevention of total

parenteral nutrition-associated liver disease. *J Pediatr* 2002;**141**:237–242.

68. Teitelbaum DH, Tracy TF, Jr., Aouthmany MM, *et al.* Use of cholecystokinin-octapeptide for the prevention of parenteral nutrition-associated cholestasis. *Pediatrics* 2005;**115**:1332–1340.

69. Abu-Elmagd KM, Costa G, Bond GJ, *et al.* Five hundred intestinal and multivisceral transplantations at a single center: major advances with new challenges. *Ann Surg* 2009;**250**:567–581.

Chapter

16

Disease of the gallbladder in infancy, childhood, and adolescence

Frank W. DiPaola and James E. Heubi

Embryologic development of the gallbladder

The hepatic rudiment appears at approximately day 18 of gestation in the human embryo. By day 25 it can be recognized as an endodermal diverticulum, which projects into the mesenchymal septum transversum. By day 30, the hepatic diverticulum enlarges and divides into the pars hepatica, cranially, and the pars cystica, caudally. The pars hepatica forms parenchymal liver components; the pars cystica differentiates into the gallbladder and cystic ducts (Figure 16.1). The gallbladder primordium is a solid structure that later in development becomes cystic, as found in the adult [1].

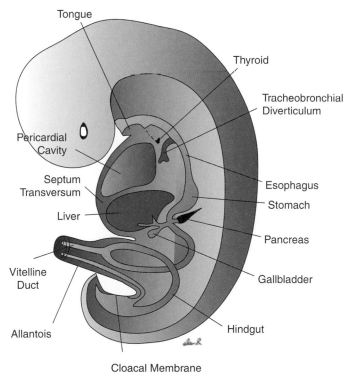

Figure 16.1 Representation of a 9 mm embryo (36 days of gestation) showing the early formation of the bile ducts and gallbladder between the liver and digestive tract. (With permission from Langman, 1990 [1].)

Congenital anomalies of the gallbladder

A variety of structural anomalies of the gallbladder has been described:

- congenital absence (agenesis) of the gallbladder
- hypoplasia of the gallbladder
- heterotopic tissue in the gallbladder (gastric, hepatic, adrenal, pancreatic, thyroid)
- multiple gallbladder formation (double gallbladder, triple gallbladder)
- septated gallbladder
- diverticuli of the gallbladder
- malposition of the gallbladder
- pendulous gallbladder ("floating gallbladder").

Congenital absence of the gallbladder long has been recognized in humans; it was known to Aristotle. Overall, the incidence of agenesis of the gallbladder has been estimated at between 1 in 7500 and 1 in 10 000 among the general population. There are a number of mammalian species lacking a gallbladder, including the horse, camel, deer, rat, and dolphin. Absence of the gallbladder may occur as an isolated anomaly or in association with other malformations. In the isolated form, absence of the gallbladder is of little clinical significance. It is believed to result from failed development of the pars cystica. Rarely, symptoms develop related to calculi formation in the biliary ductal system.

A number of anomalies have been described in association with congenital absence of the gallbladder. Extrahepatic biliary atresia is associated not uncommonly with absence of the gallbladder; situs inversus, asplenia or polysplenia, and complex congenital heart defects frequently accompany this form of biliary atresia. Imperforate anus, genitourinary anomalies, anencephaly, bicuspid aortic valves, and cerebral aneurysms are associated with agenesis of the gallbladder. Absence of the gallbladder also accompanied thalidomide embryopathy.

Hypoplasia of the gallbladder has also been described. As many as one-third of patients with cystic fibrosis may have a

---

Liver Disease in Children, Fourth Edition, ed. Frederick J. Suchy, Ronald J. Sokol, and William F. Balistreri. Published by Cambridge University Press. © Cambridge University Press 2014.

small, poorly functional gallbladder. Gallbladder hypoplasia is associated with trisomy 18.

Heterotopic tissue may be found within the gallbladder wall with gastric or hepatic tissue being the most common tissue found. Ectopic adrenal, pancreatic, and thyroid tissues have also been found. The cause of heterotopia is poorly understood. Because the ectopic tissues are all of foregut, endodermal origin, localized heteroplastic differentiation during organogenesis has been proposed. These ectopic foci within the gallbladder wall are seldom of clinical significance; however, chemical irritation secondary to "gastric" acid secretion has been reported.

The incidence of a double gallbladder has been estimated between 0.1 and 0.75 per 1000 in the general population: 28 patients with gallbladder duplication, defined as structures having two separate gallbladder cavities and two cystic ducts, have been described. The two cystic ducts may converge into a single duct forming a Y-shaped structure or may enter the biliary ductal system separately. The paired gallbladders may lie in an appropriate position in the gallbladder fossa, or the accessory gallbladder may be located under the left lobe of the liver, draining into the left hepatic ducts. Rarely, it may be found surrounded by hepatic parenchyma.

Developmentally, duplicate gallbladders are presumed to arise as diverticuli of the embryologic cystic, hepatic, or common duct. Such diverticuli commonly are seen in vertebrate embryos. If these ductal buds fail to regress, an accessory gallbladder may form, which drains into the duct from which it originated. The accessory gallbladder may be more prone to pathologic changes than a normal organ. One case report described a double gallbladder draining into the pancreatic duct of Wirsung.

A single report of a triple gallbladder has been described in the literature.

In contrast to multiple gallbladders, a single gallbladder may be divided into multiple chambers by longitudinal septa, presumably secondary to incomplete resolution of its solid phase. Conversely, small diverticuli off the body of the gallbladder may be seen. Because these diverticuli promote bile stasis, gallstones may form.

A normally formed, single gallbladder may be malpositioned. Gallbladders have been described lying beneath the left lobe of the liver, horizontally in the transverse fissure, or embedded within hepatic parenchyma. Malposition of the gallbladder may be caused by one of two mechanisms: Abnormal migration of the pars cystica could result in an aberrant gallbladder location. Alternatively, a ductal diverticulum forming a "second gallbladder," in conjunction with failed genesis of the pars cystica, could result in a single malpositioned gallbladder. Anomalous gallbladder position is clinically silent unless accompanied by cholelithiasis and cholecystitis. An increased frequency of gallstone formation in association with malposition of the gallbladder is suspected, although it has not been studied systematically.

An uncommon occurrence that may be of clinical significance is the so-called floating gallbladder. This is a gallbladder with a peritoneal coat suspending it from the undersurface of the liver. The embryogenesis is unknown, but a gallbladder-supporting membrane of this type has been seen in approximately 5% of routine autopsy examinations. This "mesentery" may cover the entire length of the gallbladder, creating a stable structure. On occasion, however, it surrounds only the cystic duct, creating a pendulous gallbladder. With this anatomic arrangement, torsion of the gallbladder may occur.

Torsion of the gallbladder is a rare clinical entity but may present a surgical emergency. Elderly women are at greatest risk, although pediatric cases have been reported. The presentation is with abrupt onset of severe, right upper quadrant abdominal pain, with nausea and vomiting. The patient is usually afebrile. On physical examination there is marked right upper quadrant tenderness and often a palpable mass. Peritoneal signs may be present. Shock may ensue. Surgical intervention reveals an infarcted gallbladder on a twisted pedicle. Rarely has the diagnosis been presumed preoperatively.

Acalculous gallbladder disease

Gallbladder disease in the absence of gallstones is being recognized with increasing frequency with the availability of newer and better ultrasound techniques. Classically, acute noncalculous gallbladder disease has been classified as either hydrops or acalculous cholecystitis; the distinction between the two syndromes may be unclear. These conditions may represent a spectrum of disease ranging from transient gallbladder distension with spontaneous resolution to acute acalculous cholecystitis with necrosis of the gallbladder wall.

Hydrops of the gallbladder

Acute hydrops is defined by marked gallbladder distension in the absence of calculi, bacterial infection, or congenital gallbladder anomaly and is associated with a normal-caliber extrahepatic biliary ductal system. The absence of a significant inflammatory component and its typically benign prognosis are the features that distinguish hydrops from acalculous cholecystitis.

Etiology and pathogenesis

Hydrops most commonly is recognized in association with Kawasaki syndrome. The incidence of gallbladder hydrops complicating Kawasaki syndrome ranges from 5 to 20%. In the most extensive series, 13.7% (16 of 117) of children with Kawasaki syndrome had hydrops when examined by ultrasound. The typical presentation included abdominal pain, vomiting, and right upper quadrant mass superimposed on the clinical features of Kawasaki syndrome (fever for longer than 5 days, conjunctivitis, oral mucosal changes, rash, and cervical adenopathy). A mild, conjugated hyperbilirubinemia may also be present. Gallbladder hydrops has also been discovered by screening ultrasonography in patients with Kawasaki syndrome in the absence of significant abdominal complaints. In the vast majority of patients, gallbladder distension is

Table 16.1 Conditions associated with gallbladder hydrops

Age group	Conditions
Infants and children	Kawasaki syndrome
	Mesenteric adenitis
	Viral hepatitis
	Streptococcal pharyngitis
	Staphylococcal infection
	Henoch–Schönlein purpura
	Hypokalemia
	Sjögren syndrome
	Nephrotic syndrome
Neonates	Sepsis
	Total parenteral nutrition
	α_1-Antitrypsin deficiency
	Fasting

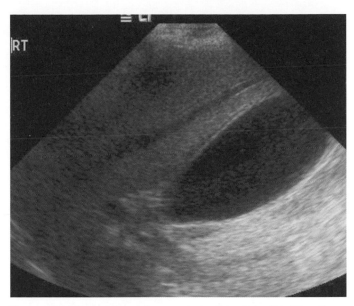

Figure 16.2 Ultrasound depicting a markedly distended gallbladder with minimal intraluminal debris and minimal wall thickening in an 8-year-old child presenting with group A β-hemolytic streptococcal pharyngitis and right upper quadrant pain.

self-limited, resolving without surgical intervention. Complications of gallbladder necrosis and perforation, however, have been reported in patients with Kawasaki syndrome. Serial clinical and ultrasonographic examinations are suggested to monitor for resolution.

The hydrops in this disorder is believed to be secondary to a vasculitic process in the gallbladder wall, with cystic duct obstruction. Perivascular leukocytic infiltration with vascular congestion has been described on pathologic examination of a hydropic gallbladder from a child with Kawasaki syndrome. Bile cultures are sterile. Enlarged lymph nodes surrounding, and perhaps obstructing, the cystic duct also have been reported. As depicted in Table 16.1, hydrops of the gallbladder has been reported in association with a variety of disorders.

Hydrops may accompany staphylococcal or streptococcal infection, with associated toxin production. Gallbladder hydrops has been described in a number of young children with antecedent upper respiratory infection (or no clear antecedent illness) in whom surgical intervention revealed enlarged mesenteric lymph nodes. Whether cystic duct obstruction secondary to adenopathy played a role in the pathogenesis of the hydrops is unclear.

Single cases of gallbladder hydrops have been reported in infants and children with Sjögren syndrome, Henoch–Schönlein purpura, viral hepatitis, and hypokalemia secondary to Bartter syndrome.

Clinical features

The child with hydrops of the gallbladder typically presents with abdominal pain and a tender right upper quadrant mass. Vomiting, fever, and stigmata of an associated illness are commonly found. The clinical picture may mimic intussusception or acute appendicitis.

The diagnosis of hydrops generally is made by ultrasonography, demonstrating a markedly distended, echo-free gallbladder and a normal-caliber biliary tree (Figure 16.2). Prior to the routine use of ultrasonography, the diagnosis typically was encountered as an unsuspected finding at laparotomy.

The mainstay of therapy is supportive, with fluid resuscitation and therapy aimed at an associated illness if indicated (such as antibiotics for streptococci). Serial ultrasound examinations are useful to confirm resolution. Surgery should be reserved for the exceedingly rare complication of gallbladder perforation. Symptomatic abdominal pain can resolve after 1 to 2 days.

Transient gallbladder distension has also been recognized with increasing frequency in neonates. Typically, the presentation is as a right upper quadrant abdominal mass in a sick neonate or premature infant. Associated conditions have included sepsis, prolonged fasting, and administration of total parenteral nutrition (TPN), likely related to the reduced cholecystokinin secretion and impaired gallbladder contraction. Gallbladder distension in neonates with cystic fibrosis (perhaps secondary to inspissation of bile) and α_1-antitrypsin deficiency (perhaps secondary to cystic duct hypoplasia) have been reported.

Ultrasonography is used to confirm that the abdominal mass is the gallbladder. Typically, with the institution of feeding, transient gallbladder distension in the neonate resolves spontaneously. It is important to remember, however, that a number of cases of culture-proven acalculous cholecystitis in neonates have been documented. Because there are no reliable ultrasound criteria for distinguishing inflammation from benign distension (thickening of the gallbladder wall is neither entirely sensitive nor specific for inflammation), failure of the abdominal mass to resolve or clinical deterioration should warrant further investigation. Surgical intervention may be required in some patients.

Acalculous cholecystitis

Acalculous cholecystitis, characterized by distension and inflammation of the gallbladder, is uncommon in infants and children. It is an important entity to recognize, however, because it may present as an abdominal emergency.

Etiology and pathogenesis

Acalculous cholecystitis has been reported at all ages from neonates to adolescents. Acalculous cholecystitis in adults commonly accompanies serious illness or trauma. Predisposing factors for the development of acalculous cholecystitis have been identified in 50% of children and include:

- postoperative state
- burns
- multiple transfusions
- trauma
- *Escherichia coli* infection of the gallbladder in neonates
- systemic infection

  - sepsis
  - leptospirosis
  - Rocky Mountain spotted fever
  - typhoid fever
  - *Cryptosporidium* infection
  - *Giardia* infection
  - cytomegalovirus infection
  - candidal infection
  - aspergillosis
- immunocompromised host
- hemophagocytic lymphohistiocytosis.

The pathophysiology of acalculous cholecystitis is poorly understood. In the postoperative or severely ill patient, the lack of enteral feeding, the administration of TPN, and the use of opiates result in gallbladder stasis. In some patients, congenital narrowing or local inflammation of the cystic duct has been demonstrated at the time of surgical intervention. Obstruction of the cystic duct with gallbladder distension and secondary bacterial invasion may lead to cholecystitis. Episodic ischemia or hypoperfusion also could play a role in the development of acalculous cholecystitis in the patient in intensive care.

Acalculous cholecystitis has been described in association with systemic infectious illness. Three patients with leptospirosis presenting as fever, pharyngitis, cervical adenopathy, and rash had tender abdominal masses that laparotomy identified as an inflamed distended gallbladder [2]. Therapy included tube cholecystostomy with good results. In a review of the experience with leptospirosis at St. Louis Children's Hospital, five of nine infections were complicated by acalculous cholecystitis requiring surgical drainage [3].

In one review of neonates with acalculous cholecystitis, 8 of 10 infants had systemic infection [4]. Bile cultures grew *Escherichia coli*, *Streptococcus viridans*, *Serratia* sp., and *Pseudomonas* sp. The two infants in whom there was no evidence of sepsis had congenital anomalies of the biliary tree with cystic duct obstruction. Another report of two neonates, one premature and one term, reported non-specific symptoms including irritability and ileus [5]. In each case, exploratory laparotomy revealed gallbladder necrosis and cultures from the gallbladder grew *E. coli*. Both infants fully recovered following cholecystectomy [5].

Gallbladder inflammation has been described with Rocky Mountain spotted fever, with rickettsial organisms demonstrated in a surgically resected gallbladder. The course of typhoid fever frequently has been complicated by acalculous cholecystitis; the first cholecystostomy was performed for acute gallbladder inflammation secondary to typhoid fever in 1901. Children with hemophagocytic lymphohistiocytosis may present with a constellation of ultrasound findings including hepatosplenomegaly, ascites, pleural effusion, periportal echogenecity, and gallbladder wall thickening.

Associated illness or anomaly is not necessary for the development of acalculous cholecystitis in the pediatric population; none of the seven patients in one series had an associated predisposing illness or documented systemic infection. Cholecystectomy was performed in all seven without postoperative complication.

Opportunistic infection may occur in the gallbladder of an immunocompromised host. Adults with HIV infection or after orthotopic liver transplant have been reported to have cholecystitis secondary to cytomegalovirus infection. Fungal infections of the gallbladder with *Candida*, *Torulopsis*, and *Aspergillus* spp. have been described. Additionally, parasitic infestation of the gallbladder with *Giardia* and *Cryptosporidium* spp. has occurred in association with HIV infection and other immunodeficiency states.

Clinical features

Patients with acalculous cholecystitis classically present with right upper quadrant abdominal pain, nausea, vomiting, and fever. Physical examination reveals right upper quadrant or generalized abdominal tenderness. A mass may be palpable. Leukocytosis is an inconsistent finding. Signs and symptoms may be less readily apparent in the neonate or the severely ill patient. The clinical presentation may be dominated by the findings of an associated illness, such as trauma or a systemic infectious process.

The differential diagnosis includes appendicitis, intussusception, infectious hepatitis, choledochal cyst, and diffuse peritonitis. Ultrasonography can demonstrate gallbladder distension, with thickening of the gallbladder wall (Figure 16.3) and echogenic intraluminal debris. Thickening of the gallbladder wall can also be demonstrated by axial CT (Figure 16.4). The reliability of excessive thickness of the gallbladder wall as an indicator of acute inflammation has been questioned. In a report by Sanders [6], a thickened gallbladder wall was present in 45% of adults with acute calculous and non-calculous

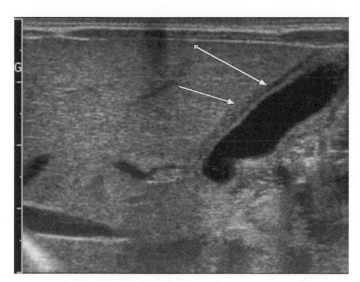

Figure 16.3 Thickening of the gallbladder wall in a 9-year-old child with leukemia and right upper quadrant pain. Longitudinal ultrasound images demonstrate striking thickening (arrows) of the gallbladder wall and pericholecystic fluid collections.

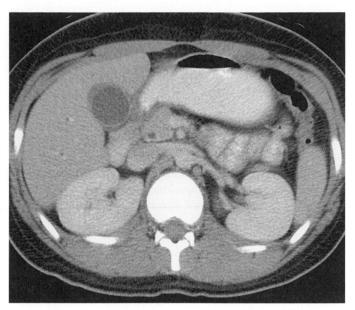

Figure 16.4 Axial CT with intravenous contrast demonstrating striking thickening of the gallbladder wall. There is also dilatation of the common bile duct as it traverses the pancreas.

cholecystitis studied by ultrasound. In a series of 793 consecutively studied infants and children, Patriquin *et al.* [7] reported that 20 patients were identified as meeting ultrasound criteria for a thick gallbladder wall (defined as >3 mm). Of these 20 patients, 16 had hypoalbuminemia, 2 had ascites, 1 had physiologic thickening associated with contraction of the gallbladder wall, and 1 had heart disease with associated systemic venous hypertension. None of the patients had clinical findings suggestive of acute cholecystitis. Of five patients with surgically proven acute cholecystitis who underwent ultrasound examinations during the study period, none had a thickened gallbladder wall. Most recently, Jeffrey and Sommer [8] evaluated 14 adults with clinically suspected acute acalculous cholecystitis but inconclusive initial abdominal ultrasounds. Four of the patients with normal gallbladder walls demonstrated progressive thickening on subsequent studies, and three of these patients had acute acalculous cholecystitis as a surgical finding. Six patients had thickened gallbladder walls at the initial ultrasound examination, but only one of these patients required a cholecystectomy after continuing to have symptoms consistent with acute acalculous cholecystitis. These data suggest that repetitive ultrasound examinations may be helpful in diagnosing acute acalculous cholecystitis. Gallbladder wall thickening may represent a local inflammatory response or may be a reflection of a systemic process; a thickened gallbladder wall depicted by ultrasound must be interpreted in the context of the clinical setting.

The diagnosis of acute acalculous cholecystitis requires a high index of clinical suspicion. Radiographic techniques can provide strong supportive evidence in the appropriate clinical setting. Ultrasound findings consistent with acute acalculous cholecystitis, however, such as gallbladder distension, gallbladder wall thickening, lack of calculi, and a poor response to cholecystokinin, can also be seen in gallbladder hydrops. Radioisotope studies with technetium-labeled mebrofenin can

be used to demonstrate patency (or lack there of) of the cystic duct. Non-filling of the gallbladder, in the presence of good hepatic uptake and intestinal excretion of radioisotope, suggests cholecystitis. Technetium cholescintigraphy had a high sensitivity for biliary obstruction in a retrospective study of adults with clinically suspected acute acalculous cholecystitis [9]. However, another study showed that scintigraphy was not specific compared with both ultrasound and CT. False positive scintigraphic results have been seen in alcoholism or in patients receiving parenteral nutrition.

Definitive therapy for acalculous cholecystitis remains controversial. Surgical intervention with tube cholecystostomy, or preferably cholecystectomy, is considered prudent in order to prevent complications such as gangrenous necrosis of the gallbladder wall, perforation, and bile peritonitis. In a published series of 12 patients, three required cholecystectomy but there was resolution without operative intervention in the other nine [10].

Other acalculous entities of the gallbladder

Another category of acalculous disease that is becoming more commonly diagnosed is gallbladder dyskinesia, also known as biliary colic. Patients presenting with this disorder often are female and have a history of right upper quadrant pain and fatty food intolerance that may have been present for longer than 1 year. Often a family history of cholelithiasis is present. Ultrasound does not show gallstones, but ultrasound or scintigraphy with cholecystokinin stimulation shows a decreased biliary ejection fraction. Dumont and Caniano [11] examined 42 children with abdominal pain and abnormal gallbladder emptying (contractility <50%) diagnosed by either ultrasound or scintigraphy with cholecystokinin. All patients were treated with cholecystectomy, and all but one improved after surgery with a mean follow-up of 20 months. Almost half of removed gallbladders had chronic inflammation. A retrospective analysis by Vegunta *et al.* [12] of 107 consecutive cholecystectomies in children at a single medical center, revealed that 62 were performed for biliary dyskinesia. Short-term relief of symptoms was observed in 85% of patients with a preoperative diagnosis of dyskinesia and approximately half of the removed gallbladders had chronic cholecystitis. Another retrospective study showed a much higher incidence of chronic cholecystitis in such patients.

Gallbladder motility has been shown to be impaired in children with Down syndrome and children and adolescents with type 1 diabetes mellitus. Fasting gallbladder volumes are increased in both conditions and contraction after a meal stimulus is reduced in Down syndrome. These abnormalities may predispose to the known increased gallstone formation in both conditions.

Other inflammatory lesions of the gallbladder

Rarely, lesions of the gallbladder accompany other systemic inflammatory disorders. A characteristic granulomatous inflammatory lesion has been demonstrated in the gallbladder wall of a patient with Crohn disease. Malacoplakia involving the gallbladder, with the formation of Michaelis–Gutmann bodies, has been reported as well. The gallbladder may be affected in patients with polyarteritis nodosa.

Tumors of the gallbladder

Neoplastic disorders of the gallbladder occur uncommonly in childhood. Adenoma of the gallbladder, a benign polypoid lesion, has been described in a child. It may present with symptoms of biliary colic; ultrasound may visualize a gallbladder polyp (Figure 16.5). Resection is recommended, because of malignant potential and association with acute acalculous cholecystitis. Gallbladder polyps also have been reported in association with Peutz–Jegher syndrome. Only three cases of adenomyomatosis of the gallbladder have been described in children. This condition may lead to abdominal pain. Although there is no consensus regarding an association with malignancy, most clinicians would recommend cholecystectomy.

Primary malignant neoplasms of the gallbladder are exceedingly uncommon in the pediatric age group. Presenting as obstructive jaundice, embryonal rhabdomyosarcoma is the most frequently encountered malignancy arising from the gallbladder and biliary tree. The prognosis is dismal because the tumor is poorly responsive to surgical and chemotherapeutic intervention.

Miscellaneous conditions

There are a number of disorders characterized by accumulation of lipids or calcium salts intraluminally or intramurally within the gallbladder. These disorders are more common in the adult population.

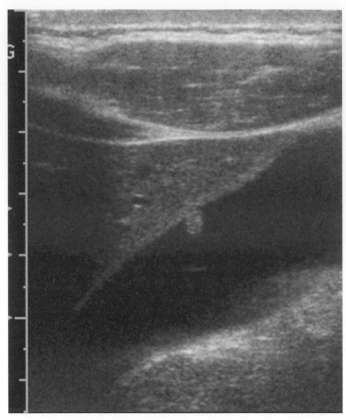

Figure 16.5 Longitudinal ultrasound demonstrating a pedunculated mass hanging from the mucosa of the gallbladder wall, which was found to be a polyp when cholecystectomy performed.

Porcelain gallbladder, an entity characterized by calcification of the gallbladder wall, occurs in association with chronic inflammation. One case has been described that was associated with extrahepatic bile duct obstruction. Cholecystectomy is advised because of the high frequency of gallbladder carcinoma reported in adults with porcelain gallbladder.

A single case of "milk of calcium" bile has been reported in the pediatric literature [15]. For unknown reasons, excessive quantities of calcium carbonate accumulate in gallbladder bile; the gallbladder is radiopaque on plain film, which appears much like a cholecystogram.

Cholesterolosis of the gallbladder involves deposition of triglycerides and cholesterol esters in macrophages within the lamina propria of the gallbladder wall. It may occur as a diffuse or localized phenomenon.

Gallbladder adenomyosis involves benign hyperplasia of the muscularis mucosa with intramucosal diverticula formation. Adenomyosis has been seen in a 16 year old whose gallbladder was resected for symptoms of cholecystitis.

Calculous gallbladder disease

Approximately 20 to 25 million North American adults have gallstones. Based upon the Framingham study, it is estimated that 12 million females and 6 million males have gallstones. Cholelithiasis is relatively uncommon in infancy and

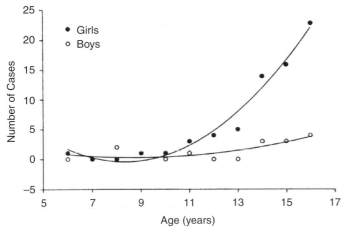

Figure 16.6 Incidence of gallstones among hospitalized Swedish children younger than 16 years of age. Note minimal incidence for both boys and girls before 11 years of age, with a sharp increase in incidence in girls and a minimal increase in boys. (Modified from Nilsson, 1966 [18] and Shaffer, 1991[14].)

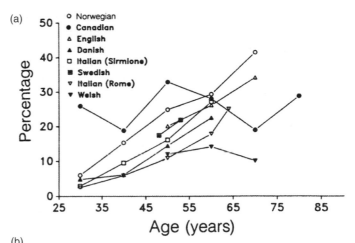

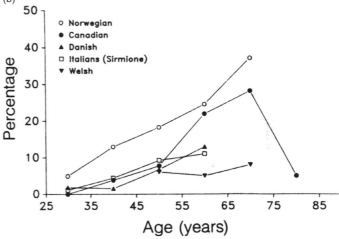

Figure 16.7 Prevalence of gallstones by surveys using ultrasonography or oral cholecystography in Caucasian women (a) and men (b) from Europe and Canada. Gallstones are more common in women and increase in frequency with increasing age. (Data from Shaffer, 1991 [14].)

childhood; however, gallstones have been detected in utero as early as after 30 weeks of gestation, and in newborns. One newborn has been described with clinical and ultrasound evidence of acute calculous cholecystitis.

Few studies have been performed that examined the incidence or prevalence of gallstone disease in children. The prevalence of gallstones among 1502 Italian males and females, 6 to 19 years of age, screened with ultrasound was 0.13% overall (0.27% in females) [16]. This compares with a prevalence of 2.9 and 1.1% among Italian females and males, respectively, between 18 and 29 years of age [17]. The incidence of gallbladder disease remains negligible in males throughout childhood and adolescence; in females there is an increase in incidence between 11 and 13 years of age [18] (Figure 16.6). The true prevalence of gallstones has been evaluated in adult Caucasians by survey with ultrasound or oral cholecystography (Figure 16.7). For both males and females, there is an increasing prevalence of gallstones with increasing age. At all ages from puberty until menopause, women have a higher frequency of stones than men [13,17,19]. Clear differences in gallstone frequency exist among ethnic backgrounds. The frequency is exceedingly low among Canadian Eskimos and east and west African natives; it reaches 30 to 70% among American Indians, Swedes, and Czechs [13]. The type of stones also varies with geographic region. Cholesterol gallstones predominate in Western cultures; pigment stones are more common among Asian populations.

Classification of gallstones

Stones may be divided into two major categories (Figure 16.8). Cholesterol stones contain more than 50% cholesterol by weight, with variable amounts of protein and calcium salts. Pigment stones (black and brown) are complex mixtures of insoluble calcium salts including calcium bilirubinate, calcium

phosphate, and calcium carbonate. Cholesterol content in pigment stones ranges from <10% in black stones to 10–30% in brown pigment stones.

Approximately 25–33% of stones removed during cholecystectomy in adults are pigment stones; as many as 72% in children are pigment stones. Less than 10% of gallstones obtained during cholecystectomy during adolescence are pigment stones; by the seventh decade of life, pigment stones are more common than cholesterol stones. Black and white adults have similar frequencies of pigment stones. Obesity does not appear to predispose to pigment stone formation.

Causes of gallstones in children

Several series have reported the cause of gallstones in children and adolescents [20–36]. Few have addressed carefully the issue of the type of stone associated with certain conditions. Friesen and Roberts [22] reviewed their hospital's experience and a total of 693 cases of pediatric gallstones reported in the literature. Based on their experience, 72% of stones were pigmented, 17% cholesterol, and 11% had unknown composition. Over the entire series, pigment stones predominated in infants and children to the age of 5 years, with cholesterol stones found more commonly between 6 and 21 years of age. Unfortunately, the composition of the stones was not known in the majority of studies, and determination of composition was based on visual inspection rather than chemical analysis. Hemolytic disease was considered the cause of gallstones in 30% of the entire series. The cause of and conditions associated with stones from the entire series are illustrated in Table 16.2. In a second smaller study, Stringer *et al.* [23] examined stone type obtained from 20 consecutive cholecystectomies for cholelithiasis in children. Of these 20, 11 had pigment stones, 2 had cholesterol stones, and 7 had calcium carbonate stones. These findings suggest that the stone composition in children differs from adults, particularly the finding of calcium carbonate stones. These stones appear to have a similar composition to pigment stones but lack bilirubinate salts. Many, but not all, had received parenteral nutrition, which may provide a potential explanation for the high frequency of calcium carbonate stones in this series.

Pigment gallstones

There are two major types of pigment stone: "black" and "brown."

In both types, pigment is present as calcium bilirubinates. In black pigment stones, pigment is cross-linked to form a black polymer that is insoluble in all solvents. In contrast, in brown pigment stones, the cross-linked polymers are present in low concentrations and the pigments are soluble in most organic solvents. Black pigment stones are found in sterile gallbladder bile. Around 50% of black pigment stones appears to be radiopaque with conventional radiographic techniques. Two-thirds of all opaque stones are pigment stones because of their high content of calcium carbonates and phosphates. Brown pigment stones generally are found in infected bile in

Table 16.2 Associated conditions by age for 693 patients with cholelithiasis reported in the literature expressed as percentage of total cases in age group

Age	Percentage total cases
0–12 months	
None	36.4
Total parenteral nutrition	29.1
Abdominal surgery	29.1
Sepsis	14.8
Bronchopulmonary dysplasia	12.7
Hemolytic disease	5.5
Malabsorption	5.5
Necrotizing enterocolitis	5.5
Hepatobiliary disease	3.6
1–5 years	
Hepatobiliary disease	28.6
Abdominal surgery	21/4
Artificial heart valve	14.3
None	14.3
Malabsorption	7.1
6–11 years	
Pregnancy	37.2
Hemolytic disease	22.5
Obesity	8.1
Abdominal surgery	5.1
None	3.4
Hepatobiliary disease	2.7
Total parenteral nutrition	2.7
Malabsorption	2.8

Source: from Friesen and Roberts, 1989 [22].

(a)

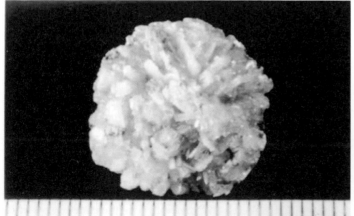

(b)

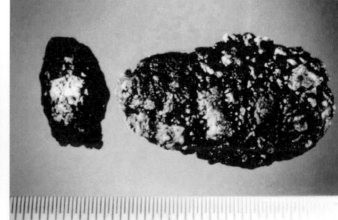

Figure 16.8 Typical appearance of a cholesterol stone with minimal bilirubin staining (a) and black pigment stone (b) removed from children. Scale, 10 mm.

intra- and extrahepatic bile ducts. They are usually radiolucent because they contain smaller amounts of calcium phosphate and carbonate than black pigment stones. Brown stones contain more cholesterol than black stones because the bile in which they develop tends to be continuously supersaturated with cholesterol. Black pigment stones are shiny, like anthracite chips, or dull, like asphalt, and relatively hard and spiculated. Brown pigment stones are soft and soap-like or greasy in consistency.

Unconjugated bilirubin is the major bile pigment in gallstones. Typically the major components of bile are bilirubin diglucuronides and two bilirubin monoglucuronide isomers. The glucuronides generally bind calcium as soluble complexes. Unconjugated bilirubin ordinarily makes up only a small fraction of normal bile pigment (1%). Most derives from endogenous enzymatic (β-glucuronidase) or non-enzymatic hydrolysis of conjugated bilirubins. Unlike the conjugates, unconjugated bilirubin is very sensitive to precipitation with ionized calcium. Although the process is still poorly understood, polymers of cross-linked bilirubin tetrapyrroles are formed in bile and serve as the basis for stone formation. The chemical initiators of the polymerization process are not known. It seems likely that polymerization is initiated by free radicals or singlet oxygen, possibly produced by the liver and secreted in bile or by macrophages or neutrophils in the gallbladder mucosa.

Calcium carbonate and phosphate are the major components of most black pigment stones; brown pigment stones do not contain appreciable amounts of these substances. Precipitation of these salts is determined by bile pH. Insoluble calcium salt formation is enhanced markedly in alkaline bile, and it is likely that black pigment stones containing calcium carbonates only form in alkaline bile. Fatty acid salts (calcium soaps) are important components of brown pigment stones. Palmitate and stearate are principal sn-1 salts of fatty acids of biliary lecithin. They generally are not found free in bile and are produced by bacterial phospholipase A_1 hydrolysis of lecithin.

Mucin glycoproteins are the framework on which pigment stones grow. Mucin is produced in the gallbladder crypts. Mucin hypersecretion by the gallbladder may play an important role in pigment stone formation.

In black pigment stone disease, bile should be supersaturated with calcium bilirubinates, calcium carbonate, and calcium phosphate. This may result from an absolute increase in the amount of unconjugated bilirubin or ionized calcium. Increased biliary unconjugated bilirubin may derive from increased pigment production and excretion in bile. In humans, the output and proportion of unconjugated bilirubin in bile may increase after a load of hemoglobin or bilirubin. Patients with spontaneous hemolysis have no more than 3% of total biliary bilirubin as the unconjugated form. Increased unconjugated bilirubin also may result from increased β-glucuronidase hydrolysis of bilirubin conjugates or reduced amounts of an inhibitor of β-glucuronidase, glutaric acid. Potential causes of increased levels of ionized calcium are

increased amounts of plasma-ionized calcium or reduced biliary calcium binders such as micellar bile salts and lecithin–cholesterol vesicles. Increased ionization of normal amounts of unconjugated bilirubin and increased bicarbonate occurs in alkaline biliary pH. Decreased biliary bile salts and cholesterol concentrations found in cirrhotic patients may lead to increased levels of ionized calcium in bile as well as reduced levels of micellar bile salt and vesicle deficiency.

Brown pigment stones require both stasis and infection. Bacterially derived β-glucuronidase, phospholipase A_1, and bile salt deconjugase produce unconjugated bilirubin, fatty acids, and unconjugated bile acids. All of these products are insoluble and precipitate as calcium salts. Ductal precipitation of these compounds together with cholesterol and mucin form soft, greasy stones shaped like the bile ducts.

Conditions predisposing to black pigment stone formation
Chronic hemolytic disease

The risk of black pigment stone formation is increased in patients with chronic hemolytic disorders including congenital spherocytosis, sickle cell (SS and SC) disease, thalassemia major and minor, pyruvate kinase deficiency, glucose-6-phosphate dehydrogenase deficiency, and autoimmune hemolytic disease. The prevalence of pigment stones in patients with hemolytic disorders increases with age, as illustrated by the age-related frequencies of gallstones in sickle cell anemia. In children younger than 10 years of age, the frequency is 14%. In those aged 10–20 years, the frequency increases to 36%. At age 22 years, the frequency is 50%, and by age 33 years it is between 60 and 85% [37–39]. Despite the identification of gallstones in over half of a cohort of patients with sickle cell disease, few are symptomatic at the time of ultrasound identification of stones. Elective laparoscopic cholecystectomy is encouraged for patients with sickle cell disease who have gallstones identified by ultrasonography. Recent studies have suggested a 12-day reduction in hospital stay with elective laparoscopic cholecystectomy compared with those undergoing emergency surgery (4 versus 16 days).

Total parenteral nutrition

The natural history of TPN-related biliary tract disease recently has been elucidated in both neonates and adults. In a prospective study of 41 neonates, 18 (44%) developed gallbladder sludge after a mean of 10 days of TPN [40]. The appearance of sludge related to prematurity, lack of enteral nutrition, and duration of TPN. In five (12%) of the neonates, sludge evolved to "sludge balls," and two developed uncomplicated gallstones. In one of these patients, the stone resolved within 6 months; in the other, the stone was still present after 1.5 years. In 84 infants and children treated with TPN, cholelithiasis was found in 11 (13%) [41]. Patients with cholelithiasis had a mean duration of TPN of 218 days, versus 115 days in patients without gallstones. Gallstones were more common in patients who had lost their ileocecal valve, had short bowel syndrome, or had more surgery. In 21 children receiving long-term TPN gallstones developed in 9 (43%) [42]. The children who developed gallstones were treated with TPN for more than twice as long as the children without gallstones: seven (78%) of children with stones received TPN for longer than 20 months, whereas patients without stones received TPN for a mean of 14 months. Several anecdotal reports have appeared that suggest that a significant proportion of stones formed during TPN remain "silent" or disappear over time. In adults treated with TPN, biliary sludge was first seen in 6% of subjects in the first 3 weeks of therapy. By 4–6 weeks of treatment, 50% had developed sludge; with increasing duration of therapy, well-circumscribed stones developed in 6 of 14 sludge-positive patients with prolonged TPN [43]. With discontinuation of TPN and resumption of oral feeding, the sludge disappeared from all patients after 5 weeks. Cholecystectomy was required for symptomatic stones in three patients, stones persisted in two, and in one patient the stones resolved spontaneously [43]. Minimal enteral nutrition or parenteral administration of cholecystokinin or its analogues may allow intermittent gallbladder contraction, reduce gallbladder stasis, and reduce the risk of gallstone formation in patients treated with TPN; however, the benefits of these interventions have been inconsistent. In a study of 95 children (mean age 20 months) [44], gallbladder sludge appeared in 22 (23%) after 1 month and 30 (32%) after 3 months of continuous TPN. With the initiation of partial oral feeding, the rate was reduced to 17% after 1 month, and sludge disappeared within 1 month of complete oral feeding. Two subjects developed gallbladder lithiasis, which disappeared with oral feeding. With both partial and total oral feeding, the plasma level of cholecystokinin increased significantly postprandially, and a significant negative correlation (r, –0.88) was found between the gallbladder sludge rate and cholecystokinin levels for any of the feeding methods used.

Cirrhosis and chronic cholestasis

Adults with cirrhosis are at increased risk for pigment gallstone formation. In autopsy studies in adults, pigment stones were more prevalent in patients with primary biliary cirrhosis (30.8%) and all patients with cirrhosis (29.4%) compared with non-cirrhotic patients (12.8%). The cause for stone formation is not currently known; it may be related, however, to hypersplenism and attendant hemolysis. The excess quantities of bilirubin produced may exceed its solubility in bile. In addition, cirrhotic patients also are prone to stone formation because their bile has limited solubilizing capability because of reduced concentrations of biliary bile acids. Patients with Wilson disease may have calcified pigment stones produced because of recurrent episodes of hemolysis. Children with progressive familial intrahepatic cholestasis type 1 appear prone to gallstone formation [45]. Pigment stones have been identified in gallbladders removed from a number of symptomatic children with cirrhosis at autopsy or at the time of orthotopic liver transplantation at the Children's Hospital of Cincinnati. Defective bile acid synthesis, as found with inborn errors of bile salt metabolism, may lead to decreased bile salt secretion, but because of attendant cholestasis patients are likely to have pigment rather than cholesterol stones. Despite reductions in biliary bile acid concentrations, the prevalence of cholesterol gallstones does not appear to be increased in cirrhosis, probably because there is a concurrent reduction in cholesterol synthesis that results in normal biliary cholesterol: bile acid ratios.

Miscellaneous conditions

A number of disparate conditions appear to be associated with sludge formation and merit discussion. Gallbladder sludge and lithiasis have been noted in infants born to morphine abusers. Ceftriaxone, a third-generation cephalosporin with broad-spectrum antimicrobial activity, is largely excreted in the bile. Up to 46% of children receiving ceftriaxone for treatment of meningitis have been found to develop gallbladder sludge, which characteristically disappears with cessation of therapy [46]. It has been proposed that excess quantities of ceftriaxone in the bile precipitates as a calcium salt, producing sludge. Use of TPN, presence of an ileal conduit, or a history of abdominal surgery places long-term survivors of childhood cancer at an increased risk for gallstone formation [47].

There are also additional conditions that may predispose to cholelithiasis but there are insufficient data to classify the stones as either pigment or cholesterol containing. Recent studies have suggested an increased frequency of gallstones in girls with Rhett syndrome, with two-thirds of girls and women younger than 43 years having stones; however, the pathophysiology of stones has not been investigated [48]. In one small series, cholelithiasis was observed in 10 of 311 infants and children (3.2%) after heart transplantation [49].

Conditions predisposing to brown pigment stone formation

Although common in children from the Pacific Rim, brown pigment stones are uncommon in the West. In the Pacific Rim, most are associated with biliary infestations with parasites such as *Ascaris lumbricoides*. Most brown pigment stones occur in obstructed bile ducts. They are rare in infants and children, although two infants have been described with biliary obstruction caused by brown pigment stones found in infected bile.

Cholesterol gallstones

Cholesterol gallstone formation results from a number of events including hepatic secretion of bile supersaturated with cholesterol, nucleation of cholesterol monohydrate crystals in the gallbladder, and impaired emptying of the gallbladder contents. Biliary supersaturation with cholesterol commonly occurs in normal individuals during a portion of the day but occurs almost universally in patients with cholesterol gallstones. Nucleation times appear to differentiate those who develop stones from those who do not.

Bile is an aqueous solution that is relatively enriched with water-insoluble hydrophobic lipids (cholesterol and

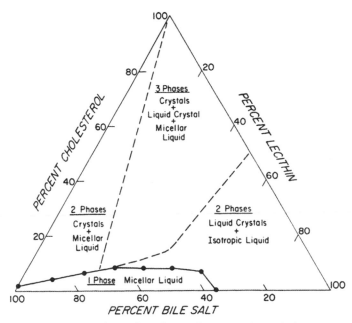

Figure 16.9 Tricoordinate phase diagram for representing a single intersecting point for the relative concentrations of cholesterol, phospholipids, and bile salts in bile [50]. Note that a clear micellar solution would be present with a composition of bile falling at the lower left of the diagram (micellar liquid). Bile with components that contain crystals would be supersaturated with cholesterol and prone to precipitate out of solution.

phospholipids) solubilized in detergents (bile acids). The dissolved solids make up about 3%, by weight, of hepatic bile. Bile salts are the predominant solute, averaging 20–30 mmol/L in hepatic bile. Phospholipid concentrations average 7 mmol/L, and cholesterol averages 2–3 mmol/L. Bilirubin normally is present at concentrations of 0.2 mmol/L. Proteins are present in concentrations of approximately 0.2% by weight. A fraction of these proteins play an important role in cholesterol crystal nucleation and gallstone formation.

The principal lipid components (phospholipid and cholesterol) are solubilized by bile salt micelles. Bile salts are extremely effective solubilizers of phospholipids. In addition, the presence of phospholipid markedly increases the extent to which bile salts can incorporate cholesterol into micelles. The relative amounts of cholesterol, phospholipid, and bile salt that may coexist in micellar solution has been determined empirically (Figure 16.9).

The maximum equilibrium solubility of cholesterol in bile can be determined from the molar ratios of cholesterol, phospholipid, and bile acids and is expressed as the cholesterol saturation index. A supersaturated bile is one in which cholesterol concentration exceeds the maximum cholesterol saturation index, and from which cholesterol monohydrate crystals precipitate.

Once cholesterol concentrations exceed their maximum equilibrium solubility, multilamellar cholesterol vesicles fuse and aggregate into a cluster that serves as a nidus for crystal formation. Nucleation may be either homogeneous or heterogeneous. Homogeneous nucleation occurs if crystallization occurs without foreign material. Heterogeneous nucleation occurs if crystallization takes place on a foreign surface such as epithelial cells, protein, calcium salts, or a foreign body. Nucleation most probably occurs through a heterogeneous pathway, because it occurs rapidly at low levels of cholesterol supersaturation.

Recently, promoters and inhibitors of cholesterol crystal formation and growth have been identified in human bile. These promoting and inhibiting factors may directly influence the "nucleating time" of bile. Biliary proteins of molecular weight 130 kDa have been proposed as potential pronucleators. In contrast, there are proteins in normal bile that inhibit nucleation. These antinucleating factors may stabilize cholesterol–phospholipid vesicles in "normal" bile and retard crystallization. Potential candidate antinucleating proteins include apolipoprotein A1 and A2.

Gallbladder mucin also may promote stone formation. Mucin causes a time- and concentration-dependent acceleration of cholesterol crystallization. Mucus hypersecretion occurs prior to gallstone formation in animals fed a gallstone-promoting diet [51]. Inhibition of mucus secretion with aspirin prevents gallstone formation but does not alter the development of diet-induced biliary cholesterol supersaturation.

Current concepts regarding gallstone formation invoke the notion that nucleation of cholesterol crystals occurs in a mucous gel through protein–lipid interactions. The rate of cholesterol crystal nucleation may be influenced by a balance between pro- and antinucleating factors.

Gallbladder stasis facilitates growth of microscopic crystals into macroscopic stones. Animal studies have suggested that a gallbladder motility defect may antedate gallstone formation. In addition, gallbladder motility worsens as stones develop. Biliary stasis complicates treatment with TPN and oral contraceptives and pregnancy.

Bile supersaturated with cholesterol may result from a deficiency of secretion of bile salts or phospholipids or a disproportionately increased secretion of cholesterol. Cholesterol stones are characteristically more common in women beyond puberty. The difference in prevalence between sexes declines after menopause. Pregnancy, which is associated with biliary cholesterol supersaturation and impaired gallbladder emptying, may contribute to the increased frequency of stones in women of childbearing age. Estrogens and oral contraceptives enhance cholesterol saturation of bile and are associated with increases in cholelithiasis. White and black American have a prevalence of cholesterol stones of 9 and 5%, respectively.

Limited information is available regarding biliary lipid composition and cholesterol saturation in normal infants and children. Bile is relatively undersaturated with cholesterol in infants and children compared with adults. This finding may be explained by the observation that the bile salt pools expand rapidly after birth, and body size-matched pools in infancy and childhood actually exceed those observed in young adults. This

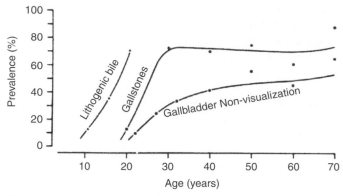

Figure 16.10 Natural history of gallstone disease in female Pima Indians. Lithogenic bile first appears in the second decade of life. The prevalence of gallstones rises approximately 10 years later, followed by non-visualization of the gallbladder, verified by two consecutive oral cholecystograms without gallbladder opacification, several years later.

may lead to a higher biliary bile salt to cholesterol secretion ratio, with less saturated bile. In the Pima Indians, a population at high risk of cholesterol cholelithiasis in adulthood, biliary lipid composition is already abnormal by 9–12 years of age, and bile becomes very supersaturated in females after puberty [52]. Nearly 90% of Pima Indian women have gallstones by the age of 65 years. The time course of development of biliary cholesterol saturation and gallstones is illustrated for this population in Figure 16.10. In populations at lower risk for cholesterol cholelithiasis and obesity, no significant changes in biliary cholesterol saturation are noted with puberty in males. In contrast, females have undersaturated bile before puberty, which becomes supersaturated after puberty [53]. Enhanced cholesterol secretion may be observed with certain drugs (estrogens, clofibrate). Most adults with gallstones have a combination of both reduced bile salt secretion and enhanced biliary cholesterol secretion.

Conditions predisposing to cholesterol gallstone formation
Obesity

Obese adults have a prevalence of cholesterol gallstones that is almost twice that of the non-obese population. Evidence has accumulated that the biliary secretion of cholesterol is increased relative to bile acid and phospholipid secretion in obese subjects. As a consequence, bile is supersaturated with cholesterol, predisposing to stone formation. Supersaturated bile may develop at puberty in women and is often associated with obesity. Unfortunately, little is known about nucleating factors in obesity. With weight loss, the cholesterol saturation actually increases. Once the individual's weight has stabilized at a lower level, the cholesterol saturation tends to decline. Little, if anything, is known about the risk of cholesterol gallstone formation in children with obesity; however, obesity appears to predispose to stone formation in adolescent females. Findings from a German study suggest that the prevalence of gallstones could be as high as 2% in obese children and adolescents. Gallstones were more common in the more

severely obese and older children with no prepubertal children having stones.

Ileal resection, jejunoileal bypass, or ileal Crohn disease

The development of gallstones when the enterohepatic circulation is interrupted may be multifactorial. With excess fecal loss of bile acids, the pool is reduced, biliary bile acid secretion declines, and bile may become supersaturated with cholesterol. Concurrently, intestinal lumenal binding of calcium to fatty acids with formation of fatty acid soaps may preclude bilirubin precipitation in the lumen, thereby allowing its reabsorption in the distal bowel with recirculation and reappearance in bile. This may produce conditions conducive to both cholesterol and pigment stone formation. Gallstone prevalence in adults with inflammatory bowel disease affecting the ileum, assessed radiographically, ranges from 28 to 34%. The increased frequency of gallstones correlates with the duration and extent of ileal disease or the interval following ileal resection. Recent studies have suggested that the incidence of gallstone disease was no greater in patients with ileal disease or resection than in appropriately age- and sex-matched control subjects. In children, anecdotal reports have appeared suggesting that children with ileal resection or disease may have an increased incidence of cholelithiasis. In most circumstances, patients have been found to have pigment rather than cholesterol stones, with stone formation associated with conditions requiring prolonged TPN and diuretics in the neonatal period. Studies of biliary lipids in children with ileal resection or dysfunction have failed to demonstrate cholesterol supersaturation; after puberty, however, biliary cholesterol supersaturation develops. It appears that children with ileal resection or dysfunction are not at increased risk of cholesterol cholelithiasis; after puberty, their biliary lipid composition is similar to adults, and they then may be prone to stone formation.

Cystic fibrosis

Autopsy series have documented the presence of radiolucent gallstones in 12.0–27.5% of patients with cystic fibrosis. The gallbladder is hypoplastic in approximately 25% of patients, and at autopsy it is filled with clear mucus. Prospective annual screening studies have shown a frequency of stones of approximately 5%. Several abnormalities of bile salt metabolism have been identified in cystic fibrosis. Initially, it was believed that increased fecal bile acid excretion led to reduced bile acid pools. Children, adolescents, and adults with cystic fibrosis were found to have high biliary cholesterol concentrations relative to bile acids and phospholipids and bile supersaturated with cholesterol. Because of the radiolucency of gallstones and the cholesterol supersaturation of bile in patients with cystic fibrosis, it was assumed that gallstones in this disease were predominantly cholesterol. More recent studies have failed to confirm some of the observations made in the 1970s. The biliary lipid composition and bile acid pools in patients with cystic fibrosis have not been shown to differ from those in control subjects. Radiolucent stones found in cystic fibrosis may be pigment stones in most circumstances [54]. Fasting and residual gallbladder volumes are increased in patients with cystic fibrosis who do not have microgallbladders. This finding, coupled with abnormalities of mucus, may predispose patients to stasis and nidus formation in the gallbladder.

Pregnancy

Women have a higher frequency of gallstones than men at all ages from puberty to menopause [17,19,22]. This suggests that hormonal influences in women may play an important role in the pathogenesis of cholesterol gallstones. Women have a smaller total bile acid pool and enhanced biliary cholesterol secretion compared with men, resulting in increased biliary cholesterol saturation. Pregnancy and the use of oral contraceptives accentuate these sex-related differences. During pregnancy, the total bile acid pool expands but there is enhanced sequestration of the pool in the intestine. Consequently, there is no change or a decline in the biliary bile acid secretion rate. Increases in gallbladder residual volume and fasting volumes, and reductions in gallbladder contractility and rate of emptying, make pregnant women and those receiving oral contraceptives particularly susceptible to gallstone formation. In two series of adolescent girls aged 14–20 years, strong associations were found between the presence of gallstones and parity and obesity; a weak, statistically non-significant association was found between oral contraceptive use and gallstones [55,56].

Miscellaneous conditions

Gallstones have been identified in at least one child with familial hypobetalipoproteinemia who presented with obstructive jaundice. In this rare condition, stones may form because of increased biliary cholesterol secretion.

Genetic predisposition to gallstones

The importance of heredity to risk for gallstone disease is becoming increasingly clear. In more than 43 000 Swedish twin pairs, the concordance rate for symptomatic gallstone disease was significantly higher in monozygotic than in dizygotic twins. In a model derived from these data, it was proposed that genetic factors were responsible for 25% of the phenotypic variation among the twins [57].

Efforts to determine the specific gene(s) involved in risk for gallstone disease are ongoing. Quantitative trait loci analysis in studies of inbred mouse strains has identified a large number of candidate lithogenic (LITH) genes. Among these, of particular interest are NR1I2 (encoding the pregnane X receptor (PXR)) and ABCG8 (encoding the hepatocanalicular cholesterol hemitransporter).

Pregnane X receptor is a nuclear receptor that is highly produced in the liver and is activated by bile acids and bile acid precursors. Knockout mice for Pxr have significantly decreased biliary concentrations of bile acids and phospholipids, resulting in an elevated cholesterol saturation index in the bile and substantial predisposition to development of cholesterol gallstones. The C57L mouse, which is a strain predisposed to cholesterol gallstones when fed a lithogenic diet, is protected from gallstone disease when treated with PXR agonists [58]. Interestingly, NR1I2 colocalizes with LITH14 on human chromosome 3q and mouse chromosome 16, suggesting that mutations in NR1I2 may be associated with risk for gallstone disease in humans as well.

Multiple human studies have clearly implicated the D19H polymorphism of ABCG8 as a susceptibility factor for gallstone disease. Genome-wide association studies of patients from Germany and Chile and linkage studies of affected sib pairs from Germany and Romania have shown a reported odds ratio for gallstone disease of 2.2 for heterozygotes and 7 for homozygotes [59,60]. These results have been replicated in Chinese patients and Swedish twin pairs [61,62].

Mutations affecting hepatocyte enzymes and membrane transporters important to bile acid and bilirubin biology also appear to be associated with risk for gallstone disease. The A105G variant of SLC10A2, encoding apical sodium dependent bile acid transporter, is associated with an odds ratio of 2 for gallstone disease [45]. Polymorphisms in UGT1A1, encoding UDP-glucuronosyltansferase, have been linked to risk for gallstone disease. One such polymorphism, the Gilbert syndrome-associated TATA box TA repeat variant, is associated with an increased risk of pigment stone formation in patients with hemolytic anemia and in patients with cystic fibrosis [64,65].

Clinical features of gallstones

In adults, gallstones may remain asymptomatic for years. The natural history of gallstones has been carefully studied. Gracie and Ransohoff [66] evaluated the outcome of gallstones in 123 male university faculty members identified 24 years earlier on pre-employment oral cholecystograms. In 16 subjects identified with asymptomatic or silent gallstones, symptoms developed that were heralded by the appearance of biliary tract pain; 3 of 13 developed biliary tract complications, 2 with acute cholecystitis and 1 with pancreatitis. If complications occurred, they were likely to follow previous episodes of biliary colic. Based on this study, it appears that the risk of serious complications associated with silent gallstones is small. Non-elective cholecystectomy is necessary in less than 5% of patients with identified silent gallstones. No studies of this type have been performed in infants and children; however, there is no reason to believe that the risk of complications with silent stones would be higher in children than adults. Non-specific dyspepsia, fatty food intolerance, and vague epigastric or right upper quadrant discomfort are common in adults with and without gallstones. In children, only recurrent right upper quadrant pain or epigastric pain would suggest gallstone disease. Typically, biliary colic is episodic and characterized by pain that is steady and lasts 1–3 hours, rather than colicky or crampy in nature. Although pain is commonly localized to

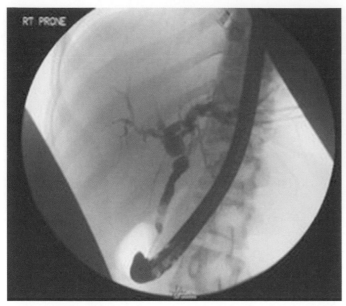

Figure 16.11 During endoscopic retrograde cholangiopancreatography, the common duct was cannulated and contrast outlines the common duct stone with proximal dilatation of the duct.

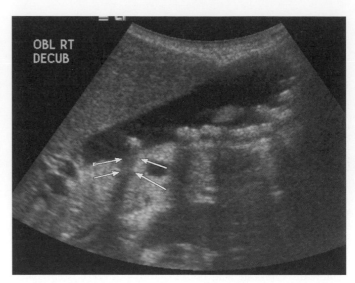

Figure 16.12 Real-time ultrasonogram demonstrating multiple, echogenic stones within the gallbladder with acoustic shadowing (arrows).

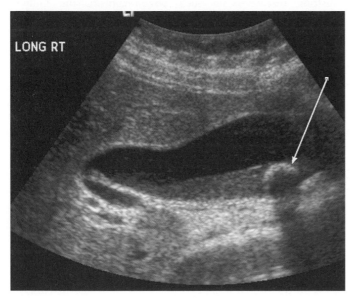

Figure 16.13 Longitudinal ultrasound of the right upper quadrant in a 16 year old with sickle cell disease abdomen, illustrating echogenic sludge in the gallbladder and a stone with acoustic shadowing (arrow).

the right upper quadrant, it may be localized to the epigastrium. Radiation of pain to the umbilicus may suggest the presence of acute appendicitis. Pain also may radiate to the right shoulder. Nausea and vomiting are common. Fever commonly is present in children younger than 15 years of age. Episodes of pain may occur irregularly over years, and the severity of attacks may vary.

The mechanism of pain is believed to relate to obstruction of the cystic duct. Pressure in the gallbladder increases in an attempt to contract against the obstruction. During an attack, there may be right upper abdomen or epigastric tenderness. Some guarding may be observed, but rebound is typically absent. Results of the physical examination even may be normal during an attack. Acute cholecystitis generally subsides spontaneously within a few days. In one-third of patients, inflammation leads to necrosis with either perforation or empyema of the gallbladder. Passage of stones into the common bile duct may cause bile duct obstruction (Figure 16.11), cholangitis, and pancreatitis.

Laboratory test results commonly are normal. The white blood cell count may be normal. In a small fraction of patients, there is transient mild elevation of serum bilirubin, aminotransferases, and alkaline phosphatase.

Ultrasonography is the safest and most sensitive and specific method for identifying gallstones (Figure 16.12). If a gallbladder can be identified by ultrasound, the stone discovery rate is as high as 98% of expected. Typically stones appear as echogenic masses with acoustic shadows. Sludge may be identified as echogenic material that layers (Figure 16.13). A thickened gallbladder wall suggests inflammation. Plain abdominal radiography identifies only stones that have a high calcium content (usually about 15% of all stones). Additional diagnostic techniques may be helpful in some circumstances. Oral cholecystography may be helpful in identifying non-calculous causes of gallbladder disease and evaluating function. Cholescintigraphy, using one of the technetium-99m-labeled acetanilide aminodiacetic acid derivatives, is currently the most accurate method for evaluating the patient with acute cholecystitis. Axial CT may also be helpful in demonstrating stones (Figure 16.14). In general, ultrasound is the method of choice for identifying gallstones in children and adolescents complaining of recurrent epigastric or right abdominal pain.

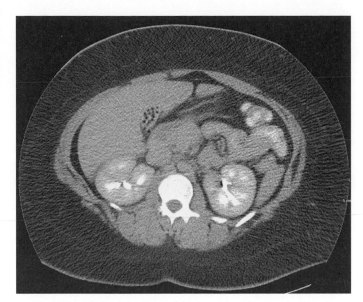

Figure 16.14 Axial CT of the abdomen demonstrating multiple cholesterol stones, which typically have a low attenuation.

Chronic cholecystitis or cholelithiasis

Generally, some inflammation accompanies cholelithiasis. In some patients, chronic inflammation leads to the development of a fibrotic and shrunken gallbladder. With fibrosis, visualization of the gallbladder and its contents may be difficult with ultrasound. As with acute cholecystitis, nuclear imaging techniques may prove helpful in diagnosing chronic cholecystitis. Failure of gallbladder visualization should suggest the presence of chronic cholecystitis.

Treatment of cholelithiasis and acute and chronic cholecystitis

Cholecystectomy is the definitive treatment for symptomatic stones. The only treatment questions that arise focus on the timing of surgery and the operative approach. In a study in which patients with gallstones were monitored carefully, 112 patients were followed who had experienced biliary pain in the previous 12 months: 60% developed recurrent pain within 2 years, and 6% required cholecystectomy [67]. Those with recurrent pain are more likely to develop significant complications and should have elective cholecystectomy without prolonged waiting.

With acute cholecystitis, emergency cholecystectomy might be warranted if complications supervene; in most patients, however, cholecystectomy can be delayed safely for between a few days and 2–3 months. The only exception to the use of cholecystectomy for treatment of gallstones might be in patients whose medical conditions make operative cholecystectomy dangerous. In chronically ill children with high-risk conditions such as severe pulmonary compromise in cystic fibrosis, cholecystotomy might be a reasonable therapeutic alternative to cholecystectomy.

Cholecystectomy is one of the most common operations performed in the USA and UK. Experience with laparoscopic cholecystectomy has demonstrated its advantage over conventional forms of operative cholecystectomy. Indications for this technique in children are the same as for open cholecystectomy, and the gallbladder should be surgically removed from patients with symptomatic cholelithiasis or children with a hemoglobinopathy and asymptomatic cholelithiasis. Several studies have demonstrated the efficacy of this technique in children with cholelithiasis caused by familial hyperlipidemia, hereditary spherocytosis, glucose-6-phosphatase deficiency, thalassemia, glycogen storage disease, and sickle cell anemia. Pediatric laparoscopic cholecystectomy has been modified from the adult procedure because the operating area is considerably smaller and children have a higher risk of having an umbilical hernia adhering to the peritoneal lining. Intraoperative cholangiography is important to exclude common bile duct stones or congenital biliary anomalies. Laparoscopic cholecystectomy allows a short postoperative recovery and is unlikely to have surgical complications. Typically, the length of hospital stay with laparoscopic cholecystectomy is 1 or 2 days in the USA and patients are able to return to work or normal activity in 1 to 2 weeks. It is believed that approximately 80% of adults requiring cholecystectomy are suitable for the laparoscopic technique. The mortality rate with the technique is less than 1%. In about 5% of patients, the surgeon must perform an open cholecystectomy because of anatomic problems or adhesions. Patients with acute cholecystitis, pancreatitis, or a high probability of upper abdominal adhesions are not considered candidates for this procedure. Reported experiences with laparoscopic cholecystectomy in children are limited. In a report of a 5-year experience from three institutions, including 110 children aged 1–16 years, there were no fatalities and the complication rate was 15.5% [68]. As experience has gained at most major pediatric centers, laparoscopic cholecystectomy has become the treatment of choice for elective cholecystectomies [68,69].

In adults with cholesterol stones, alternative non-surgical therapies have been suggested, including dissolution with chenodeoxycholic or ursodeoxycholic acids or combinations of these agents, extracorporal shock-wave lithotripsy with continued dissolution of fragments with oral bile acids, or direct instillation of cholesterol solvents into the gallbladder. The efficacies of bile acid, chenodeoxycholic acid, and ursodeoxycholic acid are similar. Because of dose-related side effects associated with the use of chenodeoxycholic acid (diarrhea, increased serum aminotransferases, and modest hypercholesterolemia), it is not used at all for gallstone dissolution. If drug therapy is used, ursodeoxycholic acid is the drug of choice for oral gallstone dissolution. Dissolution of stones can be achieved in 60% of selected patients with small gallstones. Unfortunately, cessation of therapy is associated with a recurrence rate of 10% per year. Most stones recur within 3 to 5 years after dissolution therapy. The recurrence of stones seriously limits the utility of dissolution therapy in adults and makes it particularly unsuitable for children with gallstones because of the cost of lifelong administration of oral bile acids to prevent recurrence. Oral therapy is a reasonable treatment option only for patients who are at a high surgical risk, including children.

Lithotripsy using shock waves has been used in the past to disintegrate stones after several hundred to several thousand shocks. Currently few, if any, centers use lithotripsy for stone dissolution and any discussion is only of historical interest. Patients with solitary stones were the best candidates for this therapy. Varying results have been obtained, depending on the number and size of gallstones found in the gallbladder. Large solitary stones of 2–3 cm may be dissolved in up to 90% of all patients after 13 to 18 months. The efficacy is reduced with multiple smaller stones, even though the total stone mass may be smaller than with solitary stones. Without concomitant oral bile acid therapy, gallstone recurrence rate was very high [70].

The management of asymptomatic adults with so-called silent gallstones found incidentally has changed over several decades. Silent stones do not require surgery or medical therapy because their natural history is benign. Non-surgical approaches to therapy, including oral bile acid therapy or lithotripsy, should not be considered for individuals with silent gallstones. In children, available evidence supports deferring therapy for asymptomatic stones. A review of 382 Canadian children with gallstones reported complications attributable to gallstone disease in less than 5% of the asymptomatic children, and approximately 20% of the asymptomatic children demonstrated eventual resolution of their gallstones [71]. Among the infants in the study, there was a similarly low rate of complications (8.6%) and a high rate of spontaneous resolution of gallstones (34.1%) among those infants who were followed by ultrasound [71]. With this in mind, expectant management would appear appropriate particularly for otherwise healthy infants and children with stones that are <2 cm. For patients with smaller stones, serial ultrasound examinations appear warranted to monitor for spontaneous disappearance of stones. Larger stones are more problematic. Gallstones may play a role in the development of carcinoma of the gallbladder, with larger stones (>2 cm) carrying a greater risk than small ones. Because larger stones are unlikely to disappear spontaneously, there is a reasonable argument for removing the gallbladder in an otherwise asymptomatic child because of the inherent enhanced risk of gallbladder carcinoma caused by the presence of a stone in the gallbladder over several decades.

In infants and children with known hemolytic disease, pigment stone formation will only worsen with increasing age, and cholecystectomy at time of identification of stones (even though they may be silent) appears warranted. Specifically in patients with sickle cell disease, once stones are identified the gallbladder should be removed. With increasing age, it is clear that gallstone formation and the risk of cholecystitis and attendant adhesions increases. The differentiation between biliary colic and abdominal sickle cell crisis may be more difficult with increasing age, and the risk of operative intervention increases with age; consequently, morbidity and mortality rates are lessened by early operative therapy. In patients with hemolytic disease, laporoscopic cholecystectomy should be considered prior to the development of chronic cholecystitis and potential attendant adhesions because of the lower operative morbidity rate and the reduced cost compared with operative cholecystectomy. Reports of small case series of laparoscopic cholecystectomy in children suggests that it has a similar complication and mortality rate found in adults.

Acknowledgements

The authors wish to acknowledge the valuable assistance of Janet Strife, MD, Division of Pediatric Radiology, Children's Hospital Medical Center, for supplying outstanding examples of ultrasound and CT examinations for illustration of the text. This work was supported in part by a grant from the National Center for Research Resources of the NIH UL1RR026314 and DK 068463.

References

1. Langman J. The digestive system. In *Langman's Medical Embryology*, 3rd edn. Baltimore, MD: Williams & Wilkins, 1981, pp. 217–220.

2. Ternberg JL, Keating JP. Acute acalculous cholecystitis. *Arch Surg* 1975;**110**:543–547.

3. Wong ML, Kaplan S, Dunkle LM, *et al*. Leptospirosis: a childhood disease. *J Pediatr* 1977;**90**:532–537.

4. Holcomb GW Jr., O'Neill JA, Holcomb GW III. Cholecystitis cholelithiasis and common duct stones in children and adolescents. *Ann Surg* 1980;**191**:626–635.

5. Mateos-Corral D, Garza-Luna U, Gutierrez-Martin A. Two reports of acute neonatal acalculous cholecystitis (necrotizing cholecystitis) in a 2-week-old premature infant and a term infant. *J Pediatr Surg* 2006;**41**:e3–e5.

6. Sanders R. The significance of sonographic gallbladder wall thickening. *J Clin Ultrasound* 1980;**8**:143–146.

7. Patriquin HB, DiPietro M, Barber FE, *et al*. Sonography of thickened gallbladder wall: causes in children. *AJR* 1983;**141**:57–60.

8. Jeffrey RB Jr., Sommer FG. Follow-up sonography in suspected acalculous cholecystitis: preliminary clinical experience. *J Ultrasound Med* 1993;**12**:183–187.

9. Swayne LC. Acute acalculous cholecystitis: sensitivity in detection using technetium-99m imiodiacetic acid cholescintigraphy. *Radiology* 1986;**160**:33–38.

10. Imamoglu M, Sarihan H, Sari A, Ahmetoglu A. Acute acalculous cholecystitis in children: diagnosis and treatment. *J Pediatr Surg* 2002;**37**:36–39.

11. Dumont RC, Caniano DA. Hypokinetic gallbladder disease: a cause of chronic abdominal pain in children and adolescents. *J Pediatr Surg* 1999;**34**:858–861.

12. Vegunta RK, Raso M, Pollock J, *et al.* Biliary dyskinesia: the most common indication for cholecystectomy in children. *Surgery* 2005;**138**:726–731.

13. Shaffer EA, Small DM. Gallstone disease: pathogenesis and management. *Curr Probl Surg* 1976;**13**:1–72.

14. Shaffer EA. Gallbladder disease. In Walker WA, Durie PR, Hamilton JR, *et al.* (eds.) *Pediatric Gastrointestinal Disease*, vol 2. Philadelphia, PA: Mosby, 1991, pp. 1152–1170.

15. Beauregard WG, Ferguson WT. Milk of calcium cholecystitis. *J Pediatr* 1980;**96**:876–877.

16. Palasciano G, Portincasa P, Vinciguerra V, *et al.* Gallstone prevalence and gallbladder volume in children and adolescents: an epidemiological ultrasonographic survey and relationship to body mass index. *Am J Gastroenterol* 1989;**84**:1378–1382.

17. Barbara L, Sama C, Labate AMM, *et al.* A population study on the prevalence of gallstone disease: the Sirmione Study. *Hepatology* 1987;**7**:913–917.

18. Nilsson S. Gallbladder disease and sex hormones. *Acta Chir Scand* 1966;**132**:275–279.

19. Jorgensen T. Prevalence of gallstones in a Danish population. *Am J Epidemiol* 1987;**126**:912–921.

20. Holcomb GW Jr., O'Neill JA, Holcomb GW III. Cholecystitis cholelithiasis and common duct stones in children and adolescents. *Ann Surg* 1980;**191**:626–635.

21. Takiff H, Funkalsrud EW. Gallbladder disease in childhood. *Am J Dis Child* 1984;**138**:565–568.

22. Friesen CA, Roberts CC. Cholelithiasis: clinical characteristics in children. *Clin Pediatr* 1989;**7**:294–298.

23. Stringer MD, Taylor DR, Soloway RD. Gallstone composition: Are children different? *J Pediatr* 2003;**142**:435–440.

24. Sears HF, Golden GT, Horsley JS III. Cholecystitis in adolescents. *Arch Surg* 1973;**106**:651–653.

25. Holcomb GW Jr., Holcomb GW. Cholelithiasis in infants, children and adolescents. *Pediatr Rev* 1991;**11**:268–274.

26. Pokorny WJ, Saleem M, O'Gorman RB, *et al.* Cholelithiasis and cholecystitis in childhood. *Am J Surg* 1984;**148**:742–744.

27. MacMillan RW, Schullinger JN, Santulli RV. Cholelithiasis in childhood. *Am J Surg* 1974;**127**:689–692.

28. Harned RK, Babbit DP. Cholelithiasis in childhood. *Radiology* 1975;**117**:391–393.

29. Andrassy RJ, Treadwell TA, Ratner IA. Gallbladder disease in childhood and adolescents. *Am J Surg* 1976;**132**:19–21.

30. Odom FC, Oliver BB, Kline M. Gallbladder disease in patients 20 years of age and younger. *South Med J* 1976;**69**:1299–1300.

31. Grace N, Rogers B. Cholecystitis in childhood. *Clin Pediatr* 1977;**16**:179–181.

32. Reif S, Sloven DG, Lebenthal E. Gallstones in children. *Am J Dis Child* 1991;**145**:105–108.

33. Goodman DB. Cholelithiasis in persons under 25 years old. *JAMA* 1976;**236**:1731–1732.

34. MacMillan RW, Schullinger JN, Santuli TV. Cholelithiasis in childhood. *Am J Surg* 1974;**127**:689–692.

35. Bailey PV, Connors RH, Tracy TF Jr., *et al.* Changing spectrum of cholelithiasis and cholecystitis in infants and children. *Am J Surg* 1989;**158**:585–588.

36. Strauss RT. Cholelithiasis in childhood. *Am J Dis Child* 1969;**117**:689–692.

37. Bond LR, Hatty SR, Horn MEC, *et al.* Gallstones in sickle cell disease in the United Kingdom. *Br J Med* 1987;**295**:234–236.

38. Schubert TT. Hepatobiliary system in sickle cell disease. *Gastroenterology* 1986;**90**:2013–2021.

39. Sarnaik S, Slovis TL, Corbett DP, *et al.* Incidence of cholelithiasis in sickle-cell anemia using the ultrasonic gray-scale technique. *J Pediatr* 1980;**96**:1005–1008.

40. Matos C, Avni EF, Van Gansbeke D, *et al.* Total parenteral nutrition (TPN) and gallbladder diseases in neonates. *J Ultrasound Med* 1987;**6**:243–248.

41. King DR, Ginn-Pease ME, Lloyd TV, *et al.* Parenteral nutrition with associated cholelithiasis: another iatrogenic disease of infants and children. *J Pediatr Surg* 1987;**22**:593–596.

42. Roslyn JJ, Berquist WE, Pitt HA, *et al.* Increased risk of gallstones in children receiving total parenteral nutrition. *Pediatrics* 1983;**71**:784–789.

43. Messing B, Bories C, Kunstlinger F, *et al.* Does total parenteral nutrition induce gallbladder sludge formation and lithiasis? *Gastroenterology* 1983;**84**:1012–1019.

44. Mashako NNL, Cezard J-P, Borge N, *et al.* The effect of artificial feeding on cholestasis, gallbladder sludge and lithiasis in infants: correlation with plasma cholecystokinin levels. *Clin Nutr* 1991;**10**:320–327.

45. Odievre M, Gautier M, Hadchouel M, *et al.* Severe familial intrahepatic cholestasis. *Arch Dis Child* 1973;**48**:806–812.

46. Schaad UB, Suter S, Gianella-Borradovi A, *et al.* A comparison of ceftriaxone and cefuroxime for the treatment of bacterial meningitis in children. *N Engl J Med* 1990;**522**:141–147.

47. Mahmond H, Schell M, Pui C-H. Cholelithiasis after treatment for childhood cancer. *Cancer* 1991;**67**:1439–1442.

48. Percy AK, Lane JB. Rett Syndrome: Model of neurodevelopmental disorders. *J Clin Neurol* 2005;**20**:718–721.

49. Sakopoulos AG, Gundry S, Razzouk AJ, Andrews HG, Bailey LL. Cholelithiasis in infant and pediatric heart transplant patients. *Pediatr Transplant* 2002;**6**:231–234.

50. Carey MC, Small DM. The physical chemistry of cholesterol solubility in bile: relationship to gallstone formation and dissolution in man. *J Clin Invest* 1978;**61**:998–1026.

51. Lee SP, LaMont JT, Carey MC. Role of gallstone mucous hypersecretion in the evolution of cholesterol gallstone: studies in a prairie dog. *J Clin Invest* 1981;**67**:1712–1723.

52. Bennion LJ, Knowler WC, Mott DM, *et al.* Development of lithogenic bile during puberty in Pima Indians. *N Engl J Med* 1979;**300**:873–876.

53. von Bergmann K, Becker M, Leiss O. Biliary cholesterol saturation in non-obese women and non-obese men before and after puberty. *Eur J Clin Invest* 1986;**16**:531–535.

54. Angelico M, Gandin C, Canuzzi P. Gallstones in cystic fibrosis: a critical reappraisal. *Hepatology* 1991;**14**:768–775.

55. Honore LH. Cholesterol cholelithiasis in adolescent females. *Arch Surg* 1980;**114**:62–64.

56. Buimsohn A, Albu E, Geist PH, *et al.* Cholelithiasis and teenage mothers. *J Adolesc Health Care* 1990;**11**:339–342.

57. Katiska D, Grjibovski A, Einarsson C, *et al.* Genetic and environmental influences on symptomatic gallstone disease: a Swedish study of 43 141 twin pairs. *Hepatology* 2005;**41**:1139–1143.

58. He J, Nishida S, Xu M, Makishima M, Xie W. PXR prevents cholesterol gallstone disease by regulating biosynthesis and transport of bile salts. *Gastroenterology* 2011;**140**:2095–2106.

59. Buch S, Schafmayer C, Volzke H, *et al.* A genome-wide association scan identifies the hepatic cholesterol transporter ABCG8 as a susceptibility factor for human gallstone disease. *Nat Genet* 2007;**39**:995–999.

60. Grunhage F, Acalovschi M, Tirziu S, *et al.* Increased gallstone risk in humans conferred by common variant of hepatic ATP-binding cassette transported for cholesterol. *Hepatology* 2007;**46**:793–801.

61. Kuo KK, Shin SJ, Chen ZC, *et al.* Significant association of *ABCG5* 604Q and *ABCG8* D19H polymorphisms with gallstone disease. *Br J Surg* 2008;**95**:1005–1011.

62. Katsika D, Magnusson P, Krawcyzk M, *et al.* Gallstone disease in Swedish twins: risk is associated with *ABCG8* D19H genotype. *J Intern Med* 2010;**267**:279–285.

63. Renner O, Harsch S, Schaeffeler E, *et al.* A variant of the *SLC10A2* gene encoding the apical sodium-dependent bile acid transporter is a risk factor for gallstone disease. *PLoS One* 2009;**4**: e7321.

64. Vasavda N, Menzel S, Kondaveeti S, *et al.* The linear effects of alpha-thalassemia, the *UGT1A1* and *HMOX1* polymorphisms on cholelithiasis in sickle cell disease. *Br J Haematol* 2007;**138**:263–270.

65. Wasmuth HE, Keppeler H, Herrmann U, *et al.* Coinheritance of Gilbert syndrome-associated *UGT1A1* mutation increases gallstone risk in cystic fibrosis. *Hepatology* 2006;**43**: 738–741.

66. Gracie WA, Ransohoff DF. The natural history of silent gallstones. The innocent gallstone is not a myth. *N Engl J Med* 1982;**307**:798–800.

67. Comfort MW, Gray HK, Wilson JM. The silent gallstone: a ten to twenty year follow-up of 112 cases. *Ann Surg* 1948;**128**:931–937.

68. Newman KD, Marmon LM, Attorri R, *et al.* Laparoscopic cholecystectomy in pediatric patients. *J Pediatr Surg* 1991;**26**:1184–1185.

69. Esposito C, Gonzales Sabin MA, Corcione F, *et al.* Results and complications of laparoscopic cholecystectomy in childhood. *Surg Endoosc* 2001;**15**:890–892.

70. Sackmann M, Ippisch E, Sauerbruch T, *et al.* Early gallstone recurrence rate after successful shock-wave therapy. *Gastroenterology* 1990;**98**:392–396.

71. Bogue C, Murphy AJ, Gerstle JT, Moineddin R, Daneman A. Risk factors, complications, and outcomes of gallstones in children: a single-center review. *J Pediatr Gastroenterol Nutr* 2010;**50**:303–308.

Chapter

17

Hepatitis A and hepatitis E virus infection

Philip Rosenthal

Introduction

Optimal care of children with viral hepatitis necessitates incorporation of recent advances in diagnosis, prevention, and treatment into clinical practice. Although primary viral infection of the liver has been recognized since the time of Hippocrates (460–375 BC), only since the early 1990s have significant scientific advancements allowed clinicians to alter the outcomes of these infections. Specifically, viral hepatitis can be prevented with vaccines and passive immunization and can be treated with antiviral medications. The availability of methods to detect these infections rapidly and accurately has led to changes in the epidemiology of viral hepatitis. Specifically, the absolute number of cases of acute viral hepatitis caused by the hepatitis A virus (HAV) has been reduced through the availability and expansion of vaccination efforts. Recently, a similar agent, the hepatitis E virus (HEV), has emerged as a significant pathogen.

Hepatitis A

Viral characteristics

The virion of HAV is a small spherical, particle of 27–32 nm; it does not have an envelope, contains single stranded RNA, and belongs to the hepatovirus group of picornaviruses (Figure 17.1). It is highly infectious and relatively stable to drying, ether, heat, cold storage, and denaturation by acidic conditions, making it resistant to disinfection. Inactivation of the virus can be achieved by heating food to >185°F (85°C) and treating contaminated surfaces with a 1:100 dilution of sodium hydrochloride (household bleach) in tap water. In the absence of these measures, HAV remains stable in the environment for long periods and may result in outbreaks.

There is only one serotype of HAV but there are seven genotypes based on 15–20% nucleotide diversity over a 168 base segment at the VP1/2A junction [1]. Genotype 1A predominates in the USA and western Europe [2,3]. The genome for HAV is enclosed in the nucleocapsid, which has been designated HAV antigen. It contains a linear, single-stranded molecule of RNA. The virus has been cultured in several cell lines, and the HAV genome has been cloned [4–6].

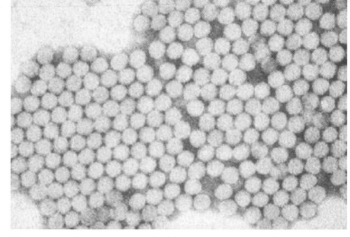

Figure 17.1 Electron micrograph of hepatitis A virus in stool.

Humans are the principal hosts for HAV. Several non-human primates may also become infected with HAV. There is no known carrier state for HAV; consequently, infection is maintained by serial transmission from acutely infected individuals to those who are susceptible [4–7]. In the USA, there were approximately 25 000 new HAV infections in 2007. However, the official number of reported cases is much lower since many people who are infected never have symptoms and are never reported to public health officials. Until 2004, HAV was the most frequently reported type of hepatitis in the USA. Currently, rates of hepatitis A in the USA are the lowest they have been in 40 years. A vaccine was introduced in 1995 and health professionals now routinely vaccinate all children, travelers to certain countries, and people at risk for the disease. Vaccination has dramatically affected rates of the disease in the USA.

Infectivity occurs primarily through fecal–oral transmission after ingestion and absorption. The ingested virus replicates in the small bowel and is transported to the liver via the portal vein. The virus enters the hepatocyte by specific receptors located on the hepatocyte plasma membrane. The viral RNA is uncoated after uptake and binds to ribosomes, causing synthesis of viral proteins. Replication of the viral genome

Liver Disease in Children, Fourth Edition, ed. Frederick J. Suchy, Ronald J. Sokol, and William F. Balistreri. Published by Cambridge University Press. © Cambridge University Press 2014.

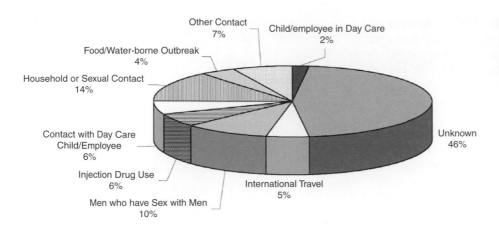

Figure 17.2 The most common sources of hepatitis A infection from 1990 through 2000; 46% of reported patients with hepatitis A could not identify a risk factor for their infection. (Adapted from Centers for Disease Control and Prevention, 2004 [8].)

occurs by RNA polymerase. The virus is subsequently secreted into the biliary tree and excreted in feces, where high concentrations of the virus may be detected. An immunologic response occurs in the liver, resulting in portal and periportal lymphocytic infiltration and liver injury.

Transmission is highest during the anicteric prodromal phase of 14–21 days after exposure, when fecal and serum viral concentrations are high. The incubation period is typically 2–6 weeks, averaging 28 days. Fecal viral excretion may last up to 3 weeks. Children may excrete virus longer than adults. Although HAV is present in serum, its concentration is several orders of magnitude less than in feces.

Epidemiology

Worldwide, HAV infection is a common illness with prevalence rates highest in areas with limited hygiene and sanitation practices. High prevalence rates are seen in Mexico, India, the Middle East, and Africa. In developing countries, where infection is endemic, most individuals are infected by 5 years of age. In developed countries, there is a large population susceptible to periodic outbreaks because of fewer exposures and infections in childhood. Better-quality sanitary standards have reduced the likelihood of fecal contamination and subsequent environmental exposure in developed countries. In recent years, with the introduction of universal childhood immunization against HAV, the number of HAV infections has been reduced in the USA. However, decreased rates of natural immunity have facilitated the ability of HAV to cause outbreaks owing to an expanding susceptible population and have shifted the burden of HAV to older populations, who are more likely to experience morbidity and mortality.

The virus is highly contagious. Factors associated with increased transmission rates include crowding, poor personal hygiene, improper sanitation, and contamination of food and water (Figure 17.2). Prominent risk factors include close contact with patients infected with HAV, spending time in child care centers, travel to endemic regions, male homosexual activity, and intravenous drug abuse. Transmission by blood transfusion or from mother to newborn (perinatal

transmission) is rare. Similarly, transmission from non-human primates has rarely been documented.

Spread of the virus usually occurs by the virus being taken in by mouth from contact with objects, food, or drinks contaminated by the feces (or stool) of an infected person. Person-to-person contact can also spread the virus when infected people do not wash their hands properly after going to the bathroom and then touch other objects or food, when parents or caregivers do not properly wash their hands after changing diapers or cleaning up the stool of an infected person, or when someone engages in certain sexual activities, such as oral–anal contact with an infected person.

Spread can also occur through eating or drinking food or water contaminated with HAV. This is more likely to occur in countries where HAV is common and in areas where there are poor sanitary conditions or poor personal hygiene. The food and drinks most likely to be contaminated are fruits, vegetables, shellfish, ice, and water. In the USA, chlorination of water kills any HAV that enters the water supply.

In the recent past, food-borne outbreaks of HAV infection in spite of apparently high hygiene standards have occurred in the USA. An outbreak of 601 people in western Pennsylvania in 2003 resulted from ingestion of salsa prepared with contaminated green onions imported from Mexico [9,10]. Three people died of liver failure during this outbreak. No ill food service workers were identified.

Many other foods have been incriminated as the vehicle for HAV delivery. A multistate food-borne outbreak of HAV infection illustrates the impact of the disease on children; 213 cases of HAV infection were reported in students attending 23 schools in Michigan and 29 cases in 13 schools in Maine [11]. This outbreak was associated with consumption of frozen strawberries served in school lunch programs. Although the agriculture standards in the USA are high, the ease of travel and shipment of produce between areas of high and low endemicity allows for ready transmission of the virus. Once contaminated products are distributed in a population without significant herd immunity, the consequences can prove fatal.

Food-borne infections and travel as sources of HAV are related. In a recent study, HAV infection among Hispanic children was associated with cross-border travel to Mexico and food-borne exposure during travel [12]. Eating foods from a taco stand or street vendor increased the risk of infection more than 17-fold, whereas eating lettuce increased the risk more than five-fold. Further, there was increased risk with higher socioeconomic status. Families that could not afford to travel were less likely to be exposed to HAV.

Day care centers have long been associated with HAV spread throughout local communities [13–16]. The high rate of spread is related to the crowded conditions, poor hygiene, and mild illness among the infected children seen in day care centers. In addition to the toddlers and staff, HAV infection can also be seen in family members. The clinical symptoms in affected children are often minimal as the majority are anicteric. The illness may be mistaken for flu or gastroenteritis. Many parents may send their children to day care centers with such clinical symptoms. Attention to hand washing and good hygiene are necessary to diminish these infections.

In the past, prior to universal childhood vaccination in the USA, the incidence of HAV infection was highest in the western states among people between 5 and 39 years of age [8]. Overall, one-third of the US population has serologic evidence of previous HAV infection [7]. The prevalence among children 6–11 years of age was 9% and among people older than 70 years it was 75%. Cyclic community-wide outbreaks of HAV infection occurring every 5–10 years were noted for decades. With the introduction and broad use of the HAV vaccine, a decreasing incidence has been most marked among the western states, which now have rates of HAV infection similar to other parts of the USA. At-risk groups, such as Native Americans, now have incidence rates below the average US rate because of implementation of an HAV vaccine strategy.

While overall the incidence has declined, there have been some groups with increased incidence. The increase in HAV infection is occurring in high-risk groups who are not receiving immunizations. These groups include drug users and men who have sex with men. This increase is reflected in an increased proportion of cases among men and an increased mean age of infection. The changing epidemiology of HAV infection is concerning because of the higher morbidity and mortality rate noted in adults.

Clinical aspects and pathogenesis

Acute HAV infection is defined as an acute illness with viral-like symptoms and jaundice or elevated serum aminotransferases (Figure 17.3). Initial clinical manifestations may present similar to a viral prodrome, with non-specific symptoms of nausea, vomiting, anorexia, fatigue, weight loss, low-grade fevers, myalgia, arthralgia, and headaches. Common signs of infection include leukopenia, hepatomegaly, and splenomegaly. Clinical features cannot reliably distinguish HAV infection from other forms of viral hepatitis and other liver diseases. The illness is usually self-limited, and the severity is age dependent. In infants and preschool-aged children, acute HAV infection may be

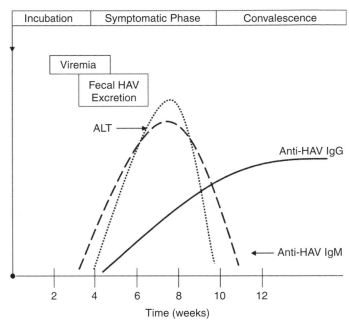

Figure 17.3 Typical course of infection with hepatitis A virus (HAV). Following exposure, an average incubation period lasts 4 weeks. During this period, viremia occurs and overlaps the early symptomatic phase. Jaundice, when present, occurs up to 6 weeks following exposure. Other symptoms may include anorexia, malaise, fever, and headache. Immediately before the symptomatic phase, fecal excretion of virions into the stool occurs. Biochemical hepatitis marked by elevation of serum alanine aminotransferase (ALT) precedes symptomatic infection. The resolution of elevated ALT typically happens after the normalization of the serum bilirubin and may take 2 months. Early infection with HAV can be detected with anti-HAV IgM antibody, and lasting immunity is indicated by a sustained elevation in anti-HAV IgG. (With permission from Balistreri, 1991 [17].)

clinically unapparent as they remain anicteric. Individuals may remain in an anicteric phase for an average of 7 days [18]. If there is progression to the icteric phase, there is dark urine secondary to excretion of bilirubin conjugates and pale-colored stools. Jaundice is present in only 10% of children younger than 6 years of age, 40% of children aged 6–14 years, and 70% of children older than 14 years of age, compared with 70–85% of adults [18]. Risk of transmission decreases 1 week after onset of jaundice. Additional symptoms may include abdominal pain, pruritus, arthralgias, rash, fever, and hepatomegaly.

Diagnosis

The diagnosis of acute HAV is dependent upon the detection of IgM anti-HAV antibodies, and can be detected in serum 5–20 days following exposure. Past infection or previous immunization is associated with serum IgG anti-HAV antibodies. Other methods to detect HAV are available but are not clinically valuable. Viral RNA can be detected in serum and stool during acute infection by nucleic acid amplification, but this is not readily available. Elevated serum aminotransferases, alkaline phosphatase, total bilirubin and direct-reacting bilirubin are observed with acute HAV. Additional laboratory studies evaluating hepatic synthetic function (international normalized ratio, albumin levels) are often necessary in the course of management.

Atypical hepatitis A

Atypical courses of HAV have been recognized and may be associated with persistence of IgM anti-HAV antibodies for as long as 6–12 months [19]. Cholestatic hepatitis and relapsing hepatitis have been reported with HAV [20]. Prolonged jaundice for greater than 3 months associated with pruritus, fever, diarrhea, and weight loss with serum bilirubin levels >10 mg/dL is defined as cholestatic hepatitis when associated with HAV. The disorder may persist for several months before spontaneous resolution. Therapy with ursodeoxycholic acid may be beneficial in reducing pruritus and improving cholestasis. Corticosteroids have been utilized in an attempt to reduce the duration of cholestasis, but data are sparse and immunosuppression may result in reactivation of HAV.

Relapsing HAV occurs in 3–20% of patients and the relapse often resembles the initial presentation. It is characterized by an episode of acute HAV followed by a remission of 4–15 weeks before a recurrence of symptoms with a high fecal HAV viral load and elevated IgM anti-HAV antibodies. The recurrent episodes may become cyclic over 3–9 months and are typically mild clinically.

Infection has also been associated with immune complex disorders including cutaneous vasculitis, arthritis, cryoglobulinemia, lupus-like syndrome, and Sjögren syndrome [21].

Acute HAV has been linked to triggering the presentation of autoimmune hepatitis and Wilson disease [22].

Chronic infection does not occur with HAV. In response to acute HAV, protective antibodies develop that provide lifelong immunity.

Infection with HAV can be a cause of fulminant liver failure. Prior to the introduction of HAV vaccine, approximately 100 individuals died from fulminant HAV infection yearly in the USA, and HAV was one of the leading indications for pediatric liver transplantation in Argentina [23]. The overall case-fatality rate is 0.3%, but it increases with older age and is 1.8% among people over 50 years of age [24]. Patients with underlying chronic liver disease, such as infection with hepatitis C virus, have an increased risk of death when superinfected with HAV [24]. Investigators have recently found that severe liver disease with HAV was associated with an insertion in *TIM1*, the gene encoding the HAV receptor, leading to addition of six amino acid residues [25]. This polymorphism has previously been shown to be associated with protection against asthma and allergic diseases and with HIV progression. This is the first genetic susceptibility factor shown to predispose to HAV-induced acute liver failure.

Treatment

The initial goal of treatment of an HAV-infected patient is to establish supportive care. There is no antiviral medication specific for its treatment. Important in the management is early detection, appropriate support and monitoring during the acute illness, recognition of the development of fulminant liver disease, and prevention of disease spread to susceptible individuals.

Acute illness

During the acute phase of HAV, bed rest may be appropriate. Specific dietary modifications are of little value. There is no demonstrable benefit for corticosteroid therapy. Hospitalization is advisable in the presence of coagulopathy, protracted vomiting, or encephalopathy.

Follow-up biochemical testing should be performed to document resolution or to exclude a progressive coagulopathy suggestive of liver failure. With HAV-associated fulminant hepatic failure, low serum aminotransferase, high serum bilirubin (>15 mg/dL), and low albumin (<2.5 g/dL) are associated with a poor outcome [26]. Listing for liver transplantation may be necessary if there is deterioration in the clinical condition.

Prevention

Keys to prevention of HAV infection include improvements in sanitation, water sources, and food preparation techniques. Personal hygiene, hand washing, and proper disposal of soiled diapers in child care settings all contribute to reducing transmission. Viral transmission can be interrupted by eliminating the virus from the population, utilizing appropriate hygiene, sanitation and isolation procedures, and the use of immunization.

Because transmission of HAV occurs before recognition of clinical infection, hygienic measures alone are often ineffective in preventing infections. The most effective method to halt transmission is immunization.

In hospitalized patients, in addition to standard precautions, contact precautions are recommended for patients who are incontinent or use diapers for at least 1 week after onset of symptoms. Children and adolescents with acute HAV infection who work as food handlers or attend or work in child care should be excluded from attending for at least 1 week after onset of symptoms.

Passive immunization

Prior to the availability of HAV vaccines, passive immunization with immunoglobulin was recommended for individuals who had household contact or intimate exposure to a patient with HAV. The use of immunoglobulin as passive immunization for pre- and postexposure prophylaxis has been refined and limited to specific age groups. The HAV protective antibody concentration in immunoglobulin varies from lot to lot and may be lower in recent preparations – the result of fewer donors having been infected with HAV. However, there are no studies demonstrating lower efficacy of immunoglobulin in preventing HAV infection when properly administered. To be effective, immunoglobulin (0.02 mL/kg) must be administered intramuscularly within 2 weeks of exposure. It is protective for up to 3 months, with 85% effectiveness. Immunoglobulin is recommended for international travelers younger than 1 year, travelers with an imminent departure who need immediate protection, adults over 40 years of age, and possibly pregnant

Table 17.1 Recommended ages and dosages of hepatitis A vaccines

Age (years)	Vaccine[a]	Dose	Volume (mL)	No doses	Schedule (months)[b]
1–18	Havrix	720 EL.U	0.5	2	0, 6–12
>18	Havrix	1440 EL.U	1.0	2	0, 6
1–17	VAQTA	25 U	0.5	2	0, 6–18
>17	VAQTA	50 U	1.0	2	0, 6
≥18	Twinrix	720 EL.U	1.0	3	0, 1, 6

EL.U, enzyme-linked immunosorbent assay units.

[a] Havrix, hepatitis A vaccine, inactivated (GlaxoSmithKline Biologicals); VAQTA, hepatitis A vaccine, inactivated (Merck); Twinrix, Havrix (720 EL.U) and hepatitis B (Engerix-B 20 µg) vaccine combination (GlaxoSmithKline Biologicals).

[b] Initial does at 0 months; subsequent numbers represent months after the initial dose.

Source: Centers for Disease Control and Prevention, 2010, 2013 [28,29].

travelers [7]. Immunoglobulin confers a dose-dependent protection; therefore, a dose of 0.06 mL/kg provides protection up to 5 months [27]. If immunoglobulin is unavailable, HAV vaccine should be given.

Active immunization

Vaccination is preferred for pre-exposure protection in all populations unless contraindicated (hypersensitivity to any vaccine components) and for postexposure prophylaxis in the majority of individuals from 12 months to 40 years of age (Table 17.1).

Currently, there are two inactivated HAV vaccines licensed by the US Food and Drug Administration for use in both children and adults beginning at 12 months of age: Havrix (GlaxoSmithKline Biologicals) and VAQTA (Merck). A combination vaccine, Twinrix (GlaxoSmithKline Biologicals), is approved for HAV vaccination as well as HBV vaccination in people over 18 years of age. The HAV portion of the three vaccines is composed of viral antigens purified from HAV-infected human diploid fibroblast cell cultures. Their antigen content is expressed for Havrix and Twinrix as enzyme-linked immunoassay units (EL.U) and for VAQTA as units of HAV antigen.

The vaccine should be administered as a primary intramuscular (deltoid) dose followed by a second dose at 6–12 months for Havrix and 6–18 months for VAQTA. Twinrix is administered according to the hepatitis B vaccine schedule of an initial dose, and additional doses are administered 1 month and 6 months later. With HAV vaccination, if the second dose is delayed, it can still be given without the need to repeat the primary dose [30].

Efficacy of the vaccine

The HAV vaccines have excellent immunogenicity such that testing for antibodies after vaccination is not required [31–35]. It is also not cost-effective to test for immunity (anti-HAV) in children in the USA and in low HAV prevalence countries before immunization [24]. High-risk population groups, such as injection drug users and immigrants from HAV-endemic countries, may be tested for evidence of immunity before HAV vaccine administration. Since the seroprevalence of anti-HAV is approximately 33% in the general population older than 40

years in the USA, screening for anti-HAV in this age group may be cost-effective [36].

The HAV vaccines are highly protective against clinical disease in immunocompetent children. A double-blind, placebo-controlled randomized trial showed 100% protective efficacy of a prototype HAV vaccine starting 18 days after the first dose in children in a New York state community at high risk for infection [37]. The vaccine was well tolerated and provided complete protective immunity against clinically apparent hepatitis A. In another large, randomized study of 40 119 school-aged children in Thailand, 94% of HAV vaccine recipients were positive for anti-HAV at 8 months and 99%, at 17 months [38]. The vaccine was highly effective in preventing clinical disease; 38 clinically apparent infections were noted in the control group compared with two in the vaccine group, a clinical efficacy of 94%.

In immunocompromised patients, the HAV vaccine is well tolerated, but immunogenicity is lower. In HIV-infected children, low CD4 cell counts have been associated with lower immunogenicity [39–41]. Lower immunogenicity of HAV vaccine was demonstrated in both adult and childhood recipients of liver transplants [42,43]. In adults with chronic liver disease, the HAV vaccine was safe but again lower immunogenicity was detected [44,45]. Several small studies in children with chronic liver disease found the vaccine to be safe and immunogenicity was close to 100% 1 month following the second dose of vaccine [46–48]. It is recommended that all children over 1 year of age, including children with chronic liver disease and those listed for liver transplant, be vaccinated with the HAV vaccine.

Limited data indicate excellent immunogenicity of HAV vaccine in seronegative infants [49]. However, for children younger than 1 year of age, passive immunization with immunoglobulin is still recommended because residual anti-HAV antibody acquired from the mother may interfere with vaccine immunogenicity [35,50–52].

Long-term immunogenicity by hepatitis A vaccine

Long-term protection and efficacy of the HAV vaccine has been reported in children up to 10 years following vaccination [53,54]. Estimates of antibody persistence derived from kinetic models indicate that protective levels of anti-HAV will persist for 20 years, without the need for periodic boosters [7,55–57]. Whether cellular memory or other immunologic mechanisms contribute to long-term protection has yet to be defined.

Adverse effects

The licensed HAV vaccines are very safe. The most common side effects in children are pain, tenderness, or warmth at the injection site, feeding issues, and headache [37,38]. No serious adverse events have been associated with HAV vaccine administration [58]. The only contraindication to vaccination is a previous allergic reaction to the vaccines or a component of the vaccines. Pregnancy is not an absolute contraindication. Although the vaccines have not been studied in pregnant women, both HAV vaccines are inactivated and so they would most likely be safe. Havrix and VAQTA are classified as pregnancy category C agents.

Recommendation for the use of hepatitis A vaccine

With the availability of a safe and efficacious HAV vaccine, and since children serve as a reservoir for transmission, routine "universal" childhood immunization against HAV has been adopted by the American Academy of Pediatrics and the Advisory Committee on Immunization Practices of the Centers for Disease Control and Prevention as the best strategy for eliminating HAV infection (Table 17.1) [58]. Universal vaccination is realistic because there is no animal reservoir of the virus, and there is no human carrier state.

Other groups recommended for HAV vaccination include people traveling to or working in countries with high or intermediate endemicity for HAV, household contacts of new international adoptees, men who have sex with men, users of injection and non-injection illicit drugs, people with occupational risk (working with non-human primates), individuals with clotting factor disorders, and people with chronic liver disease.

Employees working as food handlers or in waste management (sewerage) systems are not routinely recommended for HAV vaccination [58]. However, some restaurants and cities have adopted voluntary immunization programs for food handlers. Obviously, since HAV outbreaks can have substantial monetary implications for any restaurant, strict adherence to appropriate hand washing and personal hygiene should be mandatory.

Prevaccination testing for the presence of anti-HAV is not routinely recommended as it is not cost-effective. Exceptions would include older adolescents from high endemic populations. Further, postvaccination testing for anti-HAV is not recommended given the very high rate of vaccination response.

Public health implications of hepatitis A infection

Besides the mortality associated with HAV infection, there is significant morbidity with a significant financial burden worldwide. Cost-effective analyses clearly demonstrate the benefit of vaccination programs [59]. Estimated costs include inpatient and outpatient care, intensive care expenses for fulminant liver failure and costs associated with liver transplantation. In the USA, HAV is a reportable infectious disease. Case reporting results in costs for public health surveillance, contact investigation, outbreak response, and prophylaxis and prevention programs once an index case is identified.

Current status

An impressive decline in the incidence of HAV infection in the USA can be attributed to the sequential expansion of HAV immunization to the current institution of universal HAV vaccination in children and improved hygiene and sanitation. However, further improvements in combating this infection should be instituted. Immunization of high-risk groups continues to be underutilized. The use of the vaccine worldwide also is underemployed. Strategies to correct these situations should allow continued declines in the morbidity, mortality, and healthcare costs associated with this vaccine-preventable disease.

Hepatitis E
Viral characteristics

The hepatitis E virus is a small icosahedral, non-enveloped, RNA-containing particle 27–34 nm in dimeter that is enterically transmitted like HAV. The HEV genome is a single-stranded, positive-sense RNA of approximately 7.5 kb with three open reading frames (ORFs) [60]. It has indentations and spikes on its surface making it appear similar to calciviruses [61]. It was classified in the Calciviridae family from 1988 to 1998 [62,63] but phylogenetic analysis indicated differences in the non-structural regions that did not support this classification and it is now classified in the genus *Hepevirus* of the family Hepeviridae [64].

Using molecular techniques, HEV was found to consist of short non-coding regions at both the 5'- and 3'-ends, and three ORFs. The first consists of 1693 codons, is the largest, and encodes for non-structural proteins responsible for replication of the viral genome and processing of the viral polyprotein. The second consists of 660 codons and encodes for structural proteins. The third consists of 123 codons and encodes for a small cytoskeleton-associated phosphoprotein of uncertain function [65]. While ORF2 overlaps ORF3, neither overlap ORF1.

The virus has been characterized using molecular techniques. The presumed viral agent was serially transmitted in an animal model (macaque), resulting in typical elevation of serum aminotransferases and the detection of characteristic virus-like particles in feces and bile. Bile obtained from the gallbladder of an infected macaque was also shown to be capable of transmitting infection. The bile contained small (32–34 nm) virus-like particles serologically related to HEV, which were used to construct a library of recombinant complementary DNA (cDNAs). Differential hybridization techniques were used to identify putative HEV-cloned sequences. A single-cloned sequence (ET 1.1), absent from uninfected bile, was analyzed by sequence-independent single-primer amplification followed by hybridization probing [66]. This sequence was detected by polymerase chain reaction testing of amplified DNAs isolated from human feces obtained in five geographically disparate areas in which outbreaks of HEV had been documented; these studies suggested that HEV was the primary agent of water-borne hepatitis in these patients.

A specific antigen (HEVAg), expressed in the cytoplasm of hepatocytes in the early acute stage of infection, has been shown to induce anti-HEV in infected primates. Anti-HEV is found in acute and convalescent serum samples of patients documented to have enterically transmitted hepatitis (not caused by HAV) during outbreaks.

Although only one serotype has been recognized but extensive genomic diversity has been noted among HEV isolates [67]. Currently, HEV isolates have been designated into four genotypes [64,67]. Genotype 1 is most prevalent and accounts for most cases in Asia. In this region, the isolates have 92–99% homology [66]. The second most common genotype, genotype 2, occurs in Mexico and shares only 75% homology with genotype 1. Although HEV is found predominantly in areas with poor sanitation, it has been identified throughout the world, including the USA and Europe [68,69]. Genotypes 1 and 2 infect only humans while genotypes 3 and 4 infect both humans and animals.

Epidemiology

Epidemiologic studies have shown that HEV, like HAV, is predominantly a feces- or water-borne infection noted in developing countries, particularly in areas with inadequate public sanitation or at times of extensive flooding [66,70–76]. Outbreaks of enterically transmitted hepatitis (not caused by HAV) are often traced to contaminated water supplies. Sporadic cases of HEV infection have also been described [75]. Even in developed countries, HEV may be identified infrequently. For example, 2.6% of a control population of Japanese children were positive for anti-HEV IgG [77]; however, in this study, HEV was not associated with fulminant hepatitis and was identified in only one patient with acute hepatitis.

Hepatitis E virus is the second most common cause of sporadic hepatitis in North Africa and the Middle East [78]. In Hong Kong, HEV was shown to account for one-third of the cases of non-A, non-B, non-C hepatitis. Consequently, HEV should be suspected in travelers returning from areas of endemic disease [79].

From epidemiologic studies, it has been postulated that HEV is a zoonosis, with the swine population as a host [64,78,80]. In addition to swine, anti-HEV has been detected in cattle, dogs, rodents, and monkeys [64]. In fact, clusters of HEV in Japan have been traced to the ingestion of undercooked deer meat and pig liver [78].

The development of sensitive assays (most commonly enzyme-linked immunosorbent assays) for antibody to the HEV (anti-HEV) has confirmed that enterically transmitted HEV is also a major cause of acute sporadic and epidemic hepatitis in children in certain geographic areas [81,82].

There is considerable variability in anti-HEV seroprevalence in endemic regions. In areas of India, anti-HEV has been detected in as many as 5% of children younger than 10 years. However, in Egypt, antibodies to HEV are found in more than 60% of children by 10 years of age [78]. In India, the seroprevalence rate reaches 30–40% among adults older than 25 years [61,78,83]. In all locations, anti-HEV is less frequent than anti-HAV among young children in developing countries. This may be the result of its minimal person-to-person transmission along with other variables. In addition, HEV may be transmitted through blood transfusion [84]. Mother-to-child transmission has been documented [85]. While the data on vertical transmission of HEV are limited, when it does occur it is associated with significant morbidity and mortality [86,87].

Clinical aspects and pathogenesis

The clinical manifestations and pathologic features of HEV closely resemble those of HAV; however, there are significant differences (Table 17.2). The incubation period of HEV is somewhat longer, approximately 6 weeks (Figure 17.4). The attack rates for HEV infection are highest in adolescents and young adults (15–40 years), in both epidemic and sporadic forms. Infection is predominantly subclinical or anicteric in children [80,88].

Typically, HEV infection manifests as an acute icteric hepatitis in adolescents and adults. Initially there are flu-like symptoms, fever, chills, abdominal pain, anorexia, nausea, vomiting, diarrhea, arthralgias, and a transient macular rash. This is then followed by jaundice, dark urine, clay-colored stools, and occasional pruritus. Like HAV infection, there may be prolonged cholestasis. Physical examination reveals jaundice and hepatomegaly with or without splenomegaly. Laboratory studies include elevated serum aminotransferases, gamma-glutamyltransferase, alkaline phosphatase, and conjugated bilirubin levels.

Although the overall mortality rate is between 0.2% and 4%, the mortality rate is between 15% and 25% in pregnant women, in whom fulminant disease is highest during the third trimester [89]. Intrauterine infection with HEV has been observed, contributing significantly to perinatal morbidity and mortality [90]. As with HAV, it was felt that no risk existed for the development of chronic liver disease following acute HEV infection. However, chronic HEV infection progressing to cirrhosis has been reported in organ transplant recipients receiving immunosuppression [90,91]. Further, superinfection of HEV in individuals with underlying liver disease may cause severe hepatic decompensation [92–95].

The histology of HEV infection is somewhat characteristic, with ballooning degeneration, cholestasis, and pseudoglandular changes. Recently, it has been determined that a small proportion of US patients thought to have drug-induced liver

Table 17.2 Clinical features of hepatitis E infection

	Clinical feature
Signs and symptoms	Jaundice Fatigue Anorexia Nausea Fever Diarrhea Abdominal pain
Incubation period	Average 40 days (range, 15–60 days)
Epidemiology	Highest attack rate among young adults, 15–40 years Minimal person-to-person transmission Fecal–oral transmission (usually contaminated water) Transmission possible for 14 days after the onset of clinical symptoms Almost all US cases have been related to travel to endemic regions
People at risk for more severe infections	Pregnant women Older people
Complications	Fulminant hepatitis, severe exacerbation of underlying liver disease
Case-fatality rate	~0.2–4%, 15–25% among pregnant women
Chronic sequelae	In immunosuppressed transplant recipients

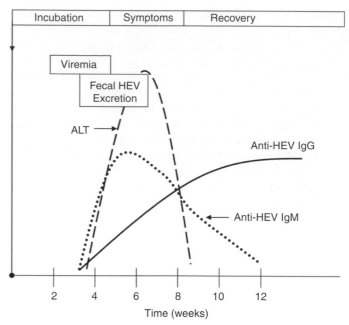

Figure 17.4 Typical course of infection with hepatitis E (HEV). The pattern is similar to that of hepatitis A but there is a mildly longer incubation period. Following exposure, an average incubation period lasts 5–6 weeks. During this period, viremia and fecal excretion of virions occur. Biochemical hepatitis, marked by elevation of serum alanine aminotransferase (ALT), precedes symptomatic infection. Early infection with HEV can be detected with anti-HEV IgM antibody, and lasting immunity is indicated by a sustained elevation in anti-HEV IgG [63].

injury actually have active or past HEV infection, based upon a study from the Drug-Induced Liver Injury Network [96].

In experimental infections of non-human primates, HEV led to variable levels of virus excretion, elevation of serum alanine aminotransferase, and histologic changes in the liver [63]. Although the exact mechanisms for pathogenesis are unknown, alanine aminotransferase elevation typically is coincident with the detection of anti-HEV in the serum and decreasing HEV antigen in hepatocytes. These findings support the role of an immune-mediated response [63]. Additionally, infiltrating lymphocytes in the liver have been found to have a cytotoxic/suppressor immunophenotype [63]. The reasons for more severe liver damage in pregnancy are not known.

Diagnosis

The diagnosis of acute HEV is dependent upon the detection of IgM anti-HEV antibodies, and these can be detected in serum 7–60 days following the onset of symptoms. Past infection is associated with serum IgG anti-HEV antibodies. Other methods to detect HEV are available but not clinically valuable. Although HEV RNA can be detected in serum and stool during acute infection by nucleic acid amplification, this method is not readily available. Elevated serum aminotransferases, alkaline phosphatase, total and direct-reacting bilirubin levels are observed with acute HEV infection. Additional laboratory studies evaluating hepatic synthetic function (international normalized ratio, albumin) are often necessary in the course of management.

Management and prevention

Currently, passive and active immunizations are not available for HEV. Therefore, the main focus is on prevention. To control infections, it is necessary to provide clean drinking water, assure proper hygiene, and dispose of sewage properly. During an epidemic, improving the water supply can rapidly decrease the number of new cases [97]. Boiling water before consumption appears to reduce the risk of acute HEV infection [98]. Because of the low person-to-person transmission rate, isolation of affected people is not indicated.

Administration of serum immunoglobulin has not been successful in reducing disease in HEV-endemic regions [63,99]. In experimental work, passive transfer of anti-HEV has alleviated HEV infection in monkeys [100]. Similarly, experimental HEV vaccines have shown some promise in experimental models [63,101,102]. Additional research is needed to further develop effective vaccines and other preventive measures.

Recently, both pegylated interferon-alfa and ribavirin have been shown to treat chronic HEV infection [103,104]. In addition, supportive therapy including restricted activity, adequate hydration and nutrition, and avoidance of hepatotoxic drugs is recommended.

References

1. Rezende G, Roque-Afonso AM, Samuel D, *et al*. Viral and clinical factors associated with the fulminant course of hepatitis A infection. *Hepatology* 2003;**38**:613–618.

2. Robertson BH, Jansen RW, Khanna B, *et al*. Genetic relatedness of hepatitis A virus strains recovered from different geographical regions. *J Gen Virol* 1992;**73**:1365–1377.

3. Fujiwara K, Yokosuka O, Fukai K, *et al*. Analysis of full-length hepatitis A virus genome in sera from patients with fulminant and self-limited acute type A hepatitis. *J Hepatol* 2001;**35**:112–119.

4. Taylor GM, Goldin RD, Karayiannis P, *et al*. In situ hybridization studies in hepatitis A infection. *Hepatology* 1992;**16**:642–648.

5. Ticehurst JR, Racaniello VR, Baroudy BM, *et al*. Molecular cloning and characterization of hepatitis A virus cDNA. *Proc Natl Acad Sci USA* 1983;**80**:5885–5889.

6. Koff RS. Hepatitis A. *Lancet* 1998;**351**:1643–1649.

7. Craig AS, Schaffner W. Prevention of hepatitis A with the hepatitis A vaccine. *N Engl J Med* 2004;**350**:476–481.

8. Centers for Disease Control and Prevention. *Hepatitis Surveillance Report 59*. Atlanta, GA: US Department of Health and Human Services, Centers for Disease Control and Prevention, 2004:1–60.

9. Centers for Disease Control and Prevention. Hepatitits A outbreak associated with green onions at a restaurant – Monaca, Pennsylvania, 2003. *MMWR Morb Mortal Wkly Rep* 2003;**52**:1155–1157.

10. Wheeler C, Vogt TM, Armstrong GL, *et al*. An outbreak of hepatitis A associated with green onions. *N Engl J Med* 2005;**353**:890–897.

11. Hutin YJF, Pool V, Cramer EH, *et al*. A multistate, foodborne outbreak of hepatitis A. *N Engl J Med* 1999;**340**:595–602.

12. Weinberg M, Hopkins J, Farrington L, *et al*. Hepatitis A in Hispanic children who live along the United States–Mexico border: the role of international travel and food-borne exposures. *Pediatrics* 2004;**114**:e68–73.

13. Hadler SC, Erben JJ, Francis DP, *et al*. Risk factors for hepatitis A in day-care centers, *J Infect Dis* 1982;**145**:255–261.

14. Benenson MW, Takafuji ET, Bancroft WH, *et al*. A military community outbreak of hepatitis type A related to transmission in a child care facility. *Am J Epidemiol* 1980;**112**:471–481.

15. Vernon AA, Schable C, Francis D. A large outbreak of hepatitis A in a daycare center: association with non-toilet-trained children and persistence of IgM antibody to hepatitis A virus. *Am J Epidemiol* 198;**115**:325–331.

16. Hadler SC, Webster HM, Erber JJ, *et al*. Hepatitis A in day care centers: a community-wide assessment. *N Engl J Med* 1980;**302**:1222–1227.

17. Balistreri WF. Viral hepatitis. *Emerg Clin North Am* 1991;**9**:365–399.

18. Leach C. Hepatitis A in the United States. *Pediatr Infect Dis J* 2004;**23**:551–552.

19. Jung YM, Park SJ, Kim JS *et al*. Atypical manifestations of hepatitis A infection: a prospective, multicenter study in Korea. *J Med Virol.* 2010;**82**:1318–1326.

20. Rachima CM, Cohen E, Garty M. Acute hepatitis A: combination of relapsing and the cholestatic forms, two rare variants. *Am J Med Sci* 2000;**319**:417–419.

21. Schiff ER. Atypical clinical manifestations of hepatitis A. *Vaccine* 1992;**10**(Suppl 1):S18–S20.

22. Ozcay F, Canan O, Akcan B, *et al*. Hepatitis A super infection as a cause of liver failure in a child with Wilson's disease. *Turk J Pediatr* 2007;**49**:199–202.

23. Ciocca M, Moreira-Silva SF, Alegria S, *et al*. Hepatitis A as an etiologic agent of acute liver failure in Latin America. *Pediatr Infect Dis J* 2007;**26**:711–715.

24. Centers for Disease Control and Prevention. Prevention of hepatitis A through active or passive immunization: recommendations of the Advisory Committee on Immunization Practices (ACIP). *MMWR Morb Mortal Wkly Rep* 1999;**48**:1–39.

25. Kim HY, Eyheramonho MB, Pichavant M, *et al*. A polymorphism in *TIM1* is associated with susceptibility to severe hepatitis A virus infection in humans. *J Clin Invest* 2011;**121**:1111–1118.

26. Arora NK, Mathur P, Ahuja A, Oberoi A. Acute liver failure. *Indian J Pediatr* 2003;**70**:73–79.

27. Amon JJ, Darling N, Fiore AE *et al*. Factors associated with hepatitis A vaccination among children 24 to 35 months of age: United States, 2003. *Pediatrics* 2006;**117**:30–33.

28. Centers for Disease Control and Prevention. *Vaccines and Immunizations.* Atlanta, GA: Centers for Disease Control and Prevention, 2010 (http://www.cdc.gov/vaccines, accessed 22 July 2013).

29. Centers for Disease Control and Prevention. *Vaccine Recommendations of the Advisory Committee for Immunization Practices.* Atlanta, GA: Centers for Disease Control and Prevention, 2013 (http://www.cdc.gov/vaccines/pubs/ACIP-list.htm, accessed 22 July 2013).

30. Landry P, Tremblay S, Darioli R, Genton B. Inactivated hepatitis A vaccine booster given ≥24 months after the primary doses. *Vaccine* 2000;**19**:399–402.

31. McMahon BJ, Williams J, Bulkow L, *et al*. Immunogenicity of an inactivated hepatitis A vaccine in Alaska native children and native and non-native adults. *J Infect Dis* 1995;**17**:676–679.

32. Horng YC, Chang MH, Lee CY, *et al*. Safety and immunogenicity of hepatitis A vaccine in healthy children. *Pediatr Infect Dis J* 1993;**12**:359–362.

33. Balcarek KB, Bagley MR, Pass RF, Schiff ER, Krause DS. Safety and immunogenicity of an inactivated hepatitis A vaccine in preschool children. *J Infect Dis* 1995;**171**(Suppl 1):S70–S72.

34. Ashur Y, Adler R, Rowe M, Shouval D. Comparison of immunogenicity of two hepatitis A vaccines – VAQTA and HAVRIX – in young adults. *Vaccine* 1999;**17**:2290–2296.

35. Letson GW, Shapiro CN, Kuehn D, *et al*. Effect of maternal antibody on immunogenicity of hepatitis A vaccine in infants. *J Pediatr* 2004;**144**:327–332.

36. Das A. An economic analysis of different strategies of immunization against hepatitis A virus in developed countries. *Hepatology* 1999;**29**:548–552.

37. Werzberger A, Mensch B, Kuter B, *et al*. A controlled trial of a formalin-

inactivated hepatitis A vaccine in healthy children. *N Engl J Med* 1992;**327**:453–457.

38. Innis BL, Snithhan R, Kunasol P, *et al.* Protection against hepatitis A by an inactivated vaccine. *JAMA* 1994;**271**:1328–1334.

39. Gouvea AF, De Moraes-pinto MI, Ono E, *et al.* Immunogenicity and tolerability of hepatitis A vaccine in HIV-infected children. *Clin Infect Dis* 2005;**41**:544–548.

40. Siberry GK, Coller RJ, Henkle E, *et al.* Antibody response to hepatitis A immunization among human immunodeficiency virus-infected children and adolescents. *Pediatr Infect Dis J* 2008;**27**:465–468.

41. Weinberg A, Gona P, Nachman SA, *et al.* Antibody-response to hepatitis A virus vaccine in HIV-infected children with evidence of immunologic reconstitution while receiving highly active retroviral therapy. *J Infect Dis* 2006;**193**:302–311.

42. Arslan M, Wiesner RH, Poterucha JJ, Zein NN. Safety and efficacy of hepatitis A vaccination in liver transplantation recipients. *Transplantation* 2001;**72**:272–276.

43. Diana A, Posfay-Barbe KM, Belli DC, Siegrist CA. Vaccine-induced immunity in children after orthotopic liver transplantation: a 12-yr review of the Swiss national reference center. *Pediatr Transplant* 2007;**11**:31–37.

44. Lee SD, Chan CY, Yu MI, *et al.* Safety and immunogenicity of inactivated hepatitis A vaccine in patients with chronic liver disease. *J Med Virol* 1997;**52**:215–218.

45. Keeffe EB, Iwarson S, McMahon BJ, *et al.* Safety and immunogenicity of hepatitis A vaccine in patients with chronic liver disease. *Hepatology* 1998;**27**:881–886.

46. Ferreira CT, da Silviera TR, Viera SM *et al.* Immunogenicity and safety of hepatitis A vaccine in children with chronic liver disease. *J Pediatr Gastroenterol Nutr* 2003;**37**:258–261.

47. El-Karaksy HM, El-Hawary MI, El-koofy NM, *et al.* Safety and efficacy of hepatitis A vaccine in children with chronic liver disease. *World J Gastroenterol* 2006;**12**:7337–7340.

48. Majda-Stanislawska E, Bednarek M, Kuydowicz J. Immunogenicity of inactivated hepatitis A vaccine in children with chronic liver disease. *Pediatr Infect Dis J* 2004;**23**:571–574.

49. Troisi CL, Hollinger FB, Krause DS, *et al.* Immunization of seronegative infants with hepatitis A vaccine (HAVRIX®; SKB): a comparative study of two dosing schedules. *Vaccine* 1997;**15**:1613–1617.

50. Piazza M, Safary A, Vegnente A, *et al.* Safety and immunogenicity of hepatitis A vaccine in infants: a candidate for inclusion in the childhood vaccination programme. *Vaccine* 1999;**17**:585–588.

51. Dagan R, Amir J, Mijalovsky A, *et al.* Immunization against hepatitis A in the first year of life: priming despite the presence of maternal antibody. *Pediatr Infect Dis J* 2000;**19**:1045–1052.

52. Fiore AE, Shapiro CN, Sabin K, *et al.* Hepatitis A vaccination of infants: effect of maternal antibody status on antibody persistence and response to a booster dose. *Pediatr Infect Dis J* 2003;**22**:354–359.

53. Hammitt LL, Bulkow L, Hennessy TW, *et al.* Persistence of antibody to hepatitis A virus 10 years after vaccination among children and adults. *J Infect Dis* 2008;**198**:1776–1782.

54. Werzberger A, Mensch B, Nalin DR, Kuter BJ. Effectiveness of hepatitis A vaccine in a former frequently affected community: 9 years' followup after the Monroe field trial of VAQTA. *Vaccine* 2002;**20**:1699–1701.

55. Chang CY, Lee SD, Yu MI, *et al.* Long-term follow-up of hepatitis A vaccination in children. *Vaccine* 1999;**17**:369–372.

56. Van Damme P, Banatvala J, Fay O, *et al.* Hepatitis A booster vacination: is there a need? *Lancet* 2003;**362**: 1065–1071.

57. Van Herckk K, Van Damme P. Inactivated hepatitis A vaccine-induced antibodies: follow-up and estimates of long-term persistence. *J Med Virol* 2001;**63**:1–7.

58. Centers for Disease Control and Prevention. Prevention of hepatitis A through active or passive immunization: recommendations of the Advisory Committee on Immunization Practices (ACIP). *MMWR Morb Mortal Wkly Rep* 2006;**55**(RR-7):1–23.

59. Rosenthal P. Cost-effectiveness of hepatitis A vaccination in children, adolescents, and adults. *Hepatology* 2003;**37**:44–51.

60. Ansari IH, Nanda SK, Durgapal H, *et al.* Cloning sequencing, and expression of the hepatitis E virus (HEV) nonstructural open reading frame 1. *J Med Virol* 2000;**60**: 275–283.

61. Krawczynski K, Aggarwal R, Kamili S. Infections of the liver. *Infect Dis Clin N Am* 2000;**14**:1–18.

62. Worm HC, van der Poel WHM, Brandstatter G. Hepatitis E: an overview. *Microbes Infect* 2002;**4**:657–666.

63. Aggarwal R, Krawczynski K. Hepatitis E: an overview and recent advances in clinical and laboratory research. *J Gastroenterol Hepatol* 2000;**15**: 9–20.

64. Ahn J-M, Kang S-G, Lee D-Y, *et al.* Identification of novel human hepatitis E virus (HEV) isolates and determination of the seroprevalence of HEV in Korea. *J Clin Microbiol* 2005;3042–3048.

65. Tam AW, Smith MM, Guerra ME, *et al.* Hepatitis E virus (HEV): molecular cloning and sequencing of the full-length viral genome. *Virology* 1991;**185**:120–131.

66. Reyes GR, Purdy MA, Kim JP, *et al.* Isolation of a cDNA from the virus responsible for enterically transmitted non-A, non-B hepatitis. *Science* 1990;**247**:1335–1339.

67. Shrestha SM, Srestha S, Tsuda F, *et al.* Genetic changes in hepatitis E virus of subtype 1a in patients with sporadic acute hepatitis E in Kathmandu, Nepal, from 1997 to 2002. *J Gen Virol* 2004;**85**:97–104.

68. Mansuy JM, Peron JM, Abravanel F, *et al.* Hepatitis E in the south west of France in individuals who have never visited an endemic area. *J Med Virol* 2004;**74**:419–424.

69. Redlinger T, O'Rourke K, Nickey L, Martinez G. Elevated hepatitis A and E seroprevalence rates in a Texas/Mexico border community. *Tex Med* 1998;**94**:68–71.

70. Aggarwal R, Naik SR. Faecal excretion of hepatitis-E virus. *Lancet* 1992;**340**:787.

71. DeCock KM, Bradley DW, Sandford NL, *et al.* Epidemic non-A, non-B hepatitis in patients from Pakistan. *Ann Intern Med* 1987;**106**:227–230.

72. Ray R, Aggarwal R, Salunke PN, *et al.* Hepatitis E virus genome in stools of hepatitis patients during large epidemic in North India, *Lancet* 1991;**338**:783–784.

73. Skidmore SJ, Yarbough PO, Gabor KA, *et al.* Hepatitis E virus: the cause of waterborne hepatitis outbreak. *J Med Virol* 1992;**37**:58–60.

74. Ticehurst J, Popkin TJ, Bryan JP, *et al.* Association of hepatitis E virus with an outbreak of hepatitis in Pakistan: serologic responses and pattern of virus excretion. *J Med Virol* 1992;**36**:84–92.

75. Chauhan A, Dilawari JB, Jameel S, *et al.* Common etiological agent for epidemic and sporadic non-A non-B hepatitis. *Lancet* 1992;**339**:1509–1510.

76. Hau CH, Hien TT, Tien NT, *et al.* Prevalence of enteric hepatitis A and E viruses in the Mekong delta region of Vietnam. *Am J Trop Med Hyg* 1998;**60**:277–280.

77. Goto K, Ito K, Sugiura T, *et al.* Prevalence of hepatitis E virus infection in Japanese children. *J Pediatr Gastroenterol Nutr* 2005;**42**:89–92.

78. Emerson SU, Purcell RH. Running like water: the omnipresence of hepatitis E. *N Engl J Med* 2004;**351**:2367–2368.

79. Bader TF, Krawczynski K, Polish LB, *et al.* Hepatitis E in a US traveler to Mexico. *N Engl J Med* 1991;**325**:1659.

80. De Groen PC. Hepatitis E in the United States: a case of "hog fever?" *Mayo Clin Proc* 1997;**72**:1197–1198.

81. Goldsmith R, Yarbough PO, Reyes GR, *et al.* Enzyme-linked immunosorbent assay for diagnosis of acute sporadic hepatitis E in Egyptian children. *Lancet* 1992;**339**:328–332.

82. Hyams KC, Purdy MA, Kaur M, *et al.* Acute sporadic hepatitis E in Sudanese children: analysis based on a new Western blot assay. *J Infect Dis* 1992;**165**:1001–1005.

83. Daniel HDJ, Warier A, Abraham P, Sridharan G. Age-wise exposure rates to hepatitis E virus in a southern Indian patient population without liver disease. *Am J Top Med Hyg* 2004;**71**:675–678.

84. Khuroo MS, Kamili S, Yattoo GN. Hepatitis E virus infection may be transmitted through blood transfusions in an endemic area. *J Gastroenterol Hepatol* 2004;**19**:778–784.

85. Singh S, Mohanty A, Joshi YK, *et al.* Mother-to-child transmission of hepatitis E virus infection. *Indian J Pediatr* 2003;**70**:37–39, 597.

86. Khuroo MS, Kamili S, Jameel S. Vertical transmission of hepatitis E virus. *Lancet* 1995;**345**:1025–1026.

87. Kumar RM, Uduman S, Rana S, *et al.* Sero-prevalence and mother-to-infant transmission of hepatitis E virus among pregnant women in the United Arab Emirates. *Eur J Obstet Gynecol Reprod Biol* 2001;**100**:9–15.

88. Arora NK, Panda SK, Nanda SK, *et al.* Hepatitis E infection in children: study of an outbreak. *J Gastroenterol Hepatol* 1999;**14**:572–577.

89. Worm HC, van der Poel WHM, Brandstatter G. Hepatitis E: an overview. *Microbes Infect* 2002;**4**:657–666.

90. Panda SK, Jameel S. Hepatitis E virus: from epidemiology to molecular biology. *Viral Hepat* 1997;**3**:227–251.

91. Kamar N, Mansuy JM, Cointault O, *et al.* Hepatitis E virus-related cirrhosis in kidney- and kidney-pancreas-transplant recipients. *Am J Transplant* 2008;**8**:1744–1748.

92. Kamar N, Garrouste C, Haagsma EB, *et al.* Factors associated with chronic hepatitis in patients with hepatitis E virus infection who have received solid organ transplants. *Gastroenterology* 2011;**140**:1481–1489.

93. Hamid SS, Atiq M, Shehzad F, *et al.* Hepatitis E virus superinfection in patients with chronic liver disease. *Hepatology* 2002;**36**:474–478.

94. Kumar A, Aggarwal R, Naik SR, *et al.* Hepatitis E virus is responsible for decompensation of chronic liver disease in an endemic region. *Indian J Gastroenterol* 2004;**23**:59–62.

95. Ramachandran J, Eapen CE, Kang G, *et al.* Hepatitis E superinfection produces severe decompensation in patients with chronic liver disease. *J Gastroenterol Hepatol* 2004;**19**:134–138.

96. Davern TJ, Chalasani N, Fontana RJ, *et al.* Acute hepatitis E infection accounts for some cases of suspected drug-induced liver injury. *Gastroenterology* 2011;**14**:1665–1672.

97. Bile K, Isse A, Mohamud O, *et al.* Contrasting roles of rivers and wells as sources of drinking water on attack and fatality rates in a hepatitis E epidemic in Somalia. *Am J Trop Med Hyg* 1994;**51**:466–474.

98. Corwin AL, Khiem HB, Clayson ET, *et al.* A waterborne outbreak of hepatitis E virus transmission in southwestern Vietnam. *Am J Trop Med Hyg* 1996;**54**:559–562.

99. Khuroo MS, Dar MY. Hepatitis E: Evidence for person-to-person transmission and inability of low dose immune serum globulin from an Indian source to prevent it. *Indian J Gastroenterol* 1992;**3**:113–116.

100. Tsarev SA, Tsareva TS, Emerson SU, *et al.* Successful passive and active immunization of cynomolgus monkeys against hepatitis E. *Proc Natl Acad Sci USA* 1994;**91**:10198–10202.

101. Tsarev SA, Tsareva TS, Emerson SU, *et al.* Recombinant vaccine against hepatitis E: dose response and protection against heterologous challenge. *Vaccine* 1997;**15**:1834–1838.

102. Kamili S. Toward the development of a hepatitis E vaccine. *Virus Res* 2011;**161**:93–100.

103. Alric L, Bonnet D, Laurent G, *et al.* Chronic hepatitis E virus infection: successful virologic response to pegylated interferon-alpha therapy. *Ann Intern Med* 2010;**153**:135–136.

104. Kamar N, Rostaing L, Abravanel F, *et al.* Ribavirin therapy inhibits viral replication in patients with chronic hepatitis E virus infection. *Gastroenterology* 2010;**139**:1612–1618.

Chapter 18

Hepatitis B virus infection

Mei-Hwei Chang

Introduction

Hepatitis B virus (HBV) infection continues to be an important health problem [1]. It may cause acute, fulminant, or chronic hepatitis; cirrhosis; and liver cancer. Although complications occur mainly during adult life, most primary HBV infection occurs during early childhood [1]. To control HBV infection and its complication, it is mandatory to understand the transmission mode and natural history starting from childhood. The age of primary infection is an important factor affecting the outcome. Infection during infancy and early childhood leads to high rates of persistent infection. Perinatal transmission from mothers who are carriers of the hepatitis B surface antigen (HBsAg) to their infants is an important route of transmission leading to chronicity in endemic areas. Before the era of universal HBV vaccination, perinatal transmission accounted for 40–50% of HBsAg carriers in Asia. Maternal HBsAg and hepatitis B e antigen (HBeAg) status affects the outcome of HBV infection in their infants. Around 90% of the infants of HBeAg-seropositive carrier mothers became HBsAg carriers. Horizontal transmission from highly infectious family members, improperly sterilized syringes, or other contaminated instruments may also occur.

This chapter details the epidemiology, transmission routes, clinical features, preventive, and therapeutic strategies for HBV infection, and also briefly introduces hepatitis delta virus (HDV) infection. The latter is a small defective RNA virus that requires HBV envelope proteins to surround the nucleocapsid complexed with the viral protein. To facilitate the discussion of HBV and HDV, a glossary of the terminology used throughout this chapter is presented in Table 18.1.

Hepatitis B virus

The virion is a partially double-stranded (long and short) DNA virus with a genome of 3200 nucleotides (Figure 18.1). It is a hepatotropic DNA virus that is classified as a member of the Hepadnaviridae. Its host range is restricted to humans and chimpanzees. The transcript of HBV contains four open reading frames (ORFs) S, C, P and X regions, encoding surface

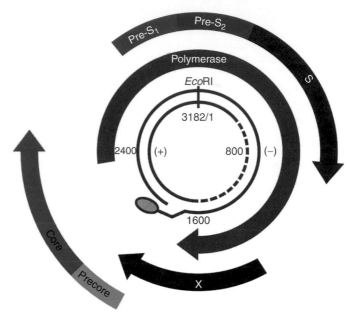

Figure 18.1 Genomic structure and open reading frames of hepatitis B virus (HBV). HBV is a partially double-stranded (long and short) DNA virus with a genome of 3200 nucleotides. The inner circles illustrate the long (—) strand and short (- -) DNA strands. The terminal protein linked to the 5'-end of the long strand is marked as a small oval ball. The transcripts of HBV contain four open reading frames, S, C, P and X regions, encoding surface protein, core protein, polymerase, and X protein, respectively.

protein, core protein, polymerase, and X protein, respectively [2]. The S ORF encodes HBsAg proteins and can be structurally and functionally divided into the pre-S$_1$, pre-S$_2$, and S regions, which encode three envelope proteins: the the major, middle, and large proteins. The C ORF encodes either the viral nucleocapsid HBV core antigen (HBcAg) or HBeAg depending on whether translation is initiated from the core or precore regions, respectively. The nucleocapsid of HBV contains a major protein, the core protein (HBcAg). The precore ORF codes for a signal peptide that directs the translation product to the host endoplasmic reticulum, where the protein is further processed to form the secreted HBeAg. This is a small secretory viral protein present in serum, which results

Liver Disease in Children, Fourth Edition, ed. Frederick J. Suchy, Ronald J. Sokol, and William F. Balistreri. Published by Cambridge University Press. © Cambridge University Press 2014.

Table 18.1 Glossary

Terminology	Definition	Significance
Hepatitis B virus (HBV)		
HBsAg	Hepatitis B surface antigen; found on the surface of the intact virus and as free particles in the serum	Presence in serum indicates acute or chronic HBV infection
HBcAg	Hepatitis B core antigen; found in the intact virion but no free particle	Detectable in liver tissue but not detectable in serum
HBeAg	Hepatitis B e antigen; a soluble antigen, translational product of precore and core gene	Presence in serum indicates active HBV infection and correlates with HBV replication; signifies high infectivity
Anti-HBs[a]	Antibody to HBsAg	A neutralizing antibody, presence in serum indicates immunity to HBV
Anti-HBc	Antibody to HBcAg	This is not a protective antibody; presence in serum of subclass IgM indicates early infection; presence in serum of subclass IgG indicates active acute or chronic infection
Anti-HBe	Antibody to HBeAg	Seroconversion of HBeAg to anti-HBe indicates resolution of active HBV replication phase in most cases
HBV DNA	DNA of HBV	Indicates HBV replication; a useful marker for infectivity and for monitoring treatment
Hepatitis D (delta) virus (HDV)		
HDVAg	Delta antigen	Presence in serum indicates HDV infection
Anti-HDV	Antibody to HDV (IgM and IgG)	Presence in serum indicates exposure to HDV
HDV RNA	RNA of HDV	Presence in serum indicates HDV replication

[a] Presence may indicate acquisition of antibody through immunoglobulin administration or protective immunity following infection or vaccination.

from proteolytic cleavage of P22C. The presence of HBeAg in serum implicates high viral replication, high viral infectivity, and possible current or later active liver disease. The P ORF encodes polymerase, which is a large protein. The HBV X ORF encodes a 16.5 kDa protein (HBxAg) that may be related to productive HBV infection and the oncogenic potential of HBV.

Replication is via reverse transcription, including protein priming by the unique extra terminal protein domain of the reverse transcriptase (the polymerase) [3]. The HBV replication cycle is summarized in Figure 18.2. The initial phase of HBV infection involves the attachment of mature virions to host cell membranes, likely involving the pre-S domain of the surface protein. After transport and entry of the viral genome into the nucleus, the single-stranded gap region in the viral genome is repaired by the viral polymerase protein, and the viral DNA is circularized to the covalently closed circular DNA form. This form of HBV DNA serves as the template for transcription of several species of genomic and subgenomic RNAs.

Hepatocytes infected by HBV usually secrete 100 to 1000 times as many empty polymers of HBV envelope proteins with spherical or filamentous shapes made mostly of small HBsAg

as infectious virions [4]. The HBsAg carries an "a" antigenic determinant, created by two "loops" of amino acids 120–160, that is recognized by most commercial assays and the epitope to which neutralizing antibody is raised.

In primary (new) HBV infection, HBsAg is the first marker detectable in the blood after an incubation period of 4 to 10 weeks, followed shortly by anti-HBc, which is predominantly of the IgM type in the early phase of self-limited infection. The typical serologic pattern of acute HBV infection is illustrated in Figure 18.3. During acute HBV infection, anti-HBc IgM appears shortly after onset of jaundice, reaches peak titers by 5 months, then subsequently declines. Serum antibody to HBsAg (anti-HBs), a protective antibody against subsequent HBV infection, may be detectable weeks to months after the elevation of aminotransferase levels and lasts for many years after infection. Anti-HBs appears within 6 months of disease onset in most patients with acute HBV infection (Table 18.2). Active hepatic inflammation, as indicated by elevated serum aminotransferases, may occur 14–60 days after HBsAg is detected in serum [6].

Viremia is established by the time HBsAg is detected in serum. The presence of HBV DNA in serum is a useful marker of viral replication and is usually associated with active liver

Table 18.2 Serologic markers and hepatitis B viral DNA levels in different phases of chronic infection[a]

Phase of infection	HBsAg	Anti-HBs	HBeAg	Anti-HBe	Anti-HBc	HBV DNA (IU/mL)	ALT	Liver histology
Early	+	−	+	−	IgM	+	↑	Acute inflammation
Recovery	−	+	−	+	IgG	−	Normal	Normal
Immune tolerance phase	+	−	+	−	IgG	$>2 \times 10^4$	Normal	Mild/minimal inflammation
Inflammatory phase					IgG, IgM	$>2 \times 10^4$	↑	Active inflammation
Inactive phase	+	−	+	−	IgG	$<2 \times 10^4$	Normal	Mild/minimal inflammation
HBeAg (−) Hepatitis	+	−	−	+	IgM/IgG	$>2 \times 10^3$	↑	Active inflammation

ALT, serum alanine aminotransferase.
[a] See Table 18.1 for other abbreviations.

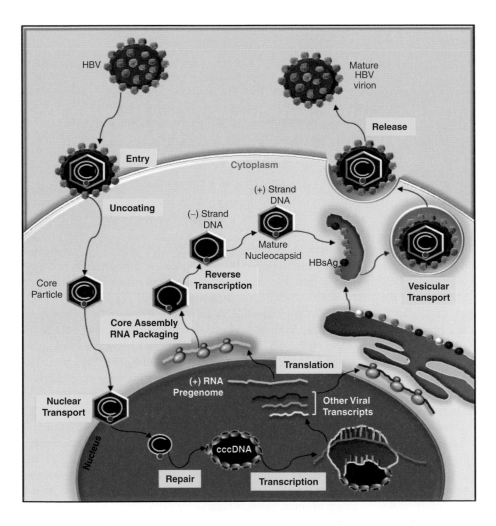

Figure 18.2 Replication cycle of hepatitis B virus (HBV). The initial phase of infection involves the attachment of mature virions to host cell membrane. After entry of the HBV genome into the nucleus, the single-stranded gap region in the genome is repaired by viral polymerase, and the viral DNA is circularized to the covalently closed circular DNA (cccDNA) form. The virus replicates via reverse transcription, including protein priming by the unique extraterminal protein domain of the reverse transcriptase (the polymerase). (Kindly drawn by Dr. Chua.)

disease and infectivity. The ranges of quantification for some commercially available HBV DNA quantitative assays are listed in Table 18.3. The serum levels of HBV DNA in primary infection are usually high, frequently in the range of 10^9 to 10^{12} copies/mL (10^8 to 10^{11} IU/mL). Circulating HBeAg can be detected in the early phase but is cleared rapidly in patients with acute HBV infection. Persistence of HBsAg in the circulation over 6 months is considered as

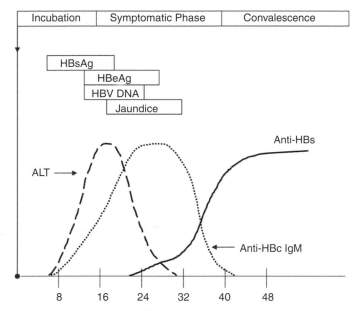

| Incubation | Symptomatic Phase | Convalescence |

Figure 18.3 Typical course of acute hepatitis B virus (HBV) infection. Primary HBV infection has an incubation period of 4–10 weeks. The earliest detectable serum marker of HBV infection is HBV surface antigen (HBsAg), which may appear between 1 and 10 weeks following exposure. Subsequently, HBV e antigen (HBeAg) and HBV DNA may be identified. HBsAg is present 2–8 weeks before the onset of symptoms, which coincide with a spike in serum alanine aminotransferase (ALT) and bilirubin, and constitutional signs. Clearance of HBsAg with the appearance of anti-HBsAg antibodies typically occurs within 6–8 months following infection. Anti-HBV core antigen (anti-HBc) IgM is present before symptomatic infection and is a marker for acute infection. (With permission from Balistreri, 1991 [5].)

Table 18.3 Comparison of the ranges of quantification for some commercially available hepatitis B viral DNA quantitative assays

Detection method	Approximate range of quantification	Commercially available assays
Signal amplification	1.4×10^5 to 1.7×10^9 copies/mL	Digene Hybrid Capture II
	2.0×10^3 to 1.0×10^8 copies/mL	Bayer Versant HBV 3.0
Target amplification	2.0×10^2 to 2.0×10^5 copies/mL	Roche Cobas Amplicor HBV
	2.0×10^2 to 1.0×10^9 IU/mL	Artus-Biotech Real Art HBV PCR
	30 to 1.1×10^8 IU/mL	Roche Cobas TaqMan
	10 to 1.0×10^9 IU/mL	Abbott Realtime PCR

Source: adapted from Andersson et al., 2009 [7].

chronic HBV infection, while loss of serum HBsAg and appearance of its antibody is considered to indicate the possibility of HBV eradication. In most patients with chronic HBV infection, viral replication continues, HBsAg remains detectable in blood, while titers of HBV DNA tend to decline gradually over time; HBeAg disappears from the blood along with seroconversion to positivity for anti-HBe. Given the short half-life of HBV virions (approximately 1 day), detectable HBV DNA levels can be sustained only by ongoing viral replication [1,4]. Anti-HBc IgG rises later and persists during chronic HBV infection as long as viral replication within the liver cell continues, or even after disappearance of HBV replication in the liver.

Global epidemiology

The prevalence of HBV infection varies in different countries and regions in the world as well as among different ethnic groups. Endemicity has been classified into three categories, high (>8%), intermediate (2–8%), and low (<2%), depending on the prevalence of (HBsAg) seropositivity. Infection with HBV is prevalent in Asia, Africa, southern Europe, and Latin America, where the HBsAg seropositivity rate ranges from 2 to 20%. Regions with a high prevalence of HBV infection also have high rates of hepatocellular carcinoma (HCC): HBV causes 60–80% of the primary liver cancer in the world, which

accounts for one of the three major causes of cancer deaths in Asia, the Pacific Rim, and Africa. Countries in the Asia–Pacific Region have the highest prevalence of endemic HBV infection. In most parts of Asia, the HBsAg carrier rate in the general population is 5–20%. Some countries in this region, such as Japan, Australia, and New Zealand, have low HBsAg prevalence rates.

In contrast, in North America, western and northern Europe, and Oceanic areas, where prevalence of HBV infection is relatively low (around 0.1%), primary HBV infection occurs mainly in adolescents and adults. Childhood HBV infection in this population is concentrated in immigrants from endemic areas and in children of high-risk groups, such as intravenous drug users. In the USA, the Third National Health and Nutrition Examination Survey (NHANES III), conducted from 1988 through 1994, revealed that the HBsAg seropositive rate was 0.41%, and the prevalence of anti-HBc was 4.9% [8]. The prevalence of HBV infection in NHANES studies was low in children until age 12 and increased thereafter in all ethnic groups. The HBsAg seroprevalence rates in Europe vary widely, ranging from 0.3% to 12%, even within a single country [9]. The most frequently reported risk factors for HBV infection in Europe include heterosexual activity, injection drug use, male homosexual activity, perinatal exposure, and household contact with infected individuals.

In endemic areas, such as Asia and Africa, most people with chronic HBV infection were infected during early childhood. Perinatal infection and household contacts with chronically infected patients during early childhood are the predominant modes of transmission. In highly prevalent areas such as Taiwan, primary HBV infection occurs predominantly during infancy and early childhood [3]. Before the implementation of the universal HBV vaccination program in Taiwan, the HBsAg seropositive (chronic HBV infection) rate in Taipei

City increased with age, ranging from 5% in infants, to 10% in children at 2 years of age and remained stationary afterward. This suggested that most chronic HBsAg carriers were infected before 2 years of age in Taiwan and other endemic areas.

In Africa, HBV transmission was considered to occur mainly horizontally during early childhood. In some countries in western Africa (e.g. Senegal and Gambia), over 90% of the population is exposed to and becomes infected with HBV during lifetime. In rural areas of west Africa, HBV infection rates increase rapidly from the age of 6 months; by the age of 2 years, 25–40% of children have been infected and 15% have developed chronic infection. By the age of 10-15 years, 80–90% of children have become infected and 20% are chronic carriers [10].

Routes of transmission

Hepatitis B virus can be transmitted via body fluids, either through mother-to-infant transmission or horizontally through blood transfusion, injection, sexual exposure, or close contact in the family or with caretakers. Perinatal transmission from highly infectious mothers to their neonates is an important route for HBV infection in Asian countries and many other endemic areas. Before the HBV vaccination era, perinatal transmission accounted for 40–50% of HBsAg carriers in endemic areas. The age of HBV infection is an important factor affecting the outcome of HBV infection. The younger the infection occurs, the higher the rate of chronic infection. Without immunoprophylaxis, more than 90% of infants who were infected by their HBeAg-positive, HBsAg-positive mothers will develop chronic HBV infection (Table 18.4) [11]. The relatively high maternal viral load transmitted to the neonate with a physiologically immature immune system during perinatal period may explain the high rate of persistent HBV infection. For those who are infected at preschool age, the chronicity rate after HBV infection decreases to approximately 25% [11]. Infection occurring in young adults results in a lower chronicity rate (<3%). In contrast to Asia, where mother-to-infant transmission is an important route, horizontal transmission in early life is considered to be the predominant mode of transmission in most of sub-Saharan Africa.

Mother-to-infant transmission

Perinatal HBV transmission from an infectious mother to her infant is an important route for HBV infection in Asian countries and other endemic areas, where it seems to account for 35–50% of carriers. Transmission can occur in utero, at the time of delivery, or after birth. Children of HBsAg-positive mothers who escaped HBV infection at the neonatal period remain at high risk of infection during early childhood. Less than 5% of neonates born to HBsAg-positive, HBeAg-negative mothers will become infected with HBV, compared with more than 90% of those born to HBsAg-positive and HBeAg-positive mothers.

Table 18.4 Age of infection and maternal hepatitis B status influence the outcome of hepatitis B virus infection in children[a]

Age of infection	Rate of persistent infection
Perinatal period	
Mother HBeAg(+), HBsAg(+)	>90%
Mother HBeAg(−), HBsAg(+)	<5%, but with risk of acute or fulminant hepatitis
Preschool age	23%
Young adults	2.7~10%

[a] See Table 18.1 for abbreviations.
Source: adapted from Beasley, 2009 [11].

The e antigen is a small viral secretory protein that can cross the placenta barrier from the mother to the infant. As both HBeAg and HBcAg are highly cross-reactive in terms of helper T-cell recognition, transplacental HBeAg may induce a specific unresponsiveness of helper T-cells to HBeAg and HBcAg in the neonates born to HBeAg-positive, HBsAg-positive mothers [12]. This may cause the high rate of chronic infection and the long-term immune tolerance status to HBV.

It is widely accepted that most perinatal HBV transmission occurs at or near the time of birth, since neonatal vaccination prevents newborn infection in 80–95% of infants. Theoretical risks for HBV transmission at delivery include exposure to cervical secretions and maternal blood. One study described a lower (9.7%) transmission rate to infants from highly infectious mothers when the infants were delivered by cesarean section than when the delivery was vaginal (24.9%) [13]. Other studies have not shown an effect of mode of delivery on the likelihood of HBV transmission and so routine cesarean section is not recommended.

Intrauterine transmission

Intrauterine HBV infection occurs rarely, in <5% of the infants of HBeAg- and HBsAg-positive mothers. In a study in Taiwan, 16 of the 665 infants born to HBeAg- and HBsAg-positive mothers were seropositive for HBsAg at birth (2.4%), suggesting intrauterine infection [14]. They remained HBsAg positive at beyond 12 months of age.

Maternal HBV DNA load is strongly associated with HBV intrauterine transmission. The possibility of HBV intrauterine HBV infection increases if maternal blood contains HBV DNA $\geq 10^8$ copies/mL. Although threatened abortion and/or threatened preterm labor appeared to increase the risk of HBV transmission in several reports, others failed to confirm this association [15].

Both HBV DNA and HBeAg are detectable in breast milk from HBeAg-positive, HBsAg-positive mothers, with lower levels of HBV in the breast milk than in serum. However, the risk of perinatal transmission does not appear to be increased in breast-fed infants. Breast-feeding is, therefore, permitted for the infants of mothers who are infected with HBV. In the era before the universal HBV vaccination program, a study enrolled 147 infants of HBsAg-positive mothers and follow them for a mean of 11 months [16]. There was no difference in the rates of chronic HBV infection in breast-fed (49% infected) versus bottle-fed (53% infected) children. If the mother has bleeding nipple lesions, caution is suggested if the mother has high levels of viremia.

After immunization with HBV vaccine and/or HBV immunoglobulin (HBIG), there is no additional risk for the transmission of HBV by breast-feeding in infants of infected mothers. The American Academy of Pediatrics has recommended that chronic HBV infection of the mother is not a contraindication to breast-feeding of infants who receive HBIG and HBV vaccine as scheduled [17].

Natural history of hepatitis B virus infection

Infection in children may follow an acute, self-limited course, a fulminant course to hepatic failure with high mortality rate, or may persist for more than 6 months and become a chronic infection. Most infected children remained asymptomatic, and only few presented with acute or fulminant hepatitis. The interaction between virus and host determines the outcome of HBV infection.

Acute infection

Acute HBV infection in children can be either symptomatic or asymptomatic; the latter is more common, particularly in infants and young children. Acute infection runs a self-limited course and recovery is marked by anti-HBs seroconversion. In symptomatic patients, the prodromal symptoms, including general malaise, anorexia, nausea, vomiting, and fever, may persist for several days to weeks. Some patients present with jaundice with or without light-colored stools. Hepatomegaly with right upper quadrant tenderness is common.

An incubation period of 40–180 days is required for virus specific cytotoxic T-lymphocytes to develop against HBV-infected hepatocytes. During this early phase, serum alanine aminotransferase (ALT) levels rise and HBsAg and HBV DNA are detectable. The preicteric phase lasts a few days to as long as a week and is followed by onset of jaundice or dark urine. The icteric phase of acute HBV infection lasts for a variable period, averaging 1–2 weeks, during which viral levels decrease. In convalescence, jaundice resolves but constitutional symptoms may last for weeks or even months. During this phase, HBsAg is cleared followed by the disappearance of detectable HBV DNA from serum.

Patients with acute HBV infection usually recover completely from the liver damage with the development of long-lasting immunity. However, persistent HBV infection may still develop in infants of HBV-carrier mothers after acute infection.

Fulminant Hepatitis B

Acute liver failure occurs in less than 1% of patients with acute HBV infection. The onset of fulminant hepatitis is typically marked by the sudden appearance of fever, abdominal pain, vomiting, and jaundice, followed by disorientation, confusion, and coma. Fulminant hepatitis B is relatively prevalent in infants below 6 months of age, particularly in endemic areas. It typically occurs in infants born to HBeAg-negative, HBsAg-positive mothers. Fulminant hepatitis B can occur as early as 2 months of age. As the diagnosis of hepatic encephalopathy is difficult to establish in infants younger than 1 year, the presence of hepatic encephalopathy is not an absolute requisite for fulminant hepatic failure in this age group [18].

Children with fulminant hepatitis B present with signs of liver failure, including coagulopathy, increasing bilirubin levels with declining aminotransferase levels, and a decreasing liver size, with or without hepatic encephalopathy, within 8 weeks after the initial symptoms of HBV infection. Both HBsAg and HBV DNA levels generally fall rapidly as liver failure develops, and some patients are HBsAg negative by the time of onset of hepatic failure. In this setting, positive titers of anti-HBs or IgM anti-HBc are important markers for diagnosis. The mortality rate for infants with fulminant hepatitis B is high; 67% of affected infants die without liver transplantation [19]. Careful monitoring and management are required for children with acute liver failure caused by HBV; they should be referred rapidly to a tertiary medical center with the availability of liver transplantation.

Precore gene mutations at nucleotide position 1896 can lead to a stop codon for HBeAg, which causes the HBV to cease production of HBeAg. Although precore mutation of HBV has been correlated with fulminant hepatitis B in adults, this could not be demonstrated in children. Precore mutation was found in 36% of children with fulminant hepatitis B and 30% of those with acute hepatitis B in a study in Taiwan [20].

Chronic infection

Chronic HBV infection is defined as persistence of HBsAg for more than 6 months. Young children with chronic HBV infection are usually HBeAg seropositive with high HBV DNA and normal aminotransferase levels. Children may gradually clear HBV DNA and HBeAg with age, and enter the HBeAg seroconversion phase [21]. This usually occurs during adolescence, or when they entered young adulthood.

HBeAg is an important marker during the natural history of chronic HBV infection. It indicates active HBV replication and high infectivity. Seroconversion of HBeAg (to anti-HBe status) is an important event during the natural history of chronic HBV infection. During the process of HBeAg seroconversion, the host immune system clears large amounts of HBV. This is accompanied by liver injury, manifested as a rise of ALT level.

The natural history of chronic HBV infection can be divided into phases according to the status of HBeAg, HBV replication, and liver injury: initial immune tolerance phase (seropositive for e antigen), inflammatory phase (seropositive for e antigen), low replicative phase (after seroconversion for e antigen), and reactivation phase (HBeAg-negative chronic infection) [22] (Table 18.2).

Initial immune tolerance phase

During the early phase of infection, the host is immune tolerant to HBV, highly infectious, with high viral DNA titers and positive HBeAg. The patients are usually asymptomatic, with normal, borderline, or mildly elevated serum ALT. This phase starts from infancy or early childhood, particularly in hyperendemic areas. Despite high levels of HBV DNA and HBeAg, liver damage in this phase is absent or minimal, as a consequence of T-cell immune tolerance to HBeAg and HBcAg. This high replication phase of HBV can persist for years to decades after primary infection.

Inflammatory (immune active) phase

When the host immune system becomes more mature to recognize HBV-related epitopes on hepatocytes, immune-mediated viral clearance and hepatocyte damage begins. This phase, which typically lasts from 2 to 7 years, is characterized by HBeAg positivity, high levels of HBV DNA and serum ALT, and active necroinflammation in the liver [21].

When children enter the inflammatory phase, most of them remain asymptomatic, or with mild non-specific symptoms such as general malaise, or poor appetite. Serum ALT is elevated and peak ALT values may fluctuate from <100 IU/L to >1000 IU/L. Severe and permanent liver damage with bridging hepatic necrosis, which may rarely progress into liver cirrhosis, does occur during childhood. Liver cirrhosis was reported in 10 of 292 (3.4%) Italian HBsAg carrier children with elevated ALT activity who were followed over a long period [23].

The natural course of HBV infection in children varies in different individuals. The HBeAg seroconversion rate is affected by age and maternal HBsAg status. Before 3 years of age, the annual HBeAg seroconversion rate is very low (<2% per year). After age 3, the annual seroconversion rate increases gradually to 3–5% [24]. Children born to HBsAg carrier mothers have a lower HBeAg seroconversion rate, whereas those without maternal HBsAg positivity tend to clear HBeAg earlier.

In patients with perinatal or early childhood infection, transition from the immune tolerance to the immune clearance phase may occur mostly during the second or third decade of life. Serial serum ALT measurements in chronic HBV-infected subjects may predict the occurrence of spontaneous HBeAg seroconversion. In a long-term follow-up study in children with chronic HBV infection, the median remaining time to spontaneous HBeAg seroconversion was observed to be 8.4, 5.1, 4.3, 4.0, and 2.8 years after the serum ALT crossed 20, 30, 40, 60, and 150 IU/L, respectively [25]. The rate of spontaneous HBeAg seroconversion within 6 months when a

subject entered the phase of serum ALT between 60 and 150 IU/L was 5.57 times that of the phase with ALT ≤60 IU/L. The rate of HBeAg seroconversion once serum ALT was >150 IU/L was 9.87 times that of the phase of ALT ≤60 IU/L. It has been suggested that serum ALT >30 IU/L could serve as a cut-off of the inflammatory phase in chronic genotype B and C HBV-infected patients [25].

Low replicative phase

After HBeAg seroconversion, serum ALT gradually returns to normal. The liver histological change in anti-HBe-positive children with chronic HBV infection is usually mild or non-specific if examined beyond 6 months after HBeAg seroconversion. Seroconversion to anti-HBe status indicates reduction of viral replication and is generally considered to be beneficial for the patients with chronic HBV infection. After HBe seroconversion, acute exacerbation with reactivation of HBV and re-elevation of ALT is uncommon in children compared with adults. Most children who undergo HBeAg seroconversion have decreased viral loads, normal serum ALT, and uneventful courses. In a prospective follow-up study of children with chronic HBV infection, only 6 of 140 (4.3%) had elevated serum ALT after HBeAg seroconversion and normalization of serum ALT. However, if severe and permanent liver damage develops during the process of HBeAg seroconversion, early HBeAg seroconversion may not reflect a good prognosis [21]. In 10 of the 72 infants with chronic HBV infection (14%) who HBeAg seroconverted early in life (before 3 years of age), two developed HCC. Each had severe liver damage, with serum ALT elevated to >500 IU/L during infancy or the second year of life, and returned to normal after 2 years of age. Serum ALT remained normal during the later follow-up period but severe liver damage persisted, and HCC developed at 10–15 years of age.

After HBeAg seroconversion, HBV DNA can be detected in sera, usually at $<2 \times 10^3$ IU/mL. In an Italian study, 32 of 37 children with HBeAg seroconversion (87%) had detectable HBV DNA by the polymerase chain reaction at the 5-year follow-up and 21 (58%) had HBV DNA at the 10-year follow-up [26]. Histologically minimal or mild hepatitis may be observed in children after HBeAg seroconversion.

Reactivation phase: e antigen-negative chronic infection

Reactivation of HBV replication and a rise in serum ALT are not common after HBeAg Seroconversion in children; however, permanent liver damage and integration of the HBV genome may develop insidiously and gradually despite clearance of HBeAg. Subsequent development of liver cirrhosis or HCC is rarely observed but does occur during childhood. In general, however, approximately 80% of childhood HCC occurs in children with anti-HBe. In an Italian long-term (29 years) follow-up study, 2% of the horizontally infected children showed progression to hepatocellular carcinoma after HBeAg seroconversion, and 6% had HBeAg-negative hepatitis [27].

Seroconversion for HBeAg is generally considered as a favorable event indicating the cessation of liver necroinflammation, and the beginning of an immune inactive status with low viral replication and minimal liver inflammation. However, HBeAg-negative hepatitis is an important cause of liver injury after HBeAg seroconversion in adults. Liver injury occurs in up to 30% of inactive adult HBV carriers during long-term follow-up without reversion of HBeAg [28]. This phase is characterized by the absence of HBeAg, the presence of anti-HBe, detectable HBV DNA levels ($>10^4$ IU/mL), serum ALT elevations, and histologically continuous necroinflammation of the liver [29]. Most patients progress to this phase after a variable duration of the inactive carrier state, but some directly progress into this phase from the immune clearance phase. The active replication of the HBV precore or basal core promoter mutants that cannot express HBeAg are thought to be the cause of HBeAg-negative chronic hepatitis in the liver observed in these patients.

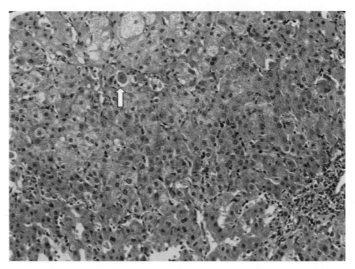

Figure 18.4 Liver biopsy showing histological features of acute hepatitis B infection in a 5-month-old boy, with lobular disarray, focal necrosis with acidophilic bodies (open arrow), and mild portal mononuclear cell infiltrate as the main findings. (Kindly provided by Professor Hey-Chi Hsu.)

Changes of hepatitis B DNA titers during chronic infection in children

Children with chronic HBV infection tends to have high viral titers and normal serum ALT initially. In a study of 58 children with chronic HBV infection and initially normal serum ALT, HBV DNA level was $10^{8.4\pm1.0}$ copies/mL at a mean age of 7 years [30]. Spontaneous HBeAg seroconversion developed during follow-up and HBV DNA decreased to $10^{2.9\pm2.0}$ copies/mL at the end of the 17-year follow-up. As opposed to the more frequent HBeAg-negative hepatitis in adults, young HBeAg seroconverters have a relatively uneventful course after HBeAg seroconversion [30]. Viral loads decrease, mean serum ALT declines to normal, and persistently abnormal serum ALT after HBeAg seroconversion is rarely found.

Spontaneous clearance of hepatitis B surface antigen

Spontaneous loss of serum HBsAg and appearance of its antibody is generally considered to indicate the possibility of HBV eradication. Although the occurrence of spontaneous HBsAg seroconversion generally reflects a favorable event, the significance and mechanism remain to be elucidated, particularly in children. Clearance of HBsAg is a rare event in children with chronic HBV infection; anti-HBs seroconversion is very uncommon. Among children with chronic HBV infection in Taiwan, the annual HBsAg clearance rate is 0.56% [31]. Clearance of HBsAg is particularly uncommon in children of HBsAg carrier mothers. Studies in adults revealed that the probability of HBsAg seroclearance correlated positively with age, the older patients having higher rates of spontaneous HBsAg clearance [32].

Patient outcome following spontaneous HBsAg seroclearance is excellent. Patients with HBsAg seroclearance have favorable biochemical, virological, and histological parameters.

However, HCC may still develop, particularly in patients with cirrhosis who had HBsAg seroclearance at an older age [32].

Liver histologic changes in children with acute or chronic infection

Liver biopsy is rarely performed in patients with acute HBV infection, particularly in children. However, as in adults, the main liver histological findings in children with acute infection include lobular disarray, focal necrosis with acidophilic bodies, and portal mononuclear cell infiltration (Figure 18.4).

Liver histological findings in children with chronic HBV infection in the immune tolerance phase generally reveal minimal or mild histologic changes with or without focal necrosis, reflecting the asymptomatic clinical manifestation and minimal serum ALT elevations. Immunohistochemical studies reveal striking expression patterns of HBV antigens in hepatocytes, with exclusive nuclear expression of HBcAg and homogeneous cytoplasmic expression of HBsAg in isolated hepatocytes, which is in sharp contrast to the frequent clustered expression of HBsAg in adults (Figure 18.5). A liver histologic study was conducted in asymptomatic children aged 4–9 years who had been born to HBeAg-positive HBsAg carrier mothers and who had chronic HBV infection and normal or minimal elevation of serum ALT [33]. Various, but mostly mild, degrees of histological abnormalities in the liver began early in life and could progress to more significant liver damage with time [21].

During the process of HBeAg seroconversion, liver lobular changes develop, with portal inflammation and various degree of fibrosis, with or without piecemeal necrosis [34]. The inflammation is mild to moderate in most occasions. Although uncommon in children, bridging hepatic necrosis may occur during an acute exacerbation [34]. Within 6 months after HBeAg seroconversion, the inflammation is less active and, beyond 6 months, it becomes inactive with mild to minimal inflammation and/or fibrosis in most children.

Liver specimens from a study of 30 children during the anti-HBe-positive stage showed inactive cirrhosis in 2 (including one with HCC), chronic hepatitis with marked fibrosis in 1,

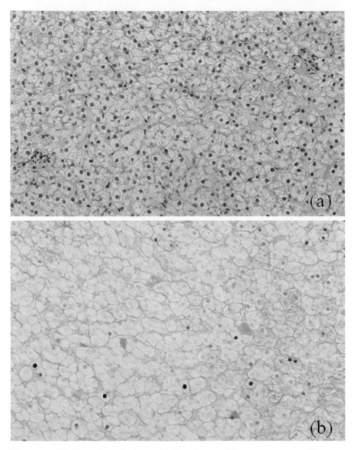

Figure 18.5 Chronic active hepatitis in a 4-year-old asymptomatic girl, perinatally infected and a carrier of hepatitis B surface antigen. (a) Liver histological features, showing minimal focal necrosis. (b) Double immunohistochemical staining reveals exclusive nuclear expression of hepatitis B core antigen (blue) and homogeneous cytoplasmic expression of hepatitis B surface antigen (brown) in isolated hepatocytes. (Kindly provided by Professor Hey-Chi Hsu.)

mild activity and moderate fibrosis in 2, mild activity with mild fibrosis in 9, and minimal histologic changes in the remaining 16 [21].

Factors affecting the natural course of infection

Interactions between virus and the host may determine the natural course of HBV infection in an individual (Table 18.5). Maternal factors may also affect the disease process in children who acquire HBV infection perinatally, leading to high rate of persistent infection. Host and viral factors may also influence the timing of HBeAg seroconversion.

Maternal factors

As mentioned above, children born to HBeAg-positive, HBsAg-positive mothers have higher rates of chronic infection and lower rates of HBeAg seroconversion during long-term follow-up. This might be a result of exposure to transplacental maternal HBeAg in utero, as suggested by the absence of T-cell response to HBcAg in children of HBeAg-positive mothers [12]. In contrast, infants of HBeAg-negative, HBsAg-positive mothers are prone to develop acute hepatitis B followed by recovery, or occasionally fulminant hepatitis [35].

Host factors

Host age

The clinical course and outcome of HBV infection is closely related to the age at infection and duration after chronic infection, as discussed above.

Host immune response

In order to maintain persistent infection in the host, HBV uses two possible mechanisms to influence the host immune system: induction of host immune tolerance and evasion of host immune surveillance with suppression of the host immune response.

After HBV infection in infancy and early childhood, an immune tolerance to HBV is induced, HBeAg being an important toleragen. Transplacental transmission of HBeAg may reduce the immune recognition signals by the infants' immune system and induce the immune tolerance status [12].

Table 18.5 Factors known to affect the clinical course of chronic hepatitis B virus infection[a]

Factors	Viral factors	Host factors
Favorable factors	Undetectable serum HBV DNA	Infection in later life
	Low HBsAg titer/HBsAg loss/HBsAg seroconversion	Horizontal transmission
	HBeAg seroconversion	Genotypes with high serum interleukin-12/ interleukin-10
Unfavorable factors	High HBV DNA titer.	Infection in early childhood
	Persistently positive HBeAg	Maternal transmission (positive maternal HBeAg)
	Genotype C or F	Immunocompromised host

[a] See Table 18.1 for abbreviations.

Subsequently, active production of HBeAg by the infected children may interfere with the cytokine production and function of cytokine, and apoptosis of the cytotoxic T-cells.

Cytokines also play roles in directly inhibiting viral replication and indirectly determining the patterns of the host immune response. Higher levels of serum interleukin-12 (>45 ng/L) and interleukin-10 (>70 ng/L) have been associated with early spontaneous HBeAg seroconversion in children. Variations in host cytokine genes may influence HBeAg seroconversion individually. The interleukin-10 1082G/G and interleukin-12β 10993C/G genotypes help to predict early spontaneous HBeAg seroconversion [36]. Additional determinant host factors need to be examined.

Viral factors

Genotypes and viral titers

Ten different HBVgenotypes (A to J) are distributed in different geographic areas. Chronic infection with each genotype may have a different clinical course and outcome. Genotypes B and C are prevalent in Asia, while genotype A and D are more common in Europe, the middle East, and India. Compared with genotypes A and B, patients with genotypes C and D have lower rates of spontaneous HBeAg seroconversion [37]. A study in children with chronic HBV infection revealed a lower HBeAg seroconversion rate in those with genotype C than with genotype B [38].

A decline in serum HBV DNA reflects a reduction in viral replication. During the natural history of chronic HBV infection, serum HBV DNA may decline to low or undetectable levels, with loss of HBeAg and appearance of anti-HBe. This generally suggests a favorable course with inactive disease [30]. Persistently high levels of serum HBV DNA into later adult life are associated with prolonged liver injury and higher risk of complication, such as liver cirrhosis or HCC [39].

Development of hepatitis B mutations during chronic infection

In order to evade the immune surveillance, HBV may mutate during the natural course of chronic infection. In the later stage of chronic HBV infection, HBV replication is gradually reduced, forming a status of latent infection, to avoid the host immune surveillance. The HBV precore stop codon mutation, basal core promoter mutation, and core gene deletion mutation may influence HBeAg seroconversion in children.

Precore and core promoter mutations

Wild-type HBV is the dominant strain during the long-term course of chronic HBV infection during childhood. An important G1896A mutation of the HBV precore gene may lead to production of a stop codon, which causes failure of HBeAg production. A long-term follow-up of 80 HBV-infected children revealed an increased proportion of the precore stop codon mutation (G1896A) from 10% during the early HBeAg-positive status to approximately 50% after HBeAg seroconversion [40]. Unlike adults, the HBV core promoter nucleotide 1762/1764 mutation does not play a major role in HBeAg seroconversion in children with chronic HBV infection in an age-matched, case–control study [41].

Core gene mutations

Because HBcAg is the target for the cytotoxic T-cell-mediated lysis of HBV infected hepatocytes, it is predisposed to mutate during the chronic infection. Mutations of the core gene may change the conformation of the core protein and allow HBV to escape or modify the immune response via loss or change of immunodominant epitopes. Mutations of the HBV core gene are more frequently seen in children with HCC. The pattern of mutation differs from that in children with chronic HBV infection. Core gene mutations at codons 74, 87, and 159 are frequently seen in HBV-infected children with HCC [42].

Treatment of hepatitis B infection in children

Children with chronic HBV infection may develop active liver inflammation and damage at any age in the presence of variable degrees of serum ALT elevation. Severe liver injury and complications, including bridging hepatic necrosis, cirrhosis, and even liver cancer, although rare, may occur in children [21]. With a long life expectancy, the risk increases over time. Whenever an ideal antiviral agent is available, treatment should be given as early as possible to eliminate the virus and prevent liver damage during chronic infection. Unfortunately, current antiviral regimens are far from effective in eradicating HBV, particularly in children with immune tolerance.

Most children with chronic HBV infection are in an immune tolerant status with high viral load and normal serum ALT. Children with normal serum ALT do not respond well to current antiviral therapy. Suppression of viral replication and prevention of active liver damage and related consequences is more feasible in children who have active viral replication and elevated serum ALT. Currently available antiviral agents are listed in Table 18.6.

The aims of antiviral therapy for chronic hepatitis B are to achieve (1) effective inhibition of viral replication, (2) reduction of liver inflammation and injury, (3) HBeAg seroconversion, and (4) prevention of liver complications, such as cirrhosis and HCC.

Indications for antiviral therapy

Children 2–17 years of age who have been HBsAg seropositive for more than 6 months, with elevated serum ALT and HBV DNA for more than 3 months may be candidates for antiviral therapy (Figure 18.6). Patients who are HBeAg seropositive with HBV DNA $>1.5 \times 10^4$ IU/mL (approximately 10^5 copies/mL), and ALT $>1.5\times$ upper limit of normal (ULN) may be considered for treatment [43]. Before entering into treatment, exclusion for other causes of abnormal serum ALT should be conducted. Patients seronegative for HBeAg but with ALT $>1.5\times$ ULN and HBV DNA $>1.5 \times 10^3$ IU/mL (10^4 copies/mL) may also be considered for treatment.

Table 18.6 Drugs for the treatment of chronic hepatitis B virus infection

Drug Approved for	Interferon-alfa	Nucleoside/nucleotide analogues
Approved for[a]		
Adults	Interferon-alfa, peginterferon-alfa	Lamivudine, adefovir dipivoxil, entecavir, telbivudine, tenofovir, disoproxil fumarate
12–17 years	–	
Children	Interferon-alfa	Lamivudine
Advantages	Finite duration, absence of resistance, higher clearance of hepatitis B surface antigen	Oral administration, no prominent adverse effects, faster decline in HBV DNA
Disadvantages	Injection pain, more adverse effects, not indicated in liver decompensation	Indefinite duration, risk of resistance

[a] Approved by the US Food and Drug Administration up to the end of 2011.

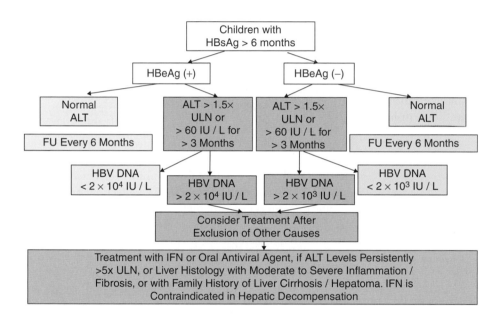

Figure 18.6 Flow chart of recommended management for children with chronic hepatitis B virus (HBV) infection. ALT, alanine aminotransferase; HbeAg, HBV e antigen; HBsAg, HBV surface antigen; IFN, interferon; FU, follow-up; ULN, upper limit of normal.

Early treatment can be considered for children with persistently abnormal ALT >5× ULN, with liver histology which reveals moderate to severe liver inflammation and/or fibrosis, or with a positive family history of liver cirrhosis or HCC.

Outside of clinical trials, interferon is the agent of choice in most cases. Growth and thyroid status should be carefully monitored. Nucleoside/nucleotide analogues can also be used in children, and development of resistance and clinical breakthrough hepatitis should be carefully monitored. Either interferon-alfa or nucleoside/nucleotide analogues (oral antiviral agents) can be considered for treatment in those without hepatic decompensation [43]. For children with positive serum HBeAg and normal serum ALT (i.e. in an immune tolerance status), there is no established benefit and thus no indication to use currently available treatment. There is also no indication

for treating children in the inactive status with negative HBeAg and normal serum ALT.

A period of 3–6 months observation is recommended before the start of therapy. However, if evidence of impending hepatic decompensation is present, therapy should be initiated as early as possible. Nucleoside/nucleotide analogues should be used, while interferon is contraindicated in patients with hepatic decompensation. Patients should be monitored carefully via serum bilirubin levels and prothrombin time.

Currently approved therapy for hepatitis B in children

Currently there are at least five oral antiviral agents and two interferons approved by US Food and Drug Administration for the treatment of adults with HBV infection. However, only conventional interferon-alfa and lamivudine are approved for use in children with hepatitis B. Adefovir dipivoxil is also approved to be used but limited to children and adolescents older than 12 years (Table 18.6).

Interferons

The advantages of interferon therapy are the well-defined treatment duration and low likelihood of emergence of resistant strains. For children, pain after injection and transient growth suppression are the main concerns during therapy. Other side effects of interferon therapy, such as fever, general malaise, leukopenia, depression, or hair loss, are less remarkable in children than adults [44].

Conventional interferon-alfa

Evidence for the efficacy of interferon therapy in children with chronic HBV is limited by the small number of children enrolled in most reported and largely uncontrolled studies. Interferon-alfa monotherapy is not effective for the induction of HBeAg seroconversion in children with normal levels of liver enzymes. In those with elevated serum ALT, the results of interferon treatment are similar to those in adults, with a higher rate of HBeAg seroconversion and normalization of serum aminotransferases in the treatment group than in the control group [44–47].

Factors that are predictive for a positive response to interferon include high pretreatment serum ALT, low pretreatment serum HBV DNA, late acquisition of HBV infection, and in the presence of hepatocellular necroinflammation. The recommended dose of conventional interferon-alfa for children with HBV infection is 0.1×10^6 U/kg (0.1 MU/kg) or $3–6\,mU/m^2$ three times a week for 6 months. Some studies in a small number of children, using higher doses, $6–10\,MU/m^2$ or longer duration, have shown a higher rate of sustained responses but also a higher rate of adverse effects [44].

A meta-analysis reported 126 treated children and 113 control children with chronic HBV infection treated with conventional interferon-alfa therapy. Clearance rate for HBeAg was 23% in the treated group and 11% in the control group [27]. Another multinational study of interferon-alfa therapy revealed an HBeAg seroconversion rate of 26% in the 70 treated children and 11% in the control group [45]. Long-term follow-up in treated and control children revealed similar HBeAg clearance rates: 60% in treated patients versus 65% in controls. The rate of HBsAg loss was 25% in the interferon responders versus 0% in controls [46,47].

Pegylated interferon-alfa

Pegylated interferon-alfa is a long-acting interferon successfully used in the treatment of chronic hepatitis C infection; it has also been used in treating HBV infection in adults. The reduced frequency of injection (once per week) has advantage over conventional interferon-alfa (three times per week), particularly in children. The safety and efficacy have been reported in studies of children with hepatitis C infection [48], but not in children with HBV.

Nucleoside/nucleotide analogues

Lamivudine

Lamivudine is a nucleoside analogue that can be used orally; it is well absorbed from the gastrointestinal tract and has a mean absolute bioavailability of 80% in adults and 68% in infants and children. The recommended daily dosage for children is 3 mg/kg, up to a maximal dose of 100 mg/day. The advantages are the convenient oral administration and the absence of prominent side effects. The main disadvantages are the high emergence rate of resistant strains and the unclear duration of treatment (Table 18.6). The efficacy of 52 weeks of lamivudine therapy was evaluated in 286 children in a multicentered placebo-controlled study [49]. At the end of therapy, a complete virologic response (evidenced by HBeAg clearance and negative HBV DNA) was achieved in 23% of the treatment group and 13% of the placebo group. The ALT normalization rate was 55% in the treatment group and 12% in the placebo group. However, only 2% in the treatment group and none in the control group lost HBsAg [49]. Higher pretreatment serum ALT and liver histological necroinflammation scores, and lower serum HBV DNA levels, predict a better treatment response.

Mutations of the HBV genome may develop to escape drug effects during therapy with nucleoside analogues but not with interferon. Mutations affecting HBV polymerase, at the reverse transcriptase (rt) region, may develop after use of lamivudine for more than 9 months. The mutations most frequently found are methionine to valine or methionine to isoleucine at the rt nucleotide 204, altering the tyrosine–methionine–aspartate–aspartate (YMDD) motif. The second common site of mutagenesis is at rt nucleotide 180, leading to a leucine to methionine substitution. In a multicenter study at week 52 after therapy, YMDD mutants were detected in 19% of patients in the lamivudine group but none in the placebo group [50]. The pretreatment serum HBV DNA tended to be higher in the patients in whom the YMDD variant was present at 52 weeks. Hepatic decompensation may occur after the emergence of the YMDD mutant.

The incidence of YMDD mutants in children at month 24 after lamivudine therapy was 49%, and rose to 64% after lamivudine therapy for 36 months [50]. Prolonged use of lamivudine did not benefit the children who did not achieve full virologic response and ALT normalization after 1 year of therapy. In total, 30% of the children achieved virologic response after 24 months of lamivudine therapy, but only 21% of children had virologic response after 36 months of lamivudine therapy. This paradoxical finding reflects the high emergence rate of lamivudine-resistant strains of HBV after prolonged therapy.

Long-term use of lamivudine after the emergence of the YMDD motif mutant may lead to an acute exacerbation.

Careful monitoring of the serum HBV DNA titer and for signs of clinical or biochemical deterioration of liver function is mandatory in children infected with mutant strains. Discontinuation of lamivudine is recommended if a biochemical exacerbation develops during therapy. Because there is no other currently approved antiviral therapy for children younger than 12 years of age other than conventional interferon-alfa, adding on or shifting to another nucleoside/nucleotide analogue is not plausible. While interferon-alfa is not suitable for those with hepatic decompensation, other effective therapy is needed for children with severe exacerbation and risk of decompensation during or after lamivudine therapy.

Adefovir dipivoxil

Adefovir dipivoxil is effective in inhibiting the replication of the YMDD motif mutants and can be used in patients with acute exacerbation of hepatic necroinflammation during lamivudine therapy. The viral suppressive effect of adefovir is less and slower than lamivudine. A median HBV DNA reduction of 3.6–4.6 $\log_{10}$ copies/mL and ALT normalization in 31–53% were observed after 1 year of therapy. Adefovir showed significant antiviral efficacy in subjects aged 12 to 17 years with HBeAg-positive chronic HBV infection but did not differ from placebo in subjects aged 2 to 11 years [51].

Entecavir

Several oral antiviral agents that have been approved for the treatment of HBV infection in adults, such as entecavir, telbivudine, or tenofovir disoproxil, are still under clinical trial and not yet approved for use in children. Entecavir is a potent and highly selective inhibitor of HBV DNA polymerase. In adults with HBeAg-positive chronic HBV infection, the rates of histologic, virologic, and biochemical improvement are significantly higher with entecavir than with lamivudine. The safety profile of the two agents is similar, and the rate of viral resistance to entecavir is much lower [52].

For adults who had HBeAg-negative chronic HBV infection and had not been previously treated with a nucleoside analogue, the rates of histological improvement, virological response, and normalization of serum ALT were significantly higher at 48 weeks with entecavir than with lamivudine [53]. Seroconversion to HBeAg after entecavir therapy occurred in 21% of the treated patients.

Long-term monitoring studies have shown low rates of resistance in nucleoside-naive patients during 5 years of entecavir, corresponding with potent viral suppression and a high genetic barrier to resistance. After 5 years of entecavir therapy in lamivudine-naive adults, low rates of viral genotypic resistance (1.2%) and virologic breakthrough (0.8%) to entecavir were detected [54]. Entecavir is superior to lamivudine in reducing serum HBV DNA in both HBeAg-positive (6.9 versus 5.4 $\log_{10}$ copies/mL) and negative adults (5.0 versus 4.5 $\log_{10}$ copies/mL), leading to much lower rate of inducing resistance strains [52,53]. These findings support entecavir as a primary therapy that enables prolonged treatment with potent viral suppression and minimal resistance [54].

Telbivudine

Telbivudine (β-l-2′-deoxythymidine) is an orally bioavailable nucleoside with potent and specific anti-HBV activity. It is shown to be more potent than lamivudine. Telbivudine has reduced wild-type HBV DNA by 5–8 $\log_{10}$ copies/mL. In both HBeAg-negative and HBeAg-positive patients, telbivudine demonstrated greater HBV DNA suppression with less resistance than lamivudine [55]. The cumulative rate of telbivudine-resistant mutations was 4.8%, 17.6%, and 34.0% for years 1, 2, and 3, respectively [56].

Tenofovir disoproxil fumarate

Tenofovir disoproxil fumarate (TDF) is a nucleotide analogue that is a potent inhibitor of HBV polymerase. In two double-blind phase III studies among adults with chronic HBV infection at week 48 of treatment, TDF had superior antiviral efficacy of viral suppression and normalization of serum ALT, with a similar safety profile to that of adefovir dipivoxil through week 48 [57]. For up to 3 years, TDF maintained a favorable safety profile and was effective in the long-term management of HBeAg-positive and HBeAg-negative adults with chronic HBV infection. Amino acid substitutions in HBV DNA polymerase that are associated with resistance to TDF were not detected in any patient. Cumulatively, 8% of HBeAg-positive patients lost HBsAg [58]. TDF has recently been approved for use in children 12–17 years of age.

Combination therapy

Combination therapies using different doses and time schedules of interferon-alfa and lamivudine have been used in pediatric studies with small number of patients and controversial results. Simultaneous use of lamivudine and interferon-alfa2a yielded a higher response and earlier anti-HBe seroconversion and viral clearance than consecutive combined therapy [59]. Further studies are needed to clarify whether the effect of combination therapy is superior to monotherapy in children.

Prevention of hepatitis B infection and its complications

Although there are several antiviral drugs to treat chronic HBV infection, it is very difficult to eradicate the infection in most patients. Prevention is the best way to control HBV infection and its complications. Among the various strategies of prevention, immunoprophylaxis is the most cost-effective way to achieve global control of HBV infection and related complications. The most important strategy has been the universal immunization program in infancy starting from the first day of life to prevent both perinatal and horizontal transmissions of HBV infection. Passive immunization using HBIG provides temporary immunity with high cost, while active immunization using vaccines provides long-term immunity and protection with much lower expense. Screening of blood products, use of disposable needles and syringes, and avoidance of unsterile instruments and utensils, which may contact blood or body fluid, are also recommended.

Active and passive immunization and the universal hepatitis B vaccination program

Prevention of mother-to-infant transmission of HBV is important because it is the main route of transmission leading to persistent HBV infection. The major preventive measures are passive immunization with HBIG and active immunization with HBV vaccines. The former contains high titers of antibody to HBsAg and provides passive protection for 3–6 months if given immediately after exposure to HBV. The principal indications for HBIG are postexposure prophylaxis, including infants of HBV carrier mothers, and patients receiving liver transplantation to prevent recurrent HBV infection.

Combined passive and active immunization with HBIG and HBV vaccine at birth has been demonstrated to reduce the risk of transmission from 70–90% to <10% among infants of HBsAg-positive, HBeAg-positive mothers [60].

Current programs for universal hepatitis B vaccination in infancy

Different vaccination schedules have been used in different countries based on their basic epidemiologic features of HBV infection and HCC, and the resources of the supporting health systems. Current programs for universal HBV vaccination in infancy can be divided into three main strategies depending on both the local epidemiologic conditions (i.e. high or low prevalence rate of HBsAg carriage in children) and the budget of the government for HBV immunization: (1) combined passive and active immunization with maternal screening for HBsAg and HBeAg, (2) combined passive and active immunization with maternal screening of HBsAg, and (3) active immunization without maternal screening of viral markers.

Combined passive and active immunization with maternal screening for hepatitis B surface and e antigens

In addition to active immunization with HBV vaccines, passive immunization with HBIG can neutralize HBV transmitted from the mother during the perinatal period. This must be given within 24 hours after birth. The first universal HBV vaccination program was launched in July 1984 in Taiwan [61]. Pregnant women were screened for HBsAg and HBeAg. All infants received four doses (0, 1, 2, 12 months of age) of plasma-derived HBV vaccine (before 1992), or three doses (0, 1, 6 months of age) of recombinant HBV vaccine (after 1992). In addition, infants of high-risk mothers with positive HBeAg and HBsAg received 0.5 mL HBIG within 24 hours after birth. The expense of all the vaccines and HBIG given to the infants was covered by the government. The coverage rate of the three-dose HBV vaccination for neonates was >95%.

Passive and active immunization with maternal screening of hepatitis B surface antigen

In some countries with adequate resources, pregnant women are screened for HBsAg but not HBeAg. All infants are recommended to receive three doses of HBV vaccines. In addition, all infants born to HBsAg-positive mothers, regardless of the HBeAg status, receive 0.5 mL HBIG within 12–24 hours of birth. This strategy saves the cost of maternal HBeAg screening but increases the cost of HBIG, which is much more costly than vaccine. The first dose of HBV vaccine is given before hospital discharge, the second is at age 1 or 2 months, and the final dose not earlier than age 24 weeks. If the maternal HBsAg status is not known, HBV vaccine is given to the newborns within 12 hours of birth and the HBsAg status of mother is determined as soon as possible. If her HBsAg is positive, HBIG is given to the infant. These infants born to HBsAg-positive mothers are recommended to be tested for anti-HBs and HBsAg at 9 to 15 months of age to determine their status.

Active immunization without maternal screening of viral markers

In areas where HBV infection prevalence is low or financial resources are limited, immunization with three doses of HBV vaccine (at 0, 1, 6 months), without antenatal screening of the mothers or administration of HBIG, is a reasonable strategy to reduce cost. Such programs have been shown to be successful in Thailand and many other countries in Asia.

World Health Organization recommendation program

In 1990, the World Health Organization recommended universal HBV immunization for all neonates in all nations. It also established the objective of reducing the incidence of new HBV carriers among children by 80% by 2001. The coverage rate with the three-dose HBV vaccines increased from 32% in 2000 to 65% in 2007. Up to 2009, a total of approximately 177 countries have followed this recommendation with a coverage rate of >80% for three doses of HBV vaccine. Some low-prevalence countries have not yet incorporated universal HBV vaccination. Universal HBV immunization programs have reduced the rate of HBV infection worldwide.

The effect of universal hepatitis B immunization on the control of liver diseases and hepatocellular carcinoma

Effective prevention of infection

A universal HBV vaccination program was begun in Italy in 1991; population surveys in 1994–1995 showed a significant decline in HBV prevalence and a 50% reduction in acute HBV infection incidence [62]. After the 1991 recommendation for universal HBV vaccination in the USA, the incidence of acute HBV infection among children in all ethnic groups declined to 1.6 per 100 000 in 2006, which represents a decline of 81% since 1990 [63]. The prevalence of chronic HBV infection in children has been reduced worldwide in areas where universal

HBV vaccination has been introduced. Generally speaking, after the universal HBV vaccination program, the HBsAg-seropositive rates were reduced to approximately one-tenth of the prevaccination rates.

Taiwan has the longest experience with universal HBV immunization in the world. Twenty years after the launch of universal HBV vaccination program, the HBsAg carrier rate decreased significantly from approximately 10% before the vaccination program to <1% in vaccinated children younger than 20 years of age [64]. The total infection rate (acute and chronic infection) was also decreased, even in those who were not vaccinated during infancy. Anti-HBc seropositivity declined from 38% to 16%, and to 4.6% in children, 15 to 20 years after the program. This universal vaccination program has transformed Taiwan from a high-endemic country to a low-endemic country.

Because of high HBV endemicity, Gambia was the first country in Africa to implement a mass HBV immunization program in infants in 1990. They demonstrated a reduced HBV burden in children, with a dramatic decrease in HBsAg prevalence from 10.0% to 0.6% [65].

Reduction of mortality from fulminant hepatitis B

Infection with HBV is the most important cause of fulminant hepatitis in children in areas endemic for HBV. Infants are particularly susceptible to fulminant hepatitis B if the mother is HBeAg seronegative but positive for HBsAg.

After the universal vaccination program in Taiwan, HBV was rarely the cause of fulminant hepatitis in children older than 1 year. In spite of the reduction in the incidence of HBV infection, HBV remains a major cause of fulminant hepatitis in infants in Asia. These infants are most likely perinatally infected from their HBeAg-negative HBsAg-positive mothers despite vaccination. The mortality rate of fulminant hepatitis in infants during 1974–1984 was 5.36 per 100 000 in Taiwan. This was reduced to 1.71 per 100 000 during 1985–1998 after the launch of the HBV vaccination program ($p < 0.001$) [66].

Reduction of hepatocellular carcinoma after the universal vaccination program

Occurrence of HCC in children is closely related to HBV infection. Current therapies for HCC are far from satisfactory. The reduction in HBV infection after the launch of universal HBV vaccination program in Taiwan was also associated with a dramatic reduction of the incidence of HCC in children. The annual incidence of HCC in children aged 6 to 14 years was reduced to one-quarter from 0.52 per 100 000 children born before the launch of universal HBV vaccination program (July 1984) to 0.13 per 100 000 children born after the program [67].

The risk of the development of HCC in the vaccinated cohorts was significantly associated with incomplete HBV vaccination, and prenatal maternal HBsAg or HBeAg seropositivity. The prevention effect for HCC by HBV vaccine extends from childhood to adolescents [68]. Failure to prevent

HCC results mostly from unsuccessful control of HBV infection transmitted by highly infectious mothers.

Long-term immunogenicity and the need for booster doses of vaccine

Long-term serial seroepidemiologic and immunologic studies of vaccinated children have provided evidence to support that universal HBV vaccination in infancy provides adequate long-term protection at least up to 20 years of age [64]. Although the vaccine remained highly efficacious in reducing the HBsAg positivity, approximately 50% of children exhibited waning humoral immunity (anti-HBs <10 mIU/mL). It is estimated that 2–10% of the vaccinated population had lost their HBV vaccine-conferred booster response. This poses the potential risk of breakthrough infection. However, the absence of an increase in HBsAg-seropositive subjects at different ages in the same birth cohort after the vaccination program strongly suggests that there is no actual increased risk of HBV infection with age.

The follow-up data from universal vaccination programs from many countries indicates that there is no scientific basis for the administration of booster doses of HBV vaccine to fully immunized individuals.

For special high-risk groups, such as liver transplant recipients, it is recommended that the serum anti-HBs level be kept in a higher titer before transplantation [69]. In the absence of adequate prophylaxis, the incidence of de novo HBV infection in pediatric orthotopic liver transplantation recipients was reported to be 15% in endemic area. An anti-HBs titer of >200 mIU/mL before transplantation may be sufficient to prevent de novo HBV infection in HBsAg-negative recipients [69].

Problems of current immunization program and strategies for a successful control of hepatitis B infection

Primary prevention by universal vaccination is the most cost-effective strategy for successful control of HBV infection and its complications. Yet several problems remain to be solved. There may be "vaccine failures." The causes of "breakthrough infection" or non-response include high maternal viral titer, intrauterine infection, mutated HBV surface proteins, poor compliance, genetic hyporesponsiveness, and immunocompromised status. Infants of HBsAg carrier mothers who are HBeAg positive and/or have a high viral load are the high-risk group for breakthrough HBV infection, in spite of immuno-prophylaxis with combination of passive (HBIG) and active (vaccine) immunization.

The rate of mutations of HBsAg occurring in HBsAg carriers born after the HBV vaccination program is increasing with time, from 7.8% before the vaccination program to 28.1% 15 years after the launch of the program [70]. The prevalence of HBV surface gene *a* determinant mutants in HBV

DNA-seropositive children with positive HBsAg or anti-HBc was higher in fully vaccinated than in unvaccinated children. Fortunately, the rate has remained unchanged (22.6%) at 20 years after initiation of the vaccination program. An HBV vaccine effective against mutant surface proteins is not urgently needed for routine HBV immunization at present, but careful and continuous monitoring for these mutants is needed.

The most important strategies of primary prevention for better control of HBV infection globally include further increasing the world coverage rates of HBV vaccines, and better methods to prevent breakthrough infection/non-responsiveness. It is important to find ways to reduce the cost of HBV vaccines and to increase funding for HBV vaccination of children living in developing countries endemic for HBV infection. It is particularly urgent in areas where HBV infection and HCC are prevalent.

Efforts to further increase the coverage rates of HBV vaccines worldwide should be made. It is important to persuade and support the policy makers of the countries that have not instituted a universal HBV vaccination program and to encourage countries which already have a program to increase the coverage rates. Further investigation into the mechanisms of breakthrough HBV infection or non-response is needed. Interventions to prevent intrauterine infection, the development of HBV vaccines against mutant surface antigens, and better vaccines for immunocompromised individuals may further reduce the incidence of new HBV infections.

Hepatitis D
Virology

Hepatitis delta virus, with a 1.7 kb single-stranded circular RNA genome, is a small defective RNA virus (Figure 18.7). It requires the help of HBV for its replication and infection and it can only infect individuals who have active HBV infection. The virion is composed of a coat of HBV envelope proteins surrounding the nucleocapsid complexed with delta antigen (HDAg), the viral protein. This HDAg has two forms, small (S) and large (L). Infection can occur either simultaneously with HBV infection (coinfection) or in chronic carriers of HBsAg (superinfection). Exacerbation of HBV infection is more frequently seen in children superinfected with HDV.

Epidemiology and route of transmission

Worldwide, more than 15 million people are coinfected with HBV and HDV. There are eight reported genotypes of HDV, with unexplained variations in their geographical distribution and pathogenicity. Prevalence is high in areas of sub-Saharan Africa, eastern Europe, the Middle East, central Asia, the South Pacific islands, the Amazon basin, and the Mediterranean basin. Hepatitis D infection is relatively prevalent in Italy. The prevalence of HDV is declining in some endemic areas but increasing in northern and central Europe, perhaps because of immigration patterns.

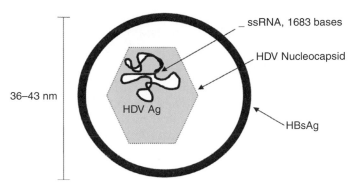

Figure 18.7 The genomic structure of delta hepatitis virus (HDV). Inside the hepatitis B virus surface envelope, there is a 19 nm HDV nucleocapsid, which contains about 60 copies of HDV antigen in its two forms (S and L) and HDV genomic single-stranded, circular RNA (ssRNA). (Centers for Disease Control and Prevention [71].)

Use of injection drug, invasive medical procedures, and promiscuous sexual activity are important risk factors for HDV infection. Perinatal transmission of HDV is uncommon.

Pathogenesis and clinical presentation

The pathogenesis of HDV infection and outcome remains unclear. HDAg is not directly cytotoxic in human hepatocytes. In the chronic phase of HDV infection, viral titer of HDV and HBV fluctuates according to the stage of viral infection.

The range of clinical presentation of HDV infection is wide, varying from mild disease to fulminant liver failure. Infection with HDV is clinically important because although it suppresses HBV replication, the presence of HDV in patients who have chronic HBV disease leads to a more rapid progression to cirrhosis, and increases the risk for HCC. There is a higher risk of liver decompensation and mortality in patients with HBV-related cirrhosis [72,73].

Twenty-three children, aged 3 to 15 years, with chronic HDV infection have been followed for 5 to 12 years to evaluate long-term outcome [74]. Although 19 (83%) had chronic hepatitis when first seen, with cirrhosis in 6 (26%), the clinical and biochemical features of the disease remained stable during observation; liver histologic findings, obtained in 14 patients, worsened in only two [74].

Prevention

After the introduction of universal HBV vaccination program in Italy, the incidence of acute HDV infection has markedly decreased. After a peak incidence of acute HDV infection in 1993 (2.8 cases per million population), the incidence decreased from 1.7 to 0.5 cases per million population during 1994 to 2004 [75]. The decrease in incidence of HDV coinfection particularly affected young adults, and it paralleled the decrease in incidence of acute HBV infection.

Efforts to increase HBV vaccine coverage in high-risk groups and to implement the safety of invasive procedures performed both inside and outside healthcare facilities are needed to control HDV infection [75].

Treatment of hepatitis D infection

Treatment of HDV is with interferon-alfa or pegylated interferon-alfa. The aims are to clear both HBV and HDV. However, interferon-alfa treatment in children with chronic HDV hepatitis has only a transient effect, and long-term treatment does not appear to induce a greater therapeutic benefit in terms of biochemical and virological response. In one study, 26 children received interferon-alfa2b $5 \, MU/m^2$ then $3 \, MU/m^2$ three times weekly for 12 (medium-term group) or 24 months (long-term group) [76]. At the end of therapy, a complete biochemical response (normalization of ALT) occurred in 12 children (5/13 in the medium-term group and 7/13 in the long-term group). Relapse occurred after stopping interferon in 10 (five in each group). No significant improvement in liver histology was seen in either group [76].

Conclusions and future prospects

Infection with HBV in infancy and early childhood leads to a high rate of persistent infection. Understanding the risk factors of perinatal transmission and the natural history of HBV infection are crucial for the better control of HBV infection.

Prevention is the most cost-effective strategy to successfully control HBV and HDV infections and their complications. Immunization for HBV has provided direct evidence to prove the oncogenic role of HBV for liver cancer. The HBV vaccine was the first example of a cancer- prevention vaccine in humans and supplies proof of principle that prevention of a virus infection may prevent its related cancer in humans.

For children with HBV infection who have not been protected by HBV immunization, antiviral therapy is needed. Better antiviral therapies are needed with high efficacy, low incidence of side effects, shorter duration of therapy, low rate of drug resistance, and durable effect.

Increased understanding of the molecular virology of HDV will be helpful to develop novel therapeutic targets are developed for this severe form of chronic viral hepatitis.

Acknowledgements

The author thanks Professor William F Balistreri for editing the manuscript, and Professor Hey-Chi Hsu, Department of Pathology, College of Medicine, National Taiwan University, for provision of Figures 18.4 and 18.5 and for expert editing of this manuscript. The author also would like to thank Dr. Hui-Hui Chua for drawing Figure 18.2.

References

1. Ganem D, Prince AM. Hepatitis B virus infection natural history and clinical consequences. *N Engl J Med* 2004;**350**:1118–1129.

2. Hsu HY, Chang MH, Chen DS, *et al.* Baseline seroepidemiology of hepatitis B virus infection in children in Taipei, 1984: a study just before mass hepatitis B vaccination program in Taiwan. *J Med Virol* 1986;**18**:301–307.

3. Nassal M. Hepatitis B viruses: Reverse transcription a different way. *Virus Research* 2008;**134**:235–249.

4. Murray JM, Purcell R, Wieland SF. The half life of hepatitis B virions. *Hepatology* 2006;**44**:1117–1121.

5. Balistreri WF. Viral hepatitis. *Emerg Clin North Am* 1991;**9**:365–399.

6. Hoofnagle JH, DiBisceglie AM. Serologic diagnosis of acute and chronic viral hepatitis. *Semin Liver Dis* 1991;**11**:73–83.

7. Andersson KL, Raymond T, Chung RT. Monitoring during and after antiviral therapy for hepatitis B. *Hepatology* 2009;**49**:S166–S173.

8. McQuillan GM, Coleman PJ, Kruszon-Moran D, *et al.* Prevalence of hepatitis B virus infection in the United States: the National Health and Nutrition Examination Surveys, 1976 through 1994. *Am J Public Health* 1999; **89**:14–18.

9. Custer B, Sullivan SD, Hazlet TK, *et al.* Global epidemiology of hepatitis B virus. *J Clin Gastroenterol* 2004;**38**: S158–S168.

10. Feret E, Larouze B, Diop B, *et al.* Epidemiology of hepatitis B virus infection in the rural community of Tip, Senegal. *Am J Epidemiol* 1987;**125**:140–149.

11. Beasley RP. Rocks along the road to the control of HBV and HCC. *Ann Epidemiol* 2009;**19**:231–234.

12. Hsu HY, Chang MH, Hsieh KH, *et al.* Cellular immune response to hepatitis B core antigen in maternal infant transmission of hepatitis B virus. *Hepatology* 1992;**15**:770–776.

13. Lee SD, Lo KJ, Tsai YT, *et al.* Role of caesarian section in the prevention of mother-to-infant transmission of the hepatitis B virus. *Lancet* 1988;**ii**:833–834.

14. Tang JR, Hsu HY, Lin HH, *et al.* Hepatitis B surface antigenemia at birth: a long-term follow-up study. *J Pediatr* 1998;**133**:374–377.

15. Li XM, Shi MF, Yang YB, *et al.* Effect of hepatitis B immunoglobulin on interruption of HBV intrauterine infection. *World J Gastroenterol* 2004;**10**:3215–3217.

16. Beasley RP, Stevens CE, Shiao IS, Meng HC. Evidence against breast-feeding as a mechanism for vertical transmission of hepatitis B. *Lancet* 1975;**2**:740–741.

17. Gartner LM, Morton J, Lawrence RA, *et al.* Breastfeeding and the use of human milk. *Pediatrics* 2005; **115**:496–506.

18. Bhaduri BR, Mieli-Vergani G. Fulminant hepatic failure: pediatric aspects. *Semin Liver Dis* 1996;**16**: 349–355.

19. Chang MH, Lee CY, Chen DS, Hsu HC, Lai MY. Fulminant hepatitis in children in Taiwan: the important role of hepatitis B virus. *J Pediatr* 1987;**111**: 34–39.

20. Hsu HY, Chang MH, Lee CY, *et al.* Precore mutant of hepatitis B virus in childhood fulminant hepatitis B: an infrequent association. *J Infect Dis* 1995;**171**:776–781.

21. Chang MH, Hsu HY, Hsu HC, *et al.* The significance of spontaneous HBeAg seroconversion in childhood: with

special emphasis on the clearance of HBeAg before three years of age. *Hepatology* 1995;**22**:1387–1392.

22. Chu CM, Karayiannis P, Fowler MJ, *et al.* Natural history of chronic hepatitis B virus infection in Taiwan: studies of hepatitis B virus DNA in serum. *Hepatology* 1985;**5**: 431–434.

23. Bortolotti F, Cadrobbi M, Crivellaro C, *et al.* Long-term outcome of chronic type B hepatitis in patients who acquire hepatitis B virus in infection in childhood. *Gastroenterology* 1990;**99**:805–810.

24. Chang MH, Sung JL, Lee CY, *et al.* Factors affecting the clearance of hepatitis B e antigen in hepatitis B surface antigen carrier children. *J Pediatr* 1989;**115**:385–390.

25. Wu JF, Su YR, Chen CH, *et al.* Predictive effect of serial serum alanine aminotransferase levels on spontaneous HBeAg seroconversion in chronic genotype B and C HBV-infected children. *J Pediatr Gastroenterol Nutr* 2012;**54**:97–100.

26. Bortolotti F, Guido M, Bartolacci S, *et al.* Chronic hepatitis B in children after e antigen seroclearance: final report of a 29-year longitudinal study. *Hepatology* 2006;**43**:556–562.

27. Bortolotti F, Wirth S, Crivellaro C, *et al.* Long-term persistence of hepatitis B virus DNA in the serum of children with chronic hepatitis B after hepatitis B e antigen to antibody seroconversion. *J Pediatr Gastroenterol Nutr* 1996;**22**:270–274.

28. Chu CM, Liaw YF. Spontaneous relapse of hepatitis in inactive HBsAg carriers. *Hep Intl* 2007;**1**:311–315.

29. Liaw YF. Natural history of chronic hepatitis B virus infection and long-term outcome under treatment. *Liver International* 2009;**29**(s1):100–107.

30. Ni YH, Chang MH, Chen PJ, *et al.* Viremia profiles in children with chronic hepatitis B virus infection and spontaneous e antigen seroconversion. *Gastroenterology* 2007;**132**:2340–2345.

31. Hsu HY, Chang MH, Lee CY, *et al.* Spontaneous loss of HBsAg in children with chronic hepatitis B virus infection. *Hepatology* 1992;**15**:382–386.

32. Chu CM, Liaw YF. HBsAg seroclearance in asymptomatic carriers of high endemic areas: appreciably high

rates during a long-term follow-up. *Hepatology* 2007;**45**:1187–1192.

33. Chang MH, Hwang LY, Hsu HC, Lee CY, Beasley RP. Prospective study of asymptomatic HBsAg carrier children infected in the perinatal period: clinical and liver histologic studies. *Hepatology* 1988;**8**:374–377.

34. Hsu HC, Lin YH, Chang MH, *et al.* Pathology of chronic hepatitis B virus infection in children: with special reference to the intrahepatic expression of hepatitis B virus antigens. *Hepatology* 1988;**8**:378–382.

35. Tseng YR, Wu JF, Ni YH, *et al.* Long-term effect of maternal HBeAg on delayed HBeAg seroconversion in offspring with chronic hepatitis B infection. *Liver Int* 2011;**31**: 1373–1380.

36. Wu JF, Wu TC, Chen CH, *et al.* Serum levels of interleukin-12 predict early, spontaneous hepatitis B virus e antigen seroconversiston. *Gastroenterology* 2010;**138**:165–172.

37. Lin CL, Kao JH. The clinical implications of hepatitis B virus genotype: Recent advances. *J Gastroenterol Hepatol* 2011;**26** (Suppl 1):123–130.

38. Ni YH, Chang MH, Wang KJ, *et al.* Clinical relevance of hepatitis B virus genotype in children with chronic hepatitis B and hepatocellular carcinoma. *Gastroenterology* 2004;**127**:1733–1738.

39. Chen CJ, Yang HI, Iloeje UH, for the REVEAL-HBV Study Group. Hepatitis B virus DNA levels and outcomes in chronic hepatitis B. *Hepatology* 2009;**49** (5 Suppl):S72–S84.

40. Chang MH, Hsu HY, Ni YH, *et al.* Precore stop codon mutant in chronic hepatitis B virus infection in children: Its relation to hepatitis B e seroconversion and natural hepatitis B surface antigen. *J Hepatol* 1998;**28**:915–922.

41. Ni YH, Chang MH, Hsu HY, Tsuei DJ. Longitudinal study on mutation profiles of core promoter and precore regions of the hepatitis B virus genome in children. *Pediatr Res* 2004;**56**:396–399.

42. Ni YH, Chang MH, Hsu HY, Tsuei DJ. Different hepatitis B virus core gene mutations in children with chronic infection versus hepatocellular carcinoma. *Gut* 2003;**52**:122–125.

43. Jonas MM, Block JM, Haber BA, *et al.* Treatment of children with chronic hepatitis B virus infection in the United States: patient selection and therapeutic options. *Hepatology* 2010;**52**: 2192–2205.

44. Torre D, Tambini R. Interferon-α therapy for chronic hepatitis B in children: a meta-analysis. *Clin Infect Dis* 1996;**23**:131–137.

45. Sokal EM, Conjeevaram HS, Roberts EA, *et al.* Interferon alfa therapy for chronic hepatitis B in children: a multinational randomized controlled trial. *Gastroenterology* 1998;**114**: 988–995.

46. Bortolotti F, Jara P, Barbera C, *et al.* Long term effect of alpha interferon in children with chronic hepatitis B. *Gut* 2000;**46**:715–718.

47. Hsu HY, Tsai HY, Wu TC, *et al.* Interferon-alpha treatment in children and young adults with chronic hepatitis B: a long-term follow-up study in Taiwan. *Liver Int* 2008;**28**: 1288–1297.

48. Schwarz KB, Gonzalez-Peralta RP, Murray KF, *et al.* The combination of ribavirin and peginterferon is superior to peginterferon and placebo for children and adolescents with chronic hepatitis C. *Gastroenterology* 2011;**140**:450–458.

49. Jonas M, Kelly DA, Mizerski J, *et al.* Clinical trial of lamivudine in children with chronic hepatitis B. *N Engl J Med* 2002;**346**:1706–1713.

50. Sokal EM, Kelly DA, Badia IB, *et al.* Long-term lamivudine therapy for children with HBeAg-positive chronic hepatitis B. *Hepatology* 2006;**43**: 225–232.

51. Jonas MM, Kelly D, Pollack H, *et al.* Safety, efficacy, and pharmacokinetics of adefovir dipivoxil in children and adolescents (age 2 to <18 years) with chronic hepatitis B. *Hepatology* 2008;**47**:1863–1871.

52. Chang TT, Gish RG, de Man R, *et al.* A comparison of entecavir and lamivudine for HBeAg-positive chronic hepatitis B. *N Engl J Med* 2006;**354**:1001–1010.

53. Lai CL, Shouval D, Lok AS, *et al.* Entecavir versus lamivudine for patients with HBeAg-negative chronic hepatitis B. *N Engl J Med* 2006;**354**:1011–1020.

54. Tenney DJ, Rose RE, Baldick CJ, *et al.* Long-term monitoring shows hepatitis B virus resistance to entecavir in nucleoside- naïve patients is rare through 5 years of therapy. *Hepatology* 2009;**49**:1503–14.

55. Lai CL, Gane E, Liaw YF, *et al.* Telbivudine versus lamivudine in patients with chronic hepatitis B. *N Engl J Med* 2007;**357**:2576–2588.

56. Seto WK, Lai CL, Fung J, *et al.* Significance of HBV DNA levels at 12 weeks of telbivudine treatment and the 3 years treatment outcome. *J Hepatol* 2011;**55**:522–528.

57. Marcellin P, Heathcote EJ, Buti M, *et al.* Tenofovir disoproxil fumarate versus adefovir dipivoxil for chronic hepatitis B. *N Engl J Med* 2008;**359**:2442–2455.

58. Heathcote EJ, Marcellin P, Buti M, *et al.* Three-year efficacy and safety of tenofovir disoproxil fumarate treatment for chronic hepatitis B. *Gastroenterology* 2011;**140**:132–143.

59. D'Antiga L, Aw M, Atkins M, *et al.* Combined lamivudine/interferon-alpha treatment in "immunotolerant" children perinatally infected with hepatitis B: a pilot study. *J Pediatr* 2006;**148**:228–233.

60. Chen HL, Lin LH, Hu FC, *et al.* Effects of maternal screening and universal immunization to prevent mother-to-infant transmission of HBV. *Gastroenterology* 2012;**142**:773–781.

61. Chen DS, Hsu NH, Sung JL, *et al.* A mass vaccination program in Taiwan against hepatitis B virus infection in infants of hepatitis B surface antigen-carrier mothers. *JAMA* 1987;**257**: 2597–2603.

62. Bonanni P, Crovari P. Success stories in the implementation of universal hepatitis B vaccination: an update on Italy. *Vaccine* 1998;**16**(Suppl):S38–S42.

63. Wasley A, Grytdal S, Gallagher K; Centers for Disease Control and Prevention (CDC). Surveillance for acute viral hepatitis: United States, 2006. *MMWR Surveill Summ* 2008;**57**:1–24.

64. Ni YH, Huang LM, Chang MH, *et al.* Two decades of universal hepatitis B vaccination in Taiwan: impact and implication for future strategies. *Gastroenterology* 2007;**132**:1287–1293.

65. Viviani S, Jack A, Hall AJ, *et al.* Hepatitis B vaccination in infancy in The Gambia: protection against carriage at 9 years of age. *Vaccine* 1999;**17**:2946–2950.

66. Kao JH, Hsu HM, Shaw WY, Chang MH, Chen DS. Universal hepatitis B vaccination and the decreased mortality from fulminant hepatitis in infants in Taiwan. *J Pediatr* 2001;**139**:349–352.

67. Chang MH, Chen CJ, Lai MS, *et al.* Universal hepatitis B vaccination in Taiwan and the incidence of hepatocellular carcinoma in children. *N Engl J Med* 1997;**336**:1855–1859.

68. Chang MH, You SL, Chen CJ, *et al.* Decreased incidence of hepatocellular carcinoma in hepatitis B vaccinees: a 20-year follow-up study. *J Natl Cancer Inst* 2009;**101**:1348–1355.

69. Su WJ, Ho MC, Ni YH, *et al.* High-titer antibody to hepatitis B surface antigen before liver transplantation can prevent de novo hepatitis B infection. *J Pediatr Gastroenterol Nutr* 2009;**48**:203–208.

70. Hsu HY, Chang MH, Ni YH, *et al.* No increase in prevalence of hepatitis B surface antigen mutant in a population of children and adolescents who were fully covered by universal infant immunization. *J Infect Dis* 2010;**201**:1192–1200.

71. Centers for Disease Control and Prevention. *Hepatitis B Slide Set.* Atlanta, GA: Centers for Disease Control and Prevention, 2006 (http://www.cdc.gov/ncidod/diseases/hepatitis/slideset/, accessed January 26, 2006).

72. Rizzetto M, Canese MG, Arico S, *et al.* Immunofluorescence detection of new antigen-antibody system (delta/anti-delta) associated to hepatitis B virus in liver and in serum of HBsAg carriers. *Gut* 1977;**18**:997–1003.

73. Fattowich G, Giustina G, Christensen E, *et al.* Influence of hepatitis delta virus infection on morbidity and mortality in compensated cirrhosis type B. *Gut* 2000;**46**:420–426.

74. Bortolotti F, Di Marco V, Vajro P, *et al.* Long-term evolution of chronic delta hepatitis in children. *J Pediatr* 1993;**122**:736–738.

75. Mele A, Mariano A, Tosti ME, *et al.* Acute hepatitis delta virus infection in Italy: incidence and risk factors after the introduction of the universal anti–hepatitis B vaccination campaign. *Clin Infect Dis* 2007;**44**:e17–e24.

76. Di Marco V, Giacchino R, Timitilli A, *et al.* Long-term interferon-alpha treatment of children with chronic hepatitis delta: a multicentre study. *J Viral Hepat* 1996;**3**:123–128.

Chapter

19

Hepatitis C virus infection

Maureen M. Jonas

Introduction

Hepatitis C virus (HCV) has emerged as an important cause of viral hepatitis in children but the actual number of infected children is underestimated. Because of the ability of this virus to establish chronic progressive infection, HCV infection is now a leading indication for liver transplantation in adults. The discovery of HCV using molecular cloning techniques in 1989 has led directly to a reduction in the number of acute HCV infections, and the establishment of detection and treatment strategies.

Virology

The virus is the prototype for the *Hepacivirus* genus of the family Flaviviridae. The virion is about 30–60 nm in diameter. The capsid is thought to be enveloped by a lipid bilayer. The envelope contains two viral glycoproteins, E1 and E2, and the nucleocapsid contained within is composed of core protein and the viral RNA genome [1].

The genome is a 9.6 kb positive, single-stranded RNA (Figure 19.1). A single open reading frame (ORF) encodes a 3011 amino acid residue polyprotein that undergoes proteolysis to yield at least 10 individual gene products. Structural proteins (core and envelope) are encoded in the 5′-quarter of the genome. The structural proteins (core, E1 and E2) are processed by host peptidase, and the non-structural (NS) proteins are subsequently cleaved by virally encoded NS2-3 and NS-3 proteases. The core protein is highly conserved and may be involved in other processes such as apoptosis, intracellular signaling, transcription, and modulation of the host immune response. Protein E2 binds specifically to host CD81, suggesting that it mediates viral entry into the cell. Unlike the core protein, E1 and E2 demonstrate considerable sequence heterogeneity from different isolates. The N-terminus of E2 contains a "hypervariable" region (HVR) HVR1 that is an important viral neutralization determinant. This region is also a T-cell determinant, able to activate helper T-cell responses during HCV infection. The sequence variability of E2 may account, at

least in part, for the ability of HCV to elude the host immune system and establish persistent infection. Downstream is a small integral membrane protein, p7, which appears to function as an ion channel but also appears necessary for efficient assembly, release, and production of infectious progeny virions from liver cells.

The 3′-region of the genome encodes seven NS proteins that participate in post-translational proteolytic processing and replication of HCV genetic material. NS3 has a multifunctional serine protease in its N-terminal domain that cleaves the remaining junctions of the HCV polyprotein. Its C-terminus contains an RNA helicase that may function during viral replication. NS4B is an integral membrane protein that alters membrane structure and contains a GTP-binding domain essential for HCV replication. NS5A is a multifunctional protein with key roles in modulating viral replication and altering the intracellular milieu in response to viral infection. Adaptive mutations that favor increased viral replication in vitro are associated with a decrease in hyperphosphorylated NS5A. Amino acid residues 2209 to 2248 of the NS5A protein have been designated as the "interferon sensitivity determining region" since mutations affecting this region are thought to be associated with variation in responsiveness to interferon therapy [3–6]. However, this designation remains somewhat controversial. NS5B is the RNA-dependent RNA polymerase that catalyzes replication of HCV. The flanking 5′- and 3′-nontranslated regions contain conserved sequences that regulate both genome replication and translation.

There is extensive genetic heterogeneity within HCV. Isolates from around the world have been divided into six major genotypes, designated 1 through 6, and more than 100 subtypes. The genomes of the most divergent HCV isolates differ by up to 35%. Genotypes 1–3 have a worldwide distribution; genotypes 4 and 5 are found principally in Africa, and genotype 6 primarily in Asia. In the USA, genotype 1 accounts for 74% (57% subtype 1a, 17% subtype 1b), genotype 2 for 15%, genotype 3 for 7%, genotype 4 for 1%, and genotype 6 for 3% of HCV infections. Within infected individuals, HCV circulates as quasispecies, a mixture of closely related but distinct

Liver Disease in Children, Fourth Edition, ed. Frederick J. Suchy, Ronald J. Sokol, and William F. Balistreri. Published by Cambridge University Press. © Cambridge University Press 2014.

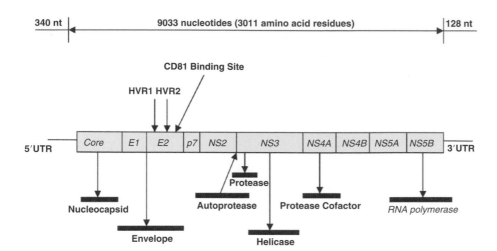

Figure 19.1 Hepatitis C virus (HCV) genome and expressed proteins. The single-stranded RNA of 9.5 kb that consists of two untranslated regions (UTRs) and a single open reading frame that encodes a 3011 amino acid residue polyprotein. The UTR at the 5'-end contains elements necessary for initiation of viral replication. The polyprotein is cleaved into single proteins by a host peptidase in the structural region, which contains the nucleocapsid core protein and two envelope proteins (E1 and E2). In the non-structural region, HCV-encoded proteases separate the remaining proteins. The E2 region contains two hypervariable regions and a binding site for CD81, an HCV receptor. The non-structural proteins include proteases, a helicase, and an RNA-dependent RNA polymerase. (With permission from Lauer and Walker, 2001 [2].)

genomes, which typically differ by 1–2%. In an infected person, quasispecies may either be present from the onset, as a result of simultaneous transmission, or may develop over time through accumulation of mutations. Such mutations may enable more efficient HCV replication or evasion of host immune responses. Certain regions of the genome are hypervariable and responsible for most, but not all, of the genomic differences in quasispecies. The HVR1 at the N-terminus of the envelope E2, at amino acid residues 384–410, is probably on the surface of the folded envelope protein and represents a neutralization epitope for humoral immunity. Appearance of antibodies against HVR1 in infected subjects is followed by emergence of new variants in the region. For these reasons, HVR1 is believed to play a role in HCV persistence and chronic HCV infection (CHC). A second hypervariable region, HVR2, is in E2 and is identified in genotype 1b isolates.

Pathology

Hepatocytes are the primary site of viral replication. Entry of HCV into the cell is mediated by a specific interaction between viral envelope protein(s) and a host cell surface receptor. The HCV E2 has been shown to bind the host cell surface protein CD81 [7], and both E1 and E2 are required for fusion. Additional host proteins other than CD81 may be required for viral entry, such as the low density lipoprotein receptor. Evidence from study of other flaviviruses supports a model in which entry via receptor-mediated endocytosis is followed by envelope fusion with the endosomal membrane to release the nucleocapsid into the cytoplasm. There, ribosome binding to the viral genome enables translation of the encoded polyprotein, with the formation of a replicative ribonucleoprotein complex. The resulting negative-strand intermediate then serves as a template for the production of positive-strand RNA. Like other flaviviruses, budding of virus likely occurs into intracellular vesicles, which release free virus from the cell by exocytosis. How HCV acquires its envelope or specifically excludes cellular proteins and RNAs during virion assembly is not known.

Immunopathogenesis of infection and viral persistence

Infection with HCV becomes chronic in at least two-thirds of those infected; the outcome (clearance versus persistent infection) is typically determined within 6 months of infection. Cell-mediated immunity seems to play a critical role, whereas the role of humoral immunity is less well understood [8]. Individuals with acute, self-limited HCV infection have early, vigorous responses with both CD4 (T helper) and CD8 (cytotoxic) T-cells. The sequences that are recognized by HCV-specific T-helper cells are immunodominant (the NS3 protein in particular) and conserved among HCV genotypes. Major histocompatibility class (MHC) haplotypes determine the presentation and recognition of a set of common viral epitopes, suggesting that these antigens may be important in development of immune reactivity. Both HCV-specific CD4 T-cells and CD8 T-cells become detectable in blood 3 to 4 weeks after infection. Infiltration of the liver with T-cells correlates with increase in serum aminotransferase (ALT) as cytotoxic lymphocytes lyse HCV-infected cells. After recovery from HCV infection, circulating HCV-specific T-helper and cytotoxic lymphocytes may be present for decades, even when the humoral response declines and HCV antibodies become undetectable [8].

Although the exact mechanism for viral persistence and the frequent development of CHC is not known, HCV-specific cytotoxic lymphocytes are found at very low levels in the blood of individuals with CHC. In contrast, patients with resolved infection have cytotoxic lymphocytes directed against a broader distribution of epitopes, and the cells exhibited stronger responses to stimulation. Both HCV-specific and non-specific CD8 T-cells are found in the liver of infected people; immune-mediated liver disease is felt to be initiated by the HCV-specific cells but amplified by the non-specific cytotoxic cells.

Mechanisms that have been postulated to explain HCV persistence include escape of innate immune response by

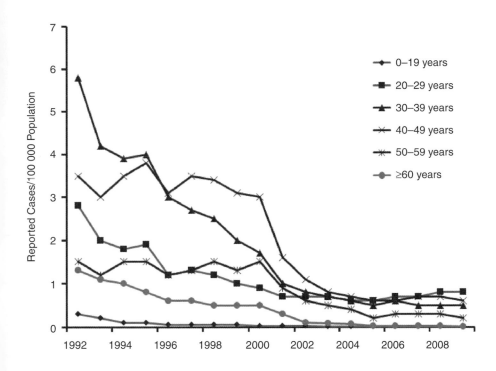

Figure 19.2 Incidence of acute hepatitis C infection in the USA, by age group, 1992–2009. Until 1995, acute hepatitis C infection was reported as "acute hepatitis, non-A/non B." (Adapted from Centers for Disease Control and Prevention, 2009 [11].)

upregulation of MHC expression on infected cells, viral sequence variations and mutations that eliminate humoral and cellular target epitopes, and lack of susceptibility of HCV to T-cell cytokines.

In 2009, three groups reported that single nucleotide polymorphisms (SNPs) located near *IL28B*, the gene encoding interleukin (IL)-28B (also known as interferon (IFN)-λ3, a type III interferon), were strongly associated with the likelihood of achieving a therapeutic effect, sustained virologic response (SVR), with combined peginterferon plus ribavirin treatment [9]. The receptors for IFNα, a type I interferon, differ from those for IL-28B, but both activate the same intracellular pathway (Jak/STAT) to result in expression of many IFN-stimulated genes.

Interleukin-28B acts again viruses by inducing the Mx proteins 2′,5′-oligoadenylate synthetase and interferon stimulated gene factor-3. Once it was recognized that *IL28B* was associated with likelihood of response to therapy, the role of this polymorphism in spontaneous control of HCV infection was studied. Genome-wide association studies have indicated that host genetic variation plays a key determinant in natural control of HCV infection. Independent studies have consistently identified variants within *IL28B* that are strongly associated with spontaneous HCV clearance [10].

Epidemiology

It is estimated that HCV affects 3% of the worldwide population, with a prevalence of 1.8% in the USA. It has also been estimated that 240 000 US children have been infected with HCV, and 68 000–100 000 have CHC. Prevalence varies considerably in subpopulations with varied risk factors. Mexican-Americans and non-Hispanic blacks have increased rates of HCV seropositivity; the odds ratios for these two populations compared with the general population are 1.6 and 1.4, respectively. Although HCV was considered a transfusion-related disease, no cases of transfusion-transmitted acute HCV infection have been detected by the Centers for Disease Control and Prevention (CDC) Sentinel Counties Viral Hepatitis Surveillance System since 1994 [11]. Even when the incidence of infections was much higher, blood transfusions accounted for no more than about 10% of all infections. Currently, the risk of HCV following a single-unit blood transfusion in the USA is less than 1 in 1 000 000.

The most important risk factor for HCV is injection drug use. For reasons that are unclear, there has been a major decline in the incidence of HCV among injection drug users, which has corresponded to the overall decrease in new HCV cases (Figure 19.2). Some have postulated that the efforts to curtail HIV infection have been responsible for a "halo effect" on the incidence of HCV. Educational programs promoting needle exchange and reducing shared needles have decreased HCV transmission. There are occasional reports of small outbreaks, such as that seen in adolescents and young adults in Massachusetts between 2002 and 2009 [12], again typically associated with injection drug use.

In addition to injection drug use, HCV infection is associated with intranasal cocaine use, high-risk sexual practices, and occupational exposure. Some infections are sporadic and community acquired, possible through non-percutaneous or covert percutaneous transmission. In the healthcare setting, HCV infection has been associated with needlestick injuries, hemodialysis, and organ transplantation. The risk of acquisition of HCV by healthcare workers following a single needlestick exposure to blood from an HCV RNA-positive patient is approximately 2%. Overall, HCV prevalence is lower among healthcare workers than in the general population. Nevertheless, nosocomial transmission of HCV is possible but has rarely been reported in the USA other than in chronic hemodialysis settings. Notable exceptions include an outbreak of HCV following intravenous immunoglobulin infusion (Gammagard, Baxter Healthcare Corporation, Glendale, CA, USA) between 1993 and 1994 [13], and another at an endoscopy center in Nevada in 2008 that was associated with use of single-dose medication vials for multiple individuals [14]. Currently, all immunoglobulin products in the USA undergo inactivation and are tested for HCV RNA before release, and guidelines for the proper use of single-dose vials have been emphasized.

Transmission of HCV by sexual or close physical contact is possible in heterosexual couples, but uncommon because the virus is inefficiently spread by this route. Bodily secretions (saliva, seminal fluid, and vaginal secretions) of people with CHC are rarely contaminated with HCV. Although chimpanzees have been experimentally infected by the injection of saliva from HCV-infected people, casual household contact and contact with saliva of infected people are very inefficient modes of transmission. Case–control studies have reported an association between exposure to a sexual contact and a history of hepatitis or to multiple sex partners and acquiring HCV infection. Other risk factors include a history of sexually transmitted disease or sex with trauma. However, 15–20% of patients with acute HCV infection have a history of sexual exposure in the absence of other risk factors. In contrast, a low prevalence of HCV infection has been reported by studies of long-term spouses of patients with CHC who had no other risk factors for infection. Similar to other blood-borne viruses, sexual transmission of HCV from males to females might be more efficient than from females to males. However, HIV-infected men who have sex with men continue to be at risk for HCV infection [15].

Many other risk factors have been examined. In the USA, there is no reported association with military service, medical/dental procedures, tattooing, acupuncture, ear piercing, or foreign travel. If transmission occurs in these settings, the frequency may be too low to detect. In the most recent surveillance report from the CDC, no risk factor was identified in 20% of cases [11]. People for whom HCV testing is indicated are listed in Table 19.1.

There have been recent data to support the contention that many children in the USA with CHC remain unidentified. One study that used crude estimates of childhood prevalence based on the National Health and Nutrition Examination Survey data and Florida public health laboratory reports of all childhood cases demonstrated that only 12% of expected cases had been identified over the last several years, and a minority of them were receiving care for this infection [16]. Similar studies are being undertaken in other US states that have viral hepatitis reporting requirements. In any case, it is likely that most

Table 19.1 Individuals who should be tested for hepatitis C infection

Testing	Demographic category
Recommended	Those with a history of illicit injection drug use
	Those with a history of persistent ALT elevation
	Those who have had a prior transfusion (blood or blood products) or recipients of organs before July 1992
	Those requiring chronic hemodialysis
	Children born to HCV-positive women
	HIV infection
	Current sexual partners of HCV-infected people
	Healthcare and public safety workers after needlestick, sharps, or mucosal exposures[a]
Not recommended	Household (non-sexual) contacts of HCV-positive individuals (without additional risk factor)
	Pregnant women without other risk factors
	International adoptees

HCV, hepatitis C virus; ALT, alanine aminotransferase.
[a] Testing of the exposure source would be indicated and subsequent testing of the exposed worker could be undertaken if needed.

children with CHC are not identified or receiving appropriate treatment and counseling.

Perinatal transmission

At present, maternal-to-neonatal transmission of HCV is the most common route of childhood infection. Worldwide, one estimate has calculated that 60 000 HCV-infected infants are born yearly [17]. With the advent of anti-HCV testing, variable rates of maternal-to-infant transmission have been reported; however, documentation of infection in early life is difficult because anti-HCV may be passively transferred from mother to child. Overall, perinatal transmission of HCV is an uncommon event; 5–6% of infants born to anti-HCV-positive women acquire HCV. Of infants born to women coinfected with HCV and untreated HIV, the rate increases to 17% (range, 5–36). The difference has been thought to be related to higher levels of HCV RNA in coinfected women. However, some studies have challenged this assumption. In a large prospective study (370 pregnancies) performed in Italy, there was a perinatal transmission rate of 5.1% but the risk of transmission was not related to viral RNA levels [18]. In this cohort, none of the mothers with HIV coinfection (4% of the cohort) transmitted HCV, but all these HIV-infected mothers received antiretroviral therapy during their pregnancies. Another study of 403 HCV-positive, HIV-negative women reported a 5% transmission rate and no relationship between viral RNA level and HCV transmission [19]. Transmission occurs with both vaginal and cesarean deliveries, although one study demonstrated a difference in HCV transmission between emergency and elective cesarean deliveries, the latter being characterized by rupture of membranes at the time of birth rather than several hours previously [20]. Rupture of membranes for longer than 6 hours before delivery was an independent risk factor for HCV transmission in a prospective study [21]. These observations indicate that it is likely that most cases of transmission of HCV from infected mothers to newborns occurs at or very near the time of delivery, and may be subject to interruption. To reduce the risk of HCV infection, the US National Institutes of Health has advised caution to avoid the use of fetal scalp monitoring and prolonged rupture of membranes [22].

Routine serologic testing of pregnant women for HCV infection is not recommended. However, women who have a history of blood transfusion before 1992, injection drug use, sexually transmitted disease, or unexplained ALT abnormality should be tested. Breast-feeding is not considered to be contraindicated in women who are infected with HCV. The American Academy of Pediatrics recommends that HCV-infected women who wish to breast-feed their infants be counseled that there appears to be no increased risk of transmission, but mothers who choose to breast-feed should consider abstaining if their nipples are cracked or bleeding [23].

Early testing of infants born to HCV-infected women is not recommended, since diagnosis may be problematic, viremia may be transient, and no intervention is available. Since maternal antibody has usually disappeared from infant's serum by 15–18 months of age (see below), testing for anti-HCV is recommended at that age for at-risk infants. A positive anti-HCV can be confirmed by further nucleic acid testing. It is estimated that up to 35% of perinatally infected children have spontaneous clearance of the virus by 3 years of age. Recently, *IL28B* genotype has been associated with the likelihood of spontaneous viral clearance in this population [24].

Neither national nor international adoptees are at increased risk of HCV infection and so routine screening is not indicated. The decision to test should be individualized if the child is born to a woman at known risk for HCV infection (e.g. an injection drug user). However, children adopted from countries where the prevalence of HCV is high, or where infection-control practices in healthcare facilities may be suboptimal, may be at risk, and testing using the antibody test (see below) should be considered in this setting.

Coinfection with HIV

In the USA, about 10% of HCV-infected people have HIV infection as well. Approximately 25% of HIV-infected people in the Western world have CHC [25]. Patients who are coinfected with HCV and HIV-1 are at increased risk for disease progression [26]. These epidemiologic data are not available for childhood infections, but the prevalence of coinfection, at least in the USA, is probably lower. Complications associated with concurrent HCV infection have emerged as one of the most frequent and complex issues in the care of patients with HIV following the introduction of potent antiretroviral therapy for HIV.

Before the advent of highly active antiretroviral therapy for HIV, deaths from liver disease in HIV infection were infrequent, ranging from 2 to 13%. Now with current treatment regimens, mortality from liver disease, chiefly related to HCV, accounts for 7–50% [27]. Even though the effect of HCV on the overall mortality of HIV infection is unclear, it is an important clinical problem in the long-term survival of HIV-infected patients. In fact, HCV infection may lessen the severity of untreated HIV infection; however, with improved survival with the administration of highly active antiretroviral therapy, treatment of HCV has assumed much greater significance. Careful consideration about the timing of both HCV and HIV treatment is necessary. In patients with advanced HIV disease, HIV treatment generally is started immediately. In coinfected patients with good immune function and/or advanced liver disease, HCV treatment may be administered first to minimize hepatotoxicity. In coinfected patients who do undergo treatment, side effects from multiple medications need to be carefully monitored and some treatment combinations are contraindicated (e.g. ribavirin and didanosine). In general, treatment of coinfected patients is similar to that of patients with isolated HCV infection, but the likelihood of therapeutic responses is lower. New direct-acting antiviral agents licensed to treat genotype 1 HCV infection in adults have not yet been approved for those with HIV coinfection, although studies are underway. Special consideration in this population needs to be given to the drug–drug interactions that are common with the new protease inhibitors (see below).

Diagnosis

The two major types of test available for laboratory diagnosis of HCV infections are antibody assays for HCV (anti-HCV) and nucleic acid tests, usually done by polymerase chain reaction (PCR) to detect HCV RNA. Interpretation of these tests is displayed in Table 19.2. Assays for IgM to detect early or acute infection are not available. The currently used immunoassay for anti-HCV is at least 97% sensitive and more than 99% specific. Negative results early in the course of acute infection can result from the prolonged interval between exposure and onset of illness and seroconversion. Within 4 months after exposure, and 5 to 6 weeks after onset of hepatitis, 80% of patients will have detectable anti-HCV. Among infants born to anti-HCV-positive mothers, passively acquired maternal antibody may persist for up to 18 months.

HCV RNA can be detected in serum or plasma within 1 to 2 weeks after exposure to the virus and weeks before onset of liver enzyme abnormalities or appearance of anti-HCV (Figure 19.3). Assays for HCV RNA are used commonly in clinical practice to confirm HCV infection in anti-HCV-positive

Table 19.2 Interpretation of hepatitis C virus (HCV) test results

Anti-HCV	HCV RNA	Interpretation
Negative	Negative	No infection
Positive	Positive	Acute or chronic infection
Negative	Positive	Early infection or chronic infection in an immunosuppressed host
Positive	Negative	Resolved infection or chronic infection or false positive antibody test

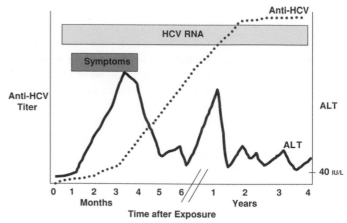

Figure 19.3 Typical sequence of events in hepatitis C virus (HCV) infection. Following viral acquisition at time 0, there is a progressive increase in serum alanine aminotransferase (ALT), indicating the onset of clinical hepatitis between 6 and 8 weeks. The appearance of HCV antibody can be detected by radioimmunoassay, with quantification of a viral antibody titer. Polymerase chain reaction can indicate infection with HCV within 1–2 weeks of exposure, well before the appearance of detectable anti-HCV, which is typical for 10–12 weeks following exposure. Because anti-HCV does not confer immunity, it can be detected in the majority of patients who progress to chronic infection. In patients who clear HCV infection, ALT values typically normalize and HCV RNA levels become undetectable; over time, anti-HCV decreases when HCV infection resolves. Although not indicated on this figure, quantitative HCV RNA levels do fluctuate through the course of acute and chronic HCV infections.

individuals, to identify infection in infants early in life (i.e. perinatal transmission) when maternal antibody interferes with ability to detect antibody produced by the infant, and to monitor patients receiving antiviral therapy. Viral RNA may be detected intermittently and, therefore, a single negative assay result is not conclusive. There are two types of HCV RNA assays, qualitative and quantitative. Quantitative assays for HCV RNA are almost as sensitive as the qualitative tests and can detect as few as 50 copies/mL in serum, but the clinical value of these quantitative assays is primarily for use in patients undergoing or about to undergo antiviral therapy.

Once HCV infection is confirmed with nucleic acid testing, the genotype can be determined. Multiple types of assays are used for this purpose. Most are quite specific, but occasionally genotype 1 HCV cannot be further characterized into subtype a or b.

Clinical features

Acute HCV infection is rarely detected in children, and fulminant hepatitis C is rare. Accordingly, there are few data regarding treatment of acute HCV in the pediatric age group. The typical sequence of virologic, clinical, and serologic events in CHC is demonstrated in Figure 19.3. While CHC is generally asymptomatic during childhood, long-term infection can lead to significant morbidity and mortality, such as cirrhosis and hepatocellular carcinoma, in later childhood or adulthood. The proportion of HCV-infected children who will suffer these serious consequences is not known, but several pediatric studies have demonstrated that the degree of hepatic fibrosis generally correlates with age and duration of infection [28,29], although progression seems to be slower than observed in those infected later in life.

Although infrequent, spontaneous HCV clearance has been well documented. In those who acquired the infection perinatally, clearance rates from 0 to 25% in the first 2–7 years have been reported. If spontaneous HCV clearance is going to occur, it appears that it does so within the first 3 years of life in the majority of instances [30]. Some investigators have concluded that children who became HCV infected via transfusion have higher rates of spontaneous clearance than those who become infected perinatally, but at least one study did not find significant differences in the clearance rates (19%)

between these modes of acquisition. Vertical transmission is associated with a high incidence of viremia and abnormal aminotransferase levels during the first 12 months [31]. Of 70 prospectively followed infants in five European centers from 1990 to 1999, 93% had abnormal serum ALT during the first 12 months, and only 19% cleared HCV RNA with normal serum ALT by 30 months of age. Clearance of viremia was independent of sex and maternal HIV coinfection. Peak serum ALT >5 × the upper limit of normal during the first 18 months and genotype 3 were more common in the patients in whom viremia resolved spontaneously.

Children with CHC are typically asymptomatic or have mild non-specific symptoms. Clinical signs of disease are present in approximately 20% of children early in infection, with 10% having hepatomegaly, and many with intermittently or persistently elevated serum ALT or aspartate aminotransferase. In a series from Japan, 45% of children who had a transfusion at the time of surgery for congenital heart disease developed CHC and chronic hepatitis, but none had cirrhosis within a 4-year follow-up period. Similarly, in a German series, 67 of 458 children who had undergone cardiac surgery (14.6%) developed serologic evidence of HCV infection, although only approximately 37 (55%) of these infected children were still infected at a mean of 19.8 years later. Only 17 of the 37 underwent liver biopsy, and three had chronic injury. Children with thalassemia or hemophilia had a high prevalence of HCV infection, but most of these individuals are now adults, and transfusion-acquired infection is no longer seen in childhood. Children treated for leukemia prior to 1990 had a high rate of

HCV infection, but in one cohort prolonged follow-up (13–27 years) did not reveal serious liver disease [32]. In contrast, an American study of individuals treated for childhood cancer revealed one death from liver disease and two deaths from hepatocellular carcinoma in the decades following HCV acquisition [33]. The same report described three patients (9%) with cirrhosis 9 to 27 years after diagnosis of the primary malignancy. It has become clear that some HCV infections acquired in childhood by transfusion are associated with serious liver disease in the decades following infection.

The rate of progression of liver disease is related to the age at acquisition, and so the development of advanced liver disease is often delayed until more than 30 years after infection in those who acquire HCV before the age of 20 years. The proportion of young patients who will eventually develop advanced fibrosis or cirrhosis at some point in their infection is not yet known. Risk factors for this progression identified so far include HIV coinfection, other immunosuppression, iron overload, and chronic alcohol ingestion. Although insulin resistance and hepatic steatosis have been implicated in the progression of fibrosis in adults with HCV [34], the role of concomitant obesity in the progression of HCV-associated liver disease in children has not been studied.

Overall, the degree of hepatitis identified in the pediatric population is less than that in adults with similar duration of infection, genotype, and serum HCV RNA. In a study of 121 children aged 2–16 years, however, 46 (38%) had moderate and 4 (3%) had severe inflammation; 5 (4%) had bridging fibrosis and 2 (1.5%) had cirrhosis [35]. The degree of inflammation correlated with the duration of the infection, and the severity of inflammation and fibrosis correlated with each other. Additionally, this analysis revealed that overweight children had more fibrosis than those who were not overweight. The conclusion was that "the positive correlation of inflammation with duration of infection and fibrosis and of obesity with fibrosis suggest that children with chronic hepatitis C will be at risk for progressive liver disease as they age and possibly acquire other comorbid risk factors." Since most children with CHC acquired the infection perinatally, one would expect that they would develop the sequelae of chronic liver disease in the second or third decade of life. In fact, hepatocellular carcinoma has been reported in adolescents, and liver transplantation for CHC-related liver disease may rarely be required prior to adulthood. As in adults receiving transplants for CHC, the outcomes are poor for children who require liver transplantation for CHC (patient and graft survival at 5 years in recipients below the age of 17 years are 71.6% and 55%, respectively).

There have been only a few case reports of hepatocellular carcinoma associated with HCV infection during childhood [36]. Liver transplantation for complications of CHC during childhood is uncommon. According to the Study of Pediatric Liver Transplantation (SPLIT) Registry, which collects data from 37 North American pediatric liver transplant centers, CHC with cirrhosis or "subacute hepatitis C" was the reason for transplant in 13 of 1378 children (1%) from 1995 through June 2003.

In addition to the physical impact of CHC on children, there is also potential for psychological impact on both the children and their families. In adults, CHC correlates with decreases in cognitive functioning and health-related quality of life. Children with CHC had worse cognitive functioning than a normative sample, but their behavioral and emotional functioning was comparable [37]. Their caregivers did, however, experience higher stress and strain on the family system.

For these reasons, the primary indications for treatment of children with HCV infection are prevention of future complications and the psychosocial benefits of eradication in this young and vulnerable population. Given the impact of CHC on children and their families, and the risk of advancing liver disease as the children age, treatment of this infection during childhood has significant potential for advantage. By the same token, the treatment itself may have adverse consequences, similar to or different from those in adults, that must be considered.

Extrahepatic manifestations

Extrahepatic manifestations of CHC are rare in children. Various non-hepatic manifestations of HCV infection have been described in adults; these include a serum sickness-like illness, autoimmune hepatitis, lymphoma, keratoconjunctivitis sicca, glomerulonephritis, lichen planus, and vasculitis with cryoglobulinemia. Many of these HCV-related manifestations are immunologically mediated (associated with circulating immune complexes) or a consequence of direct viral injury. In one study, 16 of 19 patients with type II cryoglobulinemia (immune complexes of polyclonal IgG and monoclonal IgM rheumatoid factors) had HCV viremia. The HCV RNA or anti-HCV was selectively concentrated in the cryoprecipitate, providing evidence of HCV in the pathogenesis of essential mixed cryoglobulinemia. In addition to these disorders, HCV-infected people have a high prevalence of psychological disorders such as depression and of diabetes mellitus. Most recently, CHC has been linked to non-Hodgkin B-cell lymphoma; a recent report discusses the proposed pathogenesis of this association, implicating chronic antigenic stimulation associated with HCV infection of peripheral blood B-cells [38]. In some reports, lymphoma regression with antiviral treatment has been documented.

Histologic features

According to practice guidelines, designed primarily for adults, there are three reasons to consider liver biopsy in individuals with CHC: to assess the current status of liver injury, including inflammatory and fibrosis scores; to identify features useful in the decision to treat, such as steatosis and iron overload; and to detect advanced fibrosis or cirrhosis that would necessitate surveillance for complications such as varices and hepatocellular carcinoma. It is generally felt that liver biopsy may be

(a)　　　　　　　　　　　　(b)

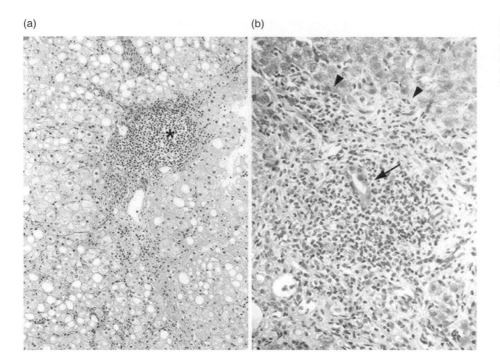

Figure 19.4 Histologic findings in chronic hepatitis C virus infection. (a) Hepatocellular steatosis and a portal lymphoid aggregate (asterisk). (b) At higher power, bile duct injury (arrow) and interface hepatitis with lymphocytes (arrowhead) can be seen.

unnecessary in those with genotypes 2 or 3 HCV, since a large majority will respond to therapy. Although advanced liver disease is uncommon during the childhood years, and childhood HCV is less commonly associated with other liver disease risk factors, sporadic cases are detected and would need to be managed accordingly. At this point, the decision to perform a liver biopsy is felt to be at the discretion of the provider, and is particularly helpful when the decision about whether to treat or defer treatment is being made. Non-invasive indicators of hepatic fibrosis, such as transient elastography, biomarkers and calculated fibrosis scores, have been studied in adults with HCV infection, but not yet in children.

The characteristic histopathologic lesions of pediatric HCV infection, including portal lymphoid aggregates or follicles, steatosis, sinusoidal lymphocytes, and steatosis (Figure 19.4), have been reported with approximately the same frequency as in adults. Although necrosis and inflammation are usually mild, at least some fibrosis is common and progresses with increasing age and duration of infection. This progressive fibrosis indicates that the natural history of HCV infection acquired in childhood may in some instances be associated with significant subsequent morbidity. In 109 Japanese children primarily infected via transfusion, the average histologic activity (Scheuer system) was 3.8 [39]. There were no cases of cirrhosis and only 3.6% of the children had bridging fibrosis with architectural distortion (stage 3). Viral genotypes were not reported, and the mean duration of infection was only 2.6 years. In contrast, although histologic activity (Scheuer and METAVIR systems) was generally mild in a series of children with HCV and abnormal ALT in the USA, portal fibrosis was described in 78% of biopsies from 40 children [28]. Fibrosis was mild in 26%, moderate in 22%, and severe in 22%;

cirrhosis was found in 8%. Two of the children with cirrhosis were young adolescents who had acquired HCV infection perinatally. In this series, 92% of children had genotype 1 HCV. The mean duration of infection in those children in whom it could be accurately determined was 6.8 years (SD, 5.3). In a series of 80 children from Italy and Spain, most of whom were infected with HCV genotype 1, and with a mean duration of infection of 3.5 years (SD, 4.3), inflammatory scores were generally low (grade 1 or 2) [40]. The frequency and severity of the bile duct damage and lymphoid follicles increased with the patient's age. Fibrosis was present in 58 (72.5%), and increased with duration of disease and patient age, just as in the American series. Only one child (1.25%) had cirrhosis.

Treatment

The main goal of therapy in CHC is to achieve sustained eradication of the HCV, defined as sustained virological response (SVR) and undetectable HCV RNA by PCR 24 weeks after the completion of therapy [41]. Secondary, and usually coincident, goals are to halt the progression of the liver disease, and prevent the development of cirrhosis and hepatocellular carcinoma. Individuals in whom an SVR is achieved enjoy durability of undetectable virus in >99% [42], a condition considered the equivalent to virologic and clinical cure. In addition, attainment of SVR has a striking effect on later liver-related morbidity and mortality [43].

Multiple factors must be considered when counseling a pediatric patient and family about treatment; some are objective, and others more subjective (Box 19.1). These include age, severity of liver disease, comorbidities, patient and family

Box 19.1 Generally accepted indications and contraindications for treatment of hepatitis C virus (HCV) infection with peginterferon and ribavirin

Therapy currently indicated

The following are accepted criteria:

- age 18 years or older
- HCV RNA positive in serum
- liver biopsy showing chronic hepatitis with significant fibrosis (bridging fibrosis or higher)
- compensated liver disease:
  - total serum bilirubin <1.5 g/dL
  - international normalized ratio <1.5
  - serum albumin >3.4 mg/dL
  - platelet count >75 × 10⁹ cells/L
- no evidence of hepatic decompensation (hepatic encephalopathy or ascites)
- acceptable hematological and biochemical indices
  - hemoglobin 13 g/dL for men and 12 g/dL for women
  - neutrophil count 1.5 × 10⁹ cells/L
  - serum creatinine <1.5 mg/dL
- willing to be treated and to adhere to treatment requirements
- no contraindications

Therapy currently contraindicated

The following criteria are contraindications for therapy:

- major uncontrolled depressive illness
- solid organ transplant (renal, heart, or lung)
- autoimmune hepatitis or other autoimmune condition known to be exacerbated by peginterferon and ribavirin
- untreated thyroid disease
- pregnant or unwilling to comply with adequate contraception
- severe concurrent medical disease such as severe hypertension, heart failure, significant coronary heart disease, poorly controlled diabetes, chronic obstructive pulmonary disease
- age less than 2 years
- known hypersensitivity to drugs used to treat HCV

Source: with permission from Ghany *et al.*, 2009 [40].

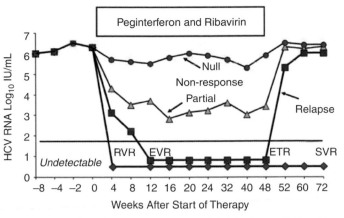

Figure 19.5 Virological responses to hepatitis C (HCV) infection. RVR, rapid virological response with clearance of HCV from serum by week 4 (as seen with a sensitive polymerase chain reaction-based assay); EVR, early virological response with a ≥2 log₁₀ IU/mL reduction in HCV RNA level compared with baseline HCV RNA, or HCV RNA negative at treatment week 12; SVR, sustained virological response, with HCV RNA negative 24 weeks after cessation of treatment; relapse, reappearance of HCV RNA in serum after therapy is discontinued; non-responder, failure to clear HCV RNA from serum after 24 weeks of therapy; partial non-responder, 2 log₁₀ IU/mL decrease in HCV RNA but still HCV RNA positive at week 24; null non-responder, failure to decrease HCV RNA by 2 log₁₀ IU/mL after 24 week of therapy. (With permission from Ghany *et al.*, 2009 [41].)

willingness, as well as drug tolerance, contraindications, and side effects.

Treated individuals should be carefully characterized by the virologic responses in the first 4–24 weeks (Figure 19.5), since recommended duration of therapy and likelihood of success are closely associated with these responses.

Standard therapy

In 2003 the US Food and Drug Administration (FDA) approved the combination of interferon and ribavirin for the treatment of CHC in children ages 3 to 17 years. Until recently, this was the only licensed treatment for children with HCV. Studies had demonstrated that response rates depended on genotype and viral load, as in adults. This was illustrated in a study of 118 children who had a 46% overall SVR rate [44].

Among children with genotype 1, the SVR rate was 48% in children who had viral levels ≤2 × 10⁶ copies/mL compared with 26% in those with >2 × 10⁶ copies/mL. Children with genotype 2 or 3 HCV had 84% SVR, and younger children had higher SVR rates than adolescents (57 versus 26%.) Similar findings had been described in an earlier smaller study.

There are now two large trials and several smaller ones that have addressed the use of pegylated interferon (peginterferon) as monotherapy or in combination with ribavirin in children. In an open-labeled, uncontrolled pilot study, 62 children and adolescents, 2–17 years of age (mean, 10.6), were treated with peginterferon-alfa2b and ribavirin for 48 weeks. The SVR rate was 59%. In 2008, the FDA approved combination therapy with peginterferon-alfa2b and ribavirin for use in children with HCV who were 3 years or older with compensated liver disease. This decision was supported by the results of a trial in which children with genotype 1 or 4, or genotype 3 with >0.6 × 10⁶ IU/mL HCV were treated for 48 weeks, and those with genotype 2, or genotype 3 with <0.6 × 10⁶ IU/mL for 24 weeks [45]. The SVR rate was 55%, in the first group and 96% in the second.

A randomized trial of peginterferon-alfa2a with or without ribavirin in children 5–17 years of age has demonstrated the superiority of combination therapy in children, with an SVR of 53% in children who received combination therapy compared with 21% in those who received monotherapy [46]. The difference was significant for both genotype 1 and non-genotype 1 infections. Analysis of the pretreatment liver biopsies in this cohort had reaffirmed the generally mild histologic disease during childhood, but instances of marked fibrosis and even cirrhosis were observed [35].

In both of these trials, peginterferon and ribavirin were generally well tolerated in these young subjects. Side effects were similar to those observed in adults, although weight loss and changes in linear growth velocity are of particular importance in children. In the peginterferon-alfa2b trial, weight loss and growth inhibition were common. In addition, 3% were treated for clinical hypothyroidism. In the peginterferon-alfa2a trial, dose reductions and early discontinuation were needed in 51% and 4%, respectively, primarily for neutropenia.

Given these considerations, peginterferon in combination with ribavirin has supplanted older therapies for children with CHC who are considered to be appropriate candidates for treatment. There are no published consensus statements or guidelines for treatment of HCV-infected children, and treatment decisions may vary with the child's age and individual disease characteristics. Examination of a liver biopsy may not be a prerequisite for treatment. It is rare to find advanced histology in young children, and the response rates of children with genotype 2 or 3 HCV are so high that baseline biopsies may provide little information regarding either likelihood of response or long-term prognosis. Exceptions are children whose parents want to know the stage of disease in considering treatment, and those with comorbid diseases in whom the results of a biopsy might influence the decision to treat. In genotype 1 infections, particularly in older children, biopsy information might be useful, since the SVR rate is not as high, and those with mild histologic changes may choose to wait for the availability of newer, more effective therapies.

Children as young as 3 years may be considered candidates for combination therapy. Decisions regarding timing of therapy are influenced by disease factors, such as degree of hepatic inflammation and fibrosis, the presence of comorbid diseases, and psychosocial factors such as school and athletic activities, family stability, availability for support, and participation in high-risk behaviors such as intravenous drug use. Treatment might be more strongly advocated for children with perinatally acquired HCV who are older than 10 years, those with at least moderate hepatic fibrosis, and in those with a comorbid disease or other features that raise concern for rapid progression. Just as in adults, obesity and insulin resistance might need to be addressed prior to HCV treatment in children, since these factors are likely to decrease the likelihood of an SVR in children [47].

Peginterferon-alfa2b ($60 \mu g/m^2$ once weekly) has been approved by the FDA for use in children 3 years and older, in combination with ribavirin (15 mg/kg daily in two divided doses). Although the peginterferon-alfa2b is most commonly available in standardized doses in a multidose injection device (PEG-Intron RediPen, Schering Plough, Kenilworth, NJ, USA), this may not be feasible to use in the smallest children. Doses may be individualized using typical vials of the drug. Ribavirin is available in an oral suspension at 40 mg/mL (Rebetol, Schering Plough) to allow for accurate dosing and adjustments. Peginterferon-alfa2a ($180 \mu g/1.73 m^2$ weekly) can also be used in combination with ribavirin; this type of interferon is approved for use in children 5 years of age and older. Peginterferon and ribavirin should be given for 24 weeks for genotype 2 and 3, and 48 weeks for genotype 1. There are insufficient data regarding other genotypes, although the longer course of therapy could be considered for genotype 4 infections, extrapolating from adult data. There are no data using a slow early virologic response (fall of at least 2 log IU/mL from baseline but not to undetectable at week 12) to substantiate the provision of 72 weeks of treatment in children with genotype 1 HCV. Once again, a case could be made for extrapolating from these recommendations in adults.

In both adults and children, clinical and laboratory adverse effects from interferon therapy are common, and appropriate monitoring is necessary. Quantitative differences in the frequency of adverse effects between interferon and peginterferon are not substantial, but the weekly administration of peginterferon does limit the fluxes in symptoms and generally limits the degree of fever, anorexia, and general flu-like symptoms. In most studies, 100% of subjects will have some adverse effects of the medication, but 80% of these are mild or moderate in severity, and generally fall into the category of "flu-like symptoms" (headache, fever, anorexia, abdominal pain, vomiting, nausea, myalgia). Such symptoms usually abate with continuing treatment and rarely warrant dose change or treatment cessation. Rarely, the interferon dosage will need to be decreased or therapy discontinued if the symptoms become intolerable. More significant adverse events occur in approximately 20–23% of subjects and include depression, irritability, alopecia, the development of autoantibodies (anti-liver, anti-thyroid), and some laboratory changes.

The development of thyroid disease is well described to be associated with both CHC and its treatment with interferon. Although studies report variable rates in children, cases of at least transient hypothyroidism are encountered in most large pediatric treatment trials. Monitoring every 3 months for thyroxine and thyroid-stimulating hormone levels is advisable, since early identification of thyroid function abnormalities allows appropriate referral and therapy in a timely fashion.

Molecular mimicry between CYP2D6 and the HCV antigens is thought to lead to viral–self immunological cross-reactivity in some subjects with CHC, leading to expression of anti-liver–kidney microsomal antibody. The presence of this autoantibody appears to be associated with an elevation in serum aminotransferases (flares) during interferon therapy, requiring prednisone treatment and potential cessation of the antiviral therapy. However, this is no longer felt to be a contraindication to antiviral therapy. Furthermore, patients with this autoantibody have similar rates of SVR as those without the antibody. Pretherapy evaluation for the presence of anti-liver–kidney microsomal antibody, and re-evaluation in the setting of a flare, should be considered.

Depression is a more common concern when treating adults; however, this should also be carefully considered and monitored for when treating children. In a large pediatric trial of 118 subjects treated with interferon-alfa/ribavirin, 15 (13%)

suffered depression during the study, 3 of these had suicidal ideation, and 1 made a suicidal attempt. Any child with a history of depression should be referred for evaluation and ongoing monitoring by a mental health professional during treatment with interferon. A history of suicidal ideation or attempt or untreated major depression should be considered a relative contraindication to treatment.

Anorexia leading to weight loss is encountered in 25–66% of subjects treated with interferons. Similarly, linear growth is impaired during treatment, but both weight and height trend back to baseline after cessation of the therapy. However, full recovery of the lost linear growth has not always been observed, at least in the short term. The Pediatric Study of Hepatitis C (PEDS-C) trial demonstrated that substantial decrements in height, weight, and body mass index (BMI) z-scores, and in percentage body fat, were observed during peginterferon-alfa2a therapy [46]. During follow-up, weight, BMI, and fat mass returned to baseline, whereas the height z-scores were still lower than baseline 24 and 48 weeks after the cessation of therapy.

Severe neurotoxicity in the form of spastic diplegia has been reported in infants treated with interferon-alfa. Although the mechanism of this neurotoxicity is not understood, the severity of the adverse effect is so significant that treatment of infants younger than 1 year should be avoided, and most pediatric hepatologists avoid the use of this medication in the first 2 years of life. Optic neuritis and retinopathies have also been observed sporadically in subjects treated with interferon-alfa, suggesting the importance of a baseline ophthalmological examination and examinations during therapy as clinically indicated.

The most common laboratory changes encountered with interferon-alfa or peginterferon therapy include neutropenia and thrombocytopenia. Serum aminotransferase elevations are less common. Significant neutropenia (absolute neutrophil count of 500–1000 cells/μL) occurs in 20–30% of treated individuals, usually within the first month of therapy. Thrombocytopenia is less common, with an acceptable threshold of 100×10^6 cells/μL. As these side effects are dose dependent, a dose reduction of 20–30% depending on the degree of cellular suppression, should be considered, with repeat laboratory analysis (weekly for peginterferon until stable) suggested. Dose adjustment without the need for treatment interruption in the setting of high compliance is generally not associated with a decrease in SVR. There are no data regarding the use of filgrastim in children who develop neutropenia in association with interferon use, although the rate of serious infection is low when the absolute neutrophil count is maintained above 500–1000 cells/μL.

Although ribavirin is associated with nausea, skin rash, cough, and shortness of breath, the most common side effect is a dose-dependent hemolytic anemia. Approximately 10% of patients experience a 1.4–1.5 g/dL decrease in hemoglobin concentration within the first 4–8 weeks of therapy, with fewer seeing a reduction to <10 g/dL. Dose adjustment is generally only considered when hemoglobin levels fall below 10 g/dL.

The use of exogenous erythropoietin has not been studied in children receiving ribavirin for CHC. Ribavirin has both teratogenic and embryotoxic effects in animal studies. Although the medication is known to be important to optimize the SVR after therapy, care must be taken in educating patients of child-bearing age as to the importance of using effective birth control while on this medication and for the 6 months after therapy. Pregnancy testing should be conducted frequently during treatment of adolescents of child-bearing potential.

It has been well demonstrated in adults that medication dose reductions and interruptions resulting in less than 80% of recommended doses are clearly associated with suboptimal responses. The success of treatment for CHC in children and adolescents is dependent not only on viral factors such as genotype and viral level and host factors such as age and histologic stage, but also on careful medical and psychosocial monitoring by the provider and medical support staff, and the availability of a supportive, engaged family. Anticipation and early intervention for side effects such as weight loss, fatigue, and behavioral changes can help to promote completion of recommended doses of these medications and ensure the highest likelihood of achieving SVR. There are no data regarding the use of hematopoietic growth factors in children receiving treatment for HCV, but most children tolerate some degree of anemia quite well, and although neutropenia was common in the clinical trials, significant infections were not observed. Interferon-associated thyroid dysfunction has been demonstrated in children, just as in adults. In one recent retrospective review, thyroid dysfunction was detected in 17% of children with HCV treated with either standard interferon or peginterferon [48]. It is prudent to monitor thyroid-stimulating hormone and promptly refer children who develop abnormalities for consideration of treatment, although it is transient in most instances.

The general management of children and adolescents with HCV infection includes more than just antiviral therapy (Table 19.3). Education about the infection, its natural history and modes of transmission, and risk factors for progression such as alcohol use, obesity, and other infections is critical to ensure optimal outcomes. In addition, the clinician can be of importance in reducing parental guilt regarding perinatal transmission and destigmatization in school and other social settings, as well as in provision of other health measures such as hepatitis A and B immunization and pregnancy prevention counseling and measures. It is also important to emphasize that children and adolescents with HCV can participate fully in school and extracurricular activities including sports without any more than the standard universal precautions that are already advocated for these settings [23].

Prognostic factors for response to therapy

The objective predictors of response to treatment in CHC include HCV RNA levels, HCV genotype, age (>40 or <40 years), and potentially BMI. Adults with a quantitative serum

Table 19.3 Counseling for hepatitis C (HCV) infection

Clinical aspect	Recommendation
To avoid transmission	HCV-infected people should avoid sharing toothbrushes and dental/shaving equipment and cover bleeding wounds
	Stop any illicit drug use; avoid sharing/reusing needles and syringes if continuing
	HCV-infected people should avoid donating blood, semen, or body tissues
	HCV-infected people should be counseled regarding sexual transmission; those in long-term relationships are at low risk for HCV transmission;[a] all others should use effective barrier methods
To minimize progressive liver disease	Assure vaccination against hepatitis A and hepatitis B viruses
	Avoid alcohol
	Minimize obesity
	In selected patients, targeted therapy for HCV will decrease risk for progressive liver disease

[a] Barrier methods can further lower risk even among individuals in long-term relationships.

HCV RNA $<1 \times 10^6$ copies/mL ($<2 \times 10^5$ IU/mL) achieve SVR with therapy more frequently than those with an elevated HCV RNA ($>5 \times 10^6$ copies/mL) [49]. Similarly, knowledge of the HCV genotype allows for better prediction of treatment response. The SVR rates to peginterferon/interferon and ribavirin treatment for genotype 2 and 3 are 60 and 80%, respectively, compared with 50% for genotype 1. Furthermore, in adults, treatment with peginterferon plus ribavirin appears to be required for only 6 months for genotype 2 or genotype 3, but for 12 months for genotype 1. Based on these findings the peginterferons are approved in children for 48 weeks for genotype 1 and 24 weeks for genotype 2 and genotype 3 infections.

The influences of gender and BMI on CHC and the response to treatment are somewhat controversial. In adults, women have milder disease and slower progression compared with men, overall. Confounding variables, such as alcohol consumption, have made this analysis complex. Similarly, some investigators have found increased treatment response among women compared with men but this finding is not consistently observed. The influence of BMI on treatment response has been demonstrated [34], with most studies detecting an improved SVR rate among adults with a BMI <28 in comparison with those with higher BMI, but this is not a universal finding. An effect of baseline BMI on response to treatment of HCV in children has recently been described; each increase of 1 unit in BMI z-score (1SD) was associated with a 12% decrease in likelihood of SVR [47]. The mechanism by which BMI could influence viral response to therapy is not yet fully understood, although the relative increase in hepatic steatosis with increased BMI and hence increase in insulin resistance could play a significant role in this pathogenesis; it is recognized that hyperinsulinemia is associated with increased genotype 1 HCV replication and poorer treatment response.

Viral kinetics during treatment may change outcomes, and there are some data to support changes in duration of peginterferon/interferon and ribavirin therapy based on early virologic responses (EVR) [50]. The EVR, defined as clearance of viremia even prior to 12 weeks, may allow prediction of SVR, and hence determination of those for whom ongoing therapy is futile. For example, the lack of an EVR at 8 weeks predicts failure of SVR better than analysis at 4 weeks of therapy (rapid virologic response (RVR)), but waiting until 12 weeks of therapy, the current standard EVR for adult treatment, may not be necessary [51]. In pediatrics, similar findings are being observed. Viral response analysis during the PEDS-C trial showed that for those patients who achieved RVR, 100% had a SVR [46]. The EVR predicted SVR in 94% of the peginterferon-alfa2a/ribavirin-treated group and 40% of the peginterferon-alfa2a/placebo-treated subjects. Similarly, 72% of subjects with EVR, but none with a $<2 \log_{10}$ IU/mL fall at 12 weeks, had SVR [52]. Many studies have observed that some children (7–14%) who do have RNA titer declines, but not to the magnitude to meet EVR definition, still achieve SVR. However, SVR is very unlikely in children with detectable RNA after 24 weeks of therapy; consequently, the current recommendation is to stop therapy if HCV RNA is detectable at 24 weeks. It is important to recognize that these predictors of response have been developed for the combination of peginterferon and ribavirin; stopping (for futility) rules will differ as new drug regimens are introduced (see below).

In 2009, it was discovered that SNPs located near *IL28B* were strongly associated with a likelihood of achieving SVR with peginterferon and ribavirin treatment [9]. The gene product IL-28B activates the same intracellular pathway as IFNα, so that many of the same interferon-stimulated genes are expressed. A particular polymorphism on chromosome 19, rs12979860, was found to be strongly associated with SVR in a number of different adult groups. Patients of European, African-American, and Hispanic ancestries with the CC genotype have a two-fold greater rate of SVR than those with the TT genotype. Heterozygotes have intermediate response rates (Figure 19.6). The effect of this polymorphism was as strong as, or stronger than, that of other host factors, such as baseline fibrosis. The C variant of this allele is most frequently present in individuals from East Asia and least common in those of African origin, and this difference has been calculated to explain approximately half of the difference that had been noted in populations according to race. *IL28B* was sequenced

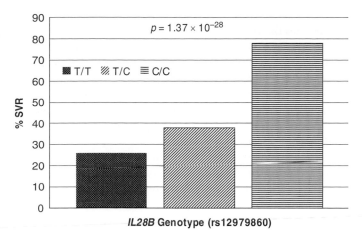

Figure 19.6 Percentage of sustained virological response (SVR) by genotypes of rs12979860 overall (combining racial and ethnic groups). (Adapted from Ge et al., 2009 [9].)

in a subset of these individuals, and two variants were highly associated with rs12979860: rs28416813 and a SNP rs8103142. There was such a high degree of correlation among the three SNPs that tests for independence, even using a large cohort of patients, were not able to resolve which is responsible for the association with SVR.

There is a minor *IL28B* allele, rs8099917, which has been associated with progression to CHC and also with lower likelihood of response to therapy. This allele has been identified in 24% of individuals with spontaneous HCV clearance, 32% of patients with CHC who responded to therapy, and 58% who did not respond [53].

It has become clear from numerous subsequent studies that host *IL28B* genotype has a profound effect on outcome of treatment, and this could be incorporated into future therapeutic trials and even, perhaps, into routine management of HCV-infected patients as testing for *IL28B* genotype has become more widely available. However, *IL28B* genotype has not yet been evaluated as a predictor of response in the pediatric population.

Other predictors of response to therapy, such as vitamin D levels and vitamin D receptor polymorphisms [54], as well as baseline proteomic profiling [55], have also recently been identified and may eventually assist in formulating individual response patterns that will more clearly define optimal types and duration of treatment.

New therapies: direct acting antiviral drugs

Studies suggest that HCV modulation of IFN induction and signaling attenuates the expression of IFN-stimulated genes, allowing HCV to escape the antiviral actions of the host response. All of the HCV enzymes are essential for HCV replication and are, therefore, potential targets for drugs. Knowledge of the structures of the NS3 protease and NS5B polymerase has allowed structure-based drug design, leading

to the development of inhibitors of these enzymes. New drug therapies, such as protease and polymerase inhibitors, designated direct-acting antiviral agents (DAAs), are under development. Inhibitors of the serine protease NS3/4A, telaprevir or boceprevir, when added to the current standard of care regimen in patients with HCV genotype 1 are associated with significantly higher SVR rates than the dual therapy of peginterferon and ribavirin. When these agents are administered as monotherapy, resistant viral variants develop rapidly. These agents have recently been licensed by the FDA for use in adults with genotype 1 HCV in combination with peginterferon and ribavirin. However, the drugs are metabolized by the cytochrome P450 system and so have important clinically significant drug interactions with inducers of that system or other agents cleared by CYP3A4/5. This may be of particular relevance to the HIV-coinfected population.

An important concept with regard to using a DAA in combination with peginterferon and ribavirin is that of response-guided therapy, in which duration of treatment is determined by early virologic responses and host *IL28B* genotype [56]. Although the same in principle, response-guided therapy with DAAs differ from those used with peginterferon and ribavirin alone. In general, response-guided therapy with DAAs is directed at non-cirrhotic patients, particularly those who are treatment naive. Specific recommendations for the use of boceprevir or telaprevir in adults with genotype 1 HCV infections have recently been incorporated into published practice guidelines [57]. Boceprevir and telaprevir may undergo pharmacokinetic and efficacy trials in children with CHC involving genotype 1.

Because of the frequent side effects and discomfort from injection, a particularly appealing treatment would be an interferon-sparing regimen that relied solely on DAA combinations. Therefore, the identification of new molecules with different mechanisms of action, having additive or synergistic effects, is an ongoing process. The goals for a DAA combination are to increase antiviral efficacy, minimize the emergence of resistance, and limit side effects. The first study of a combination of DAAs in patients was the proof-of-concept INFORM-1 study. In this randomized, placebo-controlled, double-blind trial, 87 patients with HCV genotype 1 infection were randomized to receive up to 13 days of either oral combination therapy with danoprevir (RG7227), a NS3/4A protease inhibitor, plus mericitabine (RG7128), a nucleoside polymerase inhibitor, or with matched placebo. The median reduction in HCV RNA from the baseline was $5 \log_{10}$ IU/mL, which fell below the level of detection in 88% of the patients who received the highest dose of both drugs [58]. No evidence of resistance to either compound was observed during the study and no serious adverse events were reported. The antiviral efficacy was similar in treatment-naive and treatment-experienced patients, including non-responders. Evaluation of this combination on later end-points is ongoing.

The development of HCV antiviral drugs has focused on targeting viral proteins with known enzymatic activities, such as the proteases or polymerase. However, researchers at Bristol-Myers Squibb have reported that a compound BMS-790052 with a new mechanism of action led to dramatic reductions in viral load and produced few side effects in a phase I clinical study. This compound targets NS5A, which possesses no enzymatic activity but plays a critical role in regulating viral replication and host cell interactions. Although the function of HCV NS5A is still poorly understood, the researchers have shown that small molecules targeting this protein are potent inhibitors of viral replication. Although preliminary, these data indicate that inhibitors of HCV NS5A offer considerable promise for the treatment of HCV infection. Another viral component, the p7 ion channel, can be specifically inhibited by different drugs, suggesting that this protein may be an additional target for future antiviral chemotherapy [59].

Once new DAAs become available, treatment strategies that combine several drugs with different mechanisms of action could hopefully result in interferon- and/or ribavirin-sparing regimens. Ongoing studies are directed toward demonstrating that such combinations of DAAs have synergistic antiviral potency, a low risk of resistance, and a good safety profile.

Prevention

Prevention of new HCV infections in older children requires education of preadolescents and adolescents about high-risk behaviors. Although commercial body piercing and tattooing are not clearly associated with risk, self-tattooing and self-piercing with shared needles are fairly common practices. Transmission of infection by intravenous drug use, sharing straws or other implements for intranasal cocaine administration, and the risk from sexual transmission, albeit low, may not be appreciated by teenagers.

The primary target for prevention strategies should be perinatal transmission. At the present time, universal testing of pregnant women for HCV infection is not recommended. However, if interruption of perinatal transmission can be achieved with avoidance of fetal scalp monitors and/or the selective use of cesarean delivery when the duration of amniotic membrane rupture approaches 6 hours, then identification of infected women before delivery will be a clearly indicated strategy. This is an important area of study, since major changes may become necessary in the obstetric care of infected women. Postexposure prophylaxis with immunoglobulin is not recommended for infants born to HCV-infected women. In the absence of clear data implicating breast-feeding as a means of HCV transmission, this is not considered contraindicated. There are at present no safe measures to decrease maternal HCV viremia at delivery, since currently available treatments such as interferon and ribavirin are considered contraindicated during pregnancy.

Vaccine development has been slow and difficult and HCV has been demonstrated to evade both antibody-mediated and cellular immune responses. The approaches to vaccine development have included recombinant E1 and E2 proteins, synthetic peptides, DNA, and other strategies. However, these have been largely unsuccessful for a variety of reasons. As yet, none of the products tested has been effective at inducing the appropriate neutralizing antibodies, or the CD8, CD4, and cytotoxic T-cell responses that seem to be required to provide protective immunity [60].

References

1. Brass V, Moradpour D, Blum HE. Molecular virology of hepatitis C virus (HCV): 2006 Update. *Int J Med Sci* 2006;**3**:29–34.

2. Lauer GM, Walker BD. Medical progress: hepatitis C virus infection. *N Engl J Med* 2001;**345**:41–52.

3. Enomoto N, Sakuma I, Asahina Y, *et al.* Mutations in the nonstructural protein 5A gene and response to interferon in patients with chronic hepatitis C virus 1b infection. *N Engl J Med* 1996;**334**:77–81.

4. Murakami T, Enomoto N, Kurosaki M, Izumi N, Marumo F, Sato C. Mutations in nonstructural protein 5A gene and response to interferon in hepatitis C virus genotype 2 infection. *Hepatology* 1999;**30**:1045–1053.

5. Watanabe H, Enomoto N, Nagayama K, *et al.* Number and position of mutations in the interferon (IFN) sensitivity-determining region of the gene for nonstructural protein 5a correlate with ifn efficacy in hepatitis c virus genotype 1b infection. *J Infect Dis* 2001;**183**:1195–1203.

6. Witherell GW, Beineke P. Statistical analysis of combined substitutions in nonstructural 5A region of hepatitis C virus and interferon response. *J Med Virol* 2001;**63**:8–16.

7. Pileri P, Uematsu Y, Campagnoli S, *et al.* Binding of hepatitis C virus to CD81. *Science* 1998;**282**(5390):938–941.

8. Ciuffreda D, Kim AY. Update on hepatitis C virus-specific immunity. *Curr Opin HIV AIDS* 2011;**6**:559–565.

9. Ge D, Fellay J, Thompson AJ, *et al.* Genetic variation in IL28B predicts hepatitis C treatment-induced viral clearance. *Nature* 2009;**461**:399–401.

10. Thomas DL, Thio CL, Martin MP, *et al.* Genetic variation in IL28B and spontaneous clearance of hepatitis C virus. *Nature* 2009;**461**(7265): 798–801.

11. Centers for Disease Control and Prevention. Viral Hepatitis Statistics and Surveillance. Atlanta, GA: Centers for Disease Control and Prevention, 2009 (http://www.cdc.gov/hepatitis/ Statistics/, accessed 22 July 2013).

12. Centers for Disease Control and Prevention. Hepatitis C virus infection among adolescents and young adults - Massachusetts, 2002–2009. *MMWR Morb Mortal Wkly Rep* 2011;**60**: 539–541.

13. Bresee JS, Mast EE, Coleman PJ, *et al.* Hepatitis C virus infection associated with administration of intravenous immunoglobulin. *JAMA* 1996;**276**:1563–1567.

14. Fischer GE, Schaefer MK, Labus BJ, *et al.* Hepatitis C virus infections from unsafe injection practices at an

endoscopy clinic in Las Vegas, Nevada, 2007–2008. *Clinical Infectious Disease.* 2010;**51**:267–273.

15. Centers for Disease Control and Prevention. Sexual transmission of hepatitis C virus among HIV-infected men who have sex with men: New York City, 2005–2010. *MMWR Morb Mortal Wkly Rep* 2011;**60**:945–950.

16. Delgado-Borrego A, Smith LJ, Jonas MM, *et al.* The underdiagnosis of pediatric hepatitis C: an emerging health care issue in Florida. *Gastroenterology* 2010;**138**:S779.

17. Yeung LTF, King SM, Roberts EA. Mother-to-infant transmission of hepatitis C virus. *Hepatology* 2001;**34**:223–229.

18. Conte D, Fraquelli M, Prati D, Coluci A, Minola E. Prevalence and clinical course of chronic hepatitis C virus (HCV) infection and rate of HCV vertical transmission in a cohort of 15 250 pregnant women. *Hepatology* 2000;**31**:751–755.

19. Resti M, Azzari C, Mannelli F, *et al.* Mother to child transmission of hepatitis C virus: prospective study of risk factors and timing of infection in children born to women seronegative for HIV-1. *BMJ* 1998;**317**:437–441.

20. Gibb DM, Goodall RL, Dunn DT, *et al.* Mother-to-child transmission of hepatitis C virus: evidence for preventable peripartum transmission. *Lancet* 2000;**356**:904–907.

21. Mast EE, Hwang L-Y, Seto D, Nolte FS, Kelly MG, Alter MJ. Perinatal hepatitis C virus transmission: maternal risk factors and optimal timing of diagnosis. *Hepatology* 1999;**30**:499A.

22. National Institutes of Health. National Institutes of Health Consensus Development Conference statement: management of hepatitis C. *Hepatology* 2002;**36**(5 suppl 1):S3–S20.

23. American Academy of Pediatrics. Hepatitis C. In Pickering LK (ed.) *Red Book: 2009*. Report of the Committee on Infectious Diseases. Elk Grove Village, IL: American Academy of Pediatrics, 2009, pp. 357–360.

24. Ruiz-Extremera Á, Muñoz-Gámez JA, Salmerón-Ruiz MA, *et al.* Genetic variation in interleukin 28B with respect to vertical transmission of hepatitis C virus and spontaneous clearance in HCV-infected children. *Hepatology* 2011;**53**:1830–1838.

25. Sherman KE, Rouster SD, Chung RT, Rajicic N. Hepatitis C virus prevalence among patients infected with human immunodeficiency virus: a cross-sectional analysis of the US adults AIDS Clinical Trials Group. *Clin Infect Dis* 2002;**34**:831–837.

26. Mallet V, Vallet-Pichard A, Pol S. The impact of human immunodeficiency virus on viral hepatitis. *Liver Int* 2011;**31**:135–139.

27. Weber R, Sabin CA, Friis-Moller N, *et al.* Liver-related deaths in persons infected with the human immunodeficiency virus: the D:A:D study. *Arch Int Med* 2006;**166**:1632–1641.

28. Badizadegan K, Jonas MM, Ott MJ, Nelson SP, Perez-Atayde AR. Histopathology of the liver in children with chronic hepatitis C viral infection. *Hepatology* 1998;**28**:1416–1423.

29. Guido M, Bortolotti F, Leandro G, *et al.* Fibrosis in chronic hepatitis C acquired in infancy: is it only a matter of time? *Am J Gastroenterol* 2004;**98**:660–663.

30. Jara P, Resti M, Hierro L, *et al.* Chronic hepatitis C virus infection in childhood: clinical patterns and evolution in 224 white children. *Clin Infect Dis* 2003;**36**:275–280.

31. Bortolotti F, Verucchi G, Cammà C, *et al.* Long-term course of chronic hepatitis C in children: from viral clearance to end-stage liver disease. *Gastroenterology* 2008;**134**:1900–1907.

32. Cesaro S, Bortolotti F, Petris MG, Brugiolo A, Guido M, Carli M. An updated follow-up of chronic hepatitis C after three decades of observation in pediatric patients cured of malignancy. *Pediatr Blood Cancer* 2010;**55**:108–112.

33. Strickland DK, Riely CA, Patrick CC, *et al.* Hepatitis C infection among survivors of childhood cancer. *Blood* 2000;**95**:3065–3070.

34. Sanyal AJ. Role of insulin resistance and hepatic steatosis in the progression of fibrosis and response to treatment in hepatitis C. *Liver Int* 2011;**31**:23–28.

35. Goodman ZD, Makhlouf HR, Liu L, *et al.* Pathology of chronic hepatitis C in children: liver biopsy findings in the Peds-C Trial. *Hepatology* 2008;**47**:836–843.

36. González-Peralta R, Langham MR Jr., Andres JM, *et al.* Hepatocellular carcinoma in 2 young adolescents with chronic hepatitis C. *J Pediatr Gastroenterol Nutr* 2009;**48**:630–635.

37. Rodrigue JR, Balistreri WF, Haber B, *et al.* Impact of hepatitis C virus infection on children and their caregivers: quality of life, cognitive, and emotional outcomes. *J Pediatr Gastroenterol Nutr* 2009;**48**:341–347.

38. Hartridge-Lambert SK, Stein EM, Markowitz AJ, Portlock CS. Hepatitis C and non-Hodgkin lymphoma: the clinical perspective. *Hepatology* 2011: epub November 2011 DOI 10.1002/hep.25499.

39. Kage M, Fujisawa T, Shiraki K, *et al.* Pathology of chronic hepatitis C in children. *Hepatology* 1997;**26**:771–775.

40. Guido M, Rugge M, Jara P, *et al.* Chronic hepatitis C in children: the pathological and clinical spectrum. *Gastroenterology* 1998;**115**:1525–1529.

41. Ghany MG, Strader DB, Thomas DL, Seeff LB. Diagnosis, management, and treatment of hepatitis C: an update (AASLD Practice Guideline). *Hepatology* 2009;**49**:1335–1374.

42. Nelson DR, Davis GL, Jacobson IM, *et al.* Hepatitis C virus: a critical appraisal of approaches to therapy. *Clin Gastroenterol Hepatol* 2009;**7**:397–414.

43. Alberti A. Impact of a sustained virological response on the long-term outcome of hepatitis C. *Liver Int* 2011;**31**:18–22.

44. González-Peralta R, Kelly DA, Haber B, *et al.* Interferon alfa-2b in combination with ribavirin for the treatment of chronic hepatitis C in children: efficacy, safety, and pharmacokinetics. *Hepatology* 2005;**42**:1010–1018.

45. Wirth S, Ribes-Koninckx C, Calzado MA, *et al.* High sustained virologic response rates in children with chronic hepatitis C receiving peginterferon alfa-2b plus ribavirin. *J Hepatol* 2010;**52**:501–507.

46. Schwarz KB, Gonzalez-Peralta RP, Murray KF, *et al.* The combination of ribavirin and peginterferon is superior to peginterferon and placebo for children and adolescents with chronic hepatitis C. *Gastroenterology* 2011;**140**:450–458.

47. Delgado-Borrego A, Healey D, Negre B, *et al.* Influence of body mass index on outcome of pediatric chronic hepatitis C virus infection. *J Pediatr Gastroenterol Nutr* 2010;**51**:191–197.

48. Raghunaathan KDR, Galacki DM, Quan J, Mitchell PD, Jonas MM. Prevalence and characterization of thyroid abnormalities in children and young adults treated with combination therapy for chronic hepatitis C at a single center. *Gastroenterology* 2009;**136** (Suppl 1):A808.

49. Martinot-Peignoux M, Marcellin P, Pouteau M, *et al.* Pretreatment serum hepatitis C virus RNA levels and hepatitis C genotype are the main and independent prognostic factors of sustained response to interferon alfa therapy in chronic hepatitis C. *Hepatology* 1995;**22**:1050–1056.

50. Davis GL, Wong JB, McHutchison JG, *et al.* Early virologic response to treatment with peginterferon alfa-2b plus ribavirin in patients with chronic hepatitis C. *Hepatology* 2003;**38**:645–652.

51. Fried MW, Hadziyannis SJ, Shiffman ML, Messinger D, Zeuzem S. Rapid virological response is the most important predictor of sustained virological response across genotypes in patients with chronic hepatitis C virus infection. *J Hepatol* 2011;**55**:69–75.

52. Jara P, Hierro L, de la Vega A, *et al.* Efficacy and safety of peginterferon-alfa2b and ribavirin combination therapy in children with chronic hepatitis C infection. *Pediatr Infect Dis J* 2008;**28**:1–7.

53. Rauch A, Kutalik Z, Descombes P, *et al.* Genetic variation in *IL28B* is associated with chronic hepatitis C and treatment failure: a genome-wide association study. *Gastroenterology* 2010;**138**:1338–1345.

54. Petta S, Camma C, Scazzone C, *et al.* Low serum vitamin D serum level is related to severe fibrosis and low responsiveness to interferon-based therapy in genotype 2 chronic hepatitis C. *Hepatology* 2010;**51**:1158–1167.

55. Patel K, Lucas JE, Thompson JW, *et al.* High predictive accuracy of an unbiased proteomic profile for sustained virologic response in chronic hepatitis C patients. *Hepatology* 2011;**53**:1809–1818.

56. Clark PJ, Thompson AJ, McHutchison JG. IL28B genomic-based treatment paradigms for patients with chronic hepatitis C infection: the future of personalized HCV therapies. *Am J Gastroenterol* 2011;**106**:38–45.

57. Ghany MG, Nelson DR, Strader DB, Thomas DL, Seeff LB. An update on treatment of genotype 1 chronic hepatitis C virus infection: 2011 Practice Guideline by the American Association for the Study of Liver Diseases. *Hepatology* 2011;**54**:1433–1444.

58. Gane EJ, Roberts SK, Stedman CA, *et al.* Combination therapy with a nucleoside polymerase (R7128) and protease (R7227/ITMN-191) inhibitor in HCV: safety, pharmacokinetics, and virologic results from INFORM-1. *Hepatology* 2009;**50** (Suppl):394A–395A.

59. Khaliq S, Jahan S, Hassan S. Hepatitis C virus p7: molecular function and importance in hepatitis C virus life cycle and potential antiviral target. *Liver Int* 2011;**31**:606–617.

60. Torresi J, Johnson D, Wedemeyer H. Progress in the development of preventive and therapeutic vaccines for hepatitis C virus. *J Hepatol* 2011;**54**:1273–1285.

Autoimmune hepatitis

Nanda Kerkar and Cara L. Mack

Introduction

Autoimmune hepatitis (AIH) is a progressive inflammatory disorder of unknown etiology, characterized histologically by interface hepatitis, serologically by the presence of non-organ specific autoantibodies, biochemically by elevated amino-transferases and serum IgG, and clinically by response to immunosuppressive treatment in the absence of other known causes of liver disease [1].

The spectrum of chronic inflammatory diseases of the liver extends from acute hepatitis to chronic hepatitis and finally to cirrhosis. In 1950, Waldenstrom described a form of chronic hepatitis occurring predominantly in young women with arthralgias, myalgia, hepatosplenomegaly, amenorrhea, skin rashes, fluctuating course, and invariably fatal outcome [2]. The term "lupoid" hepatitis was coined after the detection of anti-nuclear antibodies (ANAs), the then positive test for lupus erythematosus in some of these individuals. The identification of anti-smooth muscle antibody (ASMA) in 1966 led to the nomenclature of "autoimmune chronic active hepatitis" for the first time, in order to distinguish it from systemic lupus erythematosus [3]. The discovery of hepatitis A and B viruses allowed hepatitis caused by these viruses to be excluded. Histologically, the term "chronic persistent hepatitis" was used when the mononuclear inflammation was limited to the portal tracts, while the term "chronic active hepatitis" was used to characterize infiltration of the adjacent hepatic parenchyma (piecemeal necrosis) [4]. Widespread acceptance of the autoimmune basis of this condition was accepted only after controlled trials demonstrated response to immunosuppression and a link with human leukocyte antigens (HLA) HLA-B8 and HLA-DR3 was established. The discovery of hepatitis C virus in 1989 led a panel of international experts, the International Autoimmune Hepatitis Group (IAIHG), to formulate several recommendations regarding the diagnosis and classification of AIH. The IAIHG developed a scoring system to weigh each clinical, laboratory, and histological finding at presentation as well as the response to corticosteroid therapy [5].

Epidemiology

Autoimmune hepatitis is regarded as an important paradigm for the study of autoimmunity and is an important etiology of chronic hepatitis affecting both children and adults. The disease is seen in all ethnic groups and ages with a female preponderance. There is scarce epidemiological data on AIH. The reported prevalence ranges from 1.9 cases per 100 000 in Norway and 1 per 200 000 in the US general population to 20 per 100 000 in females over 14 years of age in Spain [1]. Approximately 20% of patients with chronic hepatitis among the Caucasian population of North America and West Europe have AIH. There is a significant association with the alleles *HLA-DR3* and *HLA-DR4* amongst affected patients. In Asia and Africa, the incidence of viral hepatitis secondary to hepatitis B and C viral infections is extremely high and, therefore, the proportion of chronic hepatitis secondary to AIH is much lower than in the West. In Japan, *HLA-DR4* allele is associated with AIH, in contrast to *HLA-DR3* in western countries. Extrahepatic autoimmune syndromes such as autoimmune thyroiditis, vitiligo, rheumatoid arthritis, and inflammatory bowel disease may be associated with AIH. Autoimmune hepatitis is classified into subtypes based on the presence of circulating autoantibodies: type 1 is characterized by the presence of ANA and/or ASMA and type 2 by the presence of anti-liver–kidney microsomal antibody (ALKM) or liver cytosol type 1 antibody (LC-1). The ratio of incidence of AIH type 1 and type 2 in North and South America and Japan is 6–7:1 while it is 1.5:1 in Europe and Canada. A third subtype has been designated based on the presence of autoantibodies against soluble liver antigen/liver–pancreas antigen (SLA/LP), but existence of this subtype has been a matter of debate. The presence of anti-SLA may signify a more severe form of AIH.

Pathogenesis

Liver injury in AIH occurs through uncontrolled cellular (T-cell) and humoral (B-cell) autoimmune responses targeting hepatocytes. The trigger of this autoimmune phenomenon is

Liver Disease in Children, Fourth Edition, ed. Frederick J. Suchy, Ronald J. Sokol, and William F. Balistreri. Published by Cambridge University Press. © Cambridge University Press 2014.

Table 20.1 Autoantibodies and target autoantigens in autoimmune hepatitis

Autoantibody	Autoantigen(s)
Anti-nuclear antibody (ANA)	Single-stranded/double-stranded DNA, histones, centromere
Anti-smooth muscle antibody (ASMA)	Actin, vimentin, desmin
Anti-liver–kidney microsomal antibody (ALKM)	Cytochrome P450 IID6 (CYP2D6)
Anti-soluble liver antigen/liver–pancreas antigen (anti-SLA/LP)	UGA serine transfer RNA-associated protein
Liver cytosol type 1 antibody (LC-1)	Formiminotransferase cyclodeaminase
Perinuclear anti-neutrophil cytoplasmic antibody (pANCA)	Nuclear lamina proteins
Asialoglycoprotein receptor antibody (ASGP-R)	Asialoglycoprotein receptor

not known and a leading hypothesis is that the hepatocyte injury is initiated by virus infection, followed by an abnormal autoimmune response in the genetically predisposed individual [6,7]. The identification of molecular mimicry between virus and hepatocyte proteins adds credence to this theory [8,9].

Cellular immunity

Autoimmune hepatitis occurs when there is loss of immune tolerance to hepatocyte proteins (or antigens). The inflammatory milieu within the diseased liver is composed of excessive T-lymphocytes, scattered macrophages, and plasma cells. The subsets of CD4 helper and CD8 cytotoxic T-cells are expanded and damage hepatocytes through production of proinflammatory cytokines (e.g. interferon-γ and tumor necrosis factor-α) or through granzyme-perforin mechanisms, respectively. Subsequent activation of effector cells such as macrophages and natural killer cells contributes to the ongoing hepatocyte injury [10]. Autoreactive T-cells specific to a limited number of "self" proteins have been identified and are thought to perpetuate the ongoing injury. Asialoglycoprotein receptor (ASGP-R) is expressed only in hepatocytes within the liver and is believed to be a major pathogenic antigen targeted by autoreactive T-cells. Other hepatocyte antigens that have been associated with activation of autoreactive T-cells include liver cytosolic antigen (formiminotransferase cyclodeaminase) and soluble liver antigen [11].

The ability of autoreactive T-cells to proliferate is controlled by the regulatory T-cell (Treg) subset that is characterized based on surface expression of CD4 and CD25 and nuclear expression of the forkhead transcription factor box P3. Diminished quantity and function of Tregs in patients with AIH have recently been described and this allows autoreactive T-cells to thrive and activate inflammatory responses [9,10]. A recent study in children with AIH found that quantitative deficiencies in Tregs inversely correlated with autoantibody titers. In addition, functional deficiencies of Tregs resulted in decreased ability to inhibit T-cell proliferation and interferon-γ production, resulting in increased hepatocyte injury [12].

Humoral immunity

Activation of B-cells and the subsequent generation of autoantibodies from plasma cells aids in defining AIH. A complete list of autoantibodies and the target autoantigens that have been discovered in AIH are outlined in Table 20.1. Autoantibodies function mainly as biomarkers of disease but in limited investigations have also been shown to contribute to antibody-dependent cell-mediated cytotoxicity of hepatocytes [9]. Type 1 AIH is associated with positive ANA and/or ASMA titers. However, ANA is the most non-specific autoantibody biomarker of AIH and can be positive in up to 15% of healthy people without autoimmune disease. In order to increase specificity of this antibody, serum titers of ≥1:80 are often used to define positivity. Because ASMA targets include many proteins within the cytoskeleton, like ANA, it is not specific to AIH and is found in other autoimmune diseases [6]. In AIH type 1, ANA and ASMA are both positive in approximately 50% of patients; ANA only positive occurs in 10–15% and ASMA only positive in 30–35%. The rate of autoantibody-negative AIH type 1 in well-characterized disease is <5%. Autoantibody levels vary during the course of disease and if the initial autoantibody screen is negative, repeat testing may allow for correct disease classification. Type 2 AIH is associated with ALKM-1, which are specific to the cytochrome P450 IID6 (CYP2D6) protein within the cytoplasm of hepatocytes and in proximal renal tubules [13]. Over 90% of patients with AIH type 2 are positive for ALKM-1. Approximately 50% of patients with AIH type 2 will also be positive for LC-1 but in 10% only LC-1 is detectable. The target of LC-1 is formiminotransferase cyclodeaminase, an enzyme involved in folate metabolism that is mainly expressed in the liver [14]. Levels of LC-1 correlate with disease severity (degree of hepatocyte injury, rapid progression to cirrhosis) and have been associated with other concurrent autoimmune diseases within patients [15]. An autoantibody may be present in both types of AIH, SLA/LP. The target of the anti-SLA/LP antibodies is a UGA serine transfer RNA-associated protein [13]. Anti-SLA is present in up to approximately 20% of AIH type 1 and 50% of AIH type 2; if present, it predicts a more severe course of disease. Presence of anti-SLA carries a diagnostic specificity of 99% for AIH [15]. Both types of AIH commonly have

ASGP-R (~75% of type 1 and ~40% of type 2) and this auto-antibody may be the only detectable one found in patients who are negative for the conventional autoantibodies. Elevated levels of anti-ASGP-R correlate with hepatocyte-targeted inflammation and may be a useful tool to monitor treatment efficacy [6]. Finally, perinuclear anti-neutrophil cytoplasmic antibodies (pANCA) have been identified in the majority of patients with AIH type 1 and are a heterogeneous group of antibodies that recognize a multitude of cytoplasmic proteins within neutrophils [13]. As pANCA has low specificity for AIH – it is also commonly found in primary sclerosing cholangitis (PSC) and viral hepatitis – it is not useful in the clinical setting for the diagnostic workup of AIH.

Genetic predisposition

The strongest association between genes and autoimmune diseases has been found within the *HLA* locus on the short arm of chromosome 6. Professional antigen-presenting cells (macrophages, dendritic cells, B-cells) contain HLA class II proteins (also known as major histocompatibility complex (MHC) class II) that form a complex with autoantigen(s) and present antigen to naive CD4 T-cells, leading to activation and differentiation of autoreactive T-cells. Certain HLA types are associated with AIH and increase the risk of developing disease. In the USA and Europe, the majority of adults with AIH type 1 express either *HLA-DRB1*0301* (encodes HLA-DR3) or *HLA-DRB1*0401* (HLA-DR4), or both [16]. *HLA-DRB1*0301* is also predominant in AIH type 2. Susceptibility to AIH type 2 is associated with expression of *HLA-DRB1*0701* (HLA-DR7) and *HLA-DRB1*0301*. Furthermore, *HLA-DRB1*0701* expression in AIH type 2 has been associated with a more severe form of disease [17].

Animal models of autoimmune hepatitis

Animal models of human diseases can be powerful tools in aiding understanding of disease pathogenesis and response to novel therapies. Various models have been employed to study AIH but to date no one model recapitulates all aspects of the human disease. Mouse models that affect hepatic tolerance include targeted gene deficiency (knockout mice) or autoantigen immunization strategies. Mice that are deficient in programmed death-1, a key molecule for maintenance of tolerance, and that were neonatally thymectomized to deplete Tregs, develop a severe hepatitis that mimics human AIH [18]. The hepatitis is associated with induction of ANAs, hepatic T-cell infiltrates, and lobular necrosis. This model demonstrated the significance of Tregs in disease, as replenishment of Tregs into these thymectomized mice rescued them from severe hepatitis. In another model, immunizing naive mice with supernatants from liver homogenate (autoantigen pool) resulted in experimental hepatitis that was strain dependent, suggesting genetic predisposition to disease. Adoptive transfer of activated T-cells from the diseased mice into naive recipients resulted in initiation of experimental hepatitis,

suggesting that effector T-cells play a direct pathogenic role in liver injury [18].

Based on the fact that a target autoantigen has been identified for AIH type 2, many investigators have focused on this type of AIH in order to study disease pathogenesis. One model entails immunizing mice with plasmids containing human *CYP2D6* (target of ALKM-1), human *FTCD* (target of anti-LC-1), mouse *Ctla4* (encoding cytotoxic T-lymphocyte antigen 4, which facilitates antigen uptake by antigen-presenting cells), and *Il12* (encoding interleukin-12, a Th1-skewing proinflammatory cytokine) [19]. When autoantigens and interleukin-12 were used to break tolerance, antigen-specific autoantibodies were detected, serum aminotransferases were mildly elevated, and an interface hepatitis composed of CD4 and CD8 T-cells and scattered plasma cells was observed. Another model of AIH type 2 used transgenic mice that express human CYP2D6 on hepatocytes [20]. Tolerance was broken with administration of an adenovirus-CYP2D6 vector and mice developed focal hepatocyte necrosis and a chronic hepatitis with fibrosis. The hepatic lesion was associated with a specific immune response to an immunodominant region of CYP2D6 and a cytotoxic T-cell response to adenovirus-CYP2D6-infected target cells. All of the models described above provide information on key players in the autoimmune response but none demonstrated the chronic remitting–relapsing nature of human AIH.

Diagnosis and scoring system

Diagnosis of AIH can be challenging as there is no single pathognomonic test. Early diagnosis and appropriate management is important as there is high mortality when AIH goes untreated. A significant proportion of "cryptogenic cirrhosis" is thought to be secondary to burnt out AIH and a proportion of acute liver failure of indeterminate origin is also thought to be autoimmune in origin. The original scoring system, although valuable in providing uniformity for allowing comparison of study populations in clinical trials, is cumbersome for routine clinical use. The points in the original scoring system developed by the IAIHG were assigned for "minimal" parameters including (1) female gender, (2) hepatitic biochemical profile, (3) hypergammaglobulinemia, (4) elevated autoantibody titers, (5) absence of viral hepatitis markers, (6) family history of autoimmunity, and (7) absence of drug or alcohol ingestion [5]. The "additional" parameters included (1) characteristic histology, (2) genetic factors, and (3) response to immunosuppression. A pretreatment "score" of 15 points had a sensitivity of 95%, a specificity of 97%, and a diagnostic accuracy of 67% [21]. Over the years in the course of validating the scoring system, several issues have been raised including accurate identification of antibodies, overlap with sclerosing cholangitis (SC), and specific issues pertaining to children, who largely do not imbibe alcohol or drugs nor develop primary biliary cirrhosis and where lower titer positivity of antibodies are thought to be significant. In 2008, the IAIHG

Table 20.2 Simplified diagnostic criteria for autoimmune hepatitis

Parameter	Score
Autoantibody[a]	
Anti-nuclear antibody or anti-smooth muscle antibody ≥1:40	1
Anti-nuclear antibody or smooth muscle antibody ≥1:80	2
Liver–kidney microsomal antibody ≥1:40	2
Anti-soluble liver antigen positive	2
Total serum IgG	
>ULN	1
≥1.1× ULN	2
Liver histology	
Compatible with autoimmune hepatitis: lymphocytic infiltrates, chronic hepatitis	1
Typical of autoimmune hepatitis:[b] interface hepatitis (portal tract lymphocytes and plasma cells infiltrating into parenchyma); emperipolesis;[c] hepatic rosette formation	2
Viral hepatitis absent	2
Pretreatment overall score	
Definite diagnosis	≥7
Probable diagnosis	≥6

ULN, upper limit of normal.
[a] Addition of points for all autoantibodies, maximum 2 points.
[b] Must have all three features to be considered "typical."
[c] Emperipolesis is active penetration by one cell into and through a larger cell
Source: adapted from Hennes *et al.*, 2008 [22].

used six routinely available measures including autoantibodies, total IgG, liver histology, and absence of viral hepatitis to develop a simplified scoring system (Table 20.2) [22]. A score of ≥7 points was deemed definite AIH and this simple score allowed differentiation between patients with and without AIH with a high degree of accuracy.

The overlap between AIH and SC has been controversial and several groups have used the scoring system to better delineate this group of patients. The scoring system was revised to improve exclusion of patients with biliary liver disease after it was found that more than one-third of patients with PSC fulfilled criteria for AIH. The modified scoring system was then applied to the original cohort of 114 patients with PSC and reanalysis showed that of the 38 originally classified as "probable," only 10 remained in this category, giving an overall specificity of 89.5% for exclusion of AIH in this group [23]. In pediatrics, the scoring system was applied retrospectively to 55 children with AIH or overlap syndrome with PSC [24]. Overall, 25 (89%) children with AIH as well as 15 of 23 (65%) with overlap syndrome were diagnosed as

having "definite" AIH postanalysis. The difference between the adult and pediatric studies may be because any patient with cholangiographic changes suggestive of SC was included in the adult study while only those with autoimmune markers and characteristic cholangiographic changes were included in the pediatric study. Another pediatric group modified the scoring system by removing alcohol as a diagnostic criteria and substituting gamma-glutamyltransferase for alkaline phosphatase as the latter is affected by bone growth, allowing improved categorization of the overlap group [25,26].

Clinical features

Children with AIH often present before puberty and those with AIH type 2 usually present at a very young age. There is a variable mode of presentation, ranging from being asymptomatic, and diagnosed after an incidental finding of elevated aminotransferases, to a presentation with fulminant liver failure. In more than one-third of the children, presentation can be indistinguishable from that of an acute viral hepatitis, with non-specific symptoms of malaise, anorexia, nausea, vomiting, or abdominal pain, followed by the onset of jaundice. A small percentage may present with acute liver failure, with an international normalized ratio (INR) >2 despite vitamin K therapy, with or without encephalopathy. In another third, onset may be insidious, with progressive fatigue, weight loss, and intermittent jaundice lasting for several weeks or years before diagnosis. In less than 10%, there may be no jaundice, but the patient presents with complications of portal hypertension including splenomegaly, ascites, or variceal bleeding. Children with AIH type 1 are more likely to present with cirrhosis while those with AIH type 2 present more frequently with fulminant liver failure. The course of the disease is relapsing with flares and spontaneous remissions, often resulting in a delayed or missed diagnosis.

When obtaining the history, it is important to inquire about medications the child has been taking in the past year, particularly minocycline, which is a known trigger of an "autoimmune-like hepatitis." Children with AIH may have other autoimmune disorders including thyroiditis, vitiligo, type 1 diabetes, and inflammatory bowel disease. It is essential to inquire about symptoms and observe for signs related to these associated autoimmune diseases. In addition, there is a family history of autoimmune disease in up to 40% of patients with AIH. On physical examination, children may be jaundiced with an enlarged liver or spleen. In those with decompensated disease, there may be ascites and petechiae. Laboratory tests may show evidence of hypersplenism with a low white cell count and thrombocytopenia. Biochemically, aminotransferases are elevated with or without elevated serum gamma-glutamyltransferase and total protein is high with a low/normal serum albumin. Serum IgG is typically elevated and there are increased titers of ANA, ASMA, or ALKM. It is essential to obtain a liver biopsy to establish a diagnosis of AIH. The typical histological picture is interface hepatitis: a

(a)

(b)

(c)

(d)

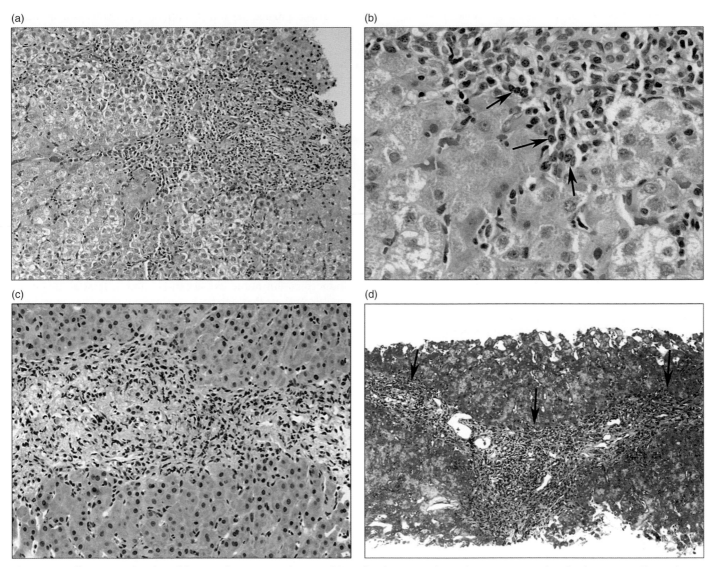

Figure 20.1 Characteristic histological features of autoimmune hepatitis. (a) Interface hepatitis with portal tracts containing lymphoplasmocytic infiltrates that extend into the lobule. (b) Interface hepatitis at higher power, showing the penetration of inflammatory cells from the portal area into the periportal parenchyma (arrows denote plasma cells). The hepatocytes show cellular swelling and degenerative changes. (c) Bridging necrosis in higher grade autoimmune hepatitis with inflammatory cells infiltrating a band of confluent necrosis. (d) Fibrosis in autoimmune hepatitis with interportal bridging fibrosis (portal tracts indicated by arrows). (a–c, hematoxylin & eosin stain; d, Trichrome stain.)

dense infiltration of the portal tracts consisting mainly of lymphocytes and plasma cells that extends into the liver lobules with destruction of the hepatocytes at the periphery of the lobule and erosion of the limiting plate. There may be bridging fibrosis or cirrhosis evident on trichrome stain (Figure 20.1).

In children with elevated serum gamma-glutamyltransferase or biliary changes on histology, it may be advisable to perform MRI studies to look for changes consistent with SC. There may be overlap between AIH and SC, which has been designated as autoimmune SC or AIH/SC overlap syndrome [24]. In this setting there are characteristic cholangiographic features of SC in combination with elevated IgG, positive autoantibodies, and interface hepatitis on liver biopsy. Although the relationship between AIH and SC is not established, one may speculate that

there is a spectrum ranging from "cholestatic" disease affecting the biliary system alone (SC) to "inflammatory" disease affecting the hepatocytes (AIH) [27]. Differences between AIH types 1 and 2 and AIH/SC overlap syndrome are illustrated in Table 20.3.

Differential diagnosis

The differential diagnosis of chronic hepatitis in children is broad, including but not limited to AIH, AIH/SC overlap syndrome, PSC, chronic infectious hepatitis (hepatitis B, hepatitis C), α_1-antitrypsin deficiency, Wilson disease, and non-alcoholic fatty liver disease. Diagnostic workup in order to exclude these non-AIH diseases includes MR cholangiopancreaticography (or endoscopic retrograde cholangiopancreatography), hepatitis

Table 20.3 Clinical, laboratory, and histologic features at presentation of autoimmune hepatitis types 1 and 2 and autoimmune hepatitis/sclerosing cholangitis overlap syndrome

Feature	Autoimmune hepatitis		Overlap syndrome[a]
	Type 1	Type 2	
Median age (years)	11	7	12
Females (%)	75	75	55
Mode of presentation (%)			
Acute hepatitis	47	40	37
Acute liver failure	3	25	0
Insidious onset	38	25	37
Complication of chronic liver disease	12	10	26
Associated immune disease (%)			
Present	22	20	48
Inflammatory bowel disease	20	12	44
Family history of autoimmune disease	43	40	37
Autoantibodies (%)			
Anti-nuclear antibody or anti-smooth muscle antibody	100	25	96
Anti-liver–kidney microsomal antibody-1	0	100	4
Perinuclear anti-neutrophil cytoplasmic antibody	45	11	74
Anti-soluble liver antigen[b]	58	58	41
Blood proteins (%)			
Increased IgG	84	75	89
Partial IgA deficiency	9	45	5
Low C4 level	89	83	70
HLA alleles, increased frequency (%)			
HLA-DR*0301	Yes	No[c]	No
HLA-DR*0701	No	Yes	No
HLA-DR*1301	No	No	Yes
Liver/biliary features (%)			
Abnormal cholangiogram	0	0	100
Interface hepatitis	66	72	35
Intrahepatic biliary features	28	6	31
Cirrhosis	69	38	15
Remission after immunosuppression (%)	97	87	89

[a] Also known as autoimmune sclerosing cholangitis.
[b] Measured by radioligand assay.
[c] But increased in *HLA-DR*0701*-negative patients.
Source: From Mieli-Vergani & Vergani, 2009 [13].

B surface antigen, hepatitis C antibody, α_1-antitrypsin level and phenotype, ceruloplasmin, and liver ultrasound.

As mentioned above, it is important to obtain a history of recent exposure to medications such as minocycline or nitrofurantoin, as these and other medications have been proposed to trigger autoimmune-like hepatitis. Mechanisms to explain this association involve covalent binding of a drug metabolite to a hepatocyte protein with resultant formation of a "neoantigen" that is recognized as foreign, eliciting an autoimmune response [28]. Minocycline-induced autoimmune-like hepatitis usually occurs acutely within 2 years after drug initiation, with a range of 3 days to 6 years. Symptoms include jaundice, lethargy, anorexia, and abdominal discomfort. In addition, signs of serum sickness (fever, rash, joint pains) may coexist. Over 90% of patients will be ANA positive with hypergammaglobulinemia, while only 25% will be ASMA positive, and ALKM positivity has not been described. Histologically, minocycline-induced autoimmune-like hepatitis mimics classical AIH, with the exception that cirrhosis at presentation has not been reported. The mainstay of treatment includes stopping the offending medication and administering corticosteroids. The overwhelming majority of patients can be weaned off immunosuppression and relapses are rare.

Autoimmune hepatitis may be associated with another underlying autoimmune disease or immunodeficiency state. The APECED (autoimmune polyendocrinopathy-candidiasis–ectodermal dystrophy) syndrome is caused by mutations of *AIRE*, encoding the autoimmune regulator. Patients with APECED syndrome present in the first decade of life with at least two of the following conditions: recurrent candidiasis, polyendocrinopathy (hypoparathyroidism, adrenal insufficiency), AIH, or dystrophy of dental enamel and nails. Up to 20% of these patients have been shown to have AIH in association with autoantibodies against cytochromes CYP1A2 and CYP2A6 [29]. This syndrome is the only one involving AIH that has an autosomal recessive pattern of inheritance. Other immune-dysregulated states associated with AIH include IPEX (immunodysregulation polyendocrinopathy enteropathy X-linked) syndrome, common variable immunodeficiency, and hyper-IgM syndrome. Common variable immunodeficiency is associated with hypogammaglobulinemia and the liver manifestation of nodular regenerative hyperplasia. Hyper-IgM syndrome is caused by mutations in genes that affect immunoglobulin class switch recombination and is associated with elevated IgM and low IgG levels. The X-linked hyper-IgM syndrome, or CD40L deficiency, is the most common and most severe form of hyper-IgM syndrome. This ligand is expressed on activated T-lymphocytes and necessary for T-cells to induce immunoglobulin isotype switching in B-cells. Typically, male infants present with recurrent bacterial and opportunistic infections. The most common liver disease found in hyper-IgM syndrome is SC with chronic *Cryptosporidia* biliary infection; however, AIH and liver and biliary tract carcinomas have also been reported [30]. Finally, types 1 and 2 AIH may have a genetically determined isolated deficiency of complement component C4, and a partial IgA deficiency has been noted in patients with type 2 AIH. The initial evaluation of AIH should, therefore, also include a complete blood cell count with differential and levels of all serum immunoglobulins (IgG, IgM, IgA).

Management

Historically there have been descriptions of early death or progression to cirrhosis complicated by portal hypertension in the absence of treatment for AIH. In the early 1970s, there were prospective controlled trials that showed the effectiveness of corticosteroids in the control of inflammatory activity in AIH (chronic active hepatitis as it was then known) [31]. It is now accepted that immunosuppression for AIH is effective in improving symptoms, resolving laboratory and histologic features, and prolonging survival. The goal of therapy is to control the autoimmune inflammatory activity and prevent progression to cirrhosis. Immunosuppressive therapy is initiated at the time of diagnosis, with the possible exception of primary transplantation as treatment for the fulminant liver failure presentation of AIH. Complete remission includes clinical recovery, biochemical normalization of serum aminotransferases, normal IgG, negative or very low autoantibody titers, and resolution of inflammation histologically [1]. The histologic response usually lags behind the biochemical response. Relapse is defined as an increase in serum aminotransferases after remission had been achieved.

Standard therapy

Corticosteroids in combination with azathioprine have been used conventionally as standard therapy in both types 1 and 2 AIH. In children, prednisone (or prednisilone) is usually administered in a dose of 1–2 mg/kg daily (60 mg maximum) in the morning with an antacid. Side effects of steroids include weight gain, cushingoid facies, acne, hirsuitism, striae, gastritis, hyperglycemia, hypertension, and deleterious effects on linear growth and development. Initiation of steroid weaning occurs after the aminotransferases have trended down consistently. The steroid dose is usually decreased by 5–10 mg every 2–3 weeks. Normalization of liver chemistries is noted after 6–9 months of therapy in 75–90% [21].

The use of azathioprine as a steroid-sparing agent is the standard of care in the USA and the majority of children can be weaned completely off corticosteroids within a few months of initiating azathioprine therapy. An alternative approach is to continue prednisone as single therapy and initiate azathioprine in the setting of rising aminotransferases during tapering of steroids or when children develop steroid-related side effects. Azathioprine is a purine analogue that is metabolized to 6-mercaptopurine and is ultimately incorporated into replicating DNA. It blocks the de novo pathway of purine synthesis, contributing to its relative specificity to lymphocytes secondary to their lack of a salvage pathway. Side effects of azathioprine include leukopenia, nausea, emesis, rash, pancreatitis, and

hepatotoxicity. Based on this risk of drug-induced hepatotoxicity, it is advised to avoid azathioprine use if the presentation of AIH is associated with acute or fulminant liver failure. The range of dosing of azathioprine is approximately 1–2 mg/kg daily. Prior to initiating azathioprine therapy, quantifying the thiopurine methyl transferase activity will ensure that the patient can appropriately metabolize azathioprine, thus decreasing the risk of significant bone marrow suppression or hepatotoxicity [32]. The dose of azathioprine needed to maintain remission will vary from patient to patient. Azathioprine metabolites can be measured in order to determine the levels of the active metabolite 6-thioguanine and hepatotoxic metabolite 6-methylmercaptopurine. The therapeutic 6-thioguanine level in the treatment of inflammatory bowel disease ranges from 235 to 260 pmol per 8×10^8 red blood cells. The therapeutic level in AIH hepatitis has not been established; however, a lower range (i.e. 150–200 pmol per 8×10^8 red blood cells) is often sufficient to maintain remission. If 6-thioguanine levels are low, then the dose of azathioprine may need to be increased, whereas if levels of the toxic 6-methylmercaptopurine are high, then the dose is reduced. When 6-thioguanine is low, but 6-methylmercaptopurine is elevated, addition of allopurinol can divert the metabolism to the 6-thioguanine pathway, allowing therapeutic levels of 6-thioguanine to be achieved [33]. 6-Mercaptopurine is a purine analogue that inhibits nucleic acid synthesis and is another active metabolite of azathioprine. It has a toxicity profile separate from azathioprine that may be secondary to variations in intestinal absorption and/or metabolism [34]. The average dosing for 6-mercaptopurine is 1–1.5 mg/kg daily and the maximum dose is 100 mg daily. 6-Mercaptopurine may be used as an alternative in those who failed standard regimen of steroids with azathioprine or were intolerant of azathioprine.

Long-term treatment with immunosuppression is required for the majority of children diagnosed with AIH. Monotherapy with azathioprine is usually successful in maintaining a sustained remission with minimal adverse events. Liver aminotransferases, autoantibodies, and total IgG are useful surrogates of disease activity and may be used to monitor response longitudinally [35]. Relapse during treatment may occur in up to 40% of patients [13] and may require a temporary increase in steroid dose. Adherence to medications is an important factor in managing AIH and non-compliance is more commonly seen in the teenage population. Subjective measures of adherence such as self-reported questionnaires by patients or caregivers are not adequate and objective methods are required to consistently monitor adherence longitudinally. Pill counts and electronic monitoring devices [36] have been used to objectively assess adherence, but blood levels of medication (i.e. 6-thioguanine) have been found to be the best measure.

It is recommended that children with type 1 AIH should have biochemical remission (normal aminotransferase levels) on monotherapy, usually azathioprine, for a minimum of 2 years prior to consideration of withdrawal of immunosuppression. In addition, documentation of histologic remission (liver biopsy) is recommended prior to weaning from immunosuppression. The majority of patients with type 2 AIH will require lifelong immunosuppression and are rarely taken off medications [37]. Discontinuation of immunosuppression is not recommended in the following situations: severe disease at presentation, recurrent relapses of disease while on therapy, or patients entering or undergoing puberty. If immunosuppression is withdrawn, it is important to monitor the aminotransferases and autoimmune markers regularly in order to detect a relapse in disease and the need to reinstitute immunosuppression.

Alternative therapies

Budesonide

Budesonide is a second-generation glucocorticoid that has a high first-pass clearance by the liver, low systemic availability, and metabolites that lack glucocorticoid activity, making it an attractive option to avoid steroid-induced side effects [38]. In a large multicenter double-blind placebo-controlled study, 203 adults with non-cirrhotic AIH were given azathioprine (1–2 mg/kg daily) with either budesonide (3 mg, two to three times daily) or prednisone (40 mg/day, tapered to 10 mg/day); 47% in the budesonide group versus 18.4% in the prednisone group achieved complete biochemical remission without predefined steroid side effects [39]. While budesonide worked well in reducing steroid-associated side effects, it is important to give the drug in combination with azathioprine to induce remission. In addition, reactivation of AIH during budesonide monotherapy has been reported [40].

Mycophenolate mofetil

Mycophenolate mofetil is another steroid-sparing agent that has been used in limited trials for the treatment of AIH. Its side effects include gastrointestinal symptoms (abdominal pain, diarrhea), bone marrow suppression, hair loss and headaches. Mycophenolate mofetil is a prodrug hydrolyzed by liver esterases to produce the active metabolite mycophenolic acid, which, in turn, inhibits de novo purine nucleotide synthesis, leading to arrest of DNA replication in T- and B-lymphocytes [41]. Success with mycophenolate mofetil in the treatment of AIH when azathioprine had failed has been reported in small cohorts of patients [42]. More recently, 26 children with AIH who had not responded or could not tolerate standard treatment with steroids/azathioprine were treated with mycophenolate mofetil at 20–40 mg/kg daily [43]. Eighteen children (70%) responded and the drug was well tolerated. Eight children in the initial cohort who had AIH/SC overlap syndrome did not respond to mycophenolate mofetil and, therefore, it should not be used as primary therapy in overlap syndrome.

Calcineurin inhibitors

Calcineurin inhibitors (cyclosporine and tacrolimus) are standard antirejection medications used in organ transplantation and have also been used successfully in the treatment of AIH. Cyclosporine has been used successfully both as primary

treatment and in those unresponsive to standard therapy [44]; however, cyclosporine trough values up to 200 μg/L were required to exert sufficient immunosuppressive effect [45]. In a multicenter study of 30 children with AIH treated with cyclosporine, 25 normalized serum ALT by 6 months and all by 1 year [46]. Tacrolimus is a macrolide antibiotic with 10–200 times the immunosuppressive effect of cyclosporine and has been shown to control autoimmune activity in adults with AIH [47]. Whether calcineurin inhibitors have any advantage over standard therapy is not clear and will require evaluation in future controlled studies analyzing not only efficacy but also long-term side effects in children.

Special considerations for management

Treatment of overlap syndrome

Children with AIH may also have histological and/or radiological features of SC leading to the terminology of AIH/SC overlap syndrome [24]. The same immunosuppressive regimen that is used in AIH is usually sufficient. The addition of ursodeoxycholic acid at a dosage of 10 mg/kg twice daily may be helpful in treating the SC component of the disease [48].

Treatment of liver failure

Children with AIH who present with liver failure are a therapeutic challenge. In a large Canadian series, 50 of 237 children with AIH developed acute (or "acute on chronic") liver failure as defined by prothrombin time >50% of baseline values. Forty-five (90%) responded to immunosuppression at a median time of 24 days. Five required liver transplantation and there were three deaths secondary to infection [49]. By contrast, the usefulness of corticosteroid therapy in the acute liver failure presentation of AIH is a matter of debate. A retrospective study examined a cohort of 16 adults with fulminant liver failure caused by AIH. Twelve (75%) received corticosteroid treatment for a median duration of 7 days and four (25%) could not be treated because of the rapid deterioration in their clinical status. The majority of patients who had received corticosteroids also needed subsequent liver transplantation (83%). Severe septic complications occurred in three while on corticosteroid therapy and in one after liver transplant. The authors concluded that corticosteroid therapy is of little benefit in the acute liver failure presentation of AIH and increases the incidence of sepsis, hence liver transplantation should not be delayed [50].

Outcomes and prognosis

The majority of children will reach remission within the first year of therapy. Lifelong treatment is necessary in the majority and one can anticipate an excellent quality of life while on low-dose maintenance medication. However, up to 40% of patients will have an episode of relapse during treatment. Risk factors associated with "on therapy" relapse include use of alternate-day steroids, puberty, and medication non-adherence [51].

Treatment failure implies worsening of clinical or laboratory parameters despite appropriate medical treatment and occurs in up to 10% of children. In an adult study, if the patient presented at an early age with an acute presentation associated with hyperbilirubinemia and the *HLA-DRB1*03* genotype, they were more likely to fail conventional therapy [52]. In children, the development of end-stage liver disease necessitating transplant has been reported in 8.5% of patients up to 14 years after diagnosis [1].

In AIH type 1, reports of sustained remission after immunosuppression withdrawal range from 20 to 40%; patients with AIH type 2 rarely can be weaned off immunosuppression. It is important to wait several years prior to considering withdrawal of therapy. In patients treated for more than 4 years before cessation of therapy, the sustained remission was 67%, compared with only 10% remission if medication was stopped in the first 2 years of treatment [53]. If relapse occurs after immunosuppression withdrawal, it usually does so within the first 18 months. There are no clinical or laboratory features that can predict who will relapse after stopping medications and, therefore, frequent monitoring of symptoms, liver tests, and autoantibodies is warranted in the first 2 years after withdrawal of immunosuppression.

Studies on mortality in pediatric AIH are limited. One report found that approximately 97% of patients treated with standard immunosuppressive therapy were alive after a median follow-up of 5 years after diagnosis [51]. The 10-year survival in children with AIH is calculated to be >90%. A recent retrospective analysis of the long-term prognosis in 34 children with AIH revealed an overall survival of 82% with a median follow-up period of 73 months [54]. Cox regression analysis revealed that weight loss, hyperbilirubinemia, prolonged INR, and positive ALKM-1 at presentation were independent risk factors associated with decreased survival. Interestingly, cirrhosis at presentation did not affect outcome. Nine patients (26%) underwent liver transplant. All deaths occurred while waiting for liver transplant (two patients) or after transplant (four patients). Chronic allograft rejection was the cause of death in all patients after transplant, and recurrent AIH was not identified in this cohort.

A potential long-term complication of chronic hepatitis is the development of hepatocellular carcinoma. The occurrence of hepatocellular carcinoma in pediatrics as a result of AIH is extremely rare and the majority of reports are in the adult population. In a retrospective study of 243 patients with AIH, hepatocellular carcinoma occurred in 15 patients (6%). All patients had AIH type 1 and hepatocellular carcinoma occurred more commonly in patients who had cirrhosis or an index gastrointestinal bleed at presentation of the AIH. The median duration from the diagnosis of AIH cirrhosis and diagnosis of hepatocellular carcinoma was 9 years [55]. Screening modalities for hepatocellular carcinoma include serum α-fetoprotein and liver ultrasound.

Liver transplantation and autoimmune hepatitis

In the USA and Europe, AIH is the indication for 2–3% of pediatric liver transplants [21]. The need for liver transplant may be acute liver failure at presentation, development of decompensated cirrhosis, or hepatocellular carcinoma. Overall approximately 10–15% of children with AIH require a transplant. Type 2 AIH and AIH/SC overlap syndrome are more often associated with the need for transplant than AIH type 1. Liver transplantation for AIH is successful, with 5- and 10-year patient survivals of approximately 75%. Recurrent post-transplant AIH may occur in up to 30% of children, with an average recurrence time of 4.6 years [21]. The incidence increases with time interval from liver transplant and is accelerated after reduction in immunosuppression. Recurrence is diagnosed when graft dysfunction is associated with biochemical (positive autoantibodies) and histological features of AIH. Additional immunosuppression after liver transplant may help to prevent recurrent AIH in the allograft. This can be achieved by a combination of low-dose calcineurin inhibitor with either azathioprine or mycophenolate mofetil.

Another form of postliver transplant AIH is known as de novo AIH. De novo AIH was first described in 1998 in pediatric liver transplant recipients who had received their transplant for non-autoimmune conditions (i.e. not AIH or PSC) and did not have hepatitis B or C. Graft dysfunction developed in 7 of 180 (4%) children, in association with elevated IgG, positive autoantibodies, and histological features of AIH, and it responded to changes in immunosuppression [56]. Since the initial description of de novo AIH, there have been several reports in the adult and pediatric literature confirming this entity, but nomenclature has been variable. The etiology is not known and mechanistic theories include molecular mimicry, calcineurin inhibitor-associated autoimmunity, and rejection as a trigger of the autoimmune response.

The management of postliver transplant recurrent AIH or de novo AIH may include a short course of corticosteroids, addition or increase in azathioprine (or mycophenolate mofetil) and a decrease in the calcineurin inhibitor. When there is failure of standard triple immunosuppressive therapy, then rapamycin may be used in place of azathioprine (or mycophenolate mofetil) to successfully control autoimmune inflammatory activity [57]. Rapamycin binds to a specific receptor called the mammalian target of RAPA (mTOR) and reduces T-cell activation by inhibiting the interleukin-2-mediated signal transduction pathway. It also inhibits B-cell stimulation and decreases antibody production. Side effects of rapamycin include hyperlipidemia, proteinuria, interstitial pneumonitis, and delayed wound healing. Rapamycin can be used safely in combination with tacrolimus provided drug levels plus serum lipid levels and urine protein/creatinine ratio are monitored. The importance of identifying post-transplant AIH lies in the fact that it responds well to immunosuppression and thereby prevents need for subsequent retransplantation. It is also important to note that while tolerance is the goal in transplant recipients, it is advisable to exercise caution while weaning immunosuppression in children who have received a transplant for AIH or in those who have developed recurrent or de novo AIH, as discontinuation of drugs may lead to recurrent AIH.

Conclusions

Autoimmune hepatitis is a chronic autoinflammatory disease of the liver that necessitates lifelong therapy in the majority of children. There are two types based on the autoantibody profile: type 1 characterized by positive ANA and/or ASMA and type 2 characterized by positive ALKM. The AIH/SC overlap syndrome (or autoimmune SC) denotes a type of autoimmune liver disease with cholangiographic features of SC along with positive autoantibodies and liver histologic features characteristic of AIH. A prompt response to immunosuppression is commonplace and the overall prognosis is excellent. Autoantibody titers and serum IgG are acceptable markers of disease activity and can be used to monitor therapy. Liver transplantation is necessary in up to 15% of children with AIH, and recurrent AIH or de novo AIH can occur posttransplant. Research focusing on the pathogenic mechanisms that trigger and perpetuate the autoimmune responses in AIH and AIH/SC overlap syndrome is required in order to be able to offer curative therapies in the future.

References

1. Mieli-Vergani G, Vergani D. Autoimmune hepatitis. *Nat Rev* 2011;**8**:320–329.

2. Waldenstrom J, Blueprotein., Nahrungseiweiss. *Dtsch Verdau Stoffwechselkr* 1950:113–119.

3. Whittingham S, Irwin J, Mackay IR, Smalley M. Smooth muscle autoantibody in "autoimmune" hepatitis. *Gastroenterology* 1966;**51**:499–505.

4. De Groote J, Desmet VJ, Gedigk P, *et al.* A classification of chronic hepatitis. *Lancet* 1968;**ii**:626–628.

5. Johnson PJ, McFarlane IG. Meeting report: International Autoimmune Hepatitis Group. *Hepatology* 1993;**18**:998–1005.

6. Manns MP, Vogel A. Autoimmune hepatitis, from mechanisms to therapy. *Hepatology* 2006;**43**(Suppl 1):S132–S144.

7. Beland K, Lapierre P, Alvarez F. Influence of genes, sex, age and environment on the onset of autoimmune hepatitis. *World J Gastroenterol* 2009;**15**:1025–1034.

8. Krawitt EL. Autoimmune hepatitis. *N Engl J Med* 2006;**354**:54–66.

9. Longhi MS, Ma Y, Mieli-Vergani G, Vergani D. Aetiopathogenesis of autoimmune hepatitis. *J Autoimmun* 2010;**34**:7–14.

10. Oo YH, Hubscher SG, Adams DH. Autoimmune hepatitis: new paradigms in the pathogenesis, diagnosis, and management. *Hepatol Int* 2010;**4**:475–493.

11. Ichiki Y, Aoki CA, Bowlus CL, *et al.* T cell immunity in autoimmune hepatitis. *Autoimmun Rev* 2005;**4**:315–321.

12. Longhi MS, Ma Y, Mitry RR, *et al.* Effect of CD4+ CD25+ regulatory T-cells on CD8 T-cell function in patients with autoimmune hepatitis. *J Autoimmun* 2005;**25**:63–71.

13. Mieli-Vergani G, Vergani D. Autoimmune hepatitis in children: what is different from adult AIH? *Semin Liver Dis* 2009;**29**:297–306.

14. Invernizzi P, Lleo A, Podda M. Interpreting serological tests in diagnosing autoimmune liver diseases. *Semin Liver Dis* 2007;**27**:161–172.

15. Czaja AJ. Autoantibodies as prognostic markers in autoimmune liver disease. *Dig Dis Sci* 2010;**55**:2144–2161.

16. Donaldson PT. Genetics in autoimmune hepatitis. *Semin Liver Dis* 2002;**22**:353–364.

17. Vergani D, Mieli-Vergani G. Aetiopathogenesis of autoimmune hepatitis. *World J Gastroenterol* 2008;**14**:3306–3312.

18. Jaeckel E, Hardtke-Wolenski M, Fischer K. The benefit of animal models for autoimmune hepatitis. *Best Pract Res Clin Gastroenterol* 2011;**25**:643–651.

19. Lapierre P, Djilali-Saiah I, Vitozzi S, Alvarez F. A murine model of type 2 autoimmune hepatitis: xenoimmunization with human antigens. *Hepatology* 2004;**39**:1066–1074.

20. Christen U, Holdener M, Hintermann E. Animal models for autoimmune hepatitis. *Autoimmun Rev* 2007; **6**:306–311.

21. Manns MP, Czaja AJ, Gorham JD, *et al.* Diagnosis and management of autoimmune hepatitis. *Hepatology* 2010;**51**:2193–2213.

22. Hennes EM, Zeniya M, Czaja AJ, *et al.* Simplified criteria for the diagnosis of autoimmune hepatitis. *Hepatology* 2008;**48**:169–176.

23. Alvarez F, Berg PA, Bianchi FB, *et al.* International Autoimmune Hepatitis Group Report: review of criteria for diagnosis of autoimmune hepatitis. *J Hepatol* 1999;**31**:929–938.

24. Gregorio GV, Portmann B, Karani J, *et al.* Autoimmune hepatitis/sclerosing cholangitis overlap syndrome in childhood: a 16-year prospective study. *Hepatology* 2001;**33**:544–553.

25. Ebbeson RL, Schreiber RA. Diagnosing autoimmune hepatitis in children: is the International Autoimmune Hepatitis Group scoring system useful? *Clin Gastroenterol Hepatol* 2004;**2**: 935–940.

26. Kerkar N. Evaluating the AIH scoring system. *J Pediatr Gastroenterol Nutr* 2005;**41**:137–138.

27. Kerkar N, Miloh T. Sclerosing cholangitis: pediatric perspective. *Curr Gastroenterol Rep* 2010;**12**:195–202.

28. Czaja AJ. Drug-induced autoimmune-like hepatitis. *Dig Dis Sci* 2011;**56**:958–976.

29. Mathis D, Benoist C. Aire. *Annu Rev Immunol* 2009;**27**:287–312.

30. Davies EG, Thrasher AJ. Update on the hyper immunoglobulin M syndromes. *Br J Haematol* 2010;**149**:167–180.

31. Cook GC, Mulligan R, Sherlock S. Controlled prospective trial of corticosteroid therapy in active chronic hepatitis. *Q J Med* 1971;**40**(158): 159–185.

32. Rumbo C, Emerick KM, Emre S, Shneider BL. Azathioprine metabolite

measurements in the treatment of autoimmune hepatitis in pediatric patients: a preliminary report. *J Pediatr Gastroenterol Nutr* 2002;**35**:391–398.

33. Dunkin D, Kerkar N, Arnon R, Suchy F, Miloh T. Allopurinol salvage therapy in pediatric overlap autoimmune hepatitis-primary sclerosing cholangitis with 6-MMP toxicity. *J Pediatr Gastroenterol Nutr* 2010;**51**:524 526.

34. Pratt DS, Flavin DP, Kaplan MM. The successful treatment of autoimmune hepatitis with 6-mercaptopurine after failure with azathioprine. *Gastroenterology* 1996;**110**:271–274.

35. Gregorio GV, McFarlane B, Bracken P, Vergani D, Mieli-Vergani G. Organ and non-organ specific autoantibody titres and IgG levels as markers of disease activity: a longitudinal study in childhood autoimmune liver disease. *Autoimmunity* 2002;**35**:515–519.

36. Kerkar N, Annunziato RA, Foley L, *et al.* Prospective analysis of nonadherence in autoimmune hepatitis: a common problem. *J Pediatr Gastroenterol Nutr* 2006;**43**:629–634.

37. Gregorio GV, Portmann B, Reid F, *et al.* Autoimmune hepatitis in childhood: a 20-year experience. *Hepatology* 1997;**25**:541–547.

38. Czaja AJ, Manns MP. Advances in the diagnosis, pathogenesis, and management of autoimmune hepatitis. *Gastroenterology* 2010;**139**:58–72 e4.

39. Manns MP, Woynarowski M, Kreisel W, *et al.* Budesonide induces remission more effectively than prednisone in a controlled trial of patients with autoimmune hepatitis. *Gastroenterology* 2010;**139**:1198–1206.

40. Lohse AW, Gil H. Reactivation of autoimmune hepatitis during budesonide monotherapy, and response to standard treatment. *J Hepatol* 2011;**54**:837–839.

41. Czaja AJ, Carpenter HA. Empiric therapy of autoimmune hepatitis with mycophenolate mofetil: comparison with conventional treatment for refractory disease. *J Clin Gastroenterol* 2005;**39**:819–825.

42. Richardson PD, James PD, Ryder SD. Mycophenolate mofetil for maintenance of remission in autoimmune hepatitis in patients resistant to or intolerant of azathioprine. *J Hepatol* 2000;**33**:371–375.

43. Aw MM, Dhawan A, Samyn M, Bargiota A, Mieli-Vergani G. Mycophenolate mofetil as rescue treatment for autoimmune liver disease in children: a 5-year follow-up. *J Hepatol* 2009;**51**:156–160.

44. Sherman KE, Narkewicz M, Pinto PC. Cyclosporine in the management of corticosteroid-resistant type I autoimmune chronic active hepatitis. *J Hepatol* 1994;**21**:1040–1047.

45. Hyams JS, Ballow M, Leichtner AM. Cyclosporine treatment of autoimmune chronic active hepatitis. *Gastroenterology* 1987;**93**:890–893.

46. Alvarez F, Ciocca M, Canero-Velasco C, *et al.* Short-term cyclosporine induces a remission of autoimmune hepatitis in children. *J Hepatol* 1999;**30**:222–227.

47. Van Thiel DH, Wright H, Carroll P, *et al.* Tacrolimus: a potential new treatment for autoimmune chronic active hepatitis: results of an open-label preliminary trial. *Am J Gastroenterol* 1995;**90**:771–776.

48. Miloh T, Arnon R, Shneider B, Suchy F, Kerkar N. A retrospective single-center review of primary sclerosing cholangitis in children. *Clin Gastroenterol Hepatol* 2009;**7**:239–245.

49. Cuarterolo ML, Ciocca ME, Lopez SI, de Davila MT, Alvarez F. Immunosuppressive therapy allows recovery from liver failure in children with autoimmune hepatitis. *Clin Gastroenterol Hepatol* 2011;**9**:145–149.

50. Ichai P, Duclos-Vallee JC, Guettier C, *et al.* Usefulness of corticosteroids for the treatment of severe and fulminant forms of autoimmune hepatitis. *Liver Transplant* 2007;**13**:996–1003.

51. Greene MT, Whitington PF. Outcomes in pediatric autoimmune hepatitis. *Curr Gastroenterol Rep* 2009;**11**:248–251.

52. Montano-Loza AJ, Carpenter HA, Czaja AJ. Improving the end point of corticosteroid therapy in type 1 autoimmune hepatitis to reduce the frequency of relapse. *Am J Gastroenterol* 2007;**102**:1005–1012.

53. Al-Chalabi T, Underhill JA, Portmann BC, McFarlane IG, Heneghan MA. Impact of gender on the long-term outcome and survival of patients with autoimmune hepatitis. *J Hepatol* 2008;**48**:140–147.

54. Radhakrishnan KR, Alkhouri N, Worley S, *et al.* Autoimmune hepatitis in children: impact of cirrhosis at presentation on natural history and long-term outcome. *Dig Liver Dis* 2010;**42**:724–728.

55. Yeoman AD, Al-Chalabi T, Karani JB, *et al.* Evaluation of risk factors in the development of hepatocellular carcinoma in autoimmune hepatitis: Implications for follow-up and screening. *Hepatology* 2008;**48**:863–870.

56. Kerkar N, Hadzic N, Davies ET, *et al.* De-novo autoimmune hepatitis after liver transplantation. *Lancet* 1998;**351**:409–413.

57. Kerkar N, Dugan C, Rumbo C, *et al.* Rapamycin successfully treats post-transplant autoimmune hepatitis. *Am J Transplant* 2005;**5**:1085–1089.

Sclerosing cholangitis

Alexander G. Miethke and William F. Balistreri

Introduction

There is a wide spectrum of etiologically obscure inflammatory disorders of the biliary tract, including the obstructive cholangiopathies that occur in infancy (biliary atresia and related entities), primary biliary cirrhosis, which is noted in adults, and primary sclerosing cholangitis (PSC), which may affect patients of all age groups, particularly those with chronic inflammatory bowel disease (IBD). These hepatobiliary disorders differ markedly in clinical expression but display substantial overlap in morphologic features, suggesting that their pathogenesis may be shared. Because the intra- and extrahepatic biliary tree may be assumed to possess a limited repertoire of reactions to injury caused by various inflammatory mechanisms, the association of PSC and IBD may provide insight into other forms of "cholangitis." The frequency of this association also presents an opportunity to trace the evolution of PSC. This chapter focuses on idiopathic forms of sclerosing cholangitis in children, the PSC–IBD complex, and related disorders.

Definition

Sclerosing cholangitis is a chronic hepatobiliary disorder characterized by inflammation of the intra- and/or extrahepatic ducts, leading to focal dilatation, narrowing, or obliteration accompanied by local periductular fibrosis. Progressive, obliterative fibrosis usually leads to biliary cirrhosis and end-stage liver disease. The structural abnormalities of larger bile ducts are best appreciated by cholangiography, which in most cases is essential in establishing the diagnosis. However, careful delineation of the histology of the hepatic parenchyma and smaller intrahepatic ducts may also suggest the diagnosis.

Sclerosing cholangitis is the most common form of chronic liver disease seen in patients with IBD, but it also may occur in the absence of IBD and in association with a wide variety of disorders (Table 21.1). The nosology remains somewhat obscure, with no consensus. By convention, sclerosing cholangitis is designated as primary regardless of the presence or absence of IBD; in either instance, cholangitis is idiopathic. Cholangitis related to chronic ascending bacterial infection,

stones, biliary tract surgery, congenital anomalies of the biliary tract, ischemic injury, neoplasia, or infectious cholangiopathy associated with immunodeficiency, particularly hyper-IgM syndrome and associated CD40L deficiency, are some of the exclusions necessary to justify the use of the term *primary cholangitis* (versus secondary cholangitis). It is assumed that prior to the onset of sclerosing cholangitis, the anatomy of the biliary tree was normal and that the condition has no relationship to disorders such as the congenital hepatic fibrosis–Caroli disease–polycystic kidney disease complex. The term *secondary sclerosing cholangitis* has been used to describe the clinical syndrome resulting from the above disorders, as well as from choledocholithiasis, postoperative stricture, or other specific ductal involvement in systemic disease (Table 21.1). Mieli-Vergani and Vergani [1] have suggested that sclerosing cholangitis be described as *primary* if it occurs (1) outside of the neonatal period, (2) without strong features of autoimmunity *and* without response to immunosuppression (as seen in so-called autoimmune sclerosing cholangitis (ASC), and (3) in the absence of complicating disorders such as immunodeficiency, Langerhans cell histiocytosis, psoriasis, cystic fibrosis, reticulum cell sarcoma and sickle cell anemia.

Spectrum of sclerosing cholangitis

The bulk of the information regarding sclerosing cholangitis has been generated through studies of adults, but since the late 1980s, an increasing number of reports of pediatric cases has been published, including several large series [2–9]. The wide spectrum of hepatobiliary lesions initially reported to affect a significant proportion of well-studied adults with IBD is now also being recognized in children with ulcerative colitis (UC) and Crohn disease, in part because of the increasingly widespread utilization of cholangiographic techniques in children.

The majority of adults with sclerosing cholangitis have an associated non-hepatic disease, indicating more than a chance occurrence; in addition to IBD, these disorders include diabetes mellitus, pancreatitis, thyroid diseases and other autoimmune disorders. These comorbidities may precede or develop subsequent to the diagnosis of sclerosing cholangitis.

Liver Disease in Children, Fourth Edition, ed. Frederick J. Suchy, Ronald J. Sokol, and William F. Balistreri. Published by Cambridge University Press. © Cambridge University Press 2014.

Table 21.1 Spectrum of sclerosing cholangitis in childhood

Types	Disorders
Prmary sclerosing cholangitis	
In association with inflammatory bowel disease	Ulcerative colitis
	Crohn disease
	Indeterminate colitis
In association with autoimmune disease	Autoimmune hepatitis–sclerosing cholangitis overlap syndrome (autoimmune sclerosing cholangitis)
	Autoimmune pancreatitis (lymphoplasmocytic sclerosing pancreatitis)
	IgG$_4$-related sclerosing disease: not reported in children to date
	Celiac disease
	Diabetes mellitus
	Thyroiditis
	Lupus
	Psoriasis
In association with other inflammatory disorders	Inflammatory pseudotumor
	Inflammatory retroperitonitis
Idiopathic	Childhood
	Neonatal sclerosing cholangitis: neonatal ichthyosis-sclerosing cholangitis syndrome (NISCH), Kabuki syndrome, with associated autoimmunity
Secondary sclerosing cholangitis	
Choledocholithiasis (sludge)	Sickle cell anemia
	Parenteral nutrition-associated
Immunodeficiency (usually associated with infectious cholangitis)	AIDS-associated cholangiopathy: cytomegalovirus, *Cryptosporidium*
	X-linked hyper-IgM/Agammaglobulinemia: *Cryptosporidium*
	Wiskott–Aldrich syndrome
	Natural killer cell deficiency: *Trichosporon*
	Agammaglobulinemia, combined variable deficiency, combined immunodeficiency: *Cryptosporidium*
	Undefined immunodeficiency: *Cryptococcus neoformans*
	Hypereosinophilia
Infection	Recurrent acute bacterial cholangitis
	Escherichia coli 0157:H7 enterocolitis
	Septic shock
	Cryptosporidium
Neoplasm	Langerhans cell histiocytosis
	Hodgkin disease
	Angioimmunoblastic lymphadenopathy
	Ductal cancer, gallbladder cancer
	Reticulum cell sarcoma
Injury	Postsurgical stenosis
	Trauma
	Caustic Injury
Other	Cystic fibrosis
	MDR3 deficiency

Similarly in children, sclerosing cholangitis may be noted in conjunction with IBD, develop in association with a wider variety of disorders, or occur in the absence of any definable associated disease (Table 21.1). One of the more common conditions associated with secondary sclerosing cholangitis is Langerhans cell histiocytosis, in which uncontrolled proliferation and dissemination of dendritic histiocytes leads to extensive infiltrates around intra- and extrahepatic bile ducts (Figure 21.1). As identification of the pathogenesis of secondary sclerosing cholangitis in systemic disease is improved, understanding of the pathobiology of biliary diseases in general, and sclerosing cholangitis in particular will improve.

Information regarding the incidence of conditions associated with sclerosing cholangitis in children was initially provided

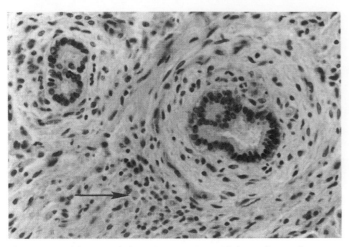

Figure 21.1 Sclerosing cholangitis in a patient with Langerhans cell histiocytosis features periductular mononuclear cells, including scattered histiocytes (arrow) (hematoxylin & eosin, original magnification ×400).

by Sisto *et al.* [8], who tabulated 78 cases, including 5 personal cases. Further reports followed: 13 cases in the UK [4], 56 children in France [3], and 32 children in Canada [9]. Three single-center studies in the USA provided a long-term follow-up of 52 children [5], a histologic study of 20 children [2], and a retrospective follow-up of 47 children with PSC [7]. In all, 106 of 180 patients (59%) were diagnosed with IBD, and overlap with autoimmune hepatitis (AIH) was found in 29% (Table 21.2). When comparing the incidence of associated autoimmune conditions, the frequencies of abnormal laboratory values and incidence of liver transplantation in these cohorts, it should be taken into consideration that some of the studies included patients with secondary sclerosing cholangitis [2,3,9], but the three US studies only enrolled subjects with PSC [5,7]. All studies probably have a referral bias in common, as they all originate from referral centers for pediatric liver transplantation.

Table 21.2 Findings associated with sclerosing cholangitis in six large pediatric series[a]

	El-Shabrawi *et al.*, 1987 [4]	Debray *et al.*, 1994 [3]	Wilschanski *et al.*, 1995 [9]	Feldstein *et al.*, 2003 [5]	Batres *et al.*, 2005 [2]	Miloh *et al.*, 2009 [7]	Total
Total No.	13	56	32	52	20	47	220
Mean age at diagnosis (years)	6	7	11	14	9	11	10
Gender (male/female)	5/8	32/24	23/9	34/18	14/6	29/18	137/83 (1.7:1)
Primary sclerosing cholangitis (No.)	13	19	30	52	19	47	180
Inflammatory bowel disease (%)[b]	69	37	56	81	53	59	59
Ulcerative colitis (%)	38	21	47	58	37	42	41
Crohn disease (%)	0	16	10	15	16	17	12
Autoimmune hepatitis (%)[b]	38	11[c]	17	35	–	25	29
Abnormal laboratory values (%)[d]							
Alkaline phosphatase	62	88	53	75	–	81	72
Gamma-glutamyltransferase	92	100	–	94	–	100	97
Aspartate aminotransferase	92	–	91	92	–	94	92
Alanine aminotransferase	–	–	–	93	–	94	94
Bilirubin	–	–	38	14	–	28	27
IgG	92	–	53	70	–	28	61
Anti-nuclear antibody	69	–	47	43	29	–	47

Table 21.2 (cont.)

	El-Shabrawi et al., 1987 [4]	Debray et al., 1994 [3]	Wilschanski et al., 1995 [9]	Feldstein et al., 2003 [5]	Batres et al., 2005 [2]	Miloh et al., 2009 [7]	Total
Anti-smooth muscle antibody	69	13	63	28	31	–	41
Anti-neutrophil cytoplasmic antibody	–	–	42	72	63	–	59

a Several studies included neonatal or secondary sclerosing cholangitis.
b Percentages given for inflammatory bowel disease and autoimmune hepatitis reflect patients with primary sclerosing cholangitis only.
c Described as "chronic active hepatitis" with positive autoantibodies.
d Laboratory values reflect the percentage abnormal of total tested cases.

Neonatal sclerosing cholangitis

The series reported by Debray et al. [3] included 15 patients with the neonatal onset of sclerosing cholangitis. All 15 had cholestasis during the first month of life, which progressed to cirrhosis. Amedee-Manesme et al. [10] originally described this entity in eight children, initially identified as having neonatal cholestasis, in whom clinical, histologic, and radiologic features compatible with sclerosing cholangitis developed. Percutaneous cholecystography demonstrated abnormal intrahepatic bile ducts with rarefaction of segmental branches, stenosis, and focal dilatation; the extrahepatic ducts were abnormal in six of the eight children. The liver biopsy samples obtained in infancy suggested bile duct obstruction; histologic examination later in life documented ductal proliferation and cirrhosis. These reports expand the spectrum of infantile cholangiopathies and beg the question as to whether these cases may represent a forme fruste of biliary atresia or an initial manifestation of progressive familial intrahepatic cholestasis type 3 (multidrug resistance-associated protein 3 (MDR3) deficiency). In a series of 48 infants younger than 100 days of age undergoing endoscopic retrograde cholangiopancreatography (ERCP) as part of a diagnostic evaluation for biliary atresia, six were diagnosed with neonatal sclerosing cholangitis, based on a patent, but abnormal biliary tree [11]. Clinical features and liver histology in all these patients were indistinguishable from biliary atresia, apart from variable presence of bile pigment in the stools. Jaundice and hepatic dysfunction improved in all subjects during follow-up. Immunostaining was performed in five children and showed MDR3 expression at the canalicular membrane, suggesting that MDR3 deficiency was not the cause for the cholangiopathy in this cohort. Neonatal sclerosing cholangitis has been identified in association with two syndromes: Kabuki syndrome (involving facial dysmorphism, developmental delay, growth hormone deficiency, skeletal anomalies, and congenital heart defects), and neonatal ichthyosis-sclerosing cholangitis syndrome, which appears to result from a claudin-1 deficiency [12]. Early age at onset, rapid progression, and association with congenital

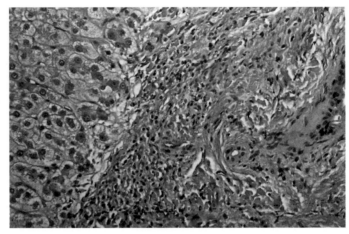

Figure 21.2 Liver biopsy in a patient with autoimmune hepatitis and primary sclerosing cholangitis shows periductular stromal edema and inflammation, along with hepatitis along portal margins (hematoxylin & eosin, original magnification ×400).

disorders suggest that neonatal sclerosing cholangitis represents a unique form of idiopathic sclerosing cholangitis.

Autoimmune hepatitis and sclerosing cholangitis

An overlap syndrome of AIH and sclerosing cholangitis has received increased attention in recent years, being described in both adults and children [5,6,9]. Such patients are defined by elevated serum immunoglobulin levels and positive serum autoantibodies (anti-nuclear antibody (ANA) or anti-smooth muscle antibody (ASMA)) in addition to histologic and radiologic findings of both autoimmune hepatitis and sclerosing cholangitis; Figure 21.2). As is true for PSC alone, the overlap syndrome often coexists with IBD, and the activity of the hepatitis does not correlate with the activity of the colitis. However, in contrast to isolated PSC, females predominate in this overlap syndrome, particularly at younger ages of presentation [6,13].

A prospective 16-year study of 55 children with AIH found radiologic evidence of sclerosing cholangitis in 50% based on screening cholangiograms [6]. Two-thirds had both intra- and extrahepatic findings, while in the remaining one-third the cholangiographic abnormalities were intrahepatic only. A biochemical and histological response to immunosuppression was shown in 89% but no cholangiographic disease regression was noted. An original diagnosis of AIH prior to cholangiography was seen in 5 of 32 patients in one series [9] and 5 of 13 in another [4]. In 2 of 56 patients in the French series, a diagnosis of both AIH and sclerosing cholangitis was made [3]. In the North American studies, the prevalence of PSC–AIH overlap syndrome ranged between 17 [9] and 35% [5]. In the study by Feldstein et al. [5], there was no difference in the clinical features, aminotransferase levels, or histologic stage of disease in the 18 children with PSC–AIH overlap syndrome when compared with those with PSC alone. However, these patients were distinguished by having higher total serum gammaglobulin levels and by the presence of ANA and/or ASMA. In a retrospective study, AIH and PSC were simultaneously diagnosed in 9 of 47 children (35%), which was defined as concomitant evidence of histologic features of AIH, specifically the presence of interface hepatitis and lymphoplasmacytic infiltration, and abnormalities of the biliary tree on imaging [7]. All patients with overlap syndrome had positive autoimmune markers (increased IgG, ANA or ASMA).

The relationship between AIH and PSC is not clear; patients with overlap may simply have concurrence of two disease processes, or they may be manifesting two features of the same disease, along a spectrum of "hepatitic" to "cholestatic" phenotypes (Figure 21.3). The term autoimmune sclerosing cholangitis has, therefore, been used interchangeably with AIH–PSC overlap syndrome; there is some suggestion that in these patients, unlike in those without evidence of autoimmunity, the progression of biliary disease might be slowed through the use of immunosuppressive therapy [13]. However, the findings in regards to response to immunosuppressive therapy in the prospective [6] and retrospective [5,7] studies need to be interpreted with caution, since subjects were typically treated with immunosuppression *and* ursodeoxycholic acid (UDCA), both of which are known to reduce serum levels of aminotransferases when used in monotherapy. In addition, control groups for treatment interventions were lacking. Importantly, the cohorts were too small to study effects of immunosuppression on hard end-points, including transplant-free survival and progression of portal hypertension, which were both shown to be poorly correlated with biochemical remission in adults with PSC [14]. Similarly, the prognosis of ASC is difficult to ascertain given the small samples sizes: compared with AIH without PSC, children with ASC appear to have a higher risk of progressing to cirrhosis requiring liver transplantation [3], whereas compared with PSC, long-term survival of patients with ASC does not differ [5]. A detailed review of autoimmune liver disease can be found in Chapter 20. It is increasingly clear that, in making the diagnosis of sclerosing cholangitis, a combination of serum markers, liver histology, and cholangiographic imaging is necessary to distinguish between the classic and autoimmune forms. Conversely, an overlap syndrome should be considered if there is an incomplete response to immunosuppressive medications or development of cholestasis in an individual diagnosed with AIH.

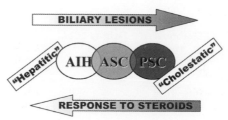

Figure 21.3 Proposed spectrum of disease and relationship between autoimmune hepatitis (AIH) and primary sclerosing cholangitis (PSC). ASC, autoimmune sclerosing cholangitis.

Furthermore, the high prevalence of AIH–PSC overlap among children may constitute an important difference in regards to pathogenesis and potentially response to immunosuppressive therapy between children and adults with PSC. Compared with an average prevalence of 29% of ASC in cohorts of children with PSC (Table 21.2), overlap with AIH was only found in 4 of 46 adults (8.7%) with PSC in a population-based study [15] and in 19 of 273 subjects (6.8%) presenting with PSC at a mean age of 32 years in a single center experience [16].

Epidemiology

The overall incidence of sclerosing cholangitis is unknown; it varies widely in geographical regions, with the highest reported cases in northern Europe and lower prevalence in southern Europe and Asia. Population-based estimates in the USA were first reported: in a study from Olmsted County, MN, a small, predominantly white community where there were 22 new cases of PSC from 1976 to 2000 [17]. The estimated age-adjusted incidence was 1.25 in 100 000 person-years in men, and 0.54 in 100 000 person-years in women. In this study, the prevalence of PSC was 20.9 per 100 000 men and 6.3 per 100 000 women; 73% of cases were associated with IBD. In a larger epidemiologic study from Calgary, Canada, 49 subjects were newly diagnosed with PSC between 2000 and 2005, of which three were younger than 18 years of age at the time of diagnosis, accounting for an incidence of 0.23 in 100 000 person-years in children, compared with 1.11 in 100 000 in adults [15]. Similar results were obtained in a population based study in the UK, in which 223 patients with PSC were identified over a period of 10 years, of whom 13 were younger than 24 years of age, with an incidence of 0.2 in 100 000 in children and young adults and a peak incidence of 1.1 in 100 000 in subjects aged 65–74 years [18].

Although these studies suggest that PSC is less common in children than in adults, the incidence of PSC in children – even those with IBD – may be underestimated because the cholangiographic anatomy of liver diseases prevalent in children is still not well defined. In published series, it is consistently more common in males in all age groups [15,17,18], with a ratio approximating 1.7:1 across the different pediatric studies (Table 21.2). It also appears that males are younger at the time of diagnosis of both PSC and UC.

Several large independent studies on the natural history of PSC have been published to date, each containing more than 100 adults [15,17,18], most recently in a cohort of 273 patients in Germany [16]. In these studies, an estimated 60–80% of patients with PSC have or will develop IBD, with UC accounting for more than 50% of the cases. An extensive literature review of 572 adults with PSC documented that the associated frequency of IBD was 76% (67% for patients with UC and 9% for Crohn disease) [19].

From 2 to 7.5% of adults with UC may simultaneously be affected with PSC [12]. In 1500 adults with UC in Sweden, there was a point prevalence of PSC at 5.5% in patients with extensive colitis, but only 0.5% in those with distal colitis [20]. A descriptive report of 36 children with PSC–IBD documented similar findings: pancolitis was present on the initial examination in 80%, along with rectal sparing in 26% [21]. Pouchitis was also common after colectomy in this study, occurring in four of five patients after ileal pouch–anal anastomosis. Recently, these findings were confirmed in a Japanese cohort, in which 29 patients with PSC were matched 1:2 with patients with UC without PSC; 69% of the patients with PSC had concomitant colitis [22]. Histopathological examination revealed more severe inflammation of the cecum and ascending colon and relative sparing of the rectum. Of note, compared with patients with PSC without IBD, subjects with the PSC–IBD complex were significantly younger and predominantly male.

There is no direct correlation between the activity of PSC and colitis in a given patient at a single time point. In fact, symptomatic PSC may occur during quiescent IBD or after colectomy [12,23]. It now appears that chronic, minimally symptomatic pancolitis may predispose to the development of PSC and, in fact, PSC might serve as a surrogate marker for chronic, asymptomatic UC [12].

In the six large published pediatric series, an average of 59% of children with PSC had IBD (Table 21.2); 41% had UC, and 12% had Crohn disease. Just as in adults with IBD and PSC, the symptoms and diagnosis of liver disease in children may precede, be coincident with, or follow the diagnosis of IBD. To determine the frequency of PSC in pediatric IBD, Hyams et al. [24] screened 555 children with IBD for evidence of liver disease based on an elevated serum alanine aminotransferase (ALT). PSC was identified in eight patients with UC (3.5% of all those with UC) and two patients with Crohn disease (0.6% of those with Crohn disease). This likely underestimates the incidence because not all patients with PSC will have elevated ALT.

Primary biliary cirrhosis is not as common in patients with Crohn disease and is seemingly limited to those with extensive colonic involvement (colitis or ileocolitis) [12]. In the study by Feldstein et al. [5], the proportion of children with Crohn disease was much higher (15%) than the 4–7% reported in adults, yet consistent with other pediatric reports (Table 21.2) [2,3,5,9,21]. The reason for this is unclear, but it may reflect the degree of colitis in Crohn disease presenting in childhood.

Clinical features

In adults, the early clinical course of PSC is similar in patients with or without documented IBD. The early course is insidious, so it may be difficult to precisely determine the onset of the disease; symptoms may be present for months before the diagnosis is made [17]. Initial symptoms consist of a gradual onset of progressive fatigue, malaise, anorexia, and weight loss. Pruritus followed by fluctuating jaundice may next occur. Clinical evidence of cholangitis, highlighted by recurrent right upper quadrant pain, fever, and hyperbilirubinemia, is often noted. The majority of patients with PSC are asymptomatic when biochemical abnormalities are first detected; this prompts further workup, including cholangiography [5,17]. Depending on the stage of disease at presentation, patients with PSC may have a normal physical examination or may exhibit some abnormality such as hepatomegaly, splenomegaly, or jaundice.

A similar insidious onset has been seen in children, with signs and symptoms of liver disease having been present for an average of 3 years before diagnosis in 56 patients in one study [3]. In another study, most of the 32 children presented with relatively non-specific complaints such as fatigue, anorexia, or pruritus [9], and 29% (15 of 52) of the patients in the study by Feldstein et al. [9] were asymptomatic at diagnosis.

The clinical features noted in children with sclerosing cholangitis are similar to those reported in adults (Table 21.3). Some features are, however, unique to childhood, including poor growth and delayed puberty. The specific clinical features occurring in a relatively large number of children have been described in the six large pediatric series [2–5,7,9]. In the series of 56 patients [3], the initial signs and symptoms included jaundice in 9, hepatomegaly in 28, splenomegaly in 1, variceal hemorrhage in 1, and abnormal liver function tests in 2 otherwise asymptomatic children. By the time of diagnosis, 25 were cholestatic, almost all had hepatomegaly, 42 had splenomegaly, and 12 had ascites. Findings in 32 patients [9] and 13 patients [4] were similar, with jaundice in 11, hepatomegaly in 30 (with coincident splenomegaly in 14), isolated splenomegaly in 1, and pruritus in 7. Of the series of 52 children [5], 15 were asymptomatic, 21 presented with abdominal pain, 14 with fatigue, and 10 with jaundice; hepatomegaly was present in 8, splenomegaly in 10, and weight loss in 9. The differences in the presentations of patients in the last study may reflect the increasing awareness of PSC and its earlier evaluation and diagnosis.

Laboratory findings

There are no specific laboratory findings of PSC. Elevated serum alkaline phosphatase is commonly noted in adults with PSC, and the vast majority will have mildly increased serum aminotransferases [5]. Approximately half have a modest increase in serum bilirubin levels, but wide variations have been noted. Hypoalbuminemia and abnormal prothrombin time are common with advanced disease.

Similarly, most children show biochemical evidence of cholestasis. However, while many children have elevated serum alkaline phosphatase, 15 of 32 had normal levels in one study [9] and 13 of 52 had normal levels in another [5].

Table 21.3 Clinical features of sclerosing cholangitis in children

	Features
Symptoms	Abdominal pain
	Fatigue
	Anorexia
	Jaundice
	Fever
	Weight loss
	Pruritus
	Delayed puberty
	Chronic diarrhea[a]
	Gastrointestinal hemorrhage
Signs	Hepatomegaly
	Hepatosplenomegaly
	Splenomegaly
	Ascites
	Xanthomas
Other	Presentation as autoimmune hepatitis poorly responsive to therapy

[a] Not necessarily associated with inflammatory bowel disease

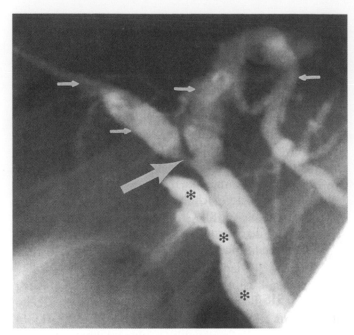

Figure 21.4 Image obtained during endoscopic retrograde cholangiopancreatography in an 18-year-old man with a 7 year history of chronic liver disease and colitis shows typical changes of sclerosing cholangitis. There is overall irregularity of the intrahepatic ducts and areas of distinct stenosis, for example the junction of the right and left hepatic ducts (large arrow); the distal intrahepatic ducts are relatively spared (small arrows). Note the unusually long cystic duct (asterisks), which is a normal variant.

Serum gamma-glutamyltransferase (GGT) appear to be more sensitive than serum alkaline phosphatase levels, with 97% of children with sclerosing cholangitis having an abnormal serum GGT at the time of diagnosis in the large series [2–5,7,9] (Table 21.2). In addition, GGT may also be more specific for hepatobiliary disease, given the wide range of normal values for alkaline phosphatase in the presence of bone growth in children. In a case series of 28 children with autoimmune liver disease, the GGT:aspartate aminotransferase (AST) ratio was found to be helpful in screening patients for overlap with PSC. Regarding biochemical evidence for hepatocellular injury, serum ALT was increased in 94% and serum AST in 92% of tested patients (Table 21.2) [2–5,7,9]. Serum aminotransferase levels tend to be higher in children than in adults, with mean AST levels >230 IU/L in two studies [5,7], compared, for example, with a mean AST of 80 IU/L in a study of adults [25]. Whether this difference is related to increased hepatocellular injury of a different pathogenesis in children, for example overlap with AIH, or an earlier stage in the disease process, is currently unknown.

Diagnosis
Imaging
The gold standard for the diagnosis of sclerosing cholangitis is cholangiography, but suspicion of disease rests on a combination of clinical signs and symptoms, laboratory data, and

characteristic liver histology. Characteristic findings on ERCP are irregular narrowing and stricture of the hepatic and common bile duct caused by fibrosing inflammation with or without involvement of the intrahepatic ducts (Figure 21.4). These areas of segmental stenosis can be widespread, diffuse, and multifocal. Strictures may be short (1–2 cm) and annular with intervening segments of apparently normal or minimally dilated ducts, which produces the characteristic beaded appearance. Focal minimal dilatation or small diverticula may be noted proximal to the stricture [26]. Band-like strictures are found in approximately 20% of adults, and diverticular outpouchings in 25%; the latter feature is suggested to be highly specific. The intrahepatic biliary tree may be the site of decreased peripheral arborization, reflecting loss of normal functioning bile ducts, imparting the "pruned tree" appearance [23,27,28]. A grading system was developed upon retrospective review of cholangiograms of 40 patients with PSC to classify the intra- and extrahepatic bile duct abnormalities [28]. In this study, cholangiographic findings of the intrahepatic ducts ranged from multiple strictures with none or minimal dilatation (grade I), over multiple strictures with saccular dilatation and decreased arborization (grade II), to severe pruning with only central bile duct being filled with contrast (grade III). Regarding the extrahepatic ducts, slight irregularities without stenosis, segmental stenosis, stenosis of almost entire length of the duct, and extremely irregular margins with diverticulum-like outpouchings were classified as grades I to IV, respectively.

In two pediatric series [3,4], all patients had irregularity of the intrahepatic ducts similar to those shown in adult series; this included duct wall irregularity, filling defects, irregular dilation, pruning of the peripheral branches, absence of opacification of some branches, beading, and confluent strictures. In the 52 children studied by Feldstein *et al.* [5], 29 (56%) of the patients had both intra- and extrahepatic bile duct involvement, 22 (42%) had isolated intrahepatic abnormalities, and only 1 (2%) had isolated extrahepatic abnormalities. In the retrospective study [7], all 47 subjects had undergone cholangiography by magnetic resonance cholangiopancreatography (MRCP) or ERCP, and abnormalities affecting intra- *and* extrahepatic bile ducts were reported for 18 (40%) of the patients. Of note, 17 (36%) of the patients displayed a normal biliary tree on imaging and were diagnosed with small-duct PSC by liver biopsy.

Recently, MRCP has been used as a non-invasive tool in the diagnosis of abnormalities of the pancreaticobiliary tree. In adults with PSC, MRI has been able to demonstrate abnormalities of both the extra- and intrahepatic biliary tree, including dilation, stenosis, beading, and pruning. In a study of 150 adults comparing ERCP with MRCP for the diagnosis of PSC, the latter showed a sensitivity of 88% and specificity of 99%. More bile duct stenoses and pruning were seen by ERCP, whereas more areas of skip dilatation were visualized by MRCP. A recent meta-analysis comparing MRCP with ERCP as the gold standard for the diagnosis of PSC, including six published studies and 456 subjects with 623 independent MRCP readings, found a sensitivity and excellent specificity of MRCP for detection of PSC across all studies of 86% and 94%, respectively [29], demonstrating that confirmation of MRCP findings by ERCP is not required.

Increasingly, MRCP is being used in children as a non-invasive means of diagnosing PSC. In one study, ERCP, MRCP, and liver biopsy were performed on 21 children with the clinical and laboratory suspicion of PSC: 13 patients (62%) showed duct abnormalities by MRCP, while 16 patients (76%) demonstrated abnormal ducts by ERCP [30]. The remaining five patients received alternative diagnoses based on liver biopsy results. In a single center case series from Canada including 19 children with an average age of 13 years, the sensitivity for MRCP in detecting PSC was 84% [31]. The primary advantages of using MRCP – particularly in a pediatric population – are that it is non-invasive, requires no radiation or contrast material, and carries a very low complication rate compared with ERCP. Use of MRCP may also visualize the biliary tract in small children in whom ERCP is not feasible, and it may be useful in following children and adults after liver transplantation to evaluate for recurrence of disease. In cases of negative or equivocal results, traditional cholangiography should be performed as it allows injection of contrast under higher pressure and better visualization of specific biliary abnormalities, for example bile duct stenosis and pruning.

In summary, in the future MRCP may be widely used in children as in adults to establish the diagnosis of PSC and to survey for complications, whereas ERCP may be reserved for therapeutic purposes, for example for dilatation of dominant strictures or evaluation for cholangiocarcinoma by brushing of the common bile duct for cytology.

Serologic markers

There are no reliable diagnostic serologic markers for PSC, although circulating non-organ-specific autoantibodies are often present. A study testing autoantibodies in 73 adults with PSC found that 97% were positive for at least one in a panel of 20, and that 81% were positive for at least three. The antibodies most frequently identified were ANA in 53%, anti-cardiolipin antibody in 66%, and anti-neutrophil cytoplasmic antibodies (ANCA) in 84% [32]. Of those tested in the pediatric series, ANCAs were positive in 59% [2,5,9]. Because of the high prevalence of perinuclear ANCA in PSC, this test is useful as a diagnostic marker when combined with other standard diagnostic tests. However, ANCAs are not specific for PSC and often occur in both UC and AIH. They are not helpful for monitoring disease activity, and their role in the pathogenesis of disease is unclear.

Based on observations that autoimmune *pancreatitis* is associated with elevated serum IgG$_4$ and responsiveness to therapy with corticosteroids, it was hypothesized that IgG$_4$ levels may also help to identify a specific subgroup of patients with PSC with distinct natural history. In 127 adults with PSC, elevated serum IgG$_4$ levels ($>$140 mg/dL) were detected in 11 (9%) [33]. These patients had higher total bilirubin and serum alkaline phosphatase; their PSC Mayo Clinic risk score was higher and the time to liver transplantation was shorter compared with patients with PSC and normal serum IgG$_4$. Whether these patients behave similarly to patients with autoimmune pancreatitis and would respond more favorably to therapy with corticosteroids requires future clinical trials. Of note, elevated IgG$_4$ levels have not been reported in children with PSC or ASC to date.

Biopsy

The histologic changes, although characteristic in many cases of PSC, tend to be less dramatic than the cholangiographic changes, perhaps because of sampling limitations and the two-dimensional nature of microscopy. The histologic hallmark is a progression of ductal lesions. Reported histologic changes range from non-specific portal edema and fibrosis and subtle pericholangitis (Figure 21.2), to severe pericholangiolar edema and sclerosis (Figure 21.5), to frank obliteration (Figure 21.6). Typically there is portal-to-portal variability. Careful review of serial biopsies, serial sections, or three-dimensional reconstructions of a single biopsy specimen is necessary in order to appreciate obliteration of ducts with sclerosis or focal duct dilatation. It may be instructive to compare the diameter of the interlobular bile ducts with that of the accompanying artery; these are normally approximately equal.

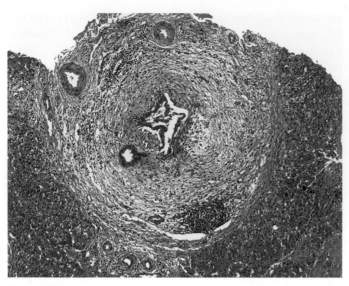

Figure 21.5 Classic "onion-skinning" periductular sclerosis in a patient with primary sclerosing cholangitis (hematoxylin & eosin, original magnification ×400).

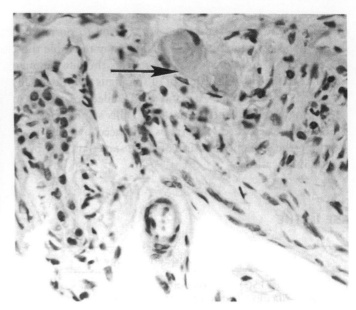

Figure 21.6 Focal fibrous obliteration of a small bile duct (arrow) in a patient with inflammatory bowel disease (hematoxylin & eosin, original magnification ×400).

The most characteristic feature found in liver specimens from patients with PSC is focal concentric edema and fibrosis ("onion-skinning") around interlobular bile ducts [2]. Synchronous or metachronous histologic changes that have been noted as sequential or concomitant lesions include bile duct proliferation, periductal fibrosis, periductal inflammation, degeneration of bile duct epithelial cells associated with inflammatory infiltration, ductal obliteration, and loss of bile ducts, along with portal edema and fibrosis, portal and periportal hepatitis, and focal parenchymal changes. The pathognomonic histologic change (fibrous-obliterative cholangitis), which occurs in the early stages, may not be present in all biopsy cores or easy to demonstrate. This lesion is succeeded over time by replacement of duct segments by solid cords of connective tissue and extensive loss of interlobular and adjacent septal bile ducts. Ultimately a local condition of bile duct paucity may develop because of the substantial reduction in the number of bile duct profiles per portal zone. However, non-obliterated ducts may proliferate, making recognition of the deficit of ducts particularly challenging. With progression, there is an increasing portal fibrosis, bridging, and progression to biliary cirrhosis. At surgery or autopsy, the extrahepatic bile ducts may appear as thickened cords without a change in duct diameter. Cross-sectional examination will reveal the lumen to be narrowed by concentric fibrous thickening of the wall (up to 10-fold), with the mucosa being unaffected [2,34].

Ludwig *et al.* [34] proposed that the histologic lesions of PSC be divided into four stages (Figure 21.7). The initial stage (I), confined to the portal tract, consists of cholangitis and portal hepatitis; fibrous obliterative cholangitis resulting in eventual loss of interlobular and adjacent septal bile ducts occurs along with lymphocytic infiltration and ductular changes (narrowing, obliteration, or proliferation). In stage II, the inflammatory process has extended beyond the portal tract to involve the periportal region, resulting in periportal fibrosis or hepatitis; the histologic features may resemble AIH. In stage III (septal stage), fibrosis of the periportal region with portal-to-portal tract bridging occurs; the histologic changes may resemble those noted in PBC in adults. Stage IV reflects the development of biliary cirrhosis. This concept of staging is not universally accepted and, because of the inherent sampling error associated with liver biopsy, it may be unreliable for following the progression of disease.

Liver biopsies from the 56 children with sclerosing cholangitis demonstrated portal fibrosis in 54, neoductular proliferation in 33, ductopenia in 4, and cirrhosis in 23 [3]. Similarly, portal fibrosis and ductular proliferation was found in all 13 patients in another series [4]. In this series, periductal fibrosis, suggestive of sclerosing cholangitis, also was seen in all 13 patients, and five had a well-developed periductal onion skin change around the bile ducts. In contrast, concentric periductular fibrosis or inflammatory infiltrate was found in only 14 of the 56 children in one study [3] and 40 of 52 in further series had liver biopsy specimens available, each demonstrating features highly suggestive of PSC [5]: ductular proliferation, ductopenia, and portal edema, and fibrosis were the most common features, occurring in 80%, 60%, and 60%, respectively. Periductal fibrosis was seen in 30%. Based on the staging criteria of Ludwig (see following discussion and Table 21.4), 46% of these patients had early disease (histologic stage I or II). In a retrospective review of 20 children diagnosed with PSC over a 20 year period [2], particular attention was given to liver histology: classic periductal concentric fibrosis was found in liver sections of only 5 patients, while features of cholangitis and duct or ductular proliferation were present in 11 (55%); 13 patients (65%) had advanced disease at presentation, 8 at stage III and 5 at stage IV.

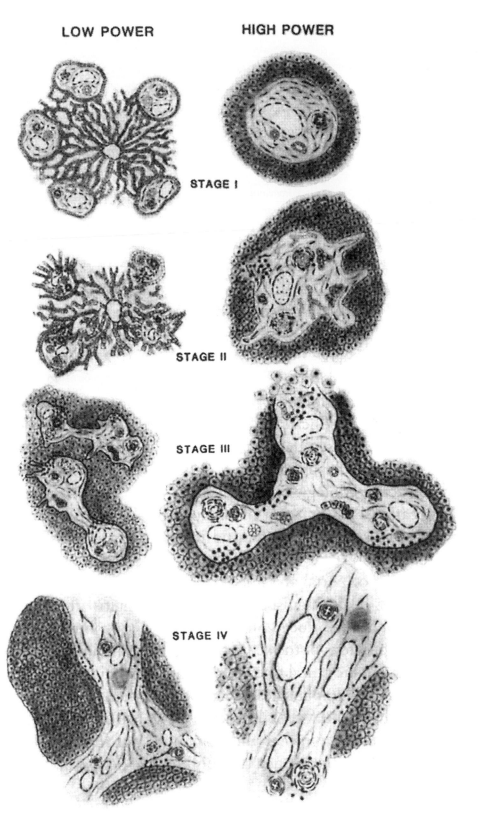

LOW POWER **HIGH POWER**

STAGE I

STAGE II

STAGE III

STAGE IV

Figure 21.7 Schematic representation of the four stages of liver disease (chronic hepatitis) associated with primary sclerosing cholangitis. In the high-power view of stage II, clusters of hepatocytes are shown within the enlarged portal tract; cholangitis is also depicted. In stage III, portal-to-portal fibrous bridging is present. The low-power view of stage IV shows a garland-shaped regenerative nodule. In stages III and IV, duct obliteration is present; the presence of these duct abnormalities would not be essential for staging. (Reprinted with permission from Ludwig, 1989 [34].)

Table 21.4 Ludwig's classification of duct disease in primary sclerosing cholangitis

Liver biopsy features	Cholangiographic findings	Suggested terminology
Typical	Not diagnostic	Small-duct PSC
Not diagnostic	Typical	Large-duct PSC (extra- or intrahepatic)
Typical	Typical	Combined large and small duct PSC (global or classic PSC)

PSC, primary sclerosing cholangitis.
Source: modified with permission from Ludwig, 1989 [34].

Patients who have negative cholangiographic findings, but nevertheless have liver histology and laboratory data consistent with PSC, are considered to have *small-duct PSC* (previously referred to as pericholangitis). In a comparison of the natural history of disease in 33 adults with small-duct PSC and 260 adults with large-duct PSC [35], patients with small-duct PSC had better survival and none developed cholangiocarcinoma during the 105 month period. By comparison, 28 patients (11%) with large-duct disease developed cholangiocarcinoma. A cohort of 32 patients with small-duct disease had only four patients who developed large-duct disease in the 63-month follow-up [36]. Although this categorization is still controversial, these results suggest that small-duct PSC may represent a unique, less aggressive subtype of PSC. Of 16 children with small-duct PSC, none progressed to large-duct disease and only two underwent liver transplantation, which meant a better graft-free survival in this subgroup compared with the patients with large-duct disease or those with overlap with AIH [7].

Pathogenesis

The initiating event and mechanisms responsible for the progressive changes of PSC are unknown, yet they appear to derive from an immune-mediated process. As is the case with many such diseases, the etiology is probably multifactorial: the process may be initiated by various triggers (e.g. infections, toxins, or ischemic injury) that adversely affect only certain, genetically susceptible individuals. Substantial research is underway to (1) define mechanisms of innate and adaptive immune responses driving initiation of hepatobiliary injury and progression of biliary fibrosis, (2) elucidate the liver-bile duct–gut interplay, and (3) better recapitulate the heterogeneity of PSC in animal models. Some of the current concepts on the pathogenesis of PSC are reviewed in Figure 21.8 [37–39].

Immunopathogenesis

Several abnormalities associated with PSC point to an immune-mediated process: (1) portal tract infiltration with T-lymphocytes, (2) genetic susceptibility associations with human leukocyte antigen (HLA) complexes driving CD4 T-cell and natural killer cell activation, (3) the presence of serum autoantibodies particularly perinuclear ANCA, and (4) the strong association with autoimmune diseases and IBD. Up to 25% of patients with PSC and IBD have one or more

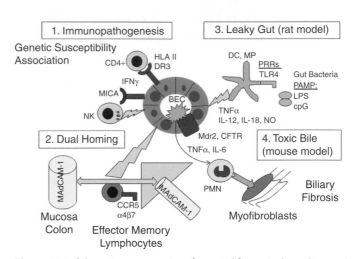

Figure 21.8 Schematic representation of potential factors in the pathogenesis of primary sclerosing cholangitis (PSC). Immunopathogenesis is supported by susceptibility to PSC with genes encoding HLA class II and class I-like proteins (MICA), determining adaptive (CD4 T-cell) and innate (natural killer (NK) cell) responses, respectively, both injuring biliary epithelial cells (BECs). The "dual homing" hypothesis is based on findings in patients with PSC–inflammatory bowel disease, showing that effector memory T-lymphocytes from the gut are recruited to the liver via mucosal addressin cell adhesion molecule (MAdCAM-1), which is expressed on portal vein/sinusoidal endothelium under inflammatory conditions [37]. The "leaky gut" hypothesis is supported by experiments showing that small bowel bacterial overgrowth in susceptible rats leads to production of proinflammatory cytokines and toxic nitric oxide (NO) by hepatic macrophages (MP) or dendritic cells (DC). Receptors on these cells, called pattern recognition receptors (PRRs), recognize invariant molecular structures (pathogen associated molecular patterns (PAMPs)), which are present, for example, on bacterial walls [38]. "Toxic bile" in *Mdr2* knockout mice, which are devoid of phospholipids, causes activation of hepatic neutrophils (PMNs), production of inflammatory cytokines, and subsequently biliary fibrosis [39]. TLR4, Toll-like receptor; LPS, lipopolysaccharide; TNF, tumor necrosis factor; IL, interleukin; CCR5, chemokine receptor type 5.

autoimmune disorders, compared with only 9% of patients with IBD without PSC. In fact, several patients have two or more autoimmune diseases, most frequently thyroid disease and diabetes mellitus. However, patients with PSC do not have a classic autoimmune phenotype, since the disease predominantly affects males, it shows poor response to immunosuppressive therapies, and the autoantibodies detected in PSC are not tissue specific and present only in a proportion of patients.

A genetic predisposition to biliary tract injury initiated by any of the postulated mechanisms must be woven into any etiopathogenetic theory, since familial occurrence of PSC has been noted in several reports and, combined with environmental factors, may account for the striking geographic clustering of PSC. A recent genome-wide association study in a primary Norwegian cohort (discovery panel) and independent verification case–control cohorts in Scandinavia, Belgium/Netherlands, and Germany showed strong associations with as subset of HLA genes and with non-HLA genes involved in bile homeostasis and macrophage activation [40]. The *HLA* genes are located on chromosome 6p21.3 and include: (1) genes A, Cw, and B encoding HLA class I antigens presenting peptides to CD8 T-cells; (2) genes *MICA/B* encoding the HLA class I chain-like (MIC) molecules, which are critical for activation of natural killer cells and γδT-cell activation; and (3) the genes *HLA-DR/HLA-DQ* and *HLA-DP* encoding class II antigens presenting peptides to CD4 T-helper (Th) cells. Several studies have identified class II haplotypes associated with PSC: *HLA-DR3*, *HLA-DQ2*, and *HLA-DR6/DQ6* are the most frequently reported. The allele *HLA-DRB1*0301* increases the risk by 2.54-fold to develop PSC, whereas *HLA-DRB1*0401* is associated with protection. Interestingly, recent high-resolution genotyping of risk alleles for DRB1 revealed how single amino acid substitutions alter the electrostatic properties of the binding groove of the class II molecule and subsequently influences the range of peptides presented to CD4 lymphocytes in patients with PSC [41]. Furthermore, results of genetic studies interrogating the *MICA* locus on chromosome 6 indicate that the innate immune system (natural killer cells and γδT-cells) may be uniquely important for initiation of PSC [42], more so perhaps than for AIH or PBC. The *MICA*008* allele has a strong positive association, and *MICA*002* confers protection from PSC. Only one pediatric series has included HLA genotyping; this found an increased incidence of *HLA-B8* and *HLA-DR2* [9]. Non-HLA-gene associations supporting an immune-mediated pathogenesis of PSC include protective polymorphisms in *K469E*, the gene encoding intercellular adhesion molecule-1 (CD54), which mediates leukocyte adhesion during immune responses. The significance of the association of PSC with variants in the gene encoding TGR5, a G protein-coupled bile acid receptor with dual function in bile acid homeostasis and control of inflammatory responses, remains in question [43].

To what extent biliary epithelial cells participate in the immune reaction is incompletely understood. They appear to act both as a target of and a participant in the immune reaction, expressing cytokines, enzymes, intercellular adhesion molecules, and HLA molecules. The fact that they aberrantly express HLA class II molecules, a classic characteristic of antigen-presenting cells, suggests that biliary epithelial cells alone might be capable of initiating an immune response by binding to autoantigens or exogenous antigens. Notably, the presence of autoantibodies to surface antigens expressed on biliary epithelial cells have been demonstrated in patients with PSC [44]. These cells were found to express the lymphocyte homing receptor (CD44) and to induce interleukin-6 production, leading to biliary epithelial cell proliferation. It is possible that persistent interleukin-6 production could account – at least in part – for the bile duct changes of PSC.

"Gut lymphocyte homing" and "leaky gut" hypotheses

Grant *et al.* [37] have proposed an intriguing mechanism of disease pathogenesis that might account for how the portal inflammation of PSC can be dyssynchronous from associated colitis. Based on their identification of gut-associated adhesion molecules (such as mucosal vascular addressin cell adhesion molecule-1 and vascular adhesion protein-1) on portal endothelium in IBD-associated liver inflammation, they posited that certain lymphocytes activated in the inflamed gut mucosa of patients with IBD develop "dual homing," acquiring the ability to bind to both mucosal and hepatic endothelium. These cells can then persist in the liver as memory T-cells, and – at some later time point – induce hepatobiliary inflammation in response to a secondary trigger. A gut-specific chemokine, CCL25, is found in the livers of patients with PSC, a finding that might help to explain how T-cells are recruited to the liver in sclerosing cholangitis [45].

An alternative theory, frequently referred to as the "leaky gut hypothesis," has held that various proinflammatory bacteria-derived products (e.g. peptides or toxic bile acids) play a role in the etiopathogenesis of hepatobiliary disease. It has been hypothesized that PSC in patients with IBD could be related to repeated episodes of low-grade bacterial infection (or portal bacteremia), suggesting that disruption of the intestinal mucosal barrier allows entry of bacteria into the portal vein. Certainly, bacterial antigens may act through molecular mimicry, whereby microbial molecules containing specific epitopes cross-react with molecules in human antigens, essentially acting as "autoantigens" to set off an inflammatory cascade in a predisposed individual.

Several microorganisms have been detected in the livers and biliary tracts of patients with sclerosing cholangitis. For example, explanted livers of patients with sclerosing cholangitis showed high bacterial positivity, with α-hemolytic streptococci making up the majority of the bacteria found. Moreover, cryptosporidiosis has long been noted in association with sclerosing cholangitis in immunodeficient patients and may occur in patients with sclerosing cholangitis without documented immunodeficiency. *Helicobacter* species have been identified in human liver samples of patients with sclerosing cholangitis, and seropositivity to chlamydial infections has been associated with PSC. However, negative studies, including the absence of portal vein bacteremia, of small bowel bacterial overgrowth, or abnormal intestinal permeability in a significant number of patients with PSC, indicate that more research needs to be done to determine how relevant recurrent bacterial infections are for disease progression of PSC.

Animal models

Investigation of the pathogenesis of PSC has been bolstered by the development of animal models for hepatobiliary injury. In one such model, lesions reminiscent of PSC (portal inflammation and bile duct proliferation) occur in genetically susceptible rats with experimental small bowel bacterial overgrowth [38]. The hepatobiliary injury noted in this model is not considered to be caused by the above postulated factors, such as septicemia or portal bacteremia; instead, it was suggested that mucosal absorption of bacterial cell wall polymers occurred and that these bacterial by-products initiated the biliary injury. Targeted disruption of the cell wall polymers prevented hepatobiliary injury [38]. Abnormally elevated levels of the bacterial endotoxin lipopolysaccharide has been demonstated in the biliary epithelium of rats with small bowel bacterial overgrowth, linking the pathogenesis of intestinal injury to that of bile duct injury in this model [46].

A second mouse model may help to define the connection between colitis and cholangitis: inflammatory cell infiltration and focal necrosis occurs in the livers of mice with dextran sulfate sodium-induced experimental colitis [47]. Cytokine analysis and mononuclear cell isolation from livers of these mice indicated a Th1-dominant immune mechanism, similar to that seen in PSC.

Furthermore, it has been noted that mice with targeted disruptions of *Mdr2*, the murine orthologue of *MDR3*, develop hepatic lesions strongly resembling the "onion-skin" cholangitis of PSC [39] (Figure 21.9). It is thought that Mdr2 deficiency reduces secretion of phospholipids across the canalicular membrane, which increases the concentration of free non-micellar bile acids ("toxic bile") in the segmental bile ducts, disrupting tight junctions and basement membranes and subsequently leading to regurgitation of bile acids, periductal inflammation, cholangitis and ultimately biliary fibrosis in these mice. Interestingly, studies in these mice also revealed that treatment with UDCA would increase biliary pressure, causing rupture of cholangioles and hepatocyte necrosis. Years later, the importance of these early animal studies was recognized when clinical observations showed that treatment with high-dose UDCA decreased graft-free survival in patients with PSC [14]. The pathogenic role of toxic bile in the disease process of PSC is further supported by experiments in Swiss albino mice showing that feeding lithocholic acid for 4 days causes bile infarcts, destructive cholangitis, activation and proliferation of myofibroblasts, and finally periductal fibrosis [48].

Studies in transgenic mice harboring mutated *CFTR*, encoding human cystic fibrosis transmembrane conductance regulator, showed that loss of CFTR in the context of dextran sodium sulfate-induced colitis affected biliary epithelial cell innate immunity and led to bacterial translocation and Toll-like receptor-mediated biliary injury and portal inflammation [49]. Although this animal model provided molecular evidence to link colitis with biliary injury, a hallmark of PSC in humans, the role of *CFTR* in PSC is still unclear. Several studies have failed to demonstrate a genetic association between *CFTR* mutations and PSC. The utility of different animal models in recapitulating various aspects of the heterogeneous disease PSC were recently reviewed by Trauner *et al.* [50]. While no

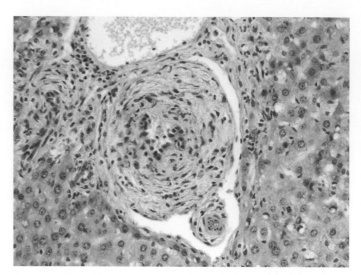

Figure 21.9 *Mdr2* knockout mice recapitulate the histologic features of primary sclerosing cholangitis and represent an excellent model to study the disease pathogenesis and response to medical therapy. Periductular fibrosis ("onion skin" appearance) in the liver of a 2-month-old *Mdr2* knockout mouse (hematoxylin & eosin, original magnification ×400).

one animal model accounts for all of the features of PSC, each has helped to shed light on elements of its pathogenesis and to identify cellular and molecular targets in the pathogenesis of PSC potentially amenable for pharmacotherapy.

Management

Determination of the efficacy of any specific therapeutic intervention for patients with PSC is bedevilled by the unpredictable natural history. The goals of therapeutic intervention for symptomatic patients with documented PSC and the treatments that have been tested are listed in Boxes 21.1 and 21.2. However, to date, there have been no published reports of large, randomized controlled trials that document an effective form of medical therapy in PSC. Non-specific management should focus on monitoring for complications, and careful assessment and management of nutritional status, including the prevention of fat-soluble vitamin deficiency.

Medications

The most widely used and studied medication for PSC is UDCA, despite inconclusive results as to its beneficial effect on the disease. This naturally occurring bile acid is a potent choleretic, immunomodulatory, and cytoprotective agent and has been shown to bring about clinical and biochemical improvement in a wide variety of hepatobiliary disorders, via enrichment of the bile acid pool and displacement of toxic bile acids. It also stimulates expression of the cellular transporters MDR3, bile salt export pump, and multidrug resistance-associated protein-4 and improves bile acid excretion. The Mayo Primary Sclerosing Cholangitis–Ursodeoxycholic Acid Study Group reported their experience in treating 105 patients with either UDCA or placebo: UDCA, in a dose of 13–15 mg/kg

Box 21.1 Goals of therapeutic intervention in the management of patients with sclerosing cholangitis

Provide symptomatic relief
  Decrease pruritus
  Improve nutrition
  - ameliorate steatorrhea
  - prevent fat-soluble vitamin deficiency

  Decrease pain (often from cholangitis)

Improve biliary drainage
  Endoscopic balloon dilation (with or without stenting)
  Choleretics (ursodeoxycholic acid): the role is currently
    unclear

Prevent/recognize/ameliorate complications
  Recurrent cholangitis and bacteremia
  Dominant stricture
  Cirrhosis (and attendant complications of portal
    hypertension)
  Cholangiocarcinoma; colonic dysplasia/carcinoma

Decrease rate of progression of underlying hepatobiliary disease
  Retard inflammation

Box 21.2 Medical and surgical modalities used to manage sclerosing cholangitis and attendant complications

Medical
  Antibiotics
  Azathioprine
  Cholestyramine
  Cladribine
  Colchicine
  Corticosteroids
  Cyclosporine
  Methotrexate
  Mycophenylate mofetil
  Penicillamine
  Pentoxifylline
  Pirfenidone
  Tacrolimus
  Ursodeoxycholic acid
  Combinations (e.g. ursodiol, prednisone and azathioprine)
  Minocycline
  Vancomycin

Surgical/endoscopic
  Intraductal lavage with steroids
  Strictures: balloon dilatation of dominant strictures (± stent
    placement)
  Resection
  Transplantation

daily, was associated with improvement in alkaline phosphatase, AST, bilirubin, and albumin levels, but not with an improvement in histology or a delay in time to treatment failure [51]. Similarly, a biochemical response to UDCA has been noted in children with PSC: 3 of 14 patients treated with UDCA had normalization of liver function tests in one series [3] and in another 27 of 52 patients undergoing medical therapy had a significant improvement in serum alkaline phosphatase, GGT, AST, and ALT with UDCA (with or without concurrent immunosuppressive therapy) [5]. The proportion of patients with symptoms also decreased after 1 year of treatment. However, these clinical and biochemical improvements have been found to be transient in most patients.

Despite results of smaller studies suggesting that UDCA at 20–25 mg/kg daily may slow the disease process in PSC, the long-term efficacy of therapy with a higher dose of UDCA (17–23 mg/kg daily) was called into question when a large 5-year randomized placebo-controlled study in 219 patients with native liver concluded that treatment with UDCA offered no benefit in either survival or prevention of cholangiocarcinoma [52]. Importantly, in a recent long-term, randomized, double blind controlled trial involving 150 patients with PSC, 76 were treated with high-dose UDCA 28–30 mg/kg daily and 74 with placebo. Higher rates of serious adverse events, particularly of variceal bleeding and need for liver transplantation, were found in the UDCA-treated group despite reduction in serum alkaline phosphatase [14]. In addition, a subgroup analysis of the same cohorts showed that patients with early-stage PSC at the time of entry into the study, defined as

histological stage I and II and/or normal serum bilirubin levels, had a higher risk of reaching the adverse clinical endpoints [53]. Based on these studies, the American Association for the Study of Liver Diseases advised in their 2010 guidelines against the use of UDCA as medical therapy in adults with PSC [54]. In summary, particularly in children, the benefit of treatment with UDCA in PSC is currently unknown and high-dose UDCA (>20 mg/kg daily) may be harmful.

Several other medications, including immunosuppressants, antifibrogenics, chelators, and antibiotics, have been used (alone or in combination) in patients with PSC, with no significant benefit (Box 21.2). Steroids have had nominal effects, with reported benefits only in patients with ASC. Drug combination regimens may hold promise.

Some agents, such as antibiotics, are currently under investigation with encouraging preliminary results. A pilot study in 16 adults with PSC showed that treatment with minocycline (100 mg twice a day) for 1 year resulted in reduction in serum alkaline phosphatase levels and Mayo Clinic risk score. However, drug therapy did not improve clinical symptoms, particularly fatigue or pruritus and, in fact, was associated with side effects, such as dizziness, in more than half of the patients. A potential problem of treatment with minocycline is that it not infrequently causes drug-induced hepatitis in children and adults. Whether the increased frequency of PSC–AIH overlap in children further aggravates the risk of adverse effects in children with PSC is not known. Davies *et al.* [55] treated 14 children with PSC and IBD with oral vancomycin and found biochemical improvement, specifically of serum ALT and GGT levels, and reduction in the ESR and clinical symptoms in all the patients. Symptoms would recur following discontinuation of the medicine. Whether prolonged therapy with vancomycin would eventually lead to enteric colonization with vancomycin-resistant bacteria (i.e. enterococci), which may predispose to complications after surgery, including liver transplantation, remains in question.

Targeting nuclear receptors and bile acid metabolism may hold promise in the near future. For example, based on experimental results in bile duct-ligated rats, a clinical trial in adults with PSC investigating combination therapy with UDCA and all-*trans*-retinoic acid is currently under way (NCT01456468 in ClinicalTrials.gov). Other targets for novel therapy may include nuclear receptors such as the farnesoid X receptor, pregnane X receptor, vitamin D receptor, and the peroxisome-proliferator-activator receptors (PPARs), as reviewed by Beuers *et al.* [56].

Supportive care of complication from chronic cholestasis focuses on supplementation of fat-soluble vitamins if deficiencies are detected, particularly in advanced disease, and treatment of pruritus. Pruritus can be severe in PSC and was found to significantly affect quality of life in observational studies in adults. Medical therapy in children, including (low-dose) UDCA, antihistamines, rifampin, and resin-binding agents such as cholestyramine or colesevelam, is similar to treatment of other cholestatic disorders in childhood [57].

Surgery

It is now recommended that biliary tract surgery be avoided if possible, as it may complicate surgery at the time of transplantation. Endoscopic balloon dilatation, however, may offer relief for patients with a focal dominant stricture without the disadvantages of a surgical approach. In fact, in selected patients with dominant strictures, endoscopic dilatation and stent placement may significantly improve symptoms and survival free of transplantation. Although dominant strictures are overall less common in children than in adults with PSC, increase in serum bilirubin, worsening pruritus, or cholangitis should prompt imaging with ultrasound and/or MRCP to evaluate for a dominant stricture amenable for therapeutic intervention by endoscopic retrograde cholangiography.

For patients with end-stage liver disease, orthotopic liver transplantation is the only therapeutic option available. Indications for transplant include cirrhosis with impaired liver function, variceal bleeding, intractable ascites, hepatic encephalopathy, and severe recurrent bacterial cholangitis. While PSC is a common reason for adult liver transplantation, it is an uncommon indication in children. A recent review of the 1995–2008 data from the Studies of the Pediatric Liver Transplantation registry showed that 79 of 2997 children (2.6%) received a transplant for PSC [58]. Transplantation for PSC traditionally involves resection of the extrahepatic biliary tree,

because of the risk of cholangiocarcinoma and recurrence of biliary strictures, and use of a Roux-en-Y loop to establish biliary drainage. However, this approach has recently been challenged and primary duct-to-duct anastomosis may be a safe alternative in patients with PSC undergoing orthotopic liver transplantation [59]. Importantly, in a recent study from UK comparing 74 liver transplant recipients with PSC–IBD with 356 patients with PSC without IBD at the time of liver transplantation, the incidence for thromboembolic events after liver transplantation, particularly for hepatic artery thrombosis, was increased in the PSC–IBD group and active colitis at the time of surgery conferred a significant risk for graft failure after liver transplantation in a multivariate analysis [60].

Prognosis

There is apparent heterogeneity in the clinical course of PSC, but inexorable progression is the rule. Some series suggest that over 80% of patients with PSC will exhibit advancing symptomatology, biochemical features of increasing liver disease, and progression on sequential biopsies. The rate of progression may be slow and insidious or relatively rapid, such that over a period of 5 to 10 years cirrhosis will develop and death will occur without liver transplantation [17,23].

Rates of progression and survival

Several large adult studies have attempted to clarify the natural history and prognosis of PSC [17,23]. In a series of 174 adults with PSC, 31% died as a result of underlying liver disease and cholangiocarcinoma, and an additional 10% were referred for liver transplantation [61]. The median survival from the time of diagnosis was 11.9 years. Multivariate analysis revealed that age, serum bilirubin and hemoglobin concentrations, the presence of IBD, and histologic stage were independent discriminators of an unfavorable outcome; high-grade strictures and diffuse strictures of the intrahepatic ducts were also indicative of a poor prognosis. In a German cohort of 273 patients with PSC, median graft-free survival was 9.6 years and persistence in rise in serum bilirubin levels for more than 3 months predicted a poor prognosis [16]. Survival rates have been similar across the largest adult studies, with the exception of a recent study of a Dutch population: median survival was 18 years, and 8% received transplants after a median disease duration of 95 months (range, 2–221). The revised Mayo Clinic risk score is commonly used in clinical practice to predict prognosis and is based on the natural history of patients with PSC; it includes the variables age, bilirubin, albumin, AST, and history of variceal bleeding (www.psc-literature.org/mrscalc.htm). Although this model performs well in predicting 5-year survival in patient cohorts, its applicability for individual patients is limited [54].

The rate of progression of childhood onset sclerosing cholangitis is still unclear.

In the series described by Batres *et al.* [2], 9 of the 20 patients required liver transplantation: two who presented with early (stage I or II) disease, and seven who presented with advanced (stage III or IV) disease. This study compared patient characteristics with liver histology and concluded that the histologic findings at diagnosis are not predictive of disease progression. In another series, only 1 of 32 children died, with 10 either listed for transplantation or having undergone transplantation [9]. Poor outcome in this group was associated with jaundice, prolongation of prothrombin time, abnormal bilirubin, and splenomegaly at presentation. In a US pediatric cohort, liver disease was progressive, and 11 of the 52 patients underwent liver transplantation during follow-up for a mean of 6.6 years (range, 0.2–16.7) [5]. The median survival without transplant was 12.7 years; low platelets, splenomegaly, and older age were variables associated with shorter survival. In the case series by Miloh *et al.* [7], orthotopic liver transplantation was performed on 9 of the 47 patients (19%) at a mean of 7 years after the diagnosis of PSC. Small-duct PSC appeared to have the best prognosis. In those with PSC–AIH overlap, 30% required a transplant even though they were biochemically responsive to therapy with corticosteroids and UDCA; the outcome in this subgroup was not better than in patients with large-duct PSC.

Post-transplantation prognosis

Post-transplant survival in adults with PSC is good, with 1-year patient survival rates of 84% to 97%. However, several post-transplantation complications occur more frequently in patients with PSC: there is evidence of an increased incidence of acute and chronic rejection, hepatic artery thrombosis, reflux cholangitis, and biliary stricturing in these patients. Recurrence of disease is now also well recognized; the reported incidence averages between 10 and 20% in the largest studies [62]. However, in a recent study of 152 adults followed after transplantation for 14 years, there was a strikingly high recurrence rate of 37% [63]. A late increase in serum alkaline phosphatase almost universally indicated biliary stricturing and disease recurrence. Factors associated with PSC recurrence in 64 adults undergoing the first orthotopic liver transplantation included presence of post-transplant UC, steroid maintenance, history of acute cellular rejection, and OKT3 (muromonab-CD3) use. Of the 11 transplant recipients in the pediatric series of Feldstein *et al.*, three had recurrence of disease [5]. An even higher rate was reported in another series, where histologic PSC recurrence after transplantation occurred in three of nine patients (1.6, 2.4, and 8.4 years postoperatively) [2]. Based on data from the Studies of the Pediatric Liver Transplantation Registry, recurrence of PSC was found in 9.8% of transplant recipients, at a mean of 18 months after transplantation [58].

Prognostic factors

There are no reliable prognostic indicators in an individual patient, but multivariate statistical survival models may be of help in identifying individual patients with PSC at low or high risk of dying [61,64]. A time-dependent Cox regression model to predict the prognosis of PSC identified bilirubin, albumin, and age at diagnosis as independent prognostic factors [64]. Genotype may also provide prognostic aid: the *HLA-DR3–HLA-DQ2* heterozygous genotype has been associated with an accelerated progression of PSC, and the *HLA-DR3–HLA-DR2* heterozygous genotype has been linked to an increased risk of death after transplantation. The prognostic value of cholangiography has also been assessed: high-grade intrahepatic strictures have been shown to be indicative of a poor prognosis [61]. The Amsterdam cholangiographic classification system combined intrahepatic and extrahepatic findings with age at first ERCP. Using this system, patient scores were found to inversely correlate with survival. Since this classification reflects disease stage, it has the potential to serve as a predictor of disease progression in patient care. However, more trials are necessary to validate this tool.

The ultimate prognosis may be altered by the fact that PSC is a premalignant condition, complicated by cholangiocarcinoma in a certain number of patients, which is often localized to the hepatic hilum (Klatskin tumor). In a prospective study of 161 adults with PSC, patients were followed until transplantation, death, or the development of cholangiocarcinoma; 11 patients (7%) developed the malignancy over a mean follow-up of 11.5 years [65]. Notably, no association was found between duration of PSC disease and the incidence of cholangiocarcinoma, despite the overwhelming majority of cases occurring in adulthood; the youngest reported case of cholangiocarcinoma was in a 14 year old with PSC and long-standing UC [66]. Transplantation may offer hope for long-term survival. Deterioration in clinical status, worsening cholestasis, and presence of a dominant strictures should prompt evaluation for cholangiocarcinoma, including serum CA19-9 level, imaging with MRCP and endoscopic retrograde cholangiography with cholangioscopy (if available) and brushing for cytology [54].

In addition to being a risk factor for biliary neoplasms, PSC also is a risk factor for colorectal cancer in those with UC. In a study of 152 adults who underwent liver transplantation for PSC, the incidence of colorectal cancer was 5.3%, compared with 0.6% in patients who underwent transplantation for non-PSC causes; pancolitis and duration of colitis greater than 10 years were risk factors [67]. Patients with UC and PSC have a significantly higher risk for the development of colorectal dysplasia and carcinoma than patients with isolated UC. In a study of pediatric PSC–IBD, 3 of 43 patients developed colonic dysplasia, with the youngest at 17 years of age [21]. Colonoscopy should be performed at the time of diagnosis of PSC, even in the asymptomatic patients, but the benefit of more intensive colonoscopic surveillance in children is currently unclear given the overall low incidence of colorectal carcinoma in children with PSC–IBD.

Summary

Primary sclerosing cholangitis is a cholangiopathy that presents as an independent entity and in association with IBD. Idiopathic forms often overlap with AIH, which should be suspected in the setting of elevated serum aminotransferases and immunoglobulins, and positive autoantibodies. Secondary forms are associated with immunodeficiencies, malignancies, and infections, among other causes. The clinical presentation of sclerosing cholangitis is similar to other cholestatic diseases, with fatigue, jaundice, and hepatosplenomegaly predominating. Abnormal laboratory findings include positive ANCA and elevated serum ALT, alkaline phosphatase, and GGT; particularly in children, elevated GGT appears to be a sensitive marker. The diagnosis is based on classic cholangiographic and histologic findings; MRCP is gaining popularity as a non-invasive diagnostic tool. Once a diagnosis is made, patients should be screened for IBD, even if they are asymptomatic. Currently, there is no medical therapy that halts progression of the disease. Treatment recommendations for UDCA, despite its potential to induce biochemical and histologic improvement, require further studies to determine its benefits over the long term. Transplantation is the only option for those with end-stage disease but may be associated with high rates of postoperative complications; the disease recurs in up to one-third of patients.

Prospective, controlled collaborative trials performed in clearly defined patient groups should lead to a better understanding of the natural history of sclerosing cholangitis in children, and ideally provide clues to the etiology of the disease, as well as its link to IBD and other disorders.

Acknowledgements

We would gratefully acknowledge the contributions of Dr. Kevin Bove, who has shared his expertise in reviewing the histologic findings of sclerosing cholangitis, as well as providing images for each edition of this text; to Professor Frank Lammert (Saarland University Hospital Homburg) for providing $mdr2^{-/-}$ mice as a generous gift to the laboratory of A.G.M.; and to Senna Adachi for assistance in preparation of the manuscript.

References

1. Mieli-Vergani G, Vergani D. Unique features of primary sclerosing cholangitis in children. *Curr Opin Gastroenterol* 2010;**26**:265–268.

2. Batres LA, Russo P, Mathews M, *et al.* Primary sclerosing cholangitis in children: a histologic follow-up study. *Pediatr Dev Pathol* 2005;**8**:568–576.

3. Debray D, Pariente D, Urvoas E, Hadchouel M, Bernard O. Sclerosing cholangitis in children. *J Pediatr* 1994;**124**:49–56.

4. El-Shabrawi M, Wilkinson ML, Portmann B, *et al.* Primary sclerosing cholangitis in childhood. *Gastroenterology* 1987; **92**(5 Pt 1):1226–1235.

5. Feldstein AE, Perrault J, El-Youssif M, *et al.* Primary sclerosing cholangitis in children: a long-term follow-up study. *Hepatology* 2003;**38**:210–217.

6. Gregorio GV, Portmann B, Karani J, *et al.* Autoimmune hepatitis/sclerosing cholangitis overlap syndrome in childhood: a 16-year prospective study. *Hepatology* 2001;**33**:544–553.

7. Miloh T, Arnon R, Shneider B, Suchy F, Kerkar N. A retrospective single-center review of primary sclerosing cholangitis in children. *Clin Gastroenterol Hepatol* 2009;**7**:239–245.

8. Sisto A, Feldman P, Garel L, *et al.* Primary sclerosing cholangitis in children: study of five cases and review of the literature. *Pediatrics* 1987;**80**:918–923.

9. Wilschanski M, Chait P, Wade JA, *et al.* Primary sclerosing cholangitis in 32 children: clinical, laboratory, and radiographic features, with survival analysis. *Hepatology* 1995;**22**:1415–1422.

10. Amedee-Manesme O, Bernard O, Brunelle F, *et al.* Sclerosing cholangitis with neonatal onset. *J Pediatr* 1987;**111**:225–229.

11. Shanmugam NP, Harrison PM, Devlin J, *et al.* Selective use of endoscopic retrograde cholangiopancreatography in the diagnosis of biliary atresia in infants younger than 100 days. *J Pediatr Gastroenterol Nutr* 2009;**49**: 435–441.

12. Floreani A, Rizzotto ER, Ferrara F, *et al.* Clinical course and outcome of autoimmune hepatitis/primary sclerosing cholangitis overlap syndrome. *Am J Gastroenterol* 2005;**100**:1516–1522.

13. Loftus EV Jr., Harewood GC, Loftus CG, *et al.* PSC-IBD: a unique form of inflammatory bowel disease associated with primary sclerosing cholangitis. *Gut* 2005;**54**:91–96.

14. Lindor KD, Kowdley KV, Luketic VA, *et al.* High-dose ursodeoxycholic acid for the treatment of primary sclerosing cholangitis. *Hepatology* 2009;**50**: 808–814.

15. Kaplan GG, Laupland KB, Butzner D, Urbanski SJ, Lee SS. The burden of large and small duct primary sclerosing cholangitis in adults and children: a population-based analysis. *Am J Gastroenterol* 2007;**102**:1042–1049.

16. Tischendorf JJ, Hecker H, Kruger M, Manns MP, Meier PN. Characterization, outcome, and prognosis in 273 patients with primary sclerosing cholangitis: A single center study. *Am J Gastroenterol* 2007;**102**:107–114.

17. Bambha K, Kim WR, Talwalkar J, *et al.* Incidence, clinical spectrum, and outcomes of primary sclerosing cholangitis in a United States community. *Gastroenterology* 2003;**125**:1364–1369.

18. Card TR, Solaymani-Dodaran M, West J. Incidence and mortality of primary sclerosing cholangitis in the UK: a population-based cohort study. *J Hepatol* 2008;**48**: 939–944.

19. Fausa O, Schrumpf E, Elgjo K. Relationship of inflammatory bowel disease and primary sclerosing cholangitis. *Semin Liver Dis* 1991;**11**:31–39.

20. Olsson R, Danielsson A, Jarnerot G, *et al.* Prevalence of primary sclerosing cholangitis in patients with ulcerative colitis. *Gastroenterology* 1991;**100**(5 Pt 1):1319–1323.

21. Faubion WA Jr., Loftus EV, Sandborn WJ, Freese DK, Perrault J. Pediatric "PSC-IBD": a descriptive report of associated inflammatory bowel disease among pediatric patients with PSC. *J Pediatr Gastroenterol Nutr* 2001;**33**:296–300.

22. Sano H, Nakazawa T, Ando T, *et al.* Clinical characteristics of inflammatory bowel disease associated with primary sclerosing cholangitis. *J Hepatobiliary Pancreat Sci* 2011;**18**:154–161.

23. Ponsioen CY, Vrouenraets SM, Prawirodirdjo W, *et al.* Natural history of primary sclerosing cholangitis and prognostic value of cholangiography in a Dutch population. *Gut* 2002;**51**: 562–566.

24. Hyams JS, Treem WR, Justinich CJ, *et al.* Characterization of symptoms in children with recurrent abdominal pain: resemblance to irritable bowel syndrome. *J Pediatr Gastroenterol Nutr* 1995;**20**:209–214.

25. Farkkila M, Karvonen AL, Nurmi H, *et al.* Metronidazole and ursodeoxycholic acid for primary sclerosing cholangitis: a randomized placebo-controlled trial. *Hepatology* 2004;**40**:1379–1386.

26. MacCarty RL, LaRusso NF, Wiesner RH, Ludwig J. Primary sclerosing cholangitis: findings on cholangiography and pancreatography. *Radiology* 1983;**149**:39–44.

27. LaRusso NF, Wiesner RH, Ludwig J, MacCarty RL. Current concepts. Primary sclerosing cholangitis. *N Engl J Med* 1984;**310**:899–903.

28. Majoie CB, Reeders JW, Sanders JB, Huibregtse K, Jansen PL. Primary sclerosing cholangitis: a modified classification of cholangiographic findings. *AJR Am J Roentgenol* 1991;**157**:495–497.

29. Dave M, Elmunzer BJ, Dwamena BA, Higgins PD. Primary sclerosing cholangitis: meta-analysis of diagnostic performance of MR cholangiopancreatography. *Radiology* 2010;**256**:387–396.

30. Ferrara C, Valeri G, Salvolini L, Giovagnoni A. Magnetic resonance cholangiopancreatography in primary sclerosing cholangitis in children. *Pediatr Radiol* 2002;**32**:413–417.

31. Chavhan GB, Roberts E, Moineddin R, Babyn PS, Manson DE. Primary sclerosing cholangitis in children: utility of magnetic resonance cholangiopancreatography. *Pediatr Radiol* 2008;**38**:868–873.

32. Angulo P, Peter JB, Gershwin ME, *et al.* Serum autoantibodies in patients with primary sclerosing cholangitis. *J Hepatol* 2000;**32**:182–187.

33. Mendes FD, Jorgensen R, Keach J, *et al.* Elevated serum IgG4 concentration in patients with primary sclerosing cholangitis. *Am J Gastroenterol* 2006;**101**:2070–2075.

34. Ludwig J. Surgical pathology of the syndrome of primary sclerosing cholangitis. *Am J Surg Pathol* 1989;**13** (Suppl 1):43–49.

35. Bjornsson E, Boberg KM, Cullen S, *et al.* Patients with small duct primary sclerosing cholangitis have a favourable long term prognosis. *Gut* 2002;**51**: 731–735.

36. Broome U, Glaumann H, Lindstom E, *et al.* Natural history and outcome in 32 Swedish patients with small duct primary sclerosing cholangitis (PSC). *J Hepatol* 2002;**36**:586–589.

37. Grant AJ, Lalor PF, Salmi M, Jalkanen S, Adams DH. Homing of mucosal lymphocytes to the liver in the pathogenesis of hepatic complications of inflammatory bowel disease. *Lancet* 2002;**359**:150–157.

38. Lichtman SN, Keku J, Clark RL, Schwab JH, Sartor RB. Biliary tract disease in rats with experimental small bowel bacterial overgrowth. *Hepatology* 1991;**13**:766–772.

39. Fickert P, Fuchsbichler A, Wagner M, *et al.* Regurgitation of bile acids from leaky bile ducts causes sclerosing cholangitis in *Mdr2* (*Abcb4*) knockout mice. *Gastroenterology* 2004;**127**: 261–274.

40. Karlsen TH, Franke A, Melum E, *et al.* Genome-wide association analysis in primary sclerosing cholangitis. *Gastroenterology* 2010;**138**: 1102–1111.

41. Hov JR, Kosmoliaptsis V, Traherne JA, *et al.* Electrostatic modifications of the human leukocyte antigen-DR P9 peptide-binding pocket and susceptibility to primary sclerosing cholangitis. *Hepatology* 2011;**53**:1967–1976.

42. Donaldson PT. Genetics of liver disease: immunogenetics and disease pathogenesis. *Gut* 2004;**53**:599–608.

43. Hov JR, Keitel V, Laerdahl JK, *et al.* Mutational characterization of the bile acid receptor TGR5 in primary sclerosing cholangitis. *PLoS One* 2010;**5**:e12403.

44. Xu B, Broome U, Ericzon BG, Sumitran-Holgersson S. High frequency of autoantibodies in patients with primary sclerosing cholangitis that bind biliary epithelial cells and induce expression of CD44 and production of interleukin 6. *Gut* 2002;**51**:120–127.

45. Eksteen B, Grant AJ, Miles A, *et al.* Hepatic endothelial CCL25 mediates the recruitment of CCR9+ gut-homing lymphocytes to the liver in primary sclerosing cholangitis. *J Exp Med* 2004;**200**:1511–1517.

46. Koga H, Sakisaka S, Yoshitake M, *et al.* Abnormal accumulation in lipopolysaccharide in biliary epithelial cells of rats with self-filling blind loop. *Int J Mol Med* 2002;**9**:621–626.

47. Numata Y, Tazuma S, Nishioka T, Ueno Y, Chayama K. Immune response in mouse experimental cholangitis associated with colitis induced by dextran sulfate sodium. *J Gastroenterol Hepatol* 2004;**19**:910–915.

48. Fickert P, Fuchsbichler A, Marschall HU, *et al.* Lithocholic acid feeding induces segmental bile duct obstruction and destructive cholangitis in mice. *Am J Pathol* 2006;**168**:410–422.

49. Fiorotto R, Scirpo R, Trauner M, *et al.* Loss of CFTR affects biliary epithelium innate immunity and causes TLR4-NF-kappaB-mediated inflammatory response in mice. *Gastroenterology* 2011;**141**:1498–508, 508 e1–5.

50. Trauner M, Fickert P, Baghdasaryan A, *et al.* New insights into autoimmune cholangitis through animal models. *Dig Dis* 2010;**28**:99–104.

51. Lindor KD. Ursodiol for primary sclerosing cholangitis. Mayo Primary Sclerosing Cholangitis–Ursodeoxycholic Acid Study Group. *N Engl J Med* 1997;**336**:691–695.

52. Olsson R, Boberg KM, de Muckadell OS, *et al.* High-dose ursodeoxycholic acid in primary sclerosing cholangitis: a 5-year multicenter, randomized, controlled study. *Gastroenterology* 2005;**129**:1464–1472.

53. Imam MH, Sinakos E, Gossard AA, *et al.* High-dose ursodeoxycholic acid increases risk of adverse outcomes in patients with early stage primary sclerosing cholangitis. *Aliment Pharmacol Ther* 2011;**34**:1185–1192.

54. Chapman R, Fevery J, Kalloo A, *et al.* Diagnosis and management of primary sclerosing cholangitis. *Hepatology* 2010;**51**:660–678.

55. Davies YK, Cox KM, Abdullah BA, *et al.* Long-term treatment of primary sclerosing cholangitis in children with

oral vancomycin: an immunomodulating antibiotic. *J Pediatr Gastroenterol Nutr* 2008;**47**:61–67.

56. Beuers U, Kullak-Ublick GA, Pusl T, Rauws ER, Rust C. Medical treatment of primary sclerosing cholangitis: a role for novel bile acids and other (post-) transcriptional modulators? *Clin Rev Allergy Immunol* 2009;**36**:52–61.

57. Ibrahim SH, Lindor KD. Current management of primary sclerosing cholangitis in pediatric patients. *Paediatr Drugs* 2011;**13**:87–95.

58. Miloh T, Anand R, Yin W, *et al.* Pediatric liver transplantation for primary sclerosing cholangitis. *Liver Transplant* 2011;**17**:925–933.

59. Damrah O, Sharma D, Burroughs A, *et al.* Duct-to-duct biliary reconstruction in orthotopic liver transplantation for primary sclerosing cholangitis: a viable and safe alternative. *Transplant Int* 2012;**25**:64–68.

60. Joshi D, Bjarnason I, Belgaumkar A, *et al.* The impact of inflammatory bowel disease post-liver transplantation for primary sclerosing cholangitis. *Liver Int* 2013;**33**:53–61.

61. Wiesner RH, Grambsch PM, Dickson ER, *et al.* Primary sclerosing cholangitis: natural history, prognostic factors and survival analysis. *Hepatology* 1989;**10**:430–436.

62. Graziadei IW. Recurrence of primary sclerosing cholangitis after liver transplantation. *Liver Transplant* 2002;**8**:575–581.

63. Vera A, Moledina S, Gunson B, *et al.* Risk factors for recurrence of primary sclerosing cholangitis of liver allograft. *Lancet* 2002;**360**:1943–1944.

64. Boberg KM, Rocca G, Egeland T, *et al.* Time-dependent Cox regression model is superior in prediction of prognosis in primary sclerosing cholangitis. *Hepatology* 2002;**35**:652–657.

65. Burak K, Angulo P, Pasha TM, *et al.* Incidence and risk factors for cholangiocarcinoma in primary sclerosing cholangitis. *Am J Gastroenterol* 2004;**99**:523–526.

66. Ross AM, Anupindi SA, Balis UJ. Case records of the Massachusetts General Hospital. Weekly clinicopathological exercises. Case 11-2003. A 14-year-old boy with ulcerative colitis, primary sclerosing cholangitis, and partial duodenal obstruction. *N Engl J Med* 2003;**348**:1464–1476.

67. Vera A, Gunson BK, Ussatoff V, *et al.* Colorectal cancer in patients with inflammatory bowel disease after liver transplantation for primary sclerosing cholangitis. *Transplantation* 2003;**75**:1983–1988.

Chapter

22

Drug-induced liver disease

Eve A. Roberts

Introduction

Drug-induced liver disease has been regarded as rare in children. Large surveys have generally failed to detect drug hepatotoxicity as a major problem in children, although adverse drug reactions (not necessarily hepatotoxic) are somewhat more frequent in preschool children and in children of any age with cancer. A study examining deaths from adverse drug reactions in children found that approximately one-sixth of such deaths involved acute liver failure, usually associated with antiepileptic or antineoplastic drugs [1]. Drug hepatotoxicity is recognized as an important cause of acute liver failure in children, as in adults [2]. Why childhood drug hepatotoxicity is otherwise relatively uncommon remains unclear. Failure to diagnose and report drug hepatotoxicity in children is a likely explanation. However, most children take relatively few medications. Recent reports of drugs most frequently causing clinically evident hepatotoxicity in adults show that a drug has to be in broad general use to end up a major offender. Although trends may change, children uncommonly take the cardiovascular, antihypertensive, or antidepressant medications commonly associated with hepatotoxicity in adults. Despite increasing prevalence of childhood overweight/obesity, most children have a lean body mass and most do not abuse ethanol or smoke cigarettes. Therefore, children are usually free of factors predisposing to drug hepatotoxicity in adults. Hepatic drug metabolism in children may be sufficiently different from that in adults to shield against drug hepatotoxicity. Indeed, old age is a risk factor for more severe hepatotoxic reactions, perhaps because the aging liver metabolizes some drugs more slowly. Capacity for hepatocellular regeneration may be greater in children than in adults. Nevertheless, drug hepatotoxicity definitely occurs in children; adolescents are probably no different from adults in their risk for drug-induced liver disease.

Drug-induced liver disease is challenging because it encompasses a wide spectrum of clinical disease. Cytotoxic processes, presenting as hepatitis, are most common, but almost every major type of hepatic pathology can occur. Hepatic drug metabolism plays an important role in hepatotoxicity in children. With many hepatotoxic drugs, a critical imbalance between generation of a toxic metabolite and detoxification processes can be identified. Focal defects in detoxification may be inherited. Toxic metabolites may alter cellular proteins to produce haptens that provoke an untoward immune response. The complicated, highly variable mechanics of the immune response influence the actual manifestation of drug-induced liver disease. Therefore pharmacogenetic and immunogenetic features are important mechanistically in most pediatric drug hepatotoxicity. Developmental changes in drug disposition and biotransformation further complicate drug hepatotoxicity in children. Making the diagnosis of drug hepatotoxicity depends largely on including it in the differential diagnosis. At the very least, drug-induced or environmental xenobiotic-induced hepatotoxicity should be considered when other etiologies of childhood liver disease are excluded. Children and adolescents taking medications known to be potentially hepatotoxic need close monitoring.

The term "drug-induced liver injury" may be preferred terminology, although injury proves difficult to define adequately. Whether it is called drug-induced liver injury or drug hepatotoxicity, the discussion relating to children differs from an overview of drug hepatotoxicity in adults. For many of the more frequent drug-induced liver injuries in children, the mechanism of the hepatotoxic process has been hypothesized and elucidated. This achievement has been important for understanding drug hepatotoxicity in patients of any age. However, our appreciation of the spectrum of possible drug hepatotoxicity in children reflects the more extensive experience in adults. Readers seeking an all-inclusive discussion of drug hepatotoxicity should consult references drawing on this adult experience [3,4] or hepatotoxicity databases (such as livertox.nlm.nih.gov).

Hepatic drug metabolism

Drug metabolism, or biotransformation, is one of the most important functions of the liver. These complex biochemical processes can be divided into two broad aspects: activation (phase I) and detoxification (phase II). Different families of enzymes perform phase I and phase II drug metabolism. With respect to hepatotoxicity, the *balance* between phase I and phase II processes is critical. Factors that influence this balance include age or stage of development, state of nutrition (mainly fasting or undernutrition; possibly obesity resulting in hepatic steatosis), coadministered drugs, and immunomodulators resulting from viral infection, for example with influenza viruses or human herpesvirus 6. Inducers (chemicals that increase the amount of functional enzymes involved in biotransformation) may affect both phase I and phase II processes, but not necessarily equally. Coadministered medications may act as inducers or inhibitors of specific drug-metabolizing enzymes. The pharmacokinetics of the drug, particularly its absorption from the gastrointestinal tract or other organs and its mode of excretion, affects hepatic biotransformation. Whether the drug is taken as a single dose or as many doses on a chronic basis may also change its hepatic metabolism. Sporadic recurrent exposure to some drugs may enhance their toxicity. Genetically determined polymorphisms of cytochromes P450 and various phase II enzymes also influence this balance.

The hemoprotein cytochromes P450, found in most body tissues, are extremely important in the liver, notably for bile acid synthesis and hormone/drug biotransformation [5,6]. They are associated with phase I reactions including hydroxylation, dealkylation, dehalogenation, and others. The common feature is that one atom of molecular oxygen is inserted into the substrate. Hence these enzymes are monooxygenases. Unlike most enzymes, many cytochromes P450 have *overlapping substrate specificity*: each is not absolutely restricted to a unique substrate. Another important feature of many hepatic cytochromes P450 is *inducibility*. In hepatocytes, various cytochromes P450 are found in the endoplasmic reticulum, mitochondria, and peroxisomes.

The cytochromes P450 are classified in families and subfamilies, which have been distinguished on the basis of primary amino acid sequence identity. With respect to human hepatic drug metabolism, cytochromes P450 in the 1A, 2B, 2C, 2D, 2E, and 3A subfamilies (abbreviated at CYP plus subfamily name) are particularly important. The CYP1A subfamily includes two major cytochromes induced by polycyclic aromatic hydrocarbons. Apart from various carcinogens and xenobiotics, caffeine and theophylline are metabolized by these cytochromes. Induction of CYP1A1 is regulated through a cytoplasmic protein, the aromatic hydrocarbon (Ah) receptor. The member of this subfamily that is exclusively hepatic is CYP1A2: it is expressed constitutively, and its induction is also regulated by the Ah receptor. The CYP2B subfamily includes cytochromes induced by phenobarbital. Some members of the CYP2B subfamily are regulated by the constitutive androstane receptor (CAR), which dimerizes with the retinoid X receptor (RXR) and then interacts with a regulatory site in the 5′-upstream region of the structural gene. CYP2E1 is the ethanol-inducible cytochrome P450, whose regulation is complex and mainly post-transcriptional. The CYP3A subfamily includes cytochromes induced by pregnenolone, glucocorticoids, rifampicin, and also phenobarbital. The most abundant

cytochrome P450 in the liver is CYP3A4, which plays an important role in the biotransformation of many drugs. It is regulated via the pregnane X receptor (PXR), which interacts with RXR to produce the functional transcriptional regulator. Various members of the nuclear receptor family (CAR, PXR, and others such as hepatocyte nuclear factor-4α) play important roles in regulating expression of hepatocellular P450s and also in regulating expression of these very receptors. Cross-talk among receptors adds a further level of complexity.

Polymorphisms for certain P450 isozymes, relating to differences in the rate of associated enzyme activities, have been identified in humans [7–9]. The first of these polymorphisms for drug oxidation to be identified involves CYP2D6. Debrisoquine 4-hydroxylation, an enzyme activity associated with this cytochrome, was found to vary significantly in the Caucasian population, some individuals being "extensive metabolizers" of debrisoquine and others "poor metabolizers." Other drugs that are substrates for CYP2D6 show the same pattern: these include antiarrhythmic agents such as encainide, beta-blockers such as metoprolol, various psychoactive agents, and codeine and dextromethorphan. The difference in metabolism between extensive and poor metabolizers appears to result from changes in the catalytic site of CYP2D6 in poor metabolizers. Poor metabolizers are at increased risk of toxic drug concentrations, possibly relevant to Ecstasy hepatotoxicity. Mephenytoin is subject to polymorphism in its metabolism, which is associated with the CYP2C subfamily. The specific isozyme involved is likely CYP2C18. The CYP3A subfamily (mainly CYP3A4 and CYP3A5) plays an important role in hepatic drug metabolism of such drugs as nifedipine, erythromycin, cyclosporine, and diltiazem; *CYP3A5* is polymorphic and tends to be expressed at a much lower level than *CYP3A4*. *CYP1A2* has some minor polymorphisms of uncertain functional importance. Polymorphisms affecting the function of proteins regulating expression of P450 enzymes may also influence hepatic drug biotransformation.

The outcome of most phase I biotransformation reactions is to make the substrate a more polar chemical with a substituent poised for further modification via a phase II reaction. Phase II detoxifying reactions are performed by a variety of enzyme types, including the glutathione *S*-transferases, UDP-glucuronosyltransferases, epoxide hydrolases, sulfotransferases, *N*-acetyltransferases, and enzymes responsible for glycine conjugation. These reactions complete the conversion of a hydrophobic chemical to a hydrophilic one, which can be excreted easily in urine or bile. Certain phase II enzymes, such as some glucuronosyltransferases, are inducible. Some are polymorphic. An important example of a phase II polymorphism involves *N*-acetylation. Arylamine *N*-acetyltransferase 2 (NAT-2) is polymorphic: individuals are either rapid or slow acetylators; a related enzyme, NAT-1, is monomorphic. These enzymes are encoded by two separate genes, and the slow acetylator phenotype of NAT-2 relates to mutations in the gene for NAT-2 causing reduced concentrations of NAT-2 in human liver. The Phase II enzyme involved in metabolism of 6-mercaptopurine, thiopurine methyltransferase, is polymorphic. Certain polymorphisms are more or less prevalent in specific ethnic groups; for example, more than 50% of Caucasians are slow acetylators. The UDP-glucuronosyltransferases are diverse and include two large subfamilies that are involved in drug metabolism (UGT1 and UGT2). Genetic abnormalities in UGT1A1 are associated with Gilbert syndrome. In Gilbert syndrome, drug metabolism may be affected, but few convincing data exist that this causes drug-induced liver injury except possibly with certain antineoplastic drugs for which UGT1A1-mediated glucuronidation is an important mode of drug disposition [10]. Additionally, glutathione S-transferases M1 and T1 are significantly polymorphic. In some metabolic diseases the activity of phase II enzymes may be abnormal. Hereditary oxoprolinemia is associated with low glutathione S-transferase activity. In hereditary tyrosinemia, glutathione S-transferase activity is abnormally low on an acquired basis because intermediates in the abnormal tyrosine pathway consume glutathione.

Hepatocellular mitochondria are increasingly recognized as playing a critical role in drug hepatotoxicity [11] since mitochondria produce energy for the cell, play an important role in fat metabolism, and mediate apoptosis. Failure to generate enough ATP may eventuate in cellular necrosis. In addition to the oxidative phosphorylation chain, mitochondria retain certain enzymes that combat oxidative stress, including superoxide dismutase 2 and glutathione peroxidase 1. Polymorphisms in the genes for these enzymes may also predispose to drug hepatotoxicity [12].

The product of a phase I reaction may be a reactive or "toxic" metabolite. A toxic metabolite is a short-lived chemically reactive species that usually cannot be detected outside of the cell. Phase II reactions usually inactivate such chemicals before they damage the hepatocyte. Conjugation with glutathione is particularly important in detoxifying electrophilic toxic metabolites and free radicals. Whether a reactive metabolite actually damages a cell depends how much reactive metabolite actually binds to cellular components, whether these organelles are critical to cell survival, and whether they can be repaired. If the toxic metabolite binds to intracellular proteins or membranes that are vital to cellular integrity, the hepatocyte may die. If it binds to a cellular protein and alters its structure, it may create a neoantigen that elicits an immune response. Damage to proteins within the bile canalicular membrane typically interferes with production of bile and thus causes cholestasis. Changes in the function of P-glycoprotein, the bile salt excretory pump, and other bile canalicular transporters that contribute to excretion of drugs and their metabolites is another mechanism of drug-induced liver injury. If the toxic metabolite binds to cellular DNA, mutagenesis or carcinogenesis may eventually ensue. In fetal tissues, binding of a toxic metabolite can also result in teratogenesis (Figure 22.1).

Hepatic drug metabolism displays complex developmental changes [13,14]. In the newborn infant, hepatic biotransformation dependent on cytochromes P450 is typically much less

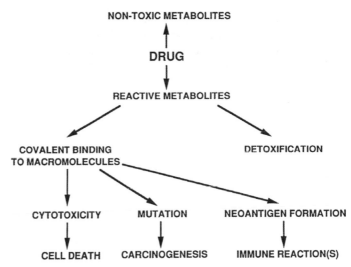

Figure 22.1 The potential fates of a toxic metabolite. Neoantigen formation includes binding of the toxic (reactive) metabolite to the cytochrome P450 which produced it.

active than that in adults. Decreased hepatic drug metabolism is particularly severe in premature infants. Metabolism and elimination of caffeine, theophylline, phenobarbital, and phenytoin are notably slow. In general, however, in early infancy, different P450 enzymes display different developmental patterns of expression. Some (CYP2A6, CYP2C9, CYP2D6, CYP2E1, and CYP3A4) are expressed and active relatively soon after birth, but others (CYP1A2, CYP2B6, and CYP2C8) take months [15]. In childhood, hepatic drug metabolism, and thus clearance of many drugs, is more rapid than in adults. Prominent examples again include theophylline, phenobarbital, and phenytoin. By puberty, adult patterns of hepatic drug metabolism appear to be well established. Caffeine, which is metabolized in part by CYP1A2, exemplifies these changes. The elimination half-life, which is very long in the newborn period, falls to approximately 3-4 hours around 6 months of age [16]. For the balance of childhood, that is until puberty, caffeine metabolism remains somewhat more rapid than in adults. In extensive metabolizers, CYP2D6 rises progressively over the first 5 years of life, and this developmental pattern appears to be independent of gestational age [17].

Phase II biotransformation processes also display developmental changes. Among phase II processes, an important example of late maturation of a detoxifying enzyme is the glucuronosyltransferase for bilirubin conjugation, which is usually deficient for a short time after birth. Sulfation tends to predominate over glucuronidation, for example in the metabolism of acetaminophen. Hepatic bile acid metabolism also shows maturational changes in the first months of life: in neonates conjugation to taurine is quantitatively more important than conjugation to glycine. Bile acid sulfation is quantitatively less important than in adults. Glutathione metabolism is also subject to developmental changes, particularly in the neonatal period. Developmental changes in the proportions of various biliary glutathione-derived thiols reflect increasing bile production over this time, as do changes in gamma-glutamyltransferase activity and other metabolic processes related to hepatic bile production.

Patterns of drug hepatotoxicity

Because the liver is anatomically and physiologically complex, drug hepatotoxicity presents clinically as a broad spectrum of biochemical, histologic, and clinical abnormalities. Most drug-induced liver disease is cytotoxic, and most often the hepatocyte is the target cell. The exact mechanism of hepatocyte death differs depending on the specific hepatotoxin. Hepatocyte damage may be zonal, reflecting metabolic specialization in the hepatic lobule. Hepatocytes in zone 3 of the Rappaport acinus have the highest concentration of cytochromes P450 and thus the greatest potential for producing toxic metabolites. Zonal hepatocellular necrosis suggests that production of toxic metabolites plays an important role in the pathogenesis of the hepatotoxicity. The cellular diversity of the liver also contributes to the diversity of drug-induced liver disease. Drug-induced injury may involve cells in the liver besides hepatocytes. Cytotoxic damage may predominate in bile duct cells (as with chlorpropamide), hepatic stellate cells (in vitamin A toxicity), or endothelial cells (with pyrrolizidine alkaloid poisoning from certain herbal teas). Damage to bile duct epithelial cells or to larger bile ducts is likely to interfere with bile flow, resulting in cholestasis.

Cytotoxicity may be modified by robustness, or inadequacy, of the cytoprotective processes or regenerative capacity of an individual's hepatocytes. It can have other effects besides cell death. Non-lethal damage to certain subcellular elements may interfere with specific metabolic functions, such as protein or lipid synthesis or energy production. Accumulation of fat or other substances in hepatocytes may then occur. Fatty liver associated with tetracycline hepatotoxicity is an example. Cholestasis can also result from injury to hepatocytes. Many drugs associated with cholestatic hepatotoxicity are substrates for the bile canalicular enzymes. They can interfere directly or indirectly with the action of the bile salt export pump or other transporters. Genetic variations in those enzymes may increase their susceptibility to drug-induced injury [18]. Whenever hepatocellular damage is sufficiently severe, some degree of cholestasis will develop, evident as clinical jaundice. Cytotoxicity may have more extensive consequences. Cirrhosis can develop. Vascular perfusion of the liver may be altered, as in veno-occlusive disease (VOD). Finally, hepatotoxicity may lead to neoplastic transformation. In some cases, toxic metabolites have been identified that are capable of binding to DNA, thus initiating carcinogenesis.

Drug hepatotoxicity is also classified in terms of the duration of the process. Acute hepatotoxic injuries develop over a relatively short time and cause a lesion without any histologic features of chronicity. Subacute hepatotoxicity refers to lesions that have developed over weeks to months, as indicated by areas of fibrosis and possible regeneration. Chronic

hepatotoxic lesions include those with fibrosis or cirrhosis, small bile duct paucity (ductopenia), vascular changes, and neoplasia.

A practical and widely used classification of drug-induced hepatotoxicity is based on clinical features. Drug-induced liver disease most often presents as a *hepatitic* process, sometimes accompanied by symptoms associated rather non-specifically with hepatitis (fatigue, anorexia, nausea, or vomiting). Drug-induced hepatitis is frequently asymptomatic, with isolated elevations in serum aminotransferases. Some drug-induced liver disease is predominantly *cholestatic*. Clinically, there is jaundice, pruritus, prominent elevation of alkaline phosphatase, and mild elevations of aminotransferases. Cholestasis associated with contraceptive steroids is a classic example of this "bland cholestasis." Some drug-induced liver disease presents a *mixed* picture, with elements of both hepatitis and cholestasis. This may be the result of injury both to hepatocytes and bile duct epithelial cells, or hepatocellular injury to the bile canalicular membrane. This *mixed hepatitic–cholestatic* process (sometimes called *hepatocanalicular jaundice*) is characteristic of hepatotoxicity caused by chlorpromazine and erythromycin.

In addition, these three basic clinical types (hepatitic, cholestatic, mixed hepatitic–cholestatic) may be associated with specific systemic syndromes. The "drug hypersensitivity syndrome" includes fever, inflammation of various organ systems (hepatitis, morbilliform rash or Stevens–Johnson syndrome, renal dysfunction, or myocarditis), lymphadenopathy, eosinophilia, and atypical lymphocytosis: hepatitis is the most frequent systemic manifestation, and acute liver failure can occur. (This constellation of findings is called DRESS syndrome – drug rash with eosinophilia and systemic symptoms – in the dermatologic literature, but the concept predates this acronym [19,20].) These features indicate an immunoallergic component, but they typically accompany drug hepatotoxicity associated with production of a toxic metabolite. Eosinophilia may not be particularly striking. In some cases intercurrent viral infection may contribute to the development of the "drug hypersensitivity syndrome." Notably, human herpesvirus 6 and 7 infection, or reactivation, may sometimes play a mechanistic role. Another classic syndrome resembles autoimmune hepatitis (so-called "chronic active hepatitis"): best nomenclature is "AIH-like." Findings in AIH-like drug hepatotoxicity include subacute or chronic course, fatigue, anorexia, variable extrahepatic findings (lupoid rash, arthralgias), elevated serum IgG, and detectable non-specific autoantibodies such as anti-nuclear antibody. In some cases, it may be difficult to exclude concurrence of drug administration and underlying autoimmune hepatitis. Drugs that have been associated with AIH-like hepatotoxicity include oxyphenisatin and α-methyldopa (both obsolete), nitrofurantoin, and minocycline. In adults, drug-induced hepatotoxicity has been associated with certain anti-liver–kidney microsomal antibodies (anti-LKM), similar to those associated with autoimmune hepatitis type 2, directed against apoproteins of specific

Table 22.1 Important clinical features of drug-induced hepatotoxicity

Type	Clinical features
Hepatic	Symptoms of hepatitis, increased serum aspartate aminotransferase and/or alanine aminotransferase
Mixed: hepatic–cholestatic	Hepatitis + cholestasis
Cholestatic	Clinical and biochemical cholestasis
Associated syndromes	
Systemic syndrome	Fever; inflammation of other organ systems (morbilliform rash, Stevens–Johnson syndrome (toxic epidermal necrolysis), renal dysfunction, myocarditis), atypical lymphocytosis, eosinophilia
"AIH-like" syndrome (mimicking autoimmune hepatitis)	Variable (acute→chronic) course + fatigue, anorexia, non-specific autoantibodies, increased IgG, variable involvement of organ systems (lupoid rash, arthralgias)

cytochromes P450. The putative reactive metabolite may bind or damage the P450 which generated it. Some P450 apoproteins can be detected on liver cell membranes.

For clinical purposes, drug-induced hepatotoxicity can be described in terms of the clinical liver disease (hepatitic, cholestatic, or hepatitic–cholestatic), with or without associated systemic syndromes (drug hypersensitivity, AIH-like) (Table 22.1), and the time course (acute, subacute, or chronic). There is no good theoretical basis for doubting that some drug-induced liver injury could be chronic. Nodular regenerative hyperplasia and ductopenia are examples of chronic drug hepatotoxicity.

Most drug hepatotoxicity is characterized in terms of *predictability*. This criterion combines mechanistic and clinical considerations. One objective is to separate chemical poisons from toxins involving host susceptibility. *Intrinsic hepatotoxicity* is differentiated from *host idiosyncrasy*. With intrinsic hepatotoxicity, the agent causes predictable hepatic damage in anyone. The toxicity is dose related, and laboratory animal models can easily be developed that exhibit the same type of hepatotoxicity. Few instances of hepatotoxicity associated with medications fit this description. Instead, most are idiosyncratic: unpredictable, infrequent, and apparently capricious. If such a reaction is accompanied by systemic features such as fever, rash, eosinophilia, atypical lymphocytosis, and possibly other major organ involvement, then classically it has been regarded as an idiosyncratic hypersensitivity reaction, with the manifest connotation of an allergic etiology.

An alternative explanation, put in its most dogmatic form, is that all drug hepatotoxicities have a biochemical basis. The problem is broadly "metabolic." Abnormal drug biotransformation leads to increased production of toxic metabolites or inadequate provision of appropriate cytoprotective defenses or both. In some cases, such abnormalities are acquired, for example by drug interaction. In many cases, the abnormality of drug biotransformation is genetic – an abnormal or defective drug-metabolizing enzyme – inherited as a genetic trait. This pharmacogenetic defect becomes apparent only if elicited by the appropriate drug. Without being strictly dose dependent, higher doses of the drug may load the biotransformation

pathway so that more toxic metabolite is produced. The target of the toxic metabolite determines the clinical features of the drug's hepatotoxicity. Damage to subcellular organelles may cause cytotoxicity directly and additionally activate immune mechanisms leading to an immunoallergic response. According to this view of drug hepatotoxicity, drug hepatotoxicities whose mechanisms we understand are predictable, even if these toxicities are rare. Animal models for such hepatotoxicities can be developed but not necessarily in conventional laboratory animals, although extensive panels of inbred strains or chimeric mice with "humanized" livers may prove informative. The importance of this biochemical concept of drug hepatotoxicity is that it provides a basis for research into, and potentially for treatment of, drug hepatotoxicity. In the case of pharmacogenetic disorders of hepatic drug biotransformation, prospective diagnosis (without in vivo drug challenge) may be possible. The importance for pediatric hepatology is that these definable abnormalities in hepatic drug biotransformation predominate among the drug hepatotoxicities most often found in children.

Biotransformation of drugs is not always the whole story, even though it is critical to generating toxic metabolites that alter cellular proteins. With many drugs, hepatocellular damage seems to be disproportional to the amount of toxic metabolite that might be formed. Therefore, it makes sense to look for amplifiers of the damage caused by the toxic metabolite. Both intracellular and extracellular processes may amplify the liver cell damage. This conceptual model is illustrated in Figure 22.2. As an extracellular amplifier, the immune response also plays an important role [21]. For many drugs, whether an individual develops liver injury – as well as its pattern of injury and severity – depends not only on the hepatic processes of drug metabolism but also on that individual's immune reactivity, which is itself dependent on genetic complexion and specifics at the time of drug exposure, such as transient stimuli from endotoxinemia. Adaptive or innate immunity may be involved. A direct connection between immune-mediated mechanisms and hepatic damage occurs when autoantibodies are expressed against specific components of hepatocytes, usually those involved in drug

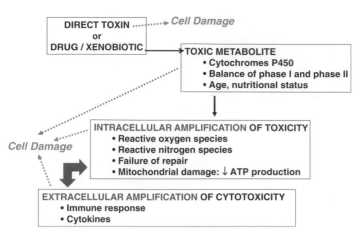

Figure 22.2 A general mechanism of severe drug hepatotoxicity. Most drugs and xenobiotics that cause liver injury elaborate a toxic metabolite within the hepatocyte or non-parenchymal liver cell. The quantity of toxic metabolite is dependent on multiple factors including features of phase I and phase II biotransformation and the balance between them. The toxic metabolite can damage the cell itself or initiate various amplifying processes within the cell or external to the cell, such as immune response. Direct toxins typically injure the liver without metabolism, but in principle amplification pathways could also be involved.

Table 22.2 Classification of hepatotoxins

Nomenclature used	Previous usage
Intrinsic hepatotoxin	Intrinsic toxin
Contingent hepatotoxin (toxic only if biotransformation[a] is abnormal, because of pharmacogenetics or acquired cause)	Metabolic idiosyncrasy
Hepatotoxin eliciting immunoallergic response[b] (implies some degree of dependence on host immunogenetics)	Hypersensitivity

[a] Generation and/or detoxification of toxic metabolite.
[b] Fever, eosinophilia, atypical lymphocytosis; or non-specific autoantibodies; or "AIH-like" (mimicking autoimmune hepatitis); or hepatic granulomatosis.

biotransformation. The targets may be cytochromes P450 or phase II enzymes such as epoxide hydrolase. The target cytochrome P450 varies with the drug: CYP1A2 for dihydralazine, CYP2E1 for halothane, and CYP2C9 for tienilic acid. Reactive metabolites may alter other hepatocellular proteins to produce neoantigens. Immune-mediated damage to hepatocytes may involve either apoptosis or necrosis. Bile acid-associated hepatocyte injury leads to apoptosis via FAS (CD95) activation. When toxic metabolites or reactive oxygen species or cytokines stimulate Kupffer cells, specific mechanisms of cell damage are set into motion involving tumor necrosis factor-α or nitric oxide produced by Kupffer cells. Nitric oxide elaborated by Kupffer cells and hepatocytes plays a role in acetaminophen hepatotoxicity. Kupffer cells can activate natural killer cells and natural killer T-cells in the liver. Cytokines such as interleukin-8 [22] and other CXC chemokines regulating leukocyte action may become involved. Kupffer cells also elaborate various factors that are cytoprotective to hepatocytes [23]. The vigor of the immune response in general, an individual's polygenic trait, most likely determines how extensively immune mechanisms contribute to drug-induced liver injury. For example, genetic polymorphisms affecting the extent of cytokine production may be relevant to diclofenac hepatotoxicity [24]. Specific *HLA* genotypes are associated with certain drug hepatotoxicities. Some components of the innate immune system, such as interleukin-10 and certain prostaglandins, are hepatoprotective. Therefore, in addition to pharmacogenetics, immunogenetics must be considered to explain drug hepatotoxicity.

Classification of chemicals that cause liver injury has to account for inevitable toxicity or for idiosyncrasy, whether from biochemical toxicity or an immune process, or some combination of the two (Table 22.2). Hepatotoxic agents can

be categorized as follows: intrinsic, contingent, and as eliciting an immunoallergic response. The intrinsic hepatotoxin is the true, predictable poison. Environmental xenobiotics usually belong in this category. The contingent hepatotoxin causes hepatotoxicity only when hepatic biotransformation is abnormal so that toxic metabolites are more likely to be generated or detoxification pathways are deficient. Hepatic biotransformation may be abnormal on an acquired or pharmacogenetic basis. This category encompasses the category denoted as "metabolic idiosyncrasy" by others. A hepatotoxin eliciting an immunoallergic response is identified when hepatotoxicity is accompanied by fever, eosinophilia, and atypical lymphocytosis or is characterized histologically by hepatic granulomatosis. Elaboration of autoantibodies, such as anti-LKM antibodies, or a fully developed AIH-like pattern is another type of immunoallergic reaction. These findings imply some degree of dependency on the host immune response. Importantly, the above categories are not mutually exclusive. Some chemicals can act as more than one type of hepatotoxin. For example, high-dose acetaminophen acts as an intrinsic hepatotoxin. By contrast, low-dose acetaminophen, normally non-toxic, acts as a contingent hepatotoxin in people in whom CYP2E1 is induced, as in chronic alcoholics. If the biochemical mechanism of hepatic biotransformation is established for a given chemical, then it is possible to predict circumstances in which that chemical would function as a contingent hepatotoxin. Currently, it is often impossible to identify abnormal hepatic biotransformation owing to a pharmacogenetic defect until after drug-induced hepatotoxicity has occurred. For the affected individual, the hepatotoxicity appears to be a chance aberration.

The clinical presentations and liver pathology of drug hepatotoxicity are extremely diverse. Drug-induced liver injury encompasses the entire spectrum of liver disease. Selected drugs and environmental toxins illustrate this broad range of drug hepatotoxicity affecting adults or children (Table 22.3). Classes of drug that predominate in causing hepatotoxicity in children, apart from acetaminophen, are antimicrobials, antiepileptics, psychoactive drugs, and those for treatment of

Table 22.3 Range of clinical and pathologic findings in hepatotoxicity from drugs or environmental toxins

Finding	Typical causative agents
Acute hepatitis	Isoniazid, halothane
Zonal liver cell necrosis	Acetaminophen
Hepatitis–cholestasis	Erythromycin, chlorpromazine, azathioprine, nitrofurantoin
Bland cholestasis	Estrogens/oral contraceptive pill, cyclosporine, haloperidol
Steatonecrosis (mimicking alcoholic hepatitis)	Perhexiline, amiodarone
Phospholipidosis	Amiodarone
Microvesicular steatosis	Valproic acid, tetracycline
Macrovesicular steatosis	L-Asparaginase
Macrovesicular fat plus fibrosis	Methotrexate
AIH-like (mimicking autoimmune hepatitis)	Minocycline, nitrofurantoin, α-methyldopa
Granulomatosis	Sulfonamides, phenylbutazone, carbamazepine
Biliary cirrhosis	Practolol, chlorpropamide
Sclerosing cholangitis	Floxuridine (administered via hepatic artery)
Gallstones	Ceftriaxone, dipyridamole
Peliosis	Estrogens, androgens
Hepatic vein thrombosis	Estrogens/oral contraceptive pill
Veno-occlusive disease	Pyrrolizidine alkaloids ("bush tea"), 6-thioguanine, busulfan, oxaliplatin
Nodular regenerative hyperplasia	Azathioprine, didanosine, 6-thioguanine
Non-cirrhotic portal hypertension	Arsenic, vinyl chloride
Liver cell adenoma	Estrogens/oral contraceptive pill, anabolic steroids
Malignant tumors (hepatocellular carcinoma, angiosarcoma)	Estrogens/oral contraceptive pill, anabolic steroids, vinyl chloride, arsenic
Porphyria	2,3,7,8-Tetrachlorodibenzo-p-dioxin, chloroquine

attention deficit disorder [25]. Drugs selected for detailed commentary here include some already encountered in clinical practice and some which may prove important in the pediatric age bracket in the future.

Acetaminophen

Acetaminophen is an effective antipyretic and analgesic. Taken in a single large dose, however, it is a potent hepatotoxin. The clinical course of this acute acetaminophen toxicity is distinctive. Immediately after the drug is taken, nausea and vomiting occur. These symptoms subside and then there is an asymptomatic interval before liver injury becomes clinically apparent. At that point, jaundice, abnormal serum aminotransferases, and coagulopathy develop. Finally hepatic failure may supervene with progressive coma. Serum aminotransferases may be extremely high in this condition, and the degree of abnormality is not necessarily predictive of outcome. In a large retrospective series of children (mainly girls) with acetaminophen overdose, prothrombin time >100 seconds (international normalized ratio, >7), hypoglycemia (<2.6 mmol/L),

serum creatinine >200 µmol/L, acidosis (pH<7.3) at any time, and progressive encephalopathy (grade 3 or 4) predicted bad outcome (death or need for liver transplant) [26]. These prognostic factors are similar to those in adults [27]. Late presentation is always problematic.

Treatment of acute acetaminophen hepatotoxicity involves the use of what is effectively an antidote, N-acetylcysteine. Whether to use N-acetylcysteine can be decided on the basis of plotting on a semilogarithmic graph the patient's plasma acetaminophen concentration against time [28]; if it falls in the zone for probable hepatic toxicity, N-acetylcysteine should be given. N-Acetylcysteine is most effective if given within 10 hours of acetaminophen ingestion, and it may be of little benefit more than 24 hours after ingestion of the acetaminophen. However, even if there is doubt as to its usefulness, it should be given anyway. Late administration of N-acetylcysteine has been associated with greater survival in adults with acute acetaminophen intoxication; no adverse side effects of the N-acetylcysteine were observed [29,30]. A 72-hour regimen of oral N-acetylcysteine appears to be as effective as the 20-hour intravenous regimen; the oral regimen may be more effective if treatment is delayed [28,31]. The dose of *N*-acetylcysteine must be appropriate for body weight because an inappropriately high dose may be toxic, causing respiratory compromise or hypotension. Other measures, such as charcoal, may be effective very early, that is, within 1 hour of ingestion; acetaminophen ingestion itself typically causes vomiting. Hemodialysis may be used early when plasma concentrations of acetaminophen are high: otherwise it is not effective. As the metabolism of acetaminophen in adolescents is similar to that of the adult, treatment should be aggressive; younger children also require *N*-acetylcysteine and supportive treatment, even when the timing and total amount of acetaminophen taken are uncertain. Liver transplantation may be required for those children in liver failure who show no improvement despite full supportive treatment. Recent experience suggests that the prognosis is good in a child if after 48 hours of treatment with *N*-acetylcysteine the prothrombin time and serum aminotransferases are all normal.

In addition to this acute type of hepatotoxicity, which is encountered in toddlers invading the medicine cabinet or in suicidal teenagers, acetaminophen hepatotoxicity in children can present more subtly, as therapeutic misadventure. This occurs through various sorts of unintentional error: actual dosing error through misunderstanding the dose or using the wrong measuring device, substitution of one formulation for another, failure to appreciate how often acetaminophen turns up in various over-the-counter medications, and the general belief that acetaminophen is "safe" for children. In typical cases, rather large doses of acetaminophen (approximately 30–70 mg/kg, less in small infants) are administered at regular intervals (usually every 2–4 hours) for 2 to 3 days, or longer, before hepatotoxicity becomes evident. This is sometimes described as "chronic" overdose, but the actual time frame is comparatively short. The liver disease presents as acute liver failure, and the systemic signs of toxicity and the asymptomatic period do not occur. Alternatively, they are neither distinctive nor noticed. Serum concentrations of acetaminophen are frequently not in a toxic range. Diagnosis is difficult unless a very meticulous drug history is taken to determine exactly what preparation of acetaminophen was used and how often. Getting the actual drug containers, even if they were discarded, may be critically important. The acute liver failure is frequently attributed to another etiology, usually acute viral hepatitis. Since its first description in this chapter, numerous cases of this type of acetaminophen hepatotoxicity have been documented [32–34]. The estimate of the lethal dose per kilogram body weight (140 mg/kg) is based on observations in adults and is probably not accurate for children in this scenario. The threshold for liver injury is highly variable from child to child. A suggested threshold on the order of 90–120 mg/kg daily with more than 1 day of drug administration is highly controversial because it impinges on the dose schedule of 15 mg/kg daily administered every 4 hours around the clock. Indeed some caution about this routine dose is appropriate: taking the "safe" dose of acetaminophen daily can cause asymptomatic

elevations of alanine aminotransferase in adults [35] and for children a maximum total dose of 75 mg/kg daily is advised. The Rumack nomogram for treatment with *N*-acetylcysteine does not apply in the situation of an infant or young child with high-dose chronic dosing. Importantly, finding a measurable serum concentration of acetaminophen 24 hours or more after the last dose should suggest the possibility of acetaminophen hepatotoxicity. The elimination half-life can be estimated from two drug levels obtained at a reasonable interval apart: if it is greater than 4 hours, it suggests hepatotoxicity. Detecting an acetaminophen protein adduct, 3-(cystein-5-yl)-acetaminophen, formed by the binding of the reactive metabolite *N*-acetyl-*p*-benzoquinoneimine (NAPQI) to glutathione, may be informative [36]. In general, it seems reasonable to treat these patients with *N*-acetylcysteine as soon as possible. Anorexia and food avoidance, which may have accompanied the underlying illness for which acetaminophen was used, may exacerbate the hepatotoxicity by causing acute depletion of glutathione stores. These children tend to present for medical assessment late in the disease course, and this may be an important reason for the poor prognosis.

The primary mechanism for acetaminophen hepatotoxicity involves the formation of a toxic metabolite. The important role of drug metabolism in this hepatotoxicity is reflected in the predominance of hepatocellular injury in Rappaport zone 3. Acetaminophen is usually metabolized via sulfation and glucuronidation (Figure 22.3). If a very large amount is taken, these pathways are saturated, and an otherwise minor pathway through cytochromes P450, including CYP1A2, CYP2E1, and CYP3A4, becomes quantitatively important. The product of this pathway is a highly reactive species, NAPQI, a potent electrophile. It is conjugated by glutathione, provided that sufficient glutathione is available, to form mercapturic acid, which is excreted in the urine. Otherwise NAPQI reacts with cellular proteins, causing cell damage and cell death. Intracellular processes amplifying cellular damage contribute to the liver injury, which may seem to be disproportionate to the amount of toxic metabolite produced. It appears that NAPQI initiates oxidative stress caused by reactive-oxygen and reactive-nitrogen species. This entails mitochondrial damage, apparently downregulating the oxidative phosphorylation chain, which itself becomes self-perpetuating and results in failure to produce ATP [37,38]. An intracellular antioxidant response mediated by the nuclear transcription factor NF-E2-related factor is also activated [39]. Apart from glutathione, other cytoprotective metabolic pathways dependent on diet may be important [40]. As part of an extracellular enhancement mechanism, various cytokines can increase or decrease the liver injury. CD44 plays an important role in the hepatotoxic mechanism: subnormal expression of CD44 may tip the balance toward increased proinflammatory cytokine signaling [41]. Polymorphonuclear leukocytes do not appear to enhance the injury, perhaps in part because there is less migration as a result of the decreased CD44 signal. By providing substrate for making more glutathione, *N*-acetylcysteine

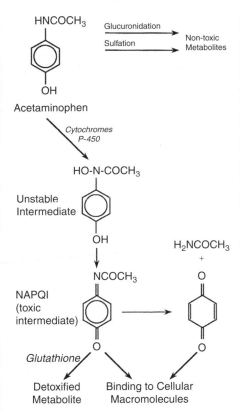

Figure 22.3 Hepatic metabolism of acetaminophen. Intracellular amplification mechanisms include mitochondrial damage downregulating the oxidative phosphorylation chain and inhibiting ATP production, as well as generation of reactive oxygen and reactive nitrogen species. Extracellular amplification mechanisms include action of proinflammatory cytokines, possibly enhanced by subnormal expression of CD44.

can minimize hepatotoxicity if given early enough. It does not reverse the toxic effects of the toxic metabolite once they have occurred. *N*-Acetylcysteine may also promote hepatocellular recovery by enhancing oxygen delivery to the liver tissue.

Young children appear to be resistant to hepatotoxicity from acute acetaminophen overdose and tend to recover when it does occur [42]. The incidence of hepatotoxicity was 5.5% in a study of 417 children aged 5 years or younger, compared with 29% in adolescents and adults at comparable toxic blood levels [43]. Various studies of acetaminophen pharmacokinetics, metabolism, and toxicity in children suggest a biochemical basis for this difference. The elimination half-life is essentially the same in children and adults, although with interindividual variation it ranges as much as 1–3.5 hours [44]. The elimination half-life is somewhat longer (2.2–5.0 hours) in neonates. The profile of metabolites differs greatly in early childhood from that in adolescence and adulthood: sulfation predominates over glucuronidation. The switch to the adult pattern seems to occur around 12 years of age. However, even in newborns, urinary metabolites reflecting cytochrome P450-generated intermediates can be found; therefore, the capacity for producing toxic metabolites seems to be present from an extremely early age. In vitro studies with fetal human hepatocytes have shown that the cytochrome P450-generated intermediates can be formed and conjugated to glutathione as early as at 18 weeks of gestation, but the rate of formation is approximately 10% of that in adult human hepatocytes; sulfation, but not glucuronidation, of

acetaminophen also can be detected in the human fetal liver cells. Human infants may also have a greater capacity for synthesis of glutathione than adults and so can produce enough new glutathione to inactivate toxic metabolites of acetaminophen more effectively.

Despite this relative resistance to this type of hepatotoxicity, very young children can develop severe hepatotoxicity from acetaminophen. Some of these reports represent acute poisoning [45]. Therapeutic misadventure from inappropriate dosing is more frequent in this age group: 22 of 47 cases reviewed in the largest published series were children aged 3 years or younger, and 6 of these 22 were infants aged 6 months or younger [32]. Some of this acetaminophen-associated hepatotoxicity might be avoided by clear instructions to parents about dosing and use of conservative dosage guidelines. Hepatotoxicity and extreme prolongation of the elimination half-life of acetaminophen have also been found in infants born after maternal self-poisoning with acetaminophen.

Some children may have innate defects in acetaminophen detoxification, but this has been difficult to pinpoint mechanistically. Children with 5-oxoprolinuria, who cannot produce glutathione efficiently, are at increased risk of liver injury from acetaminophen. The possibility that patients with Crigler–Najjar syndrome or Gilbert syndrome are more susceptible to acetaminophen hepatotoxicity is a complex pharmacologic question based on data from the Gunn rat: it requires further investigation. Whether drugs such as zidovudine, phenytoin, and phenobarbital increase acetaminophen hepatotoxicity is disputed [46]. Mercury poisoning through exposure to elemental mercury apparently enhanced acetaminophen hepatotoxicity in one child; however, mercury is itself hepatotoxic [47]. The experience in adults of chronic alcohol abuse with consequent induction of CYP2E1 may be relevant to acetaminophen hepatotoxicity in some adolescents [48]. The sum effect of drug interactions over the entire range of acetaminophen hepatotoxicity is likely complex and highly individualistic. Attention to these modifiers may be important in the pediatric age group.

The implications for liver injury of new formulations of acetaminophen, such as sustained-release tablets, remain uncertain. Confusing the sustained-release tablet dosage schedule (every 8 hours) with the conventional dosage schedule (every 4–6 hours) might result in hepatotoxicity. Combining acetaminophen with a potentially habituating analgesic might result in excessive chronic use of acetaminophen. The plethora of over-the-counter medications that contain acetaminophen increases risk of liver injury. Acetaminophen rectal suppositories are used in children, and these pose unique problems of drug absorption and bioavailability depending on the composition of suppository matrix. Severe liver damage in a child was reported attributed to high-dose acetaminophen exposure with rectal suppositories [49]. Although several other potentially hepatotoxic drugs were also administered, this attribution is credible. Oro-dispersible tablets (which melt in the mouth) are designed for children's use and may increase the risk of childhood hepatotoxicity [50].

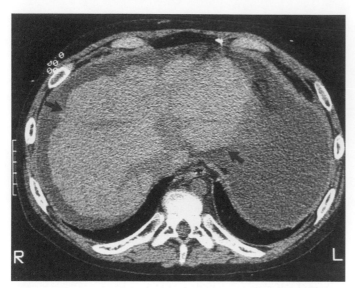

Figure 22.4 CT of the liver in chronic amiodarone administration. The increased density of the liver (appears white) results from the iodine in the amiodarone accumulated in hepatocytes. (Courtesy of Dr. Paul Babyn, Department of Diagnostic Imaging, the Hospital for Sick Children, Toronto.)

Amiodarone

Amiodarone is an iodinated benzofuran derivative used for the treatment of cardiac arrhythmias. Although reserved for more severe disease, it is used from time to time in children. Asymptomatic elevations of serum aminotransferases may occur. Phospholipidosis is associated with progressive liver damage in some patients. Although iodine accumulation in the liver may produce striking hepatic parenchymal density on CT (Figure 22.4), it is not in itself a sign of hepatotoxicity.

Amiodarone-induced hepatotoxicity, characterized by hepatomegaly and abnormal aminotransferases, may develop within a month of treatment or after 1 year of treatment. Asymptomatic elevations in aminotransferases are frequent, occurring in one-quarter to one-half of patients treated; these abnormalities may return to normal spontaneously, even if the drug is not discontinued. Alternatively, progressive chronic liver disease occurs in some patients. Severe amiodarone hepatotoxicity has been reported in a child [51]. It presented as rapidly progressive hepatic failure beginning after 2 months of treatment at a relatively high dose of amiodarone (9 mg/kg daily): clinical presentation was described as Reye-like because of vomiting and progressive stupor but no jaundice.

The mechanism of amiodarone hepatotoxicity remains undetermined, but it may involve abnormal hepatic biotransformation. Amiodarone may also interfere with mitochondrial beta-oxidation and oxidative phosphorylation.

Antineoplastic drugs

Many drugs used to treat neoplasia can cause hepatotoxicity [52]. Potential for liver damage in children may vary from the experience in adults. Moreover, these drugs are rarely used separately and patients receiving them are usually at risk for multiple types of liver injury. A hepatitic pattern, often asymptomatic with elevation in serum aminotransferases and no other evidence of severe liver toxicity, is common. Antineoplastic drugs, which frequently produce this reaction, include nitrosoureas, 6-mercaptopurine, cytosine arabinoside, cisplatinum, and dacarbazine. With cis-platinum the mechanism of liver injury appears to involve oxidative stress [53,54]. For both cis-platinum and dacarbazine, induction of CYP2E1 might enhance the risk of liver damage. Cyclophosphamide may cause a dose-related drug hepatitis [55]. Carmustine and 6-mercaptopurine can also cause severe cholestasis [56]. Adriamycin, dactinomycin, and vinca alkaloids are infrequently associated with hepatotoxicity. However, several patients treated with dactinomycin at the Hospital for Sick Children, Toronto, have developed severe hepatic dysfunction, with extremely elevated serum aminotransferases and coagulopathy, all of which resolved spontaneously when off the drug. Similar experience has been reported in treatment of Wilms tumor [57]. Irradiation may enhance hepatotoxicity of dactinomycin. Adriamycin given together with 6-mercaptopurine may increase the hepatotoxic potential of 6-mercaptopurine. Steatosis or portal fibrosis has been found on liver biopsies from children with acute lymphoblastic leukemia treated with various anticancer drugs [58].

L-Asparaginase is associated with severe hepatic injury characterized by severe steatosis, hepatocellular necrosis, and fibrosis, which is usually reversible after the L-asparaginase is stopped [59,60]. Severe microvesicular steatosis has been reported. The most likely mechanism for this hepatotoxicity is a profound interference with hepatocellular protein metabolism. Thrombocytopenia and acute liver failure were reported in an 18-year-old patient receiving carboplatin [61].

Toxic microvascular injury, mainly reported as VOD, is an important pattern of hepatotoxicity associated with antineoplastic drugs. An alternative term to VOD, sinusoidal obstruction syndrome, draws attention to the role of damage to sinusoidal endothelial cells in its etiology [62]. Acute presentation of VOD is with an enlarged tender liver, ascites or unexplained weight gain, and jaundice; serum aminotransferases may be elevated. In surviving patients, the liver disease may progress to cirrhosis, with hepatic venular sclerosis and sinusoidal fibrosis. Patients with a more subacute course may show splenomegaly and thrombocytopenia. Although 6-thioguanine is a classic cause of VOD, other antineoplastic drugs such as cytosine arabinoside, busulfan, dacarbazine, carmustine, dactinomycin, and oxaliplatin have been associated with VOD at conventional or high doses, and drug interactions may enhance their propensity for causing this type of liver injury [63]. Currently, VOD most frequently develops after allogeneic bone marrow (stem cell) transplant [64]; however, it has been reported with other regimens used for treatment of childhood solid tumors [65,66]. It has been disputed whether VOD is a consequence of chemotherapeutic conditioning regimens or part of the spectrum of liver injury caused by graft-versus-host disease, and in some individual patients it may, in fact, be difficult to make this distinction. In some cases, cholestasis or cytokines released as part of graft-versus-host disease might contribute to the development of VOD or increase its severity. Irradiation by itself can lead to VOD, possibly because endothelial cells lining hepatic sinusoids are more sensitive to radiation than hepatocytes. The combination of irradiation and chemotherapy in conditioning regimens appears to accelerate development of VOD compared with the effect of a single injurious agent (irradiation or chemical) [67]. Methotrexate plus cyclosporine (used as prophylaxis for graft-versus-host disease) in patients prepared for bone marrow transplant by a regimen using busulfan and cyclophosphamide led to a higher incidence of jaundice and VOD disease than methylprednisolone and cyclosporine prophylaxis in similarly prepared patients [68]. In general, most antineoplastic drugs carry some risk of provoking VOD.

Clinical predictors of likelihood for development of VOD in children have not yet been identified; however, ongoing hepatitis, such as chronic viral hepatitis, before transplant increases susceptibility to hepatic damage [69]. Development of multiorgan failure presages poor survival. Polymorphisms affecting glutathione S-transferases appear to correlate with increased risk [70]; risk associated with other phase II enzymes is less established [71]. In many patients, the process resolves, but in a sizable proportion, the process is fatal or leads to chronic liver damage [72,73]. Treatment has generally been aimed at interfering with thrombosis, such as defibrotide [74] or other agents [75], but given the disease mechanism, early treatment with glutathione replacement might be appropriate. Anecdotal evidence suggests its efficacy [76,77].

The pathogenesis of VOD involves primary injury to sinusoidal endothelial cells. There is secondary subendothelial hemorrhage, hepatocellular necrosis, and hepatic vein obliteration. Liver injury progresses from congestion in the sinusoids to parenchymal extinction. With dacarbazine, VOD involves damage to sinusoidal endothelial cells by toxic metabolite(s) produced in the endothelial cells; glutathione appears to protect against toxicity [78]. In contrast, with VOD caused by cyclophosphamide, the toxic metabolites are produced in hepatocytes [79]. In a rat model in which monocrotaline was the toxic chemical, glutathione depletion and decreased hepatic production of nitric oxide contribute to the disease mechanism [80]. Among cytokines that may play a role in the disease mechanism, vascular endothelial growth factor has been shown to be elevated in children who develop severe VOD [81].

6-Thioguanine has recently been found to cause nodular regenerative hyperplasia in patients with inflammatory bowel disease, and in one patient VOD was also present [82]. A long-term follow-up study of children with 6-thioguanine hepatotoxicity revealed that 7 of 10 had clinically significant portal hypertension; however, the nature of the underlying chronic lesion was not determined [83].

Aspirin

Hepatotoxicity has been associated with high-dose aspirin treatment. The hepatotoxicity appears to be dose dependent, and patients without rheumatoid disease can develop hepatotoxicity. However, most cases are reported in patients with rheumatoid diseases. Approximately 60% of the 300 reported cases have been in patients with juvenile rheumatoid arthritis (not necessarily all children), and a further 10% have occurred in children with acute rheumatic fever. A prospective study of aspirin hepatotoxicity in adults with rheumatoid arthritis or osteoarthritis revealed that 5% of those taking aspirin developed asymptomatic elevations of serum aspartate aminotransferase. The preponderance of cases in patients with rheumatologic diseases, however, raises the possibility that these patients have a predisposition to this toxicity. A single case of apparent hepatotoxicity associated with low-dose aspirin therapy in a young child after liver transplant has been reported; there were essentially asymptomatic elevations of serum aminotransferases, and liver biopsy revealed zonal, but periportal, hepatocellular necrosis [84].

In most cases, salicylate hepatotoxicity has hepatitic features, with anorexia, nausea, vomiting, abdominal pain, and elevated serum aminotransferases [85]. Hepatomegaly is usually present, and the liver may be tender. Progressive signs of liver damage such as jaundice and coagulopathy are rare. Even in uncomplicated cases, serum aminotransferase levels may be >1000 IU/L. In some cases encephalopathy (not related to Reye syndrome) has been present. Clinical and laboratory abnormalities resolve when aspirin is stopped. Liver histology typically shows a non-specific picture with acute, focal hepatocellular necrosis.

Reye syndrome may be considered a type of aspirin-associated hepatotoxicity, and its incidence has fallen precipitously since treatment of febrile illnesses with aspirin has been abandoned. Given its dose dependency, aspirin may be an intrinsic toxin. Additionally, given the role of viral infection in some patients and disordered immune function in others, it may also be classified as a contingent hepatotoxin. Aspirin appears to inhibit mitochondrial function.

Atomoxetine

Atomoxetine is a possible treatment for attention deficit disorder and, therefore, could find broad utility in children. It undergoes extensive hepatic biotransformation, mainly by CYP2D6 but also by CYP2C19 or other P450 enzymes [86]. Severe liver injury with features of hepatitis has occurred in adults and children, including acute liver failure in a child. An AIH-like pattern of injury has been reported [87]. The hepatotoxic mechanism is not known, but it appears to involve metabolic idiosyncrasy. Individuals with the CYP2D6 polymorphism are at increased risk. Atomoxetine is, therefore, a contingent hepatotoxin capable of eliciting an immunoallergic response.

Azathioprine

Azathioprine is a potent immunosuppressive drug that consists of 6-mercaptopurine linked to an imidazole side-chain. In effect, it is a prodrug for 6-mercaptopurine. Since its introduction in the 1960s, azathioprine has been associated with hepatotoxicity, including in children, but these early studies are confounded by underdiagnosed concomitant viral liver disease. In adults, azathioprine hepatotoxicity has been characterized mainly by cholestasis or a hepatitic–cholestatic picture. Liver biopsy in one patient showed centrilobular ballooning of hepatocytes and canalicular cholestasis [88]. Azathioprine hepatotoxicity has been described in orthotopic liver transplant recipients: endothelial cell damage, as well as hepatocyte damage and cholestasis, was noted [89]. In addition, several cases of nodular regenerative hyperplasia associated with azathioprine have been reported [90]. Nodular regenerative hyperplasia is more common than previously appreciated and is an important pattern of injury with azathioprine. Chronic use has been associated with cirrhosis in some cases. Polymorphisms affecting thiopurine methyltransferase are associated with myelosuppression and may predispose to hepatotoxicity.

6-Mercaptopurine has been associated more directly with liver toxicity and causes a mixed hepatitic–cholestatic reaction [91]. Hepatic accumulation of 6-mercaptopurine metabolites was postulated in four children who developed hepatotoxicity from 6-mercaptopurine during treatment for acute lymphoblastic leukemia; one child had severe cholestatic hepatitis [56]. High concentration of the 6-mercaptopurine metabolite 6-methylmercaptopurine nucleotide predicts hepatotoxicity [92]: consequently, complex metabolic pathways affected by multilocus genetic polymorphisms, and possibly age, are important.

Carbamazepine

Carbamazepine is a dibenzazepine derivative, similar structurally to imipramine in that it has fundamentally a tricyclic chemical structure. Hepatotoxicity is uncommon. In children, the usual clinical picture has been hepatitis, often associated with a drug hypersensitivity syndrome similar to that of phenytoin. Two children presented with a mononucleosis-like illness consisting of rash, lymphadenopathy, hepatosplenomegaly, and neutropenia. A child treated at the Hospital for Sick Children, Toronto, also presented with fever, rash, incipient liver failure, lymphopenia, and eosinophilia. Rechallenge of her lymphocytes in vitro with metabolites of carbamazepine provided evidence of defective detoxification mechanisms [93].

Even more severe hepatotoxicity has been reported in children. One child died of progressive liver failure when carbamazepine was not stopped [94]. Four children with fatal acute liver failure were taking carbamazepine, phenytoin, and primidone [95]. Severe hepatitis has been reported in three children taking only carbamazepine: one recovered with corticosteroid treatment but the others died or required liver transplant [96]. Another child developed severe hepatitis with coagulopathy 5 months after beginning treatment with carbamazepine; she survived with prednisone treatment [97].

Like phenytoin and phenobarbital, carbamazepine may be metabolized via arene oxides. These metabolites are ordinarily detoxified by the phase II enzyme epoxide hydrolase. People with an inherited metabolic idiosyncrasy, possibly involving an abnormal epoxide hydrolase, may be unable to detoxify active metabolite(s) of carbamazepine and thus develop hepatotoxicity. The same metabolic idiosyncrasy creating susceptibility to carbamazepine hepatotoxicity may set up cross-susceptibility to phenytoin and phenobarbital hepatotoxicity [98]. This may explain the fatal hepatotoxicity reported in some children taking multiple antiepileptic drugs because primidone contains phenobarbital. Immunogenetics also influences susceptibility to carbamazepine hypersensitivity syndrome, including liver injury: namely, *HLA-A*3101* allele in Northern European ethnicity [99]. *HLA-B*1502* allele in Han Chinese and other Asian ethnicities appears related mainly to dermatological reactions.

Oxcarbazepine can cause similar hepatotoxicity in children [100], and in one case acute liver failure occurred [101].

Cocaine

Cocaine hepatotoxicity has not yet been reported in children or adolescents. A clinically severe hepatitic reaction has been reported in five young adults: the predominant histologic finding was extensive zonal necrosis of hepatocytes in Rappaport zone 3 with zone 1 steatosis [102]. The mechanism of this hepatotoxicity remains undetermined. The histologic pattern of hepatic injury in humans is consistent with generation of a toxic metabolite, probably by cytochromes P450. Such a toxic metabolite might be similar to that in the mouse or a potent electrophile. Glutathione appears to protect against cocaine-induced hepatic injury. CYP3A subfamily enzymes are important in biotransformation of cocaine. Ethanol and phenobarbital-type inducers appear to increase cocaine hepatotoxicity, as may endotoxin.

Cyclosporine

Cyclosporine has a novel cyclic structure composed of 11 amino acid residues and is extremely lipophilic. It is metabolized in humans by CYP3A4 and is, therefore, susceptible to predictable drug interactions that might affect its hepatotoxic potential. Although at high dosage a mixed hepatitic–cholestatic picture may develop, the more frequent hepatic abnormality is mainly bland cholestasis: direct hyperbilirubinemia without other evidence of hepatocellular damage [103]. Cyclosporine inhibits the bile salt excretory pump [104], and it affects gene expression [105] and alters canalicular membrane fluidity in rats [106].

Ecstasy

The synthetic amphetamine 3,4-methylenedioxymethamphetamine is generally known as "Ecstasy" and continues to be a popular "recreational" drug, despite being potentially very hazardous. Deaths have occurred with ingestion of only one tablet. It can cause severe hyperthermia with rhabdomyolysis, cardiac damage with arrhythmias, disseminated intravascular coagulation, and acute renal failure. Hepatotoxicity, reported mainly in young adults, led to death or liver transplantation in several; recent reports of severe hepatotoxicity included some adolescents [107–110]. There may be a few days between taking Ecstasy and becoming unwell, or patients may be found "collapsed" within hours of taking it. Some patients have coagulopathy and hypoglycemia without developing full-blown acute liver failure. Liver histology is variable with Ecstasy hepatotoxicity. The spectrum ranges from focal to extensive hepatocellular necrosis, with variable degrees of cholestasis, sometimes microvesicular steatosis. Interindividual variation in susceptibility is a prominent feature of Ecstasy hepatotoxicity; hyperthermia itself, impure drug, or coadministered recreational drugs or ethanol may contribute to the liver damage in some cases. Genetic predisposition involves the CYP2D6 variants with decreased activity. Certain drugs (such as paroxetine, fluoxetine, and certain protease inhibitors) inhibit CYP2D6, and indeed Ecstasy inhibits its own biotransformation by this cytochrome P450. The mechanism of liver injury includes CYP3A4 as well as CYP2D6, interaction of drug with PXR regulating CYP3A4 and cellular stress responses, and glutathione as the principal phase II detoxifier; in vitro data indicate that Ecstasy or its metabolites can mobilize cytokine-mediated immune responses [111]. The occurrence of Ecstasy hepatotoxicity with acute liver failure in adolescents depends on emerging trends for teenage usage. Public education on the risks of using Ecstasy is urgently required.

Other less acute or less severe patterns of clinical liver disease may occur [112]. A teenager with chronic hepatitis caused by Ecstasy showed giant cell hepatitis on liver biopsy, possibly a manifestation of an AIH-like process [113].

Erythromycin

All forms of erythromycin, not just erythromycin estolate, are potentially hepatotoxic [114–116]. The clinical presentation is similar regardless of which erythromycin ester is involved: anorexia, nausea, jaundice, and abdominal pain, predominantly in the right upper quadrant. Pruritus caused by cholestasis has been reported in adults. The overall clinical appearance is that of a mixed hepatitic–cholestatic process, although the cholestatic component may be prominent enough to suggest biliary tract obstruction. Hepatomegaly, sometimes with splenomegaly, appears to be common in children. A single report of erythromycin ethylsuccinate hepatotoxicity in a child indicated relatively mild, self-limited disease [115]. Histologic findings include prominent cholestasis and focal necrosis of hepatocytes, both of which tend to be worse in acinar zone 3. Eosinophils are prominent in portal infiltrates and in the sinusoids [114]. The zonality suggests the action of a toxic metabolite.

The mechanism of erythromycin hepatotoxicity remains obscure. Erythromycin and other macrolide antibiotics are metabolized in the liver by the CYP3A subfamily. Hepatocellular damage may be caused by a toxic metabolite, but this is by no means proved.

Other macrolide antibiotics are also associated with hepatotoxicity. Azithromycin was associated with cholestatic liver injury in two children, severe in one [25]. Azithromycin does not inhibit P450 enzymes and the hepatotoxic mechanism has not been determined. It is likely a contingent hepatotoxin, certainly capable of eliciting immunoallergic response. Severe cholestatic liver injury associated with clarithromycin was reported in a 15-year-old girl; it was unresponsive to treatment with ursodiol but subsided with prednisone [117]. Whether nimesulide contributed to this hepatotoxicity is uncertain. Cholestatic liver injury has been reported in adults [118]. Telithromycin, a ketolide antibiotic active against resistant pneumococci, may cause early-onset severe hepatitis with abdominal pain, jaundice and ascites, which was fatal in 4 and required liver transplantation in 1 of 42 adults reported [119]. It is contraindicated in myasthenia gravis. Its safety in children has not been established.

Estrogens: oral contraceptive pill

Cholestasis is a well-recognized complication of estrogens administered in oral contraceptives pills. Estrogen inhibits the bile salt export pump; mutations or polymorphisms in *ABCB11* may render the pump more susceptible to inhibition [18]. Estrogen-induced changes in bile composition may lead to gallstone formation and diminished gallbladder function.

Hepatic vein thrombosis (Budd–Chiari syndrome) has been associated with use of oral contraceptives [120]. Importantly, it occurs in adolescents. Other disorders associated with hepatic vein thrombosis, such as paroxysmal nocturnal hemoglobinuria, circulating lupus anticoagulant, and congenital disorders of coagulation proteins, should be excluded. Early diagnosis is important for a good outcome, but clinical presentation may be subtle: only gradual increase in abdominal girth caused by ascites and non-specific changes in liver function tests.

Liver cell adenoma is the principal neoplasm associated with prolonged use of oral contraceptives. Rarely hepatocellular carcinoma has been found [121]; oral contraceptive-associated adenomas may progress to hepatocellular carcinoma. Uncomplicated liver cell adenomas may regress when the oral contraceptive pill is stopped. Peliosis hepatis, which is focal dilatation of the hepatic sinusoids, is another lesion associated with chronic use of oral contraceptives.

Felbamate

Felbamate is a relatively new anticonvulsant sometimes used for treating seizures in Lennox–Gastaut syndrome and thus available for use in children. It has been associated with serious adverse effects: aplastic anemia and, less commonly, acute liver failure. Severe hepatotoxicity has occurred in young children [122]. The mechanism of this hepatotoxicity is not established but may involve P450-generated reactive metabolite(s), which then bind to and modify cellular proteins and initiate an immune reaction [123]. CYP2E1 and CYP3A4 appear to play an important role in hepatic biotransformation of felbamate. One reactive metabolite, 2-phenylpropenal, is detoxified by glutathione but is also capable of inhibiting certain glutathione-S-transferases. Felbamate is apparently a contingent hepatotoxin capable of causing an immunoallergic reaction, dependent in part on both the pharmacogenetic and immunogenetic complexion of the individual taking the drug.

Haloperidol

Haloperidol may be associated with hepatotoxicity, shown by elevated serum aminotransferases [124]. Cholestasis may dominate the clinical picture, although some degree of hepatocellular damage and eosinophilia may be present. A prolonged severe bland cholestatic reaction, mimicking extrahepatic bile duct obstruction, may develop in children.

Halothane

Halothane hepatotoxicity is classically hepatitic. It may manifest as asymptomatic hepatitis, indicated only by abnormal serum aminotransferases in the first or second week after anesthetic exposure, or as severe hepatitis with extensive hepatocyte necrosis and liver failure. Predictors for developing halothane hepatotoxicity in adults include older age, female sex, obesity, and multiple exposures to halothane. Hepatitis associated with halothane is infrequent in children although halothane is often used in pediatric anesthetic practice. Based on large retrospective studies in children, the incidence is approximately 1 in 80 000–200 000, in contrast to an incidence of 1 in 4000–30 000 in adults. One study suggests that halothane hepatotoxicity is less common in both adults and children [125]. Certainly halothane hepatitis occurs in children. Ten cases have been documented in detail in children aged 11 months to 15 years, all of whom had multiple exposures to halothane. Three children died of fulminant liver failure but all the others recovered [126,127]. In addition, three cases of halothane hepatitis were found retrospectively [128,129] as well as three additional children who succumbed to fulminant hepatic failure after halothane [130]. Other reports of hepatitis or hepatic failure in children after halothane anesthesia are difficult to evaluate because of inadequate data or the presence of complicated, and thus confounding, systemic disease; these may amount to an additional nine cases.

Halothane is metabolized by various P450 enzymes and toxic metabolites are generated [131,132]. Oxidative or reductive metabolic pathways predominate, depending on the prevailing tissue oxygen tension (Figure 22.5). Reductive metabolism generates a toxic intermediate, identified as a chlorotrifluoroethyl radical, that leads to lipid peroxidation,

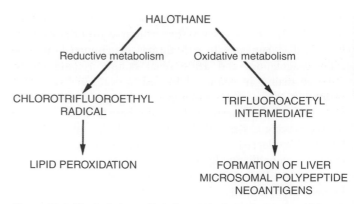

Figure 22.5 Metabolic fates of halothane. Whether reductive or oxidative metabolism predominates depends on the tissue oxygen tension. Formation of neoantigens is associated exclusively with the oxidative pathway.

and oxidative metabolism generates a trifluoroacetyl intermediate that can acetylate cellular membranes, thus generating trifluoroacetyl adducts. The contribution of these complex metabolic systems to human hepatotoxicity remains a matter of some dispute. However, the oxidative pathway is probably predominant in humans. Recent work shows that CYP2A6 and CYP3A4 are associated with the reductive metabolism and CYP2A6 and CYP2E1 (mainly the latter) are associated with the oxidative pathway.

The mechanism of halothane hepatotoxicity involves a connection between cytotoxic damage from reactive metabolites and immunologic phenomena often associated with this hepatotoxicity. The oxidative pathway appears to be associated with hepatocellular membrane damage and immune phenomena typical of the clinical hepatotoxicity syndrome. Patients surviving halothane hepatotoxicity were found to have an antibody to altered hepatocyte membrane constituents. Antibodies to these neoantigens have now been identified in sera from patients with halothane hepatitis [133]. Further studies showed that neoantigens, analogous to neoantigens derived from halothane-treated animals, are expressed in human liver in individuals exposed to halothane [134]. Only one of these neoantigens has been purified and identified; this particular trifluoroacetylated protein is a microsomal carboxylesterase [135]. Kupffer cells may play a role in the process by which the trifluoroacetyl adducts initiate an immune response.

Herbal medications

The hepatotoxic potential of herbal medications is important. The pharmacology of these drugs (active ingredient, metabolism, potential drug interactions) is frequently not well understood. Some herbals alter hepatic drug metabolism. The purity and strength of the actual drug used may not be known. How the herbal preparation is actually manufactured can affect potency and potential toxicity. Patients, including adolescents, may take herbal medications intermittently, and they may not report using herbals to physicians. Some may have underlying liver disease: for example, children with chronic hepatitis C are known to take herbal drugs frequently. Since some herbals are administered to promote weight loss, increased use of these agents in children may be encountered, given the current "epidemic" of childhood obesity. Little is known about the effect of hepatic steatosis on the biotransformation of these drugs. Use of herbal medications also displays cultural biases. Herbals may be administered to children to promote good health. Finally, herbal medications can be bought nowadays over the Internet such that a wide range of agents are available, particularly to adolescents.

Among herbal preparations, the toxicity of certain bush teas containing pyrrolizidine alkaloids, which can cause VOD, are best known. Comfrey is also hepatotoxic because it contains pyrrolizidine alkaloids [136]. Fatal VOD associated with an unspecified herbal medication has been reported in a child [137]. Germander hepatotoxicity [138] appears to be mediated by diterpenoid toxic metabolites formed through biotransformation by CYP3A4 [139,140].

Kava kava, which is used to treat anxiety and promote relaxation, has been removed from the market in some countries because of severe hepatotoxicity [141]. In one instance, a 14-year-old girl required liver transplantation [142]. Some controversy persists as to the real risk of hepatotoxicity, which may depend in part on how the kava is extracted. Kavalactones are capable of inhibiting certain hepatic P450 enzymes [143].

Other herbals established as hepatotoxic include chaparral leaf [144,145], jin bu huan [146], and ma huang (ephedra) [147]. Echinacea may have some hepatotoxic potential. Acute liver failure was reported in a child who received a medication containing various herbs and metals [148].

Infliximab

Infliximab is a humanized monoclonal antibody that is increasingly recognized as causing hepatotoxicity in adults: it causes an AIH-like liver disorder [149,150] or cholestatic hepatitis [151]. Occasionally liver injury is severe enough to require liver transplantation [149,152]. No cases have been reported in children as yet, but AIH-like injury was reported in a 22 year old [153]. More cases have been identified than currently published. It is possible that infliximab-associated AIH-like hepatotoxicity could be mistakenly diagnosed as autoimmune hepatitis sometimes associated with inflammatory bowel disease, an important distinction as management differs.

Isoniazid

Isoniazid has been associated with a wide spectrum of hepatotoxicity in adults. It is an important cause of drug hepatotoxicity wherever tuberculosis is highly prevalent. The most frequent abnormality is asymptomatic elevation of serum aminotransferases. Overt symptoms of hepatitis (fatigue, anorexia, nausea, and vomiting) indicate severe disease; mortality is greater than 10% in patients with jaundice [154]. On histologic examination, isoniazid hepatotoxicity frequently looks exactly like acute viral hepatitis. Submassive hepatic necrosis or an AIH-like pattern can occur. Hepatocellular damage sometimes has a zonal pattern, which suggests hepatotoxicity involving drug metabolism.

Isoniazid hepatotoxicity is generally considered to be more common in adults than in children; however, there have been numerous reports of isoniazid hepatotoxicity, including fatal hepatitic necrosis, in children being treated for, or receiving prophylaxis for, tuberculosis [154,155]. In large studies of children receiving isoniazid alone as prophylaxis against tuberculosis, hepatotoxicity (indicated by abnormal serum aminotransferases) had a 7% incidence in a series of 369 children and a 17.1% incidence in 239 patients aged 9–14 years [156]. These findings are nearly equivalent to those in adults, in whom the incidence of transiently elevated serum aminotransferases is estimated at 10–20%. The overall incidence of symptomatic isoniazid hepatitis in children is 0.1–7.1% [157]. Evidence from small studies suggests that hepatic dysfunction occurs in children being treated with isoniazid and rifampicin for tuberculosis, with severe hepatitis in approximately 30–40%. Children under 2 years of age may be at greater risk. The contribution of brief sequential courses of streptomycin and ethambutal to the hepatotoxicity of isoniazid plus rifampicin is difficult to determine. Inducers of cytochromes P450 may enhance isoniazid hepatotoxicity. Severe isoniazid hepatotoxicity has been found in children treated concurrently with isoniazid and carbamazepine [158]. As in adults, hepatotoxicity typically develops in the first 2–3 months of treatment; in most children, mild biochemical disturbance resolves with either no change in dose or else a modest dose reduction. Hepatitis with jaundice necessitates drug withdrawal. Children with more severe tuberculosis seem to be at greater risk for hepatotoxicity, particularly if tuberculous meningitis is present. Malnourished children may be at greater risk of hepatotoxicity.

Isoniazid hepatotoxicity appears to be caused by a toxic metabolite. Candidate toxic metabolites include acetylhydrazine and hydrazine; isoniazid itself may cause hepatocellular damage [159]. Acetylation via NAT-2 is important in isoniazid metabolism. Acetylisoniazid or its derivatives have been proposed as toxic, and recent studies indicate that acetylhydrazine, derived from acetylisoniazid, undergoes biotransformation by cytochromes P450, principally CYP2E1, to produce these reactive metabolites. Genetically determined activity of CYP2E1 influences whether hepatotoxicity develops. Likewise, slow acetylators in the NAT-2 polymorphism appear to be a greater risk. Reports in children have failed to show a clear pattern of hepatotoxicity in relation to acetylator status but most were underpowered. Other data suggest that CYP2E1 activity is a more important determinant for hepatotoxicity than acetylator status [160]. Chronic use of alcohol leading to induction of CYP2E1 is known to increase the risk of isoniazid hepatotoxicity. Moreover, isoniazid acting as a nucleophile can activate macrophages. Therefore, isoniazid is a classic contingent hepatotoxin capable of causing an immunoallergic reaction.

Monitoring with frequent measurement of serum amino-transferases and direct inquiry for hepatitic symptoms is necessary during at least the first 3 months of treatment. If typical hepatitic symptoms develop, isoniazid must be discontinued promptly. Extra caution appears required if the child is taking an antiepileptic drug concurrently.

Ketoconazole

In contrast to amphotericin, which is rarely associated with hepatotoxicity, the oral antifungal drug ketoconazole was found to cause significant hepatotoxicity soon after it was introduced for general use. The initial large review of ketoconazole hepatotoxicity in the USA included two children (a 17-year-old boy and a 5-year-old boy, both with chronic mucocutaneous candidiasis) among 54 reported occurrences, of which 33 (including both children) were judged as probable or possible cases of ketoconazole-induced hepatotoxicity [161]. Similar series from the UK and the Netherlands included no children. Presenting symptoms included jaundice and hepatitis (anorexia, nausea, vomiting, and malaise) and occurred on average after 6–8 weeks of treatment (range: 5 days to 6 months). Peripheral eosinophilia was noted in only one patient in the British series, in 10% of the Dutch patients and in none of the US patients. A patient who developed fulminant hepatitis associated with ketoconazole also had no eosinophilia or rash; other adults with fatal hepatotoxicity have since been reported. In all series, the hepatic lesion was mainly hepatocellular necrosis, often with a centrilobular predominance, or a mixed hepatocellular–cholestatic injury, but some patients had mainly cholestatic features. One report described protracted jaundice caused by a predominantly cholestatic lesion. Some patients have also been noted to have asymptomatic elevations of serum aminotransferases, which returned to normal when the drug was stopped.

The prevailing interpretation of these clinical observations is that ketoconazole-induced hepatotoxicity results from metabolic idiosyncrasy. A toxic metabolite has been postulated but not defined; no abnormality of drug detoxification has been specifically demonstrated

Lamotrigine

Lamotrigine is an anticonvulsant drug that can cause the drug hypersensitivity syndrome classically associated with phenytoin [162–164]. Severity of liver damage is variable, but severe acute hepatitis, including acute liver failure, can occur. Lamotrigine can be shown to generate an arene oxide intermediate, which is a candidate for mediating this hepatotoxicity. Children may be more likely to produce this intermediate via cytochrome P450 particularly with rapid dose escalation. Therefore, it is a contingent hepatotoxin that is capable of eliciting an immunoallergic response. Cross-sensitivity to phenytoin, carbamazepine, and phenobarbital may be present. Ingestion of lamotrigine by a 3-year-old child resulted in rash and elevated serum aminotransferases [165].

Methotrexate

Chronic low-dose treatment with methotrexate, as used in psoriasis or certain connective tissue diseases, frequently causes hepatic fibrosis with steatosis [166]. The histologic appearance may be similar to that of alcoholic hepatitis with fibrosis. Hepatic fibrosis has occasionally been found in children with juvenile rheumatoid arthritis. It is difficult to screen for liver damage by biochemical testing. Serum aminotransferases may not reflect ongoing liver damage and may be normal even after the development of cirrhosis or fibrosis. Using an aggregate of aminotransferase determinations (percentage abnormal over 6 or 12 months) may compensate for the relative insensitivity of these measurements [167]. Risk factors for the likely development of liver disease proposed for adults (advanced age, chronic ethanol use, obesity, diabetes mellitus, and renal insufficiency) have limited utility for children, except obesity. Although daily administration of methotrexate appears more prone to cause hepatotoxicity, weekly pulse doses are also associated with the development of hepatic fibrosis. Higher cumulative doses are more likely to be associated with hepatotoxicity, but liver damage has sometimes been found at low cumulative doses. The cumulative dose at which hepatotoxicity becomes likely in children has not been determined.

Because of the difficulty in predicting the likelihood of methotrexate-induced liver damage and in detecting it biochemically, regular histologic examination of the liver by liver biopsy has been customary. Liver biopsy before treatment and at regular, often yearly, intervals during prolonged treatment has been advised, but this may involve a considerable number of invasive procedures for a child. The need for such stringent surveillance has been questioned, particularly for children with juvenile rheumatoid arthritis. The risk of methotrexate hepatotoxicity in this group appears to be comparatively low. No child in a cross-sectional study of 14 children with juvenile rheumatoid arthritis who had received a methotrexate cumulative dose >3000 mg or >4000 mg/1.73 m^2 body surface area had significant fibrosis and only one had moderate-to-severe hepatocellular, fatty, inflammatory, or necrotic changes on liver biopsy. In a large study of 37 liver biopsies from 25 patients with juvenile rheumatoid arthritis, most were normal or near-normal; four had moderate-to-severe fatty or inflammatory changes, and two had mild portal fibrosis. Weak but significant correlations were found between abnormal histology and percentage of aminotransferase elevations and body mass index [168]. In similar previous studies, normal or near-normal liver histology was found [169,170]. Two patients with juvenile rheumatoid arthritis treated with methotrexate have been reported as developing some degree of liver fibrosis [171].

The surveillance strategy must be individualized for each patient. Children with juvenile rheumatoid arthritis taking methotrexate should have serum aminotransferases checked frequently (monthly or bimonthly). Those with elevated aspartate aminotransferase or alanine aminotransferase on 40% or more tests in 1 year should be considered for liver biopsy. Those with other risk factors such as obesity or diabetes mellitus should also be considered for liver biopsy surveillance. Performing a liver biopsy after a large cumulative dose of methotrexate has been taken may be judicious, particularly if continued treatment is anticipated. The merits of a pretreatment liver biopsy should not be disregarded because several studies indicate that hepatic abnormalities may be present before treatment, which would otherwise be (wrongly) attributed to methotrexate hepatotoxicity. This is particularly important if the child is overweight or obese. Children with other indications for methotrexate, such as psoriasis or inflammatory bowel disease, may require closer surveillance, because these guidelines may not apply to other diseases. The *C677T* polymorphism in methylenetetrahydrofolate reductase may predispose to hepatotoxicity [172]: the utility of this determination in children requires further investigation.

Methotrexate is also associated with acute hepatitis. High-dose methotrexate treatment used in some antineoplastic treatment regimens may produce acute hepatitis, as shown by a sudden rise in aminotransferases [173]. After chronic treatment for malignancy, usually at comparatively low doses, hepatic damage may be relatively mild, with some steatosis and fibrosis; however, severe liver disease with ascites, hepatosplenomegaly, and transient jaundice has been reported.

The mechanism of methotrexate toxicity remains undetermined although a toxic metabolite has been postulated. The poorly soluble metabolite 7-hydroxymethotrexate has been detected after treatment with high-dose regimens and may be associated with renal toxicity from methotrexate. Direct cytotoxicity is another possibility. Studies in rats suggest that methotrexate can damage the bile canalicular transporter multidrug resistance-associated protein-2 (MRP2), possibly contributing to hepatotoxicity. The mechanism of chronic hepatotoxicity may differ from that of acute toxicity.

Minocycline

Microvesicular steatosis caused by tetracycline administered intravenously is currently rare. Minocycline, a tetracycline derivative, used to treat acne in adolescents, has greater potential for causing liver damage than generally appreciated. Specifically, minocycline hepatotoxicity causes AIH-like liver injury. Several cases have been reported in teenagers: hepatitic symptoms, jaundice, elevated serum aminotransferases, and positive anti-nuclear antibodies were common [174–176]. Another typical presentation was polyarthritis with biochemical hepatitis; jaundice was present when hepatitis was severe. Histologic features resembling AIH may be found on liver biopsy. In many patients, liver damage resolved when the drug was discontinued. Oral prednisone may be administered, analogous to treatment for typical AIH: response is usually favorable and steroids can be tapered and stopped completely after adequate treatment (ordinarily 1–2 years). Alternatively, acute hepatotoxicity may occur. Two cases of acute liver failure

in adolescents have been reported [177,178]: one died before transplant, and the other underwent liver transplant. Careful monitoring of liver function is indicated whenever minocycline is used chronically. The mechanism of hepatotoxicity is undetermined but includes immunoallergic features.

Nevirapine

The antiretroviral drug nevirapine has been utilized as prophylaxis against mother-to-infant transmission of HIV. This non-nucleoside reverse transcriptase inhibitor can cause significant hepatotoxicity in pregnant women receiving it, and it also can cause liver injury in the neonate [179]: longer treatment protocols are more likely to cause hepatotoxicity and a drug hypersensitivity syndrome may be present. A genetic abnormality in *ABCB1*, encoding P-glycoprotein, namely the single-nucleotide polymorphism C3435T, was associated with hepatotoxicity, as well as variations in *CYP2B6* and *CYP3A5* [180].

Non-steroidal anti-inflammatory drugs

The non-steroidal anti-inflammatory drugs (NSAIDs) are a chemically disparate group of anti-inflammatory drugs, defined here as excluding aspirin. It is difficult to assess their hepatotoxic potential in adults or children. Many NSAIDs have little or no risk of hepatic toxicity. Review of several large registries for adverse drug reactions (mainly in adults) revealed diclofenac, sulindac, ibuprofen, naproxen, piroxicam, and nimesulide as most reported to cause hepatotoxicity, in that order [181]. Yet, two widely used NSAIDs, ibuprofen and naproxen, have been associated with liver injury rather infrequently relative to their widespread use. A study of adverse effects associated with NSAIDs in children revealed a variety of adverse side effects, but liver injury was not prominent [182]. Sulindac, diclofenac, and nimesulide are noteworthy for hepatotoxicity. Hepatic biotransformation of NSAIDs, mainly via the CYP2C subfamily, may play an important role the mechanism of their liver injury.

Sulindac can cause important hepatotoxicity as a hepatitic–cholestatic reaction, which may be accompanied by systemic involvement including fever and rash [154,183]. Diclofenac causes elevated serum aminotransferases in 10–15%, but it also causes severe liver injury in rare patients, usually at least 1–3 months into chronic treatment. This is typically a mixed hepatitic–cholestatic injury. Serum aminotransferases are greatly elevated, and in some cases features of the drug hypersensitivity syndrome or an AIH-like injury are present. Diclofenac appears to be a contingent hepatotoxin that can sometimes elicit immunoallergic features. Biotransformation via CYP3A4 and CYP2C9 can produce two quinoneimine toxic metabolites, or an arene oxide can be produced. Higher doses tend to be more toxic. Glucuronidated metabolites excreted into bile via MRP2 can damage the bile canalicular excretory apparatus (variants in CYP2C8, UGT27 *and* ABCC2 are associated with increased risk); because it is a weak acid, it can act as an uncoupler of mitochondrial ATP production. Environmental factors that may enhance hepatotoxicity include concurrent medication with other CYP3A4 substrates and systemic inflammatory disease [184].

Nimesulide is a highly efficacious selective cyclooxygenase 2 inhibitor, which is less likely than some NSAIDs to cause renal or gastrointestinal damage. It is related to sulfonamides. It appears to be somewhat more hepatotoxic than most other NSAIDs [185], with greater severity of liver injury. So far children have not been affected except an adolescent simultaneously treated with clarithromycin. Oxidative injury to mitochondria may play a role in the mechanism of hepatotoxicity, and genetically determined differences in hepatocellular defenses could contribute to susceptibility.

Pemoline

Pemoline, used for the treatment of attention deficit disorders, has been associated with hepatotoxicity ranging from asymptomatic elevation of serum aminotransferases to acute liver failure [186,187]. Other cases of acute liver failure have been reported to regulatory agencies, and several children have now required liver transplantation. The drug has largely been withdrawn from the market. If pemoline is used, serum aminotransferases and other liver function tests must be followed at least monthly throughout the first year of treatment and frequently thereafter because onset of hepatotoxicity may be late in the course of treatment, possibly because it inhibits its own biotransformation. An autoimmune basis for hepatotoxicity seems unlikely. When pemoline is associated with elevated aminotransferases, it must be discontinued promptly. Among alternative therapies, methylphenidate has rarely been associated with some hepatotoxicity, whereas hepatotoxicity has been problematic with atomoxetine.

Penicillins

Semisynthetic derivatives of penicillin have been associated with liver injury. Oxacillin has been associated with hepatitis; oxacillin, cloxacillin, and flucloxacillin have all caused severe cholestasis. Amoxicillin–clavulanic acid may pose the greatest risk of hepatotoxicity among antibiotics [188]. It has been associated with cholestasis or a mixed hepatitic–cholestatic reaction. Cholestatic hepatitis has been reported in one child [189]. Hepatitis with a drug hypersensitivity syndrome occurred in a 13-year-old girl [190]. Acute liver failure with amoxicillin–clavulanic acid has been reported in a few adults [191]. Susceptibility relates to HLA class II markers for certain penicillin derivatives [192,193]. With prolonged cholestasis, the development of small bile duct paucity (ductopenia) has been observed. Notably, ductopenia with severe cholestasis has been reported in a 3-year-old boy treated briefly with amoxicillin–clavulanic acid; severe progressive disease mandated liver transplantation [194].

Phenobarbital

In view of how widely phenobarbital is used, hepatitis is rare. When it occurs, it is usually associated with a multisystemic drug hypersensitivity syndrome, but liver involvement may dominate the clinical picture. Relatively more frequent occurrence in children reflects use of phenobarbital in the pediatric age group. In most children with clinically significant hepatotoxicity, jaundice began within 8 weeks of starting phenobarbital, along with generalized rash and fever [195]. Eosinophilia and other systemic involvement may occur. Usually the liver disease was moderately severe but self-limited; however, two children died of fulminant hepatic failure [196]. One child developed chronic liver disease.

The mechanism of phenobarbital-induced hepatotoxicity remains unclear. Results from in vitro rechallenge of lymphocytes indicate an inherited defect in detoxification of an active metabolite.

Those who develop hepatotoxicity with phenobarbital typically develop adverse reactions with other barbiturates, such as with sedation. Susceptibility to drug hepatotoxicity with carbamazepine or phenytoin may be present. Therefore, substituting either of these latter anticonvulsants may worsen the hepatitis.

Phenytoin

Diphenylhydantoin has been associated with a broad range of adverse effects. Phenytoin-induced hepatitis is not infrequent in children; the incidence is estimated at 2–4 per 100 000 exposures. It was the only drug-induced hepatitis mentioned specifically among adverse drug reactions in a large prospective study of adverse drug reactions in children. Numerous pediatric cases of phenytoin hepatotoxicity have been reported [197], along with an additional nine children in whom hepatic dysfunction was incidental to other organ system involvement [93]. At least six more children were described as having DRESS syndrome, where liver involvement varied from mild to severe.

Phenytoin hepatotoxicity presents as a hepatitic process associated with a drug hypersensitivity syndrome. Aminotransferases are elevated, and the patient may be moderately jaundiced. In severe cases, clinical features of hepatic failure (coagulopathy, ascites, altered level of consciousness) are also present. The drug hypersensitivity syndrome typically includes fever, rash (such as morbilliform rash, Stevens–Johnson syndrome (toxic epidermal necrolysis)), lymphadenopathy, leukocytosis, eosinophilia, and atypical lymphocytosis. Histopathologic examination of the liver shows spotty necrosis of hepatocytes, along with features reminiscent of mononucleosis in some case or of viral hepatitis in others; cholestasis may complicate more severe hepatocellular injury, and granulomas are sometimes found [198]. Reports of a diphenylhydantoin-induced cholestatic hepatitis are unconvincing. In severe cases, treatment with high-dose corticosteroids has been effective in some patients, although this has not been tested in a controlled trial and anecdotal reports have not consistently shown clear benefit. Current opinion favors steroid treatment.

A toxic metabolite may be the cause of phenytoin hepatotoxicity. Phenytoin is metabolized via an arene oxide intermediate, which is ordinarily metabolized and detoxified by epoxide hydrolase [199]. This hypothesis has been investigated in vitro with lymphocytes, which are easy to isolate and retain most phase II biotransformation pathways. When lymphocytes from individuals who have developed the drug hypersensitivity syndrome to phenytoin are incubated in vitro with phenytoin and a murine microsomal system to generate the intermediate metabolites of phenytoin, these lymphocytes are killed to a greater extent than lymphocytes from normal control subjects [200]. Studies of parents indicate an intermediate sensitivity to the toxic metabolite(s), consistent with an inherited defect in drug detoxification. Instead of only causing cell death, the toxic metabolite may bind to certain cellular proteins and thus create haptens for initiating an immune response. This may account for the features of a drug hypersensitivity syndrome or granuloma formation. Phenytoin, therefore, appears to be a contingent hepatotoxin that is capable of eliciting an immunoallergic response.

Three of four children reported with fatal diphenylhydantoin hepatotoxicity were taking phenobarbital at the same time. The same problem has been reported when phenytoin and carbamazepine are used concurrently [98]. The potential for this cross-susceptibility was established by in vitro studies [93]. The prevalence of this cross-sensitivity is approximately 40–50% in those with intolerance for one of these antiepileptic drugs. In general, patients experiencing hepatotoxicity from phenytoin should not be treated with phenobarbital, carbamazepine, or lamotrigine.

Propylthiouracil

Hepatitis is a rare, but potentially dangerous, complication of propylthiouracil treatment for hyperthyroidism. Numerous cases, some very severe, have been reported in children; several have required liver transplantation [201]. Propylthiouracil hepatotoxicity appears to be more frequent in girls, and overall females predominate 8:1. The clinical presentation includes non-specific symptoms of hepatitis, such as anorexia, nausea, vomiting, and jaundice. Serum aminotransferases are moderately elevated. Symptoms typically begin within 2–3 months of starting treatment, but intervals of 9–15 months between starting treatment and onset of hepatotoxicity have occurred. Because asymptomatic elevation of aminotransferases may be the earliest sign of hepatotoxicity, these should be checked regularly throughout treatment. A mixture of hepatitic and cholestatic features has been reported in some adults with propylthiouracil hepatotoxicity. Liver histology shows mild to severe hepatocellular necrosis, characterized as submassive in three cases.

Propylthiouracil is classified as a drug capable of causing AIH-like liver injury; however, given the available data, it is difficult to confirm these as true cases of drug-induced AIH-like

injury, and the association of propylthiouracil hepatotoxicity with this pattern in reported adult cases remains problematic. In contrast, a more convincing case of propylthiouracil hepatotoxicity associated with this AIH-like liver injury has been reported in one child who developed urticaria during treatment with methimazole and non-icteric hepatomegaly with elevated aminotransferases after more than 1 year of treatment with propylthiouracil [202]. Liver biopsy revealed portal inflammation and moderate piecemeal necrosis; treatment with corticosteroids and stopping the propylthiouracil led to prompt clinical improvement in the liver disease. Because thyroid disease is more likely to accompany AIH type 2, the presence of ALKM antibodies should be sought in any child in whom propylthiouracil-induced AIH-like hepatitis is suspected.

Neonatal hepatitis attributed to lymphocyte sensitization during gestation while the mother was taking propylthiouracil during pregnancy occurred in one child [203]. Neonatal methimazole hepatotoxicity was reported [204].

Retinoids

Vitamin A taken chronically in excess is a well-known cause of hepatotoxicity, with changes in hepatic stellate (Ito) cells, steatosis, and fibrosis. The retinoids currently in clinical use are isotretinoin and etretinate. Severe teratogenicity has been the major adverse side effect. Hepatotoxicity associated with these compounds has been variable, generally with a hepatitic pattern, as evidenced by asymptomatic elevations in serum aminotransferases. Of the two, etretinate shows greater potential for liver toxicity [205], possibly because it is more lipophilic than isotretinoin and accumulates in the liver with chronic administration. On liver biopsy, there have been variable degrees of hepatocellular necrosis; rare patients have developed cirrhosis.

Risperidone

Risperidone is an antiepileptic drug that is also used in autism spectrum disorders; it may be associated with elevations of serum aminotransferases. Its overall hepatotoxic potential is difficult to determine and has been disputed. It causes weight gain and fatty liver may develop. A report of risperidone hepatotoxicity in two children may actually have been concurrence of non-alcoholic steatohepatitis and drug toxicity [206]. Cholestatic hepatitis has been reported in one adult [207]. However, it has become evident that severe liver injury may occur in some children [208]. Children taking risperidone should have serum aminotransferases and bilirubin monitored regularly; tracking body mass index and waist circumference may also be worthwhile.

Sulfonamides

Any sulfonamide can cause hepatotoxicity. Children are most commonly treated with these drugs for otitis media, upper respiratory infections, or inflammatory bowel disease. Sulfanilamide, trimethoprim–sulfamethoxazole, and pyrimethamine-sulfadoxine have all been reported as causing significant hepatotoxicity [209]. Sulfasalazine has been associated with severe liver disease in adolescents and young adults, including acute liver failure, sometimes fatal [210]. The spectrum of sulfa-associated liver toxicity also includes asymptomatic elevation of serum aminotransferases [211] and granulomatous hepatitis. A bland cholestatic pattern has sometimes been reported. In general, sulfa hepatotoxicity is associated with a systemic drug hypersensitivity reaction. Fever, significant rash, periorbital edema, atypical lymphocytosis, lymphadenopathy, and renal dysfunction with proteinuria all may occur; myocarditis may be prominent. Dapsone resulting in acute liver failure with typical features of the sulfa drug hypersensitivity syndrome occurred in a child treated for leprosy [212].

Sulfonamide hepatotoxicity results from elaboration of an electrophilic toxic metabolite in the liver. The reactive species appears to be derived from the hydroxylamine metabolite of the particular sulfonamide [213,214]. The hydroxylamine metabolite of sulfamethoxazole has been identified in humans. Some patients who developed sulfa hepatotoxicity have been shown to be slow acetylators (in the rapid/slow polymorphism for NAT-2) as well as being unable to detoxify this reactive metabolite. Upon in vitro rechallenge of their lymphocytes with sulfonamide and a metabolite-generating system, the patient's lymphocytes show significantly more cytotoxicity than control lymphocytes [209]. Glutathione appears to be important for detoxifying the toxic metabolite.

Valproic acid

Valproic acid is an eight-carbon, branched fatty acid. Its systemic and hepatic toxicity remains an important problem [215]. It causes two main patterns of liver injury. A certain proportion of patients, estimated at 11–30%, develop elevated serum aminotransferases usually within a short time of starting treatment. This is a dose-responsive biochemical abnormality that resolves when the dose of valproic acid is decreased. It may be an example of "adaptation" where compensatory metabolic or biotransformation mechanisms take over and mitigate the hepatotoxic effect. Much more rarely, patients develop progressive liver failure that may resemble Reye syndrome clinically [216]. This severe form of hepatotoxicity usually does not improve when the drug is withdrawn and is frequently fatal in children [217,218]. It cannot be predicted by regular monitoring of serum aminotransferases and other liver function tests. The time from initiating treatment with valproic acid and onset of liver disease is usually less than 4 months, but longer duration of treatment does not preclude hepatotoxicity. Severe valproic acid hepatotoxicity occurs more often in children than in adults. Specific risk factors in children include age under 2 years, multiple anticonvulsant treatment along with valproic acid, coexistent medical problems such as mental retardation, developmental delay, or congenital abnormalities. In such children, the risk of fatal hepatotoxicity is 1:600. Valproic acid appears to alter medium-chain fatty acid metabolism by mitochondria in an age-dependent fashion [219]. Hyperammonemia, not associated with liver failure, is another adverse metabolic effect; it is rarely associated with encephalopathy [220,221] but it mandates stopping valproic acid treatment.

The severe hepatotoxicity typically presents with a hepatitis-like prodrome, mainly malaise, anorexia, nausea, and vomiting. A noteworthy feature is that seizure control may deteriorate over the same time period. A febrile illness may appear to trigger the onset of liver failure. Coagulopathy is often present early; jaundice typically develops later, along with other signs of progressive hepatic insufficiency such as ascites and hypoglycemia. Hypoglycemia indicates a poor prognosis. Death from liver failure, complicated by renal failure or infection, is frequent. One child with valproic acid-induced acute liver failure also had an unusual skin eruption (lichenoid dermatitis). Liver histology reviewed in one large series [217] showed hepatocellular necrosis, which may be zonal, with outright loss of hepatocytes and moribund hepatocytes remaining. Acidophilic bodies, ballooned hepatocytes, and small duct reaction may be present. Microvesicular steatosis is the most common finding overall and is often present in addition to features of cell necrosis. Hepatocellular mitochondria may be sufficiently prominent on light microscopy to make hepatocytes look granular and excessively eosinophilic. In patients presenting clinically like Reye syndrome, fever, coagulopathy, progressive loss of consciousness, severe acidosis, and variably abnormal aminotransferases are present, but the patient is not jaundiced. Hepatocellular necrosis, as well as microvesicular fat, is found on histologic examination of the liver, unlike the characteristic histologic findings of Reye syndrome. The succinate dehydrogenase stain, reflecting mitochondrial function, is negative in Reye syndrome but positive in drug-induced Reye-like hepatotoxicity (Figure 22.6). On electron microscopic examination, the mitochondrial changes associated with valproic acid hepatotoxicity differ from those of Reye syndrome.

Valproic acid is extensively metabolized in the liver [222], mainly by glucuronidation. Because it is a fatty acid, valproic acid also can undergo mitochondrial or peroxisomal beta-oxidation. Mitochondrial metabolism is the more important. Valproic acid passes through the mitochondrial membrane spontaneously and is converted to its coenzyme A thioester in the mitochondrial matrix; the major product of mitochondrial metabolism, 2-propylpentanoyl-CoA, can be hydrolyzed to form valproic acid again or conjugated to carnitine and excreted [223]. Two other pathways, omega- and omega-1-hydroxylation, involve cytochromes P450.

The mechanism of severe valproic acid hepatotoxicity appears to involve generation of toxic metabolite(s) plus some type of metabolic idiosyncrasy. Metabolic idiosyncrasy is probable not only because severe hepatotoxicity is rare but because toxic ingestions do not necessarily lead to liver necrosis.

(a) (b)

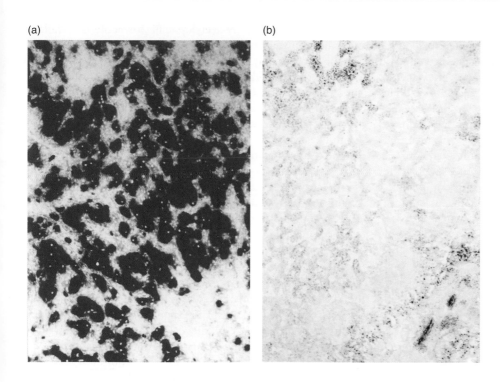

Figure 22.6 Comparison of liver biopsies processed histochemically for the mitochondrial enzyme succinic acid dehydrogenase in Reye-like hepatotoxicity caused by valproic acid and in Reye syndrome. (a) Liver lobule from a patient with valproic acid toxicity: note positive cytoplasmic staining indicative of normal succinic acid dehydrogenase activity (magnification × 250). (b) Liver lobule from a patient with Reye syndrome: note virtual absence of staining for succinic acid dehydrogenase in that only a few hepatocytes in zones 1 and 3 show weak staining (magnification × 250). (Courtesy of Dr. M. James Phillips, Department of Pathology, the Hospital for Sick Children, Toronto.)

Valproic acid – and more specifically its partially unsaturated metabolite 4-en-valproic acid – are related structurally to two known hepatotoxins which both cause microvesicular steatosis: hypoglycin, responsible for Jamaican vomiting sickness, a Reye-like hepatopathy, and 4-pentenoic acid, which inhibits beta-oxidation (Figure 22.7). Valproic acid itself is capable of inhibiting mitochondrial beta-oxidation; some of its metabolites also have this effect. 4-en-Valproic acid is produced by P450-related omega-oxidation and has been detected in patients with liver failure developing on valproic acid treatment. Similarities and differences in these metabolic toxicities compared with hypoglycin and 4-pentenoic acid merely reflect the complexity of this metabolic system. Moreover, the beta-oxidation metabolite of 4-en-valproic acid ((*E*)-2,4-dien-valproic acid) may also act as a toxic metabolite. Urinary levels of thiol conjugates of these two metabolites were elevated in children under 7 years of age receiving valproic acid monotherapy and also in older children if they were receiving treatment with an antiepileptic drug capable of inducing P450 enzymes along with the valproic acid [224]. Concentrations of the thiol conjugates of (*E*)-2,4-dien-valproic acid were higher than those of 4-en-valproic acid.

Investigations of valproic acid metabolism in patients with severe hepatotoxicity indicate that beta-oxidation is inhibited in these patients [225]; however, biochemical abnormalities consistent with inhibition of beta-oxidation have also been found in children on valproic acid treatment at low risk for hepatotoxicity [226]. There is interindividual variation in the exact step in beta-oxidation blocked [225]. Increased amounts of 4-en-valproic acid have been measured in some patients. In

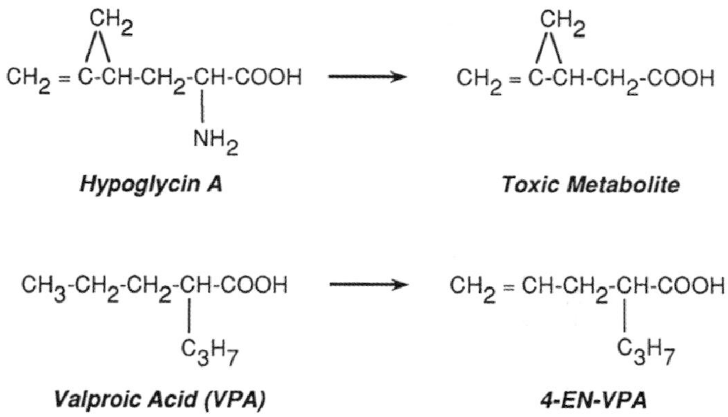

$$CH_2 = \overset{\overset{\displaystyle CH_2}{\diagup\diagdown}}{C}\text{-CH-CH}_2\text{-}\underset{\underset{\displaystyle NH_2}{|}}{CH}\text{-COOH} \longrightarrow CH_2 = \overset{\overset{\displaystyle CH_2}{\diagup\diagdown}}{C}\text{-CH-CH}_2\text{-COOH}$$

Hypoglycin A   *Toxic Metabolite*

$$CH_3\text{-}CH_2\text{-}CH_2\text{-}\underset{\underset{\displaystyle C_3H_7}{|}}{CH}\text{-COOH} \longrightarrow CH_2 = CH\text{-}CH_2\text{-}\underset{\underset{\displaystyle C_3H_7}{|}}{CH}\text{-COOH}$$

Valproic Acid (VPA)   *4-EN-VPA*

Figure 22.7 Similarity in the chemical structures of the toxic metabolite of hypoglycin A and the metabolite of valproic acid, 4-en-valproic acid.

one patient, increased propylglutaric acid, the product of a P450-associated pathway, was found, as was evidence of decreased beta-oxidation [225]. These observations suggest a combination of inhibited fatty acid beta-oxidation and mobilized alternative pathways (e.g. involving cytochromes P450) is required to produce hepatotoxic metabolites. Recent experimental evidence suggests that oxidative stress plays a secondary role [227,228].

Valproic acid appears to be a contingent hepatotoxin. It is likely that some people have anomalous mitochondrial beta-oxidation that renders them more susceptible to adverse metabolic effects of valproic acid. An intercurrent problem, such as a viral illness, might additionally inhibit beta-oxidation. If such a person were also taking drugs that strongly induce P450 enzymes (such as phenytoin, phenobarbital, or carbamazepine), the effect of inhibiting mitochondrial beta-oxidation and shunting into cytochrome P450-associated pathways would be magnified. Someone who develops severe valproic acid hepatotoxicity may not be able to make metabolic adjustments to detoxify these metabolites or subsequent toxic intermediates before significant mitochondrial damage occurs. The metabolic idiosyncrasy reflects a functional defect in the mitochondrion itself. Experimental data in the ornithine transcarbamylase-deficient mouse support the hypothesis of an intrinsic metabolic defect in the mitochondrion. The ornithine transcarbamylase-deficient mouse develops hepatocellular necrosis and microvesicular steatosis at doses of valproic acid that do not affect the normal control adversely. Ornithine transcarbamylase deficiency may be one such definable abnormality and has been suspected in some patients. Cytochrome c oxidase deficiency may predispose to valproic acid hepatotoxicity. Valproic acid hepatotoxicity has been reported in an adult with Friedreich ataxia [229].

The connection between inherent mitochondrial dysfunction and valproic acid hepatotoxicity is further strengthened by the apparently high incidence of valproic acid hepatotoxicity in children with Alpers syndrome, caused by abnormalities in the mitochondrial DNA polymerase-γ [230,231]. Individuals at risk may not have clinically apparent Alpers syndrome. Recent findings show that heterozygous genetic variation in *POLG*, encoding polymerase-γ, appeared to predispose to valproic acid hepatotoxicity, mainly through a p.Q1236H substitution [232]. The toxic mechanism in such cases appears to be suppression of hepatocellular regeneration, not a simple change in mitochondrial metabolism. Genetic testing of *POLG* is of benefit before initiating treatment, at least with certain seizure disorders [233].

Decreased serum carnitine has been found in valproic acid hepatotoxicity. Serum carnitine is also low in patients treated chronically, without any clinical evidence of hepatotoxicity [234]. Conjugation to carnitine is a minor metabolic pathway for valproic acid. It is not known whether this pathway is important for the development of hepatotoxicity. Equally, the value of carnitine repletion as treatment for severe hepatotoxicity is controversial [235]. A retrospective study indicated efficacy if carnitine is started very early in the course of severe hepatotoxicity [236].

Principles of treatment

Once the drug responsible is stopped, most drug-induced liver disease resolves spontaneously. Liver injury with prominent cholestasis may take longer to resolve. Severe chronic changes may not regress. However, bridging necrosis on liver biopsy does not indicate aggressive chronic liver damage in drug-induced liver disease. Specific antidotes are available for some hepatotoxins, such as N-acetylcysteine in acetaminophen hepatotoxicity. Use of N-acetylcysteine for acute liver failure not caused by acetaminophen, but possibly by another hepatotoxic drug, was beneficial in adults with grade 1–2 hepatic coma. A recent study indicated that its use was not beneficial for this indication in children. The use of steroids in drug-induced liver disease is controversial. High-dose steroid treatment has merit when severe acute hepatitis dominates a multisystem drug hypersensitivity reaction or DRESS syndrome. Administration of intravenous corticosteroids in these circumstances may reduce mortality. Prednisone treatment of AIH-like drug hepatotoxicity, in addition to stopping the offending drug, appears beneficial, and in general a circumscribed course of treatment is effective.

Drug hepatotoxicity is an important cause of acute liver failure in all ages. Liver transplantation may be necessary. The general management of acute liver failure in drug hepatotoxicity is essentially the same as with viral hepatitis. The prognostic rule that predicting a case-fatality rate >10% for drug-induced liver disease featuring significantly elevated serum aminotransferases plus clinically evident jaundice has not been validated for children but deserves attention.

What then becomes the most important question is how to diagnose drug-induced liver disease. A high index of suspicion is exceedingly important. The history of the illness must be comprehensive, with detailed attention to all drugs taken, including over-the-counter and herbal preparations. Potential exposure to environmental or industrial toxins must be sought by direct questioning. The possibility that the child has taken a parent's or grandparent's medication must be considered. In children, it is important to ensure that the appropriate dosage was actually given. With acetaminophen, for example, this may involve examining the actual medication bottle used and determining how the care-giver understood the dosing regimen. Liver biopsy is often informative and sometimes definitive. It may discriminate between ordinary AIH and AIH-like drug injury [237]. Electron microscopy may reveal abnormalities highly suggestive of drug hepatotoxicity. Algorithms for determining the likelihood of an adverse drug reaction [238,239] may be helpful. The Naranjo algorithm is easier to use than others. Drug rechallenge in the patient is potentially risky and may not be definitive; consequently, it appears to have no role in pediatric practice. In vitro rechallenge may sometimes be informative.

A pre-emptive approach to hepatotoxicity may be possible in the near future. Methods are being developed for cell-based screening of prospective drugs. Genomic and bioinformatics technologies may also permit novel methods to identify potential hepatotoxicity early in drug development. Various new methodologies, including toxicogenomics and metabolomics, permit better delineation of the pharmacogenetic and immunogenetic profiles which relate to the hepatotoxicity of specific drugs. They may permit a truly individualized approach to drug therapy in the future. Avoiding drug-induced liver injury is certainly a legitimate goal of "personalized medicine."

References

1. Clarkson A, Choonara I. Surveillance for fatal suspected adverse drug reactions in the UK. *Arch Dis Child* 2002;**87**:462–467.

2. Squires RH Jr., Shneider BL, Bucuvalas J, *et al.* Acute liver failure in children: the first 348 patients in the pediatric acute liver failure study group. *J Pediatr* 2006;**148**:652–658.

3. Zimmerman HJ. *Hepatotoxicity: The Adverse Effects of Drugs and Other Chemicals on the Liver*. Philadelphia, PA: Lippincott, Williams & Wilkins, 1999.

4. Kaplowitz N, DeLeve L. *Drug-induced Liver Disease*. Waltham, MA: Academic Press, 2013.

5. Ingelman-Sundberg M. Human drug metabolising cytochrome P450 enzymes: properties and polymorphisms. *N Schmied Arch Pharmacol* 2004;**369**:89–104.

6. McGraw J, Waller D. Cytochrome P450 variations in different ethnic populations. *Expert Opin Drug Metab Toxicol* 2012;**8**:371–382.

7. Weinshilboum R. Inheritance and drug response. *N Engl J Med* 2003;**348**:529–537.

8. Cascorbi I. Genetic basis of toxic reactions to drugs and chemicals. *Toxicol Lett* 2006;**162**:16–28.

9. Russmann S, Jetter A, Kullak-Ublick GA. Pharmacogenetics of drug-induced liver injury. *Hepatology* 2010;**52**:748–761.

10. Burchell B, Soars M, Monaghan G, *et al.* Drug-mediated toxicity caused by genetic deficiency of UDP-glucuronosyltransferases. *Toxicol Lett* 2000;**112–113**:333–340.

11. Pessayre D, Fromenty B, Berson A, *et al.* Central role of mitochondria in drug-induced liver injury. *Drug Metab Rev* 2012;**44**:34–87.

12. Lucena MI, Garcia-Martin E, Andrade RJ, *et al.* Mitochondrial superoxide dismutase and glutathione peroxidase in idiosyncratic drug-induced liver injury. *Hepatology* 2010;**52**:303–312.

13. Hines RN, McCarver DG. The ontogeny of human drug-metabolizing enzymes: phase I oxidative enzymes. *J Pharmacol Exp Ther* 2002;**300**:355–360.

14. Kearns GL, Abdel-Rahman SM, Alander SW, *et al.* Developmental pharmacology: drug disposition, action, and therapy in infants and children. *N Engl J Med* 2003;**349**:1157–1167.

15. Tateishi T, Nakura H, Asoh M, *et al.* A comparison of hepatic cytochrome P450 protein expression between infancy and postinfancy. *Life Sci* 1997;**61**:2567–2574.

16. Aranda JV, Collinge JM, Zinman R, Watters G. Maturation of caffeine elimination in infancy. *Arch Dis Child* 1979;**54**:946–949.

17. Treluyer JM, Gueret G, Cheron G, Sonnier M, Cresteil T. Developmental expression of CYP2C- and CYP2C-dependent activities in the human liver: in-vivo/in-vitro correlation and inducibility. *Pharmacogenetics* 1997;**7**:441–452.

18. Lang C, Meier Y, Stieger B, *et al.* Mutations and polymorphisms in the bile salt export pump and the multidrug resistance protein 3 associated with drug-induced liver injury. *Pharmacogenet Genomics* 2007;**17**:47–60.

19. Walsh SA, Creamer D. Drug reaction with eosinophilia and systemic symptoms (DRESS): a clinical update and review of current thinking. *Clin Exp Dermatol* 2011;**36**:6–11.

20. Cacoub P, Musette P, Descamps V, *et al.* The DRESS syndrome: a literature review. *Am J Med* 2011;**124**:588–597.

21. Jaeschke H, Gores GJ, Cederbaum AI, *et al.* Mechanisms of hepatotoxicity. *Toxicol Sci* 2002;**65**:166–176.

22. James LP, Farrar HC, Darville TL, *et al.* Elevation of serum interleukin 8 levels in acetaminophen overdose in children and adolescents. *Clin Pharmacol Ther* 2001;**70**:280–286.

23. Ju C, Reilly TP, Bourdi M, *et al.* Protective role of Kupffer cells in acetaminophen-induced hepatic injury in mice. *Chem Res Toxicol* 2002;**15**:1504–1513.

24. Aithal GP, Ramsay L, Daly AK, *et al.* Hepatic adducts, circulating antibodies, and cytokine polymorphisms in patients with diclofenac hepatotoxicity. *Hepatology* 2004;**39**:1430–1440.

25. Molleston JP, Fontana RJ, Lopez MJ, *et al.* Characteristics of idiosyncratic drug-induced liver injury in children: results from the DILIN prospective study. *J Pediatr Gastroenterol Nutr* 2011;**53**:182–189.

26. Mahadevan SB, McKiernan PJ, Davies P, Kelly DA. Paracetamol induced hepatotoxicity. *Arch Dis Child* 2006;**91**:598–603.

27. Makin AJ, Wendon J, Williams R. A 7-year experience of severe acetaminophen-induced hepatotoxicity (1987–1993). *Gastroenterology* 1995;**109**:1907–1916.

28. Smilkstein MJ, Knapp GL, Kulig KW, Rumack BH. Efficacy of oral N-acetylcysteine in the treatment of acetaminophen overdose. *N Engl J Med* 1988;**319**:1557–1562.

29. Harrison PM, Keays R, Bray GP, Alexander GJ, Williams R. Improved outcome of paracetamol-induced fulminant hepatic failure by late administration of acetylcysteine. *Lancet* 1990;**335**:1572–1573.

30. Keays R, Harrison PM, Wendon JA, *et al.* Intravenous acetylcysteine in paracetamol induced fulminant hepatic failure: a prospective controlled trial. *BMJ* 1991;**303**:1026–1029.

31. Yarema MC, Johnson DW, Berlin RJ, *et al.* Comparison of the 20-hour intravenous and 72-hour oral acetylcysteine protocols for the treatment of acute acetaminophen poisoning. *Ann Emerg Med* 2009;**54**:606–614.

32. Heubi JE, Barbacci MB, Zimmerman HJ. Therapeutic misadventures with acetaminophen: hepatoxicity after multiple doses in children. *J Pediatr* 1998;**132**:22–27.

33. Walls L, Baker CF, Sarkar S. Acetaminophen-induced hepatic failure with encephalopathy in a newborn. *J Perinatol* 2007;**27**:133–135.

34. Savino F, Lupica MM, Tarasco V, *et al.* Fulminant hepatitis after 10 days of acetaminophen treatment at recommended dosage in an infant. *Pediatrics* 2011;**127**:e494–e497.

35. Watkins PB, Kaplowitz N, Slattery JT, *et al.* Aminotransferase elevations in healthy adults receiving 4 grams of acetaminophen daily: a randomized controlled trial. *JAMA* 2006;**296**:87–93.

36. Webster PA, Roberts DW, Benson RW, Kearns GL. Acetaminophen toxicity in children: diagnostic confirmation using a specific antigenic biomarker. *J Clin Pharmacol* 1996;**36**:397–402.

37. Jaeschke H, Knight TR, Bajt ML. The role of oxidant stress and reactive

nitrogen species in acetaminophen hepatotoxicity. *Toxicol Lett* 2003;**144**:279–288.

38. Fannin RD, Russo M, O'Connell TM, *et al.* Acetaminophen dosing of humans results in blood transcriptome and metabolome changes consistent with impaired oxidative phosphorylation. *Hepatology* 2010;**51**:227–236.

39. Goldring CE, Kitteringham NR, Elsby R, *et al.* Activation of hepatic Nrf2 in vivo by acetaminophen in CD-1 mice. *Hepatology* 2004;**39**:1267–1276.

40. Liu HH, Lu P, Guo Y, *et al.* An integrative genomic analysis identifies Bhmt2 as a diet-dependent genetic factor protecting against acetaminophen-induced liver toxicity. *Genome Res* 2010;**20**:28–35.

41. Harrill AH, Watkins PB, Su S, *et al.* Mouse population-guided resequencing reveals that variants in CD44 contribute to acetaminophen-induced liver injury in humans. *Genome Res* 2009;**19**: 1507–1515.

42. Peterson RG, Rumack BH. Age as a variable in acetaminophen overdose. *Arch Intern Med* 1981;**141**:390–393.

43. Rumack BH. Acetaminophen overdose in young children. Treatment and effects of alcohol and other additional ingestants in 417 cases. *Am J Dis Child* 1984;**138**:428–433.

44. Peterson RG, Rumack BH. Pharmacokinetics of acetaminophen in children. *Pediatrics* 1978;**62**:877–879.

45. Hickson GB, Altemeier WA, Martin ED, Campbell PW. Parental administration of chemical agents a cause of apparent life threatening events. *J Pediatr* 1989;**83**:772–776.

46. Rumack BH. Acetaminophen misconceptions. *Hepatology* 2004;**40**:10–15.

47. Al-Sinani S, Al-Rawas A, Dhawan A. Mercury as a cause of fulminant hepatic failure in a child: case report and literature review. *Clin Res Hepatol Gastroenterol* 2011;**35**:580–582.

48. Zimmerman HJ, Maddrey WC. Acetaminophen (paracetamol) hepatotoxicity with regular intake of alcohol: analysis of instances of therapeutic misadventure. *Hepatology* 1995;**22**:767–773.

49. Bruun LS, Elkjaer S, Bitsch-Larsen D, Andersen O. Hepatic failure in a child after acetaminophen and sevoflurane

exposure. *Anesth Analg* 2001;**92**: 1446–1448.

50. Ceschi A, Hofer KE, Rauber-Luthy C, Kupferschmidt H. Paracetamol orodispersible tablets:a risk for severe poisoning in children? *Eur J Clin Pharmacol* 2011;**67**:97–99.

51. Yagupsky P, Gazala E, Sofer S. Fatal hepatic failure and encephalopathy associated with amiodarone therapy. *J Pediatr* 1985;**107**:967–970.

52. Floyd J, Mirza I, Sachs B, Perry MC. Hepatotoxicity of chemotherapy. *Semin Oncol* 2006;**33**:50–67.

53. Pratibha R, Sameer R, Rataboli PV, Bhiwgade DA, Dhume CY. Enzymatic studies of cisplatin induced oxidative stress in hepatic tissue of rats. *Eur J Pharmacol* 2006;**532**:290–293.

54. Lu Y, Cederbaum AI. Cisplatin-induced hepatotoxicity is enhanced by elevated expression of cytochrome P450 2E1. *Toxicol Sci* 2006;**89**:515–523.

55. Honjo I, Suou T, Hirayama C. Hepatotoxicity of cyclophosphamide in man:pharmacokinetic analysis. *Res Commun Chem Pathol Pharmacol* 1988;**61**:149–165.

56. Berkovitch M, Matsui D, Zipursky A, *et al.* Hepatotoxicity of 6-mercaptopurine in childhood acute lymphocytic leukemia: pharmacokinetic characteristics. *Med Pediatr Oncol* 1996;**26**:85–89.

57. Hazar V, Kutluk T, Akyuz C, *et al.* Veno-occlusive disease-like hepatotoxicity in two children receiving chemotherapy for Wilms' tumor and clear cell sarcoma of kidney. *Pediatr Hematol Oncol* 1998;**15**:85–89.

58. Topley J, Benson J, Squier MV, Chessells JM. Hepatotoxicity in the treatment of acute lymphoblastic leukemia. *Med Pediatr Oncol* 1979;7:393–399.

59. Pratt CB, Johnson WW. Duration and severity of fatty metamorphosis of the liver following L-asparaginase therapy. *Cancer* 1971;**28**:361–364.

60. Sahoo S, Hart J. Histopathological features of L-asparaginase-induced liver disease. *Semin Liver Dis* 2003;**23**: 295–299.

61. Hruban RH, Sternberg SS, Meyers P, *et al.* Fatal thrombocytopenia and liver failure associated with carboplatin therapy. *Cancer Invest* 1991;**9**:263–268.

62. DeLeve LD, Shulman HM, McDonald GB. Toxic injury to hepatic sinusoids: sinusoidal obstruction syndrome (veno-occlusive disease). *Semin Liver Dis* 2002;**22**:27–42.

63. D'Antiga L, Baker A, Pritchard J, Pryor D, Mieli-Vergani G. Veno-occlusive disease with multi-organ involvement following actinomycin-D. *Eur J Cancer* 2001;**37**:1141–1148.

64. Barker CC, Anderson RA, Sauve RS, Butzner JD. GI complications in pediatric patients post-BMT. *Bone Marrow Transplant* 2005;**36**:51–58.

65. Sulis ML, Bessmertny O, Granowetter L, Weiner M, Kelly KM. Veno-occlusive disease in pediatric patients receiving actinomycin D and vincristine only for the treatment of rhabdomyosarcoma. *J Pediatr Hematol Oncol* 2004;**26**:843–846.

66. Elli M, Pinarli FG, Dagdemir A, Acar S. Veno-occlusive disease of the liver in a child after chemotherapy for brain tumor. *Pediatr Blood Cancer* 2006;**46**:521–523.

67. McDonald GB, Sharma P, Matthews DE, *et al.* The clinical course of 53 patients with veno-occlusive disease of the liver after marrow transplantation. *Transplantation* 1985;**39**:603–608.

68. McDonald GB, Slattery JT, Bouvier ME, *et al.* Cyclophosphamide metabolism, liver toxicity, and mortality following hematopoietic stem cell transplantation. *Blood* 2003;**101**:2043–2048.

69. El-Sayed MH, El-Haddad A, Fahmy OA, Salama II, Mahmoud HK. Liver disease is a major cause of mortality following allogeneic bone-marrow transplantation. *Eur J Gastroenterol Hepatol* 2004;**16**:1347–1354.

70. Srivastava A, Poonkuzhali B, Shaji RV, *et al.* Glutathione S-transferase M1 polymorphism: a risk factor for hepatic venoocclusive disease in bone marrow transplantation. *Blood* 2004;**104**: 1574–1577.

71. Stoneham S, Lennard L, Coen P, Lilleyman J, Saha V. Veno-occlusive disease in patients receiving thiopurines during maintenance therapy for childhood acute lymphoblastic leukaemia. *Br J Haematol* 2003;**123**:100–102.

72. Reiss U, Cowan M, McMillan A, Horn B. Hepatic venoocclusive disease in blood and bone marrow transplantation in children and young adults: incidence,

risk factors, and outcome in a cohort of 241 patients. *J Pediatr Hematol Oncol* 2002;**24**:746–750.

73. Ravikumara M, Hill FG, Wilson DC, *et al.* 6-Thioguanine-related chronic hepatotoxicity and variceal haemorrhage in children treated for acute lymphoblastic leukaemia-a dual-centre experience. *J Pediatr Gastroenterol Nutr* 2006;**42**:535–538.

74. Corbacioglu S, Greil J, Peters C, *et al.* Defibrotide in the treatment of children with veno-occlusive disease (VOD): a retrospective multicentre study demonstrates therapeutic efficacy upon early intervention. *Bone Marrow Transplant* 2004;**33**:189–195.

75. Shin-Nakai N, Ishida H, Yoshihara T, *et al.* Control of hepatic veno-occlusive disease with an antithrombin-III concentrate-based therapy. *Pediatr Int* 2006;**48**:85–87.

76. Ringden O, Remberger M, Lehmann S, *et al.* N-Acetylcysteine for hepatic veno-occlusive disease after allogeneic stem cell transplantation. *Bone Marrow Transplant* 2000;**25**:993–996.

77. Lee AC, Goh PY. Dactinomycin-induced hepatic sinusoidal obstruction syndrome responding to treatment with N-acetylcysteine. *J Cancer* 2011;**2**:527–531.

78. DeLeve LD. Dacarbazine toxicity in murine liver cells: a model of hepatic endothelial injury and glutathione defense. *J Pharmacol Exp Ther* 1994;**268**:1261–1270.

79. DeLeve LD. Cellular target of cyclophosphamide toxicity in the murine liver: role of glutathione and site of metabolic activation. *Hepatology* 1996;**24**:830–837.

80. DeLeve LD, Wang X, Kanel GC, *et al.* Decreased hepatic nitric oxide production contributes to the development of rat sinusoidal obstruction syndrome. *Hepatology* 2003;**38**:900–908.

81. Iguchi A, Kobayashi R, Yoshida M, *et al.* Vascular endothelial growth factor (VEGF) is one of the cytokines causative and predictive of hepatic veno-occlusive disease (VOD) in stem cell transplantation. *Bone Marrow Transplant* 2001;**27**:1173–1180.

82. Geller SA, Dubinsky MC, Poordad FF, *et al.* Early hepatic nodular hyperplasia and submicroscopic fibrosis associated with 6-thioguanine therapy in

inflammatory bowel disease. *Am J Surg Pathol* 2004;**28**:1204–1211.

83. Rawat D, Gillett PM, Devadason D, Wilson DC, McKiernan PJ. Long-term follow-up of children with 6-thioguanine-related chronic hepatoxicity following treatment for acute lymphoblastic leukaemia. *J Pediatr Gastroenterol Nutr* 2011;**53**:478–479.

84. Chen TC, Ng KF, Jeng LB, Yeh TS, Chen CM, Aspirin-related hepatotoxicity in a child after liver transplant. *Dig Dis Sci* 2001;**46**:486–488.

85. Hamdan JA, Manasra K, Ahmed M. Salicylate-induced hepatitis in rheumatic fever. *Am J Dis Child* 1985;**139**:453–455.

86. Garnock-Jones KP, Keating GM. Atomoxetine: a review of its use in attention-deficit hyperactivity disorder in children and adolescents. *Paediatr Drugs* 2009;**11**:203–226.

87. Lim JR, Faught PR, Chalasani NP, Molleston JP, Severe liver injury after initiating therapy with atomoxetine in two children. *J Pediatr* 2006;**148**:831–834.

88. DePinho RA, Goldberg CS, Lefkowitch JH. Azathioprine and the liver. Evidence favoring idiosyncratic, mixed cholestatic-hepatocellular injury in humans. *Gastroenterology* 1984;**86**:162–165.

89. Sterneck M, Wiesner R, Ascher N, *et al.* Azathioprine hepatotoxicity after liver transplantation. *Hepatology* 1991;**14**:806–810.

90. Seiderer J, Zech CJ, Diebold J, *et al.* Nodular regenerative hyperplasia: a reversible entity associated with azathioprine therapy. *Eur J Gastroenterol Hepatol* 2006;**18**:553–555.

91. Lennard L. The clinical pharmacology of 6-mercaptopurine. *Eur J Clin Pharmacol* 1992;**43**:329–339.

92. Adam de Beaumais T, Fakhoury M, Medard Y, *et al.* Determinants of mercaptopurine toxicity in paediatric acute lymphoblastic leukemia maintenance therapy. *Br J Clin Pharmacol* 2011;**71**:575–584.

93. Shear NH, Spielberg SP. Anticonvulsant hypersensitivity syndrome. In vitro assessment of risk. *J Clin Invest* 1988;**82**:1826–1832.

94. Zucker P, Daum F, Cohen MI. Fatal carbamazepine hepatitis. *J Pediatr* 1977;**91**:667–668.

95. Smith DW, Cullity GJ, Silberstein EP. Fatal hepatic necrosis associated with multiple anticonvulsant therapy. *Aust N Z J Med* 1988;**18**:575–581.

96. Hadzic N, Portmann B, Davies ET, Mowat AP, Mieli-Vergani G. Acute liver failure induced by carbamazepine. *Arch Dis Child* 1990;**65**:315–317.

97. Morales-Diaz M, Pinilla-Roa E, Ruiz I. Suspected carbamazepine-induced hepatotoxicity. *Pharmacotherapy* 1999;**19**:252–255.

98. Sierra NM, Garcia B, Marco J, *et al.* Cross hypersensitivity syndrome between phenytoin and carbamazepine. *Pharm World Sci* 2005;**27**:170–174.

99. McCormack M, Alfirevic A, Bourgeois S, *et al.* HLA-A*3101 and carbamazepine-induced hypersensitivity reactions in Europeans. *N Engl J Med* 2011;**364**:1134–1143.

100. D'Orazio JL. Oxcarbazepine-induced drug reaction with eosinophilia and systemic symptoms (DRESS). *Clin Toxicol* 2008;**46**:1093–1094.

101. Bosdure E, Cano A, Roquelaure B, *et al.* [Oxcarbazepine and DRESS syndrome: a paediatric cause of acute liver failure.] *Arch Pediatr* 2004;**11**:1073–1077.

102. Wanless IR, Dore S, Gopinath G, *et al.* Histopathology of cocaine hepatotoxicity. Report of four cases. *Gastroenterology* 1990;**98**:497–501.

103. Kassianides C, Nussenblatt R, Palestine AG, Mellow SD, Hoofnagle JH. Liver injury from cyclosporine A. *Dig Dis Sci* 1990;**35**:693–697.

104. Stieger B, Fattinger K, Madon J, Kullak-Ublick GA, Meier PJ. Drug- and estrogen-induced cholestasis through inhibition of the hepatocellular bile salt export pump (Bsep) of rat liver. *Gastroenterology* 2000;**118**:422–430.

105. Bramow S, Ott P, Thomsen Nielsen F, *et al.* Cholestasis and regulation of genes related to drug metabolism and biliary transport in rat liver following treatment with cyclosporine A and sirolimus (Rapamycin). *Pharmacol Toxicol* 2001;**89**:133–139.

106. Yasumiba S, Tazuma S, Ochi H, Chayama K, Kajiyama G. Cyclosporin A reduces canalicular membrane fluidity and regulates transporter function in rats. *Biochem J* 2001;**354**:591–596.

107. Brauer RB, Heidecke CD, Nathrath W, *et al.* Liver transplantation for the

treatment of fulminant hepatic failure induced by the ingestion of ecstasy. *Transplant Int* 1997;**10**:229–233.

108. Andreu V, Mas A, Bruguera M, *et al.* Ecstasy: a common cause of severe acute hepatotoxicity. *J Hepatol* 1998;**29**: 394–397.

109. Greene SL, Dargan PI, O'Connor N, Jones AL, Kerins M. Multiple toxicity from 3,4-methylenedioxymethamphetamine ("ecstasy"). *Am J Emerg Med* 2003;**21**:121–124.

110. Smith ID, Simpson KJ, Garden OJ, Wigmore SJ. Non-paracetamol drug-induced fulminant hepatic failure among adults in Scotland. *Eur J Gastroenterol Hepatol* 2005;**17**: 161–167.

111. Antolino-Lobo I, Meulenbelt J, van den Berg M, van Duursen MB. A mechanistic insight into 3,4-methylenedioxymethamphetamine ("ecstasy")-mediated hepatotoxicity. *Vet Q* 2011;**31**:193–205.

112. Ellis AJ, Wendon JA, Portmann B, Williams R. Acute liver damage and ecstasy ingestion. *Gut* 1996;**38**: 454–458.

113. Munoz P, Drobinska A, Bianchi L, Zuger C, Pirovino M. [Acute giant cell hepatitis in a 17-year old man.] *Schweiz Rundsch Med Prax* 2004;**93**:2109–2112.

114. Zafrani ES, Ishak KG, Rudzki C. Cholestatic and hepatocellular injury associated with erythromycin esters. Report of nine cases. *Dig Dis Sci* 1979;**24**:385–396.

115. Phillips KG. Hepatotoxicity of erythromycin ethylsuccinate in a child. *CMAJ* 1983;**129**:411–412.

116. Principi N, Esposito S. Comparative tolerability of erythromycin and newer macrolide antibacterials in paediatric patients. *Drug Saf* 1999;**20**:25–41.

117. Giannattasio A, D'Ambrosi M, Volpicelli M, Iorio R. Steroid therapy for a case of severe drug-induced cholestasis. *Ann Pharmacother* 2006;**40**:1196–1199.

118. Fox JC, Szyjkowski RS, Sanderson SO, Levine RA. Progressive cholestatic liver disease associated with clarithromycin treatment. *J Clin Pharmacol* 2002;**42**:676–680.

119. Brinker AD, Wassel RT, Lyndly J, *et al.* Telithromycin-associated hepatotoxicity: clinical spectrum and

causality assessment of 42 cases. *Hepatology* 2009;**49**:250–257.

120. Lewis JH, Tice HL, Zimmerman HJ. Budd–Chiari syndrome associated with oral contraceptive steroids. Review of treatment of 47 cases. *Dig Dis Sci* 1983;**28**:673–683.

121. Neuberger J, Nunnerley HB, Davis M, *et al.* Oral-contraceptive-associated liver tumours: Occurrence of malignancy and difficulties in diagnosis. *Lancet* 1980;**i**:273–276.

122. Pellock JM. Felbamate. *Epilepsia* 1999;**40**(Suppl 5):S57–S62.

123. Popovic M, Nierkens S, Pieters R, Uetrecht J. Investigating the role of 2-phenylpropenal in felbamate-induced idiosyncratic drug reactions. *Chem Res Toxicol* 2004;**17**:1568–1576.

124. Gaertner I, Altendorf K, Batra A, Gaertner HJ. Relevance of liver enzyme elevations with four different neuroleptics: a retrospective review of 7263 treatment courses. *J Clin Psychopharmacol* 2001;**21**:215–222.

125. Lo SK, Wendon J, Mieli-Vergani G, Williams R. Halothane-induced acute liver failure: continuing occurrence and use of liver transplantation. *Eur J Gastroenterol Hepatol* 1998;**10**: 635–639.

126. Kenna JG, Newberger J, Mieli-Vergani G, Mowat AP, Williams R. Halothane hepatitis in children. *BMJ* 1987;**294**:1209–1211.

127. Hassall E, Israel DM, Gunasekaran T, Steward D. Halothane hepatitis in children. *J Pediatr Gastroenterol Nutr* 1990;**11**:553–557.

128. Wark HJ. Postoperative jaundice in children. *Anaesthesia* 1983;**38**:237–242.

129. Warner LO, Beach TP, Gariss JP, Warner EJ. Halothane and children: the first quarter century. *Anesth Analg* 1984;**63**:838–840.

130. Psacharopoulos HJ, Mowat AP, Davies M, *et al.* Fulminant hepatic failure in childhood: an analysis of 31 cases. *Arch Dis Child* 1980;**55**:252–258.

131. Farrell GC. Mechanism of halothane-induced liver injury: is it immune or metabolic idiosyncrasy? *J Gastroenterol Hepatol* 1988;**3**:465–482.

132. Pohl LR, Satoh H, Christ DD, Kenna J. The immunologic and metabolic basis of drug hypersensitivities. *Annu Rev Pharmacol Toxicol* 1988;**28**: 367–387.

133. Kenna JG, Satoh H, Christ DD, Pohl LR. Metabolic basis for a drug hypersensitivity: antibodies in sera from patients with halothane hepatitis recognize liver neoantigens that contain the trifluoroacetyl group derived from halothane. *J Pharm Exp Ther* 1988;**245**:1103–1109.

134. Kenna JG, Neuberger J, Williams R. Evidence for expression in human liver of halothane-induced neoantigens recognized by antibodies in sera from patients with halothane hepatitis. *Hepatology* 1988;**8**:1635–1641.

135. Satoh H, Martin BM, Schulick AH, *et al.* Human anti-endoplasmic reticulum antibodies in sera of patients with halothane-induced hepatitis are directed against a trifluoroacetylated carboxylesterase. *Proc Natl Acad Sci USA* 1989;**86**:322–326.

136. Rode D. Comfrey toxicity revisited. *Trends Pharmacol Sci* 2002;**23**: 497–499.

137. Zuckerman M, Steenkamp V, Stewart MJ. Hepatic veno-occlusive disease as a result of a traditional remedy: confirmation of toxic pyrrolizidine alkaloids as the cause, using an in vitro technique. *J Clin Pathol* 2002;**55**: 676–679.

138. Laliberte L, Villeneuve JP. Hepatitis after the use of germander, a herbal remedy. *CMAJ* 1996;**154**:1689–1692.

139. Lekehal M, Pessayre D, Lereau JM, *et al.* Hepatotoxicity of the herbal medicine germander: metabolic activation of its furano diterpenoids by cytochrome P450 3A depletes cytoskeleton-associated protein thiols and forms plasma membrane blebs in rat hepatocytes. *Hepatology* 1996;**24**: 212–218.

140. Fau D, Lekehal M, Farrell G, *et al.* Diterpenoids from germander, an herbal medicine, induce apoptosis in isolated rat hepatocytes. *Gastroenterology* 1997;**113**:1334–1346.

141. Clouatre DL. Kava kava: examining new reports of toxicity. *Toxicol Lett* 2004;**150**:85–96.

142. Campo JV, McNabb J, Perel JM, *et al.* Kava-induced fulminant hepatic failure. *J Am Acad Child Adolesc Psychiatry* 2002;**41**:631–632.

143. Anke J, Ramzan I. Pharmacokinetic and pharmacodynamic drug interactions with Kava (*Piper methysticum* Forst. f.). *J Ethnopharmacol* 2004;**93**:153–160.

144. Batchelor WB, Heathcote J, Wanless IR. Chaparral-induced hepatic injury. *Am J Gastroenterol* 1995;**90**:831–833.

145. Sheikh NM, Philen RM, Love LA. Chaparral-associated hepatotoxicity. *Arch Intern Med* 1997;**157**:913–919.

146. Horowitz RS, Feldhaus K, Dart RC, Stermitz FR, Beck JJ. The clinical spectrum of Jin Bu Huan toxicity. *Arch Intern Med* 1996;**156**:899–903.

147. Skoulidis F, Alexander GJ, Davies SE. Ma huang associated acute liver failure requiring liver transplantation. *Eur J Gastroenterol Hepatol* 2005;**17**: 581–584.

148. Webb N, Hardikar W, Cranswick NE, Somers GR. Probable herbal medication induced fulminant hepatic failure. *J Paediatr Child Health* 2005;**41**: 530–531.

149. Tobon GJ, Canas C, Jaller JJ, Restrepo JC, Anaya JM. Serious liver disease induced by infliximab. *Clin Rheumatol* 2007;**26**:578–581.

150. Goldfeld DA, Verna EC, Lefkowitch J, Swaminath A. Infliximab-induced autoimmune hepatitis with successful switch to adalimumab in a patient with Crohn's disease: the index case. *Dig Dis Sci* 2011;**56**:3386–3388.

151. Moum B, Konopski Z, Tufteland KF, Jahnsen J. Occurrence of hepatoxicity and elevated liver enzymes in a Crohn's disease patient treated with infliximab. *Inflamm Bowel Dis* 2007;**13**:1584–1586.

152. Kinnunen U, Farkkila M, Makisalo H. A case report: ulcerative colitis, treatment with an antibody against tumor necrosis factor (infliximab), and subsequent liver necrosis. *J Crohns Colitis* 2012;**6**:724–727.

153. Mancini S, Amorotti E, Vecchio S, Ponz de Leon M, Roncucci L. Infliximab-related hepatitis: discussion of a case and review of the literature. *Intern Emerg Med* 2010;**5**:193–200.

154. Zimmerman HJ. Update of hepatotoxicity due to classes of drugs in common clinical use: Non-steroidal drugs, anti-inflammatory drugs, antibiotics, antihypertensives, and cardiac and psychotropic drugs. *Sem Liver Dis* 1990;**10**:322–338.

155. Wu SS, Chao CS, Vargas JH, *et al.* Isoniazid-related hepatic failure in children: a survey of liver transplantation centers. *Transplantation* 2007;**84**:173–179.

156. Spyridis P, Sinantios C, Papadea I, *et al.* Isoniazid liver injury during chemoprophylaxis in children. *Arch Dis Child* 1979;**54**:65–67.

157. Palusci VJ, O'Hare D, Lawrence RM. Hepatotoxicity and transaminase measurement during isoniazid chemoprophylaxis in children. *Pediatr Infect Dis J* 1995;**14**:144–148.

158. Campos-Franco J, Gonzalez-Quintela A, Alende-Sixto MR. Isoniazid-induced hyperacute liver failure in a young patient receiving carbamazepine. *Eur J Intern Med* 2004;**15**:396–397.

159. Metushi IG, Cai P, Zhu X, Nakagawa T, Uetrecht JP. A fresh look at the mechanism of isoniazid-induced hepatotoxicity. *Clin Pharmacol Ther* 2011;**89**:911–914.

160. Vuilleumier N, Rossier MF, Chiappe A, *et al.* CYP2E1 genotype and isoniazid-induced hepatotoxicity in patients treated for latent tuberculosis. *Eur J Clin Pharmacol* 2006;**62**:423–429.

161. Lewis JH, Zimmerman HJ, Benson GD, Ishak KG. Hepatic injury associated with ketoconazole therapy. Analysis of 33 cases. *Gastroenterology* 1984;**86**:503–513.

162. Schlienger RG, Knowles SR, Shear NH. Lamotrigine-associated anticonvulsant hypersensitivity syndrome. *Neurology* 1998;**51**:1172–1175.

163. Fayad M, Choueiri R, Mikati M. Potential hepatotoxicity of lamotrigine. *Pediatr Neurol* 2000;**22**:49–52.

164. Overstreet K, Costanza C, Behling C, Hassanin T, Masliah E. Fatal progressive hepatic necrosis associated with lamotrigine treatment: a case report and literature review. *Dig Dis Sci* 2002;**47**:1921–1925.

165. Zidd AG, Hack JB, Pediatric ingestion of lamotrigine. *Pediatr Neurol* 2004;**31**:71–72.

166. Kremer JM, Lee RG, Tolman KG. Liver histology in rheumatoid arthritis patients receiving long-term methotrexate therapy. A prospective study with baseline and sequential biopsy samples. *Arthritis Rheum* 1989;**32**:121–127.

167. Kremer JM, Furst DE, Weinblatt ME, Blotner SD. Significant changes in serum AST across hepatic histological grades:prospective analysis of 3 cohorts receiving methotrxate therapy for rheumatoid arthritis. *J Rheumatol* 1996;**23**:459–461.

168. Hashkes PJ, Balistreri WF, Bove KE, Ballard ET, Passo MH. The relationship of hepatotoxic risk factors and liver histology in methotrexate therapy for juvenile rheumatoid arthritis. *J Pediatr* 1999;**134**:47–52.

169. Graham LD, Myones BL, Rivas-Chacon RF, Pachman LM. Morbidity associated with long-term methotrexate therapy in juvenile rheumatoid arthritis. *J Pediatr* 1992;**120**:468–473.

170. Kugathasam S, Newman AJ, Dahms BB, Boyle JT. Liver biopsy findings in patients with juvenile rheumatoid arthritis receiving long-term, weekly methotrexate therapy. *J Pediatr* 1996;**128**:149–151.

171. Keim D, Ragsdale C, Heidelberger K, Sullivan D. Hepatic fibrosis with the use of methotrexate for juvenile rheumatoid arthritis. *J Rheumatol* 1990;**17**:846–848.

172. Fisher MC, Cronstein BN. Metaanalysis of methylenetetrahydrofolate reductase (*MTHFR*) polymorphisms affecting methotrexate toxicity. *J Rheumatol* 2009;**36**:539–545.

173. Locasciulli A, Mura R, Fraschini D, *et al.* High-dose methotrexate administration and acute liver damage in children treated for acute lymphoblastic leukemia. A prospective study. *Haematologica* 1992;**77**:49–53.

174. Malcolm A, Heap TR, Eckstein RP, Lunzer MR. Minocycline-induced liver injury. *Am J Gastroenterol* 1996;**91**:1641–1643.

175. Gough A, Chapman S, Wagstaff K, Emery P, Elias E. Minocycline induced autoimmune hepatitis and systemic lupus erythematosus-like syndrome. *BMJ* 1996;**312**:169–172.

176. Bhat G, Jordan J Jr., Sokalski S, *et al.* Minocycline-induced hepatitis with autoimmune features and neutropenia. *J Clin Gastroenterol* 1998;**27**:74–75.

177. Davies MG, Kersey PJW. Acute hepatitis and exfoliative dermatitis associated with minocycline. *BMJ* 1989;**298**:1523–1524.

178. Boudreaux JP, Hayes DH, Mizrahi S, *et al.* Fulminant hepatic failure, hepatorenal syndrome, and necrotizing pancreatitis after minocycline hepatotoxicity. *Transplant Proc* 1993;**25**:1873.

179. McKoy JM, Bennett CL, Scheetz MH, *et al.* Hepatotoxicity associated with

long- versus short-course HIV-prophylactic nevirapine use: a systematic review and meta-analysis from the Research on Adverse Drug events And Reports (RADAR) project. *Drug Saf* 2009;**32**:147–158.

180. Ciccacci C, Borgiani P, Ceffa S, et al. Nevirapine-induced hepatotoxicity and pharmacogenetics: a retrospective study in a population from Mozambique. *Pharmacogenomics* 2010;**11**:23–31.

181. Agundez JA, Lucena MI, Martinez C, et al. Assessment of nonsteroidal anti-inflammatory drug-induced hepatotoxicity. *Expert Opin Drug Metab Toxicol* 2011;**7**:817–828.

182. Titchen T, Cranswick N, Beggs S. Adverse drug reactions to nonsteroidal anti-inflammatory drugs, COX-2 inhibitors and paracetamol in a paediatric hospital. *Br J Clin Pharmacol* 2005;**59**:718–723.

183. Whittaker SJ, Amar JN, Wanless IR, Heathcote J. Sulindac hepatotoxicity. *Gut* 1982;**23**:875–877.

184. Boelsterli UA. Diclofenac-induced liver injury: a paradigm of idiosyncratic drug toxicity. *Toxicol Appl Pharmacol* 2003;**192**:307–322.

185. Merlani G, Fox M, Oehen HP, et al. Fatal hepatoxicity secondary to nimesulide. *Eur J Clin Pharmacol* 2001;**57**:321–326.

186. Marotta PJ, Roberts EA. Pemoline hepatotoxicity in children. *J Pediatr* 1998;**132**:894–897.

187. Rosh JR, Dellert SF, Narkewicz M, Birnbaum A, Whitington G. Four cases of severe hepatotoxicity associated with pemoline: possible autoimmune pathogenesis. *Pediatrics* 1998;**101**:921–923.

188. Gresser U. Amoxicillin-clavulanic acid therapy may be associated with severe side effects review of the literature. *Eur J Med Res* 2001;**6**:139–149.

189. Stricker BH, Van den Broek JW, Keuning J, et al. Cholestatic hepatitis due to antibacterial combination of amoxicillin and clavulanic acid (augmentin). *Dig Dis Sci* 1989;**34**:1576–1580.

190. Yu MK, Yu MC, Lee F. Association of DRESS syndrome with chylous ascites. *Nephrol Dial Transplant* 2006;**21**:3301–3303.

191. Fontana RJ, Shakil AO, Greenson JK, Boyd I, Lee WM. Acute liver failure due to amoxicillin and amoxicillin/clavulanate. *Dig Dis Sci* 2005;**50**:1785–1790.

192. Daly AK, Donaldson PT, Bhatnagar P, et al. *HLA-B*5701* genotype is a major determinant of drug-induced liver injury due to flucloxacillin. *Nat Genet* 2009;**41**:816–819.

193. Lucena MI, Molokhia M, Shen Y, et al. Susceptibility to amoxicillin-clavulanate-induced liver injury is influenced by multiple HLA class I and II alleles. *Gastroenterol* 2011;**141**:338–347.

194. Chawla A, Kahn E, Yunis EJ, Daum F. Rapidly progressive cholstasis: an unusual reaction to amoxicillin/clavulinic acid in a child. *J Pediatr* 2000;**136**:121–123.

195. Roberts EA, Spielberg SP, Goldbach M, Phillips MJ. Phenobarbital hepatotoxicity in an 8-month-old infant. *J Hepatol* 1990;**10**:235–239.

196. Li AM, Nelson EA, Hon EK, et al. Hepatic failure in a child with anti-epileptic hypersensitivity syndrome. *J Paediatr Child Health* 2005;**41**:218–220.

197. Bessmertny O, Hatton RC, Gonzalez-Peralta RP. Antiepileptic hypersensitivity syndrome in children. *Ann Pharmacother* 2001;**35**:533–538.

198. Mullick FG, Ishak KG. Hepatic injury associated with diphenylhydantoin therapy. *Am J Clin Pathol* 1980;**74**:442–452.

199. Spielberg SP, Gordon GB, Blake DA, Mellits ED, Bross DS. Anticonvulsant toxicity in vitro:possible role of arene oxides. *J Pharmacol Exp Ther* 1981;**217**:386–389.

200. Spielberg SP, Gordon GB, Blake DA, Goldstein DA, Herlong HF. Predisposition to phenytoin hepatotoxicity assessed in vitro. *N Engl J Med* 1981;**305**:722–727.

201. Rivkees SA, Mattison DR. Propylthiouracil (PTU) hepatoxicity in children and recommendations for discontinuation of use. *Int J Pediatr Endocrinol* 2009;**2009**:1320–1341.

202. Maggiore G, Larizza D, Lorini R, et al. PTU hepatotoxicity mimicking autoimmune chronic active hepatitis in a girl. *J Pediatr Gastroenterol Nutr* 1989;**8**:547–548.

203. Hayashida CY, Duarte AJ, Sato AE, Yamashiro-Kanashiro EH. Neonatal hepatitis and lymphocyte sensitization by placental transfer of propylthiouracil. *J Endocrinol Invest* 1990;**13**:937–941.

204. Loomba-Albrecht LA, Bremer AA, Wong A, Philipps A. Neonatal cholestasis due to hyperthyroidism: an unusual case and clinical implications. *J Pediatr Gastroenterol Nutr* 2012;**54**:433–434.

205. Fallon MB, Boyer JL. Hepatic toxicity of vitamin A and synthetic retinoids. *J Gastroenterol Hepatol* 1990;**5**:334–342.

206. Kumra S, Herion D, Jacobsen LK, Briguglia C, Grothe D. Case study: risperidone-induced hepatotoxicity in pediatric patients. *J Am Acad Child Adolesc Psychiatry* 1997;**36**:701–705.

207. Krebs S, Dormann H, Muth-Selbach U, et al. Risperidone-induced cholestatic hepatitis. *Eur J Gastroenterol Hepatol* 2001;**13**:67–69.

208. Copur M, Erdogan A. Risperidone rechallenge for marked liver function test abnormalities in an autistic child. *Recent Pat Endocr Metab Immune Drug Discov* 2011;**5**:237–239.

209. Shear NH, Spielberg SP, Grant DM, Tang BK, Kalow W. Differences in metabolism of sulfonamides predisposing to idiosyncratic toxicity. *Ann Intern Med* 1986;**105**:179–184.

210. Besnard M, Debray D, Durand P, et al. [Fulminant hepatitis in two children treated with sulfasalazine for Crohn disease.] *Arch Pediatr* 1999;**6**:643–646.

211. Karpman E, Kurzrock EA. Adverse reactions of nitrofurantoin, trimethoprim and sulfamethoxazole in children. *J Urol* 2004;**172**:448–453.

212. Bucaretchi F, Vicente DC, Pereira RM, Tresoldi AT. Dapsone hypersensitivity syndrome in an adolescent during treatment of leprosy. *Rev Inst Med Trop Sao Paulo* 2004;**46**:331–334.

213. Rieder MJ, Uetrecht J, Shear NH, et al. Diagnosis of sulfonamide hypersensitivity reactions by in-vitro "rechallenge" with hydroxylamine metabolites. *Ann Intern Med* 1989;**110**:286–289.

214. Cribb AE, Spielberg SP. Hepatic microsomal metabolism of sulfamethoxazole to the hydroxylamine. *Drug Metab Dispos* 1990;**18**:784–787.

215. Sztajnkrycer MD. Valproic acid toxicity: overview and management. *J Toxicol Clin Toxicol* 2002;**40**:789–801.

216. Suchy FJ, Balistreri WF, Buchino J, *et al.* Acute hepatic failure associated with the use of sodium valproate. Report of two fatal cases. *N Engl J Med* 1979;**300**:962–966.

217. Zimmerman HJ, Ishak KG. Valproate-induced hepatic injury: Analysis of 23 fatal cases. *Hepatology* 1982;**2**:591–597.

218. Koenig SA, Siemes H, Blaker F, *et al.* Severe hepatotoxicity during valproate therapy: an update and report of eight new fatalities. *Epilepsia* 1994;**35**:1005–1015.

219. Price KE, Pearce RE, Garg UC, *et al.* Effects of valproic acid on organic acid metabolism in children: a metabolic profiling study. *Clin Pharmacol Ther* 2011;**89**:867–874.

220. McCall M, Bourgeois JA. Valproic acid-induced hyperammonemia: a case report. *J Clin Psychopharmacol* 2004;**24**:521–526.

221. Gerstner T, Buesing D, Longin E, *et al.* Valproic acid induced encephalopathy – 19 new cases in Germany from 1994 to 2003: a side effect associated to VPA-therapy not only in young children. *Seizure* 2006;**15**:443–448.

222. Eadie MJ, Hooper WD, Dickinson RG. Valproate-associated hepatotoxicity and its biochemical mechanisms. *Med Toxicol Adverse Drug Exper* 1988;**3**:85–106.

223. Li X, Norwood DL, Mao L-F, Schulz H. Mitochondrial metabolism of valproic acid. *Biochemistry* 1991;**30**:388–394.

224. Gopaul S, Farrell K, Abbott F. Effects of age and polytherapy, risk factors of valproic acid (VPA) hepatotoxicity, on the excretion of thiol conjugates of (E)-2,4-diene VPA in people with epilepsy taking VPA. *Epilepsia* 2003;**44**:322–328.

225. Eadie MJ, McKinnon GE, Dunstan PR, MacLaughlin D, Dickinson RG. Valproate metabolism during hepatotoxicity associated with the drug. *Q J Med* 1990;**77**:1229–1240.

226. Kossak BD, Schmidt-Sommerfeld E, Schoeller DA, *et al.* Impaired fatty acid oxidation in children on valproic acid and the effect of L-carnitine. *Neurology* 1993;**43**:2362–2368.

227. Tong V, Teng XW, Chang TK, Abbott FS. Valproic acid I: time course of lipid peroxidation biomarkers, liver toxicity, and valproic acid metabolite levels in rats. *Toxicol Sci* 2005;**86**:427–435.

228. Tong V, Teng XW, Chang TK, Abbott FS. Valproic acid II: effects on oxidative stress, mitochondrial membrane potential, and cytotoxicity in glutathione-depleted rat hepatocytes. *Toxicol Sci* 2005;**86**:436–443.

229. Konig SA, Schenk M, Sick C, *et al.* Fatal liver failure associated with valproate therapy in a patient with Friedreich's disease: review of valproate hepatotoxicity in adults. *Epilepsia* 1999;**40**:1036–1040.

230. Schwabe MJ, Dobyns WB, Burke B, Armstrong DL. Valproate-induced liver failure in one of two siblings with Alpers disease. *Pediatr Neurol* 1997;**16**:337–343.

231. Kayihan N, Nennesmo I, Ericzon BG, Nemeth A. Fatal deterioration of neurological disease after orthotopic liver transplantation for valproic acid-induced liver damage. *Pediatr Transplant* 2000;**4**:211–214.

232. Stewart JD, Horvath R, Baruffini E, *et al.* Polymerase gamma gene *POLG* determines the risk of sodium valproate-induced liver toxicity. *Hepatology* 2010;**52**:1791–1796.

233. Saneto RP, Lee IC, Koenig MK, *et al.* POLG DNA testing as an emerging standard of care before instituting valproic acid therapy for pediatric seizure disorders. *Seizure* 2010;**19**:140–146.

234. Beghi E, Bizzi A, Codegoni AM, Trevisan D, Torri W. Valproate, carnitine metabolism, and biochemical indicators of liver function. *Epilepsia* 1990;**31**:346–352.

235. Lheureux PE, Hantson P. Carnitine in the treatment of valproic acid-induced toxicity. *Clin Toxicol* 2009;**47**:101–111.

236. Bohan TP, Helton E, McDonald I, *et al.* Effect of L-carnitine treatment for valproate-induced hepatotoxicity. *Neurology* 2001;**56**:1405–1409.

237. Suzuki A, Brunt EM, Kleiner DE, *et al.* The use of liver biopsy evaluation in discrimination of idiopathic autoimmune hepatitis versus drug-induced liver injury. *Hepatology* 2011;**54**:931–939.

238. Naranjo CA, Busto U, Sellers EM, *et al.* A method for estimating the probability of adverse drug reactions. *Clin Pharmacol Ther* 1981;**30**:239–245.

239. Garcia-Cortes M, Stephens C, Lucena MI, Fernandez-Castaner A, Andrade RJ. Causality assessment methods in drug induced liver injury: strengths and weaknesses. *J Hepatol* 2011;**55**:683–691.

Liver disease in immunodeficiencies

Nedim Hadžić

Introduction

Man and microbes are committed to a perennial evolutionary conflict in which the human immune system represents a powerful tool of protection against invasion. The liver plays an important role in the immune defense because of its central position adjacent to the gastrointestinal tract, representing the first line of defense against ingested or translocated pathogens and various antigens from food.

There are two types of immune response: innate and adaptive. Innate immunity represents the first line of immune defense in which cells such as phagocytes, natural killer (NK) cells, and NK T-cells recognize highly conserved antigens from the invading microorganisms and provide a prompt non-specific inflammatory response. The principal intrahepatic defenders are Kupffer cells – resident macrophages, strongly supported by the action of NK cells, previously also known as Pit cells, which represent approximately 50% of the lymphocyte pool in a healthy liver. In contrast, the adaptive immune system is more phylogenetically advanced and includes highly specialized cells such as T- and B-lymphocytes, produced and differentiated in the lymphoid organs. On stimulation, these cells undergo sophisticated processes of immune diversification enabling them to mount specific immune responses to different invading antigens from the environment. These events are much slower and involve mechanisms such as cell-to-cell interaction, proliferation of B-cells, production of antibodies and cytokines, and activation of effector cytotoxic cells.

Historically, the adaptive immune response has been divided into two types: the humoral arm, mediated by B-cells capable of producing antibodies and responsible for mounting defense against bacterial and fungal infections, and the cellular arm, predominantly controlling viral, protozoan, mycobacterial, and other intracellular pathogens. In reality, this distinction is relatively artificial because the immune system, in order to control the infection, must have both of the components activated. This is achieved through a network of complex feedback mechanisms affecting both arms, orchestrated by CD4 T-cells via various costimuli on the lymphocyte surface and serine mediators such as acute phase proteins, cytokines, and complement components.

Role of the liver in immune defenses

The main immunologic functions of the liver include participation in the acute inflammatory response, production of acute phase proteins, induction of tolerance to various antigens, tumor surveillance, and elimination of activated lymphocytes [1]. These are achieved through a complex interaction between macrophages, antigen-presenting cells, hepatocytes and effector cells of the innate and adaptive immune system trafficking through the liver. The portal vein is a principal supplier of the liver of massive amount of lymphocytes and antigens from the intestine, which come into close contact with the endothelial cells through an extensive sinusoid network. Kupffer cells control the influx of microorganisms and toxins from the gastrointestinal tract by ensuring that the majority of the pathogens are eliminated via phagocytosis before entering the systemic circulation. The hepatocytes are a major production site for components of the systemic inflammatory response, such as C-reactive protein, fibrinogen, α_1-antitrypsin, α_1-antichymotrypsin, mannose-binding lectin, amyloid, and ceruloplasmin [1]. These acute phase reactants assist in infection control and clearance of the pathogens. Finally, most of the activated lymphocytes, after fulfilling their immunologic duties, are destroyed by the hepatic elements of the reticuloendothelial system or via apoptosis. Consequently, the term "immunologic graveyard" has been coined for the liver [2].

An intriguing physiologic function inherent to the liver, encompassing elements from both innate and adaptive immunity, is immunologic tolerance. To distinguish between self- and foreign antigens, the immune system undergoes perpetual sophisticated mechanisms of T-cell clonal selection in the thymus and at the periphery. The key players in maintaining mechanisms of "central" and "peripheral" tolerance are T regulatory cells. In addition, the intrahepatic antigen-presenting cells, including Kupffer cells, dendritic cells, sinusoidal endothelial cells, and stellate cells, are heavily involved in

Liver Disease in Children, Fourth Edition, ed. Frederick J. Suchy, Ronald J. Sokol, and William F. Balistreri. Published by Cambridge University Press. © Cambridge University Press 2014.

the processes of induction and maintenance of immunologic tolerance [1–3]. This critical role of the liver may help in understanding its relatively immune-privileged position and the lesser degree of tissue compatibility required for successful liver transplantation.

A variety of immunologic disturbances have been observed as a consequence of both acute liver failure [4] and chronic liver disease [5]. These include upregulation of various cytokines, such as interleukin (IL)-1, IL-6, tumor necrosis factor-α, and interferon-γ, and abnormal synthesis of acute phase reactants and complement components [6]. It is noteworthy that despite the frequent overproduction of immunologic components, the overall immune function remains impaired, suggesting a lack of cross-talk or immunologic coordination. This immune paresis often adds to the infection-related mortality in liver disorders, particularly in acute liver failure [4]. Conversely, inborn defects of the immune function per se can also contribute to both acute and chronic liver disorders, a fact particularly relevant from the pediatric perspective because these conditions tend to present in childhood.

Defects in the defense mechanisms can be divided in *primary* immunodeficiencies in which there is a genetic cause of the impaired immunity and *secondary* immunodeficiencies in which the presence of viruses, such as HIV, or some major medical intervention, such as chemotherapy or immunosuppressive medications, render the immune responses abnormal. Much of our current understanding of the physiology of the immune reactions originates from recognition of clinical patterns of immune dysfunction in immunodeficient patients and the identification of specific types of microorganisms isolated from them. Developments in immunogenetics have helped to define genotype/phenotype patterns which exist.

Primary immunodeficiencies

Primary immunodeficiencies (PIDs) are rare but potentially fatal disorders of the innate and adaptive immune systems. More than 130 PIDs have been identified at a clinical or genetic level, with an estimated incidence of approximately 1 in 10 000 live births [7,8].

Broadly speaking, PIDs can be divided into disorders of innate and adaptive immunity. Since the 1980s, the diagnosis and management of PIDs have been dramatically improved because of advances in immunogenetics, better anti-infectious strategies, and the earlier and more effective use of hematopoietic stem cell transplantation (HSCT) as a definitive treatment [7].

Secondary immunodeficiencies, related to HIV infection, chemotherapy, post-organ transplantation immunosuppression, or immune ablation, are also better controlled because of the use of modern anti-infectious strategies. In particular, progression of HIV infection has been significantly reduced by the advent of combination antiviral treatment [9].

The PIDs are inherited in either an autosomal recessive or an X-linked manner. Therefore, boys are more likely to be affected by PIDs. A simplified classification of PIDs is presented in Table 23.1. A majority of children with significant PIDs present early in infancy, when passive protection from transplacentally and breast milk-acquired immunoglobulins starts to wane. Life-threatening chest infections, often caused by *Pneumocystis jiroveci*, are a typical clinical presentation for children with severe combined immunodeficiency (SCID) or hyper-IgM syndrome. Milder forms of PIDs could be diagnosed following investigation into chronic diarrhea; recurrent chest, skin, or ear infections; or failure to thrive. Many children come from consanguineous families. Some have a positive family history of unexplained neonatal and infantile deaths in siblings or maternal relatives because of the X-linked pattern of inheritance in some PIDs [7,8].

The main clinical problems in the management of immunodeficiencies are recurrent and opportunistic infections. In addition, these patients have an increased lifelong risk of developing malignancies and autoimmune disorders [7]. Frequently, the type of infection broadly indicates whether the problem affects the humoral (e.g. recurrent pyogenic pathogens: bacteria, fungi) or the cellular (e.g. opportunistic pathogens: viruses, atypical bacteria, protozoa) arm of the immune system. For example, isolation of protozoan *P. jiroveci* from the bronchial aspirate suggests a likely problem in cellular immunity, while identification of *Staphylococcus aureus* from a liver abscess points to neutrophil dysfunction. However, in most immunodeficiencies, both cellular and humoral pathways are affected to some degree. For example, the X-linked form of hyper-IgM syndrome – CD40 ligand deficiency, an inborn immunoglobulin defect in class-switch recombination that renders the patients unable to produce other than IgM forms of immunoglobulin – is caused by abnormal interaction between activated lymphocytes and B-cells [10]. Consequently, early antibiotic prophylaxis, subcutaneous immunoglobulin, or intravenous immunoglobulin (IVIg) replacement therapy is indicated for the majority of PIDs. This therapeutic approach, by reducing the incidence of infections, has greatly improved the quality of life of children with PIDs, although there are no data yet regarding their impact on the longer term incidence of complications.

Liver complications in children with immunodeficiencies

Hepatic complications in children with immunodeficiencies can be related to chronic infections unaffected by antimicrobial prophylaxis, drugs used to control the infections, or complications before or after HSCT. Approximately 25% of children with PIDs are estimated to have some form of liver involvement [11]. By far the most common hepatic complication of the PIDs is sclerosing cholangitis (discussed in detail in Chapter 21) [11]. Typically, immunodeficient children with sclerosing cholangitis do not present with classical symptoms of cholangiopathy such as jaundice, fatigue, or pruritus. Elevation of liver enzymes (aspartate aminotransferase,

Table 23.1 Common primary immunodeficiencies

Condition	Chromosome, gene	Gene product	Function
X-linked immunodeficiency			
X-linked SCID	Xq13, *IL2RG*	Common γ chain	T-cell and natural killer cell development, T- and B-cell function
X-linked agammaglobulinemia (Bruton)	Xq22, *BTK*	Bruton tyrosine kinase (Btk)	Pre-B-cell maturation
X-linked hyper-IgM syndrome (CD40 ligand deficiency)	Xq26, *CD40LG*	CD40 ligand (CD154)	Isotype switching, T-cell function
Wiskott–Aldrich syndrome	Xp11, *WASP*	WASP	Cytoskeletal defect affecting hematopoietic stem cell derivatives
X-linked chronic granulomatous disease	Xp21, *CYBB*	gp91^{phox}	Component of NADPH oxidase–phagocytic burst
X-linked lymphoproliferative disease type 1 (Duncan syndrome)	Xq25, *SH2D1A*	Signaling lymphocytic activation molecule (SLAM)-associated protein (SAP)	T-cell response to EBV
X-linked lymphoproliferative disease type 2	Xq25, *XIAP* (*BIRC4*)	X-linked inhibitor-of-apoptosis (XIAP)	T-cell response to EBV
Properdin deficiency	Xp21	Properdin	Component of complement cascade
Autosomal recessive immunodeficiency: SCID type			
Adenosine deaminase deficiency	20q12-13, *ADA*	Adenosine deaminase	Removal of toxic metabolites from purine salvage pathway
Purine nucleoside phosphorylase deficiency	14q11, *PNP*	Purine nucleoside phosphorylase (PNP)	Removal of toxic metabolites from purine salvage pathway
Recombinase activating gene deficiency	11p13, *RAG1*, *RAG2*	Recombination-activating protein 1 and 2	Defective DNA recombination
JAK3 deficiency (T–B+NK SCID)	19p13, *JAK3*	JAK3	Abnormal T- and NK-cell development
Zap70 deficiency	2q12, *ZAP70*	ZAP70	Abnormal intrathymic T-cell selection
Autosomal recessive immunodeficiency: non-SCID type			
Leukocyte adhesion deficiency type 1	21q22, *ITGB2*	CD11/CD18	Defective leukocyte adhesion and migration
Chronic granulomatous disease	7q11, *NCF1*	p47^{phox}	Defective respiratory burst and phagocytic intracellular killing
	1q25, *NCF2*	p67^{phox}	
	16p24, *CYBA*	p22^{phox}	
Chediak–Higashi syndrome	1q42, *LYST*	LYST	Abnormalities in lysosomal protein trafficking
MHC class I deficiency	6p21, *TAP1*, *TAP2*	Transporter associated with antigen processing (TAP1 and TAP2)	Abnormal presentation of HLA class I molecules
MHC class II deficiency	16p13, *MHC2TA*	MHC class II transactivator (CIITA)	Defective regulation of MHC II molecule expression
	19p12, *RFXANK*	RFXANK	
	1q21, *RFX5*	RFX5	
	13q13, *RFXAP*	RFXAP	

Table 23.1 (*cont.*)

Condition	Chromosome, gene	Gene product	Function
Autoimmune lymphoproliferative syndrome	10q24, *FAS*	APT1 (Fas)	Defective apoptosis
Ataxia telangiectasia	11q22, *ATM*	ATM (protein kinase)	Cell cycle control and DNA repair responses

SCID, severe combined immunodeficiency

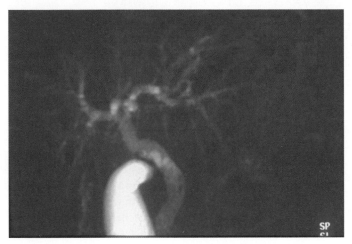

Figure 23.1 MR cholangiopancreatography demonstrating advanced intrahepatic and extrahepatic cholangiopathy in a patient with combined immunodeficiency.

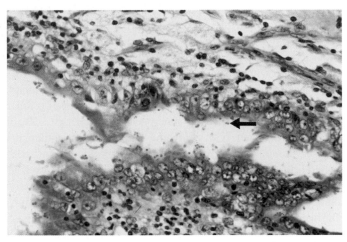

Figure 23.2 Cryptosporidium oocysts (arrow) in the section of the liver biopsy of the patient with hyper-IgM syndrome and sclerosing cholangitis (hematoxylin & eosin, ×150).

gamma-glutamyltransferase, or alkaline phosphatase) may be trivial or absent. Expert ultrasonography could indicate mild dilatation of the extrahepatic or, less frequently, intrahepatic bile ducts and splenomegaly. In the presence of biochemical or ultrasound changes, further evaluation with liver biopsy and cholangiography is indicated. The increased sensitivity of magnetic resonance cholangiopancreatography (MRCP) has reduced the requirement for the more invasive direct cholangiographic techniques, such as endoscopic retrograde cholangiopancreatography (ERCP) and percutaneous transhepatic cholangiography. One study has reported a good concordance between MRCP and ERCP in diagnosing cholangiopathy when the disease is advanced [11] (Figure 23.1). However, subtle radiologic changes may be missed on MRCP. The same study indicated a good correlation but a slightly increased sensitivity of radiologic compared with histologic methods for diagnosing PID-related sclerosing cholangitis in children [11].

Role of opportunistic infections in the development of sclerosing cholangitis

Sclerosing cholangitis has been described in a number of immunodeficiencies, predominantly of the combined cellular and humoral type [12,13]:

- hyper-IgM syndrome
- combined immunodeficiency
- common variable deficiency
- Wiskott–Aldrich syndrome
- MHC class II deficiency
- interferon-γ deficiency
- DiGeorge syndrome
- immunoglobulin subclass deficiency.

The most common association is with hyper-IgM syndrome [14]. In a significant proportion of these patients, *Cryptosporidium* spp. is identified, in particular with the use of more sensitive detection approaches, such as polymerase chain reaction-based assays [15]. Standard microscopy, following a modified acid-fast stain, can often overlook the focal presence of *Cryptosporidium* oocysts in the gastrointestinal tract, where the microbe usually resides in the intestinal and biliary epithelium. Rarely, *Cryptosporidium* can be identified in liver biopsy specimens at the surface of the biliary epithelium by light microscopy (Figure 23.2). There are 10 *Cryptosporidium* species, with *C. parvum* representing the most common human pathogen. Two distinct genotypes of *C. parvum* relevant to humans – human type 1 and bovine type 2 – have been identified. In immunocompetent individuals, this ubiquitous organism can cause small waterborne outbreaks of diarrhea, but it has not been associated with cholangiopathy. The pathogenic role of *C. parvum* in immunodeficiency has not been fully elucidated, but animal models of *Cryptosporidium*-related cholangiopathy have been described [16]. Interferon-γ knock-out mice appear to be particularly susceptible to *Cryptosporidium* infection, suggesting that this cytokine plays a critical role in the immune defense against this pathogen [16]. Biliary damage in humans appears to be caused by a direct cytopathic effect of *C. parvum* via apoptotic mechanisms [17]. In addition, *C. parvum* can induce cholangiopathy in HIV infection [18] and after organ transplant [19]. Other intracellular parasites such as *Microsporidium* spp., *Mycobacterium avium intracellulare*, and cytomegalovirus (CMV) have also been reported in association with cholangiopathy in adults infected with HIV [18]. It is possible that the particularly fast evolution of *C. parvum* cholangiopathy in patients with HIV results from the synergistic effect of multiple biliary infections [18].

Children with chronic cholangiopathy have been reported to have an increased number of gastrointestinal malignancies, including cholangiocarcinoma, lymphoma, and hepatocellular carcinoma. One multicenter study has reported that 55% of patients with hyper-IgM syndrome and sclerosing cholangitis had cryptosporidiosis [14]. One 18-year-old patient with hyper-IgM syndrome, undergoing curative sequential liver and stem cell transplantation, was found to have dysplastic biliary changes in the explanted liver (Figure 23.3) [20]. Similar histologic appearances have been noted in patients with HIV infection [18]. Therefore, it is conceivable that the failure of antimicrobials to clear *C. parvum* or other protozoans from the biliary tract could lead to chronic cholangiopathy, dysplastic changes, and, ultimately, biliary malignancies. The mechanisms for other described immunodeficiency-associated malignancies, such as lymphoma and hepatocellular carcinoma, however, remain less than clear, although it can be speculated that inability to mount an effective immune surveillance against potentially neoplastic antigens or clones could play a role.

Hyper-IgM syndrome

Hyper-IgM syndrome is a paradigm for immunodeficiency-associated sclerosing cholangitis, which, if not corrected, progresses to chronic biliary disease and cirrhosis in the majority of the patients. In addition, children with hyper-IgM suffer from neutropenia, opportunistic infections, chronic mouth ulcers, chronic diarrhea, failure to thrive, and poorly defined chronic encephalopathy [10,21]. The estimated incidence is between 1 in 500 000 and 1 in 1 000 000 live births [7,10]. One study reported only 20% survival at 20 years of age in this condition, with life-threatening opportunistic infections and progressive hepatobiliary complications being the main cause of death [14]. Hyper-IgM syndrome is caused by absence of CD40 ligand on activated lymphocytes and lack of interaction with CD40 molecules from B-cells in the X-linked form (CD40 ligand deficiency), or defective expression of activation-induced cytidine deaminase on B-cells in the autosomal recessive form of the disease [10]. Therefore, in both forms, B-cells are unable to direct physiologic IgM class switching to other

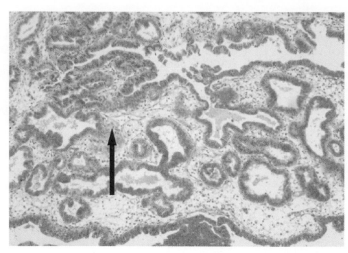

Figure 23.3 Dysplastic changes (arrow) in the biliary epithelium of the explanted liver of a patient with CD40 ligand deficiency and end-stage chronic liver disease (hematoxylin & eosin, ×400).

immunoglobulin types. It is important to note that serum IgM levels are not always elevated in this condition.

In the past, the majority of children with hyper-IgM syndrome presented to the hepatologist with well-established signs of advanced liver disease, such as biochemical abnormalities and portal hypertension. An increased awareness of the hepatic involvement in PIDs among immunologists in recent years has led to earlier referrals and preventive measures, with a consequent reduction in presentations with severe liver involvement. Many children with hyper-IgM syndrome may remain clinically asymptomatic well into the second decade of life, when progression of the liver disease typically occurs. Therefore, pediatricians and parents alike have felt uneasy about considering mortality-associated transplantation options in children with hyper-IgM syndrome, who often have a near normal quality of life on immunoglobulin replacement and anti-infectious prophylaxis. Recently, a partial improvement in the immune function was observed following serial infusions of recombinant CD40 ligand in three children [22].

Liver transplantation has been attempted for end-stage biliary disease in hyper-IgM syndrome, but fatal cholangiopathy recurs within months after the operation [23]. The recurrence may well be accelerated by the effect of post-transplant immunosuppression on quiescent infections of the gastrointestinal tract. It has become clear that correction of the immune defect is essential for patient and graft survival. Although HSCT is able to correct the immunodeficiency [24], associated hepatic complications such as sinusoidal obstruction syndrome (also known as veno-occlusive disease), drug hepatotoxicity, and graft-versus-host-disease significantly reduce survival [25]. Therefore, a reduced intensity conditioning approach that avoids irradiation and uses less hepatotoxic chemotherapeutics, for example, melphalan, and a smaller amount of infused cells, has been introduced for HSCT in the presence of significant pre-existing organ (lungs, liver, or heart) damage. This modified gentler approach has been termed non-myeloablative or "mini" HSCT [26,27]. A sequential approach with combined liver and "mini" HSCT 1 month later has proved successful in a teenager with decompensated biliary cirrhosis secondary to hyper-IgM syndrome [20]. Some children with less advanced liver disease can survive isolated non-myeloablative HSCT, but generally patients with hyper-IgM should be identified and screened for a matched donor for HSCT early, while the liver involvement is absent or minimal. The use of umbilical cord grafts has expanded the availability of donors for the correction of this and other immune defects.

Management of cryptosporidiosis and sclerosing cholangitis in immunodeficient patients

Cryptosporidiosis represents a frequent problem in patients with PIDs [11,15] but has also been described after solid organ transplantation [19]. Infected patients often have vague abdominal symptoms with watery diarrhea and fever, but may also be completely asymptomatic [11,15]. Jejunal biopsy can increase the diagnostic yield in suspected *C. parvum* infection, showing non-specific features such as mild to moderate villous atrophy, submucosal inflammatory infiltrate, and crypt hyperplasia [19]. Some studies have observed a disproportionate elevation of alkaline phosphatase in HIV-positive patients with *C. parvum*-associated cholangiopathy [18].

Although most commonly seen in hyper-IgM syndrome and its variant CD40 ligand deficiency, sclerosing cholangitis, often in conjunction with cryptosporidiosis, has also been described in patients with other PIDs (Table 23.1) [11,28]. Therefore, this condition needs to be considered in all immunodeficient patients with abnormal hepatic biochemical markers, regardless of their primary diagnosis.

The medical management of cryptosporidiosis is not satisfactory. Clearly, the critical therapeutic maneuver is to increase the immune competence of the host whenever possible. Despite availability of several drugs effective against *Cryptosporidium*, their efficacy is uncertain, particularly in the setting of chronic immunosuppression. Paromomycin, azithromycin, letrazuril, and recombinant interleukin-2 have been investigated in HIV-positive patients, but without convincing evidence about their benefits [29,30]. Intravenous paromomycin poses considerable risks for inducing conductive deafness, even when the serum levels are kept within the therapeutic range. Nitazoxanide is a novel drug with a proven activity in cryptosporidial diarrhea of immunocompetent patients [31], but no information is available in the immunodeficiency setting.

It is prudent to initiate prophylaxis against *C. parvum* with oral medications, effective in the intestinal lumen, and the boiling of drinking water in all children with hyper-IgM syndrome. The standard choice is paromomycin 250–500 mg twice daily. Once *C. parvum* has penetrated the hepatic barriers, any treatment short of re-establishing the immunity is likely to be futile. We also recommend starting choleretic treatment with ursodeoxycholic acid (20 mg/kg daily) [32] in the hope that it will reduce the likelihood of *C. parvum* ascending from the gut into the biliary tract.

Children with PIDs who have evidence of persistent hepatic biochemical derangement, even only of a mild degree, should be promptly considered for HSCT because these changes are likely to progress. In the presence of more advanced liver involvement, clinically documented by dilated ducts on ultrasound, splenomegaly, or mild jaundice, each patient should be evaluated individually to assess the relative risks for HSCT. Availability of a well-matched donor, lack of evidence for *C. parvum* colonization, satisfactory renal and lung function, and absence of neutropenia increase the chances of a successful outcome. Finally, if the patient with PID presents with end-stage chronic liver disease (coagulopathy, hypoalbuminemia, or ascites) the only viable option is sequential liver and HSCT. The reverse order for these procedures is unlikely to succeed because the decompensated liver would probably not tolerate the effects of pre-HSCT conditioning. Furthermore, the risks of early post-HSCT complications such as sinusoidal obstruction syndrome, acute graft-versus-host disease, or reactivation of quiescent pathogens are much higher with end-stage liver damage [11,25]. The same concerns would apply to a theoretically possible simultaneous living-related liver and HSCT.

Miscellaneous immunodeficiencies and liver disease

Several rare metabolic liver-based conditions have been associated with immunodeficiency, such as adenosine deaminase deficiency [33], lysinuric protein intolerance [34], and propionic acidemia [35]. Their immune phenotype may vary from SCID in adenosine deaminase deficiency to a slightly increased frequency of infections in propionic acidemia. The hepatic damage is thought to be inflicted by accumulation of toxic metabolites and appears to improve with pegylated-adenosine deaminase supplements in adenosine deaminase deficiency [33]. Another rare association is SCID and multiple intestinal atresia with ensuing parental nutrition-induced liver damage [36]. In this otherwise fatal condition, one report suggested amelioration of the immune phenotype following a liver–small bowel transplant, possibly related to the transfer of the peripheral stem cells into the heavily immunosuppressed host during the operation [37].

A recent report has described an intriguing association between common variable immunodeficiency, which typically presents outside pediatric age group, and nodular regenerative hyperplasia associated with portal hypertension [38]. The authors have postulated autoimmune etiology, as these patients often had low-titer serum autoantibodies and 90% had intrasinusoidal lymphocytic infiltrate in the liver histology. They have also confirmed the presence of epitheloid granulomas, known to be associated with various forms of immunodeficiency, in 43% of their patients [38].

Chronic viral hepatitis in patients with immunodeficiencies

Immunodeficient patients often have abnormal responses to viral pathogens. Given their common long-term requirements for blood products, they may have been exposed to hepatotropic viruses despite the much improved safety of such products. Moreover, these patients are less likely to mount an adequate immune response to vaccines, when they are available, as is the case for hepatitis B virus (HBV). Longer term, chronic viral infections in immunodeficient patients could have a more aggressive clinical course, particularly in the setting of coinfection. One study from Italy found evidence of HBV and hepatitis C (HCV) in 6 of 11 children with PIDs and liver disease, with a 5-year survival of 60% [39].

HIV infection

Liver disease in HIV infection

It was estimated that 34 million adults and 2.5 million children worldwide were infected with HIV at the end of 2009 (http://www.unaids.org). The majority of children acquire the infection vertically from their HIV-infected mothers. The advent of highly active antiretroviral therapy (HAART) in 1996 considerably modified the natural history of this infection in geographic regions where the treatment is affordable [9]. Compared with adults with HIV infection, the survival time in children is significantly shorter even with the use of long-term HAART. Unfortunately, this treatment has also created a frustrating dual scenario; in the developed world, HIV infection has become a potentially controllable chronic disease with improved medium-term morbidity, whereas it remains a major killer in the developing countries where HAART is unavailable. An 81% decrease in mortality of children who were HIV positive diagnosed in the USA between 1987 and 1999 has been reported, albeit with no significant change in morbidity [40]. The median age at death of children infected with HIV was 5 years, with hepatic causes contributing in only 4% [40].

The gastrointestinal tract is a common port of entry for HIV. The term "HIV enteropathy" has been coined to describe characteristic histologic changes including monocytic mucosal inflammation and an increased number of intraepithelial lymphocytes caused by invasion of the lamina propria and intestinal macrophages by HIV. As the CD4 cell count declines, further histologic changes follow, such as crypt hyperplasia and villous atrophy. Activated lymphocytes release a variety of cytokines, such as interferon-γ and tumor necrosis factor-α, causing further disturbances in the life cycle and function of the enterocytes [41]. Diverse ultrastructural changes, including irregular, broadened, and short microvilli, mitochondrial swelling, and deposition of intracytoplasmic inclusion bodies in the various cellular organelles, have been described [41]. Inevitably, these chronic morphologic changes

in the intestinal tract give rise to clinical symptoms of chronic diarrhea, malnutrition, and weight loss [9]. Breast-feeding may play a role in reducing the rate of progression in countries where HAART is not available [9]. As HIV infection progresses further, the virus spreads to Kupffer cells in the liver, where it can be detected in a characteristically scattered appearance [42]. More advanced disease, reflected in an increased viral load and lower CD4 cell counts, overwhelms the macrophage scavenger control in the lungs and in the liver, frequently leading to opportunistic infections in the respiratory and gastrointestinal tract, including the liver.

The hepatic pathology in HIV infection in children shares some similarities with the findings in adults, such as nonspecific portal inflammation, Kupffer cell hyperplasia, and high incidence of opportunistic infections, including CMV, *Mycobacterium avium* complex, *Cryptococcus*, and *Cryptosporidium* [42]. However, some intriguing differences have been reported, such as decreased incidence of granulomas and fatty change, more prominent giant cell transformation of the hepatocytes, cholestasis, and occasional presence of diffuse lymphoplasmocytic infiltrate associated with lymphoid interstitial pneumonitis [43,44]. Moreover, children from the developing world appear to have more prominent inflammatory features and increased incidence of opportunistic infections, contributing to earlier deaths than those observed in their peers from the developed world [43]. Because most of the pediatric studies have been based on autopsy material, the role of liver biopsy in the clinical management of HIV-positive patients with minor biochemical abnormalities is uncertain [44]. Less invasive tests for the diagnosis of opportunistic infections, which are the most common reason for the liver involvement, are available.

Opportunistic infections and HIV cholangiopathy

During the pre-HAART era, HIV-related cholangiopathy associated with *Cryptosporidia*, *Microsporidia*, and CMV was frequently reported from both adults and children [45]. This condition, clinically and radiologically similar to sclerosing cholangitis in PIDs, is still the most common hepatic feature of HIV infection, although it is less frequent, with a better preserved immunocompetence of the HIV-infected patients achieved through HAART [9]. Clinical symptoms include abdominal pain, scleral icterus, hepatomegaly, and diarrhea. Mild to moderate elevation of serum alkaline phosphatase, gamma-glutamyltransferase, aspartate aminotransferase, and bilirubin is common. Abdominal ultrasonography often demonstrates a mild dilatation of the bile ducts, enlarged gallbladder, and abnormal echo pattern of the liver with minimal splenomegaly [46]. Although MRCP may be useful in documenting suspected HIV cholangiopathy, ERCP is preferred because of the additional possibility of bile sampling to identify the pathogens and of therapeutic biliary stenting or papillotomy in the presence of distal biliary stricture or papilary stenosis, respectively [45].

Table 23.2 Hepatobiliary disorders described with HIV infection

Disorder	Associated condition
Viral hepatitis	Chronic hepatitis B Chronic hepatitis C Adenovirus Cytomegalovirus Epstein–Barr virus
Cholangiopathy	*Cryptosporidium parvum* *Microsporidium* Cytomegalovirus
Opportunistic infections	*Mycobacterium avium intracellulare* *Histoplasma capsulatum* *Cryptococcus neoformans* *Pneumocystis jiroveci*
Malignancies	Non-Hodgkin B-cell lymphoma Kaposi sarcoma Hepatoblastoma Acute B-cell lymphoblastic leukemia Burkitt lymphoma
Secondary to antiretroviral treatment	Mitochondrial injury Mitochondrial DNA depletion syndrome Pancreatitis
Miscellaneous	Peliosis hepatis Acalculous cholecystitis

Management of HIV-related hepatic involvement in children is limited. A range of liver disorders has been described in association with HIV infection (Table 23.2). Often, presence of the liver complications simply reflects the general clinical condition of the patient. Therefore, it is hoped that the wider use of effective antiretroviral treatment will arrest their development. By analogy to prevention of cholangiopathy in PIDs, where protozoans such as *C. parvum* or *Microsporidium* spp. are also frequently implicated, it is prudent to initiate antiprotozoal prophylaxis with azythromycin or paromomycin as soon as a decline in peripheral CD4 cell count is observed. At present, however, there are no controlled data to endorse this suggestion. Choleretic treatment with ursodeoxycholic acid (20 mg/kg daily) may be of benefit when evidence of cholangiopathy is present [32].

Some research indicates that HAART treatment per se may be hepatotoxic [47,48]. In addition to the liver involvement, affected patients may have profound lactic acidosis, myopathy, hypercapnia, organic aciduria, anemia, and a range of neurologic symptoms. The underlying mechanism for these symptoms appears to be mitochondrial injury resulting in depletion of mitochondrial DNA in the liver and muscle. On withdrawal of nucleoside analogues, the clinical symptoms have been reported to reverse, with normalization of mitochondrial DNA content in the muscle [47,48].

Following the success of HAART, HIV infection has ceased to be a contraindication for liver transplantation. Short-term transplant results in adults are comparable to other indications, although the longer term outcome is likely to be affected by progression of associated pathologies, such as recurrent HCV infection [49].

Coinfection with HIV and other hepatotropic viruses

Evolution of chronic liver disease caused by hepatotropic viruses (HBV and HCV) in the presence of HIV infection appears to be accentuated [50–52]. The prolonged survival of the coinfected children requires tailored therapeutic strategies. It has been suggested that children with HIV and HCV coinfection need to be treated early, while immune competence of the host is preserved [52]. However, this is less clear for children coinfected with HIV and HBV. It is conceivable that impaired cytotoxic, HBV-specific, T-cell function may result in a lesser degree of hepatocyte damage despite ongoing HBV replication. Whether HIV infection-related decline in immune competence is associated with reduced liver injury is possible, but unproven. There is an increased risk of HBV-related acute liver failure observed in adults coinfected with HIV [51]. Of note, the nucleoside analogue lamivudine and the nucleotide inhibitor adefovir, which have proven suppressive activity against HBV, are frequent components of the combined antiretroviral regimens, together with some other novel antivirals such as tenofovir and emtricitabine. Studies in individuals coinfected with HIV and HCV show that combination therapy with pegylated interferon and ribavirin is safe, but that the response is less than in patients infected with HCV alone [52].

Hepatitis B virus and primary immunodeficiency

Chronic HBV infection is rarely diagnosed in children with PIDs. There are two primary reasons for this: (1) the countries where PIDs are predominantly diagnosed have a lower incidence of HBV; and (2) to inflict hepatocellular injury to HBV-infected hepatocytes, cytotoxic T-lymphocytes, sensitized against cells expressing HBV-related peptides, need to be fully operational, which is often not the case in children with PIDs. Therefore, their HBV DNA titers and amount of HBVe antigen could be high, but the liver damage remains minimal because of the lack of host immune response required to cause injury to the hepatocytes.

No published data on the long-term outcome of HBV-positive patients with PIDs are available, but some analogy can be drawn from HBV/HIV coinfected adults who, despite the earlier postulate, appear to have an accelerated course of HBV [53]. In a study of adults coinfected with HBV and HIV dating from a pre-HAART era, the histologic features of hepatitis were less advanced as HIV infection progressed [51]. More recent studies indicate reduced rates of anti-HBV e antigen (HBVeAg) and anti-HBV surface antigen (HBVsAg) seroconversion, with a higher incidence of decompensated end-stage cirrhosis [53]. Antiretroviral treatment can trigger anti-HBeAg and anti-HBsAg seroconversion and enhance immune control of HBV replication by restoring T-cell integrity, but may also induce flares of hepatitis. Current recommendations suggest the use of interferon, adefovir, or entecavir in HBV/HIV-coinfected drug-naive patients who do not require antiretroviral treatment. Combination of tenofovir with the nucleoside analogues lamivudine or emtricitabine has been proposed as potentially effective treatment for both viruses [54].

If immunity is restored, for example after successful HSCT, there is a danger of overwhelming hepatitis B. Therefore, the use of lamivudine or adefovir is recommended for the HBV-positive patients undergoing HSCT. It has been reported that using donors positive for anti-HBV core antigen may lead to a transfer of adoptive HBV immunity after HSCT [55]. This approach should minimize the likelihood of post-HSCT acute hepatitis B.

Hepatitis C virus and primary immunodeficiency

Evidence of HCV infection in patients with PIDs should be sought by measuring serum HCV RNA because of the patients' frequently assumed deficiency in producing antibodies. Nevertheless, one study suggested that 8 of 18 adults with various primary impairments of antibody production, such as common variable immunodeficiency, hyper-IgM syndrome, and IgG subclass deficiency, were able to produce anti-HCV antibodies [56].

Chronic hepatitis C has an accelerated course in individuals with immunodeficiencies [57]. When compared with immunocompetent individuals, immunodeficient patients have significantly higher HCV RNA titers during acute hepatitis. Before 1990, there were several well-documented outbreaks of HCV infection in patients with immunodeficiencies caused by contaminated immunoglobulins and leading to progressive liver disease, often requiring liver transplantation [57,58]. The results of transplantation were largely disappointing with prompt recurrence and fatal infectious complications [58]. It is likely that post-transplant immunosuppression played a significant contributory role in these adverse outcomes. However, an adult with common variable immunodeficiency has been reported to have cleared the virus after liver transplantation, but aggressive recurrence with severe cholestatic hepatitis and liver failure prompted withdrawal of immunosuppression. Five years after the transplant, he remained well on low-dose immunosuppression, subsequently reintroduced [59].

There are no data on whether immunodeficient patients should be treated early with the emerging more efficient anti-HCV strategies. Early treatment would appear logical, although it is unlikely that there will ever be a sufficient number of immunodeficient patients to endorse this speculation through a formal trial. The same would apply to children perinatally coinfected by HIV and HCV in view of the highly effective antiretroviral therapy now available.

Hemophagocytic lymphohistiocytosis

Hemophagocytic lymphohistiocytosis (HLH) is a hyperinflammatory syndrome characterized by high fever, pancytopenia, hypercytokinemia, and coagulopathy [60,61]. Cardinal clinical features are hepatosplenomegaly, ascites, respiratory failure, skin infiltrates, and central nervous system involvement. Frequent laboratory findings are hypofibrinogenemia, hyperferritinemia, hypertriglyceridemia, and elevated serum lactate dehydrogenase [61]. Hallmark of the disease is the presence of hemophagocytosis in activated macrophages in the bone marrow, ascitic, or cerebrospinal fluid (Figure 23.4). This diagnostic feature may not be seen at presentation and cytologic examination of the bone marrow or ascitic fluid may need to be repeated if clinically indicated. At autopsy, the hemophagocytic infiltrates can be found in the liver, lungs, skin, kidneys, and brain [60,61]. This systemic disease is often triggered by infection and may progress to hepatic and renal failure. The microorganisms reported in association with HLH include viruses (Epstein–Barr virus (EBV), herpes simplex and zoster, CMV, HIV, avian flu), bacteria, and fungi, but often no organism is identified [60,62]. Children with HLH who present with liver involvement and multiorgan failure have a high mortality rate [62]. The most recent clinical diagnostic criteria are presented in Box 23.1. To diagnose HLH either a molecular genetic confirmation or fulfillment of five out of the eight clinical criteria listed are required [63].

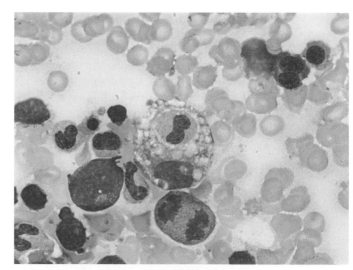

Figure 23.4 Phenomenon of hemophagocytosis demonstrated by a large histiocyte (center) engulfing two smaller cells in the bone marrow aspirate.

Box 23.1 Diagnostic criteria for hemophagocytic lymphohistiocytosis (HLH)

1. A molecular diagnosis consistent with HLH

   or

2. Diagnostic criteria for HLH (5 of the 8 criteria fulfilled)
   - fever
   - splenomegaly
   - cytopenias (affecting $\geq$2 of 3 lineages in the peripheral blood):
     - hemoglobin (<90 g/L) (in infants <4 weeks, <100 g/L)
     - platelets (<100 $\times$ 10^9/L)
     - neutrophils (<1.0 $\times$ 10^9/L)

   - hypertriglyceridemia and/or hypofibrinogenemia (fasting triglycerides $\geq$3.0 mmol/L (i.e. $\geq$265 mg/dL, fibrinogen $\leq$1.5 g/L)
   - hemophagocytosis in bone marrow, ascitic fluid, liver, spleen, or lymph nodes; no evidence of malignancy
   - low or absent natural killer cell activity (according to local laboratory reference)
   - ferritin $\geq$500 µg/L
   - soluble CD25 (i.e. soluble interleukin-2 receptor) $\geq$2400 U/mL

Source: modified from Henter, 2004 [63].

Despite its recognition more than 50 years ago [64] and recent progress in understanding its pathogenesis [65], HLH remains underdiagnosed, probably because of its non-specific clinical features and often fulminant progression. Its incidence is estimated to be approximately 1 in 50 000 live births [60,61].

Most patients with HLH will have abnormal NK cell function, with evidence of impaired granule-dependent cytotoxic pathways. Perforin is a 60 kDa polypeptide secreted by cytoplasmic granules of NK cells and cytotoxic lymphocytes. Its physiologic role, on stimulation, is to form "pores" or perforations in the membrane of the target cells, allowing other mediators of cell death (i.e. granzyme) to enter the cell and facilitate osmotic cell lysis [60,65]. The ongoing yet inefficient stimulation of the immune system via various complex pathogenic mechanisms results in overexpression of proinflammatory cytokines, such as tumor necrosis factor-α, IL-6, IL-8, IL-12, IL-18, interferon-γ, and macrophage inhibitory protein 1α, but also of a number of hemopoietic growth factors released by the overstimulated lymphocytes and macrophages [65]. Consequently, the physiological contraction of the immune response does not occur.

Approximately 70–80% of the patients with HLH, predominantly presenting in infancy, have an autosomal recessive primary immune defect (primary or familial form of HLH (FHL)), often unmasked by an acute infection [60]. Only 20–30% of these children have documented mutations affecting perforin [60,61], and it is speculated that other modifiers or yet unrecognized defects of cytotoxicity could play a role in the remaining patients. In older patients with HLH, the "overstimulation" of the immune system may also be triggered by a microbial stimulus (secondary form). Consanguinity is not a common feature, but this sporadic form of HLH can be seen in association with malignancy, autoimmune disorders, or after organ transplant [66]. "Macrophage activation syndrome" is an alternative term sometimes used in rheumatology to describe a phenomenon similar to HLH.

Familial HLH is a heterogeneous syndrome with possibly different degrees of clinical severity. There are now at least five variants of familial HLH for which a number of mutations in the genes involved in the intracellular perforin- and granzyme-related intracellular killing homeostasis have been identified in children from various ethnic groups, with some preliminary suggestions of genotype–phenotype correlations (Table 23.3) [67–71]. The best documented are the defects in perforin synthesis (FHL2) in which absence of perforin-1 in the cytotoxic granules of NK cells can also be demonstrated immunohistochemically [68]. Expression of perforin in peripheral lymphocytes using a fluorescence activated cell sorter technique can be used as a simple and rapid screening test for confirmation of perforin deficiency in a child with clinically suspected HLH [72]. Some laboratories have recently broadened this "fast track" flow cytometry testing by screening for markers of other forms of impaired cytotoxicity (Munc and syntaxin) and X-linked proliferative syndromes, which could have clinical presentation similar to FHL2 [7].

Griscelli syndrome is another autosomal recessive form of HLH associated with variable pigment distribution, ranging from hair hypopigmentation and albinism to hyperpigmentation of sun-exposed areas. The underlying genetic defect is mutation in *RAB27A*, located at chromosome 15q21, encoding several Rab proteins involved in melanin synthesis by melanosomes in the skin melanocytes and intracellular killing in the lymphocytes [7].

A milder clinical phenotype of HLH has recently been described in patients with lysinuric protein intolerance [34]. Hyperammonemia and aminoaciduria may be suggestive of this metabolic condition, but in children presenting with acute liver failure, these findings are not helpful. A recent study demonstrated that 8 out of 29 patients with lymphoma had one or two *PRF1* mutations in the gene area linked to FHL1 [73]. This observation suggests that there is some overlap between primary and secondary HLH; some forms of secondary HLH could be related to missense mutations or polymorphisms in the perforin or other cytotoxicity genes. Production of the polypeptides may normally be unaffected but could become impaired and clinically significant in the presence of overwhelming infection, malignancy, or chronic connective tissue disorder, where secondary forms of HLH have been occasionally observed [60]. Therefore, further insight into genetic background of the late-onset forms of HLH will be required to determine whether the distinction between primary and secondary forms remains justified.

Table 23.3 Genetic variants of familial hemophagocytic lymphohistiocytosis (FHL)

	Locus	Gene	Function	Reference
FHL1	9q21.3-22	Unknown		Ohadi et al. [67]
FHL2	10q21-22	PERFORIN 1 (PRF1)	Perforin synthesis	Dufourcq-Lagelouse et al. [68]
FHL3	17q25	UNC13D	Munc 13-4 synthesis, granule priming	Feldmann et al. [69]
FHL4	6q24	STX11	Synthaxin 11 synthesis, vesicle trafficking, membrane fusion	zur Stadt et al. [70]
FHL5		STXBP2	Syntaxin- binding protein 2, Munc 18-2	Côte et al. [71]

Treatment of hemophagocytic lymphohistiocytosis

The clinical manifestations of acute HLH are invariably associated with infection [61,63]. However, the majority of symptoms are related to the effects of the overstimulated immune system and antimicrobial treatment may have a limited role [62]. Therefore, the main aim of treatment is to neutralize the effects of the ongoing overwhelming, yet inefficient, inflammatory response. Paradoxically, the initial treatment of these patients, including those who could have a primary immune defect, is with immunosuppressive agents such as epidophyllotoxin etoposide, corticosteroids and cyclosporine, in conjunction with a high-dose IVIg [63,74].

The recently modified HLH-94 treatment protocol recommends 8 weeks of initial therapy with epidophyllotoxin etoposide (150 mg/m^2 twice weekly for 2 weeks and then weekly), with daily oral cyclosporin aiming at trough levels of 200 µg/L, and dexamethasone (initially 10 mg/m^2 for 2 weeks followed by 5 mg/m^2 for 2 weeks, 2.5 mg/m^2 for 2 weeks, 1.25 mg/m^2 for 1 week, and 1 week of tapering). From week 9 onward, the maintenance therapy includes dexamethasone pulses (10 mg/m^2 for 3 days every second week) and epidophyllotoxin etoposide infusions (150 mg/m^2) on alternate weeks. Full details of the treatment protocol are available elsewhere [63]. Some children with milder forms may respond to this treatment, but severe and primary forms may require consideration for antithymocyte globulin with intrathecal methotrexate, if deemed safe on clinical grounds [74].

Children who present with liver involvement and HLH are often critically ill and need intensive supportive management [62]. Aggressive broad-spectrum antibiotic, antiviral, and antifungal treatment is given while awaiting culture results. Liposomal amphotericin B is the antifungal of choice because it is also effective against *Leishmania* sp., a common trigger for HLH in some geographic areas. Assisted mechanical ventilation is required early because of lung involvement and development of central nervous system complications. Renal support with hemofiltration or dialysis is often indicated because of impending renal failure.

In parallel with the intensive medical management, children with HLH need to be assessed for urgent diagnosis of PID and consideration for HSCT [75,76]. Familial HLH is universally relapsing and search for a familial or an unrelated donor must start immediately after diagnosis. Secondary HLH usually responds to medical treatment and does not require HSCT

[76]. Of note, asymptomatic relatives of children with primary HLH secondary to perforin deficiency (FHL2) have reduced perforin expression in their lymphocytes [72]. There is a possibility that some of these prospective donor siblings may be in a preclinical phase of the same disease, which could then be accelerated by post-HSCT immunosuppression. Therefore, unrelated donors are preferable, particularly in the absence of convincingly better results of HSCT from the familial donors [76,77]. Overall, survival at 1–3 years after HSCT is approximately 30–75% [75–77], but one single-center study reported 100% survival in 12 children with more than 2 years of follow-up [76]. Another series also reported no fatalities in 12 children, including three with mild liver involvement, after non-myeloablative HSCT [77].

Liver transplantation has traditionally been considered to be contraindicated in the acute phase of HLH because of the hyperactivated immune system, multiorgan failure, and the critical condition of the patient. The assumption was that the abnormality of the immune system would recur and promptly affect the liver graft. A case report by Matthes-Martin et al. [78] has broadened the discussion about familial HLH. A 4-month-old girl presenting with HLH-related acute liver failure initially received a living-related liver transplant from her mother, followed by myeloablation and haploidentical stem cell grafting from the same donor 70 days later. Two months later, a complete donor chimerism was obtained after a further maternal T-cell infusion, which led to a complete withdrawal of immunosuppression. The child is alive and well 5 years later (Dr. Helmut Gadner, personal communication).

X-linked lymphoproliferative disease

X-linked lymphoproliferative (XLP) disease is a rare familial condition; affected males present with fulminant, often fatal, infectious mononucleosis, B-cell lymphomas or progressive dysgammaglobulinaemia. The condition was described in the 1970s in a large US family, the Duncan kindred, in which six of the boys but none of the girls were affected, which led to the initial name (Duncan disease) [79]. In the majority, but not in all patients, the disease becomes symptomatic on acquiring EBV infection [80].

Clinically, children usually present with fever; liver involvement including hepatitis, hepatosplenomegaly, or frank liver failure; and lymphadenopathy. Female carriers can have a milder involvement. Less frequently, XLP disease can present with lymphomas and autoimmune disorders such as colitis, vasculitis, psoriasis, or Wegener granulomatosis in children younger than 5 years [81]. Histologically, the affected organs exhibit a polyclonal infiltration by EBV-infected cells, but also reactive CD4 and CD8 T-cells and sometimes hemophagocytosis [81]. Therefore, XLP disease should also be considered in the differential diagnosis of the HLH syndrome.

X-linked lymphoproliferative disease is caused by mutations in the Src homology 2 (SH2) domain-containing gene 1A (*SH2D1A*), encoding a cytoplasmic adapter called signaling lymphocytic activation molecule (SLAM)-associated protein (SAP) [82]. Cytoplasmic adapters are intracellular molecules modulating intracellular signaling processes. Aberrant reactivity within the SAP pathway induces a severe disruption of cytotoxic T-cell function, which, when triggered by EBV, leads to uncontrolled B-cell proliferation [80,82]. By positional cloning, XLP disease has been mapped to a single locus at chromosome Xq24–25 [83]. A new form called XLP2 has been reported, where mutations in XIAP (or BIRC4) encoding the X-linked inhibitor-of-apoptosis were identified in boys from three families [84]. It has been suggested that the individuals with the classic XLP (XLP1) have a more severe clinical course, including episodes of hemophagocytosis and development of lymphomas, while the patients with XLP2 are more commonly found to have splenomegaly and hemorrhagic colitis [85].

Occurrence of XLP disease may not always been triggered by EBV infection. Measles virus and *Neisseria meningitidis* have also been implicated [81]. The immune response against EBV is controlled by the primary and memory CD8 cytotoxic T-lymphocyte (CTL) reaction toward major histocompatibility complex–peptide complexes produced with EBV latent proteins: EBNA-3A, EBNA-3B, and EBNA-3C. The CTL function is genetically determined via various mechanisms, including the SAP-dependent pathway, possibly explaining the variable individual clinical response against infectious mononucleosis in immunocompetent individuals. In patients with XLP disease, the failure of CTLs to control ongoing EBV-driven B-cell proliferation may ultimately give rise to lymphoid malignancies [7].

The treatment options for XLP disease are limited. Characterization of the immune defect in an acutely unwell child usually takes longer than the fulminant course of the disease. In families with a previous positive history, it is possible to perform elective HSCT before the affected boys are exposed to EBV [7]. Novel treatments with anti-B-cell monoclonal antibodies have been shown to induce clinical benefits in patients with XLP disease [86].

A better understanding of the interaction between invading pathogens, SLAM and SAP proteins, and activation of cytotoxic T-cells will help not only in the understanding of the pathogenesis of XLP disease but potentially also of post-transplant lymphoproliferative disorder, for which EBV also represents a common trigger.

Chronic granulomatous disease

Chronic granulomatous disease is a primary neutrophil disorder caused by a defect in the production of the respiratory oxidative burst, leading to ineffective phagocytosis. About two-thirds of affected patients are boys with a mutation at chromosome Xp21, and the remaining children have a less severe, autosomal recessive form of the disease with mutations at 7q11, 1q25, or 16p25 [7,8].

Patients with chronic granulomatous disease are particularly susceptible to infections caused by catalase-producing bacteria and fungi. The failure to eradicate these infections leads to granuloma formation in the skin, liver, bone, brain, or gut. Approximately 25% of children with chronic granulomatous disease will present with hepatic abscesses [87]. One series from the UK reported a 33% incidence of newly diagnosed chronic granulomatous disease among children with pyogenic liver abscesses [88]. The diagnosis is made via a simple nitroblue–tetrazolium test in which a failure of intracytoplasmic granules to change color suggests abnormal neutrophil function. Carriers, including mothers of children with X-linked disease, will often have a history of recurrent mouth ulcers or prolonged infections and mildly abnormal nitroblue–tetrazolium tests. Following the diagnosis in a proband, the whole family should undertake screening with this test because the disease could be initially asymptomatic [7]. It is strongly recommended that chronic granulomatous disease is excluded in any child presenting with a liver abscess even in the absence of a history of pyogenic skin lesions or recurrent infections [88].

Hepatic abscesses require aspiration both for diagnostic and therapeutic purposes. The most common isolated microorganism in children is *S. aureus* [88]. Intravenous antibiotics often need to be given for several months until ultrasonographic resolution is evident and until fever and inflammatory markers, such as leukocytosis and C-reactive protein, normalize. Resistant infections may be considered for interferon-gamma treatment and infusions of purified white cells. Indefinite antimicrobial prophylaxis with itraconazole and septrin is mandatory, sometimes in association with subcutaneous interferon-gamma [87]. If this strategy fails, HSCT is increasingly being performed with satisfactory results [89].

New developments in pharmacologic manipulation of the immune response

Advances in immunopharmacology have improved the treatment of several serious conditions with presumed immune pathogenesis. Most of the new products are recombinant, thus removing past fears about incidental transmission of infectious agents. Historically, intramuscular and then IVIg supplementation was the first to modify the clinical course and prognosis of many PIDs. Immune manipulation now plays a significant role in the management of several immune-mediated conditions relevant for pediatric hepatologists, including neonatal hemochromatosis, also known as gestational alloimmune liver disease [90], aplastic anemia associated with acute liver failure [91], and giant cell Coombs-positive hepatitis [92]. In addition, the clinical phenotype of neonatal hemochromatosis has been shown to be ameliorated by maternal antenatal prophylaxis with IVIg [93]. Some transplant centers monitor serum immunoglobulin levels and aim to replace massive gastrointestinal losses after small bowel or liver transplantation with IVIgs (unpublished observation). Furthermore, IVIg is occasionally considered in sepsis or multiorgan failure complicating acute liver failure, although a recent large international study failed to observe the beneficial effects on the sepsis outcome following their use in neonates [94]. Data from the North American Studies of Pediatric Liver Transplantation group suggested that using IVIg within the first week after liver transplant leads to a reduced rate of rejection, improved graft survival and a decreased number of retransplants [95]. However, this observation has not been universally accepted and requires confirmation in further prospective studies, as its cost implications are considerable.

In the field of liver transplantation, where immune manipulation leading to immune tolerance remains an ongoing aim, use of monoclonal antibodies blocking some of the activation pathways has shown some, but not spectacular, results [96]. Between 1996 and 2006, the use of monoclonal antibodies has approximately doubled in solid organ transplantation methodology [96]. The OKT3 antibodies, targeting CD3-positive cells, were the first in use since the 1980s. Their main side effect is significant cytokine-release syndrome, characterized by fever, headaches, and gastrointestinal and neurological symptoms [96]. They have been gradually replaced by polyclonal anti-CD3 antibodies, namely anti-thymocyte globulin and anti-lymphocyte globulin. These are purified preparations of gamma-immunoglobulins raised in rabbits or horses against human thymocytes. They have been used in liver transplantation as a calcineurin inhibitor-sparing induction therapy [97] or as a rescue treatment of chronic rejection [98]. Anti-thymocyte globulin and anti-lymphocyte globulin have also been used for severe forms of aplastic anaemia, which develop in about one-third of children with cryptogenic acute liver failure [91,99], in particular in the absence of matched donors for stem cell transplantation [99]. Anecdotally, this treatment has been used for immune ablation of the donors, where severe post-hematopoietic stem cell immunological reactions were anticipated. Clearly, risks of fulminant infections short term and secondary malignancies medium to long term [100] are of concern, but better efficacy of newer anti-infective prophylaxis regimens could reduce at least the former of the problems.

Anti-IL-2 receptor antagonists (anti-CD25) such as basiliximab or daclizumab have been used for steroid- or renal-sparing effects and for enhancing immune tolerance in ABO-incompatible transplantation and retransplantation [101]. They block the α-chain of the IL-2 receptor, targeting specifically activated lymphocytes of the donor and theoretically retaining the pre-existing immune competence of the recipient [102]. One prospective study after pediatric liver transplantation compared use of the basiliximab induction with standard steroid-based antirejection protocol and reported less cellular rejection (68% versus 88%) occurring later (median 28.5 versus 10 days postoperatively). However, the infection rate was increased (72% versus 50%) and the 1-year graft survival was 6% inferior in the basiliximab cohort [103].

Anti-CD52 monoclonal antibodies (alemtuzumab, Campath-1H) are humanized preparations directed against CD52 glycoprotein receptor on the membrane of T- and B-lymphocytes, macrophages, eosinophils, NK cells, and dendritic cells. This suggests they would be ideal agents for conditioning before HSCT. Campath-1H has also been used for resistant cellular and chronic rejection after solid organ transplantation, resistant forms of giant cell Coombs-positive hepatitis of infancy [104], and steroid-resistant acute [105] and chronic [106] graft-versus-host disease. Its depletory effects on the immune cells are long lasting, often for several years. The data on prospective studies after liver transplantation are limited. The only published pediatric study using historic controls reported a reduced rate of acute rejection following induction therapy with alemtuzumab (66% versus 100%) and a much prolonged median time to acute rejection (333 days versus 25 days) [107]. In one randomized controlled study in adults, clear outcome benefits were not observed because of an increased incidence of infectious complications in the alemtuzumab cohort [108].

Rituximab (Mabtera) is a chimeric anti-CD20 monoclonal antibody that induces rapid depletion of CD20 B-lymphocytes, predominantly through the process of antibody-dependent cell-mediated cytotoxicity [109]. It has been increasingly used as adjuvant treatment for lymphomas, autoimmune and connective tissue disorders, where a key role of ongoing B-cell proliferation is assumed [110,111]. In pediatric hepatology, rituximab has become a standard treatment for EBV-driven post-transplant lymphoproliferative disease [112], but also for some presumed autoimmune conditions such as giant cell Coombs-positive hepatitis of infancy [92,113], autoimmune hemolytic anemia [114], and immune thrombocytopenia [115,116] observed postliver transplantation. Rituximab could also be considered as a rescue treatment for a newly observed phenomenon of recurrent postliver transplantation bile salt export pump deficiency-related cholestasis [117] and for refractory forms of autoimmune liver disease [110,118]. However, non-critical use of rituximab is not without its perils; late-onset neutropenia [119], HBV reactivation, and transient hypogammaglobulinemia [120] have been described after rituximab treatment, potentially rendering recipients susceptible to dramatic infectious complications such as *P. jiroveci* pneumonia [121]. It is thought that B-cell depletion after rituximab lasts approximately 6 months and is followed by a new B-cell ontogeny characterized by the appearance of immature (CD38++,CD10+,CD24+) and naive (CD27+) B-cells [110]. To minimize this temporary humoral immunity impairment, some centers advocate monitoring serum immunoglobulins after rituximab use and, if required, using short-term IVIg supplementation with *P. jiroveci* prophylaxis (unpublished personal experience). The cost–effectiveness of this strategy remains contentious.

The role of pathogen-specific, "hyperimmune," immunoglobulins in prevention or treatment of conditions such as HBV or CMV infection is not well defined [122]. There is a well-established regimen for prophylaxis of perinatally acquired HBV transmission by administering anti-HBV immunoglobulin to offspring of HBeAg-positive mothers within 2 to 3 days after the birth. Guidelines on preventing HBV reactivation from the HBV-positive liver grafts have not been established. Anti-HBV immunoglobulin is given using different expensive schedules, but recently much more in combination with various antiviral drugs.

Immune modulation is an increasingly dynamic area where technology advances will continue to offer an even more targeted manipulation of the immune response. This could be associated with risks of infectious complications in the short term and development of malignancies long term. For example, post-transplant lymphoproliferative disorder has been described more often in children exposed to immune ablation post-transplant [100]; consequently, use of immune modulation has to be carefully balanced against potential deleterious downstream effects.

References

1. Mackay IR. Hepatoimmunology: a perspective. *Immunol Cell Biol* 2002;**80**:36–44.

2. Crispe IN, Dao T, Klugewitz K, *et al.* The liver as a site of T-cell apoptosis: graveyard, or killing field? *Immunol Rev* 2000;**174**:47–62.

3. Weiler-Normann C, Rehermann B. The liver as an immunological organ. *J Gastroenterol Hepatol* 2004;**19**:S279–S283.

4. Rolando N, Wade J, Davalos M, *et al.* The systemic inflammatory response syndrome in acute liver failure. *Hepatology* 2000;**32**:734–739.

5. Tilg H, Wilmer A, Vogel W, *et al.* Serum levels of cytokines in chronic liver diseases. *Gastroenterology* 1992;**103**:264–274.

6. Izumi S, Hughes RD, Langley PG, *et al.* Extent of the acute phase response in fulminant hepatic failure. *Gut* 1994;**35**:982–986.

7. Notarangelo L. Primary immunodeficiencies. *J Allergy Clin Immunol* 2010;**125**:S182–S194.

8. Jones AM, Gaspar HB. Immunogenetics: changing the face of immunodeficiency. *J Clin Pathol* 2000;**53**:60–65.

9. Hammer SM. Management of newly diagnosed HIV infection. *N Engl J Med* 2005;**353**:1702–1710.

10. Davies EG, Thrasher AJ. Update on the hyper immunoglobulin M syndromes. *Br J Haematol* 2010;**149**:167–180.

11. Rodrigues F, Davies ED, Harrison P, *et al.* Liver disease in primary immunodeficiencies. *J Pediatr* 2004;**145**:333–339.

12. Record CO, Shilkin KB, Eddleston ALWF, Williams R. Intrahepatic sclerosing cholangitis associated with a familial immunodeficiency syndrome. *Lancet* 1973;**ii**:18–20.

13. Davis JJ, Heyman MB, Ferrell L, *et al.* Sclerosing cholangitis associated with chronic cryptosporidiosis in a child with a congenital immunodeficiency disorder. *Am J Gastroenterol* 1987;**82**:1196–1202.

14. Hayward AR, Levy J, Facchetti F, *et al.* Cholangiopathy and tumours of the pancreas, liver and biliary tree in boys with X-linked immunodeficiency with hyper-IgM. *J Immunol* 1997;**158**: 977–983.

15. McLauchlin J, Amar CFL, Pedraza-Diaz S, *et al.* Polymerase chain reaction-based diagnosis of infection with Cryptosporidium in children with primary immunodeficiencies. *Pediatr Inf Dis J* 2003;**22**:329–334.

16. Stephens J, Cosyns M, Jones M, Hayward A. Liver and bile duct pathology following *Cryptosporidium parvum* infection of the immunodeficient mice. *Hepatology* 1999;**30**:27–35.

17. Chen XM, Levine SA, Tietz P, *et al.* *Cryptosporidium parvum* is cytopathic for cultured human biliary epithelia via an apoptotic mechanism. *Hepatology* 1998;**28**:906–913.

18. Cello JP. Acquired immunodeficiency syndrome cholangiopathy: spectrum of disease. *Am J Med* 1989;**86**: 539–546.

19. Gerber DA, Green M, Jaffe R, Greenberg D, *et al.* Cryptosporidial infections after solid organ transplantation in children. *Pediatr Transplant* 2000;**4**:50–55.

20. Hadzic N, Pagliuca A, Rela M, *et al.* Correction of the hyper IgM-syndrome after liver and bone marrow transplantation. *N Engl J Med* 2000;**342**:320–324.

21. Winkelstein JA, Marino MC, Ochs H, *et al.* The X-linked hyper-IgM syndrome. Clinical and immunological features of 79 patients. *Medicine* 2003;**82**:373–384.

22. Jain A, Kovacs JA, Nelson DL *et al.* Partial immune reconstitution of X-linked hyper IgM syndrome with recombinant CD40 ligand. *Blood* 2011;**118**:3811–3817.

23. Martinez Ibanez V, Espanol T, Matamoros N, *et al.* Relapse of sclerosing cholangitis after liver transplantation in patients with hyper-IgM syndrome. *Transplant Proc* 1997;**29**:432–433.

24. Thomas C, De Saint BG, Le Deist F, *et al.* Brief report: correction of X-linked hyper-IgM syndrome by allogeneic bone marrow transplantation. *N Engl J Med* 1995;**333**:426–429.

25. Khawaja K, Gennery AR, Flood TJ, *et al.* Bone marrow transplantation for CD40 ligand deficiency: a single centre experience. *Arch Dis Child* 2001;**84**:508–511.

26. Amrolia P, Gaspar HB, Hassan A, *et al.* Nonmyeloablative stem cell transplantation for congenital immunodeficiencies. *Blood* 2000;**96**:1239–1246.

27. Jacobsohn DA, Emerick KM, Scholl P, *et al.* Nonmyeloablative hematopoietic stem cell transplant for X-linked hyper-immunoglobulin M syndrome with cholangiopathy. *Pediatrics* 2004;**113**:122–127.

28. Kahn K, Sharp H, Hunter D, Kerzner B, *et al.* Primary sclerosing cholangitis in Wiskott–Aldrich syndrome. *J Pediatr Gastroenterol Nutr* 2001;**32**:95–99.

29. Blanshard C, Shanson DC, Gazzard BG. Pilot studies of azithromycin, letrazuril and paromomycin in the treatment of Cryptosporidiosis. *Int J STD AIDS* 1997;**8**:124–129.

30. Nachbaur D, Kropshofer G, Feichtinger H, *et al.* Cryptosporidiosis after CD34-selected autologous peripheral blood stem cell transplantation (PBSCT). Treatment with paromomycin, azithromycin and recombinant human interleukin-2. *Bone Marrow Transplant* 1997;**19**:1261–1263.

31. Rosignol JF, Ayoub A, Ayers MS. Treatment of diarrhea caused by *Cryptoporidium parvum*: a prospective randomized, double-blind, placebo-controlled study of nitazoxanide. *J Infect Dis* 2001;**184**:103–106.

32. Gilger MA, Gann ME, Opekun AR, Gleason WA Jr. Efficacy of ursodeoxycholic acid in the treatment of primary sclerosing cholangitis in children. *J Pediatr Gastroenterol Nutr* 2000;**31**:136–141.

33. Bollinger ME, Arredondo-Vega FX, Santisteban I, *et al.* Brief report: hepatic dysfunction as a complication of adenosine deaminase deficiency. *N Engl J Med* 1996;**334**:1367–1371.

34. Bader-Meunier B, Parez N, Muller S. Treatment of hemophagocytic lymphohistiocytosis with cyclosporin A and steroids in a boy with lysinuric protein intolerance. *J Pediatr* 2000;**136**:134.

35. Raby RB, Ward RB, Herrod HG. Propionic academia and immunodeficiency. *J Inherit Metab Dis* 1994;**17**:250–251.

36. Moreno LA, Gottrand F, Turck D, *et al.* Severe combined immunodeficiency syndrome associated with autosomal recessive familial multiple gastrointestinal atresias: study of a family. *Am J Med Genet* 1990;**37**: 143–146.

37. Gilroy RK, Coccia PF, Talmadge JE, *et al.* Donor immune reconstitution after liver-small bowel transplantation for multiple intestinal atresia with immunodeficiency. *Blood* 2004;**103**:1171–1174.

38. Malamut G, Ziol M, Suarez F, *et al.* Nodular regenerative hyperplasia: the main liver disease in patients with primary hypogammaglobulinemia and hepatic abnormalities. *J Hepatol* 2008;**48**:74–82.

39. Fiore M, Ammendola R, Gaetaniello L, *et al.* Chronic unexplained liver disease in children with primary immunodeficiency syndromes. *J Clin Gastroenterol* 1998;**26**:187–192.

40. Selik RM, Lindegren ML. Changes in deaths reported with human immunodeficiency virus infection among United States children less than thirteen years old, 1987 through 1999. *Pediatr Infect Dis J* 2003;**22**:635–641.

41. Fontana M, Boldorini R, Zuin G, *et al.* Ultrastructural changes in duodenal mucosa of HIV-infected children. *J Pediatr Gastroenterol Nutr* 1993;**17**:255–259.

42. Duffy LF, Daum F, Kahn E, *et al.* Hepatitis in children with acquired immune deficiency syndrome: histopathologic and immunocytologic features. *Gastroenterology* 1986;**90**: 173–181.

43. Morotti RA, Tata M, Drut R, *et al.* Liver pathology in children with AIDS: a comparison between the South American and North American population. *Pediatr Pathol Mol Med* 2001;**20**:537–545.

44. Lacaille F, Fournet JC, Blanche S. Clinical utility of liver biopsy in children with acquired immunodeficiency syndrome. *Pediatr Infect Dis J* 1999;**18**:143–147.

45. Bouche H, Housset C, Dumont JL, *et al.* AIDS-related cholangitis: diagnostic features and course in 15 patients. *J Hepatol* 1993;**17**:34–39.

46. Chung CJ, Sivit CJ, Rakusan TA, *et al.* Hepatobiliary abnormalities on sonography in children with HIV infection. *J Ultrasound Med* 1994;**13**:205–210.

47. Clark SJ, Creighton S, Portmann B, *et al.* Acute liver failure associated with antiretroviral treatment for HIV: a report of six cases. *J Hepatol* 2002;**36**:295–301.

48. Church JA, Mitchell WG, Gonzales-Gomes I, *et al.* Mitochondrial DNA depletion, near-fatal metabolic acidosis, and liver failure in an HIV-infected child treated with combination antiretroviral therapy. *J Pediatr* 2001;**138**:748–751.

49. Neff GW, Bonham A, Tzakis AG, *et al.* Orthotopic liver transplantation in patients with human immunodeficiency virus and end-stage liver disease. *Liver Transplant* 2003;**9**:239–247.

50. Martin P, DiBisceglie AM, Kassianides C, *et al.* Rapidly progressive non-A non-B hepatitis in patients with human immunodeficiency virus infection. *Gastroenterology* 1989;**97**:1559–1561.

51. Housset C, Pol S, Carnot F, *et al.* Interactions between human immunodeficiency virus-1, hepatitis delta virus and hepatitis B virus infections in 260 chronic carriers of hepatitis B virus. *Hepatology* 1992;**15**:578–583.

52. Resti M, Azzari C, Bortolotti F. Hepatitis C virus infection in children coinfected with HIV: epidemiology and management. *Pediatr Drugs* 2002;**4**:571–580.

53. Puoti M, Torti C, Bruno R, *et al.* Natural history of chronic hepatitis B in co-infected patients. *J Hepatol* 2006;**44**: S65–S70.

54. Benhamou Y. Treatment algorithm for chronic hepatitis B in HIV-infected patients. *J Hepatol* 2006;**44**:S90–S94.

55. Lau G, Suri D, Liang R, *et al.* Resolution of chronic hepatitis B and anti-HBs seroconversion in humans by adoptive transfer of immunity to hepatitis B core antigen. *Gastroenterology* 2002;**122**:614–624.

56. Quinti I, Pandolfi F, Paganelli R, *et al.* HCV infection in patients with primary defects of immunoglobulin production. *Clin Exp Immunol* 1995;**102**:11–16.

57. Bjoro K, Froland SS, Yun Z, *et al.* Hepatitis C infection in patients with primary hypogammaglobulinemia after treatment with contaminated immune globulin. *N Engl J Med* 1994;**331**: 1607–1611.

58. Smith MSH, Webster DB, Dhillon AP, *et al.* Orthotopic liver transplantation for chronic hepatitis in two patients with common variable immunodeficiency. *Gastroenterology* 1995;**108**:879–884.

59. Gow PJ, Mutimer D. Successful outcome of liver transplantation in a patient with hepatitis C and common variable immune deficiency. *Transplant Int* 2002;**15**:380–383.

60. Filipovich AH. Hemophagocytic lymphohistiocytosis and other hemophagocytic disorders. *Immunol Allergy Clin N Am* 2008;**28**:293–313.

61. Freeman HR, Ramanan AV. Review of haemophagocytic lymphohistiocytosis. *Arch Dis Child* 2011;**96**:688–693.

62. Hirst WJ, Layton DM, Singh S, *et al.* Haemophagocytic lymphohistiocytosis: experience at two U.K. centres. *Br J Haematol* 1994;**88**:731–739.

63. Henter JI, Horne A, Arico M, *et al.* HLH-2004: diagnostic and therapeutic guidelines for hemophagocytic lymphohistiocytosis. *Pediatr Blood Cancer* 2007;**48**:124–131.

64. Farquhar JW, Claireaux AE. Familial haemophagocytic reticulosis. *Arch Dis Child* 1952;**27**:519–525.

65. Arico M, Danesino C, Pende D, Moretta L. Pathogenesis of haemophagocytic lymphohistiocytosis. *Br J Haematol* 2001;**114**:761–769.

66. Chisuwa H, Hashikura Y, Nakazawa Y, *et al.* Fatal hemophagocytic syndrome after living-related liver transplantation: a report of two cases. *Transplantation* 2001;**72**:1843–1846.

67. Ohadi M, Lalloz MR, Sham P, *et al.* Localization of a gene for familial hemophagocytic lymphohistiocytosis at chromosome 9q21.3–22 by homozygosity mapping. *Am J Hum Genet* 1999;**64**:165–171.

68. Dufourcq-Lagelouse R, Jabado N, Le Deist F, *et al.* Linkage of familial hemophagocytic lymphohistiocytosis to 10q21–22 and evidence for heterogeneity. *Am J Hum Genet* 1999;**64**:172–179.

69. Feldmann J, Callebaut I, Raposo G, *et al.* Munc13-4 is essential for cytolytic granules fusion and is mutated in a form of familial hemophagocytic lymphohistiocytosis (FHL3). *Cell* 2003;**115**:461–473.

70. zur Stadt U, Schmidt S, Kasper B, *et al.* Linkage of familial hemophagocytic lymphohistiocytosis (FHL) type-4 to chromosome 6q24 and identification of mutations in syntaxin 11. *Hum Mol Gen* 2005;**14**:827–834.

71. Côte M, Ménager MM, Burgess A, *et al.* Munc18-2 deficiency causes familial hemophagocytic lymphohistiocytosis type 5 and impairs cytotoxic granule exocytosis in patient NK cells. *J Clin Invest* 2009;**119**:3765–3773.

72. Kogawa K, Lee SM, Villanueva J, *et al.* Perforin expression in cytotoxic lymphocytes from patients with hemophagocytic lymphohistiocytosis and their family members. *Blood* 2002;**99**:61–66.

73. Clementi R, Locatelli F, Dupre L, *et al.* A proportion of patients with lymphoma may harbor mutations of the perforin gene. *Blood* 2005;**105**:4424–4428.

74. Stephan JL, Donadieu J, Ledeist F, *et al.* Treatment of familial hemophagocytic lymphohistiocytosis with antithymocyte globulins, steroids, and cyclosporin A. *Blood* 1993;**82**: 2319–2323.

75. Fischer A, Cerf-Bensussan N, Blanche S, *et al.* Allogeneic bone marrow transplantation for erythrophagocytic lymphohistiocytosis. *J Pediatr* 1986;**108**:267–270.

76. Durken M, Horstmann M, Bieling P, *et al.* Improved outcome in haemophagocytic lymphohistiocytosis after bone marrow transplantation from related and unrelated donors: a single-centre experience of 12 patients. *Br J Haematol* 1999;**106**:1052–1058.

77. Cooper N, Rao K, Gilmour K, *et al.* Stem cell transplantation with reduced intensity conditioning for haemophagocytic lymphohistiocytosis. *Blood* 2006;**107**:1233–1236.

78. Matthes-Martin S, Peters C, Koningsrainer A, *et al.* Successful stem cell transplantation following liver transplantation from the same haploidentical family donor in a girl with hemophagocytic lymphohistiocytosis. *Blood* 2000;**96**:3997–3999.

79. Purtilo DT, Cassel CK, Yang JPS, *et al.* X-linked recessive progressive combined variable immunodeficiency (Duncan's disease). *Lancet* 1975;**i**: 935–941.

80. Howie D, Sayos J, Terhorst C, Morra M. The gene defective in X-linked lymphoproliferative disease controls T cell dependent immune surveillance against Epstein–Barr virus. *Curr Opin Immunol* 2000;**12**:474–478.

81. Nichols KE, Ma CS, Cannons JL, *et al.* Molecular and cellular pathogenesis of X-linked lymphoproliferative disease. *Immunol Rev* 2005;**203**:180–199.

82. Sayos J, Wu C, Morra M, *et al.* The X linked lymphoproliferative: disease gene product SAP regulates signals induced through the co-receptor SLAM. *Nature* 1998;**395**:462–469.

83. Skare JC, Sullivan JL, Milunsky A. Mapping the mutation causing the X-linked lymphoproliferative syndrome in relation to restriction fragment length polymorphisms on Xq. *Hum Genet* 1989;**82**:349–353.

84. Rigaud S, Fondaneche MC, Lambert N, *et al.* XIAP deficiency in humans causes an X-linked lymphoproliferative syndrome. *Nature* 2006;**444**:110–114.

85. Paclopnik Schmid J, Canioni D, Moshous D, *et al.* Clinical similarities and differences of patients with X-linked lymphoproliferative syndrome type 1 (XLP-1/SAP deficiency) versus type 2 (XLP-2/XIAP deficiency). *Blood* 2011;**117**:1522–1529.

86. Milone MC, Tsai DE, Hodinka RL, *et al.* Treatment of primary Epstein–Barr virus infection in patients with X-linked lymphoproliferative disease using B-cell-directed therapy. *Blood* 2005;**105**:994–996.

87. Finn A, Hadzic N, Morgan G, Strobel S, Levinsky RJ. Prognosis of chronic granulomatous disease. *Arch Dis Child* 1990;**65**:942–945.

88. Muorah M, Hinds R, Verma A, *et al.* Liver abscesses in children in the developed world: a single centre experience. *J Pediatr Gastroenterol Nutr* 2006;**42**:201–206.

89. Gungor T, Halter J, Klink A, *et al.* Successful low toxicity hematopoietic stem cell transplantation for high-risk adult chronic granulomatous disease patients. *Transplantation* 2005;**79**:1596–1606.

90. Rand EB, Karpen SJ, Kelly S, *et al.* Treatment of neonatal hemochromatosis with exchange transfusion and intravenous immunoglobulin. *J Pediatr* 2009;**155**:566–571.

91. Tung J, Hadzic N, Layton M, *et al.* Bone marrow failure in children with acute liver failure. *J Pediatr Gastroenterology Nutr* 2000;**31**:557–561.

92. Maggiore G, Sciveres M, Fabre M, *et al.* Giant cell hepatitis with autoimmune hemolytic anemia in early childhood: long-term outcome in 16 children. *J Pediatr* 2011;**159**:127–132.

93. Whitington PF, Kelly S. Outcome of pregnancies at risk for neonatal hemochromatosis is improved by treatment with high-dose intravenous immunoglobulin. *Pediatrics* 2008;**121**: e1615–e1621.

94. INIS Collaborative Group. Treatment of neonatal sepsis with intravenous immune globulin. *N Engl J Med* 2011;**365**:1201–1211.

95. Bucuvalas JC, Anand R; Studies of the Pediatric Liver Transplantation Research Group. Treatment with immunoglobulin improves outcome for pediatric liver transplant recipients. *Liver Transplant* 2009;**15**:1564–1569.

96. Krischock L, Marks SD. Induction therapy: why, when, and which agent? *Pediatr Transplant* 2010;**14**:298–313.

97. Soliman T, Hetz H, Burghuber C, *et al.* Short-term induction therapy with anti-thymocyte globulin and delayed use of calcineurin inhibitors in orthotopic liver transplantation. *Liver Transplant* 2007;**13**:1039–1044.

98. Kerkar N, Morotti RA, Iyer K, *et al.* Anti-lymphocyte therapy successfully controls late "cholestatic" rejection in pediatric liver transplant recipients. *Clin Transplant* 2011;**25**:E584–E591.

99. Hadžić N, Height S, Ball S, *et al.* Evolution in the management of acute liver failure-associated aplastic anaemia in children: a single centre experience. *J Hepatol* 2008;**48**:68–73.

100. Norin S, Kimby E, Ericzon BG, *et al.* Posttransplant lymphoma: a single-center experience of 500 liver transplantations. *Med Oncol* 2004;**21**:273–284.

101. Hale DA. Biological effects of induction immunosuppression. *Curr Opin Immunol* 2004;**16**:565–570.

102. Spada M, Petz W, Bertani A, *et al.* Randomized trial of basiliximab induction versus steroid therapy in pediatric liver allograft recipients under tacrolimus immunosuppression. *Am J Transplant* 2006;**6**:1913–1921.

103. Rovelli A, Corti P, Beretta C, *et al.* Alemtuzumab for giant cell hepatitis with autoimmune hemolytic anemia. *J Pediatr Gastroenterol Nutr* 2007;**45**:596–599.

104. Schub N, Günther A, Schrauder A, *et al.* Therapy of steroid-refractory acute GVHD with CD52 antibody alemtuzumab is effective. *Bone Marrow Transplant* 2011;**46**:143–147.

105. Gutierrez-Aguirre CH, Cantu'-Rodriguez OG, Borjas-Almaguer OD, *et al.* Effectiveness of subcutaneous low-dose alemtuzumab and rituximab combination therapy for steroid-resistant chronic graft-versus-host disease. *Haematologica* 2012;**97**:717–722.

106. Kato T, Selvaggi G, Panagiotis T, *et al.* Pediatric liver transplant with campath 1H induction: preliminary report. *Transplant Proc* 2006;**38**:3609–3611.

107. Levitsky J, Thudi K, Ison MG, *et al.* Alemtuzumab induction in non-hepatitis C positive liver transplant recipients. *Liver Transplant* 2011;**17**:32–37.

108. Taylor RP, Lindorfer MA. Immunotherapeutic mechanisms of anti-CD20 monoclonal antibodies. *Curr Opin Immunol* 2008;**20**:444–449.

109. Cooper N, Arnold DM. The effect of rituximab on humoral and cell mediated immunity and infection in the treatment of autoimmune diseases. *Br J Haematol* 2010;**149**:3–13.

110. Gobert D, Bussel JB, Cunningham-Rundles C, *et al.* Efficacy and safety of rituximab in common variable immunodeficiency-associated immune cytopenias: a retrospective multicentre study on 33 patients. *Br J Haematol* 2011;**155**:498–508.

111. Messahel B, Taj MM, Hobson R, *et al.* Single agent efficacy of rituximab in childhood immunosuppression related lymphoproliferative disease: a United Kingdom Children's Cancer Study Group (UKCCSG) retrospective review. *Leuk Lymphoma* 2006;**47**:2584–2589.

112. Miloh T, Manwani D, Morotti R, *et al.* Giant cell hepatitis and autoimmune hemolytic anemia successfully treated with rituximab. *J Pediatr Gastroenterol Nutr* 2007;**44**:634–636.

113. Czubkowski P, Williams M, Bagia S, Kelly D, Gupte G. Immune-mediated hemolytic anemia in children after liver and small bowel transplantation. *Liver Transplant* 2011;**17**:921–924.

114. Shores D, Kobak G, Pegram LD, Whitington PF, Shneider BL. Giant cell hepatitis and immune thrombocytopenic purpura: reversal of liver failure with rituximab therapy. *J Pediatr Gastroenterol Nutr* 2011.

115. Miloh T, Arnon R, Roman E, *et al.* Autoimmune hemolytic anemia and idiopathic thrombocytopenic purpura in pediatric solid organ transplant recipients, report of five cases and review of the literature. *Pediatr Transplant* 2011;**15**:870–878.

116. Siebold L, Dick AA, Thompson R, *et al.* Recurrent low gamma-glutamyl transpeptidase cholestasis following liver transplantation for bile salt export pump (BSEP) disease (posttransplant recurrent BSEP disease). *Liver Transplant* 2010;**16**:856–863.

117. Tsuda M, Moritoki Y, Lian ZX, *et al.* Biochemical and immunologic effects of rituximab in primary biliary cirrhosis patients with an incomplete response to ursodeoxycholic acid. *Hepatology* 2012;**55**:512–521.

118. Wolach O, Shpilberg O, Lahav M. Neutropenia after rituximab treatment: new insights on a late complication. *Curr Opin Hematol* 2012;**19**:32–38.

119. Cambridge G, Leandro MJ, Teodorescu M, *et al.* B cell depletion therapy in systemic lupus erythematosus: effect on autoantibody and antimicrobial antibody profiles. *Arthritis Rheum* 2006;**54**:3612–3622.

120. Kolstad A, Holte H, Fossa A, Lauritzsen GF, Gaustad P, Torfoss D. Pneumocystis jirovecii pneumonia in B-cell lymphoma patients treated with the rituximab-CHOEP-14 regimen. *Haematologica* 2007;**92**:139–140.

121. Green M, Michaels MG, Katz BZ, *et al.* CMV-IVIG for prevention of Epstein–Barr virus disease and posttransplant lymphoproliferative disease in pediatric liver transplant recipients. *Am J Transplant* 2006;**6**:1906–1912.

122. Patterson SJ, Angus PW. Post-liver transplant hepatitis B prophylaxis: the role of oral nucleos(t)ide analogues. *Curr Opin Organ Transplant* 2009;**14**:225–230.

Chapter

24

Laboratory diagnosis of inborn errors of metabolism

Piero Rinaldo

Introduction

Inborn errors of metabolism are recognized with increasing frequency as a cause of disease manifestations in every organ and at every life interval from the fetus to the geriatric patient. Yet, their collective incidence is often underestimated, and diagnostic errors often occur, leading to devastating consequences for patients and their families, including criminal charges [1]. Among an increasing number of single gene disorders that are currently recognized, inborn errors of the intermediate metabolism of amino acids, carbohydrates, and fatty acids deserve special attention. The majority of these diseases have been identified within the past 30 years, primarily through the detection of endogenous metabolites abnormally accumulating in biologic fluids [2]. This chapter will focus predominantly on the laboratory diagnosis of three major groups of metabolic diseases: organic acidurias, congenital lactic acidemias, and disorders of fatty acid oxidation (FAO). Aspects of urea cycle defects and amino acid disorders will be covered to a lesser extent.

The inborn errors listed in Table 24.1 share a common natural history, which is the occurrence of either acute life-threatening illness in early infancy or unexplained developmental delay with intercurrent episodes of metabolic decompensation in later childhood. Unfortunately, the clinical presentations of these diseases are often attributed to a variety of other causes:

- accidental ingestion
- cerebral palsy
- child abuse (including Munchausen-by-proxy syndrome)
- cyclic vomiting syndrome
- developmental delay
- intraventricular brain hemorrhage
- Reye syndrome
- seizure disorder
- sepsis
- sudden infant death syndrome
- sudden unexpected death in early life (attributed to infections)
- murder.

Table 24.1 Most common inborn errors of metabolism associated with acute life-threatening illness

	Types/examples
Organic acidurias	Defects of branched-chain amino acid metabolism
Congenital lactic acidemias	Pyruvate oxidation defects Gluconeogenesis defects Krebs cycle defects Respiratory chain defects
Disorders of fatty acid transport and oxidation	Defects of membrane-bound enzymes and transporters Defects of mitochondrial matrix enzymes
Urea cycle disorders	Ornithine transcarbamylase, carbamylphosphate synthetase deficiency
Amino acid disorders	Maple syrup urine disease Non-ketotic hyperglycinemia

Indeed, once a patient is properly diagnosed with a metabolic condition, it is not uncommon to retrospectively find that a sibling within the same family presented with similar symptoms but had passed away without a precise diagnosis, not to mention criminal proceedings.

Two major misconceptions stand behind the frequent failure of correctly diagnosing a metabolic disorder: (1) that a high degree of specialization is needed in order to suspect and initially manage acutely ill patients with inborn errors of metabolism, and (2) that very expensive analytical instruments are required to undertake a diagnostic challenge of this apparent magnitude. However, even today, in what has been called the genomic era, specific training in metabolic genetic diseases receives marginal coverage in the curriculum of medical students and pediatric residents at many academic institutions. This situation is disconcerting because newborns and infants

Liver Disease in Children, Fourth Edition, ed. Frederick J. Suchy, Ronald J. Sokol, and William F. Balistreri. Published by Cambridge University Press. © Cambridge University Press 2014.

with life-threatening illnesses of the type covered here are initially placed under the responsibility of either a general practitioner or a pediatric subspecialist, and rarely immediately into the hands of a metabolic specialist.

The aim of this chapter is to emphasize that a methodical use of routine laboratory tests supplemented by one or two specialized investigations should allow a prompt biochemical diagnosis of patients affected with one of these metabolic diseases, preventing serious sequelae or almost inevitable death. Although effective treatment for many metabolic disorders remains unavailable or unaffordable in terms of financial requirements, ample evidence has demonstrated that a growing number of these diseases can be treated effectively and efficiently [3]. Therefore, high morbidity and mortality should not be systematically assumed in reference to these inborn errors of intermediate metabolism.

Recognition of signs and symptoms

The clinical aspects of metabolic disorders with primary hepatic disease are specifically addressed in Section IV of this book. For a better understanding of the diagnostic process generally pertinent to these and other conditions, a brief recapitulation of the cardinal clinical findings of these disorders is necessary to put the laboratory analyses to be described in a practical perspective.

Although the final diagnosis of a specific inborn error of metabolism is a laboratory process, several clinical elements should effectively raise the level of suspicion in that diagnostic direction. Saudubray [4] delineated several pathophysiologic patterns of clinical presentation, the recognition of which may provide valuable diagnostic signs. The clinical picture in a newborn or infant that is dominated by severe neurologic deterioration is more informative than might be assumed from the notion that limited, stereotyped responses are evoked by several different causes (sepsis, encephalitis, ingestion, Reye syndrome, and others). In the neonatal period, a patient who becomes rapidly comatose after a variable (hours to days) symptom-free period could be clinically categorized as being in an intoxication-type of neurologic distress. By comparison, the absence of a symptom-free period associated with a delayed evolution of coma is rather indicative of an energy-deficit type of neurologic distress. In both cases, a failure to respond to symptomatic therapy, followed by rapid deterioration of an infant's general status, is a typical manifestation of certain types of metabolic disease. Many organic acidemias, urea cycle disorders, and selected disorders of amino acid metabolism belong to the former category, and primary lactic acidemias, mitochondrial FAO disorders pertain to the latter. Additional stratification of clinical symptoms can also be beneficial: the presence of cardiac failure and other functional heart disorders are characteristic for FAO disorders and mitochondrial diseases. Lastly, if persistent hypoglycemia and liver

dysfunction are the most prominent features observed for a patient, these findings would suggest a possible disorder of carbohydrate metabolism, such as glycogenosis type I or III, fructose intolerance, or galactosemia. These disorders are discussed elsewhere in this book.

Routine laboratory investigations

Table 24.2 lists the basic laboratory investigations that are recommended when a clinical picture compatible with an inborn error of metabolism has been recognized. Recognition of a diagnostic pattern, potentially within hours from the time of admission, may allow the implementation of adequate therapeutic measures pending confirmation of the preliminary diagnosis by specialized laboratory investigations [2]. Although blood gases, electrolytes, and glucose are routinely part of the evaluation of any acutely ill child, ammonia, lactate, and pyruvate are not consistently requested at admission. In urine, the qualitative determination of 3-keto acids by a commercial dip strip (e.g. Chemstrip; Roche Diagnostics, Basel, Switzerland) and 2-keto acids by the dinitrophenylhydrazine test can be performed at bedside in the early stage of evaluation of an acutely ill patient. A guideline for diagnostic orientation by routine laboratory investigations is shown in Table 24.3 and discussed in the context of each specific group of disorders. Obviously, partial deviations from a model pattern are always possible, in light of the variable nature of a particular metabolic block, and the role that environmental factors play in individual patients.

Other simple manual tests that could aid the differential diagnosis of other disorders in acutely ill patients include the detection in urine of reducing substances and sulfites. A positive reducing substances test (Clinitest, Bayer AG, Leverkusen, Germany) may be indicative for galactosemia or hereditary fructose intolerance. Gross galactosuria, however, also may occur in patients with severe liver disease of any origin, and false negative reactions for reducing substances have been observed in symptomatic newborns with galactosemia [5]. Qualitative detection of sulfites in fresh urine (Merkoquant 10013 Sulfit Test or Macherey-Nagel Quantofix

Table 24.2 Routine laboratory investigations in the initial evaluation of patients with inborn errors of metabolism

Medium	Tests
Serum	Blood gases, electrolytes
	Glucose, ammonia, uric acid
	Lactic acid, pyruvic acid (L:P ratio)
	Ketone bodies (3-hydroxybutyrate/acetoacetate ratio)
Urine	Ketone bodies (3-keto acids)
	2-Keto acids (dinitrophenylhydrazine test)
	Reducing substances
	Sulfites
	Dinitrophenylhydrazine

Table 24.3 Interpretation of routine laboratory investigations for the diagnosis of inborn errors of metabolism

	Organic acidurias	Primary lactic acidemias				Fatty acid oxidation disorders	Urea cycle disorders	Amino acid disorders	
		Pyruvate oxidation	Gluconeogenesis	Pyruvate carboxylase	Respiratory chain			MSUD	NKHG
Approximate number of IEMs	>50	7	3	3	>100	23	8	4	1
Neurologic distress	I	ED	ED	ED	ED	ED	I	I	I
Metabolic acidosis	+++	+++	+++	+++	+++	+	–	–	–
3-Keto aciduria (ketone bodies)	+++	–	+	++	++	–	–	+	–
2-Keto aciduria (DNPH positive)	–	+++	–	+	–	–	–	+++	–
Hyperammonemia	+	+	+	+++	+	+	+++	–	–
Hypoglycemia	+	–	+++	+	+	+++	–	–	–
Lactic acidemia	+	+++ (permanent)	+++ (intermittent (fasting))	+++ (permanent)	+++ (permanent (fed))	+	–	–	–
Lactate:pyruvate ratio		<15	>20	>30	>50				
3-Hydroxybutyrate/ acetoacetate ratio		>2	>2	<1	>3				

DNPH, dinitrophenylhydrazine; IEM, inborn error of metabolism; MSUD, maple syrup urine disease; NKHG, non-ketotic hyperglycinemia; I, intoxication type; ED, energy deficiency type of neurologic distress; +, possibly present; +++, typically present with high diagnostic significance; –, not typically present.

SO3, Gallard Schlesinger, New York, USA) from a patient presenting with severe neurologic distress, lactic acidosis, and hypouricemia is indicative of a diagnosis of molybdenum cofactor deficiency [6].

Specialized laboratory investigations

On admission, special consideration should be given to the immediate collection and proper storage of urine and blood samples from patients in severe decompensation. These samples may not be available postmortem, or material collected even after a partial recovery may not show certain diagnostic abnormalities otherwise detectable, or more easily detectable, under acute conditions. Any volume of urine (stored at –20°C with no preservatives, or even a wet diaper obtained at the emergency room) and plasma/serum (≤0.5 mL, stored at –20°C) should be considered adequate for testing. Alternatively, a blood spot on filter paper could provide enough material for one or more of the specialized laboratory investigations described later in this chapter. In case of death, collection of body fluids and tissues should be secured according to available protocols [7].

Quantitative profiling of amino acids, carnitine, and acylcarnitines in plasma, as well as urine organic acids and acylglycines, is the analysis of choice to reach a biochemical diagnosis for the vast majority of these disorders. There are, of course, indications, advantages, and limitations to these tests in the differential diagnosis of each group of inborn errors of metabolism. Furthermore, the provision of a detailed interpretation is essential [8], because a biochemical genetics service differs from a conventional clinical chemistry laboratory in the expectation to provide an overview of abnormal and relative negative results (i.e. ketotic versus non-ketotic dicarboxylic aciduria, methylmalonic aciduria with or without homocystinuria), to quantify pertinent abnormal compounds whenever possible, correlate available clinical information, explain the elements of the differential diagnosis, provide recommendations for additional biochemical testing and in vitro confirmatory studies (enzyme assay, molecular analysis), give the name and phone number of key contacts who may provide these studies, and provide a phone number for the laboratory director in case a referring physician has additional questions.

Group I: organic acidurias

Organic acids are water-soluble compounds containing one or more carboxyl groups as well as other functional groups (keto, hydroxy) and form the intermediate metabolites of all major groups of organic cellular components: amino acids, lipids, carbohydrates, nucleic acids, and steroids. Organic acidurias are a biochemically heterogeneous group of inborn errors of metabolism biochemically characterized by the accumulation of metabolites that either are not present under physiologic conditions (formed from activation of alternative pathways in response to the loss of function of a specific gene product) or are pathologic amounts of normal metabolites [9]. These disorders share a common natural history, which is the occurrence of either acute life-threatening illness in early infancy or unexplained developmental delay with intercurrent episodes of metabolic decompensation in later childhood. The incidence of individual inborn errors of organic acid metabolism varies from 1 in 10 000 to less than 1 in 1 000 000 live births. However, their collective incidence approximates 1 in 3000 live births. This estimation does not include other inborn errors of metabolism (i.e. amino acid disorders, urea cycle disorders, congenital lactic acidemias) for which diagnosis and monitoring also require organic acid analysis. All possible disease entities included, the incidence of conditions in which informative organic acid profiles could be detected in urine is likely to approach 1 in 1000 live births.

A situation of severe and persistent metabolic acidosis of unexplained origin, elevated anion gap, and severe neurologic manifestations should always be considered as a strong diagnostic indicator for one of these diseases, findings that warrant immediate verification and should not be postponed, as occurs frequently, when more common causes have been ruled out. The presence of ketonuria, occasionally massive, provides an important clue toward the recognition of disorders such as methylmalonic aciduria, propionic aciduria, and isovaleric aciduria, particularly in the neonatal period. Hyperammonemia, hypoglycemia, and hyperlactacidemia are frequently associated findings, particularly during acute episodes of metabolic decompensation. Plasma amino acid analysis may provide only limited and generally non-specific information for enzyme deficiencies affecting distal steps of amino acid catabolism. Therefore, the biochemical diagnosis of individual organic acidemias ultimately relies on urine organic acid analysis by gas chromatography/mass spectrometry (GC/MS) [9]. Detection, positive identification, and eventually quantification of pathognomonic organic acids by GC/MS could be available in a matter of hours if the analysis is performed at a local laboratory. Otherwise, results from a referral laboratory should be available within 24 hours for an urgent case.

A large proportion of organic acidurias known to date affect the intermediate metabolism of the essential branched-chain amino acids isoleucine, leucine, and valine. The diagnostic specificity of organic acid analysis under acute and asymptomatic conditions is outlined for individual defects in Table 24.4 [10]. Informative profiles may not always be detected in disorders where the excretion of diagnostic metabolites depends on the residual activity of the defective enzyme, the dietary load of precursors, or the anabolic status of a patient. In some cases, methods with higher specificity and sensitivity, such as acylcarnitine determination by electrospray ionization-tandem MS [11] and acylglycine determination by GC/MS stable isotope dilution analysis [9], can overcome the limitations of standard organic acid analysis to assess patients who are not acutely ill. However, these tests are rarely needed to diagnose the most frequent and acute organic acidurias.

Group II: congenital lactic acidemias

A classification of enzyme defects leading to a primary lactic acidemia is shown in Table 24.5. In addition to a clinical picture of energy deficiency neurologic distress [4], a marked elevation in blood or cerebrospinal fluid (CSF) lactate concentrations warrant special attention. This should not be assumed to indicate a phenomenon secondary to sepsis, peripheral hypoxia, or merely suboptimal sampling of a patient under severely compromised conditions. Any unexplained occurrence of hyperlactacidemia should be systematically investigated by evaluation of the parameters shown in Table 24.2, particularly the simultaneous determination of serum lactate and pyruvate.

Obtaining a plasma lactate:pyruvate (L:P) ratio (normal values in fed state, <15) [12] may be highly informative in acutely ill patients. However, a reliable measurement demands accurate specimen sampling for both lactate and pyruvate obtained at the same time as well as laborious processing of collected specimens. Lactic acidemia with a normal L:P ratio is indicative of disorders of the pyruvate dehydrogenase (PDH) complex; lactic acidemia with a high L:P ratio is indicative of either pyruvate carboxylase deficiency, one of four known gluconeogenesis defects, or a mitochondrial respiratory chain defect. In the latter, the L:P ratio could be markedly elevated. A possible diagnosis of pyruvate carboxylase deficiency may be corroborated by documenting a decreased 3-hydroxybutyrate: acetoacetate ratio (normal values in fed state, 1.0–1.5), which occurs from the consequence of forced accumulation of reducing equivalents (NADH) in the cytosolic compartment via malate–aspartate shuttling. The oxidized status of the mitochondrial matrix halts the reduction of acetoacetate to 3-hydroxybutyrate, a functional block reflected by a decrease of their relative ratio in blood. In respiratory chain disorders affecting the liver, the 3-hydroxybutyrate:acetoacetate ratio is typically elevated.

Ketonuria is more commonly observed in a primary rather than secondary lactic acidemia, and hyperammonemia can be a key element in the recognition of the cross-reacting material-negative form of pyruvate carboxylase deficiency [13], a defect of gluconeogenesis with typical diagnostic features also at the amino acid level, as described below. Other gluconeogenesis defects present with hypoglycemia as the dominant sign in

Table 24.4 Organic acidurias: diagnostic significance of organic acid, acylcarnitine, and acylglycine analysis[a]

Common name	Enzyme deficiency	Organic acids (also newborn screening)		Acylcarnitines	Acylglycines[b]
		Acute	Asymptomatic		
Branched-chain amino acid metabolism					
Isovaleric aciduria	Isovaleryl-CoA dehydrogenase	+	+	+	+
3-Methylcrotonylglycinuria	3-Methylcrotonyl-CoA carboxylase	+	–	+	+[c]
3-Methylglutaconic aciduria	3-Methylglutaconyl-CoA hydratase	+	+	+	0
3-Hydroxy 3-methylglutaric aciduria	3-Hydroxy 3-methylglutaryl-CoA lyase	+	+	+	0
2-Methylacetoacetic aciduria	2-Methylacetoacetyl-CoA thiolase	+	–	+	+
3-Hydroxyisobutyric aciduria	3-Hydroxyisobutyryl-CoA dehydrogenase	+	+	0	0
	Methylmalonyl/malonyl semialdehyde dehydrogenase	+	–	0	0
Propionic aciduria	Propionyl-CoA carboxylase	+	+	+	+
Methylmalonic aciduria	Methylmalonyl-CoA mutase	+	+	+	+[d]
Methylmalonic aciduria	Cobalamin metabolism (multiple defects)	+	+	+	+[d]
	Succinyl-CoA transferase	+	+	0	0
Malonic aciduria	Malonyl-CoA decarboxylase	+	–	+	0
Miscellaneous					
Ethylmalonic encephalopathy	ETHE1 (unknown function)	+	+	+	+
Glutaric aciduria type I	Glutaryl-CoA dehydrogenase	+	+	+	+
D-2-Hydroxy glutaric aciduria	Unknown	+	–	0	0
L-2-Hydroxyglutaric aciduria	Unknown	+	–	0	0
2-Ketoadipic aciduria	2-Ketoadipic dehydrogenase	+	–	0	0
4-Hydroxybutyric aciduria	Succinic semialdehyde dehydrogenase	+	–	0	0
Hyperoxaluria type I	Alanine:glyoxylate aminotransferase	+	+	0	0
Hyperoxaluria type II	D-Glyceric dehydrogenase	+	+	0	0
Glyceroluria	Glycerol kinase	+	+	0	0
Pyroglutamic aciduria	Glutathione synthetase	+	+[e]	0	0
Alcaptonuria	Homogentisic acid oxidase	+	+	0	0
Mevalonic aciduria	Mevalonic synthetase	+	+	0	0

[a] Acute analysis of a urine sample collected during an episode of metabolic decompensation; asymptomatic, analysis of a urine sample collected in clinical remission; +, diagnostic profile; –, possible occurrence of an uninformative urinary organic acid profile in asymptomatic patients, depending on the clinical status and effectiveness of therapy; 0, test not informative.
[b] Stable isotope dilution analysis of the metabolites (acylglycines and organic acids) listed in Table 24.7.
[c] 3-Methylcrotonylglycine independently measured by gas chromatography/mass spectrometry (GC/MS) stable isotope dilution analysis.
[d] Propionylglycine independently measured by GC/MS stable isotope dilution analysis.
[e] If applicable, exclude transient pyroglutamic aciduria in response to acetaminophen intake [10].

association with lactic acidemia, hepatomegaly, and liver disease. The more pronounced and apparent are symptoms such as hypoglycemia and hepatomegaly, the more distal a defect is to pyruvate carboxylase in the gluconeogenic pathway.

Beyond the varied clinical signs and symptoms, some of which bear high diagnostic specificity [4], amino acid and organic acid analysis may provide precise laboratory information for the diagnosis of the lactic acidemias (Table 24.5).

Table 24.5 Congenital lactic acidemias: diagnostic significance of clinical information and specialized laboratory investigations

	Clinical findings	Urine organic acids	Plasma amino acids
Disorders of gluconeogenesis			
Glucose-6-phosphatase deficiency	+	–	–
Fructose-1,6-diphosphatase deficiency	–	–	–
Phosphoenolpyruvate carboxykinase deficiency	–	–	–
Pyruvate carboxylase deficiency	+	+	–
Apoenzyme deficiency			
CRM-positive	–	+	–
CRM-negative	–	+	+
Coenzyme deficiency			
Holocarboxylase deficiency	+	+	–
Biotinidase deficiency	+	+	–
Disorders of pyruvate metabolism (PDH complex)			
Pyruvate decarboxylase (E1 subunit of PDH) deficiency			
α-Subunit deficiency (X-linked)	+	+	–
β-Subunit deficiency	+	+	–
E1 phosphatase deficiency	–	–	–
Dihydrolipoyl transacetylase (E2 subunit) deficiency	–	–	–
Dihydrolipoyl dehydrogenase (E3 subunit) deficiency	–	+	+
Krebs cycle disorders			
α-Ketoglutarate dehydrogenase deficiency	–	+	+
Fumarase deficiency	–	+	–
Aconitase deficiency	–	+	–
Respiratory chain defects (partial list)			
NADH–coenzyme Q reductase (complex I)			
Myopathy	+	+	–
Encephalomyopathy	+	+	–
MELAS	+	+	–
Succinate dehydrogenase (complex II)	–	+	–
Coenzyme Q–cytochrome *c* reductase (complex III)			
Myopathy	+	–	–
Encephalopathy	+	–	–
Cytochrome *c* oxidase (complex IV)			
Myopathy			
Fatal infantile myopathy	+	–	+[a]
Benign infantile myopathy	+	–	–
Encephalopathy			
Leigh syndrome			
Kearns–Sayre syndrome	+	–	–

Table 24.5 (cont.)

	Clinical findings	Urine organic acids	Plasma amino acids
MERRF	+	–	–
ATP synthase (complex V)	+	+	–

ATP, adenosine triphosphate; CRM, cross-reacting material; MELAS, mitochondrial encephalopathy lactic acidosis stroke-like episodes; MERRF, myoclonus epilepsy with ragged red fibers; NADH, nicotinamide adenine dinucleotide (reduced); PDH, pyruvate dehydrogenase; +, typical clinical findings or informative profiles by either urine organic acid or plasma amino acid analysis; –, not informative beyond a possible elevated plasma alanine level.
[a] Generalized amino aciduria (Fanconi syndrome).

The presence of elevated plasma alanine concentration is a common feature of these defects and could actually corroborate a potential diagnosis of primary lactic acidemia in early diagnostic stages. The cross-reacting material-negative form of pyruvate carboxylase deficiency presents with elevated plasma concentration of citrulline and lysine [14]. A defect of the E3 subunit of the PDH complex also compromises the catalytic function of 2-ketoglutarate and branched-chain amino acid dehydrogenase complexes, with the accumulation of valine, isoleucine, leucine, and allo-isoleucine to an extent that this disorder was once thought to be a variant of maple syrup urine disease [15]. Additionally, elevated plasma glutamic acid concentrations have been reported in isolated 2-ketoglutarate dehydrogenase deficiency [16], although incorrect sample handling is a much more frequent cause of the same finding [17]. Moreover, generalized amino aciduria concurrent with lactic acidemia is an important element in the recognition of cytochrome c oxidase deficiency with renal involvement and Fanconi syndrome [18].

Significant lactic acidemia is typically accompanied by an increased excretion of 2-hydroxybutyric acid, observable by an organic acid analysis, and is a signature finding much like an observed elevation of plasma alanine. Marked elevations of Krebs cycle intermediates (succinate, fumarate, and malate) have been quantitatively reported in patients with pyruvate carboxylase deficiency [19]. Although these findings have been found in additional cases with pyruvate carboxylase deficiency confirmed by enzyme assays, an increased excretion of Krebs cycle intermediates is often overlooked, possibly because of the broad reference values for these organic acids between different age groups [12]. Patients with multiple carboxylase deficiencies give a typical urine organic acid profile characterized by the presence of 3-hydroxyisovaleric acid, 3-methylcrotonylglycine, propionylglycine, 3-hydroxy propionic acid, and methylcitric acid [20]. As discussed above, PDH complex defects show a characteristic elevation of both lactate and pyruvate; 2-ketoglutaric acid, and the 2-keto-2-hydroxyorganic acids that originate from branched-chain amino acid metabolism are present in urine from patients with an E3 subunit defect of the PDH complex. Organic acid analysis is obviously the method of choice for the recognition of fumarase deficiency and 2-ketoglutarate dehydrogenase deficiency, two disorders primarily affecting the Krebs cycle and whose key compounds, fumarate, and 2-ketoglutarate, respectively, are found in massive levels in urine. Moreover, an elevated excretion of succinic acid could be an indication of succinate dehydrogenase deficiency [21]. However, this compound is also elevated in urine from dietary and medication factors, and even in bacterial contamination, and these artefacts must be ruled out. Abnormal excretions of 3-hydroxyisobutyric acid, 2-ethylhydracrylic acid, 2-methyl-3-hydroxybutyric acid, and tiglylglycine have been reported in a handful of patients with NADH–CoQ reductase (complex I) deficiency [22]. However, they are general abnormalities associated with an increase in the NADH:NAD ratio and are the consequence of the inhibition of NAD-requiring dehydrogenases found in the mitochondria.

Group III: disorders of fatty acid oxidation

Fatty acid oxidation plays a major role in energy production during periods of fasting. At the cellular level, long-chain fatty acids are oxidized to acetyl-coenzyme A (acetyl-CoA) in mitochondria following transport through the cell membrane and carnitine-mediated mitochondrial import [23]. Under fasting conditions, acetyl-CoA fuels the hepatic synthesis of ketone bodies, which are used by extrahepatic tissues as alternative substrates for energy production.

Inherited FAO disorders represent a more widely recognized class of metabolic diseases [24]. Symptoms may appear at any age, from birth [25] to adult life [26], frequently leading to life-threatening episodes of metabolic decompensation after a period of inadequate caloric intake or intercurrent illness. Typical manifestations include hypoketotic hypoglycemia, liver disease, or cardiomyopathy.

During an acute episode of metabolic decompensation, routine laboratory tests may reveal non-ketotic hypoglycemia, a characteristic feature of many FAO disorders. However, there have been several reports of patients unexpectedly presenting with ketonuria [27]. Liver function tests, ammonia, and creatine phosphokinase may be markedly abnormal. Serum lactate is often increased under acute conditions, particularly in patients with disorders of long-chain fatty acid metabolism. Once a suspicion of an FAO disorder has been raised, it is necessary to rely on specialized biochemical investigations to formulate a more specific diagnosis. For this purpose, the collection of plasma and urine specimens

Table 24.6 Disorders of fatty acid transport and oxidation: diagnostic significance of specialized investigations

	Carnitine		Acylcarnitines	Organic acids	Acylglycines[a]
	FC	AC/FC			
Disorders of membrane-bound enzymes					
Long-chain fatty acid transport defect	N to low	–	–	–	–
Carnitine transport defect	Very low	–	–	–	–
Carnitine palmitoyltransferase I deficiency (liver)	High	–	–	–	–
Carnitine acylcarnitine translocase deficiency	N to low	High	+	–	–
Carnitine palmitoyltransferase II deficiency					
Neonatal onset (liver, heart, kidney)	N to low	High	+	–	–
Late onset (skeletal muscle)	N to low	High	+	–	–
VLCAD deficiency	N to low	High	+	+(acute)	–
ETF-ubiquinone oxidoreductase deficiency	N to low	High	+	+	+
TFP deficiency					
LCHAD deficiency	N to low	High	+(acute)	+(acute)	–
α-TFP deficiency	N to low	High	+(acute)	+(acute)	–
β-TFP deficiency	N to low	High	+	+(acute)	–
Defects of mitochondrial matrix enzymes					
MCAD deficiency	N to low	High	+	+(acute)	+
M/SCHAD deficiency	N to low	High	+	+(acute)	–
MCKAT deficiency	N to low	High	?	+(acute)	+
SCAD deficiency	N to low	High	+	+(acute)	+
Myopathic form	N to low	High	+	–	–
Systemic form	N to low	High	+	+(acute)	–
Hepatic form	N to low	High	?	+(acute)	–
Glutaric acidemia type II					
α-ETF deficiency	N to low	High	+	+	+
β-ETF deficiency	N to low	High	+	+	+
Riboflavin responsive form	N to low	High	+	+(acute)	+
2,4-Dienoyl-CoA reductase deficiency	N to low	High	+	–	–

AC, esterified fraction (acylcarnitines); FC, free carnitine; ETF, electron transport flavoprotein; LCHAD, long-chain 3-hydroxyacyl-CoA dehydrogenase; MCAD, medium-chain acyl-CoA dehydrogenase; MCKAT, medium-chain ketoacyl-CoA thiolase; M/SCHAD, medium- and short-chain 3-hydroxyacyl-CoA dehydrogenase; SCAD, short-chain acyl-CoA dehydrogenase; TFP, trifunctional protein; VLCAD, very-long-chain acyl-CoA dehydrogenase; +, diagnostic profile; +(acute), possible occurrence of an uninformative profile of urinary organic acids in asymptomatic patients, depending on clinical status and effectiveness of therapy; –, test not informative; N, normal; ?, insufficient information available to establish diagnostic significance.
[a] Stable isotope dilution analysis of the metabolites (acylglycines and organic acids) listed in Table 24.7.
Source: modified with permission from Rinaldo *et al.*, 1998 [28].

at the earliest possible stage of an acute episode is strongly recommended.

Table 24.6 summarizes the characteristic biochemical findings in plasma and urine of patients with individual disorders [28]. The correct identification of FAO disorders is an increasingly complex process that can hardly be achieved by a single test but requires the performance of multiple analyses and their integrated interpretation. Moreover, uninformative metabolite profiles occur frequently in affected patients because of their clinical and nutritional status and, therefore, should not be taken as sufficient evidence to exclude the possibility of an underlying FAO disorder in a patient with clinical evidence of fasting intolerance.

In urine, analysis of organic acids and acylglycines, performed by GC/MS, is recommended [12]. Organic acid

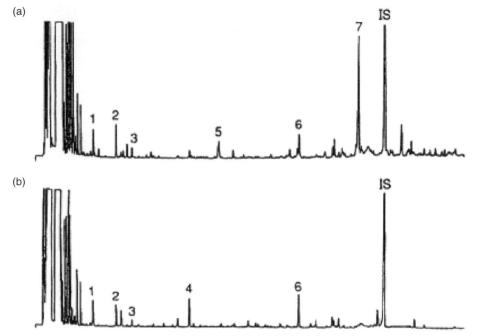

Figure 24.1 Urine organic acid profiles in asymptomatic patients with fatty acid beta-oxidation disorders. Capillary gas chromatographic profiles of organic acid trimethylsilyl derivatives. (a) A 7-year-old boy with medium-chain acyl-CoA dehydrogenase deficiency (diagnosed by acylglycine determination and confirmed by molecular analysis performed in the laboratory of Dr. Kay Tanaka, Yale University). (b) A 3-day-old boy with electron transfer flavoprotein subunit β deficiency (diagnosed prenatally by immunoblot analysis, pulse-labeling experiments, and metabolite analysis in amniotic fluid). 1, lactic acid; 2, oxalic acid; 3, 3-hydroxy isobutyric acid; 4, 4-deoxythreonic acid; 5, adipic acid; 6, 4-hydroxy phenylacetic acid; 7, hippuric acid; IS, internal standard (pentadecanoic acid). All peak identifications were confirmed by gas chromatography–mass spectrometry.

profiles may vary significantly from one defect to another and are dependent on the clinical status of the patient. A signature pattern of hypoketotic medium-chain dicarboxylic acidemia ($C_6 > C_8 > C_{10}$) with multiple unsaturated species ($C_{8:1} < C_8$, $C_{10:1} > C_{10}$) is seen in patients with the three most common FAO disorders: medium-chain acyl-CoA dehydrogenase deficiency, very-long-chain acyl-CoA dehydrogenase deficiency, and long-chain 3-hydroxyacyl-CoA dehydrogenase deficiency. In the last, C_6 to C_{14} 3-hydroxydicarboxylic aciduria is often a more prominent feature. However, supportive therapy may alleviate the need for FAO as an energy source and this rapidly diminishes the excretion of characteristic organic acids.

Figure 24.1 presents two profiles obtained from asymptomatic patients, one with electron transfer flavoprotein subunit β deficiency and the other with medium-chain acyl-CoA dehydrogenase deficiency. In both patients, the organic acid profiles were essentially normal. Profiles such as these underscore the fact that a diagnosis of FAO disorders could be missed if a standard organic acid analysis is the only biochemical test performed, particularly when a patient is free of clinical symptoms (e.g. when an abnormal result of newborn screening is reported) or even shortly after recovery from an acute episode of metabolic decompensation. One test indicated for the recognition of patients with mild or intermittent biochemical phenotypes, which may be missed by organic acid analysis, is the quantitative analysis of acylglycines by stable isotope dilution methods (Table 24.6) [12]. Table 24.7 summarizes the patterns of excretion of acylglycine compounds in eight different disorders and three common circumstances related to dietary or pharmacologic treatment. The acylglycine profile is particularly effective for the differential diagnosis of

ethylmalonic acidemia, a biochemical phenotype that could be linked to multiple disorders [29].

In plasma, carnitine (total and free) and acylcarnitines are necessary components of the laboratory workup of a patient suspected of having an FAO disorder. Despite the higher significance of acylcarnitine profiling, plasma carnitine determination cannot be overlooked because it offers the only method to biochemically recognize patients affected with a carnitine uptake deficiency without performing a tissue biopsy [30]. Indeed, it may also offer an important clue in the differential diagnosis of disorders such as carnitine palmitoyltransferase type 1 deficiency, which lacks a characteristic metabolite pattern in plasma acylcarnitines or organic acids [9,11].

The analysis of acylcarnitines is best performed by tandem MS [8,11]. The commercial availability of relatively affordable bench-top triple quadrupole mass spectrometers and the reliability of liquid chromatography–MS interface based on electrospray ionization have made the application of these techniques a cornerstone of the clinical biochemical genetics laboratory. Likewise, tandem MS is at the forefront of technology revolutionizing US state and national newborn screening programs aimed at identifying inborn errors of metabolism [31].

Disorders of FAO frequently manifest with sudden and unexpected death [7]. Figure 24.2 summarizes a diagnostic protocol that allows detection of multiple disorders based on the evaluation of independent diagnostic criteria [32]. If parental permission to perform an autopsy is not granted, an immediate effort should be made to retrieve specimens that may still be available: if death occurred in a nursery or hospital setting, the laboratory should be immediately contacted and asked to hold any unused portions of blood or urine specimens previously

Table 24.7 Diagnostic specificity of acylglycine and organic acid determination by stable isotope dilution analysis for the differential diagnosis of acyl-CoA dehydrogenase deficiencies, physiological ketosis and iatrogenic conditions

Metabolite	SCAD	EMA encephalopathy	ETF-QO	MCAD	MCKAT	GDH	IVDH	2MBCAD	KET	MCT	VALP
Ethylmalonic acid	+++	+++	+++	–	–	–	–	–	+	–	–
Methylsuccinic acid	+	+	+	–	–	–	–	–	–	–	–
Glutaric acid	–	–	+++	–	–	+++	–	–	+	–	–
Isobutyrylglycine	–	+++	+	–	–	–	–	–	+	–	–
Butyrylglycine	+	+	+	–	–	–	–	–	+	+	+
2-Methylbutyrylglycine	–	+++	+	–	–	–	–	+++	–	–	+
Isovalerylglycine	–	+	+++	–	–	–	+++	–	–	–	–
Hexanoylglycine	+	+++	+++	+	–	–	–	–	–	–	+
Octanoylglycine	–	–	+	+	–	–	–	–	–	+	–
Phenylpropionylglycine	–	–	–	+++	–	–	–	–	–	–	–
Suberylglycine	–	–	+	+++	–	–	–	–	+	+	–
Dodecanedioic acid	–	–	+	–	+++	–	–	–	+	–	–
Tetradecanedioic acid	–	–	+	–	+++	–	–	–	–	–	–
Hexadecanedioic acid	–	–	+	–	+++	–	–	–	–	–	–

2MBCAD, 2-methyl branched-chain acyl-CoA dehydrogenase deficiency; EMA, ethylmalonic acid; ETF, electron transport flavoprotein deficiency, ETF-QO, ETF ubiquinone-oxidoreductase deficiency; GDH, glutaryl-CoA dehydrogenase deficiency; IVDH, isovaleryl-CoA dehydrogenase deficiency; MCAD, medium-chain acyl-CoA dehydrogenase deficiency; MCKAT, medium-chain 3-ketoacyl-CoA thiolase deficiency; SCAD, short-chain acyl-CoA dehydrogenase deficiency; KET, physiological ketosis; MCT, medium chain triglycerides (diet supplemented with); VALP, valproic acid therapy; +++, high diagnostic significance; +, possibly present; –, not typically present.

collected for routine tests. If available, these specimens should be subjected to a complete metabolic workup as described above. If death occurs at home after discharge, retrieval of any unused portion of the patient's blood spot card, collected for newborn screening, could be arranged via a request submitted by a physician to the state laboratory. Blood spots may be sent for acylcarnitine analysis by electrospray tandem MS or for DNA isolation for mutation analysis. If the acylcarnitine profile is not informative, testing of parental plasma carnitine levels for biochemical markers of heterozygosity may also be indicated, particularly if the aim of testing is to rule out the possibility that the patient died from a carnitine uptake defect [30].

Group IV: urea cycle disorders

In urea cycle disorders [33], routine laboratory investigations (Table 24.3) are often dominated by the presence of hyperammonemia and respiratory alkalosis. However, in some cases, such as argininemia, blood ammonia may be within normal range and there have been conflicting reports about significance of respiratory alkalosis. Indeed, it has been reported that patients presenting with urea cycle disorders may be either acidotic or alkalotic during acute episodes of metabolic decompensation [34]. Therefore, an organic acid analysis could be of benefit to definitively rule out whether hyperammonemia in a patient is secondary to an underlying organic aciduria.

Plasma amino acids and urine orotic acid are required for a differential diagnosis, which can be effectively achieved according to established protocols [35]. High glutamine and alanine concentrations are typical but not diagnostic for these disorders, reflecting a non-specific consequence of cellular nitrogen accumulation. A low or absent citrulline concentration is consistent with either ornithine transcarbamylase or carbamylphosphate synthetase deficiencies. Indeed, these two disorders can be differentiated by testing orotic acid in urine, which is only elevated in ornithine transcarbamylase deficiency. Therefore, the diagnosis of carbamylphosphate synthetase deficiency is made biochemically by the step-by-step exclusion of other disorders. While a more than 20-fold increase in citrulline concentration (normal values <50 μmol/L) indicates a defect of argininosuccinic synthetase, a condition commonly known as citrullinemia type I, a two- to five-fold elevation of plasma citrulline in the presence of argininosuccinic acid in urine is indicative of argininosuccinase deficiency. Clinical and more detailed diagnostic aspects of urea cycle defects are discussed in Chapter 38.

Group V: amino acid disorders

Two disorders will be briefly considered in this last section: maple syrup urine disease and non-ketotic hyperglycinemia, which should always be contemplated in the context of a differential diagnosis among those inborn errors listed in Tables 24.1 and 24.3.

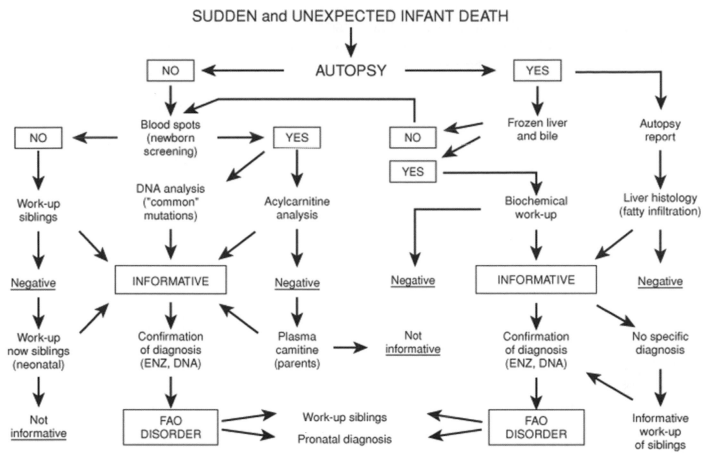

Figure 24.2 Protocol for the postmortem screening of fatty acid oxidation disorders. DNA, molecular analysis; ENZ, enzymatic assay; FAO, fatty acid oxidation. (Reprinted with permission from Rinaldo *et al.*, 1999 [32].)

Maple syrup urine disease is caused by a defect of one of the three components of the branched-chain 2-keto acid dehydrogenase complex [36]. In untreated or decompensated patients, a diagnosis of maple syrup urine disease could be suspected by a positive dinitrophenylhydrazine test or simply by the presence of a characteristically sweet smell in urine or earwax, the latter in older patients. A diagnosis is more reliably substantiated by either plasma amino acid or urine organic acid analysis. Through the keto–enol tautomerization of (2S)-2-keto-3-methylvaleric acid to its (2R)-enantiomer (mirror image), L-alloisoleucine is formed in vivo [37]. The detection of L-alloisoleucine in plasma or dried blood spots [38] is a pathognomonic finding of maple syrup urine disease, along with a high concentration of the three branched-chain amino acids (particularly leucine). Their accumulation results from the freely reversible transamination of 2-keto acids (2-ketoisocaproic acid, 2-keto-3-methylvaleric acid, and 2-ketoisovaleric acid) to the corresponding amino acid. 2-Hydroxyisovaleric acid may also be present in large amounts. When organic acids are analyzed by GC/MS [12], the 2-keto acids should first be stabilized by oximation with hydroxylamine hydrochloride or other equivalent reagents.

Non-ketotic hyperglycinemia is a severe condition caused by a defect of the mitochondrial glycine cleavage system [39]. The key element that raises the suspicion of this disorder is the sum of all uninformative results by routine laboratory investigations in a child with progressive neurologic symptoms (Table 24.3) and the observation that plasma and CSF amino acid analysis reveals high concentrations of glycine in plasma (frequently >1000 μmol/L, normal values <500 μmol/L in newborns and <300 μmol/L in older infants) and in CSF (>30 μmol/L, normal values <10 μmol/L). The calculation of a CSF:plasma glycine concentration ratio (>0.09, normal <0.04) is critical in the differential diagnosis of this condition [40]. Of course, the reliability of this parameter hinges on the fact that both the plasma and CSF specimens must be collected simultaneously. No other abnormalities are detectable by amino acid or organic acid analysis for this disorder.

Newborn screening for disorders of amino acid, organic acid, and fatty acid metabolism

The natural history of most of the conditions described in this chapter has changed dramatically since the implementation in recent years of the uniform newborn screening panel of conditions [41,42]. In this of 55 conditions, 42 are metabolic disorders detected by analysis of amino acid and acylcarnitine profiles in dried blood spots using tandem MS [43]. The sensitivity and specificity of the markers detected with the primary screening is variable, and when less than adequate these could be improved by the application of second-tier tests to the same specimen, thus not requiring further patient contact [38,44,45]. Further improvement has been achieved by the definition of analyte disease ranges and cut-off target ranges [46]; a large-scale collaborative effort has culminated with the introduction of a novel approach for the postanalytical interpretation of newborn screening results without analyte cut-off values based on a multivariate pattern recognition software [47]. It is likely that more conditions will be added to the recommended panel [48,49], but only after a rigorous evidence review process of the natural history of the condition, available screening test(s), and efficacy of early intervention has been completed and deemed to be sufficient to justify the inclusion.

There exist many more investigations – in vivo provocative tests, in vitro enzyme assays, and molecular methods – available for the diagnosis of inborn errors of metabolism. These procedures have not been considered here for the sole reason that they have no significant impact on the way physicians confront the occurrence of a life-threatening episode of metabolic decompensation at the bedside. In the very critical initial hours, the diagnosis of an inborn error of metabolism must rely on the kind of routine and specialized biochemical laboratory investigations described within this chapter.

References

1. Eminoglu TF, Tumer L, Okur I, *et al.* Very long-chain acyl CoA dehydrogenase deficiency which was accepted as infanticide. *Forensic Sci Int* 2011;**210**:e1–3.

2. Blau N, Duran M, Gibson KM (eds.). *Laboratory Guide to the Methods in Biochemical Genetics.* Berlin: Springer-Verlag, 2008.

3. Saudubray JM, van der Berghe G, Walter JH (eds.) *Inborn Metabolic Diseases: Diagnosis and Treatment.* Berlin: Springer-Verlag, 2012.

4. Saudubray JM. Clinical approach to inborn errors of metabolism in pediatrics. In Saudubray JM, van der Berghe G, Walter JH (eds.) *Inborn Metabolic Diseases: Diagnosis and Treatment.* Berlin: Springer-Verlag, 2012, pp. 4–54.

5. Crushell E, Chukwu J, Mayne P, Blatny J, Treacy EP. Negative screening tests in classical galactosaemia caused by S135L homozygosity. *J Inherit Metab Dis* 2009;**32**:412–415.

6. Johnson JL, Duran M. Molybdenum cofactor deficiency and isolated sulfite oxidase deficiency. In Valle D, Beaudet AL, Vogelstein B, *et al.* (eds.) *The Online Metabolic & Molecular Bases of Inherited Disease.* (http://www.ommbid.com, accessed 22 July 2013).

7. Rinaldo P. Postmortem investigations. In Hoffman GF, Zschocke J, Nyhan WL (eds.) *Inherited Metabolic Diseases.* Berlin: Springer-Verlag, 2010, pp. 335–338.

8. Rinaldo P, Cowan TM, Matern D. Acylcarnitine profile analysis. *Genet Med* 2008;**10**:151–156.

9. Rinaldo P. Organic acids. In Blau N, Duran N, Gibson KM (eds.) *Laboratory Guide to the Methods in Biochemical Genetics.* Berlin: Springer-Verlag, 2008, pp. 137–170.

10. Pitt JJ, Hauser S. Transient 5-oxoprolinuria and high anion gap metabolic acidosis: clinical and biochemical findings in eleven subjects. *Clin Chem* 1998;**44**:1497–1503.

11. Matern D. Acylcarnitines, including in vitro loading tests. In Blau N, Duran N, Gibson KM (eds.) *Laboratory Guide to the Methods in Biochemical Genetics.* Berlin: Springer-Verlag, 2008, pp. 171–206.

12. Vassault A. Lactate, pyruvate, acetoacetate and 3-hydroxybutyrate. In Blau N, Duran N, Gibson KM (eds.) *Laboratory Guide to the Methods in Biochemical Genetics.* Berlin: Springer-Verlag, 2008, pp. 35–51.

13. Wang D, De Vivo D. Pyruvate carboxylase deficiency. In Pagon RA, Bird TD, Dolan CR, Stephens K (eds.) *GeneReviews.* Seattle, WA: University of Washington, Seattle, 1993– (website, updated July 2011; accessed March 13, 2012).

14. Coude FX, Ogier H, Marsac C, *et al.* Secondary citrullinemia with hyperammonemia in four neonatal cases of pyruvate carboxylase deficiency. *Pediatrics* 1981;**68**:914.

15. Munnich A, Saudubray J-M, Taylor J, *et al.* Congenital lactic acidosis, α-ketoglutaric aciduria and variant form of maple syrup urine disease due to a single enzyme defect: dihydrolipoyldehydrogenase deficiency. *Acta Paediatr Scand* 1982;**71**:167–171.

16. Bonnefont JP, Chretien D, Rustin P, *et al.* Alpha-ketoglutarate dehydrogenase deficiency presenting as congenital lactic acidosis. *J Pediatr* 1992;**121**:255–258.

17. Shih VE. Amino acid analysis. In Blau N, Duran M, Blaskovics ME, *et al.* (eds.) *Physician's Guide to the Laboratory Diagnosis of Metabolic Diseases.* 2nd edn. Berlin: Springer-Verlag, 2003, pp. 11–26.

18. Tein I. Neonatal metabolic myopathies. *Semin Perinatol* 1999;**23**:125–151.

19. Chalmers RA. Organic acids in urine of patients with congenital lactic acidosis: an aid to differential diagnosis. *J Inherit Metab Dis* 1984;**7**(suppl 1):79–89.

20. Cowan TM, Blitzer MG, Wolf B. Technical standards and guidelines for the diagnosis of biotinidase deficiency. *Genet Med* 2010;**12**:464–470.

21. Bourgeron T, Rustin P, Chretien D, *et al.* Mutation of a nuclear succinate dehydrogenase gene results in mitochondrial respiratory chain deficiency. *Nat Genet* 1995;**11**:144–149.

22. Bennett MJ, Sherwood WG, Gibson KM, *et al.* Secondary inhibition of multiple NAD-requiring dehydrogenases in respiratory chain complex I deficiency: possible metabolic markers for the primary defect. *J Inherit Metab Dis* 1993;**16**:560–562.

23. Strauss AW, Andresen BS, Bennett MJ. Mitochondrial fatty acid oxidation defects. In Sarafoglu K, Hoffman GF, Roth KS (eds.) *Pediatric Endocrinology and Inborn Errors of Metabolism.* New York: McGraw Hill Medical, 2009, pp. 51–70.

24. Rinaldo P, Matern D. Disorders of fatty acid transport and mitochondrial

oxidations. In Rimoin DL, Connor MJ, Pyeritz RE, Korf BR (eds.) *Emery and Rimoin's Principles and Practice of Medical Genetics*, 5th edn, vol 3. Philadelphia, PA: Churchill Livingstone-Elsevier, 2007, pp. 2285–2295.

25. Rinaldo P, Stanley CA, Sanchez LA, *et al.* Sudden neonatal death in carnitine transporter deficiency. *J Pediatr* 1997;**131**:304–305.

26. Raymond K, Bale AE, Barnes CA, *et al.* Medium-chain acyl-CoA dehydrogenase deficiency: sudden and unexpected death of a 45 year old woman. *Genet Med* 1999;**1**:293–294.

27. Patel JS, Leonard JV. Ketonuria and medium-chain acyl-CoA dehydrogenase deficiency. *J Inherit Metab Dis* 1995;**18**:98–99.

28. Rinaldo P, Raymond K, al-Odaib A, Bennett MJ. Fatty acid oxidation disorders: clinical and biochemical features. *Curr Opin Pediatr* 1998;**10**:615–621.

29. Drousiotou A, DiMeo I, Mineri R, *et al.* Ethylmalonic encephalopathy: application of improved biochemical and molecular diagnostic approaches. *Clin Genet* 2011;**79**:385–390.

30. Stanley CA, DeLeeuw S, Coates PM, *et al.* Chronic cardiomyopathy and weakness or acute coma in children with a defect in carnitine uptake. *Ann Neurol* 1991;**30**:709–716.

31. Vogeser M, Seger C. A decade of HPLC-MS/MS in the routine clinical laboratory: goals for further developments. *Clin Biochem* 2008;**41**:649–662.

32. Rinaldo P, Yoon HR, Yu C, *et al.* Sudden and unexpected neonatal death: a protocol for the postmortem diagnosis of fatty acid oxidation disorders. *Semin Perinatol* 1999;**23**:204–210.

33. Summar ML. Urea cycle disorders. In Sarafoglu K, Hoffman GF, Roth KS (eds.) *Pediatric Endocrinology and Inborn Errors of Metabolism*. New York, McGraw Hill Medical, 2009, pp. 141–152.

34. Bachmann C, Colombo JP. Acid-base status and plasma glutamine in patients with hereditary urea cycle disorders. In Soeters PB, Wilson JHP, Meijer AJ, *et al.* (eds.) *Advances in Ammonia Metabolism and Hepatic Encephalopathy*. Amsterdam: Elsevier, 1988, pp. 72–78.

35. Dietzen DJ, Rinaldo P, Whitley RJ, *et al.* National Academy of Clinical Biochemistry laboratory medicine practice guidelines – Follow up testing for metabolic diseases identified by expanded newborn screening using tandem mass spectrometry. *Clin Chem* 2009;**55**:1615–1626.

36. Chuang DT, Wynn RM, Shih VE. Maple syrup urine disease (branched-chain ketoaciduria). In Valle D, Beaudet AL, Vogelstein B, *et al.* (eds.) *The Online Metabolic & Molecular Bases of Inherited Disease* (http://www.ommbid. com, accessed 22 July 2013).

37. Matthews DE, Ben-Galim E, Haymond MW, *et al.* Alloisoleucine formation in maple syrup urine disease: isotopic evidence for the mechanism. *Pediatr Res* 1980;**14**:854–857.

38. Oglesbee D, Sanders KA, Lacey JM, *et al.* 2nd-tier test for quantification of alloisoleucine and branched-chain amino acids in dried blood spots to improve newborn screening for maple syrup urine disease (MSUD). *Clin Chem* 2008;**54**: 542–549.

39. Dulac O, Rolland MO. Nonketotic hyperglycinaemia (glycine encephalopathy). In Saudubray JM, van den Berghe G, Walter JH (eds.) *Inborn Metabolic Diseases: Diagnosis and Treatment*. Berlin: Springer-Verlag, 2012, pp. 349–356.

40. Hamosh A, Johnston MV. Nonketotic hyperglycinemia. In Valle D, Beaudet AL, Vogelstein B, *et al.* (eds.) *The Online Metabolic & Molecular Bases of Inherited Disease* (http://www.ommbid. com, accessed 22 July 2013).

41. Watson MS, Mann MY, Lloyd-Puryear MA, Rinaldo P, Howell RR. Newborn screening: toward a uniform screening panel and system. *Genet Med* 2006;**8** (Suppl):1S–11S.

42. Rinaldo P, Matern D. Newborn screening for inherited metabolic diseases. In Hoffman GF, Zschocke J, Nyhan WL (eds.) *Inherited Metabolic Diseases*. Berlin: Springer-Verlag, 2010, pp. 251–262.

43. Turgeon C, Magera MJ, Allard P, *et al.* Combined newborn screening for succinylacetone, amino acids, and acylcarnitines in dried blood spots. *Clin Chem* 2008;**54**:657–664.

44. Tortorelli S, Turgeon CT, McHugh DMS, *et al.* Two-tier approach to the newborn screening of methylene tetrahydrofolate reductase deficiency and other re-methylation disorders by tandem mass spectrometry. *J Pediatr* 2010;**157**:271–275.

45. Turgeon CT, Magera MJ, Cuthbert CD, *et al.* Simultaneous determination of total homocysteine, methylmalonic acid, and 2-methylcitric acid in dried blood spots by tandem mass spectrometry. *Clin Chem* 2010;**56**: 1686–1695.

46. McHugh DMS, Cameron CA, Abdenur JE, *et al.* Clinical validation of cutoff target ranges in newborn screening of metabolic disorders by tandem mass spectrometry: A worldwide collaborative project. *Genet Med* 2011;**13**:230–254.

47. Marquardt G, Currier R, McHugh DMS, *et al.* Enhanced interpretation of newborn screening results without analyte cutoff values. *Genet Med* 2012; **14**:648–655.

48. Green NS, Rinaldo P, Brower A, *et al.* Committee report: advancing the current recommended panel of conditions for newborn screening. *Genet Med* 2007;**9**:792–796.

49. Calonge N, Green NS, Rinaldo P, *et al.* Committee report: method for evaluating conditions nominated for population-based screening of newborns and children. *Genet Med* 2010;**12**:153–159.

25 α_1-Antitrypsin deficiency

David H. Perlmutter

Introduction

Homozygous (PiZZ phenotype) α_1-antitrypsin (α_1-AT) deficiency is a relatively common genetic disorder, affecting 1 in 3000 live births [1]. It is an autosomal codominant disorder associated with 85–90% reduction in serum concentrations of α_1-AT. A single amino acid substitution results in an abnormally folded protein that is unable to traverse the secretory pathway. The mutant α_1-antitrypsin Z (α_1-ATZ) protein is retained in the endoplasmic reticulum (ER) rather than secreted into the blood and body fluids.

α_1-Antitrypsin is an approximately 55 kDa secretory glycoprotein that inhibits destructive neutrophil proteases, elastase, cathepsin G, and proteinase 3. Plasma α_1-AT is derived predominantly from the liver and increases three- to five-fold during the host response to tissue injury or inflammation. It is the archetype of a family of structurally related circulating serine protease inhibitors called serpins.

Nationwide prospective screening studies by Sveger and coworkers [2,3] in Sweden have shown that only 8–10% of the PiZZ population develops clinically significant liver disease over the first 20 years of life. Nevertheless, this deficiency is the most frequent genetic cause of liver disease in children and the most frequent genetic disease for which children undergo orthotopic liver transplantation. It also causes chronic hepatitis, cirrhosis, and hepatocellular carcinoma in adults [4].

Although the condition does not affect children, many α_1-AT-deficient individuals develop destructive lung disease and emphysema as adults. Most of the data in the literature indicate that emphysema results from a loss-of-function mechanism whereby decreased numbers of α_1-AT molecules within the lower respiratory tract allow unregulated elastolytic attack on the connective tissue matrix of the lung [5]. Oxidative inactivation of residual α_1-AT as a result of smoking accelerates lung injury. Moreover, the elastase–antielastase theory for the pathogenesis of emphysema is based on the concept that oxidative inactivation of α_1-AT as a result of cigarette smoking plays a key role in the emphysema of α_1-AT-sufficient individuals, the vast majority of patients with emphysema [5].

Liver disease in this deficiency appears to involve a gain-of-toxic function mechanism whereby retention of mutant α_1-ATZ molecule in the ER of liver cells eventually exacts hepatotoxic effects. This has been best demonstrated by the development of hepatic fibrosis [6] and carcinoma [7] in mice with transgenic expression of mutant α_1-ATZ [8].

The diagnosis of α_1-AT deficiency is based on the altered migration of the abnormal α_1-ATZ molecule in serum specimens subjected to isoelectric focusing gel analysis. Treatment of α_1-AT deficiency-associated liver disease is mostly supportive. Liver transplantation has been used successfully for severe liver injury. Although the clinical efficacy has not been demonstrated, many patients with emphysema caused by α_1-AT deficiency are being treated by intravenous and intratracheal aerosol administration of purified plasma α_1-AT. An increasing number of patients with severe emphysema have been undergoing lung transplantation. Several new pharmacologic and genetic strategies for prophylaxis of both liver and lung disease are under development for clinical application.

Clinical manifestations
Liver disease

Liver involvement is often noticed first at 1–2 months of age, because of persistent jaundice (Table 25.1). Conjugated bilirubin levels in the blood and serum aminotransferase levels are mildly to moderately elevated. Blood levels of alkaline phosphatase and gamma-glutamyltransferase also may be elevated. The liver may be enlarged. There is a tendency for some affected infants to be small for gestational age. Because these clinical and laboratory characteristics are similar to other causes of liver injury in the newborn period, these infants may initially be given the diagnosis of neonatal hepatitis syndrome and subjected to a diagnostic evaluation for various disorders including α_1-AT deficiency [9]. Infants also may be evaluated initially for α_1-AT deficiency because of an episode of gastrointestinal bleeding, bleeding from the umbilical stump, or bruising. A small number of affected infants,

Liver Disease in Children, Fourth Edition, ed. Frederick J. Suchy, Ronald J. Sokol, and William F. Balistreri. Published by Cambridge University Press. © Cambridge University Press 2014.

Table 25.1 Liver disease associated with α₁-antritrypsin deficiency

	Liver features
Clinical features	Prolonged jaundice in infants Neonatal hepatitis syndrome Mild elevation of aminotransferases in toddler Portal hypertension in child/adolescent Severe liver dysfunction in child/adolescent Chronic hepatitis in adult Cryptogenic cirrhosis in adult Hepatocellular carcinoma in adult
Diagnostic features	Diminished serum levels of α₁-antitrypsin Abnormal mobility of α₁-antitrypsin in isoelectric focusing Periodic acid–Schiff positive, diastase-resistant globules in liver cells

approximately 10% of the deficient population, have hepatosplenomegaly, ascites, and liver synthetic dysfunction in early infancy. An even smaller number have severe fulminant liver failure in infancy [9]. A few infants are recognized initially because of a cholestatic clinical syndrome characterized by pruritus and hypercholesterolemia. The clinical picture in these patients resembles extrahepatic biliary atresia, but histologic examination shows paucity of intrahepatic bile ducts.

Liver disease associated with α₁-AT deficiency may also be discovered first in late childhood or early adolescence, when the affected individual develops abdominal distension from hepatosplenomegaly or ascites, has splenomegaly, or has upper intestinal bleeding caused by esophageal variceal hemorrhage. In some of these patients, there is a history of unexplained prolonged obstructive jaundice during the neonatal period. In others, there is no evidence of any previous liver injury, even if the neonatal history is carefully reviewed (Table 25.1).

Deficiency of α₁-AT should be considered in the differential diagnosis of any adult who presents with chronic hepatitis, cirrhosis, portal hypertension, or hepatocellular carcinoma of unknown origin. An autopsy study in Sweden showed a higher risk of cirrhosis in adults with α₁-AT deficiency than was previously suspected and that α₁-AT deficiency has a strong association with primary liver cancer [4]. Moreover, the risk of liver cancer was greater than could be accounted for by the known increase associated with cirrhosis alone [4]. Interestingly, cirrhosis and liver cancer may be initially diagnosed in a patient with little in the way of clinical manifestations of liver disease, perhaps only asymptomatic hepatomegaly or elevated aminotransferases or bilirubin levels. Primary liver cancer is also observed in the absence of cirrhosis in some patients with α₁-AT deficiency [10]. The histology of the hepatic cancer can be characteristic of hepatocellular carcinoma or cholangiocarcinoma, or have features of both [10]. Although it has been said that heterozygotes are at increased risk of primary liver

cancer, it has not been possible to prove that the cancers in these patients are caused by the allelic variant itself.

The only prospective data on the natural history of α₁-AT deficiency-associated liver injury is the Swedish nationwide screening study done by Sveger [2]. In this study, 200 000 newborn infants were screened, and 127 individuals with PiZZ were identified. Of these 127 infants, 14 had prolonged cholestatic jaundice, and 9 of the 14 had severe liver disease, as indicated by clinical and laboratory criteria. Another eight of the PiZZ infants had mild abnormalities of serum bilirubin or serum aminotransferase levels or hepatomegaly. Approximately 50% of the remainder of the 127 had only abnormal aminotransferase levels [2]. Published follow-up studies of the original cohort of 127 children with PiZZ at 26 years of age showed that more than 85% had persistently normal serum aminotransferase levels with no evidence of liver dysfunction [3]. Issues not addressed by the Sveger study included whether 26 year olds with α₁-AT deficiency had persistent subclinical histologic abnormalities, despite lack of clinical or biochemical evidence of liver injury, and whether liver disease eventually becomes clinically evident during adulthood.

It still is not clear what clinical manifestations or abnormal laboratory test results can be used to predict a poor prognosis for individuals with α₁-AT deficiency-associated liver disease. Even children with cirrhosis and portal hypertension can lead relatively healthy lives for years without the need for liver transplantation, or for years before the transplant procedure is needed [11]. Timing of liver transplantation should depend more on overall life functioning rather than any single clinical or biochemical determination.

Evidence that the heterozygous (MZ) genotype of α₁-AT by itself causes liver disease is weak. All of the studies of this issue are biased in ascertainment because the index population is derived from a pathologic registry or some other type of clinical database. Furthermore, existing studies do not include concurrent prospective controls [12]. For this reason it is always important to exclude other causes when evaluating patients with liver disease who are heterozygous for the Z allele. Because of clinical experience over the years in which there is no other explanation for severe liver disease in MZ heterozygotes despite exhaustive diagnostic evaluation, I suspect that the lack of evidence for predisposition to liver disease in heterozygotes is because of difficulties in study design more than anything else.

Liver disease has been described for several other allelic variants of α₁-AT. Children with compound heterozygosity type PiSZ are affected by liver injury in a manner similar to PiZZ children [2,3]. There are several reports of liver disease in the α₁-AT deficiency variant PiM_malton. These are particularly interesting associations because the mutant PiM_malton and PiSZ α₁-AT molecules have been shown to undergo polymerization and retention within the ER [12]. Liver disease has been detected in single patients with several other α₁-AT allelic variants – such as PiM_Duarte, Pi_W, and Pi_FZ [12] – but it is not clear whether other causes of liver injury for which we have more sophisticated diagnostic assays, such as infection with hepatitis C and autoimmune hepatitis, have been excluded completely in these patients.

Lung disease

The incidence and prevalence of emphysema in α_1-AT deficiency have not been studied prospectively. Autopsy studies suggest that 60–65% of people with homozygous PiZZ α_1-AT deficiency develop clinically significant lung injury [1,5]. There are smokers with α_1-AT deficiency however, who do not have any symptoms of lung disease or evidence of pulmonary function abnormalities until the seventh or eighth decade of life [1].

The typical person with lung disease is a man and a cigarette smoker. Onset of dyspnea is insidious in the third to fourth decade of life. About 50% of affected people develop cough and recurrent lung infections. The disease progresses to a severe limitation of airflow. A reduction in the forced expiratory volume, an increase in total lung capacity, and a reduction in diffusing capacity occur. Chest radiographs demonstrate hyperinflation with marked lucency at the lung bases. Histopathologic studies demonstrate panacinar emphysema, more prominent in the lower lung [1,5].

It is rare for emphysema to affect an α_1-AT-deficient patient during childhood. A number of patients have been described in the literature, but for each of these, an alternative explanation can be offered [12]. A number of infants with α_1-AT deficiency have had pulmonary function testing suggesting a subtle degree of hyperinflation. Another study, however, did not detect any significant difference between the pulmonary function of PiZZ children between the ages of 13 and 17 and that of an age-matched control group [12]. These data indicate that it is extremely rare for α_1-AT deficiency to cause emphysema in individuals aged younger than 25 years.

The destructive effect of cigarette smoking on the outcome of lung disease in α_1-AT deficiency has been demonstrated in many studies. Actuarial studies suggest that cigarette smoking reduces median survival by more than 20 years in deficient people. The rate of decline in forced expiratory volume is four times greater in smoking than in non-smoking people with α_1-AT deficiency [1,5].

There is still limited information about the incidence of liver disease in α_1-AT-deficient individuals with emphysema. In one study of 22 patients with PiZZ and emphysema, there was elevated serum aminotransferase in 10 patients, and cholestasis was present in one patient [13]. Liver biopsies were not done in this study; they may be necessary to determine accurately the extent of liver injury in these patients.

Pathophysiology
Structure of α_1-antitrypsin

α_1-Antitrypsin is a single-chain polypeptide, approximately 52–55 kDa, with 394 amino acid residues, and with three asparagine-linked complex carbohydrate side-chains. There are two major isoforms in serum, depending on the presence of a biantennary or triantennary configuration for the carbohydrate side-chains. It has a globular shape and a highly ordered internal domain composed of two central β-sheets surrounded by a small β-sheet and nine α-helices. The dominant structure is the five-stranded β-pleated sheet termed the A sheet [9].

α_1-Antitrypsin is the archetype of the serpins (serine protease inhibitors), including antithrombin III, α_1-antichymotrypsin, C1 inhibitor, α_2-antiplasmin, protein C inhibitor, heparin cofactor II, plasminogen activator inhibitors 1 and 2, protease nexin 1, ovalbumin, angiotensinogen, corticosteroid-binding globulin, and thyroid-binding globulin, among others [9]. These proteins share about 25–40% primary structural homology, with higher degrees of regional homology in functional domains. Most serpins function as suicide inhibitors by forming equimolar complexes with a specific target protease. Other serpins are not inhibitory. For example, corticosteroid- and thyroid hormone-binding globulins, which are thought to represent carriers for corticosteroid and thyroid hormone, respectively, form complexes but do not inactivate their hormone ligands.

A comparison of α_1-AT with other members of the serpin supergene family has generated several important concepts about the structure and function of α_1-AT. For example, the reactive site, P1 residue, of α_1-AT is localized to a canonic loop that rises above the gap in the center of the A sheet [9] (Figure 25.1) [14]. This loop may provide a certain degree of flexibility to the functional activity of the inhibitor. The reactive loop conformation of serpins is also thought to make them susceptible to proteolytic cleavage by thiolenzymes and metalloenzymes. The P1 residue itself is the most important determinant of functional specificity for each serpin molecule. This concept was confirmed dramatically by the discovery of α_1-AT Pittsburgh, a variant in which the P1 residue of α_1-AT, Met 358, is replaced by Arg. In this variant, α_1-AT functions as a thrombin inhibitor, and severe bleeding diathesis results [15].

The C-terminal fragment of α_1-AT and the other serpins also bears important structural and functional characteristics. There is a much higher degree of sequence homology among serpins in the C-terminus. A small fragment at this terminus is cleaved during formation of the inhibitory complex with serine protease. This C-terminal fragment possesses chemotactic activity [9]. Moreover, this fragment bears the receptor-binding domain for cell surface binding, internalization of α_1-AT–elastase and other serpin–enzyme complexes, and activation of a signal-transduction pathway for upregulation of α_1-AT gene expression [9].

α_1-Antitrypsin is encoded by a 12.2 kb gene (*SERPINA1*) (Figure 25.2) located on human chromosome 14q31-32.2 [9]. The first two exons and a short 5′-segment of the third exon code for 5′-untranslated regions of the α_1-AT mRNA. Most of the fourth exon and the remaining three exons encode the protein sequence of α_1-AT. A 72 base sequence constitutes the 24 amino acid residue sequence forming the N-terminus. The three sites for Asn-linked carbohydrate attachment are at

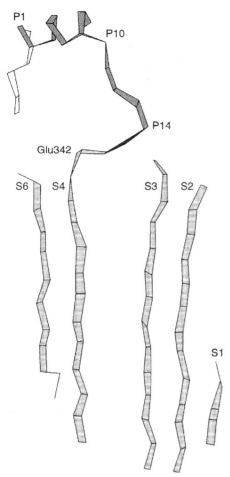

Figure 25.1 Ribbon diagram of the A sheet and reactive center loop of native α₁-antitrypsin. Because the native protein has not been crystallized, this ribbon diagram is generated by computer models based on the crystal structures of cleaved α₁-antitrypsin and native ovalbumin. The reactive center loop is shown in black. Residues P10 and P14 are numbered from the reactive-site methionine P1. The C-terminal fragment is shown as white ribbons. β-helices of the A sheet are shown as gray ribbons and referred to as S1, S2, S3, S5, and S6. The Glu 342 residue, which is replaced by Lys in α₁-ATZ PIZ α₁-antitrypsin is designated. (Adapted with permission from Carrell et al., 1991 [14].)

residues 46, 83, and 247. The active site, the so-called P1 residue, Met 358, is encoded in the seventh exon. It is not yet known whether the two exons, also called short open-reading frames, in the upstream untranslated region of the gene are involved in translational regulation of its expression [9]. There is a "sequence-related gene" about 12 kb downstream from the gene for α₁-AT. Because no evidence exists that the sequence-related gene is expressed, it is considered a pseudogene. The genes for two other serpins, α₁-antichymotrypsin and corticosteroid-binding globulin, also are linked closely on chromosome 14 [9]. The α₁-AT mRNA expressed in liver is 1.4 kb long. In macrophages, the α₁-AT mRNA is slightly longer. In fact, there are three forms of α₁-AT mRNA in macrophages, depending on transcription initiation sites in two upstream exonic structures (exons IA and IB) [16].

Structural variants of α₁-AT in humans are classified according to the protease inhibitor phenotype system as defined by agarose electrophoresis or isoelectric focusing of plasma [12]. The Pi classification assigns a letter to variants according to position of migration of α₁-AT in these gel systems, using alphabetic order from low to high isoelectric point. For example, the most common normal variant migrates to an intermediate isoelectric point, designated *M*. People with the most common severe deficiency have an α₁-AT allelic variant that migrates to a high isoelectric point, designated *Z*.

More than 100 allelic variants of α₁-AT have been reported [5]. Structural variants of α₁-AT not associated with changes in serum concentration or functional activity from the normal range are termed *normal allelic variants* and include the M1, M2, M3, M1 (Ala 213), X, Christchurch, and P_Saint Alban's alleles

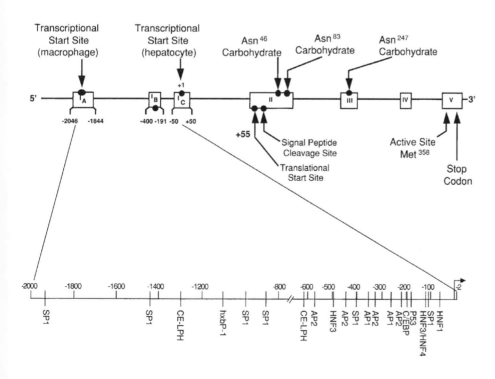

Figure 25.2 Schematic representation of the structure of the gene for α₁-antitrypsin (not to scale) and map of potential regulatory elements based on its sequence.

Table 25.2 Null variants of α_1-antitrypsin

| | Defect | | Clinical disease | | |
			Liver	Lung	Cellular defect
Null$_{Granite\ Falls}$	Single base deletion	Tyr 160	−	+	No detectable RNA
Null$_{Bellingham}$	Single base deletion	Lys 217	−	+	No detectable RNA
Null$_{Mattawa}$	Single base insertion	Phe 353	−	+	IC degradation?
Null$_{Hong\ Kong}$	Dinucleotide deletion	Leu 318	−	+	IC accumulation
Null$_{Ludwigshafen}$	Single base substitution	Ile 92–Asp	−	+	Dysfunctional protein (EC degradation?)
Null$_{Clayton}$	Single base insertion	Glu 363	−	+	IC degradation?
Null$_{Bolton}$	Single base deletion	Glu 363	−	+	IC degradation?
Null$_{Isola\ di\ Procida}$	Deletion	Exons II–V	−	+	Unknown
Null$_{Riedenburg}$	Deletion	Exons II–V	−	+	Unknown
Null$_{Newport}$	Single base substitution	Gly 115–Ser	−	+	Unknown
Null$_{Bonny\ Blue}$	Intron deletion		−	+	Unknown
Null$_{New\ Hope}$	Two base substitutions	Gly 320–Glu Glu 342–Lys	− −	+	Unknown
Null$_{Trastavere}$	Single base substitution	Trp 194–stop	−	+	Unknown
Null$_{Kowloon}$	Single base substitution	Tyr 38–stop	−	+	Unknown
Null$_{Saarbruecken}$	Single base insertion	Pro 362–stop	−	+	Unknown
Null$_{Lisbon}$	Single base substitution	Thr 68–Ile	−	+	Unknown
Null$_{West}$	Intron deletion		−	+	Unknown

IC, intracellular; EC, extracellular.

[5]. In each case examined, a single relatively conservative substitution is present. The α_1-AT variants in which α_1-AT is not detectable in serum are called *null allelic variants* (Table 25.2) and, if inherited with another null variant or deficiency variant, are associated with premature development of emphysema [5]. Several types of defect, including insertions and deletions, appear to be responsible for these variants (Table 25.2). In two instances, α_1-AT Null$_{Isola\ di\ Procida}$ and α_1-AT Null$_{Reidenburg}$, there is deletion of all α_1-AT coding regions. In two other cases, α_1-AT Null$_{Bellingham}$ and α_1-AT Null$_{Granite\ Falls}$, α_1-AT mRNA is undetectable. Three other null alleles result in truncated proteins that are degraded in the ER: Null$_{Mattawa}$, Null$_{Hong\ Kong}$, and Null$_{Clayton}$ [12].

Several variants of α_1-AT associated with a reduction in serum concentrations of α_1-AT have been described and are called *deficiency variants* (Table 25.3). Some of these variants are not associated with clinical disease, such as the S variant [5]. Other deficiency variants are associated with emphysema [5,12] such as M$_{Heerlen}$, M$_{Procida}$, M$_{Malton}$, M$_{Duarte}$, M$_{Mineral\ Springs}$, P$_{Lowell}$, and W$_{Bethesda}$. In two people with M$_{Malton}$ and one with M$_{Duarte}$, hepatocyte α_1-AT inclusions and liver disease have been reported [12]. In one person with the deficiency variant S$_{Iiyama}$, emphysema and hepatocyte inclusions were reported, but this person did not have liver

disease [12]. Dysfunctional variants of α_1-AT include α_1-AT Pittsburgh [15]. There also is a decrease in serum concentration and functional activity for α_1-AT M$_{Mineral\ Spring}$ [12]. For several variants that have been identified in compound heterozygotes such as α_1-AT F, α_1-AT Null$_{Newport}$, and α_1-AT Z$_{Wrexham}$, it is not clear whether the variants result in normal, null, deficient, or dysfunctional changes [12].

Function of α_1-antitrypsin

α_1-Antitrypsin is an inhibitor of serine proteases in general, but its most important targets are neutrophil elastase, cathepsin G, and proteinase 3: proteases released by activated neutrophils. Several lines of evidence suggest that inhibition of these neutrophil proteases is the major physiologic function of α_1-AT [5]. First, individuals with α_1-AT deficiency are susceptible to premature development of emphysema, a lesion that can be induced in experimental animals by instillation of excessive amounts of neutrophil elastase. These observations have led to the concept that destructive lung disease may result from perturbations of the net balance of elastase and α_1-AT within the local environment of the lung. Second, the kinetics of association for α_1-AT and neutrophil elastase are more favorable, by several orders of magnitude, than those for

Table 25.3 Deficiency variants of α₁-antitrypsin

	Defect		Clinical disease		Cellular defect
			Liver	Lung	
Z	Single base substitution M₁ (Ala 213)	Glu 342–Lys	+	+	IC accumulation
S	Single base substitution	Glu 264–Val	–	–	IC accumulation
M$_{Heerlen}$	Single base substitution	Pro 369–Leu	–	+	IC accumulation
M$_{Procida}$	Single base substitution	Leu 41–Pro	–	+	IC accumulation
M$_{Malton}$	Single base deletion	Phe 52	?	+	IC accumulation
M$_{Duarte}$	Unknown	Unknown	+?	+	Unknown
M$_{Mineral Springs}$	Single base substitution	Gly 57–Glu	–	+	No function; EC degradation?
S$_{Iiyama}$	Single base substitution	Ser 53–Phe	–	+	IC accumulation
P$_{Duarte}$	Two base substitution	Arg 101–His Asp 256–Val	+?	+	Unknown
P$_{Lowell}$	Single base substitution	Asp 256–Val	–	+	IC accumulation; reduced function
W$_{Bethesda}$	Single base substitution	Ala 336–Thre	–	+	EC degradation?
Z$_{Wrexham}$		Ser19–Leu	?	?	Unknown
F	Single base substitution	Arg 223–Cys	–	–	Unknown
T	Single base substitution	Glu 264–Val	–	–	Unknown
I	Single base substitution	Arg 39–Cys	–	–	IC accumulation; reduced function
M$_{Palermo}$	Single base deletion	Phe 51	–	–	Unknown
M$_{Nichinan}$	Single base deletion and single base substitution	Phe 52 Gly 148–Arg	–	–	Unknown
Zausburg	Single base substitution	Glu 342–Lys	–	–	Unknown

IC, intracellular; EC, extracellular.

α₁-AT and any other serine protease. Third, α₁-AT constitutes more than 90% of the neutrophil elastase inhibitory activity in the one body fluid that has been examined, pulmonary alveolar lavage fluid.

α₁-Antitrypsin acts competitively by allowing its target enzymes to bind directly to a substrate-like region within its reactive center loop [9]. The reaction between enzyme and inhibitor is essentially second order, and the resulting complex contains one molecule of each of the reactants. A reactive-site peptide bond within the inhibitor is hydrolyzed during formation of the enzyme–inhibitor complex. Hydrolysis of this bond, however, does not proceed to completion. An equilibrium, near unity, is established between complexes in which the reactive-site peptide bond of α₁-AT is intact (native inhibitor) and those in which this peptide bond is cleaved (modified inhibitor). The complex of α₁-AT and serine protease is a covalently stabilized structure that is resistant to dissociation by denaturing compounds, including sodium dodecyl sulfate and urea. The interaction between α₁-AT and serine protease is suicidal in that the modified inhibitor is no longer able to bind with or inactivate the enzyme.

The net functional activity of α₁-AT in complex biologic fluids may be modified by several factors [5,9]. First, the reactive-site methionine may be oxidized and thereby rendered inactive as an elastase inhibitor. In vitro, α₁-AT is oxidatively inactivated by activated neutrophils and by oxidants released by alveolar macrophages of cigarette smokers. Second, the functional activity of α₁-AT may be modified by proteolytic inactivation. Several members of the metalloprotease family – including collagenase and *Pseudomonas* elastase – and of the thiol protease family can cleave and inactivate α₁-AT.

Although α₁-AT from the plasma or liver of individuals with PiZZ α₁-AT deficiency is functionally active [5,9], there may be a decrease in its specific elastase inhibitory capacity. Ogushi *et al.* [17] have shown that the kinetics of association with neutrophil elastase and the stability of complexes with neutrophil elastase were decreased significantly for α₁-AT isolated from PiZZ plasma. There was no decrease in the functional activity of α₁-AT from PiSS individuals.

α₁-Antitrypsin has also been shown to protect experimental animals from the lethal effects of tumor necrosis factor [18]. Most of the evidence from these studies indicates that this protective effect results from inhibition of the synthesis and release of platelet-activating factor from neutrophils, presumably through the inhibition of neutrophil-derived proteases.

Several studies indicate that α_1-AT has functional activities other than inhibition of serine protease. The C-terminal fragment of α_1-AT, which can be generated during the formation of a complex with serine protease or during proteolytic inactivation by thiol- or metalloproteases, is a potent neutrophil chemoattractant [9]. Furthermore, it has been shown to prevent cellular entry of HIV [19,20].

Although effects on lymphocyte activities and immune and inflammatory function have been attributed to α_1-AT [21], there are inherent conflicts in some of the reports, and the data have not been duplicated. There is no evidence that the immune response is altered systematically in α_1-AT-deficient individuals.

Biosynthesis of α_1-antitrypsin

The predominant site of synthesis of plasma α_1-AT is the liver. This is most clearly shown by conversion of plasma α_1-AT to the donor phenotype after orthotopic liver transplantation [9]. It is synthesized in human hepatoma cells as a 52 kDa precursor; undergoes post-translational, dolichol phosphate-linked glycosylation at three asparagine residues and undergoes tyrosine sulfation. It is secreted as a 55 kDa native single-chain glycoprotein with a half-time for secretion of 35 to 40 minutes [9].

Tissue-specific expression of α_1-AT in human hepatoma cells is directed by structural elements within a 750-nucleotide region upstream of the hepatocyte transcriptional start site in exon Ic. Within these regions are structural elements that are recognized by hepatocyte nuclear transcription factors (HNFs), including HNF1α, HNFβ, HNF4, and HNF3 plus CCAAT/enhancer binding protein (C/EBP) [9]. HNF1α and HNF4 appear to be particularly important for expression of human *SERPINA1* (encoding α_1-AT). Two distinct regions within the proximal element bind these two transcription factors. In fact, substitution of five nucleotides within the region of nucleotides (–77 through –72) disrupts binding of HNF1α and dramatically reduces production of the human α_1-AT in the liver of transgenic mice [9]. Substitution of four nucleotides at positions (–118 through –115 disrupts the binding of HNF4 but does not alter expression of the human gene for α_1-AT in the liver of adult transgenic mice. The latter mutation does result in a reduction in the production of human α_1-AT in the liver during embryonic development. HNF1α and HNF4 have a synergistic effect on expression of the gene for α_1-AT in hepatocytes and enterocytes [12].

Plasma concentrations of α_1-AT increase three- to five-fold during the host response to inflammation or tissue injury [9]. Because the source of this additional α_1-AT has been thought to be the liver, α_1-AT is known as a positive hepatic acute phase reactant. Synthesis of α_1-AT in human hepatoma cells (HepG2, Hep3B) is upregulated by interleukin-6 but not by interleukin-1 or tumor necrosis factor. Plasma concentrations

of α_1-AT also increase during oral contraceptive therapy and pregnancy [9].

α_1-Antitrypsin is also synthesized and secreted in primary cultures of human blood monocytes and bronchoalveolar and breast milk macrophages [22]. Expression of α_1-AT in monocytes and macrophages is influenced by products generated during inflammation, such as bacterial lipopolysaccharide and interleukin-6 [9].

Production of α_1-AT is also regulated by a feed-forward mechanism in which elastase–α_1-AT complexes mediate an increase in synthesis of α_1-AT through the interaction of a pentapeptide domain in the C-terminal tail of α_1-AT with a novel cell surface receptor [9]. This class of receptor molecules is now referred to as serpin–enzyme complex (SEC) receptors because they recognize the highly conserved domains of other SECs, such as antithrombin III–thrombin, α_1-antichymotrypsin–cathepsin G, and, to a lesser extent, C1 inhibitor–C1s and tissue plasminogen activator–plasminogen activator inhibitor 1 complexes, as well as that of elastase–α_1-AT complexes [9]. Substance P, several other tachykinins, bombesin, and the amyloid-β peptide bind to the SEC receptor through a similar pentapeptide sequence [9]. The SEC receptor can mediate endocytosis of soluble amyloid-β peptide, but it does not recognize the aggregated form of amyloid-β peptide, which is toxic to neurons and other cell types [12]. The SEC receptor may play a role in preventing amyloid-β peptide from accumulating in the amyloid deposits associated with Alzheimer disease.

α_1-Antitrypsin mRNA has been isolated from multiple tissues in transgenic mice [23,24], but in many cases it has not been possible to distinguish whether this mRNA is in ubiquitous tissue macrophages or other cell types. α_1-Antitrypsin is synthesized in enterocytes and Paneth cells, as indicated by studies in intestinal epithelial cell lines, ribonuclease protection assays of human intestinal RNA, and in situ hybridization analyses in cryostat sections of human intestinal mucosa [12]. Production of α_1-AT in enterocytes increases during differentiation from crypt to villus, in response to interleukin-6 and during inflammation in vivo. It is also synthesized by pulmonary epithelial cells [12]. Interestingly, synthesis of α_1-AT in pulmonary epithelial cells is less responsive to regulation by interleukin-6 than by a related cytokine, oncostatin M [12].

Clearance and distribution

The half-life of α_1-AT in plasma is approximately 5 days [5]. It is estimated that the daily production rate of α_1-AT is 34 mg/kg body weight, with 33% of the intravascular pool of α_1-AT degraded daily. There is a slight increase in the rate of clearance of radiolabeled α_1-ATZ compared with wild-type α_1-AT if infused into PiMM individuals, but this difference does not account for the decrease in serum levels of α_1-AT in deficient individuals [5].

α_1-Antitrypsin diffuses into most tissues and is found in most body fluids [5]. Its concentration in lavage fluid from the lower respiratory tract is approximately equivalent to that in serum; it is also found in feces, and increased fecal concentrations of α_1-AT correlate with the presence of inflammatory lesions of the bowel [12]. In each case, it has been assumed that α_1-AT was derived from serum. Local sites of synthesis, however, such as macrophages and epithelial cells, also may make important contributions to the α_1-AT pool in these tissues and body fluids. It has been reported that the rate of fecal α_1-AT clearance is higher in patients with homozygous PiZZ α_1-AT deficiency than in normal people [12]. Because the former have only 10–15% of the normal serum concentrations of α_1-AT, a local intestinal source for fecal α_1-AT is implicated. One possible explanation is that the bulk of α_1-AT in feces is derived from sloughed enterocytes. Increased fecal α_1-AT in those with homozygous PiZZ α_1-AT deficiency would result from intracellular accumulation of the abnormal α_1-AT molecule in enterocytes that are being sloughed at the usual rate. Increased fecal α_1-AT in normal PiMM people with inflammatory-related, protein-losing enteropathy would result from increased sloughing of enterocytes alone.

Mechanism for deficiency of α₁-antitrypsin in PiZZ individuals

The mutant α_1-ATZ molecule is characterized by a single nucleotide substitution that results in an amino acid substitution, Lys for Glu 342 [9]. There is a selective decrease in the secretion of α_1-AT, with the mutant protein accumulating in the ER [9]. The defect is not specific for liver cells; it also affects extrahepatic sites of α_1-AT synthesis, such as macrophages and transfected cell lines [9]. Site-directed mutagenesis studies have shown that this single amino acid substitution is sufficient to produce the cellular defect [9]. Once translocated into the lumen of the ER, the mutant α_1-AT protein is unable to traverse the remainder of the secretory pathway because it is folded abnormally.

Studies by Lomas and colleagues showed for the first time that the α_1-ATZ protein was prone to polymerization and aggregation [25] and these authors proposed a mechanism for polymerization that involved a unique loop-sheet insertion phenomenon. More recent studies that elucidated the crystal structure of a stable serpin dimer have provided the basis for an interesting new model in which a domain-swapping mechanism explains the formation of polymers and insoluble aggregates of α_1-ATZ [26]. In contrast to the loop-sheet insertion model, this mechanism of polymerization is not unique, having been described for a number of other proteins. This model predicts that the final step in folding of the serpin molecule is the incorporation of strand s5a into the central β-sheet A. The substitution of Lys for Glu 342 that characterizes the α_1-ATZ molecule lies within strand s5a and this substitution disrupts the usual intramolecular interaction with Lys 290 on strand s6a and Thr 203 within strand s5a. As a result the region that would otherwise be destined to form strand s5a in the α_1-ATZ protein is flexible and unstructured

in a way that favors domain swapping of s5a together with the reactive center loop/strand s4a between adjacent α_1-ATZ molecules. Presumably this leads to progressive linear polymerization. Finally, the unfolding event that leads to domain swapping is predicted to expose a 30 residue helical linker region. Because this linker is hydrophobic, it is plausible to envision lateral association between linear polymers that would produce tangled aggregates that are seen in the ER of liver cells in α_1-AT deficiency. This model provides explanations for several phenomena that have been somewhat mysterious in the past: how the α_1-ATZ molecule transitions from a relatively normally folded intermediate into polymers and insoluble aggregates; how a small proportion of newly synthesized α_1-ATZ molecules (10–15%) are kinetically capable of folding into a conformation that can traverse the secretory pathway; and how accumulation of polymerized α_1-ATZ in the ER does not activate the unfolded protein response (UPR), presumably because the structure of the polymer closely resembles the relaxed conformation of the normally folded monomer.

Two series of studies have suggested that polymerization of α_1-ATZ is the cause of its retention in the ER, including, most notably, studies in which its secretion is partially corrected by introduction of a second mutation that suppresses loop-sheet polymerization [26]. However, these studies have not excluded the possibility that retention is caused by a distinct abnormality in folding that is partially corrected by the second, experimentally introduced mutation. Indeed, several recent observations militate against the idea that polymerization is the cause of ER retention. First, naturally occurring variants of α_1-AT in which the C-terminal tail of α_1-AT is truncated, including a double mutant with the substitution that characterizes the Z allele and the substitution that results in C-terminal truncation, are retained in the ER even though they do not polymerize [27]. Second, only approximately 18% of the intracellular pool of α_1-ATZ at steady state is in the form of polymers in model cell lines characterized by marked ER retention [27,28]. A greater degree of polymerization is thought to be prevented by the activity of ER chaperones. Most of the cellular pool of α_1-ATZ in the ER in vivo is in heterogeneous soluble complexes with multiple ER chaperones (Figure 25.3) [28,29], a state that cannot be modeled by studies of purified α_1-ATZ in vitro. These observations suggest the possibility that polymerization of α_1-ATZ in the ER is an effect, rather than a cause, of the retention. This possibility does not preclude a specific role of polymers in the pathogenesis of tissue injury. In fact, three new lines of evidence argue for the specific role of polymers in injury to the liver. The first of these is the discovery that an inherited form of progressive dementia is associated with mutations in neuroserpin that have effects on the structure of that molecule that are almost identical to the effects of the Z mutation on α_1-AT [30]. Second, there is now evidence suggesting that polymers that accumulate in the ER are degraded by a mechanism distinct from that of polymers, autophagic as distinct from proteosomal

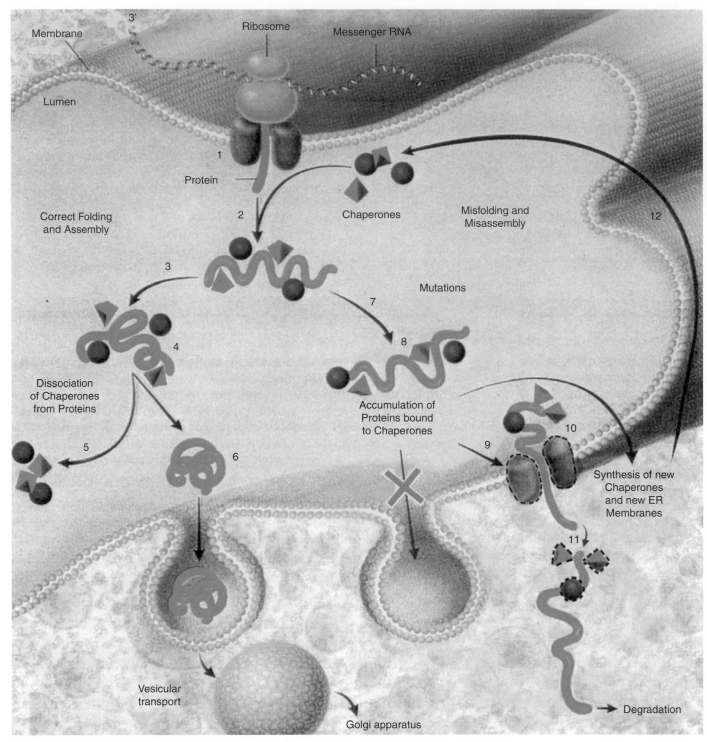

Figure 25.3 The fate of polypeptides in the endoplasmic reticulum (ER). Secretory and membrane proteins are cotranslationally translocated into the lumen of the ER through the import channel associated with Sec61p (1). These polypeptides transiently interact with several chaperones (2) to facilitate folding (3). Once folding is completed (4), there is dissociation of chaperones (5) and vesicular transport out of the ER (6). In the cases of mutant proteins (7) that remain misfolded even after interaction with chaperones (8), there is accumulation of misfolded proteins bound to their chaperones. The quality control apparatus of the ER mediates transport of these misfolded proteins, free or bound to chaperones, to the ER membrane (9) or through a channel, perhaps even through the import channel associated with Sec61p (10), into the cytoplasm (11) for degradation. The accumulation of misfolded proteins induces the synthesis of new chaperones and new ER membrane to accommodate the increased load of misfolded proteins and thereby protect the cells (12). (Adapted with permission from Kuznetsov and Nigam, 1998 [29].)

degradation [31]. Third, recent studies indicate that accumulation of the polymerogenic mutant α₁-ATZ activates cellular signaling pathways that are distinct from those activated by non-polymerogenic α₁-AT mutants [31].

Cellular adaptive responses to mutant α₁-antitrypsin Z retained in the endoplasmic reticulum

We now know that cells have elaborate mechanisms for degrading mutant proteins that are retained in the ER. The pathways by which retained α₁-ATZ is degraded are also candidates for genetic variations that predispose some homozygotes or protect other homozygotes from liver injury by the gain-of-toxic function mechanism. One study has provided a substantiation of this concept by showing that there is a lag in ER degradation of α₁-ATZ after gene transfer into cell lines derived from susceptible hosts, homozygotes with liver disease, when compared with cell lines from protected hosts, homozygotes completely free of liver disease [32].

Several pathways appear to be involved in the ER degradation of α₁-ATZ. The proteosomal system was implicated first and has since been demonstrated in a number of model systems [31]. Both the classical ubiquitin-dependent and the ubiquitin-independent proteosomal pathways play a role. The mechanism by which molecules like mutant α₁-ATZ that are found in the lumen of the ER reach the proteosome in the cytoplasm has been called ER-associated degradation (ERAD) and involves some type of retrograde translocation mechanism. A multiprotein complex that includes luminal and membrane-bound chaperones, membrane-spanning transport proteins, and cytoplasmic ubiquitin ligases has been implicated in the ERAD pathway for model luminal ERAD substrates. A mechanism in which the proteosome directly mediates extraction of substrates from the ER membrane is also favored as a part of the mechanism by which ERAD mediates its actions.

Nevertheless, there was evidence from studies of the proteasomal pathway in mammalian cell lines, cell-free microsomal translocation systems, and yeast that this pathway could not completely account for disposal of α₁-ATZ. Autophagy was first implicated in α₁-AT deficiency when a marked increased in autophagosomes were observed in fibroblast cell lines engineered for expression of α₁-ATZ [33]. Increased autophagosomes were observed in the liver of PiZ mice and in liver biopsy specimens from patients [33].

Autophagy is a catabolic process by which the cell digests its internal constituents to generate amino acids in response to nutrient starvation and other stress states. It also appears to play a role in homeostasis, cell growth, and differentiation. It begins with the formation of a membranous platform around a targeted region of the cell. This platform becomes a double-membrane vesicle as it envelopes cytoplasm together with parts of or entire subcellular organelles. Eventually this autophagosome fuses with the lysosome for degradation of its contents.

Therefore, the presence of abundant autophagosomes in the liver in α₁-AT deficiency and its models raised the possibility that autophagy could be involved in degrading the mutant α₁-ATZ that is retained in the ER. Indeed the initial study went on to show that disposal of α₁-ATZ was partially abrogated by chemical inhibitors of autophagy, including 3-methyladenine, wortmannin, and LY-294002 [33]. However, because these drugs have other cellular effects and so cannot be considered specific for autophagy, genetic evidence that autophagy participated in disposal of α₁-ATZ was sought. An embryonic fibroblast cell line (MEF) from an ATG5-null mouse was engineered for expression of α₁-ATZ [34]. The results showed a marked delay in degradation of α₁-ATZ in the ATG5-null compared with the wild type MEF cells. Furthermore in the ATG5-null cell line it became possible to observe massive accumulation of α₁-ATZ with very large inclusions throughout the cytoplasm. Therefore, in addition to providing definitive evidence that autophagy contributes to the disposal of α₁-ATZ, these studies suggest that it plays a "homeostatic" role in the α₁-AT-deficient state by preventing toxic cytoplasmic accumulation of α₁-ATZ through piecemeal digestion of insoluble aggregates.

A study by Kruse et al. [35] using a completely different strategy also demonstrated the importance of autophagy in disposal of α₁-ATZ. Human α₁-ATZ was expressed in a library of yeast mutants and screened for mutants that were impaired for degradation of α₁-ATZ. One of the mutants corresponded to the yeast homologue of mammalian ATG6. In the absence of this ATG6 homologue or the homologue of ATG16 there was a marked delay in disposal of human α₁-ATZ. These studies were particularly revealing because delay in degradation of α₁-ATZ was most apparent in the autophagy-deficient yeast strains when α₁-ATZ was produced at high levels. At lower levels of production, α₁-ATZ was degraded at a rate not significantly different from that in wild-type yeast. These results are consistent with the notion that at lower levels of production α₁-ATZ in the ER is predominantly soluble and can be degraded by the proteasome whereas at higher levels it is more likely to transition to insoluble polymers/aggregates that require autophagy for disposal.

Kruse et al. [36] also discovered that a mutant subunit of fibrinogen that forms insoluble aggregates in the ER of liver cells in an inherited form of fibrinogen deficiency depends on autophagy for disposal. This type of fibrinogen deficiency has been associated with a chronic liver disease characterized by distinct fibrillar aggregates in the ER of liver cells. These results substantiate the concept that chronic liver disease can be caused by accumulation of an aggregation-prone protein in the ER and that autophagy is specialized for the disposal of aggregation-prone proteins that accumulate in the ER.

Several lines of evidence suggest that there are one or more other pathways that contribute to disposal of α₁-ATZ. A pathway that depends on a tyrosine phosphatase activity has been described [37]. The studies of Kruse et al. [35] indicated that α₁-ATZ could be transported to the trans-Golgi and then targeted to the lysosome of yeast but a comparable pathway has not been described in mammalian cells.

In addition to degradation mechanisms, cells appear to have a number of other mechanisms by which they attempt to adapt to, or protect themselves, from proteins that are retained in the ER. Because differences in an adaptive response could theoretically explain variation in the liver disease phenotype, we have recently begun a series of studies designed to characterize how cells respond to ER retention of α_1-ATZ using cell line and transgenic mouse model systems with tetracycline-inducible expression of the mutant gene. These models permit us to see the earliest responses and to separate them from compensatory adaptations that arise later. Because the relative expression of the mutant gene can be regulated in this kind of model system, it is also possible to determine the effect of the mutant gene product at specific concentrations, at specific stages of development, and for specific intervals.

Accumulation of α_1-ATZ in the ER is sufficient to activate the autophagic response. This was demonstrated by mating two types of transgenic mice: the Z mouse, with liver-specific inducible expression of α_1-ATZ in which α_1-ATZ accumulates in the ER of hepatocytes only when doxycycline is removed from the drinking water [34], and the GFP-LC3 mouse, in which autophagosomes have green fluorescence because LC3 is an autophagosomal membrane-specific protein. Although green fluorescent autophagosomes are only seen in the liver of the GFP-LC3 mouse when it is starved, they are seen in the liver of the Z × GFP-LC3 mouse simply by removing doxycycline from the drinking water and inducing the accumulation of mutant α_1-ATZ in the ER of hepatocytes [34]. This is a particularly important observation because it represents the first evidence that a single protein can activate the autophagic response. Although there is much still to learn about how accumulation of α_1-ATZ in the ER activates autophagy, recent studies have shown that the regulator of G signaling 16 may play a role in mediating this effect. This regulator is an antagonist of Gαi3, which ordinarily inhibits hepatic autophagy [31]. Hidvegi et al. [38] have shown that the regulator of G signaling 16 is markedly upregulated when α_1-ATZ expression is induced and that this effect could de-repress the autophagic response.

Surprisingly, accumulation of α_1-ATZ in the ER does not activate the UPR. The UPR is a signaling pathway that activates a number of genes in response to accumulation of unfolded proteins in the ER [31]. In addition to new synthesis of ER chaperones, such as BiP (GRP78), and enzymes that facilitate disulfide bond formation, other processes occur, including bolstering the protein-folding capacity of the ER, increasing lipids for synthesis of new ER membrane required to handle the increased protein load, increasing synthesis of proteins that participate in degradative and other cellular translocation mechanisms. There is also a decrease in initiation of translation in such a way that only specific mRNAs can be translated, thereby preventing the de novo synthesis of proteins that will further accumulate in the ER [31]. Although we do not detect activation of the UPR when α_1-ATZ accumulates in the ER, we do detect it when truncated non-polymerogenic α_1-AT variants accumulate in the ER [39], suggesting that the failure to activate the UPR is specific for the α_1-ATZ variant [39]. With what is known about the mechanisms by which the UPR is initiated, it has always been relatively easy to understand how polymerized or aggregated proteins would not elicit this response. Results of structural studies provide an explanation for why soluble monomeric α_1-ATZ might not be recognized by the UPR sensing apparatus [26]. These results suggested that the monomeric α_1-ATZ intermediate adopts a conformation that resembles the wild-type molecule and, therefore, would not be recognized as unfolded. The lack of UPR signaling in cells that accumulate α_1-ATZ is likely to be an important part of how liver cells behave in vivo in α_1-AT-deficient-patients, perhaps partially accounting for the chronic, slowly progressing nature of the disease. A liver picture dominated by hepatocyte apoptosis and fulminant liver failure would be likely if the UPR was being activated.

In contrast, the ER overload pathway and its signature target nuclear transcription factor kappa B (NF-κB) is activated when α_1-ATZ accumulates in the ER [39]. The ER overload pathway was first described as activation of NF-κB in response to the type of "ER stress" that is generated by treatment of cells with brefeldin A or by experimental accumulation of adenovirus E3 protein in the ER [39]. The fact that ER accumulation of α_1-ATZ activates NF-κB but not the UPR provides strong corroborating evidence for the previously held contention that the ER overload pathway was distinct from the UPR. Activation of NF-κB has potentially important implications for target organ injury in α_1-AT deficiency. In particular it plays an important role in inflammation-associated carcinogenesis and this appears to be related to its effect on cell proliferation [31].

Using cell line and mouse model systems with inducible expression of mutant α_1-ATZ two other signal transduction pathways associated with ER stress have been investigated. Accumulation of α_1-ATZ in the ER led to cleavage and activation of the ER caspases: caspase-12 in mouse cells and caspase-4 in human cells [39]. These results indicate that both the mitochondrial and ER caspase pathways are activated in α_1-AT deficiency. Accumulation of α_1-ATZ in the ER also specifically mediated cleavage and activation of BAP31 (B-cell receptor-association protein 31) [39], an integral membrane protein of the ER that is involved in the ER retention of several proteins and appears to mediate proapoptotic signals from the ER to mitochondria. This last may provide a mechanistic basis for the mitochondrial dysfunction that has been found in cell line and transgenic mouse models as well as in the liver of α_1-AT-deficient patients [40].

Genomic analysis of the liver from our mouse model with inducible expression of mutant α_1-ATZ demonstrated several other cellular response pathways that are specifically activated, including the lipogenic and sterolgenic signaling pathways that are mediated by transforming growth factor-β, extracellular regulated kinase 2, and the sterol regulatory element-binding proteins [38]. The transforming growth factor-β signaling pathway plays a dominant role in tissue fibrosis and can explain the primary pathological effect of α_1-ATZ accumulation on the liver.

Modifiers that affect the function of any of these pathways could increase susceptibility to liver disease according to our theory. Indeed, a single nucleotide polymorphism (SNP) in the downstream flanking region of ER mannosidase I has been implicated in early-onset liver disease among α_1-AT-deficient individuals [41]. Because ER mannosidase I plays a role in ERAD, a polymorphism that affects its function would be a prime candidate for a modifier of liver disease in α_1-AT deficiency. However, further epidemiological studies are needed to determine if this SNP is truly affecting liver disease susceptibility and further cellular studies are needed to identify how it alters the fate of the mutant protein.

An SNP in the upstream flanking region of the gene for α_1-AT itself has also been implicated in liver disease susceptibility [42]. There is no reason to believe that this SNP would affect the disposal of α_1-ATZ. The logical explanation for the effect of this polymorphism would be to increase production of α_1-ATZ, but the published results did not substantiate that notion. Furthermore, the study could have led to an entirely different conclusion with a legitimate alternative way of classifying one of the patient groups.

Pathogenesis of liver injury in α₁-antitrypsin deficiency

There are several theories for the pathogenesis of liver injury in α_1-AT deficiency [9]. According to the immune theory, liver damage results from an abnormal immune response to liver antigens. This theory is based on the observation that peripheral blood lymphocytes from PiZZ infants are cytotoxic for isolated hepatocytes; however, this is probably a non-specific effect of liver injury in that peripheral blood lymphocytes from PiMM infants with a similar degree of liver injury caused by idiopathic neonatal hepatitis syndrome are also cytotoxic for isolated hepatocytes. More recent studies have indicated an increase in the *HLA-DR3-HLA-DW25* haplotype in α_1-AT-deficient individuals with liver disease [9]. There is no difference, however, in the expression of class II major histocompatibility complex (MHC) antigen in the livers of these individuals compared with normal control subjects [9]. Moreover, an increase in the prevalence of a particular *HLA-DR* haplotype in the affected population does not by itself imply altered immune function. Because of the linkage disequilibrium displayed by genes within the MHC, it is possible that increased susceptibility is caused by the products of unrelated but linked genes. For example, the MHC contains genes for several heat shock/stress proteins, proteins that play an important role in the biogenesis and transport of other proteins through the secretory pathway.

The accumulation theory, in which liver damage is thought to be caused by accumulation of mutant α_1-AT molecules in the ER of liver cells, is the most widely accepted. Experimental results in transgenic mice are most consistent with this theory and completely exclude the possibility that liver damage is caused by "proteolytic attack" as a consequence of diminished serum of α_1-AT concentrations. Transgenic mice carrying the mutant Z allele of human *SERPINA1* develop periodic acid–Schiff-positive, diastase-resistant intrahepatic globules and liver injury early in life [8]. Because there are normal levels of α_1-AT and presumably other antielastases in these animals, as directed by endogenous murine genes, the liver injury cannot be attributed to proteolytic attack.

Some have argued that the histologic characteristics of the liver in the transgenic mouse model are not identical to those in humans. Detailed histologic characterization of the liver in one transgenic mouse model by Geller *et al.* [43] has shown that there are focal areas of liver cell necrosis, microabcesses with an accumulation of neutrophils and regenerative activity in the form of multicellular liver plates, and focal nodule formation during the neonatal period. Nodular clusters of altered hepatocytes that lack α_1-AT-immunoreactivity are also seen during the neonatal period. With aging, there is a decrease in the number of hepatocytes containing α_1-ATZ globules; there is also an increase in the number of nodular aggregates of α_1-AT-negative hepatocytes and development of periosinusoidal fibrosis [44]. Within 6 weeks, there are dysplastic changes in these aggregates. Adenomas occur within 1 year, and invasive hepatocellular carcinoma is seen between 1 and 2 years of age [44]. Recent studies have shown that liver injury in another transgenic mouse model, the PiZ mouse, is most prominently characterized by fibrosis [6] and carcinogenesis [7]. Together with minimal inflammation, mild steatosis [6], and glycogen depletion [45], this liver pathology very closely phenocopies what is seen in humans affected by the deficiency.

Data from individuals who have null alleles of α_1-AT and, therefore, negligible serum levels of α_1-AT have also been used as evidence against the proteolytic attack theory. These individuals do not develop liver injury – at least not sufficiently to result in clinical detection. However, only a few individuals with null alleles have been reported, and each has a different allele. Based on data in PiZZ individuals showing that only 10–15% of these individuals develop clinically significant liver injury, it might be necessary to evaluate seven to eight individuals with each null allele before detecting one with liver injury.

The recognition that several other naturally occurring variant alleles of α_1-AT associated with deficiency can undergo polymerization has provided some support for the accumulation theory. The most important of these is the compound heterozygous α_1-ATSZ phenotype. Mahadeva *et al.* [46] have shown that α_1-ATS and α_1-ATZ may form heteropolymers. A nationwide study of α_1-AT deficiency in Sweden found that the incidence of liver disease among individuals with the PiSZ phenotype is similar to that of individuals with the PiZZ phenotype [2,3]. It is also known that the PiM$_{Malton}$ allele undergoes polymerization, and several of the patients carrying this have been reported to have α_1-AT globules in their liver and liver injury [12]. However, there is a report of an individual with PIS$_{\text{Iiyama}}$ allele having hepatocyte α_1-AT globules but no liver injury [12]. Other variants that are thought to undergo aggregation have not been associated with liver damage. It is also not clear how many of the patients with very rare variants have been thoroughly examined for liver disease, infection with hepatitis C virus, or evidence for autoimmune or alcoholic hepatitis. Again, on the basis of what is known about the PiZZ and PiSZ phenotype, at least seven to eight individuals with each of these alleles would need to be examined to detect one with liver injury and there are probably no more than that many of the rare variants together that have been identified to date.

It has been difficult to reconcile the accumulation theory with the observations of Sveger [2,3], which showed that only a subset of PiZZ α_1-AT-deficient individuals develop significant liver damage. We have predicted that a subset of the PiZZ population is more susceptible to liver injury by virtue of one or more additional inherited traits or environmental factors that exaggerate the intracellular accumulation of the mutant Z α_1-AT protein or exaggerate the cellular pathophysiologic consequence of mutant α_1-AT accumulation. To address this prediction experimentally, skin fibroblasts from α_1-AT PiZZ individuals, with or without liver disease, were transduced with amphotropic recombinant retroviral particles designed for constitutive production of mutant α_1-AT [32]. Human skin fibroblasts do not produce endogenous α_1-AT but, presumably, express other genes involved in the postsynthetic processing of secretory proteins. The results show that expression of mutant human gene for α_1-AT was conferred on each fibroblast cell line. Compared with the same cell line transduced with the wild-type *SERPINA1*, there was selective intracellular retention of the mutant α_1-ATZ protein in each case. However, there was a marked delay in degradation of the mutant α_1-ATZ protein after it accumulated in the fibroblasts from PiZZ individuals with liver disease (susceptible hosts) compared with those without liver disease (protected hosts) (Figure 25.4) [47]. These data provide evidence that other factors affecting the fate of the mutant α_1-ATZ molecule, such as a lag in ER degradation, at least in part determine susceptibility to liver disease.

The lag in ER degradation of α_1-ATZ in susceptible hosts may involve several distinct mechanisms. In one susceptible host, the retained α_1-ATZ interacts poorly with calnexin [32]. In the liver cells of this host, there is likely to be only a very little polyubiquitinated calnexin–α_1-ATZ complex that can be recognized for proteolysis by the proteasome. In several other susceptible hosts, the retained α_1-ATZ interacts well with calnexin but is degraded slowly. These hosts may have a defect in calnexin that prevents its ubiquitination or a defect in either the ubiquitin system or a component of the proteasome.

The molecular basis for liver cell injury in α_1-AT deficiency is still largely undefined. Detailed studies of liver pathology in the PiZ mouse model demonstrated significant increases in mitochondrial damage and dysfunction as well as caspase-3 activation in situ [40,48]. Similar alterations were noted in the liver of α_1-AT-deficient patients. Mitochondrial depolarization

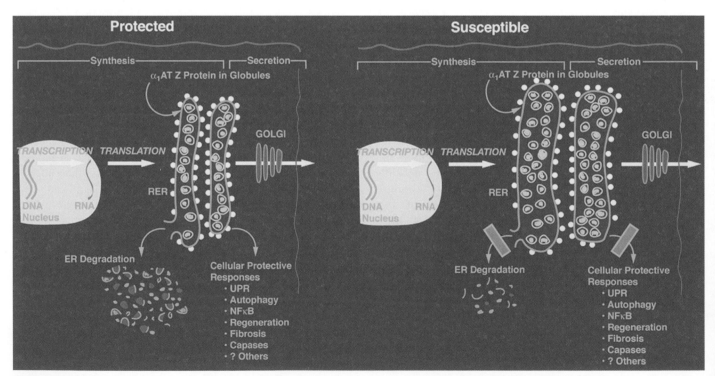

Figure 25.4 Difference in endoplasmic reticulum degradation of α_1-antitrypsin Z (ATZ) in protected and susceptible hosts. The block in degradation in susceptible hosts is represented by a small dark bar. UPR, unfolded protein response. (Adapted with permission from Teckman and Perlmutter, 1995 [47].)

followed induction of *SERPINA1* expression in a cell line model [40]. Most importantly, mitochondrial damage and stress-induced mortality were profoundly abrogated by treatment with cyclosporine but not by tacrolimus [40]. Both of these drugs modulate the immune response but only cyclosporine antagonizes mitochondrial depolarization and so these data provide further evidence for the concept that mitochondrial dysfunction is a sequella of the primary cellular defect in α₁-AT deficiency. It is not known whether mitochondrial dysfunction is a direct effect of the changes that occur in the ER or an indirect effect, perhaps involving the heightened autophagic response and mitophagy.

Hepatic regeneration and carcinogenesis in α₁-antitrypsin deficiency

To begin to understand how the liver is injured and how it regenerates in α₁-AT deficiency, Rudnick *et al.* [49] used the PiZ mouse model of α₁-AT deficiency and measured the degree of injury by bromodeoxyuridine labeling to quantify hepatocellular proliferation. These studies showed that there was increased hepatocellular proliferation in the liver of the PiZ mouse at baseline. Although the increase was five- to tenfold above the control mice and highly statistically significant, there was still a relatively low number of bromodeoxyuridine-positive hepatocytes at one time (2–3% detected over 72 hours of continuous labeling). These data indicate that liver injury in the mouse model is relatively mild and appropriately corresponds to the slowly progressing liver disease that is seen in most α₁-AT-deficient patients. The increase in hepatocellular proliferation was entirely accounted for by globule-devoid hepatocytes. It is not known how these globule-devoid hepatocytes arise, but they are known to have less total α₁-ATZ per cell and less polymerized α₁-ATZ per cell compared with the globule-containing hepatocytes [50]. These studies of Rudnick *et al.* [49] show that globule-devoid hepatocytes have a selective proliferative advantage and that is why zones of the liver that have no globule-containing hepatocytes are seen in every liver biopsy from patients with α₁-AT deficiency and in liver from the mouse models of α₁-AT deficiency and why these zones without globule-containing hepatocytes increase with age [31,43,44]. This also why hepatic cancers appear to predominantly arise from the zones of globule-devoid hepatocytes [51,52]. Furthermore, the degree of proliferation of the globule-devoid hepatocytes is directly proportional to the number of globule-containing hepatocytes [49]. We have speculated that these globule-devoid hepatocytes are younger cells that eventually go on to be globule-containing hepatocytes, but there is a continuous supply of younger cells as a part of the ongoing regenerative activity [53]. The globule-containing hepatocytes have more aggregated α₁-ATZ, activated autophagy, and activated NFκB. They are relatively impaired in regeneration and although they are undergoing cell death [54] it is at a relatively low rate and so they could be said to be also relatively impaired in death as well. The term

"relative" is used to describe the impairment in proliferation and death because these globule-containing cells will proliferate and die at higher rates after partial hepatectomy, a much more powerful regenerative stimulus than the proteotoxic state that is elicited by chronic intracellular accumulation of α₁-ATZ.

Based on these observations, David Rudnick and I have theorized that the globule-containing hepatocytes are "sick but not dead" and are responsible for regenerative signaling, but the globule-devoid hepatocytes are the predominant ones that can respond to these signals [53]. This theory has been validated, at least in part, by recent studies in which normal hepatocytes repopulate the livers of PiZ mice [55]. Wild-type donor hepatocytes spontaneously repopulated the livers of PiZ mice, replacing 20–98% of mutant host hepatocytes. The normal cells were shown to initially divide almost exclusively around globule-containing hepatocytes. Later they replaced globule-devoid hepatocytes presumably because these cells are "sick" compared with the normal donor cells even though they are "less sick" than the original globule-containing hepatocytes.

In essence, the theory [53] envisions that cross-talk between the globule-containing and globule-devoid cells perpetuates chronic hepatocellular proliferation, eventually leading to carcinogenesis within globule-devoid zones. The relative impairment in cell death in the globule-containing hepatocytes could account for the small number of cancers that do arise in these cells [7,52].

Diagnosis

Diagnosis is established by serum α₁-AT phenotype determination in isoelectric focusing or by agarose electrophoresis at acid pH. The phenotype should be determined in neonatal hepatitis or unexplained chronic liver disease in older children, adolescents, and adults. It is particularly important in the neonatal period because it may be very difficult to distinguish patients with α₁-AT deficiency from those with biliary atresia. Moreover, it is not uncommon for neonates with a PiZZ phenotype to have no biliary excretion on scintographic studies [12]. There is one report of α₁-AT deficiency and biliary atresia in a single patient [12]. We have had several patients with homozygous PiZZ α₁-AT deficiency and cholestasis and no biliary excretion of technetium-labeled mebrofenin, but in each of these, with more prolonged observation, cholestasis remitted, and it was obvious that the patient did not also have biliary atresia.

Serum concentrations of α₁-AT may be helpful, if used with phenotype, to distinguish individuals who are homozygous for the *Z* allele from *SZ* compound heterozygotes, both of whom may develop liver disease. In some cases, phenotype determinations of parents or other relatives are also necessary to ensure the distinction between *ZZ* and *SZ* allotypes, a distinction that is important for genetic counseling. Serum concentrations of α₁-AT occasionally are misleading. For example, serum α₁-AT concentrations may increase during the host response to inflammation, even in homozygous PiZZ individuals, giving a falsely reassuring impression.

Pathology

The distinctive histologic feature of homozygous PiZZ α_1-AT deficiency, periodic acid–Schiff-positive, diastase-resistant globules in the ER of hepatocytes substantiates the diagnosis (Figure 25.5). According to some observers, these globules are not as easy to detect in the first few months of life [12]. The presence of these inclusions should not be interpreted as diagnostic of α_1-AT deficiency. Similar structures occasionally are observed in PiMM individuals with other liver diseases. The inclusions are eosinophilic, round to oval, and 1–40 μm in diameter. They are most prominent in periportal hepatocytes but also may be seen in Kupffer cells and cells of biliary ductular lineage. There may be evidence of variable degrees of hepatocellular necrosis, inflammatory cell infiltration, periportal fibrosis, or cirrhosis. There is often evidence of bile duct epithelial cell destruction, and occasionally there is a paucity of

intrahepatic bile ducts. Our studies have shown that there also may be an intense autophagic reaction detected by electron microscopic examination of liver biopsy specimens, with a full array of nascent and degradative-type autophagic vacuoles [33].

Treatment

The most important principle in the treatment of α_1-AT deficiency is avoidance of cigarette smoking. Cigarette smoking markedly accelerates the destructive lung disease that is associated with α_1-AT deficiency, reduces the quality of life, and significantly shortens longevity of these individuals [5].

There is no specific therapy for α_1-AT deficiency-associated liver disease. Clinical care largely involves supportive management of symptoms resulting from liver dysfunction and the prevention of complications (Chapter 9). Although ursodeoxycholic acid and vitamin E have been mentioned in the literature, the clinical efficacy of these medications/nutriceuticals has not been investigated in a controlled clinical trial.

(a)

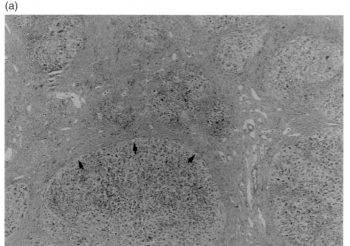

(b)

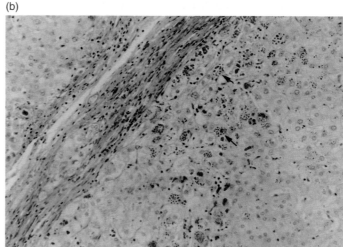

(c)

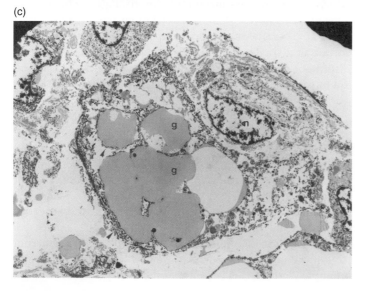

Figure 25.5 Hepatic histology in homozygous PiZZ α-antitrypsin deficiency. (a) Micrograph of liver biopsy specimen deficiency demonstrating increased fibrous tissue deposition (arrowheads) and nodular transformation. (periodic acid–Schiff (PAS)–diastase staining, 4× magnification.) (b) Micrograph of liver biopsy demonstrating the PAS-positive, diastase-resistant globules. (Two of the hepatocytes with globules are indicated by arrows.) (PAS–diastase staining, 40× magnification.) (c) Electron micrograph of same biopsy specimen demonstrating globules in endoplasmic reticulum. n, nucleus; g, globules; arrowheads, ribosomes.

Orthotopic liver transplantation

Progressive liver dysfunction and liver failure has been treated by orthotopic liver transplantation, with survival rates approaching 92% at 1 year and 90% at 5 years in children, and 89% at 1 year and 83% at 5 years in adults [56]. Nevertheless, a number of PiZZ individuals with severe liver disease, even cirrhosis or portal hypertension, may have relatively low rates of disease progression and lead relatively normal lives for extended periods of time [11]. With the availability of living related donor transplantation techniques, it may be possible to manage these patients expectantly for some time. Children with α₁-AT deficiency and mild liver dysfunction (elevated aminotransferase levels or hepatomegaly) without functional impairment may never need liver transplantation.

Pharmacologic strategies

Clincal trials of pharmacologic therapy for α₁-AT deficiency have been limited. Patients have been given the synthetic androgens danazol or stanozolol because of the dramatic effects of these agents in hereditary angioedema, which is a deficiency of the homologous serine proteinase inhibitor C1 inhibitor, and because danazol initially was found to increase serum levels of α₁-AT in PiZZ individuals [12]. Further evaluation, however, demonstrated that danazol increases serum levels of α₁-AT in only 50% of α₁-AT-deficient people, and the magnitude of the effect is small [12]. Moreover, it was not clear from any of the studies whether the effect of androgens occurred at the level of synthesis and might, therefore, also be associated with increased accumulation of α₁-ATZ in the ER, with potential hepatotoxic consequences. A pilot trial of 4-phenylbutyric acid was carried out [57] after it was demonstrated that it could enhance secretion of α₁-ATZ in the PiZ mouse model [58]. Treatment with 4-phenylbutyric acid did not result in increased serum levels of α₁-ATZ in humans [57] but it is important to note that this outcome could have been explained by the inability of patients to tolerate the relatively large dosage that may be necessary for the salutary effect. 4-Phenylbutyric acid was tested in the mouse model because it was thought to have chemical chaperone activity but it also has histone deacetylase inhibitory activity and recent studies have suggested that histone deacetylase inhibitors may profoundly facilitate the translocation of proteins through the secretory pathway. Other drugs with histone deacetylase inhibitor and/or chemical chaperone activity are likely to be tested soon.

Several iminosugar compounds may be useful for chemoprophylaxis of liver and lung disease in α₁-ATZ. These compounds are designed to interfere with oligosaccharide side-chain trimming of glycoproteins and have been investigated as potential therapeutic agents for viral hepatitis and other types of infections [12]. Several of these compounds were initially examined to determine the effect of inhibiting glucose or mannose trimming from the carbohydrate side-chain of α₁-ATZ on its fate in the ER. Surprisingly, a glucosidase inhibitor, castanospermine, and two α-mannosidase I inhibitors, kifunensine and

deoxymannojiromicin, mediate increased secretion of α₁-ATZ and the secreted molecules are functionally active [59]. Kifunensine and deoxymannojiromicin are not as attractive as castanospermine as a basis for chemoprophylaxis because these compounds also mediate a decrease in intracellular degradation of α₁-ATZ. The mechanism of action of castanospermine on α₁-ATZ is unknown. An interesting hypothesis for the action of kifunensine and deoxymannojiromicin has mutant α₁-ATZ interacting with ERGIC-53 for transport from ER to Golgi when mannose trimming is inhibited.

A novel strategy of increasing intracellular degradation of α₁-ATZ has been recently investigated [6]. Carbamazepine, one of a group of drugs that have recently been shown to enhance autophagy, could decrease the hepatic load of α₁-ATZ and influence the evolution of fibrosis in the liver of the PiZ mouse model. Autophagy was targeted because it appears to be specialized for degradation of aggregation-prone proteins and because it is specifically activated when α₁-ATZ accumulates in cells. Carbamazepine was selected because it has been used safely for many years as an anticonvulsant and mood stabilizer. The study showed that oral administration of carbamazepine to PiZ mice for 2 weeks reduced the hepatic α₁-ATZ load and markedly decreased hepatic fibrosis [6]. In mammalian cell line models, carbamazepine enhanced autophagic degradation of α₁-ATZ but, surprisingly, it affected other mechanisms of degradation of α₁-ATZ, including the proteasomal mechanism and perhaps an as yet undefined degradation mechanisms [6]. This drug is now being tested in patients with severe liver disease in α₁-AT deficiency using a double-blind randomized placebo-controlled design.

Several other autophagy enhancer drugs have been identified as candidates for treatment of liver disease in α₁-AT deficiency using a newly developed *Caenorhabditis elegans* model of α₁-AT deficiency in a high-content screening platform [60]. Six hit compounds met the stringent criteria of this screening, including a four-fold reduction in α₁-ATZ accumulation on multiple screening and individual drug trials. Interestingly, all of these have autophagy enhancer activity even though the screen was designed to detect drugs that would reduce α₁-ATZ accumulation by other mechanisms. Two of the hit compounds, fluphenazine and pimozide, are mood stabilizers, raising the possibility that a common mechanism is responsible for the autophagy enhancer activity.

Treatment of emphysema or destructive lung disease

Patients with α₁-AT deficiency and emphysema have undergone replacement therapy with purified and recombinant plasma α₁-AT, either by intravenous or by intratracheal aerosol administration [5]. This therapy is associated with improvement in serum concentrations of α₁-AT and in α₁-AT and neutrophil elastase inhibitory capacity in bronchoalveolar lavage fluid, without significant side effects. Although initial studies have suggested that there is a slower decline in forced expiratory volume in patients on replacement therapy, this only occurred in a subgroup of patients, and the study was not randomized [61].

Protein replacement therapy is designed only for individuals with established and progressive emphysema. It is not being considered for individuals with liver disease because there is no information to support the notion that deficient serum levels of α_1-AT are related mechanistically to liver injury.

A number of patients with severe emphysema from α_1-AT deficiency have undergone lung transplantation since the late 1980s. The latest data from the St. Louis International Lung Transplant Registry show that 91 patients with emphysema and α_1-AT deficiency had undergone single or bilateral lung transplantation by 1993. Actuarial survival for patients in this category who underwent transplantation between 1987 and 1994 is approximately 50% for 5 years. Lung function and exercise tolerance is significantly improved [62].

Gene replacement therapy

Several advances in gene replacement therapy have recently been published. Cruz et al. [63] showed that siRNA delivered within a recombinant adeno-associated virus and injected into the portal vein of the PiZ mouse model could reduce total α_1-ATZ levels in the liver but there was no change in the amount of insoluble polymerized α_1-ATZ. More recently, Li et al. [64] used a serotype 8 adeno-associated virus to deliver a signal DNA construct that encoded a short hairpin RNA to knock down endogenous production of α_1-ATZ together with a wild-type α_1-AT cassette to restore production of the normal protein. Administration of this recombinant virus into the PiZ mouse model appeared to decrease hepatic load of the mutant protein, decrease liver injury, and deliver normal human α_1-AT into the bloodstream. However, the reproducibility of these results and the effects over a long-term interval have not yet been demonstrated.

Other strategies

Because transplanted hepatocytes can repopulate the diseased liver in several mouse models, cell transplantation has become possible therapy for liver disease. Ding et al. [55] recently showed that normal mouse hepatocytes could spontaneously repopulate the liver of the PiZ mouse model of α_1-AT deficiency, replacing from 20 to 98% of the native hepatocytes. The possibility of cell transplantation therapy for α_1-AT deficiency has also been greatly advanced by a recent study showing that induced pluripotent stem cells from patients with α_1-AT deficiency could be subjected to targeted gene correction using zinc finger nucleases differentiated into hepatocytes, and then those cell lines could repopulate the uPa mouse model of liver disease [65]. Together these studies form an exciting basis for autologous cell-based therapies for α_1-AT deficiency.

Prevention

It is not clear how prenatal diagnosis for this deficiency should be used and how families should be counseled regarding the diagnosis. Data indicate that 80–85% of people with α_1-AT deficiency do not have evidence of liver disease at age 18 years and that PiZZ people may not develop emphysema or even pulmonary function abnormalities until age 60–70 years. These data could support a counseling strategy in which amniocentesis and abortion are discouraged. The only other data on this subject suggest a 78% chance that a second PiZZ child will have serious liver disease if the older sibling had serious liver disease [66]. This study, however, is retrospective and heavily influenced by bias in ascertainment of patients. The issue will not be resolved until studied prospectively, as, for example, in the Swedish population [2,3].

Several recent studies have suggested that population screening for α_1-AT deficiency would be efficacious. First, there is now evidence that knowledge of and counseling regarding the consequences of α_1-AT deficiency is associated with a reduced rate of smoking among affected adolescents [67]. Second, there were no significant negative psychosocial consequences in early adulthood from neonatal screening for α_1-AT deficiency in Sweden [68]. These data should give new momentum to reconsideration of screening programs for α_1-AT deficiency.

References

1. Silverman EK, Sandhaus RA. Clinical practice. Alpha1-antitrypsin deficiency. *N Engl J Med* 2009; **360**:2749–2757.

2. Sveger T. Liver disease in α_1-antitrypsin deficiency detected by screening of 200 000 infants. *N Engl J Med* 1976;**294**:1216–1221.

3. Piitulainen E, Carlson J, Ohlsson K, *et al.* Alpha-1-antitrypsin deficiency in 26-year-old subjects: lung, liver and protease/protease inhibitor studies. *Chest* 2005;**128**:2076–2081.

4. Eriksson S, Carlson J, Velez R. Risk of cirrhosis and primary liver cancer in alpha-1-antitrypsin deficiency. *N Engl J Med* 1986;**314**:736–739.

5. Crystal RG. Alpha-1-antitrypsin deficiency, emphysema and liver disease: genetic basis and strategies for therapy. *J Clin Invest* 1990;**95**: 1343–1352.

6. Hidvegi T, Ewing M, Hale P, *et al.* An autophagy-enhancing drug promotes degradation of mutant α_1-antitrypsin Z and reduces hepatic fibrosis. *Science* 2010;**329**:229–232.

7. Marcus NY, Brunt EM, Blomenkamp K, *et al.* Characteristics of hepatocellular carcinoma in a murine model of alpha-1-antitrypsin deficiency. *Hepatol Res* 2010;**40**: 641–653.

8. Carlson JA, Rogers BB, Sifers RN, *et al.* Accumulation of PiZ antitrypsin causes liver damage in transgenic mice. *J Clin Invest* 1988;**83**:1183–1190.

9. Teckman JH, Qu D, Perlmutter DH. Molecular pathogenesis of liver disease in α_1-antitrypsin deficiency. *Hepatology* 1996;**24**:1504–1516.

10. Zhou H, Fischer H-P. Liver carcinoma in PiZ alpha-1-antitrypsin deficiency. *Am J Surg Pathol* 1998;**22**: 742–748.

11. Volpert D, Molleston JP, Perlmutter DH. Alpha1-antitrypsin deficiency-associated liver disease progresses slowly in some children. *J Pediatr Gastro Nutr* 2000;**31**:258–263.

12. Perlmutter DH. Alpha-1-antitrypsin deficiency. In Schiff ER, Sorrell MF, Maddrey WC (eds.) *Schiff's Diseases of the Liver*, 11th edn. Oxford: Wiley-Blackwell, 2011, pp. 835–867.

13. Schonfeld JV, Brewer N, Zotz, R, *et al.* Liver function in patients with pulmonary emphysema due to severe alpha-1-antitrypsin deficiency (PiZZ). *Digestion* 1996;**57**:165–169.

14. Carrell RW, Evans DL, Steen DE. Mobile reactive centre of serpins and the control of thrombosis. *Nature* 1991;**353**:376.

15. Owen MC, Brennan SO, Lewis JH, *et al.* Mutation of antitrypsin to antithrombin: alpha-1-antitrypsin Pittsburgh (358 Met-Arg), a fatal bleeding disorder. *N Engl J Med* 1983;**309**:694–698.

16. Hafeez W, Ciliberto G, Perlmutter DH. Constitutive and modulated expression of the human alpha-1-antitrypsin gene: different transcriptional initiation sites used in three different cell types. *J Clin Invest* 1992;**89**:1214–1222.

17. Ogushi F, Fells GA, Hubbard RC, *et al.* Z-type α₁-antitrypsin is less competent than M1-type α₁-antitrypsin as an inhibitor of neutrophil elastase. *J Clin Invest* 1987;**89**:1366–1374.

18. Camussi G, Tetta C, Bussolino F, *et al.* Synthesis and release of platelet-activating factor is inhibited by plasma α₁-proteinase inhibitor or α₁-antichymotrypsin and is stimulated by proteinases. *J Exp Med* 1988;**168**: 1293–1306.

19. Munch J, Standker L, Adermann K, *et al.* Discovery and optimization of a natural HIV-1 entry inhibitor targeting the g41 fusion peptide. *Cell* 2007;**129**:263–275.

20. Forssmann WG, The H-K, Stoll K, *et al.* Short-term monotherapy in HIV-infected patients with a virus entry inhibitor against the gp41 fusion peptide. *Sci Transl Med* 2010;**2**: 63–66.

21. Janciauskiene SM, Bals R, Koczulla R, *et al.* The discovery of α₁-antitrypsin and its role in health and disease. *Resp Med* 2011;**105**:1129–1139.

22. Perlmutter DH, Cole FS, Kilbridge P, *et al.* Expression of the α₁-proteinase inhibitor gene in human monocytes and macrophages. *Proc Natl Acad Sci USA* 1985;**82**:795–799.

23. Koopman P, Povey S, Lovel-Badge RH. Widespread expression of human alpha-1-antitrypsin in transgenic mice revealed by in situ hybridization. *Genes Dev* 1989;**3**:16–25.

24. Carlson JA, Rogers BB, Sifers RN, *et al.* Multiple tissues express alpha-1-antitrypsin in transgenic mice and man. *J Clin Invest* 1988;**82**:26–36.

25. Yamasaki M, Li W, Johnson DJD, *et al.* Crystal structure of a stable dimer reveals the molecular basis of serpin polymerization. *Nature* 2008;**455**: 1255–1258.

26. Sidhar SK, Lomas DA, Carrell RW, *et al.* Mutations which impede loop-sheet polymerization enhance the secretion of human α₁-antitrypsin deficiency variants. *J Biol Chem* 1995;**270**:8393–8396.

27. Lin L, Schmidt B, Teckman J, Perlmutter DH. A naturally occurring non-polymerogenic mutant of α₁-antitrypsin characterized by prolonged retention in the endoplasmic reticulum. *J Biol Chem* 2001;**276**:33893–33898.

28. Schmidt BZ, Perlmutter DH. GRP78, GRP94 and GRP170 interact with α1 AT mutants that are retained in the endoplasmic reticulum. *Am J Physiol Gastrointest Liver Physiol* 2005;**289**: G444–G455.

29. Kuznetsov G, Nigam SK. Folding of secretory and membrane proteins. *N Engl J Med* 1998;**339**:1688–1695.

30. Davis RL, Shrimpton AE, Holohan PD, *et al.* Familial dementia caused by polymerization of mutant neuroserpin. *Nature* 1999;**401**:376–379.

31. Perlmutter DH. Alpha-1-antitrypsin deficiency: Importance of proteasomal and autophagic degradative pathways in disposal of liver disease-associated protein aggregates. *Annu Rev Med* 2011;**62**:4.1–4.13.

32. Wu Y, Whitman I, Molmenti E, *et al.* A lag in intracellular degradation of mutant α₁-antitrypsin correlates with the liver disease phenotype in homozygous PiZZ α₁-antitrypsin deficiency. *Proc Natl Acad Sci USA* 1994;**91**:9014–9018.

33. Teckman JH, Perlmutter DH. Retention of mutant α₁-antitrypsin Z in endoplasmic reticulum is associated with an autophagic response. *Am J Physiol* 2000;**279**:G961–G974.

34. Kamimoto T, Shoji S, Mizushima N, *et al.* Intracellular inclusions containing mutant α1 ATZ are propagated in the absence of autophagy. *J Biol Chem* 2006;**281**:4467–4476.

35. Kruse KB, Brodsky JL, McCracken AA. Characterization of an *ERAD* gene as VPS30/ATG6 reveals two alternative and functionally distinct protein quality control pathways: one for soluble α1 PiZ and another for aggregates of α1 PiZ. *Mol Biol Cell* 2006;**17**: 203–212.

36. Kruse K, Dear A, Kaltenbrun ER, *et al.* Mutant fibrinogen cleared from the endoplasmic reticulum via endoplasmic reticulum-associated protein degradation and autophagy: an explanation for liver disease. *Am J Pathol* 2006;**168**:1300–1308.

37. Cabral CM, Choudhury P, Liu Y, Sifers RN. Processing by endoplasmic reticulum mannosidases partitions a secretion-impaired glycoprotein into distinct disposal pathways. *J Biol Chem* 2000;**275**:25015–25022.

38. Hidvegi T, Mirnics K, Hale P, *et al.* Regulator of G signaling 16 is a marker for the distinct endoplasmic reticulum stress state associated with aggregated mutant α1-antitrypsin Z in the classical form of α1-antitrypsin deficiency. *J Biol Chem* 2007;**282**:27769–27780.

39. Hidvegi T, Schmidt BZ, Hale P, Perlmutter DH. Accumulation of mutant α₁-antitrypsin Z in the ER activates caspases-4 and -12, NFκB and BAP31 but not the unfolded protein response. *J Biol Chem* 2005;**280**: 39002–39015.

40. Teckman JH, An JK, Blomenkamp K, *et al.* Mitochondrial autophagy and injury in the liver in α₁-antitrypsin deficiency. *Am J Physiol* 2004;**286**: G851–G862.

41. Pan S, Huang L, McPherson J, *et al.* Single nucleotide polymorphism-mediated translational suppression of endoplasmic reticulum mannosidase I modifies the onset of end-stage liver disease in alpha-1-antitrypsin

deficiency. *Hepatology* 2009;**50**: 275–281.

42. Chappell S, Hadzic N, Stockley R, *et al.* A polymorphism of the alpha-1-antitrypsin gene represents a risk factor for liver disease. *Hepatology* 2008;**47**:127–132.

43. Geller SA, Nichols WS, Dycacio MJ, *et al.* Histopathology of α_1-antitrypsin liver disease in a transgenic mouse model. *Hepatology* 1990;**12**:40–47.

44. Geller SA, Nichols WS, Kim SS, *et al.* Hepatocarcinogenesis is the sequel to hepatitis in Z#2 α_1-antitrypsin transgenic mice: histopathological and DNA ploidy studies. *Hepatology* 1994;**19**:389–397.

45. Hubner RH, Leopold PL, Kiura M, *et al.* Dysfunctional glycogen storage in a mouse model of α_1-antitrypsin deficiency. *Am J Respir Cell Mol Biol* 2009;**40**:239–247.

46. Mahadeva R, Chang W-SW, Dafforn TR, *et al.* Heteropolymerization of S, I, and Z α_1-antitrypsin and liver cirrhosis. *J Clin Invest* 1999;**103**:999–1006.

47. Teckman JH, Perlmutter DH. Conceptual advances in the pathogenesis and treatment of childhood metabolic liver disease. *Gastroenterology* 1995;**108**:1263–1279.

48. Teckman JH, An J-K, Loethen S, Perlmutter DH. Effect of fasting on liver in a mouse model of α_1-antitrypsin deficiency: constitutive activation of the autophagic response. *Am J Physiol* 2002;**283**:61117–61124.

49. Rudnick DA, Liao Y, An JK, *et al.* Analyses of hepatocellular proliferation in a mouse model of α1-antitrypsin deficiency. *Hepatology* 2004;**39**: 1048–1055.

50. An JK, Blomenkamp K, Lindblad D, *et al.* Quantitative isolation of alpha-1-AT mutant Z protein polymers from human and mouse livers and the effect of heat. *Hepatology* 2005;**41**:160–167.

51. Hadzic N, Quaglia A, Mieli-Vergani G. Hepatocellular carcinoma in a 12-year-old child with PiZZ α_1-antitrypsin deficiency. *Hepatology* 2006; **43**:194.

52. Zhou H, Ortiz-Pallardo ME, Ko Y, Fischer H-P. Is heterozygous alpha-1-antitrypsin deficiency type PiZ a risk factor for primary liver cancer. *Cancer* 2000;**88**:2668–2676.

53. Rudnick DA, Perlmutter DH. Alpha-1-antitrypsin deficiency: A new paradigm for hepatocellular carcinoma in genetic liver disease. *Hepatology* 2005;**42**: 514–521.

54. Lindblad DA, Blomenkamp K, Teckman J. Alpha-1-antitrypsin mutant Z protein content in individual hepatocytes correlates with cell death in a mouse model. *Hepatology* 2007;**46**:1228–1235.

55. Ding J, Yannam GR, Roy-Chowdhury N, *et al.* Spontaneous hepatic repopulation in transgenic mice expressing mutant human α_1-antitrypsin by wild-type donor hepatocytes. *J Clin Invest* 2011;**121**:1930–1934.

56. Kemmer N, Kaiser T, Zacharias V, Neff GW. Alpha-1-antitrypsin deficiency: outcomes after liver transplantation. *Transplant Proc* 2008;**40**:1492–1494.

57. Burrows JAJ, Willis LK, Perlmutter DH. Chemical chaperones mediate increased secretion of mutant α_1-antitrypsin (α_1-AT) Z: a potential pharmacological strategy for prevention of liver injury and emphysema in α_1-AT deficiency. *Proc Natl Acad Sci USA* 2000;**97**: 1796–1801.

58. Teckman JH. Lack of effect of oral 4-phenylbutyrate on serum alpha-1-antitrypsin in patients with alpha-1-antitrypsin deficiency: a preliminary study. *J Pediatr Gastroenterol Nutr* 2004;**39**:34–37.

59. Marcus NY, Perlmutter DH. Glucosidase and mannosidase inhibitors mediate increased secretion of mutant α_1-antitrypsin Z. *J Biol Chem* 2000;**275**:1987–1992.

60. Gosai SJ, Kwak JH, Luke CJ, *et al.* Automated high-content live animal drug screening using *C. elegans* expressing the aggregation prone serpin α_1-antitrypsin Z. *PLOS one* 2010;**5**: e15460.

61. Abboud RT, Ford GT, Chapman KR. Emphysema in alpha1antitrypsin deficiency: Does replacement therapy affect outcome? *Treat Respir Med* 2005;**4**:1–8.

62. Burton CM, Milman N, Carlsen J, *et al.* The Copenhagen National Lung Transplant group: survival after single lung, double lung and heart-lung transplantation. *J Heart Lung Transplant* 2005;**24**:1834–1843.

63. Cruz PE, Mueller C, Cossette TL, *et al.* In vivo post-transcriptional gene silencing of alpha-1-antitrypsin by adeno-associated virus vectors expressing siRNA. *Lab Invest* 2007;**87**:893–902.

64. Li C, Xiao P, Gray SJ, *et al.* Combination therapy utilizing shRNA knockdown and an optimized resistant transgene for rescue of diseases caused by misfolded proteins. *Proc Natl Acad Sci USA* 2011;**108**:14258–4263.

65. Yusa K, Rashid T, Strick-Marchand H, *et al.* Targeted gene correction of α_1-antitrypsin deficiency in induced pluripotent stem cells. *Nature* 2011;**478**:391–394.

66. Psacharopoulos HT, Mowat AP, Cook PJL, *et al.* Outcome of liver disease associated with alpha-1-antitrypsin deficiency (PiZ). *Arch Dis Child* 1983;**58**:882–887.

67. Wall M, Moe E, Eisenberg J, *et al.* Long-term follow-up of a cohort of children with alpha-1-antitrypsin deficiency. *J Pediatr* 1990;**116**:248–251.

68. Sveger T, Thelin T, McNeil TF. Young adults with α_1-antitrypsin deficiency identified neonatally: their health, knowledge about and adaptation to the high-risk condition. *Acta Paediatr* 1997;**86**:37–40.

Chapter

26

Cystic fibrosis liver disease

Meghana Sathe and Andrew P. Feranchak

Introduction

Cystic fibrosis (CF) is a genetic disorder characterized by epithelial electrolyte transport abnormalities, elevated sweat Cl^- concentrations, pancreatic insufficiency, and chronic lung disease in most patients. It is the most common potentially fatal genetic disorder in the Caucasian population, affecting 1 in 2400–3500 live births [1,2]. It is an autosomal recessive disorder caused by a mutation in the gene *CFTR* encoding the cystic fibrosis transmembrane conductance regulator (CFTR), a membrane channel protein. The clinical significance of hepatobiliary disease in CF has not been well characterized primarily because of two factors: (1) pulmonary involvement leads to early mortality in a majority of patients, and (2) the clinical identification of CF-associated liver disease has been difficult because, although it is progressive, liver involvement is often asymptomatic until the appearance of end-stage complications. Recently, with improved pulmonary treatments, median life expectancy now exceeds 30 years and CF-associated hepatobiliary disease is recognized and characterized more comprehensively. Liver disease is now the third major cause of death in CF (after pulmonary disease and complications of lung transplant). In recent years, advances in our understanding of the function of CFTR in bile duct epithelia have provided a stronger scientific basis for the pathogenesis of the disease, leading to insights concerning potentially novel therapeutic approaches.

The earliest reports of CF probably date to the Middle Ages, with reports of malnourished and "sickly" children that tasted "salty" when kissed. In 1905, Landsteiner published the first description of an abnormal pancreas and meconium ileus in CF, although it was Anderson's description in 1938 that gave us a more modern description of "cystic fibrosis of the pancreas" [3]. In 1953, di Sant'Agnese described the abnormal sweat electrolyte concentrations forming the basis for the diagnostic sweat test, which served as the basis of the diagnosis until the recent availability of genetic analysis. On a cellular level, meticulous studies of the sweat duct led Quinton to describe the Cl^- transport defect [4]. Finally, it was the discovery of the responsible gene in 1989 by Riordan, Tsui, and Collins that permitted critical breakthroughs in the understanding of CF pathogenesis [5]. It was hoped that the gene discovery would herald a quick and forthcoming cure for CF, and although this dream has not been realized to date, the intense study of the role of CFTR in cell and organ function has advanced our knowledge of basic cellular physiology enormously.

Cystic fibrosis transmembrane conductance regulator

Action as a channel

CFTR is located on the long arm of chromosome 7. It contains 250 000 base pairs with 27 exons and encodes a polypeptide product of 1480 amino acid residues CFTR. The protein belongs to a family of transmembrane proteins known as ATP-binding cassette (ABC) proteins, which all contain transmembrane sequences and hydrolyze ATP for activation. CFTR contains two domains, capable of spanning the membrane six times, separated by regulatory cytoplasmic domains consisting of two consensus nucleotide-binding domains and an intervening regulatory domain (Figure 26.1). It is now well established that CFTR functions as a cyclic adenosine monophosphate (cAMP)-dependent Cl^- channel in the apical membrane of secretory epithelia. CFTR-associated Cl^- channels have a small unitary conductance of approximately 8 picosiemens and a linear current–voltage relation. Under normal conditions, cAMP-dependent protein kinase A phosphorylates CFTR, causing channel opening and transport of Cl^-.

Action as a regulator

There is increasing evidence to suggest that, in addition to its role as a Cl^- channel, CFTR, as the name implies, also functions as a *regulator* of other membrane proteins and channels [6]. This was first suggested by the observation that, in addition to abnormal Cl^- and HCO_3^- transport, CF tissues display other transport abnormalities such as defective regulation of outwardly rectified Cl^- channels and increased Na^+

Liver Disease in Children, Fourth Edition, ed. Frederick J. Suchy, Ronald J. Sokol, and William F. Balistreri. Published by Cambridge University Press. © Cambridge University Press 2014.

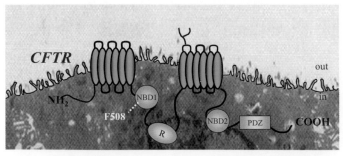

Figure 26.1 Putative monomeric structure for the cystic fibrosis transmembrane conductance regulator (CFTR). The 1480 amino acid residues are arranged into 12 membrane-spanning domains. The first six transmembrane domains are followed by an intracellular regulatory domain, or R-domain, containing phosphorylation sites for protein kinase A. Transmembrane segments 6 and 12 are followed by sequences containing ATP-binding domains or nucleotide-binding domains (NBD). The most common CF-associated mutation (ΔF508) results from a base pair deletion in exon 10, causing a deletion of phenylalanine at position 508 in the first NBD region. The C-terminal end of the protein contains PDZ-domains that may facilitate protein–protein interactions.

absorption through epithelial Na^+ channels [7]. Expression of wild-type CFTR not only corrects the cAMP-dependent Cl^- conductance but leads to normalization of outwardly rectified Cl^- channel regulation and epithelial Na^+ channel activity.

In other secretory epithelia, CFTR has been shown to regulate glutathione transport, mucin secretion, water transport through aquaporins, and ATP permeability [8]. In addition to its effect on membrane transport activity, CFTR appears to play a role in vesicular transport and pH regulation of intracellular organelles. How CFTR regulates these membrane proteins and transport activities is not currently known. The finding that CFTR contains specific sequences that bind integral membrane proteins and cytoskeletal elements raises the possibility of *membrane regulatory complexes* in the apical domain of epithelial cells. Studies demonstrate that the intracellular portion of CFTR binds to protein modules referred to as PSD-95/Discs-large/ZO-1 (PDZ) domains, which promote protein–protein interactions. Several PDZ-domain-containing proteins have been shown to bind to CFTR including EBP50 and E3KARP, which are both expressed in cholangiocytes and may be important regulators of ductular bile formation [9]. Understanding the nature of these interactions is an area for future investigation and may serve as the basis for novel therapies for CF. Overall, these observations suggest that CFTR is multifunctional, serving as both an ion channel and as a protein that regulates other ion channels.

Role in liver function

In human liver, CFTR is expressed on the apical membrane of bile duct cells (cholangiocytes) and gallbladder epithelia but is not expressed in hepatocytes or other cells of the liver [10]. In the mouse (and probably humans), CFTR is found predominantly in the medium to large sized intrahepatic bile ducts, but not in the small intrahepatic ducts. Its location on the apical (luminal) membrane of cholangiocytes, as well as the large

increase in cAMP-stimulated CFTR activity observed with secretory agonists, suggests an important role of CFTR in bile formation [11].

The formation of bile by the liver depends on complementary interactions between hepatic parenchymal cells (hepatocytes) and intrahepatic bile duct cells (cholangiocytes). Both of these cell types work in a complementary manner to initiate and modify bile flow. Bile formation is initiated at the hepatocyte canalicular membrane through the transport of bile acids, organic and inorganic solutes, electrolytes, and water. Subsequently, bile flows into the lumen of the intrahepatic bile ducts where it undergoes alkalinization and dilution as a result of cholangiocyte secretion. Although cholangiocytes constitute <5% of the nuclear mass of the liver, they form an extensive branching network and account for approximately 40% of bile flow in humans; demonstrating a prodigious capacity for secretion.

Studies in isolated cholangiocytes, biliary epithelial monolayers, and isolated bile duct segments have helped to elucidate the basic mechanisms of constitutive and stimulated secretion in biliary epithelium [12]. One of the current working models is shown in Figure 26.2. Intracellular Cl^- accumulation occurs via uptake of Cl^- at the basolateral membrane by a bumetadine-sensitive $Na^+/K^+/2Cl^-$ cotransporter. While the intracellular accumulation of Cl^- leads to values above the electrochemical equilibrium, the Cl^- permeability of the apical membrane under basal conditions is low. However, exposure to agonists, such as secretin, that increase intracellular cAMP levels leads to a rapid series of events including (1) opening of Cl^- channels in the apical membrane and efflux of Cl^- into the duct lumen, (2) an increase in Cl^-–HCO_3^- exchange activity with a resultant increase in ductal HCO_3^- concentration, and (3) movement of water out of the cell through water channels or aquaporins. The findings that CFTR is localized to the apical membrane of cholangiocytes and secretin-stimulated Cl^- channels have properties analogous to CFTR support a working model that postulates a role for CFTR in the regulation of ductular secretion. According to this model, the secretin-stimulated increase in Cl^- and HCO_3^- permeability is through protein kinase A-dependent activation of CFTR. The generation of a lumen-negative potential favors movement of Na^+ into the bile duct through a paracellular pathway and water through aquaporins. Additionally, two K^+ channels (SK2, IK1) have been identified in the basolateral membrane of cholangiocytes and play an important role in maintaining the membrane potential difference necessary for continued transepithelial secretion [13]. Therefore, CFTR contributes to normal bile formation and alkalinization through the regulation of Cl^-, HCO_3^-, and water transport (Figure 26.2). Although this model implies a prominent role for CFTR in normal bile formation, it fails to explain why only a minority of patients with CF develop liver disease despite the fact that they all have abnormal or absent CFTR in bile duct epithelia. This observation suggests that CFTR may not be the predominant pathway for Cl^- secretion in cholangiocytes.

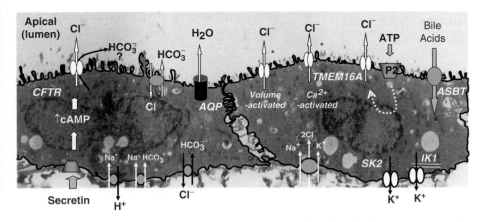

Figure 26.2 Model of cholangiocyte bile formation highlighting channels involved in secretion. Stimulation of basolateral receptors by secretin results in increases in cAMP and protein kinase A-dependent stimulation of Cl^- efflux through CFTR. The transmembrane Cl^- gradient drives Cl^-/HCO_3^- exchange. Alternatively, HCO_3^- may enter bile through a conductive manner or through CFTR itself. Water is transported via aquaporin (AQP) proteins. The increase in HCO_3^- and water secretion leads to alkalinization and dilution of bile. Other Cl^- channels, including volume-sensitive, P2 receptor-linked, and TMEM16A, a Ca^{2+}-activated Cl^- channel, have been identified. Lumenal ATP and bile acids may also stimulate Cl^- efflux. An apical transporter for bile acids has been identified (ASBT). On the basolateral membrane, Na^+/H^+ exchange, Na^+-dependent Cl^-/HCO_3^- exchange, and Na^+/HCO_3^- symport help to maintain intracellular pH and HCO_3^- concentrations. Uptake of Cl^- is mediated by a $Na^+/K^+/2Cl^-$ cotransporter. The Ca^{2+}-activated K^+ channels (SK2, IK1) have been identified in the basolateral membrane and work in parallel with apical Cl^- channels to hyperpolarize the membrane and provide the driving force for continued secretion. See text for details. P2, purinergic receptor; *, location (apical versus basolateral) not definitively established.

Alternative channels and cholangiocyte secretion

In addition to CFTR, cholangiocytes express several other Cl^- channels, including a Ca^{2+}-activated Cl^- channel, a purinergic receptor-linked Cl^- channel, and a volume-stimulated Cl^- channel (Figure 26.2) [14]. However, their regulation and overall contribution to biliary secretion is largely unknown at present. It is attractive to speculate, however, that these alternative Cl^- channels may compensate for the CF secretory defect in the liver in CF. In fact, in the $Cftr^{-/-}$ mouse model, increased expression of Ca^{2+}-activated Cl^- channels in tracheal epithelial cells is associated with mild pulmonary disease [15]. Recently, a Ca^{2+}-activated Cl^- channel, TMEM16A, has been identified in liver, where it is localized predominantly on the apical membrane of cholangiocytes [16]. This represents the only other Cl^- channel, besides CFTR, identified on a molecular basis in biliary epithelium and, therefore, it may be an attractive therapeutic target for new choleretic agents.

A potential role for mechanosensitive pathways is supported by the observation that secretion mediated by extracellular nucleotides (e.g. ATP) acting on purinergic (P2) receptors on the luminal membrane of biliary epithelial cells is functionally important [17]. ATP is present in bile, and binding of ATP to P2 receptors increases Cl^- efflux from isolated cholangiocytes and dramatically increases transepithelial secretion in biliary epithelial monolayers [18]. Indeed, the magnitude of the secretory response to ATP is two- to three-fold greater than that observed with cAMP. With recent studies demonstrating that the mechanical effects of fluid-flow and/or shear stress at the apical membrane of biliary epithelial cells is a robust stimulus for ATP release, a model emerges in which mechanosensitive ATP release and Cl^- secretion is a dominant pathway regulating biliary secretion [19]. If these observations apply to in vivo conditions, a decrease in bile flow associated with CF may be accompanied by alterations in these mechanosensitive pathways, which may further exacerbate abnormalities in Cl^- secretion and bile formation.

Summary

In summary, CFTR is a cAMP-dependent Cl^- channel expressed on the apical membrane of cholangiocytes that contributes to ductular secretion. However, the possible role of other membrane Cl^- channels is yet to be determined. Intriguing studies have established that CFTR, in addition to its role as a Cl^- channel, is in fact a "transmembrane regulator" modulating other membrane permeability pathways. Further study of CFTR function and regulation may help to elucidate the mechanisms of cholangiocyte function and bile formation. The remainder of this chapter focuses on the hepatobiliary effects of abnormal CFTR function, namely, CF-associated liver disease.

CFTR mutations

There are now more than 2000 recognized mutations in *CFTR* (CFTR Mutation Data Base: http://www.genet.sickkids.on.ca/cftr). Worldwide, the ΔF508 mutation accounts for 66% of the described mutations while G542X and G551D, the next two most common mutations, account for 2.4% and 1.6%, respectively (CFTR Mutation Data Base). The incidence of CF in the Caucasian population corresponds to a carrier frequency of approximately 5%. This high carrier frequency in a lethal genetic disease suggests the possibility of a survival advantage for heterozygotes. In fact, it has been suggested that the absent or unresponsive Cl^- channel associated with *CFTR* mutations may have protected infants during epidemics of cholera, which causes secretory diarrhea through toxin-mediated,

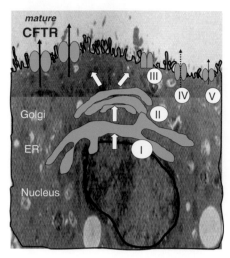

Figure 26.3 Classification of *CFTR* mutations. Class I mutations (nonsense and frameshift) result in abnormal mRNA production and no CFTR protein. Class II mutations (amino acid deletion, missense) result in abnormal CFTR protein trafficking with subsequent degradation. Class III mutations (missense) result in a mature CFTR protein that is refractory to normal activation. Class IV mutations (missense) result in a CFTR protein that localizes normally, but with a reduction in single-channel conductance. Class V mutations (alternative splicing, missense) result in a decreased full-length mRNA and a decrease in the number of functional CFTR channels at the apical membrane. ER, endoplasmic reticulum.

cAMP-dependent activation of Cl⁻ channels. The $Cftr^{-/-}$ mouse has been shown to be resistant to the effects of cholera infection, providing some evidence for this theory [20].

Mutations are classified into five groups according to their effect on CFTR protein function (Figure 26.3). Class I mutations (such as G542X and R553X) cause impairment of CFTR mRNA production. Class II mutations result in defective processing or trafficking of CFTR protein to the apical membrane. The most common mutation, ΔF508, is of this class and results in a base pair deletion in exon 10 with a consequent deletion of phenylalanine at position F508 in the first nucleotide-binding domain of the protein [5]. The F508-CFTR protein does not fold correctly and is subsequently diverted from normal trafficking to the apical membrane and degraded by the ubiquitin–proteosome pathway. Class III mutations (G551D and others) are associated with defective regulation of CFTR, which locates correctly to the apical membrane but does not respond to cAMP agonists. Class IV mutations (R117H and others) demonstrate some residual Cl⁻ conductance but at a significantly decreased amplitude. Class V mutations (A455E, P574H, and others) lead to abnormal splicing of CFTR with partial reduction in the number of functioning Cl⁻ channels. Mutations of classes I, II, and III are considered severe because they result in an absence of functioning CFTR at the plasma membrane, whereas class IV and V are "mild" mutations with some residual CFTR activity demonstrated. The report from the Cystic Fibrosis Foundation (CFF) registry, which records data from USA CF centers, reveals that ΔF508/ΔF508 homozygotes account for 50.6% and F508/other heterozygotes account for 37.9% of the mutations reported in the registry.

Overall, although specific gene mutations have been associated with the severity of pancreatic involvement, there is no correlation between specific genotype and clinically detectable liver disease in patients with CF. However, there appears to be a lower frequency of liver disease in pancreatic-sufficient patients, who generally have milder mutations. Because all patients with CF have abnormal CFTR in the biliary tree, it is unclear why significant liver disease does not develop in all patients. Because patients with CF and identical *CFTR* mutations exhibit variable onset and severity of liver disease, it is postulated that there are other modifying genetic or environmental factors that determine whether clinically significant hepatobiliary involvement will occur.

Pathogenesis of liver injury

The pathophysiology underlying the development of CF-associated liver disease is still only speculative. Definitive studies directly assessing the effects of abnormal CFTR in the liver are lacking. Several proposed pathways in the pathogenesis of CF liver disease are shown in Figure 26.4. One leading hypothesis is that impaired secretory function of cholangiocytes results in a decrease in bile flow (cholestasis) and thickened, inspissated secretions in the bile ductules. The subsequent bile duct obstruction leads to liver cell injury and the development of fibrosis and cirrhosis. The histologic finding of inspissated eosinophilic material in bile ducts, a pathognomonic lesion in CF, provides some morphologic evidence for this "bile duct plugging" theory. Theoretically, abnormal viscosity of bile could result from several factors including defective transport of Cl⁻, HCO₃⁻, and mucins; Na⁺ reabsorption; altered composition of the bile acid pool; or a combination of these. Bile duct plugging would be anticipated to initiate a series of secondary steps including cholangiocyte injury, release of inflammatory mediators, and stellate cell activation with subsequent deposition of collagen, ultimately leading to fibrosis and cirrhosis.

Alternatively, the initiating step may be direct cholangiocyte injury from an abnormal CFTR protein. As mentioned above, the most common mutation ΔF508 results in protein misfolding and subsequent degradation by the ubiquitin–proteosome pathway. The misfolded protein can potentially form aggresomes, which may lead to cellular injury as seen in other diseases. This suggests a possible role of chaperone proteins, which are responsible for quality control mechanisms in the cell by targeting and degrading abnormal or misfolded proteins in the disease pathogenesis.

Although the initiating event in the development of liver disease is unknown, it appears that a progressive fibrogenic process ultimately leads to cirrhosis in a subset of patients. It is felt that this continuum, from cholestasis to focal biliary obstruction and ultimately to cirrhosis, may progress over many years. Genetic and environmental factors may modify any and all components of the pathway and may explain the heterogeneity in the liver response to abnormal CFTR

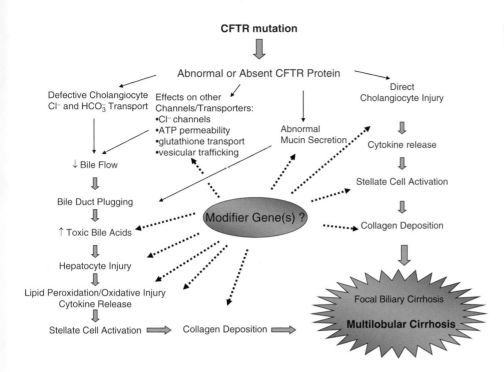

Figure 26.4 A proposed model of the pathogenesis of cystic fibrosis liver disease.

function. Several potential factors that have been proposed to contribute to, or modify, the liver injury in CF include altered mucin secretion, accumulation of toxic bile acids, abnormal oxidant–antioxidant balance, stellate cell activation, and fat accumulation (steatosis).

Mucins

Hypersecretion of mucus is a major contributor to the lung pathology in CF. If similar factors are operable in the bile duct, then one potential etiology of increased bile viscosity would be altered mucin secretion. The viscous properties of mucus are determined in large part by mucin glycoproteins. The role of mucins in the bile duct is not defined, and there is conflicting evidence linking CFTR and mucin secretion. However, CFTR may contribute to normal mucin gel formation through effects on HCO_3^- secretion. The normal expansion of mucins, once secreted from the cell, is dependent on HCO_3^- and, therefore, the abnormal HCO_3^- transport associated with CF may promote mucin aggregation and plugging of the lumen as recently proposed by Quinton [21].

Toxic bile acids

Patients with CF may have an altered bile acid pool, with an increase in hydrophobic and a decrease in hydrophilic bile acids. In fact, a study examining bile acid profiles in patients with CF found a higher level of endogenous biliary ursodeoxycholic acid (UDCA) in patients with CF but no liver disease compared with those with CF-associated liver disease [22]. The authors suggested that the elevated UDCA in these patients without liver disease may play a possible protective role. In addition to a decrease in hydrophilic bile acids, retaining hydrophobic bile acids may be responsible for subsequent hepatocyte injury, as seen in other cholestatic disorders.

Antioxidants

Several studies have suggested that there is an imbalance between oxidant injury and antioxidant defenses in cystic fibrosis. This imbalance may result from malabsorption of dietary antioxidants such as vitamin E, tocopherols, beta-carotene, and other carotenoids, or through direct effects of CFTR on the transport of antioxidants such as glutathione. In the liver, a decrease in lipid-soluble antioxidant activity may potentially result in increased free radical production and oxidative hepatic injury. Antioxidants may counteract these effects on the mitochondrial membrane and this suggests other potential novel therapies for CF-associated liver disease.

Stellate cells

Hepatic stellate cells have been implicated in the pathogenesis of cystic fibrosis and may play a role in the progressive fibrosis characteristic of this disorder [23]. Potentially, activation of stellate cells could occur through direct cholangiocyte or indirect hepatocyte injury with subsequent release of proinflammatory cytokines. In liver biopsy specimens of patients with CF, stellate cells have been found located in the periportal regions of the liver and their activation has been correlated with areas of collagen deposition and fibrosis [23]. Additionally, the acquisition of a robust actin-based cytoskeleton in activated stellate cells imparts a contractile phenotype and appears to contribute to the pathogenesis of portal hypertension, a prominent clinical manifestation of liver disease in CF. Elucidation of the role of stellate cells in the progressive fibrosis associated with liver disease, may suggest novel therapies targeting these cells.

Steatosis

Hepatic steatosis is a common finding in CF, although it is unclear whether it results from the abnormal CFTR and the cholangiocyte transport defect or represents a separate, secondary entity. Several factors may contribute to hepatic steatosis in CF, including malnutrition, essential fatty acid deficiency, and elevated circulating levels of cytokines. The mechanism by which intracellular fat accumulation causes liver disease is an ongoing area of investigation. It may be that fat accumulation provides an increased substrate for lipid peroxidation and oxidative injury. It is unclear whether hepatic steatosis progresses to fibrosis or multilobular cirrhosis; however, the progressive nature of other disorders associated with fat accumulation (non-alcoholic fatty liver disease) suggests that steatosis may not be as benign a condition in CF as once thought.

Summary

Further studies into the pathogenesis of CF liver disease are clearly needed. It is hoped that the use of novel models of biliary epithelium and animal models will help to further our knowledge. Recently, several animal models, including mouse, pig, and ferret, have been developed that develop liver disease similar to that observed in humans and may provide important insight into the factors responsible for the development and progression of CF liver disease.

Potential genetic modifiers

Family studies suggest that factors independent of CFTR contribute to the development of liver disease and have led to intense scrutiny of the role of modifier genes in the pathogenesis of CF liver disease. Several associations or risk factors for the development of liver disease in CF have been described, including a history of meconium ileus, human leukocyte antigen (HLA) type, and heterozygosity for mutations in genes responsible for other liver diseases or in genes involved in mediating the response to liver injury.

Meconium ileus

Several studies have suggested that a history of meconium ileus as an infant is a risk factor for the subsequent development of liver disease. However, in a large study of genetic modifiers of liver disease in CF, no association between meconium ileus and the development of liver disease was observed [24]. In fact, the prevalence of meconium ileus in patients with liver disease was similar to the prevalence of those with pancreatic insufficiency and, therefore, may not represent an independent risk factor.

Immune system and antioxidant status

Several studies have shown an association between certain HLA types and susceptibility for liver disease in CF. A higher frequency of HLA-DQw6 has been reported in British patients with CF liver disease compared with those without liver disease. Duthie et al. [25] found HLA-DQ6 in 66% of patients with liver disease but in only 33% without it. Two other antigens, HLA-DR15 and HLA-B7, with linkage disequilibrium with this locus, were also significant risk factors. It is interesting to note that the association was greater in males than in females, and only in males when the phenotype was restricted to portal hypertension (representing more severe disease). These findings suggest a possible immune contribution to the pathogenesis of hepatobiliary injury or, alternatively, another susceptibility gene linked with specific haplotypes lies at or near the *HLA-DQ* locus.

Other ion channels

It has been proposed that other Cl^- channels may modify phenotypic expression of CF. Several mouse models of CF have demonstrated the importance of other Cl^- channels in modulating organ-level disease expression. Clarke et al. [15] demonstrated that expression of Ca^{2+}-activated Cl^- channels in the lung of $Cftr^{-/-}$ mice may explain the mild pulmonary disease in these animals; while modulation of the severity of the gastrointestinal disease may also be affected by alternative channels on intestinal enterocytes. The role of other ion channels and transporters in normal bile formation as well as the pathogenesis of CF liver disease remains to be established.

Other genetic modifiers

Recently, the Z allele of *SERPINA1* (encoding α_1-antitrypsin) was identified as a marker for the development of severe liver disease in patients with CF [24]. The α_1-antitrypsin protein is mainly expressed in the liver and is a serine protease inhibitor. Deficiency of the α_1-antitrypsin is associated with an increased risk of chronic lung disease. In the liver, the normal protein (coded by the *M* allele) is secreted into the plasma, while the abnormal protein (coded by the *Z* allele) folds abnormally and accumulates in the endoplasmic reticulum. The accumulation of this abnormal protein leads to hepatocyte apoptosis, fibrosis, and ultimately cirrhosis. Therefore, the mechanism by which α_1-antitrypsin modifies liver disease in CF is likely by rendering the hepatocyte more susceptible to injury in the presence of abnormal CFTR and ongoing biliary obstruction.

Two additional genes, *PAI1* (encoding plasminogen activator inhibitor 1) and *TIMP1* (encoding tissue inhibitor of metalloproteinase 1 (TIMP1)) were shown by cDNA array analysis to be downregulated from liver tissue from patients with CF liver disease versus normal patients and patients with non-CF cholestatic liver disease [26]. Both of these genes encode proteins that normally inhibit matrix metalloproteinases. Therefore, a decrease in plasminogen activator inhibitor 1 and TIMP1 activity would be predicted to increase matrix metalloproteinase activity and lead to increased matrix turnover [26]. Interestingly, plasminogen activator inhibitor 1 has been classified recently as SERPINE1, a serine protease inhibitor, like α_1-antitrypsin, and both *PAI1* and *CFTR* are located on the long arm of chromosome 7.

While smaller cohort studies have suggested possible associations of polymorphisms in other genes and CF liver disease, including genes for transforming growth factor-β, mannose-binding lectin, and glutathione *S*-transferase, larger screening studies have not been able to confirm these associations.

Prevalence of cystic fibrosis liver disease

Determining the true prevalence of CF liver disease has been difficult because (1) no universally accepted definition has been established, (2) many patients with significant liver disease are compensated and remain asymptomatic, and (3) there are no sensitive and specific markers for the diagnosis of CF liver disease.

The most recent data (from 2006) from the CFF registry reported elevated liver enzymes in 1052 of 13,319 patients younger than 18 years of age (7.9%) and in 757 of 10,369 patients 18 years or older (7.3%), whereas liver cirrhosis was reported in 1.4% of patients seen in US CF centers. It should be noted that these numbers rely on self-reporting and, therefore, appear to underestimate significantly the true prevalence of liver disease. Although retrospective analyses have reported prevalence figures between 4.2 and 24%, with a slight predominance in males and a peak in adolescence, autopsy data indicate a progressive increase in prevalence with age from 10% in infants to 72% in adults [27].

Four large prospective studies from different countries have been performed and may help to provide more accurate estimates of the true prevalence of clinically significant CF-associated liver disease. A prospective study of 153 patients with CF in Australia revealed the presence of hepatomegaly in 30% of patients, whereas 13% had multilobular cirrhosis defined by biochemical, clinical, and imaging criteria [28]. A prospective study from Sweden in 124 patients with CF, followed over a 15-year period, revealed abnormal biochemical markers of liver disease in 25% of children and the development of cirrhosis in 10% as confirmed by liver biopsy [29]. In this study, severe liver disease occurred predominantly by preadolescence or adolescence. Additionally, no risk factors for the development of liver disease were identified. However, deficiency of essential fatty acids was associated with steatosis. A prospective study from Italy followed 177 patients with CF up to a median of 14 years [30]. Significant liver disease (defined by persistent hepatomegaly, elevated liver enzymes on two consecutive visits, and ultrasound abnormalities) developed in 47 patients (26.5%) with an incidence rate of 1.8/100 patient-years. Cirrhosis was present

in 5 (10%) and developed in 12 other patients, giving an incidence rate of 4.5/100 liver disease patient-years. In this study, meconium ileus, male sex, and severe *CFTR* mutations were associated with the development of liver disease. Lastly, a study from Canada reported a prevalence of 18% at 2 years, 29% at 5 years, and 41% at 12 years [31]. Cirrhosis developed in 7.8% of patients at a median of 10 years, and the development of liver disease was independently associated with a history of meconium ileus and pancreatic insufficiency. The high prevalence rates in this study may reflect the more lenient definition of liver disease used (the findings on more than one occasion of either abnormal liver enzymes or abnormal ultrasound imaging). Together, based on these prospective studies, the best current estimate for clinically significant liver disease in children with CF is approximately 10–26%, with cirrhosis occurring in approximately 7–13%. Additionally, in contrast to the autopsy data, which suggest that there is an increase in the development of liver disease over time, most prospective studies revealed that liver disease developed before or during adolescence, suggesting that most patients who will develop clinically significant liver disease will do so at an early age.

Clinical manifestations of cystic fibrosis liver disease

The two most common clinical presentations of liver disease in CF are (1) an abnormal liver on physical examination (hepatomegaly or a small hard liver) or (2) elevated serum liver enzymes on routine screening. A small, hard liver on examination or signs of portal hypertension suggest cirrhosis. It should be noted that patients with CF can present with end-stage liver disease and even cirrhosis with few, if any, outward signs to suggest chronic liver disease. Hepatomegaly suggests steatosis or focal biliary cirrhosis but may also suggest congestive hepatopathy associated with cor pulmonale and right heart failure. These distinct clinical manifestations including hepatic steatosis, neonatal cholestasis, focal biliary cirrhosis, and multilobular cirrhosis have been described based on clinical or histologic criteria and have variable prevalence rates. (Table 26.1)

Congestive hepatopathy

Although hepatic congestion is not a direct result of defective CFTR protein in bile duct epithelial cells, it nonetheless should be considered a clinically significant cause of hepatomegaly in CF. Chronically elevated right-sided heart pressures or cor pulmonale may lead to congestive hepatopathy through increased hepatic vein and sinusoidal pressures. The elevated sinusoidal pressure is thought to cause hepatocyte injury and necrosis. Eventually this can progress to "cardiac cirrhosis" with the development of bands of fibrosis extending between centrilobular areas with intervening normal portal areas. The diagnosis should be considered in those patients with CF with

Table 26.1 Hepatobiliary manifestations of cystic fibrosis

Condition	Percentage affected
Asymptomatic elevation of liver enzymes	10–46
Liver	
Hepatomegaly	30
Hepatic steatosis	20–60
Neonatal cholestasis	2–38
Focal biliary cirrhosis	10–72
Multilobular cirrhosis	7–20
Hepatocellular carcinoma	Very rare
Biliary tract	
Microgallbladder	20–30
Cholelithiasis	1–10
Common bile duct stenosis	<2
Sclerosing cholangitis	<1
Cholangiocarcinoma	Very rare

(a)

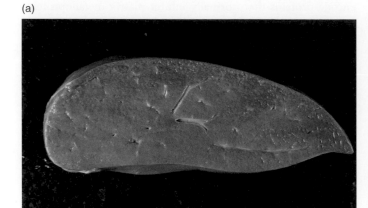

(b)

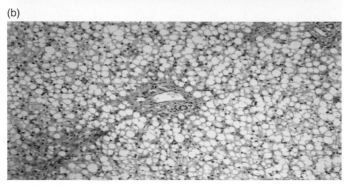

Figure 26.5 Steatosis in cystic fibrosis. (a) Cut section of the liver revealing extensive fatty infiltration. The liver is large and soft. (b) Photomicrograph of a histologic section from the liver above. Histology reveals extensive micro- and macrovesicular fat (hematoxylin & eosin stain.) (Courtesy of Dr. Arthur Weinberg, University of Texas Southwestern Medical Center, Dallas, Texas.)

chronic lung disease, clinical signs of cor pulmonale, a large liver (and sometimes tender) on examination, and dilated hepatic veins on ultrasound examination. Ultrasonography with Doppler and echocardiography are, therefore, the main modalities that aid in the diagnosis. Additionally, Doppler ultrasonography or angiography can be helpful to exclude other vascular complications such as thrombosis of hepatic veins or inferior vena cava. Biochemical analysis usually reveals serum aminotransferase levels that are only mildly elevated (<2× to 3× times normal), and a prothrombin time that is normal or only slightly prolonged (<5 seconds prolonged). If aminotransferases are >3× normal, consideration should be given to the co-occurrence of other liver disorders. It is important to exclude hepatic congestion as a cause of hepatomegaly before any consideration of a percutaneous liver biopsy because the dilated hepatic veins associated with this condition increase the risk of bleeding; consequently, a transjugular or surgical approach should be considered in that circumstance. Treatment of this disorder relies on improving the underlying cardiac or lung disease.

Neonatal cholestasis

Prolonged neonatal cholestasis may be quite common in newborns with CF. In one CF report, 35% of infants with CF had evidence of hepatomegaly or cholestasis within the first few months of life, and autopsy data has revealed histologic evidence of obstructive cholestasis in 38% of patients younger than 3 years with CF. Infants with CF and cholestasis should be evaluated thoroughly to exclude other cholestatic liver diseases, such as biliary atresia. On examination, hepatomegaly may be present and biochemical evaluation reveals elevation of serum direct bilirubin and gamma-glutamyltransferase concentrations. Stools may be acholic as in other cholestatic disorders, such as biliary atresia. Coexistent factors such as

abdominal surgery, parenteral nutrition, or infection may contribute to prolonged cholestasis. There does not appear to be an increased risk for the long-term development of cirrhosis with an early history of neonatal cholestasis. It is important, however, to consider the diagnosis of CF in infants who present with cholestasis. A sweat test or genotype testing should, therefore, be performed as part of the evaluation of neonatal cholestasis.

Steatosis

Hepatic steatosis is characterized by a large, soft liver on palpation (Figure 26.5a), but other signs of chronic liver disease or portal hypertension are usually not present. Histologic examination reveals hepatic parenchymal cells filled with micro-and macrovesicular fat (Figure 26.5b). Ultrasound has been used to aid in the diagnosis; however, the true sensitivity or specificity of this modality to determine the presence of steatosis and exclude other causes is still unknown. Other imaging studies such as CT or MRI have also been used to reveal fat density of the liver, although once again the sensitivity of these modalities to diagnosis steatosis in CF is unknown. This lesion is relatively common in CF, occurring in 20 to 60% of affected patients depending on the study. It is unclear

(a)

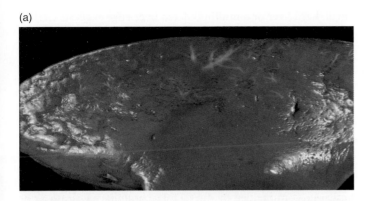

(b)

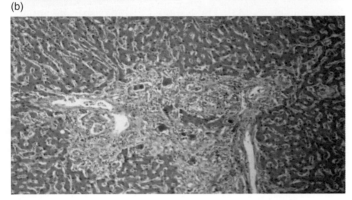

Figure 26.6 Focal biliary cirrhosis in cystic fibrosis. (a) The surface of the liver displays focal areas of scarring and furrowing. Large areas of normal preserved hepatic architecture are present. (b) Photomicrograph of a histologic section from liver above. The portal tract is expanded with bile duct proliferation and plugging of ducts with "eosinophilic material." Cholestasis and significant bands of fibrosis are present. (Hematoxylin & eosin staining.) (Courtesy of Dr. Arthur Weinberg, University of Texas Southwestern Medical Center, Dallas, Texas.)

whether this is a result of abnormal CFTR function in cholangiocytes or reflects a secondary effect of malnutrition or deficiency of trace element or minerals. Steatosis may resolve with improved nutritional status and correction of trace mineral, vitamin, or fatty acid deficiencies. Although this lesion is felt to be benign and non-progressive, the recent interest in non-alcoholic steatohepatitis as a cause of cirrhosis in adults may lead to a reappraisal of this belief.

Focal biliary cirrhosis and multilobular cirrhosis

Focal biliary cirrhosis is characterized histologically by focal areas of portal inflammation and fibrosis, bile duct obstruction and proliferation, and the inclusion of eosinophilic material in bile ductules (Figure 26.6). This lesion is considered pathognomonic of CF liver disease. The focal areas of fibrosis may give the liver a furrowed appearance (Figure 26.6a). The pink-staining eosinophilic material seen in the bile ductules, as well as the focal nature of the lesion, provides more evidence for the "bile duct plugging" hypothesis as contributing to the pathogenesis of this disease. The clinical diagnosis of focal biliary cirrhosis is difficult as both the physical examination and biochemical evaluation may be normal. Additionally,

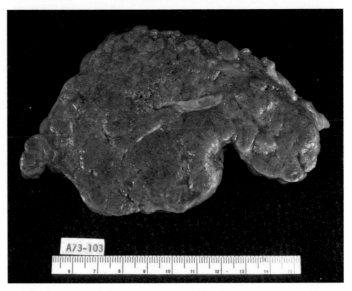

Figure 26.7 Multilobular cirrhosis in cystic fibrosis. Cut section of the liver revealing significant lobulation, fibrosis, scarring, and cirrhosis. (Courtesy of Dr. Arthur Weinberg, University of Texas Southwestern Medical Center, Dallas, Texas.)

ultrasound examination has not proved to detect this lesion reliably. Given the silent nature of this lesion, the prevalence of focal biliary cirrhosis can only be estimated from autopsy series. Autopsy studies indicate an increasing incidence of this lesion with increasing age, and focal biliary cirrhosis may progress into the more severe multilobular cirrhosis with portal hypertension or liver failure. It is not known why a subset of patients with focal biliary cirrhosis will progress to more severe liver disease and eventually multilobular cirrhosis.

Multilobular cirrhosis is characterized histologically by extensive, broad bands of fibrosis extending between portal areas (Figure 26.7). The liver is extensively lobulated, and within the individual lobules, both focal areas of scarring and intervening areas of normal hepatocyte parenchyma are present. Physical examination reveals a multilobulated and firm liver; in fact, the extensive lobulation is characteristic of this lesion. Signs of chronic liver disease such as clubbing, spider angiomata, and palmar erythema may be present. The identification of splenomegaly or ascites may herald the development of portal hypertension. Prospective studies have suggested prevalence rates of multilobular cirrhosis as high as 17%, and the majority of patients identified were younger than 14 years of age [32]. Studies have confirmed that the majority of patients with significant CF liver disease develop it by early adolescence [30]. Patients with multilobular cirrhosis are at risk from complications of end-stage liver disease and portal hypertension, including esophageal varices, ascites, encephalopathy, fatigue, splenomegaly, hypersplenism, and coagulopathy. In fact, complications from portal hypertension cause the majority of morbidity with this liver lesion. Impaired bile flow may lead to fat malabsorption and fat-soluble vitamin deficiencies. Treatment is based on correction of these deficiencies, optimizing nutritional status, and therapy with UDCA.

Biliary tract disease

Biliary abnormalities are common in CF, although it is unclear how a defective or absent CFTR protein results in the biliary manifestations such as gallbladder atrophy or bile duct stenosis. These findings may suggest even another potential role of CFTR, namely, as a developmental regulator of the biliary tree and gallbladder. A small or microgallbladder is present in 20–30% of patients with CF, and although it appears to be a benign condition without clinical sequelae, the finding in an infant should at least raise the suspicion of biliary atresia, which has been described in patients with CF.

Cholelithiasis is found in 1–10% of patients; however, clinical symptoms of cholecystitis have been reported to occur in less than 4% of cases, usually in older children. The main component of gallstones in CF is calcium bilirubinate, which is resistant to dissolution by UDCA therapy. Cholecystectomy is, therefore, the treatment of choice for gallstones in symptomatic patients. The approach is not as clearly defined in the asymptomatic patient, in whom stones are identified with routine ultrasound, although consideration should be given to elective cholecystectomy if pulmonary function is stable, because these stones increase the risk of cholecystitis and future complications.

Diagnosis and screening

It is important to note that at present there are no established diagnostic criteria universally accepted to establish the presence of CF liver disease. The diagnosis is usually established by a constellation of findings, including (1) an abnormal physical examination (hepatomegaly; a small, hard liver; splenomegaly; signs of portal hypertension; other signs of chronic liver disease), (2) persistently elevated liver enzymes (>3× normal on two or more sequential occasions), (3) abnormal imaging studies (abnormal ultrasound or other imaging modality demonstrating multilobular cirrhosis), or (4) abnormal liver histology.

Physical examination

A meticulous clinical examination is the fundamental means for detecting and following the progression of liver disease in CF. A careful liver examination should be performed at every clinic. An abnormal examination suggests underlying pathology and warrants further evaluation. Hepatomegaly is the most important finding to suggest the presence of liver disease. However, simply noting the degree that the liver edge is below the rib margin may be misleading because of the lung hyperinflation often present in CF; therefore, the entire span should be carefully measured and recorded. Hepatomegaly should be defined as a liver size above the upper limit of normal for age. If hepatomegaly is confirmed, then consideration should be given to the predominant lesion present (steatosis, focal biliary cirrhosis, or congestive hepatopathy secondary to chronic pulmonary or cardiac disease). Conversely, the presence of a small, hard liver or a multilobulated liver edge suggests cirrhosis. In this setting, portal hypertension is suggested by splenomegaly and dilated abdominal wall vasculature. Examination for other signs of chronic liver disease (palmar erythema, clubbing, or spider nevi) should always be conducted. A complete nutritional assessment should be performed in conjunction with a dietician, including an evaluation for any clinical signs of fat-soluble deficiency.

Biochemical evaluation

Serum liver enzyme analysis should be performed on a yearly basis as recommended by the CFF Hepatobiliary Disease Consensus guidelines [33]. These should include aspartate aminotransferase, alanine aminotransferase, bilirubin (total and direct), alkaline phosphatase, and gamma-glutamyltransferase. It should be noted that none of the biochemical measures have been shown to correlate with the degree of hepatic fibrosis in CF. In fact, patients may have completely normal liver enzymes in the presence of cirrhosis. Conversely, elevations in serum liver enzymes are common in CF, occurring in 10–46% of patients, and may not represent true liver disease [34]. Therefore, the diagnosis of CF liver disease cannot rely solely on elevated liver enzymes at one point in time. Based on these uncertainties in the evaluation of serum liver enzymes, the CFF Hepatobiliary Consensus Group has proposed a strategy for the interpretation of these tests (Figure 26.8). If a value is >1.5× the upper limit of normal for age, it is recommended that that value should be repeated in 3–6 months. If the level remains elevated for more than 6 months, without another explanation, it is indicative of possibly clinically significant liver involvement. At any time, if a value is >3× normal, tests of liver synthetic function, including prothrombin time, total protein, albumin, blood ammonia, cholesterol, and glucose, should be performed and further evaluation into the etiology performed. Exclusion of other causes of aminotransferase elevation, such as drugs, toxins, infectious hepatitis, biliary atresia, α_1-antitrypsin deficiency, autoimmune hepatitis, or other metabolic liver diseases, should be made when appropriate. It should be noted that, in large series of patients with suspected CF liver disease, other liver diseases, such as biliary atresia and α_1-antitrypsin deficiency, have been reported.

Ultrasonography

One of the most helpful imaging studies is ultrasonography of the liver and biliary tract. The CFF Hepatobiliary Consensus Group has recommended obtaining an ultrasound in all patients with CF in whom liver disease is suspected [33]. Ultrasound is presently the modality of choice to screen for biliary tract abnormalities in CF (biliary obstruction or stricture, gallstones, gallbladder abnormalities). Additionally, combined with Doppler, ultrasound is helpful in evaluating the vasculature. Reversal of flow (hepatofugal) in the portal vein usually indicates portal hypertension. Likewise, dilated hepatic veins suggest cor pulmonale or right heart failure. Some recent

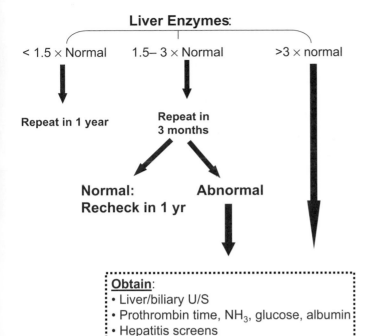

Liver Enzymes:

< 1.5 × Normal   1.5– 3 × Normal   >3 × normal

Repeat in 1 year   Repeat in 3 months

Normal: Recheck in 1 yr   Abnormal

Obtain:
- Liver/biliary U/S
- Prothrombin time, NH_3, glucose, albumin
- Hepatitis screens
- Exclude other liver diseases

Figure 26.8 Serum liver enzyme screening protocol for the detection of cystic fibrosis liver disease. Based on the Cystic Fibrosis Foundation Hepatobiliary Disease Consensus Guidelines. Assumes physical examination is normal and patient has no clinical evidence of liver disease. Serum liver enzymes should be obtained annually. If levels are persistently >1.5× normal (on at least two consecutive occasions) or >3× normal, then further evaluation is indicated. See text for further description.

studies suggest that ultrasound may be useful in the initial screening to determine the predominant lesion present as well as for following the progression of liver disease. A large study of 195 patients with CF found a correlation between ultrasound findings of cirrhosis and abnormal liver enzymes [35]. In a follow-up study of this original cohort, the ultrasound examination was repeated in the 106 patients originally without findings of liver disease [36]; after 10 years, 19 of the 106 (18%) had developed abnormal ultrasound changes with 8 having signs of portal hypertension. Overall, the majority of studies revealed a disparity between ultrasound findings and serum liver enzyme levels. Nonetheless, observations from these long-term studies suggest that routine ultrasound may be a valuable marker of early liver disease; however, findings may be subjective and operator dependent, and the true sensitivity and specificity of this test to detect clinically significant liver disease has not been determined.

Other imaging studies

Other imaging studies that have been evaluated in small numbers of patients with CF include abdominal CT and MRI. Computed tomography is very effective at identifying cirrhosis from any cause including multilobular cirrhosis associated with CF. Additionally, CT may be of benefit in identifying fat density of the liver associated with hepatic steatosis. The

accuracy of CT in detecting early liver changes associated with CF is not known, and the radiation exposure makes CT unsuitable for screening purposes. Like CT, MRI is effective in detecting findings associated with cirrhosis and portal hypertension, although its sensitivity in the detection of early changes is unknown. Magnetic resonance cholangiopancreatography has become a valuable modality for the imaging of the biliary tree.

Transient elastography

Transient elastography (Fibroscan) is a newer non-invasive modality which has been utilized to evaluate tissue stiffness as an indicator of liver fibrosis. An ultrasound transducer probe mounted on a vibrator is utilized to take measurements of wave propagation through the liver, and fibrosis is assessed as liver stiffness by calculating the velocity of wave propagation. It has been suggested that this technology may aid in assessing the degree of fibrosis and decrease intraoperator variability. Liver elastography has been utilized in patients with CF to detect fibrosis and may help guide clinical decisions regarding further evaluation for esophageal varices. However, additional studies are needed to determine the efficacy of this promising new, non-invasive tool for the evaluation of cirrhosis in CF-associated liver disease.

Liver biopsy

The role of liver biopsy in the evaluation of suspected liver disease in the patient with CF is controversial. Arguments in favor of performing a liver biopsy include: (1) it is the most accurate means to define the predominant lesion present (steatosis or focal biliary cirrhosis); (2) it may help to quickly exclude other causes; and (3) it will help to determine the degree of fibrosis present. Arguments against performing a liver biopsy include: (1) the recognized risk of sampling error because of the heterogeneous distribution of liver lesions, (2) patients may be at a higher risk for complications (pneumothorax from lung hyperexpansion or bleeding from dilated hepatic veins secondary to cor pulmonale), and (3) no definitive treatment exists and, therefore, there is no reason to make an accurate diagnosis. At this time, the decision to perform a liver biopsy must be an individual determination based on the clinical scenario. If a percutaneous liver biopsy is felt to be indicated, ultrasound should always be performed immediately before the procedure to exclude dilated hepatic veins and ascites and to locate an appropriate spot with special care to avoid the lower lobe of the lung. If dilated hepatic veins or ascites are present, a percutaneous liver biopsy should not be performed and consideration should be given to a surgical or transjugular biopsy if indicated. Given the elusive nature of the diagnosis of CF liver disease, it is strongly advised to obtain a surgical liver biopsy, if it can be done without difficulty or additional significant risk, during abdominal surgery for any reason in the patient with CF.

Biomarkers

Given the difficulty in identifying the presence and severity of liver disease in CF, serum biomarkers of early disease have been sought, including bile acid profiles, inflammatory markers, matrix remodeling proteins, and functional tests of hepatic reserve.

In one recent study comparing patients with CF with and without liver disease, significant correlations were seen among serum cholic acid levels (or the ratio of serum cholic acid to chenodeoxycholic acid) and hepatic fibrosis [22]. The use of serum bile acid profiles in the early detection of CF liver disease warrants further study.

Several markers of hepatic injury and inflammation, including glutathione S-transferase B1 activity, high-molecular-mass alkaline phosphatase, and serum hyaluronic acid, have been shown to be elevated in subsets of patients with CF with liver disease. Additionally, serum markers to detect liver fibrosis have been evaluated in CF. Both collagen VI and serum prolyl hydroxylase have been shown to be increased in a small number of patients with CF compared with those without liver disease. One study analyzed the serum of 36 patients with CF-associated liver disease, 30 patients with CF without liver disease, and 39 control patients for several markers of hepatic fibrosis, including TIMP1, collagen type IV, matrix metalloproteinase 2, hyaluronic acid, and prolyl hydroxylase [37]; TIMP1, prolyl hydroxylase, and collagen IV were increased in patients with CF with liver disease compared with those without (or control subjects), and the TIMP1 and prolyl hydroxylase levels correlated negatively with fibrosis score. In this study, collagen IV and TIMP1 differentiated patients with CF with and without liver disease. Although studies of serum markers of fibrosis and matrix remodeling appear promising in the detection of liver disease, one concern is that these markers may be affected by growth as well as by the airway epithelial cell remodeling associated with chronic lung disease. The use of these serum markers of liver injury, inflammation, and fibrosis, therefore, require further study to determine the usefulness in screening programs.

Treatment

Once the presence of liver disease has been identified, the predominant lesion defined, and other diseases excluded, consideration should be given to treatment. A multidisciplinary approach is recommended for the management of liver disease in CF involving all members of the CF care team, including a hepatologist, surgeon, and radiologist.

Hepatic steatosis

The fundamental treatment of hepatic steatosis is nutritional rehabilitation, normalizing biochemical parameters of micronutrients, and maximizing growth. It is essential to optimize intake of protein, fat, and energy; institute pancreatic enzyme replacement therapy; and identify and correct any trace element, mineral, or vitamin deficiencies. Biochemical evaluation of essential fatty acids and fat-soluble vitamins should be carried out and these replaced if found to be inadequate. It is important to exclude contributing factors such as ethanol, hepatotoxic medications, and other drugs or toxins. Lastly, given the recent interest of insulin resistance in the development of hepatic steatosis, consideration should be given to evaluation of diabetes by glucose tolerance testing.

Focal biliary cirrhosis and multilobular cirrhosis

Ursodeoxycholic acid, a hydrophilic bile acid normally produced in small quantities by the human liver, has been shown to improve bile flow and biochemical parameters of liver injury in CF. However, no treatment, including UDCA, has yet been shown to alter the progression of liver disease or the development of cirrhosis in CF. Ursodeoxycholic acid may have several potential mechanisms of action, including enrichment of the hydrophilic bile acid pool [38], stimulation of Cl^- and HCO_3^- transport [38,39], and direct cytoprotective and immunomodulatory effects. Prospective clinical trials of UDCA, at doses of 10–20 mg/kg daily for 6–12 months, have shown improvements in serum liver enzyme levels in children with CF liver disease [40]. In a 2-year, uncontrolled study, UDCA therapy improved the liver histology, with less inflammation and bile duct proliferation, in 7 of 10 patients with CF-related liver disease [41]. A 10-year prospective study in 70 patients with CF liver disease suggested that UDCA (20 mg/kg daily) may improve the ultrasound appearance of the liver [42]. Despite these findings, there is still no long-term data to prove that UDCA alters the natural course of liver disease in patients with CF. However, given the improved biochemical parameters, ultrasound findings, and, perhaps, histologic data, the CFF Hepatobiliary Disease Consensus Group has recommended it is "prudent to treat patients with CF who have cholestasis-fibrosis-cirrhosis" [33]. Another recent guidelines statement recommended UDCA for all patients with CF-associated liver disease [43]. However, it should be noted that the initial recommendation was on the basis of lack of harm and potential benefit in CF-associated liver disease based on reported benefits of UDCA in other cholestatic liver diseases including primary biliary cirrhosis and primary sclerosing cholangitis. However, UDCA did not demonstrate any benefit in terms of morbidity and mortality in one large study in primary sclerosing cholangitis [44] and a recent Cochrane review of primary biliary cirrhosis [45]. Furthermore, the study found an increased risk of the development of colorectal neoplasia in patients with ulcerative colitis and primary sclerosing cholangitis who were treated with high-dose UDCA [44]. While a recent European Consensus statement recommends the use of UDCA for patients with CF and liver disease [43], a follow-up letter to the editor poignantly summarized the current controversies surrounding the use of UDCA in CF by stating that "the role and use of UDCA is controversial and the evidence for and against its use requires critical appraisal. ...Simply put, at present, there are no convincing data to demonstrate that UDCA is efficacious or harmful in CFLD" [46].

Long-term clinical trials to determine the ultimate effect of UDCA on morbidity and mortality are needed. Therefore, ideally, patients receiving UDCA therapy should be enrolled in clinical trials. It will be important to determine whether early treatment will alter the natural progression of the disease and decrease the occurrence of cirrhosis and the complications associated with portal hypertension. At present, there are no studies to promote the routine, prophylactic use of UDCA in all patients with CF. Clearly, this would result in overtreatment in a significant portion of patients. Once again, this highlights the need for research into the basic pathogenesis of the disease to identify risk factors and markers for screening.

Patients in whom liver disease is identified should receive counseling and education concerning the promotion of "liver health" including the avoidance of alcohol, liver-toxic medications, herbal therapies, and obesity. Additionally, patients should receive vaccines against hepatitis A and B viruses.

Nutritional management

An important component of the management of liver disease in CF is maintenance of a normal nutritional state. Patients with CF may require energy intake that exceeds recommendations by 20–40% because of the continued fat malabsorption, increased caloric expenditure from chronic lung disease, and the increased oxygen consumption associated with cholestasis. Protein intake should not be restricted in children with CF unless decompensated hepatic failure with encephalopathy and hyperammonemia are present. Infants with significant cholestasis may require formulae containing medium-chain triglyceride to promote intestinal absorption of dietary lipid. Attention should be given to the optimization of pancreatic enzyme replacement therapy in those patients with pancreatic insufficiency. Dosing of pancreatic enzyme replacement therapy should ideally be based on dietary composition with a goal to minimize fat malabsorption and steatorrhea while maximizing growth and weight gain. High doses ($>3000\,U$ lipase/kg per meal) should be avoided because these have been associated with the development of fibrosing colonapathy. The CFF Consensus Committee on Pancreatic Enzyme Replacement Therapy has recommended lipase dosage ranges of 1000–2500 U/kg per meal for up to 4 years of age and 500–2500 U/kg per meal for ages 4 and older in patients with CF and pancreatic insufficiency. Monitoring fat-soluble vitamin status is even more important in the presence of liver disease than in the patient with CF who has pancreatic insufficiency alone. A multidisciplinary approach including physicians, nurses, dieticians, nutritionists, and pharmacists is essential to the successful management of the complex nutritional issues facing the patient with CF liver disease.

Portal hypertension and liver transplantation

Cystic fibrosis-associated liver disease rarely causes acute liver failure; rather it leads to the complications of end-stage liver disease, namely, those associated with portal hypertension. A long-term study of 40 patients with CF liver disease. reported the development of portal hypertension in 10 (25%), all of whom had variceal hemorrhage [47]. Prevention of recurrent variceal hemorrhage with the use of beta-blockers may be contraindicated in patients with CF because of adverse effects on bronchial reactivity. Surgical portosystemic shunt and transjugular portosystemic shunt may be indicated for the management of portal hypertension in these patients, allowing for prolonged survival, a bridge to liver transplant, or both. Partial splenectomy was used in the past management of hypersplenism in patients with CF with liver disease; however, this procedure has been abandoned in favor of other approaches. Partial splenic embolization has been used to treat hypersplenism and extreme splenomegaly with success in other conditions, and using smaller volume embolization reduces the morbidity associated with this procedure.

Liver transplantation should be offered to those patients with life-threatening complications of portal hypertension or severe functional impairment and who have adequate pulmonary function, good compliance with care, and no other contraindications. Some controversy has existed regarding the possible adverse role of pulmonary infections in patients with CF before liver transplant. A recent review of the US United Network for Organ Sharing database highlights several important observations: (1) liver transplantation for CF is rare, (2) compared with their counterparts without CF, children with CF who underwent liver transplantation had a lower survival at 30 days, and (3) a clear survival advantage was observed for patients undergoing liver transplantation versus those on the waiting list [48]. Additionally, experience with combined lung–liver transplantation or small bowel–liver transplantation is limited but has been performed in patients with CF. Selection of the most appropriate intervention (repeated sclerotherapy or banding, portosystemic shunt, partial splenectomy, or liver transplantation) for the management of end-stage CF liver disease and portal hypertension must be individualized in as much as there is insufficient data to support a best practices approach.

Future therapies

Based on our growing knowledge of CFTR function in cellular physiology, potentially new and exciting therapies may be developed for the treatment and prevention of CF. Strategies to correct the basic biliary defect, target and correct the abnormal CFTR trafficking, activate other Cl^- channels or transport pathways, and treat the progressive fibrosis through antioxidants or antifibrotic therapies are all being evaluated.

Gene therapy

One fundamental goal of treatment strategies has been to correct the basic gene defect through the use of somatic gene transfer. Successful insertion of normal *CFTR* into normal and CF bile duct cell lines in culture has been achieved and has been performed experimentally by retrograde infusion into the biliary tree of the rat [49]. It is doubtful that this approach will be successful in humans because of the invasive nature of endoscopic retrograde cholangiopancreatography. Strategies for clinically feasible approaches for gene transfer to the biliary tree (e.g. appropriate vector development) will need to be developed and validated before clinical application of this novel approach becomes feasible.

Correctors and potentiators of CFTR

New pharmacologic treatments are being studied that target specific CFTR mutant proteins to correct protein structure, folding, or trafficking [50]. For example, class I mutations, associated with a premature stop signal and, therefore, producing no functional CFTR protein, can be corrected in vitro by certain aminoglycoside antibiotics, which cause the aberrant stop signal to be skipped. Class II mutations (e.g. ΔF508) result in an unstable protein that does not traffic to the apical membrane correctly. The protein can potentially be restored to a normal pathway by manipulation of chaperone protein–CFTR interactions. This has been accomplished in vitro using chemical chaperones or drugs, such as butyrate or adenosine receptor antagonists, that affect modulation of protein folding. Class III mutations result in CFTR with reduced Cl^- secretory capacity; genistein, a flavonoid compound, and milrinone, a phosphodiesterase inhibitor, can partially restore the decreased Cl^- conductance associated with the class IV mutations. At present, all of these approaches require significant further development, and their potential application to the treatment of liver disease is unknown. Although further studies are warranted, given the suggestion that "non-CFTR factors" may determine the development of liver disease, these strategies to correct an abnormal CFTR protein may be of limited benefit in the treatment of CF liver disease.

Alternative channels

Understanding the basic mechanisms involved in cholangiocyte transport and secretion may suggest other areas of intervention to modulate bile flow. Indeed, the apical membrane of cholangiocytes contains several other Cl^- channels, which at least in single cell or epithelial monolayer studies, have a larger unitary conductance than CFTR itself [18]. The presence of alternative channels may modify organ-level disease expression in CF. For example, the mild lung disease in the CF mouse may be explained by the high expression of Ca^{2+}-activated Cl^- channels in the epithelial airway cells of these animals [15]. Recently, a Ca^{2+}-activated Cl^- channel has been identified in the liver and contributed importantly to biliary secretion in response to extracellular ATP [16]. Understanding the regulation of these alternative channels may provide strategies to bypass the secretory defect associated with CF.

Choleretic agents

Currently, although UDCA is the only choleretic agent that may be beneficial in CF liver disease, other bile acids or analogues are being developed. One such synthetic bile acid is 24-norursodeoxycholic acid, a side-chain-shortened C23 homologue of UDCA. This agent has recently been studied in *ABCB4* (encoding multidrug resistance protein 2) knockout mice ($Mdr2^{-/-}$), a model of primary sclerosing cholangitis, where it improved biliary HCO_3^- secretion and hepatic fibrosis. Therefore, modification of UDCA may increase the hydrophilicity of the bile acid and increase HCO_3^--rich bile flow. Further studies in other cholestatic conditions, including CF, are warranted. Another novel approach for the treatment of cholestatic liver disorders is to increase expression of bile acid transporters by the use of nuclear receptor agonists. Although the use of these agents is potentially an exciting therapeutic modality, studies are clearly needed to determine the safety and efficacy of nuclear receptor agonists in cholestatic liver conditions such as CF.

Antioxidants

Given a possible imbalance in oxidants versus antioxidants in CF, there may be a rationale for exploring the use of antioxidants as a therapeutic strategy. In early clinical trials, aerosolized glutathione has been delivered to the lung in patients with CF and was shown to increase airway glutathione levels, but it only had a modest effect on markers of oxidant injury. Although *N*-acetylcysteine, a substrate for glutathione production, has been used in an acetaminophen-induced liver injury, its role in the treatment of other liver diseases is unknown; and a recent multicenter study of *N*-acetylcysteine in the treatment of acute liver failure failed to demonstrate any beneficial effect. Therefore, while results of antioxidant treatment in experimental models of oxidative liver injury appear promising, there is no direct clinical evidence to support this therapy for CF liver disease at this time.

Antifibrotic agents

Understanding the role of the hepatic stellate cell in the progressive fibrosis associated with CF may lead to new treatment strategies to prevent ongoing cellular injury and interrupt fibrogenesis. Although a number of antifibrogenic agents that target stellate cells are in the development phase and may prove to be beneficial in the future, the role of antifibrotic agents in the treatment of CF liver disease warrants further study.

Conclusions

The pathogenesis of CF liver disease continues to be a mystery. However, our knowledge of CFTR structure, function, and regulation in novel models of biliary epithelium continues to increase at a rapid rate. In the future, it is anticipated that this knowledge will translate into therapeutic strategies for the successful treatment and prevention of CF liver disease.

Acknowledgements

Research was supported by the Cystic Fibrosis Foundation and the National Institute of Diabetes, Digestive and Kidney Diseases of the National Institutes of Health (DK078587).

References

1. Kosorok MR, Wei WH, Farrell PM. The incidence of cystic fibrosis. *Stat Med* 1996;**15**:449–462.

2. Dodge JA, Morison S, Lewis PA, *et al.* Incidence, population, and survival of cystic fibrosis in the UK, 1968–95. UK Cystic Fibrosis Survey Management Committee. *Arch Dis Child* 1997;**77**:493–496.

3. Anderson D. Cystic fibrosis of the pancreas and its relation to celiac disease: a clinical and pathological study. *Am J Dis Child* 1938;344–399.

4. Quinton PM. Chloride impermeability in cystic fibrosis. *Nature* 1983;**301** (5899):421–422.

5. Riordan JR, Rommens JM, Kerem B, *et al.* Identification of the cystic fibrosis gene: cloning and characterization of complementary DNA. *Science* 1989;**245** (4922):1066–1073.

6. Schwiebert EM, Benos DJ, Egan ME, Stutts MJ, Guggino WB. CFTR is a conductance regulator as well as a chloride channel. *Physiol Rev* 1999; **79**(1 Suppl):S145-S166.

7. Gabriel SE, Clarke LL, Boucher RC, Stutts MJ. CFTR and outward rectifying chloride channels are distinct proteins with a regulatory relationship. *Nature* 1993;**363**(6426):263–268.

8. Braunstein GM, Roman RM, Clancy JP, *et al.* Cystic fibrosis transmembrane conductance regulator facilitates ATP release by stimulating a separate ATP release channel for autocrine control of cell volume regulation. *J Biol Chem* 2001;**276**:6621–6630.

9. Fouassier L, Duan CY, Feranchak AP, *et al.* Ezrin-radixin-moesin-binding phosphoprotein 50 is expressed at the apical membrane of rat liver epithelia. *Hepatology* 2001;**33**:166–176.

10. Cohn JA, Strong TV, Picciotto MR, *et al.* Localization of the cystic fibrosis transmembrane conductance regulator in human bile duct epithelial cells. *Gastroenterology* 1993;**105**: 1857–1864.

11. Fitz JG, Basavappa S, McGill J, Melhus O, Cohn JA. Regulation of membrane chloride currents in rat bile duct epithelial cells. *J Clin Invest* 1993;**91**:319–328.

12. Fitz JG. Cellular mechanisms of bile secretion. In Zakim D, Boyer TD (eds.) *Hepatology*, 3rd edn. Philadelphia, PA: Saunders, 1996, pp. 362–376.

13. Dutta AK, Khimji AK, Sathe M, *et al.* Identification and functional characterization of the intermediate-conductance Ca(2+)-activated K(+) channel (IK-1) in biliary epithelium. *Am J Physiol Gastrointest Liver Physiol* 2009;**297**:G1009-G1018.

14. Feranchak AP, Sokol RJ. Cholangiocyte biology and cystic fibrosis liver disease. *Sem Liv Disease* 2001;**21**:471–488.

15. Clarke LL, Grubb BR, Yankaskas JR, *et al.* Relationship of a non-cystic fibrosis transmembrane conductance regulator-mediated chloride conductance to organ-level disease in Cftr($^{-/-}$) mice. *Proc Natl Acad Sci USA* 1994;**91**:479–483.

16. Dutta AK, Khimji AK, Kresge C, *et al.* Identification and functional characterization of TMEM16A, a Ca^{2+}-activated Cl$^-$ channel activated by extracellular nucleotides, in biliary epithelium. *J Biol Chem* 2011;**286**: 766–776.

17. Feranchak AP, Fitz JG. Adenosine triphosphate release and purinergic regulation of cholangiocyte transport. *Semin Liver Dis* 2002;**22**:251–262.

18. Dutta AK, Woo K, Doctor RB, Fitz JG, Feranchak AP. Extracellular nucleotides stimulate Cl$^-$ currents in biliary epithelia through receptor-mediated IP3 and Ca^{2+} release. *Am J Physiol Gastrointest Liver Physiol* 2008;**295**:G1004–G1015.

19. Woo K, Dutta AK, Patel V, Kresge C, Feranchak AP. Fluid flow induces mechanosensitive ATP release, calcium signalling and Cl$^-$ transport in biliary epithelial cells through a PKCzeta-dependent pathway. *J Physiol* 2008;**586** (Pt 11):2779–2798.

20. Gabriel SE, Brigman KN, Koller BH, Boucher RC, Stutts MJ. Cystic fibrosis heterozygote resistance to cholera toxin in the cystic fibrosis mouse model. *Science* 1994;**266**(5182):107–109.

21. Quinton PM. Role of epithelial HCO3 transport in mucin secretion: lessons from cystic fibrosis. *Am J Physiol Cell Physiol* 2010;**299**:C1222-C1233.

22. Smith JL, Lewindon PJ, Hoskins AC, *et al.* Endogenous ursodeoxycholic acid and cholic acid in liver disease due to cystic fibrosis. *Hepatology* 2004;**39**:1673–1682.

23. Lewindon PJ, Pereira TN, Hoskins AC, *et al.* The role of hepatic stellate cells and transforming growth factor-beta(1) in cystic fibrosis liver disease. *Am J Pathol* 2002;**160**:1705–1715.

24. Bartlett JR, Friedman KJ, Ling SC, *et al.* Genetic modifiers of liver disease in cystic fibrosis. *JAMA* 2009;**302**: 1076–1083.

25. Duthie A, Doherty DG, Donaldson PT, *et al.* The major histocompatibility complex influences the development of chronic liver disease in male children and young adults with cystic fibrosis. *J Hepatol* 1995;**23**:532–537.

26. Pereira TN, Lewindon PJ, Greer RM, *et al.* A transcriptional basis for cystic fibrosis liver disease: pilot study of differentially expressed genes associated with hepatic fibrosis. *J Pediatr Gastroenterol Nutr* 2012;**54**:328–335.

27. Vawter GF, Shwachman H. Cystic fibrosis in adults: an autopsy study. *Pathol Annu* 1979;**14**:357–382.

28. Gaskin KJ, Waters DL, Howman-Giles R, *et al.* Liver disease and common-bile-duct stenosis in cystic fibrosis. *N Engl J Med* 1988;**318**:340–346.

29. Lindblad A, Glaumann H, Strandvik B. Natural history of liver disease in cystic fibrosis. *Hepatology* 1999;**30**: 1151–1158.

30. Colombo C, Battezzati PM, Crosignani A, *et al.* Liver disease in cystic fibrosis: A prospective study on incidence, risk factors, and outcome. *Hepatology* 2002;**36**:1374–1382.

31. Lamireau T, Monnereau S, Martin S, *et al.* Epidemiology of liver disease in

cystic fibrosis: a longitudinal study. *J Hepatol* 2004;**41**:920–925.

32. Colombo C, Apostolo MG, Ferrari M, *et al.* Analysis of risk factors for the development of liver disease associated with cystic fibrosis. *J Pediatr* 1994;**124**:393–399.

33. Sokol RJ, Durie PR. Recommendations for management of liver and biliary tract disease in cystic fibrosis. Cystic Fibrosis Foundation Hepatobiliary Disease Consensus Group. *J Pediatr Gastroenterol Nutr* 1999;**28**(Suppl 1): S1–S13.

34. Sokol RJ, Carroll NM, Narkewicz MR *et al.* Liver blood tests during the first decade of life in children with cystic fibrosis identified by newborn screening. *Pediatr Pulm* 1994;**10**:275.

35. Patriquin H, Lenaerts C, Smith L, *et al.* Liver disease in children with cystic fibrosis: US-biochemical comparison in 195 patients. *Radiology* 1999;**211**: 229–232.

36. Lenaerts C, Lapierre C, Patriquin H, *et al.* Surveillance for cystic fibrosis-associated hepatobiliary disease: early ultrasound changes and predisposing factors. *J Pediatr* 2003;**143**: 343–350.

37. Pereira TN, Lewindon PJ, Smith JL, *et al.* Serum markers of hepatic fibrogenesis in cystic fibrosis liver disease. *J Hepatol* 2004;**41**: 576–583.

38. Heuman DM. Hepatoprotective properties of ursodeoxycholic acid. *Gastroenterology* 1993;**104**: 1865–1870.

39. Shimokura GH, McGill JM, Schlenker T, Fitz JG. Ursodeoxycholate increases cytosolic calcium concentration and activates Cl⁻ currents in a biliary cell line. *Gastroenterology* 1995;**109**: 965–972.

40. Colombo C, Crosignani A, Assaisso M, *et al.* Ursodeoxycholic acid therapy in cystic fibrosis-associated liver disease: a dose-response study. *Hepatology* 1992;**16**:924–930.

41. Lindblad A, Glaumann H, Strandvik B. A two-year prospective study of the effect of ursodeoxycholic acid on urinary bile acid excretion and liver morphology in cystic fibrosis-associated liver disease. *Hepatology* 1998;**27**: 166–174.

42. Nousia-Arvanitakis S, Fotoulaki M, Economou H, Xefteri M, Galli-Tsinopoulou A. Long-term prospective study of the effect of ursodeoxycholic acid on cystic fibrosis-related liver disease. *J Clin Gastroenterol* 2001;**32**:324–328.

43. Debray D, Kelly D, Houwen R, Strandvik B, Colombo C. Best practice guidance for the diagnosis and management of cystic fibrosis-associated liver disease. *J Cyst Fibros* 2011;**10**(Suppl 2):S29–S36.

44. Lindor KD, Kowdley KV, Luketic VA, *et al.* High-dose ursodeoxycholic acid for the treatment of primary sclerosing cholangitis. *Hepatology* 2009;**50**: 808–814.

45. Gong Y, Huang ZB, Christensen E, Gluud C. Ursodeoxycholic acid for primary biliary cirrhosis. *Cochrane Database Syst Rev* 2008;(**8**): CD000551.

46. Ooi CY, Nightingale S, Durie PR, Freedman SD. Ursodeoxycholic acid in cystic fibrosis-associated liver disease. *J Cyst Fibros* 2012;**11**:72–73.

47. Efrati O, Barak A, Modan-Moses D, *et al.* Liver cirrhosis and portal hypertension in cystic fibrosis. *Eur J Gastroenterol Hepatol* 2003;**15**: 1073–1078.

48. Gridelli B. Liver: benefit of liver transplantation in patients with cystic fibrosis. *Nat Rev Gastroenterol Hepatol* 2011;**8**:187–188.

49. Yang Y, Raper SE, Cohn JA, Engelhardt JF, Wilson JM. An approach for treating the hepatobiliary disease of cystic fibrosis by somatic gene transfer. *Proc Natl Acad Sci USA* 1993;**90**: 4601–4605.

50. Becq F, Mall MA, Sheppard DN, Conese M, Zegarra-Moran O. Pharmacological therapy for cystic fibrosis: from bench to bedside. *J Cyst Fibros* 2011;**10**(Suppl 2): S129–S145.

Inborn errors of carbohydrate metabolism

Rana F. Ammoury and Fayez K. Ghishan

Introduction

Inborn errors of carbohydrate metabolism that lead to hepatic dysfunction are represented mainly by galactosemia, hereditary fructose intolerance (HFI), and glycogen storage disease (GSD) types I, III, and IV. The clinical presentation of such patients includes varying degrees of hypoglycemia, acidosis, growth failure, and hepatic dysfunction. Appropriate steps in obtaining clinical history, physical examination, and laboratory evaluation support a definitive diagnosis. Advances in biochemistry and molecular biology, which have made significant contributions toward better understanding of the molecular defects underlying these disorders, are anticipated to eventually result in the development of newer treatment strategies. This chapter highlights current knowledge.

Disorders of galactose metabolism

In 1935, Mason and Turner provided the first detailed characterization of a galactose-intolerant individual [1]. Since then, three distinct disorders of galactose metabolism and several variant forms of the disease have been identified. These disorders are transmitted by autosomal recessive inheritance and are expressed as a cellular deficiency of one of three enzymes in the metabolic pathway through which galactose is converted to glucose: galactose-1-phosphate uridyl transferase, galactokinase, and uridine diphosphate (UDP) galactose-4-epimerase. Since each of these conditions results in milk-induced galactosemia but represents three distinct biochemical entities, the terms *transferase-deficiency galactosemia*, *galactokinase-deficiency galactosemia*, and *epimerase-deficiency galactosemia* have traditionally been used to distinguish between the various forms of the disease. Each enzymatic defect associated with galactosemia results in a distinctive clinical presentation. Clinical manifestations of toxicity in transferase-deficiency galactosemia, the classic form of the disease, include malnutrition, growth failure, cataract formation, progressive liver disease, mental retardation, and ovarian failure [2]. Galactokinase deficiency, originally described by Gitzelmann in 1967, results primarily in cataract formation and galactosuria [3]. In most cases of UDP-galactose-

4-epimerase deficiency, the defect is limited to erythrocytes and leukocytes; therefore, affected individuals display no clinical or laboratory manifestations of galactosemia [4]. In a variant form of epimerase deficiency galactosemia identified by Holton and colleagues in 1981, however, the defect is more generalized and results in a severe clinical presentation resembling the classic form of the disease [5].

Treatment of galactosemia has remained essentially unchanged since the disorder first was described more than 60 years ago. Confidence in dietary strategies that effectively minimize galactose intake in affected individuals, however, has declined significantly since the late 1990s. This coincides with recognition that long-term complications such as learning difficulties, speech disorders, ovarian failure, and ataxia syndromes commonly occur in well-treated patients. It is now clear that development of new treatment strategies is necessary to positively impact the ultimate outcome of this disorder. To this end, future research efforts should be focused on developing a complete understanding of the molecular and biochemical basis of galactosemia, particularly as they relate to the pathogenesis of these long-term complications [6].

Biochemistry of galactose metabolism

Galactose is a monosaccharide that is derived from the hydrolysis of lactose, the sugar in dairy products. Lactose is hydrolyzed into glucose and galactose by the disaccharidase lactase in the brush border membranes of the enterocytes. Galactose is transported across the brush border membrane of the enterocyte through the sodium-dependent glucose–galactose transporter [7]. Galactose is metabolized to glucose in a series of reactions as depicted in Figure 27.1. The first step in galactose metabolism involves phosphorylation of galactose by ATP utilizing the enzyme galactokinase. This enzyme is present in bacteria, yeast, and mammalian tissues [8]. Galactokinase in the human liver shows developmental changes, with progressive increase from the seventh week of gestation until term [9]. The level of activity in the red blood cells is higher in the newborn than in the adult. The enzyme, however, is not regulated by galactose.

Liver Disease in Children, Fourth Edition, ed. Frederick J. Suchy, Ronald J. Sokol, and William F. Balistreri. Published by Cambridge University Press. © Cambridge University Press 2014.

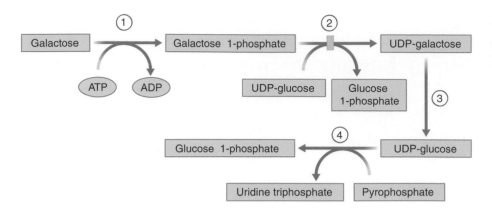

Figure 27.1 Galactose metabolism. 1, Galactokinase; 2, galactose 1-phosphate uridyltransferase; 3, uridine diphosphate galactose-4-epimerase; 4, uridine diphosphate glucose pyrophosphorylase.

The second step in galactose metabolism involves the reaction of galactose 1-phosphate with UDP-glucose, which is catalyzed by the enzyme galactose-1-phosphate uridyltransferase. The enzyme is present in most mammalian tissues including the liver. This reaction results in the formation of UDP-galactose and glucose 1-phosphate. The complementary DNA (cDNA) encoding for the human transferase enzyme is 1295 bases in length and encodes a 43 kDa protein [10].

The third step in galactose metabolism involves the interconversion of UDP-galactose to UDP-glucose catalyzed by UDP-galactose-4-epimerase. The fourth step in galactose metabolism involves the generation of glucose 1-phosphate from UDP-glucose by UDP-glucose pyrophosphorylase. This enzyme has been crystallized from the mammalian liver and appears to play a role in the synthesis of UDP-glucose from UDP and glucose.

Alternative pathways of galactose metabolism involve reduction to galactitol through two enzymes: aldose reductase and L-hexonate dehydrogenase. The existence of this alternative pathway explains the presence of galactitol in the urine of patients with both transferase and galactokinase deficiencies. The other pathway involves oxidation of galactose to galactonate. Patients with transferase deficiency excrete galactonate in their urine.

Humans are capable of metabolizing large quantities of galactose, as evidenced by the rapid clearance of galactose from blood [11]. Elevation of plasma glucose occurs shortly after galactose infusion as a result of conversion of galactose to glucose. Tracer studies indicate that as much as 50% of galactose may be found in glucose pools within 30 minutes of injection [11]. The removal mechanism of galactose from the blood is saturated at plasma levels of about 50 mg/dL secondary to the limited ability of galactokinase to phosphorylate the sugar [12]. When blood levels increase by 30–40 mg/dL, urinary losses become substantial [12]. During infancy, 40% of calories are derived from the hydrolysis of lactose to galactose and glucose. Therefore, the conversion of galactose to glucose is of importance to maintain euglycemia, and enzymatic defects of this pathway are most likely to produce clinical signs and symptoms as well as marked elevations of blood and urine galactose levels during a crucial period of development.

Transferase-deficiency galactosemia

The first described defect leading to galactosemia results from deficient activity of the enzyme required for the second of four steps in galactose metabolism (Figure 27.1). The consequences of this defect are much more severe than those of the other two defects, galactokinase deficiency and UDP-galactose-4-epimerase deficiency.

Molecular basis of transferase-deficiency galactosemia

Transferase deficiency is an autosomal recessive disorder. The sequences of the homologous proteins from *Escherichia coli*, from *Saccharomyces cerevisiae*, and from humans have been reported and show overall sequence identity of 35% [13]. The cDNA encoding the human transferase enzyme is 1295 bases in length and predicts a 43 kDa protein [10]. The gene (*GALT*) has been mapped to chromosome 9p18, spans 4 kb, and has 11 exons. The amino acids histidine (164)–proline–histidine (166) form an active site sequence that is essential for activity of the enzyme [14]. Southern, northern, and western blot experiments suggested that the majority of the patients with galactosemia have missense mutations that result in low or undetectable enzymatic activity [15]. So far more than 219 mutations have been identified [16].

The two most commonly characterized mutations lead to glutamine 188 substitution by arginine (Q188R) and lysine 285 by asparagine (K285N), which account for 75% of all mutations in Caucasian and Hispanic populations [17]. Substitution of arginine 333 by tryptophan (R333W) occurs at a highly conserved domain in the homologous enzymes from *E. coli*, yeast, and humans. Several other mutations have been described, such as valine 44 to methionine (V44M) and methionine 142 to lysine (M142K). Leucine substitution by serine (L135S) occurs mostly in African-Americans while asparagine substituted by aspartic acid (N314D) that occurs in Caucasians, Asians as well as African-Americans and is the basis for the Duarte variant. This variant is benign as the transferase expresses diminished but adequate enzyme activity [18]. These other mutations result in low or total loss of activity of the transferase. Therefore, it appears that transferase-deficiency galactosemia results from missense mutations that tend to occur in regions that are highly conserved throughout evolution while polymorphisms occurring in non-conserved domains result in normal enzymatic function [19].

Clinical presentation

Since its first description in 1935, numerous patients with transferase-deficiency galactosemia have been followed for years and reports of variable clinical presentations, growth, and developmental patterns, and long-term prognosis have been published. These reports, coupled with case descriptions published since 1935, have established clearly the clinical entity of this disease.

The disease varies in severity from an acute fulminant illness characterized by abdominal distension, vomiting, diarrhea, anorexia, and hypoglycemia after the first milk feeding to a more common subacute illness (such as jaundice and failure to thrive) beginning within the first few days of life. In milder cases, moderate intestinal upset after galactose ingestion may be the only manifestation. Most certainly, the great variation in clinical characteristics among patients with this complex disorder ultimately will be elucidated through correlation of genotypic and phenotypic features [18]. Failure to thrive is the most common presenting symptom and occurs in almost all patients. Vomiting or diarrhea may occur in 95%. Jaundice and hepatomegaly develop almost as frequently after the first week of life. Severe hemolysis and erythroblastosis may occur in some patients and may accentuate jaundice caused by intrinsic liver disease. Prolonged conjugated hyperbilirubinemia is a common presenting symptom in infants with this form of galactosemia. Urine tests for reducing sugars should be performed in all infants presenting with this symptom. Ascites may develop within 2 to 5 weeks after birth, as a result of continued galactose ingestion and is present in most infants who succumb to the disease.

Cataracts may develop early within the postnatal period, or they may be present at birth if the mother ingested generous amounts of dairy products late in pregnancy. These punctate lesions in the nucleus of the lens may be so small that slit-lamp examination is required for visualization. Signs of increased intracranial pressure and cerebral edema also have been observed as a presenting feature [20]. Mental retardation may become apparent after several months.

In 1977, Levy and associates identified a direct correlation between galactosemia and neonatal E. coli sepsis. In their review of over 700 000 infants screened during a 12-year period, four of eight infants were diagnosed with septicemia and transferase-deficiency galactosemia during the second week of life; three of the four died [21]. Thirty-five more patients with classic galactosemia were identified through further review of data from routine screening of over 2.5 million infants from eight other US states. E. coli sepsis was documented in 10 of the 35 patients, and nine of these died despite antibiotic therapy. Systemic infection seems to develop at approximately 7 to 14 days of age and appears to be directly associated with continued galactose ingestion secondary to inhibition of leukocyte bactericidal activity by the sugar [22]. As a result of these important clinical observations, neonates diagnosed with galactosemia or E. coli sepsis should undergo further evaluation to rule out the alternative condition.

Mild symptoms of vomiting or diarrhea following milk ingestion may be the only presenting symptoms in mild forms of the disease. A few individuals have been found to be entirely asymptomatic on milk feedings. These patients, who are usually black, are homozygous for the disease and may have the ability to metabolize moderate amounts of galactose [23].

Lactose-free formulae have become increasingly accessible, and feeding trials with these products often are employed in infants who experience recurrent vomiting and growth failure early in life. Because these are the most common presenting symptoms of galactosemia, a child with the disorder may display improvement in symptoms without recognition of the underlying defect. In such patients, galactosemia may remain undetected through the first several months of life until motor retardation, hepatomegaly, or cataracts develop [24]. Still others may be diagnosed after several years of life. These individuals usually suffer from mental retardation and visual disturbances caused by cataracts and frequently have a history of vomiting after milk intake managed by reduced intake or use of milk substitutes [24].

Laboratory findings

Aberrant laboratory findings may be varied but include elevated blood and urinary levels of galactose, hyperchloremic acidosis, albuminuria, aminoaciduria, hypoglycemia, and blood changes reflecting deranged liver function. Occasionally, infants may have severe and prolonged hypoglycemia. It apparently is caused by the inhibition of glucose release from glycogen [25]. In addition there is an inhibition of glucose formation through gluconeogenesis [26]. The galactosuria may be intermittent because of poor food intake or may disappear within 3 or 4 days of intravenous feeding. Therefore, if the urine is not tested for reducing sugar during a period of galactosuria, the diagnosis may not be suspected. The finding of a urinary reducing substance that does not react with the glucose oxidase test should be suspicious for galactosemia. This finding does not establish the diagnosis, because several other conditions such as fructosuria, lactosuria (from deficient intestinal lactase), and severe liver disease of any origin may impair the clearance of blood galactose and result in the presence of urinary reducing sugar that is not glucose [24].

Biochemical features and pathogenesis of toxicity

Pathologic changes that accompany galactosemia affect the liver, lens of the eye, brain, and kidney. Toxicity seems to result primarily from accumulation of two by-products of galactose metabolism, galactose 1-phosphate and galactitol (Figure 27.2). The biochemical causes of toxicity in individual organs may differ, depending on the metabolic patterns and functions of the involved organs.

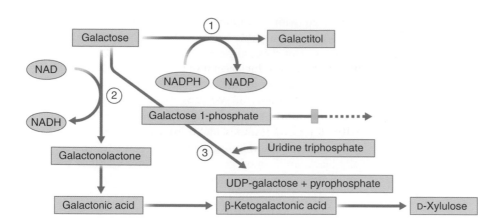

Figure 27.2 Alternative pathways of galactose metabolism. 1, aldose reductase or l-hexonate dehydrogenase; 2, galactose dehydrogenase; 3, uridine diphosphate galactose pyrophosphorylase.

Liver

Hepatic changes associated with transferase-deficiency galactosemia result entirely from abnormal galactose metabolism. In affected individuals, galactose ingestion results in elevated levels of both galactose 1-phosphate and galactitol in the liver. Other findings, however, suggest that one or more additional metabolites act alone or together to produce the liver damage seen in this form of the disease. For example, liver damage does not occur in normal laboratory animals fed diets rich in galactose, despite hepatic galactitol accumulation in chicks [27] and hepatic accumulation of galactose 1-phosphate in rats [28]. Furthermore, humans with galactokinase deficiency accumulate large amounts of galactitol but develop no liver damage. The amount of galactosamine, which is known to stimulate hepatocellular changes in animals, was found to be increased in one patient with galactosemia [29].

Kidney

Individuals with transferase-deficiency galactosemia develop renal tubular dysfunction following galactose ingestion; over time, levels of galactose 1-phosphate and galactitol accumulate in the kidneys [29]. Alteration in kidney function appears to result primarily from increased galactose 1-phosphate levels, because patients with galactokinase deficiency who characteristically excrete large amounts of galactitol do not develop renal impairment. Galactose 1-phosphate accumulation also may produce the aminoaciduria seen in this disorder through secondary inhibition of amino acid accumulation by the tubules [30]. The inhibition is non-competitive and similar to that seen in human intestine [31].

Lenticular changes

The specific mechanisms for cellular changes in the eye are more clearly understood than in other organs. Changes in the lens seem to result primarily from galactitol accumulation, which initially was reported by van Heyningen in 1959 [32]. Later, Kinoshita and colleagues demonstrated that a concomitant increase in water content occurred with galactitol build-up caused by oncotic pressure exerted by the alcohol [33]. Poor diffusion of galactitol from these tissues leads to further damage and cataract formation. Application of an osmotically balanced incubation medium prevents opacification [33].

Nutrient supplementation has been shown to alter the rate of cataract formation in animals. Biochemical changes induced by galactose feeding include decreases in several enzymatic reactions, amino acid transport, protein synthesis, and alterations in ion fluxes. These occur simultaneously as cataract formation takes place [33–35]. As little as 2 days of galactose ingestion can reduce glycolysis and lenticular respiration by approximately 30%, and this reduction is sustained until cataracts are formed. Nutrient imbalances and changes in lenticular water content resulting from galactitol accumulation are principal initiators of lenticular opacification.

Brain

Galactitol accumulates in higher concentrations in brain tissue of humans and rats fed galactose than in any other tissue except the lens [28]. Therefore, galactitol appears to be a factor in the development of brain function abnormalities seen in transferase-deficiency galactosemia. On the other hand, damage from galactitol accumulation in patients with galactokinase deficiency seems to be limited to the lens.

Pathologic alterations in brain tissue of individuals with transferase-deficiency galactosemia may not be completely reversible through dietary galactose restriction. Considerable attention has been paid to defining the specific mechanism for galactose-induced brain damage. Studies in chick brain showed that galactose administration diminished ATP, reduced brain glucose and glycolytic intermediates, redistributed hexokinase, enhanced fragility of neural lysosomes, and decreased fast axoplasmic transport [36,37]. The effects could be temporarily reversed by glucose [38]. Changes in the chick brain appear to be related to several factors such as hyperosmolality, alterations in energy metabolism, abnormal serotonin levels, and interference with active uptake of glucose into the neurons [36,37,39]. It remains to be determined whether these changes in chicks are similar to galactose-induced abnormalities in patients with transferase deficiencies.

Intestine

Although intestinal epithelium of patients with galactosemia is also deficient in transferase activity, this deficiency does not appear to alter intestinal transport of galactose [31]. Many infants develop intestinal symptoms of vomiting and diarrhea after galactose ingestion, but it is unclear whether this is a direct effect on the intestine or secondary to the effects of galactose on the central nervous system.

Gonads

Among galactosemic females, 90% have ovarian failure, which is present shortly after birth. Biochemically, follicular-stimulating hormone is high whereas antimullerian hormone is low compared with controls (hypergonadotropic hypogonadism) [40]. However, Badik and colleagues demonstrated that 100% of girls with Duarte galactosemia had no apparent decrease in antimullerian hormone or increase in follicular-stimulating hormone, suggesting that these girls are not at increased risk for premature ovarian insufficiency [41]. Males with galactosemia have normal testicular function. The mechanism underlying ovarian failure in galactosemic women is not known, although galactose toxicity has been implicated. Despite the documented ovarian failure in most of the affected patients, successful pregnancies have been reported [42].

Pathology

Early hepatic lesions, present in the first weeks of life, consist of cholestasis and diffuse fatty vacuolation with little to no inflammatory reaction. The fatty changes are extensive and generalized throughout the lobule. Later, disorganization of the liver cells with pseudoductular and pseudoglandular formation occurs. This tendency toward pseudoglandular orientation of cells has been described as characteristic of galactosemia but is relatively non-specific. As the disease progresses, delicate fibrosis appears, first in the periportal regions and eventually extending to bridge adjacent portal tracts. Regenerating nodules and hepatic fibrosis are late features that, with continued galactose ingestion, progress to cirrhosis similar in many respects to the cirrhosis of ethanol abuse. Death usually occurs in the first year of life unless galactose intake is decreased or curtailed. Frank cellular necrosis is unusual but may occur with large amounts of dietary galactose. Despite the severity of the hepatic lesion, there is a remarkable lack of infiltration of inflammatory cells [43].

Except for cataract formation in the lens, other tissues show only minor changes. Kidneys show dilation of tubules at the corticomedullary junction. The spleen enlarges as a result of portal hypertension. Lesions in the brain are subtle, with minor loss of nerve cells and gliosis in the dentate nucleus and gliosis in the cerebral cortex and gray matter [44].

Genetics

Investigations of red blood cell and leukocytic transferase activities in family members indicate that the disorder is transmitted as an autosomal recessive trait [45]. Heterozygotes have about 50% of normal activity, and genotype detection is more accurate when the transferase to galactokinase ratio is determined [46]. Population studies indicate that the incidence of heterozygosity for galactosemia is between 0.9 and 1.25% and that between 8 and 13% carry the Duarte gene [47]. Incidences of transferase-deficiency galactosemia derived from large-scale screening in neonatal nurseries have been between 1:10 000 and 1:70 000 live births [48].

Diagnosis

The presence of urinary reducing sugar that does not react with glucose oxidase reagents in an infant with vomiting and growth failure on milk feedings supports a presumptive diagnosis of galactosemia. During the first 2 weeks of life, some normal premature and term infants excrete up to 60 mg/dL of galactose in urine. Furthermore, it should be remembered that lactose, fructose, and pentose can produce the same urine test result, and that the specific sugar may be identified only by paper or gas–liquid chromatography. Paper impregnated with galactose oxidase makes screening for galactosuria easier. Regardless, galactose restriction should be instituted promptly if no other dietary carbohydrate is identified. Confirmation of the diagnosis should be made through direct measurement of transferase activity. Xu and colleagues developed a highly sensitive radiochemical assay that can detect galactose 1-phosphate uridyltransferase activity as low as 0.1% of normal in erythrocytes and leukocytes [49]. Galactose tolerance tests should never be employed for this purpose, because it has been suggested that a single exposure to a large quantity of galactose may produce brain injury resulting from prolonged severe hypoglycemia.

Measurement of red cell UDP-glucose consumption has been employed extensively as a diagnostic test for galactosemia since the late 1980s [24]. It is based on quantification of UDP-glucose before and after incubation of galactose 1-phosphate using added red cell hemolysate as the enzyme source. Results are obtained through spectrophotometric measurement of nicotinamide adenine dinucleotide (NAD), which is formed from hepatic NAD through the conversion of UDP-glucose to UDP-glucuronic acid by UDP-glucose dehydrogenase. Homozygous patients exhibit complete absence of red cell transferase activity. Heterozygous carriers typically display intermediate levels of enzyme activity. Infants with 50% of normal enzyme activity should undergo further tests to identify the presence of a specific variant of the disease [50].

With the advent of screening for galactosemia, multiple variants of this disease have become apparent, the variants being more prevalent than classic transferase-deficiency galactosemia [50]. There are three homozygotic types.

1. "Classic" galactosemia is autosomal recessive, and there is no transferase activity in erythrocytes, fibroblasts, liver, and presumably in any other tissue. In heterozygotic, unaffected carriers, activity is 50% of normal.

2. The Duarte variant is the most common form of galactosemia and is only detected by enzyme screening, because these infants are asymptomatic. Red cell transferase activity is 50% of normal, and on starch gel electrophoresis the enzyme migrates faster than normal. Red cells of patients who have this variant produce two distinct bands rather than the single normal transferase band. In addition, red cells of a parent of a Duarte-homozygous patient have three bands for the variant enzyme. Homozygotic Duarte erythrocytes have 50% of normal enzyme activity; heterozygous Duarte erythrocytes have 75% of normal activity. Duarte-variant galactosemia may occur in 10–15% of the population. The Duarte gene is apparently allelic with the normal and galactosemic genes, because the most frequently detected abnormality on neonatal screening tests is the compound heterozygous state, consisting of classic galactosemia with the Duarte variant. Two protein bands are present on protein electrophoresis, and erythrocyte transferase activity is 25% of control. Although some of these infants appear asymptomatic at birth and remain so during infancy, others have systemic symptoms with metabolic manifestations of galactosemia.

3. In the "Negro" variant, erythrocytic transferase activity is absent, but 10% of normal activity is present in liver and intestine. The Duarte and the Negro variants may be asymptomatic despite galactose ingestion, although patients with the variant may develop a galactose toxicity syndrome in the neonatal period.

In addition to the homozygotic variants, several heterozygotic variants have been identified.

1. Indiana variant, in which erythrocytic transferase activity is approximately 35% of normal and is highly unstable (mobility on starch gel electrophoresis is slower than normal);

2. Rennes variant, which has about 7–10% of normal transferase activity (this variant also travels more slowly than normal by electrophoresis);

3. Los Angeles variant, which has erythrocytic transferase activity higher than normal (about 140%); this has been detected in six families. Electrophoretic mobility of this variant of the enzyme is similar to that of the Duarte variant. West German and Chicago variants have also been identified by screening procedures.

Screening for galactosemia

The rationale for genetic screening is three-fold: (1) to detect disease at its incipient stage and thereby offset harmful expression of the mutant genotype through appropriate medical treatment; (2) to identify a variant genotype for which reproductive options (family planning) may be provided; and (3) to identify gene frequency or biologic significance and natural history of variant phenotypes.

Various screening methods for galactosemia have been used [51]. The original Guthrie test used filter-paper blood samples from which a microbiologic assay detected elevated galactose levels. The newer Beutler test assays the erythrocyte transferase activity directly from dried filter paper, and the Paigen assay is an improved bacteriologic method that includes detection of elevated levels of galactose and galactose 1-phosphate. Measurements of elevated galactose require that the infant receive sufficient dietary galactose or a false negative test will result. Conversely, the normal enzyme may become inactive in a hot or humid climate, and a false positive (negative enzyme activity) may be reported.

In utero assay for galactosemia is indicated in pregnant women with a family history of galactosemia. Cultured fibroblasts from amniotic fluid can be assayed for transferase activity. Additionally, the technique of chorionic villus sampling has been used to detect galactosemia during the 10th week of gestation [52]. Cloning of the cDNA encoding for the transferase enzyme and the finding that the majority of galactosemic patients have missense mutations have allowed for rapid molecular approaches using the polymerase chain reaction to detect common mutations.

Treatment

Although the cause of the entire toxicity syndrome in transferase deficiency is uncertain, there is no disagreement that elimination of galactose intake reverses the biochemical manifestations of transferase-deficiency galactosemia. Some patients seem to have increasing tolerance to galactose with advancing age; however, studies using [14C]-galactose do not support the clinical impression that alternative pathways of galactose metabolism develop at puberty, nor is there any indication that any drug will increase galactose oxidation, although some patients with variant forms of transferase deficiencies can oxidize limited amounts of galactose [23,24].

The only acceptable treatment at present is elimination of dietary galactose. Permissible diets are described in at least two publications [11,53]. Preparations used in treating infants are Pregestimil, Nutramigen, and the soybean milk preparations. Both Pregestimil and Nutramigen are prepared from casein and may contain small amounts of lactose, but this amount of lactose does not appear to be sufficient to impair therapeutic efficacy. The soybean formulae contain small amounts of galactose in raffinose and stachyose, and other dietary constituents contain small amounts of galactosides, but these carbohydrates are not digested by human intestinal enzymes and should not affect the efficacy of treatment [53]. Because of the frequent addition of milk to a number of proprietary food items, strict attention must be given to the diet during and after weaning. Concern has been raised regarding the presence of galactose in grains, fruits, and vegetables [54]. These foods contain significant amounts of soluble galactose, although newer information related to substantial endogenous production of galactose has minimized this concern [55].

It is important to be aware that asymptomatic heterozygotic mothers may have elevated serum galactose levels after ingestion of diets high in milk. Infants delivered of such mothers may have the galactosemic syndrome at birth. For this reason, restriction of galactose during the pregnancies of women who have previously borne children with galactosemia is recommended [23,24,53]. The use of uridine and aldose reductase inhibitors in galactosemic patients has not been shown to be effective despite their theoretical advantage [56,57]. Boxer *et al.* [58] have been able to generate a small molecule capable of selectively inhibiting galactokinase thus preventing conversion of galactose to galactose 1-phosphate. This has not been tested in vitro or vivo yet.

Prognosis

When untreated, galactosemia results in early deaths of many affected children and is attended by the prospect of mental retardation of those who survive. In a series of 43 galactosemic patients, there were 13 neonatal deaths, which occurred at an average age of 6 weeks and were usually attributed to infection [53]. Levy and coworkers noted that 9 of 35 patients died of *E. coli* infections and strongly recommended early cultures and institution of antibiotics effective against *E. coli* in any infant with galactosemia who appears ill [21].

Treatment of galactosemic patients with a galactose-free diet results in survival with reversal of the acute symptoms, normal growth, and complete recovery of liver function; however, the long-term outcome (particularly for intellectual development) is not entirely certain. Experience gained in the long-term follow-up of 59 patients in the Los Angeles area indicates that many patients have developed very well and have attained college-level educations [53]. Others who were equally well treated with galactose restriction have had various intellectual deficiencies, including verbal dyspraxia, reduced intelligence, learning disabilities, and neurologic deficits [59]. The causes of the variability in the responses to treatment need further exploration. Impairment of speech affects a significant number of patients with galactosemia, appears in early childhood, and persists into adulthood [60]. The pattern of speech impairment may allow labeling as apraxia of speech. In many cases, impaired speech is related to decreased IQ.

Osteoporosis is a frequent complication among females with galactosemia. The mechanisms underlying this complication may relate to low calcium intake, lack of sex hormones associated with ovarian failure, and an independent defect in collagen synthesis resulting in disturbances in bone mineralization [61]. Treatment with hormone replacement and vitamin D therapy (1000 IU daily) has resulted in the onset of menarche and increased bone density in two 28-year-old galactosemic twins when treatment was started at 25 years of age [61].

Although genetic and social factors may influence results of intelligence tests, such factors do not explain all the differences observed. The association of thyroid dysfunction with galactosemia may have some role in the outcome [62]. A factor that definitely affects outcome is the age of the patient at diagnosis. Evidence supports the previous impression that a more favorable outcome can be expected when a patient is treated at an early age. For example, the mean IQ of 16 patients treated before 7 days of age was 99.5, whereas that of patients treated between 4 and 6 months of age was 62. It is generally desirable to institute treatment at the earliest possible age, and neonatal screening is an important step in this direction.

Galactokinase-deficiency galactosemia

Galactokinase deficiency is less common than classic transferase deficiency, with an incidence of about 1 in 10 000 [24]. It does not result in progressive liver disease and mental retardation, but galactose exposure may result in cataract formation [3]. It is appropriate to compare this entity with transferase deficiency because it affects the first reaction (kinase) and the transferase the second reaction of the galactose pathway (Figure 27.1). Comparison of patients with these defects and those with a defect involving the third reaction (epimerase) has helped to define some of the mechanisms of toxicity in several organs, including the development of cataracts. With galactokinase deficiency, there is no accumulation of galactose 1-phosphate, and usually no systemic manifestations. Cataract formation is related to synthesis of galactitol in the lens and osmotic disruption of lens fiber architecture, as discussed above. An early start of a galactose-restricted diet resulted in regression or prevention of cataracts [63], but slight cataracts without visual impairment occurred in 50% of the patients, 56% of whom were non-compliant. Clinical symptoms of hypoglycemia, mental retardation, microcephaly, and failure to thrive, were associated with non-compliance [63]. Maternal galactokinase deficiency may result in fetal cataract formation [24]. Because of the potential for cataract formation, lifelong elimination of galactose is suggested. The gene (*GALK1*) has been mapped to chromosome 17q24, and 20 mutations have been described in the gene for galactokinase, resulting in loss of the activity of the enzyme [64].

Galactose epimerase-deficiency galactosemia

Galactose epimerase catalyzes the third reaction of galactose metabolism (Figure 27.1). Epimerase deficiency was discovered incidentally while screening for galactosemia and has an incidence of about 1 in 46 000 in Switzerland. Patients have normal erythrocyte transferase activity but elevated levels of galactose 1-phosphate [4]. One form of this condition is apparently caused by a decreased stability of the epimerase and leads to enzyme deficiency in those cells in which its turnover is slow or absent, such as erythrocytes [65]. It is, therefore, considered to be a benign illness in as much as the enzyme deficiency is limited to leukocytes and red blood cells. Affected people with the form limited to leukocytes and red blood cells have no symptoms, but patients with generalized epimerase deficiency have been described and these patients have signs and symptoms identical to transferase-deficiency galactosemia [5].

By contrast with transferase deficiency, in which UDP-galactose can be formed from UDP-glucose, one patient with generalized epimerase deficiency was unable to synthesize the galactose precursor necessary for synthesis of glycoproteins and glycolipids. These glycosylated compounds are necessary for cell membrane integrity, particularly in the central nervous system. Therefore, in contrast to patients with transferase deficiency, the rare patient with systemic epimerase deficiency may require small quantities of galactose for normal growth and development. One patient with epimerase deficiency continued to show slightly elevated levels of galactose 1-phosphate in red cells even with dietary restriction of galactose. Appropriate treatment of this disorder, therefore, requires frequent monitoring of erythrocyte galactose 1-phosphate levels in order best to determine the optimal dietary level of galactose.

Disorders of fructose metabolism

There are three recognized disorders of fructose metabolism. Until the mid 1950s, the only identified defect was the benign disorder essential fructosuria [66]. This results from fructokinase deficiency, which converts fructose to fructose 1-phosphate. It was first revealed in a patient checked for glycosuria while being investigated for possible diabetes [67]. Fructose, although, containing no aldehyde group, becomes a reducing sugar in basic solution and will give a positive urine test for reducing substances but a negative reaction on glucose oxidase testing.

In 1956, it was noted in some patients that ingestion of fructose was followed by vomiting, severe hypoglycemia, and liver disease [68]. A year later, this illness was characterized and named hereditary fructose intolerance and was found to be due to a deficiency in fructose-1-phosphate aldolase [69]. A third disorder of fructose metabolism, caused by fructose-1,6-diphosphatase (FDPase) deficiency was identified in 1970. It was associated with fasting-induced as well as diet-induced hypoglycemia, but more strikingly, both fasting and dietary fructose caused lactic acidosis [70]. These three disorders are distinct both clinically and biochemically. Essential fructosuria does not cause liver injury. Patients with FDPase deficiency may show transient fatty infiltration of the liver. In contrast, liver injury may be a significant feature of HFI.

Biochemistry of fructose metabolism

Fructose is a monosaccharide that belongs to the ketose group and is a widely distributed compound in nature. Free fructose is found in fruits and in honey. A major source of fructose is the disaccharide sucrose, which is hydrolyzed into fructose and glucose by the disaccharidase sucrase at the brush border membrane of enterocytes. Fructose is transported across the intestinal and liver plasma membranes via a carrier protein called GLUT5, a sodium-independent transporter [71]. Once absorbed, fructose is utilized mainly by the liver, kidney, and small intestine. Approximately 75% of fructose is taken up by the liver; the kidney and small intestine take up the remaining 25%. These tissues possess specialized enzymes involved in fructose metabolism. These enzymes are fructokinase aldolase B and triokinase (Figure 27.3).

The first step in fructose metabolism involves fructokinase, which catalyzes the phosphorylation of fructose to fructose 1-phosphate. The next step involves fructoaldolase. Three

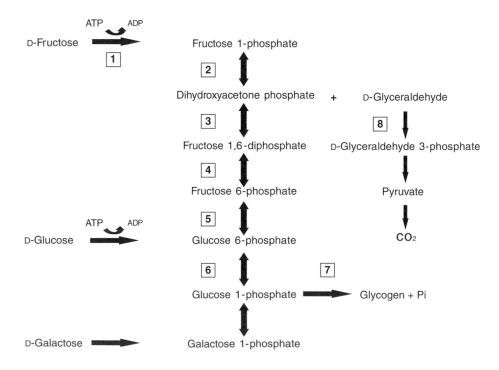

Figure 27.3 Fructose metabolism. 1, Fructokinase; 2, fructoaldolase; 3, fructose-1,6-diphosphate aldolase; 4, fructose-1,6-biphosphatase; 5, phosphohexose; 6, phosphoglucomutase; 7, glycogen phosphorylase; 8, triokinase.

aldolase isozymes have been identified. Aldolase B is present in the liver, kidney, and small intestine and acts on fructose 1-phosphate to produce D-glyceraldehyde and fructose 1,6-diphosphate to produce dihydroxyacetone phosphate. The two other aldolases are aldolase A, found in the muscle, and aldolase C, found in the brain. Both aldolase A and C have much greater activity against fructose 1,6-diphosphate than aldolase B. The presence of these two enzymes allows gluconeogenesis and glycolysis to continue even in the absence of aldolase B. The cDNA encoding for human and rat aldolase B has been cloned [72] and the gene is localized to chromosome 9q22.3 [73]. The resulting D-glyceraldehyde is converted into D-glyceraldehyde 3-phosphate by triokinase.

Other enzymes involved in fructose metabolism include FDPase, which catalyzes the splitting of fructose 1,6-diphosphate to fructose 6-phosphate and phosphate. This process is irreversible but the reverse reaction is catalyzed by phosphofructokinase. Alternative pathways of fructose metabolism involve the conversion of fructose directly to fructose 6-phosphate by hexokinase and glucokinase. The affinity of these two enzymes for fructose, however, is several-fold lower than that for glucose.

Hereditary fructose intolerance

In 1956, Chambers and Pratt described HFI in a young woman who complained of vomiting after ingestion of fruit or sugar [74]. The authors recognized the variation in symptoms from those of essential fructosuria and speculated that the illness resulted from accumulation of a toxic intermediate. In 1957, Froesch and associates [75] reported the syndrome in two siblings and two relatives and proposed that aldolase deficiency was the causative factor, based on the results of two liver biopsies. The defect was later characterized as an inability of aldolase to split fructose 1-phosphate [76].

Molecular basis

The frequency of HFI is 1 in 20 000 individuals. It has a recessive mode of inheritance and is caused by a deficiency of aldolase B, which is normally present in the liver, kidneys, and small intestine. The enzymatic activities of aldolase A in muscle and aldolase C in brain are normal [77]. The activity of tissue aldolase B is reduced to less than 15% of normal values. The three isoenzymes are related and are derived from a single ancestral gene.

The aldolase B gene (ALDOB) has been sequenced and is mapped to human chromosome 9q13-q32 [78]. The gene has 14 500 bp, nine exons, and encodes 364 amino acid residues [78]. The first mutation described was a G to C transversion in exon 5, which resulted in alanine substitution by proline at position 149 of the protein (A149P) within a region critical for substrate binding. The G to C transversion created a new recognition site for the restriction enzyme Aha II [79]. The alanine at position 149 is a conserved amino acid because it is present in aldolase B of humans, rats, and chickens [80]. The

substitution of proline is likely to disrupt the spatial configuration of juxtaposed residues in aldolase B and adversely affect its catalytic activity. The mutation resulting in A149P was found in 33 of 50 patients (67%) with HFI [81]. The mutation is encountered more frequently in patients from northern than from southern Europe. Several other mutations have been described, such as that leading to alanine substitution by aspartic acid at position 174 (A174D) and asparagine substitution by lysine at position 334 (N334K) [82]. The molecular defects in aldolase B alleles were characterized in 31 North Americans with HFI [83]: 59% had A149P, 11% had A174D, and 2% had N334K. Nine subjects (29%) had HFI alleles that were not these common, missense mutations [83]. So far, more than 40 disease-causing mutations have been reported. The missense mutations could be classified into two groups: catalytic mutants with retained tetrameric structure but altered kinetic properties (W147R, R303W, and A337V) and structural mutations in which heterotetramers dissociate into subunits with impaired enzymatic activity (A149P, A174D, N334K) [84]. Mutations upstream of the protein-coding region of ALDOB were first reported in an analysis of 61 patients with HFI that revealed single base mutations in the promoter, intronic enhancer, and first exon, which is entirely untranslated. These novel mutations represent 2% of alleles in American patients with HFI [85].

Clinical presentation

Patients with HFI may be extremely ill and may die after continuous exposure to fructose. However, affected patients are generally healthy and symptom free so long as they do not ingest fructose or fructose-containing foods [86]. For this reason, symptoms do not arise until breast milk or cow's milk formulae are supplemented with fructose-containing foods. In fortunate children, fructose is not introduced until after an affected infant is 5–6 months of age. By this time, the child is likely to associate nausea, vomiting, and symptoms of hypoglycemia with sweet-tasting food. In such cases, aversion to sweets is probably life saving, and the diagnosis may go undetected until adulthood. When this occurs, the diagnosis may be suspected on the basis of a careful history that recognizes the extreme aversion to dietary "sweets." Symptoms associated with HFI may be categorized as resulting from acute or chronic exposure to fructose leading to the accumulation of fructose 1-phosphate in tissues in which aldolase B is normally present:

- acute
  - nausea, vomiting
  - tremor
  - dizziness
  - lethargy, coma
- chronic
  - failure to thrive
  - jaundice, cirrhosis

- vomiting and diarrhea
- feeding difficulties.

The largest single collection of patients consists of 55 patients diagnosed between 1961 and 1977 as having HFI [87]. Fifty had become symptomatic because of dietary fructose, and five were diagnosed shortly after birth because an older sibling of each infant was known to have HFI. Fourteen patients received fructose in their first feedings, and symptoms usually appeared within a few days. The remaining patients received a fructose-free diet (breast milk or cow's milk formula). Their symptoms began immediately after introduction of dietary fructose or sucrose. Of the 50 patients, 32 (64%) were diagnosed as having HFI at less than 6 months of age, 12 (24%) between 6 and 12 months of age, and 6 (12%) after 1 year of age. The younger patients were usually admitted to the hospital on an emergency basis with acute liver impairment, sepsis, bleeding diathesis, shock, or dehydration. Patients younger than 6 months of age developed a triad of jaundice, edema, and bleeding tendency. Older patients were admitted more often because of liver enlargement, ascites, or both. Vomiting and hepatomegaly were observed in all patients, and about half had anorexia, weight retardation, and bleeding tendency. About a third had jaundice, diarrhea, edema or ascites or both, and growth retardation. An aversion to sweet foods was developed by 13 (26%), occurring as early as 3 months of age and in two children resulted in continued breast-feeding until 9 months of age. Vomiting and diarrhea in the young children were sometimes severe enough to cause dehydration.

With greater awareness, more cases of HFI in children are being diagnosed, and the condition is arrested by feeding fructose-restricted diets. One cautionary note is that a number of proprietary milks, primarily the soy-based formulae, contain sucrose as a significant source of the carbohydrate calories. The remaining carbohydrate is usually a glucose oligosaccharide. Hypoglycemia and seizures may not be a problem in affected infants fed these formulae because the remaining carbohydrate is glucose. The liver disease caused by fructose ingestion may be progressive, however, and infants fed these formulae may simply fail to thrive, have hepatomegaly and vomiting, or progress to chronic liver failure and death. Acute liver failure in fructose intolerance is exceedingly unusual, and the absence of hepatomegaly in an infant who has severe liver disease and has reducing sugar in the urine should make one doubt the diagnosis of HFI. Follow-up studies of infants and recognition of older patients with HFI indicate a normal life expectancy. Patients retain their sensitivity to dietary fructose as adults, but the hypoglycemic response to fructose may be somewhat more delayed in adults than in infants (45–60 minutes in infants; 60–90 minutes in adults). The sensitivity to fructose may be life threatening for adults. For example, patients with known HFI have been given sorbitol intravenously after surgery. Because sorbitol is metabolized to fructose, one patient died of complications from the sorbitol infusion [88].

Biochemical features and pathogenesis of fructose toxicity

The clinical and biochemical abnormalities seen in patients with HFI result from decreased fructose 1-phosphate, aldolase B, and fructose-1,6-phosphate aldolase activity in liver:

- renal tubular dysfunction: increased urine losses of fructose, glucose, amino acids, proteins, urate, bicarbonate, phosphate
- blood
- hematologic: anemia, thrombocytopenia
- liver: conjugated hyperbilirubinemia, prolonged prothrombin time
- metabolic: hypoglycemia, hypophosphatemia, hypomagnesemia, lactic acidosis, hyperuricemia

Aldolase B is normally present in the liver, renal tubular cells, and intestinal mucosa [89]. It catalyzes the conversion of fructose 1-phosphate to D-glyceraldehyde and dihydroxyacetone phosphate (reaction 2 in Figure 27.3). The metabolic consequences of this enzymatic deficiency are accumulation of large amounts of fructose 1-phosphate in the liver and depletion of inorganic phosphate (Pi) and ATP. The inability to metabolize fructose 1-phosphate in cells of affected patients leads to sequestration of large amounts of Pi. One of the many effects secondary to this sequestration of Pi is an inability to regenerate ATP, a process that depends on the presence of Pi. The clinical and laboratory features of HFI can be understood on the basis of this simple scheme (Figure 27.4).

Patients with HFI have been shown to have levels of activity of aldolase ranging from 0 to 12% of normal [90]. In addition, most patients have reduced levels of activity of hepatic aldolase B ranging from 25 to 85% of normal [90]. The differential between the activities of the two aldolase reactions (converting fructose 1-phosphate and fructose 1,6-phosphate) suggests that they are separate protein moieties. However, Gurtler and Leuthardt have crystallized human liver aldolase and have shown that both enzymatic activities are attributable to a single liver aldolase [91]. In addition, slight alterations of the aldolase molecule, such as splitting off an end-terminal residue, may change the ratio of its affinity for fructose 1-phosphate or fructose 1,6-diphosphate [92].

Patients with HFI produce a protein that has the immunologic properties of fructose 1-phosphate aldolase but is biologically inactive [93]. On the basis of these findings, it seems probable that a mutation of the structural gene is responsible for the enzyme defect in HFI. More recent studies suggest that the mutation in HFI affects aldolase B function by decreasing substrate affinity, maximal velocity, and/or enzyme activity [94].

Accumulation of fructose 1-phosphate apparently causes the major manifestations of the disease through inhibition of other enzymatic reactions. Two metabolic pathways studied most extensively are gluconeogenesis and glycogenolysis. Their inhibition by fructose 1-phosphate explains fructose-induced hypoglycemia. Concentrations of fructose 1-phosphate in

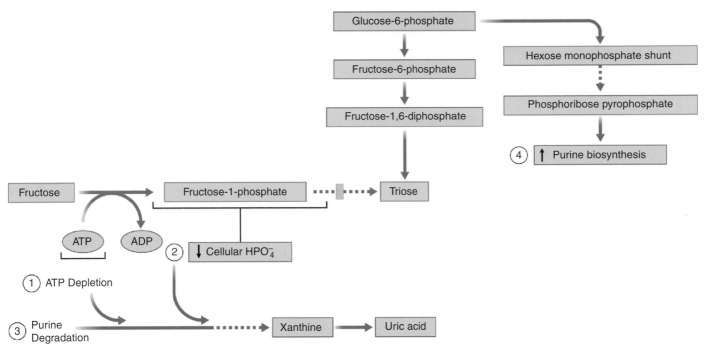

Figure 27.4 Mechanism of hyperuricemia and hypophosphatemia in aldolase B deficiency. Because of aldolase B defect, ATP is consumed in the fructokinase reaction, leading to ATP depletion. Fructose 1-phosphate accumulation inhibits ATP generation from anaerobic glycolysis. Phosphate is trapped in fructose 1-phosphate, leading to depletion of intracellular phosphate. Both depletions favor degradation of purines to uric acid.

excess of 10 mmol/L completely inhibit fructose-1,6-diphosphate aldolase activity in vitro [95]. This finding suggests that fructose 1-phosphate inhibits gluconeogenesis at this enzymatic step. Inhibition at this site is further supported by the finding that fructose-induced hypoglycemia is not prevented by simultaneous infusions of gluconeogenic precursors such as dihydroxyacetone or glycerol. In addition, liver specimens from patients with HFI do not form labeled glucose from [^{14}C]-glycerol when fructose is present but oxidation of [^{14}C]-glycerol is apparently unaffected by fructose (reaction 2) [96].

Patients with HFI apparently also have inhibition of glycogenolysis after fructose intake. This inhibition occurs above the level of phosphoglucomutase. In support of this idea was the finding that when galactose is administered together with fructose, hypoglycemia is less pronounced and does not last as long as when fructose is given alone (reaction 3) [86]. Therefore, a defect in the phosphorylation of glycogen to glucose 1-phosphate is incriminated. Several studies of normal liver indicate that depletion of Pi as well as accumulation of fructose 1-phosphate may contribute to an almost complete failure of glycogen mobilization [97]. In addition, depletion of intracellular ATP levels may contribute to the lack of glycogen degradation to glucose 1-phosphate [98].

A variant of fructose intolerance has been described in which the red cell galactose 1-phosphate uridyltransferase activity was normal but galactose as well as fructose caused hypoglycemia [99]. The nature of this finding is unclear, because a re-evaluation of these patients 12 years later showed normal blood glucose responses to fructose and galactose [100].

Results of studies in newborn infants delivered at term suggest that they have less capacity for fructose metabolism in the first few days of life compared with later in life [101]. This is believed to be caused by the immaturity of the enzymes for handling fructose. In these studies, a rapid infusion of fructose caused a prompt but transient decrease in blood glucose and suppressed the glucagon-induced elevation of blood glucose. Although hepatic aldolase was not measured, the findings suggest that until further studies are completed, the use of fructose or sorbitol as a calorie source (as in total parenteral nutrition (TPN)) for term infants in the first few days of life may not be justified. Enzymatic maturation may take longer in premature infants, although definitive studies have not been reported.

Laboratory findings

The primary laboratory features of HFI are fructose-induced hypoglycemia and hypophosphatemia and/or chronic liver disease. In addition, serum and urinary urate levels may be increased.

Odievre and colleagues showed that the laboratory findings in HFI were actually variable [87]. Liver tests were severely deranged in the younger patients in their series. Deficiency of clotting factors and elevated alanine aminotransferase were present in all but one of the patients younger than 6 months of age. Two patients also had serum albumin of 2.8 g/dL. Fifteen patients had aminoaciduria; the predominant amino acids were tyrosine and methionine in three of these. All patients showed complete resolution of laboratory abnormalities in response to removal of fructose from the diet during a succeeding 2-week period.

Hypoglycemia

Hypoglycemia induced by dietary or intravenous fructose is a characteristic of the illness. The hypoglycemia is not caused by excess circulating insulin [95,102]. Sorbitol provokes hypoglycemia before substantial amounts of fructose are released into the circulation and is evidence against a direct effect of fructose on blood glucose levels. More likely, the adverse effects of fructose result from intracellular accumulation of a fructose metabolite, such as fructose 1-phosphate [95]. This metabolite impairs both gluconeogenesis and glycogenolysis (reactions 2 and 3 in Figure 27.3). Studies with [^{14}C]-glucose indicate a complete cessation of hepatic glucose release after fructose infusion [102]. Also, glucagon does not increase blood glucose after fructose-induced hypoglycemia, even in the presence of normal to slightly elevated hepatic glycogen content [103].

Hypophosphatemia

Hypophosphatemia is the second prominent feature of fructose-induced hypoglycemia (Figure 27.4). The reduction of Pi precedes that of glucose and may be the only abnormal finding when a small dose of fructose is administered. Hypophosphatemia appears to be a consequence of binding and sequestration of phosphorus in the form of fructose 1-phosphate within the hepatocytes [104]. The first step in fructose metabolism is phosphorylation of the sugar by ATP. With large doses of fructose, ATP is depleted rapidly. With deficient activity of aldolase, as occurs in HFI, Pi is not released back into the cell. To compensate, phosphate from the serum is sequestered by the liver, with a resulting reduction in available circulating phosphate. Phosphorylation of fructose decreases intracellular phosphate in normal individuals, but the phosphate sequestered in normal liver is made available by further metabolism of fructose 1-phosphate. Therefore, changes in serum phosphate are extremely transient in a normal individual and depend on the amount of fructose ingested.

Elevation of serum levels of hepatic enzymes

Elevation of serum levels of hepatic enzymes appears to be the direct effect of increased hepatic fructose 1-phosphate. Within 1.5 hours of a large dose of fructose, serum aminotransferase levels may increase more than two-fold. The mechanism of liver cell damage is not clear, but it may result from a combination of depletion of ATP and a direct toxic effect of elevated levels of the phosphorylated hexose.

Hyperuricemia and increased urate excretion

Hyperuricemia and increased urate excretion appear to result from depletion of intracellular ATP and Pi. This depletion of ATP and Pi increases the rate of purine degradation to uric acid (Figure 27.4) [98].

Other laboratory findings

Other findings are less consistent. Some patients show substantial decreases in serum potassium and increases in serum magnesium after fructose intake. Some have increases in serum lactate and pyruvate [86,90]. These changes appear to be related to the extent of liver damage and the severity of hypoglycemia. Granulocytosis may be noted with chronic fructose ingestion. As blood glucose declines after fructose ingestion, insulin and insulin-like activity decrease and levels of glucagon, epinephrine, and growth hormone increase. In response to these hormonal changes, the non-esterified fatty acids in plasma increase more than two-fold, a response not observed in normal subjects [86,90,105].

Renal tubular acidosis and a Fanconi-like syndrome with renal tubular reabsorptive defects have been reported [87]. In one patient, renal tubular acidosis persisted despite restriction of dietary fructose. The renal tubular acidosis is normalized in most patients as soon as fructose intake ceases [106]. Fructose-1-phosphate aldolase is normally present in the renal tubules but it is absent in patients with HFI. Hence, the transient renal disturbance in affected patients may be from accumulation of fructose 1-phosphate in renal tubular cells after fructose intake [89].

Diagnosis

Because the clinical presentation of HFI is highly variable and many of its characteristic features commonly occur with other disorders, the differential diagnosis may include hepatitis, intrauterine infection, septicemia, hemolytic uremic syndrome, galactosemia, tyrosinosis, Wilson disease, and other storage disorders. A detailed nutritional history correlating onset of symptoms with intake of fructose-containing foods is often a key component in the diagnostic process. Suspicion is fostered by the presence of reducing substances in urine. Although various conditions may be associated with hypoglycemia, most of them are associated with fasting. Hypoglycemia after eating should be a clue to the possibility of HFI. Other diseases that are associated with hypoglycemia following ingestion of food include deficiency of FDPase, galactosemia, and leucine intolerance.

Traditionally, direct measure of fructose 1-phosphate aldolase in hepatic or small intestine tissue samples has been employed in the diagnosis of HFI. The liver is the preferred source for biopsy specimens because an assessment of tissue damage, as indicated by the presence of limited and scattered necrosis of hepatocytes, intralobular and periportal fibrosis, and diffuse fatty vacuolization resulting from fructose 1-phosphate accumulation, can be made simultaneously [87]. Assay of enzyme activity in serum and blood cells shows only slightly reduced levels and is of little diagnostic value. Currently, more than 95% of patients with HFI can be diagnosed through amplification of DNA with a limited number of allele-specific oligoneuclotides, circumventing the need for tissue biopsy [81].

Treatment

A diet containing no fructose alleviates all the symptoms and liver dysfunction associated with HFI [81,84,86]. It is important that children and their parents receive detailed dietary counseling about which foods contain fructose. Older children commonly may associate discomfort with specific foods and regularly avoid them. However, infants are completely dependent on dietary selections made by their parents. Sorbitol also must be eliminated, because of its conversion to fructose in the human body. The common practice of adding small amounts of sugar to processed foods demands almost constant attention to avoid substantial fructose intake.

Prognosis

Patients maintained on fructose-free diets have developed entirely normally, with normal lifespans, although most continue to have slight hepatomegaly with hepatic steatosis [87]. Even infants with severely deranged liver function and substantial hepatic fibrosis can achieve remarkable recoveries once fructose is removed from their diets.

Fructose diphosphatase deficiency

In 1970, Baker and Winegrad described a patient who had a third type of genetic defect in fructose metabolism [70]. The predominant clinical findings were hepatomegaly and fasting-induced hypoglycemia with lactic acidosis. The patient was shown later to have deficient hepatic FDPase activity. Other patients with similar clinical and laboratory findings have subsequently been reported [107]. The primary difference between patients with FDPase deficiency and patients with HFI is that fasting as well as dietary fructose induces symptoms in these patients. Several patients have been found to have "partial" FDPase deficiencies. These patients do not have lactic acidosis but develop hypoglycemia during fasting or secondary to dietary intake of fructose or glycerol. The deficiency of FDPase is inherited as an autosomal recessive trait. The diagnosis can be made by measurement of FDPase in cultured lymphocytes and confirmed by detections of mutations in FBP1 (encoding FDPase) [108].

Glycogen storage diseases

Glycogen, a polysaccharide, is the primary carbohydrate storage compound in animals. It is present in virtually all animal cells and is particularly abundant in liver and muscle tissue. It undergoes depolymerization through phosphorolysis and hydrolysis to release free glucose as needed to sustain cellular processes and to maintain normal blood glucose concentrations during fasting. The formation and degradation of glycogen are highly regulated processes involving at least eight enzymes. Deficiencies of each enzyme have been identified in humans and result in the recognized forms of GSD (Figure 27.5). In most types of GSD, the glycogen content of liver or muscle or both is excessive. In unusual cases, the glycogen content may be less than normal, the molecular structure of glycogen may be abnormal, or both may occur. Despite differences in the specific enzymatic defects, most of the syndromes are not readily distinguishable on clinical grounds alone, and tissue analyses for glycogen content and enzymatic activity are

necessary to confirm the diagnoses. The discussion here is limited to types I (defect in glycogenosis), III (amylo-1,6-glucosidase deficiency), and IV (α-1,4 glucan-6-glycosyl transferase deficiency) because their clinical expressions primarily involve the liver; however, the clinical features of all GSDs are provided in Table 27.1 [109].

Biochemistry of glycogen metabolism

Glycogen is a polymer of glucose units linked between the C-1 of one D-glucopyranosyl residue and the hydroxyl at C-4 of the adjacent residue (1,4-linkage). Short chains of glucose residues linked through the hydroxyl groups at C-6 of some of the residues (α-1,6-linkage) represent 7 to 8% of the glycogen, which allows a highly branched structure. The role of glycogen in the liver is to provide glucose to the blood for various organs. At times of stress or if blood glucose levels fall, the liver rapidly releases glucose into the bloodstream, which carries it to organs such as the brain. Glycogen in the muscle serves as a reserve of glycolytic fuel to be used locally if oxygen or glucose availability declines.

Glycogen is synthesized from and degraded to glucose (Figure 27.5). Glycogen synthesis occurs through the action of glycogen synthase and branching enzymes. Hydrolysis occurs through phosphorylase and amylo-1,6-glucosidase. Glycogen synthase catalyzes the synthesis of glycogen from UDP-glucose. Several protein kinases can phosphorylate glycogen synthase. Branching of glycogen is carried out by the transfer of α-1,4-linked glucosyl units from the outer chains of glycogen into a 1,6-position. Glycogen phosphorylase is an interconvertible enzyme, with the α and β forms representing the active and inactive forms, respectively. The phosphorylase enzyme catalyzes the transfer of a glucose unit at the non-reducing end of α-1,4-glucosyl chain glycogen to liberate glucose 1-phosphate. Activation of this enzyme by epinephrine and glucagon plays a major role in controlling glycogenolysis. After extensive phosphorylase action on glycogen, the molecule contains four glucose residues in α-1,4-glucosidic bonds attached by an α-1,6-link. This unit is termed *phosphorylase limit dextrin*. The enzyme oligo-(1,4→1,4)-glucan transferase removes three of the four glucose residues, exposing the 1,6-linkages to be acted upon by the amylo-1,6-glucosidase enzyme to yield free glucose. Both enzymes represent the catalytic activity of the debrancher enzyme.

Because glycogen contains 8% branch points (1,6-links), glycogen degradation by phosphorylase and debrancher enzymes yields about 8% free glucose. The major end-product of glycogen hydrolysis by phosphorylase is glucose 1-phosphate, which is acted on by the enzyme phosphoglucomutase to yield glucose 6-phosphate. There is no known deficiency of the enzyme phosphoglucomutase. Glucose-6-phosphatase (G6Pase) is responsible for the formation of the majority of glucose from gluconeogenesis and glycogenolysis; it is a microsomal enzyme that catalyzes the hydrolysis of glucose 6-phosphate into glucose and phosphate. Glucose-

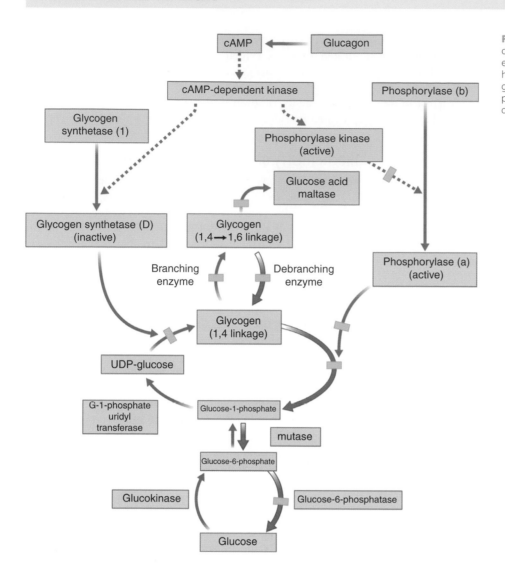

Figure 27.5 Pathway for glycogen synthesis and degradation to glucose. Broken lines indicate enzymatic activation after glucagon stimulation; heavy arrows indicate glycogen degradation from glucagon infusion; and boxes across lines indicate points in the metabolic sequence where enzymatic defects have been identified.

6-phosphatase is present in the liver and kidney and in intestinal mucosa.

The control of glycogen metabolism is mediated by several factors that control glycogen synthesis and degradation by the enzymes glycogen synthetase and phosphorylase, respectively. Control of these enzymes occurs through several factors, including hormonally mediated changes in the concentrations of glucose and glycogen [110]. During feeding, high glucose concentration in the sinusoids allows glucose to bind to the phosphorylase enzyme and causes conversion of active phosphorylase into inactive phosphorylase, resulting in a halt in glycogenolysis. Because active phosphorylase is an inhibitor of the synthetase, its inactivation allows glycogen synthesis to proceed. During fasting, a hormonally mediated (glucagon) increase in cAMP allows activation of protein kinase, which converts inactive to active phosphorylase, initiating glycogenolysis. High glycogen content also favors glycogenolysis by inhibiting glycogen synthetase.

Glycogen storage disease type IA

In 1929, von Gierke published detailed reports of autopsies of two young children in which the most remarkable findings were excessive glycogen accumulation in hepatic and renal tissues, resulting in three-fold and two-fold increases, respectively, in organ size [111]. In the 1950s, further investigation by Cori and Cori showed that hepatic G6Pase activity was deficient in patients with von Gierke disease [112]. In 1954, von Gierke disease was classified as GSD-I [113]. It is the most commonly diagnosed form of hepatic glycogenosis, representing approximately 25% of all cases.

In GSD-I, there is a defect in conversion of glucose 6-phosphate to glucose as in normal glycogenolysis and gluconeogenesis. Originally, GSD-I was thought to represent four subtypes: GSD-IA, a deficiency in G6Pase, GSD-IB, a deficiency in glucose 6-phosphate transporter, GSD-IC, a deficiency in a phosphate transporter and GSD-ID, a deficiency in glucose transporter [114]. Recent studies confirmed the molecular identity of GSD-IA

Table 27.1 Glycogen storage diseases

Disease type	Enzyme	Clinical manifestations
IA	Glucose-6-phosphatase	Hepatomegaly, hypoglycemia, acidosis
IB	Glucose-6-phosphatase transporter	Hepatomegaly, hypoglycemia, infection
II	Lysosomal acid α-glucosidase	Muscle hypotonia
III	Debrancher	Hepatomegaly
IV	Brancher	Liver cirrhosis
V	Muscle phosphorylase	Muscle cramps
VI	Liver phosphorylase	Hepatomegaly
Phosphorylase kinase deficiency	Liver α-subunit	Hepatomegaly
	Muscle α-subunit	Muscle cramps
	Liver β subunit	Hepatomegaly
	Liver γ-subunit	Hypoglycemia, liver fibrosis
	Muscle γ-subunit	Muscle cramps
Fanconi–Bickel syndrome	Glucose transporter 2	Hepatomegaly, renal Fanconi syndrome
Glycogen synthase deficiency	Liver glycogen synthase 2	Ketotic hypoglycemia

Source: adapted with permission from Elpeg, 1999 [109].

and IB; however the identity of GSD-IC and ID have not been defined and indeed they may represent mutations affecting the glucose 6-phosphate transporter, suggesting that this transporter may also translocate glucose 6-phosphate and phosphate [115]. Figure 27.6 represents schematically the different GSD subtypes [116].

Molecular basis

The cDNA encoding the murine G6Pase was cloned by screening a mouse liver cDNA library differentially with mRNA populations representing the normal and the albino deletion mouse known to express markedly reduced level of G6Pase [117]. This discovery allowed the cloning of the human G6Pase cDNA by homology screening. The human gene (*G6PC*) spans 12.5 kb, composed of five exons, and encodes for a protein of 357 amino acid residues [118]. The gene has been localized to chromosome 17q21. To date, more than 84 mutations have been identified in the gene in patients with GSD-IA [118,119]. The two most common mutations give rise to R83C and Q347X, which account for more than 70% of mutations in Caucasian populations [120]. The common mutated form Q347X has a protein truncation of the last 10 C-terminal amino acids that contain the signal for retention of the enzyme in the endoplasmic reticulum.

Clinical presentation

The expression of clinical and biochemical symptoms of GSD-I varies considerably among patients, even in the absence of differences in age, measurable enzyme activity, or treatment. Some individuals require frequent hospitalizations as a result of marked metabolic abnormalities. Others may experience

only mild symptoms and slightly delayed growth. Still others may succumb to the disease during infancy or early childhood.

Children with GSD-I are generally of short stature more so in GSD-IB than GSD-IA where impaired growth hormone secretion is associated with reduced insulin growth factor-1 [121]. They are also prone to adiposity, but without disproportionate head circumference or limb or trunk lengths. Bone films may reveal delayed bone age and osteoporosis [122]. On physical examination, increased fat deposition is most notable on cheeks, breasts, buttocks, and the backs of arms and thighs. A protuberant abdomen and lumbar lordosis result from hepatomegaly, which may be detected as early as 2 months of age. The spleen is usually normal in size. Profound hypoglycemia after relatively short periods of fasting, and severe hepatomegaly, are the most striking features of the disorder. Except in severe cases, hypoglycemia may not become apparent during the first several weeks of life, in which the infant feeds every 2 to 3 hours; however, septicemia may lead to earlier recognition of this symptom, particularly in patients with GSD-IB. Metabolic acidosis resulting from hypoglycemia may cause weakness, malaise, headache, increased respiratory rate, and fruity breath; a few patients experience recurrent fevers with these symptoms [123]. Hypoglycemic convulsions and severe metabolic acidosis may result in death. In other patients, severe hypoglycemia may occur without clinical symptoms. This phenomenon is presumably caused by concomitantly high blood lactate levels, which provide an alternative source of energy for the brain [124].

Liver abnormalities usually include only slight elevations in serum aminotransferases, which improve quickly with stabilization of the blood glucose concentration to between 70 and

449

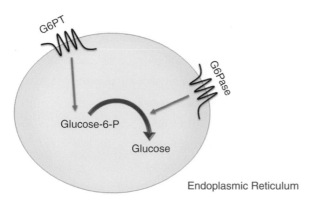

Defect in G6Pase leads to GSD-IA
Defect in G6PT leads to GSD-IB

Figure 27.6 Schematic model of hepatic microsomal glucose-6-phosphatase (G6Pase). Glucose 6-phosphate entry into the endoplasmic reticulum is via a transport protein (G6PT). Hydrolysis occurs by the catalytic subunit of the glucose-6-phosphatase. (Adapted from Boyer *et al.*, 2011 [116].)

110 mg/dL. There is no hepatic cirrhosis or liver failure in GSD-I. However, by the age of 15 years most patients develop hepatic adenomas, and these have been documented by ultrasound as early as 3 years of age. Solitary hepatocellular carcinomas within individual nodules also have been found in a number of patients [125]. The kidneys show no abnormalities beyond substantial enlargement caused by excessive glycogen accumulation and the inability to release free glucose. Individuals who survive puberty, however, may develop progressive nephropathy and gouty complications secondary to persistent hyperuricemia [126].

Biochemical characteristics

Hypoglycemia

The most consistent and life-threatening feature of GSD-I is the low blood glucose levels that result from relatively short periods of fasting. Fasting for as short a time as 2–4 hours is almost always associated with decreases in blood glucose to <70 mg/dL, and it is not uncommon to observe levels of 5–10 mg/dL after 6–8 hours of fasting. In normal individuals, blood glucose levels are maintained within a relatively narrow range by hepatotropic agents such as glucagon, which releases glucose either from stored glycogen or by gluconeogenesis. In GSD-I, degradation of glycogen can occur, or lactate or other gluconeogenic precursors can be converted to glucose 6-phosphate, but in the absence of G6Pase, glucose is not released, and blood glucose levels continue to decline. Blood hormone measurements indicate that, during periods of hypoglycemia, insulin levels are appropriately low and glucagon levels are high. After a glucose load, there is a substantial although somewhat delayed insulin release, with concomitant decreases in glucagon and alanine levels [127]. Therefore, the hormonal response to changes in the blood glucose concentrations appears appropriate.

In 1969, Havel and colleagues used [^{14}C]-glucose as a marker to show that two adults with GSD-I had near-normal basal rates of glucose production [128]. This observation was confirmed in patients of all ages by several investigators who used deuterated glucose as the isotopic marker [129]. These studies defined several features of the illness that have important therapeutic implications:

1. Patients with GSD-I can release glucose into the circulation at close to normal basal rates.
2. Patients cannot increase glucose release during hypoglycemia or after a pharmacologic dose of glucagon; therefore, their basal rates of glucose production are also their maximal rates of production.
3. Maximal glucose production is variable between patients but is not related to residual activity of hepatic G6Pase. However, the tendency for fasting-induced hypoglycemia and severity of the clinical illness is directly related to maximal rates of glucose production.
4. Endogenous glucose production is not inhibited unless an exogenous source of glucose is provided at a rate of 8 mg/kg per min, an amount that maintains blood glucose levels at about 90 mg/dL.
5. The improvement in ability to fast for a longer time after the second decade of life appears to result from a decrease in glucose utilization rather than an increase in glucose production.

Lactic acidosis

Under normal circumstances, most circulating lactate is generated by muscle glycolysis during exercise. Removal and metabolism of this lactate are efficiently performed by the liver. However, much of the circulating lactate in patients with GSD-I is generated by hepatic glycolysis [130]. This phenomenon is apparently the result of hepatic stimulation to release glucose from glycogen in combination with inefficient gluconeogenesis. Excess glucose 6-phosphate formed during glycogenolysis cannot be hydrolyzed to free glucose because of the lack of G6Pase activity. Instead, glucose 6-phosphate is diverted through the glycolytic pathway. This metabolic diversion appears to be the basis for enhancement of lactate formation, as illustrated in Figure 27.7.

Hyperlipidemia

Elevation of plasma lipids is a consistent and striking abnormality [131]. Levels of triglyceride may reach 6000 mg/dL, with associated cholesterol levels of 400–600 mg/dL. Free fatty acid levels are also usually elevated. Around puberty, xanthomas can appear over extensor surfaces, but they may also appear in childhood, with involvement of the nasal septum. Those located on the septum may contribute to the frequency of prolonged nosebleeds seen in some patients.

As with lacticemia, elevated levels of triglyceride and cholesterol appear to be a consequence of increased rates of glycogenolysis and glycolysis. Excess hepatic glycolysis may increase

Type I glycogen storage disease

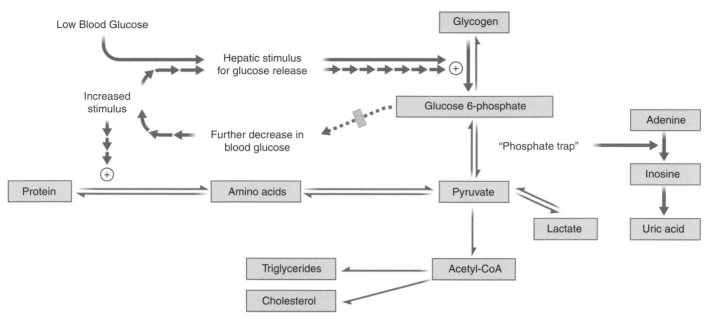

Figure 27.7 Biochemical basis for the primary laboratory findings in patients with glucose-6-phosphatase deficiency (indicated by the solid rectangle). The increased production of glucose 6-phosphate that results from continuous stimulation of glycogen breakdown apparently increases glycolysis, which, in turn, results in a net increase (indicated by dark arrows) in the production of lactate, triglyceride, cholesterol, and uric acid. Both glycogenolysis and gluconeogenesis are involved in the overproduction of substrate.

hepatic levels of NADH, nicotinamide-adenine dinucleotide phosphate (NADPH), and acetyl-coenzyme A (acetyl-CoA), three compounds important in fatty acid and cholesterol synthesis [130]. Thus, increases in glycerol 3-phosphate and acetyl-CoA generated by the glycolytic pathway, together with high levels of reduced cofactors, could sustain an increased rate of triglyceride and cholesterol synthesis [132]. In addition to this apparent increased rate of lipid synthesis, an event concomitant with hypoglycemia is lipolysis from peripheral lipid stores. This further augments the tendency for hyperlipidemia and hepatic steatosis to occur by increasing circulating free fatty acids [131,132].

Hyperuricemia

Although blood levels of uric acid and the tendency to develop gouty arthritis and nephropathy vary in different patients, those who survive puberty often have gouty complications [133]. Hyperuricemia was originally attributed to the increased levels of serum lactate and lipid, which competitively inhibit urate excretion. However, the high level of urate excretion together with the rate of incorporation of [^{14}C-l]-glycine into plasma and urinary urate indicates that an increased rate of purine synthesis de novo is probably more important in the genesis of hyperuricemia than is a decrease in urate excretion [134]. The rate of purine synthesis can be influenced by at least two mechanisms: (1) alteration of the substrate (precursor) concentration (i.e. phosphoribosyl pyrophosphate (PRPP) and glutamine levels), and (2) alteration of the end-product

(purine) concentration (i.e. low intracellular purine levels increase purine synthesis) [135]. In support of the former, two substrates, PRPP and glutamine, are necessary for the first committed reaction. This reaction transfers the amine from l-glutamine to PRPP to form 5-phosphoribosyl-1-amine and is apparently rate limiting for the entire sequence of purine synthesis. Although tissue glutamate and glutamine levels have not been measured, blood levels of the two substrates obtained from hyperuricemic patients with GSD-I are three- to eightfold higher than are values obtained after urate is normalized by glucose infusion [132]. In addition to the possibility of increased availability of glutamine, the high levels of glucose 6-phosphate produced during periods of hypoglycemia and excessive glycogenolysis may increase synthesis of the second important substrate in purine synthesis, ribose 5-phosphate [133]. These findings suggest that an apparent increased availability of purine precursors, glutamine, and ribose 5-phosphate may cause a secondary increase in PRPP and thus increase the rate of purine synthesis. Studies using human leukocytes indicate, however, that an increase in availability of glutamine and ribose 5-phosphate alone will not increase the generation of PRPP [136]. Assuming this is true in liver, the second mechanism, alteration of end-product concentration, should be more important in modulating the increased rate of purine synthesis in patients with GSD-I.

In support of the second mechanism for hyperuricemia, a decreased concentration of purine ribonucleotides would favor an increase in the rate of purine biosynthesis by releasing the glutamine pyrophosphate-ribose-phosphate amidotransferase from end-product inhibition [137]. Although hepatic nucleotide levels during hypoglycemic episodes have not been determined directly, indirect evidence suggests that, in patients with GSD-I, hypoglycemia can reduce adenyl ribonucleotide levels. Such a conclusion is based on measured values of hepatic ATP before and after simulating the effects of hypoglycemia with intravenous glucagon administration [138]. Seven patients had a three-fold decrease in hepatic ATP levels with concomitant 1.3-fold decrease in ADP. Such a reduction in ATP has been shown to favor the rapid degradation of adenyl or guanyl ribonucleotides to xanthine and uric acid. The latter set of reactions is also favored by low intracellular phosphate levels, which apparently occur through phosphate trapping of the phosphorylated sugar. Normally, this accumulation of glucose 6-phosphate is prevented by the action of G6Pase [139].

These observations suggest that the increase in urate production is secondary to recurrent episodes of hypoglycemia, which result in compensatory glucagon release. This hepatotropic agent stimulates glycogen degradation to glucose 6-phosphate. The absence of G6Pase activity results in a phosphate-trapping effect and lowering of ATP levels, which in turn promotes degradation of preformed purines to uric acid [139,140]. Finally, the decrease in end-product (purine) concentration promotes a high rate of purine biosynthesis.

Hypophosphatemia

Low serum phosphate levels generally are seen during hypoglycemic episodes. Glucagon injection in patients with GSD-I is followed by a decrease in serum phosphate level. Because glucose 6-phosphate cannot be converted to glucose, phosphate is trapped within the compound, resulting in intracellular depletion of phosphate and a compensatory shift of extracellular phosphate into the cell. A similar phenomenon has been well documented in patients with HFI.

Recurrent fever

A few patients have recurrent fever in association with acidosis and hypoglycemia. In these patients, the fever can be reproduced by intravenous injection of glucagon if the patient is already slightly hypoglycemic (blood glucose 35–55 mg/dL) and acidotic (arterial blood pH 7.28–7.36). The febrile response begins 8–12 minutes after glucagon injection (0.1 mg/kg given over 3 minutes), and usually peaks 12–16 minutes later. If the low blood glucose level is corrected by intravenous administration of glucose and the acidosis is corrected by sodium bicarbonate, the temperature usually returns to normal within 45 minutes of glucagon infusion.

The febrile response may represent an uncoupling of oxidative phosphorylation secondary to lack of Pi. The glucagon results in the excessive formation of glucose 6-phosphate from glycogen. Because of the G6Pase deficiency, a burst of glycolysis results in excess production of reduced cofactors, which normally produce high-energy phosphates. Because of low intracellular phosphate levels, oxidative phosphorylation, were

it to occur, would have to be uncoupled, leading to production of heat rather than chemical energy in the form of ATP.

Platelet dysfunction

Patients with GSD-I usually have prolonged bleeding times secondary to abnormal platelet aggregation. Corby and coworkers examined platelet function in 13 patients, each with deficient hepatic activity of one of the following enzymes: G6Pase, debrancher enzyme, phosphorylase, or phosphorylase kinase [140]. Only the seven patients with G6Pase deficiencies had abnormal platelet aggregation, and four of these also had abnormal platelet adhesiveness. The defect appears to be intrinsic, because cross-over and resuspension studies using patients' platelets in normal plasma and normal platelets in patients' plasma did not alter in vitro platelet function. Two such patients had the ADP content of affected platelets measured, and in both instances it was normal. Nevertheless, the release of ADP from platelets in response to added collagen and epinephrine was markedly impaired. These observations suggest that the functional defect is an impairment of the ability of the platelet membrane to release ADP. A similar defect in ADP release from platelets with elevated cholesterol content has been shown [141]. The elevated cholesterol content impaired fluidity of the membrane, causing secondary impairment of ADP and epinephrine-induced aggregation.

Hepatic adenomas and carcinomas

Most patients with GSD-I who are more than 15 years of age are now found to develop adenomas. This is at variance with the previously held view that they occur only infrequently. Adenomas develop in most patients during the second decade of life, but they may be found in 3-year-old children. The nodules, which are best demonstrated by ultrasonography and radioisotopic scanning, show increased echodensity and decreased isotope uptake. At laparotomy, they appear as discrete, pale nodules that range in number from one to many and in size from 1 to 5 cm. A number of patients have been found to have solitary hepatocellular adenocarcinomas in individual nodules [142]. The mechanism causing the adenomas or their malignant degeneration is not known, but treatment with portacaval shunting does not prevent their development. The pathogenesis of hepatic adenomas is not known but they are believed to be secondary to chronic stimulation of the liver by hepatotrophic agents such as glucagon. Our own experience with two patients who had adenomas prior to nocturnal feeding showed resolution of these adenomas after 3 years of treatment [143]. A significant difference in progression to hepatocellular adenoma has been shown between two groups based on 5-year mean serum triglyceride concentrations: those with ≤500 mg/dL having slower progression than those with >500 mg/dL [144].

The tendency for adenoma formation and malignant transformation is highest in young adults with GSD-I and appears to be a consequence of supportive therapy, which currently ensures survival into childhood and young adulthood. The mechanism leading to hepatic malignancy is unknown. A similar progression has been observed in experimental hepatocarcinogenesis from exposure to *N*-nitrosomorpholine. The progression from normal hepatocytes to malignancy appears to be as follows. First, multifocal areas of cells containing excessive glycogen develop. The cells in these areas also show decreased G6Pase activity. Second, the focal cluster of cells develops a gradual reduction in glycogen content and a concomitant increase in ribosomes, reflected as basophilia by hematoxylin and eosin (H&E) staining. Finally, the foci enlarge and acquire the phenotypic markers of hepatocellular carcinoma. These experimental observations, coupled with the findings in patients with GSD-I, led Bannasch and associates to postulate that the metabolic disturbance leading to hepatocellular glycogenesis is fixed at the genetic level in both the experimental animals and the patients and is causally related to the neoplastic transformation [145]. An examination of the distinct genomic and genetic characteristics of hepatocellular adenoma associated with GSD-IA indicated that chromosome 6 alterations could be an early event in the liver tumorigenesis in GSD-I [146].

Diagnosis

Accurate diagnosis of GSD-I has become crucial for the development of an effective approach to treatment. Direct assay of hepatic enzyme activity (hydrolysis by G6Pase) in a fresh liver biopsy specimen is advocated. In order to provide some selectivity in the application of this procedure, determination of serial blood glucose and lactate levels during a 4- to 6-hour fast as well as maximum blood glucose response to glucagon is recommended. A deficiency of phosphorylase kinase, which is not routinely measured in liver tissue samples, should be suspected if blood glucose rises more than 30 mg/dL [123].

Traditionally, glucagon, galactose, fructose, and glucose tolerance tests were used to diagnose GSD. Glucagon administration typically fails to produce an increase in blood glucose in these patients. Within 20 minutes after administration, however, patients may experience a substantial decrease in blood glucose, followed by development of severe metabolic acidosis. Patients with GSD-I are unable to convert galactose and fructose to free glucose. Administration of either of these sugars results in a flat blood glucose curve. The use of these tests has the advantage of avoiding risks associated with more invasive diagnostic techniques; however, a substantial blood volume is required for completion, and results frequently fail to yield a definitive diagnosis.

In GSD-I, the liver cells are distended with glycogen and often contain medium-sized to large lipid vacuoles. The lipid content in the liver of an untreated patient is substantially greater than that in the liver of a patient who has been treated, but in either instance, hepatic steatosis is a prominent morphologic feature. The liver cells are pale-staining and have prominent plasma membranes.

It is not possible to distinguish between normal and elevated levels of cytoplasmic glycogen in the liver in any of the

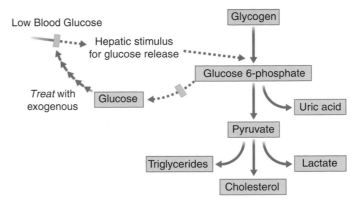

Figure 27.8 A biochemical basis for management of patients with glucose-6-phosphatase deficiency (indicated by solid rectangle). By preventing the decrease in blood glucose with an exogenous supply of glucose, excessive glycolysis and gluconeogenesis are prevented. This results in a net decrease in production of circulating triglyceride, cholesterol, lactate, and uric acid.

forms of glycogenosis through the use of periodic acid–Schiff (PAS) stain [147]. Therefore, a quantitative determination is necessary to make a diagnosis of excessive glycogen content.

Treatment

Present recommendations for treatment of GSD-I stem primarily from the studies by Folkman and associates who first illustrated the reversal of most biochemical abnormalities after TPN [148]. Their observation that both TPN and portacaval shunting delivered nutrients primarily into the systemic circulation suggested that hepatic exposure to nutrients was important in the pathogenesis of many of the biochemical abnormalities [149]. Nevertheless, it was later demonstrated that the same beneficial effect seen with TPN or portacaval shunting could be achieved with an intragastric infusion of a nutrient solution similar in content to that used for TPN [150]. This suggested that bypassing the liver with nutrients was not the most important factor in reversing the abnormalities. The similarity in the three types of treatment (i.e. portacaval shunting, TPN, and continuous intragastric infusion of glucose) was that a hormonal stimulus to the liver to produce glucose was decreased or averted. Specifically, both TPN and continuous intragastric feeding prevented a hepatic stimulus for glucose release by maintaining blood glucose levels in the range 90–150 mg/dL, whereas the portacaval shunt prevented such a stimulus by diverting pancreatic and enteric blood into systemic circulation. On this basis, the hypothesis for treatment illustrated in Figure 27.8 was formulated.

The hypothesis states that, as blood glucose falls below a critical level, compensatory mechanisms cause glycogen degradation to glucose 6-phosphate. In the absence of G6Pase, glucose 6-phosphate is not hydrolyzed to release free glucose, and the hepatic stimulus for glycogenolysis results in formation of other intermediates such as lactate, triglycerides, and cholesterol. To interrupt the stimulus, treatment with an exogenous source of glucose inhibits the release of hepatotropic stimuli and thus the excess glycogenolysis. If this postulate is correct, any method of treatment that maintains blood glucose above a critical level should also prevent, or at least alleviate, biochemical manifestations of the illness. In addition, the hypothesis suggests that diversion of portal vein blood flow should dilute hepatotropic agents in the systemic circulation. This dilution should result in less stimulation of glycogenolysis.

Theoretically, either portacaval shunting or continuous infusion of a high-glucose diet should be effective in reversing most manifestations of the illness, with the exception that portacaval shunting should have little or no beneficial effect on hypoglycemia. Consequently, portacaval shunting is not recommended as a sole form of treatment for those patients who are expected to have frequent episodes of very low blood glucose or for small children in whom shunts may be more likely to close spontaneously.

Although TPN and continuous intragastric infusion of glucose are effective treatment modalities for GSD-I, they are impractical on a long-term basis. A more practical method was devised to maintain blood glucose at physiologic concentrations or at levels that would prevent stimulation of excess glycogenolysis and glycolysis. This treatment consisted of a high-glucose diet given to simulate TPN. This was given enterally either by nasogastric tube or by gastrostomy during night-time sleep, along with a high-starch diet that was consumed at frequent intervals while the patient was awake. Such a regimen has successfully maintained a large number of patients relatively symptom free for more than 10 years and has provided normal or near-normal growth and development [151].

A number of patients can maintain normal blood glucose levels by taking cold, uncooked cornstarch (2 g/kg) at 6-hour intervals [152]. This regimen has been used by a number of patients to avoid the continuous nocturnal feedings. A number of younger children have not been able to maintain normal glucose and lactate levels with the cornstarch regimen as well as they had with the continuous nocturnal feeding regimen [153]. In the author's experience, growth rates were less with the raw starch regimen than with continuous feedings, and one patient consumed such large quantities of cornstarch that protein intake was insufficient to maintain normal secretory proteins (albumin, transferrin, and retinol-binding protein). Therefore, although the cornstarch feedings can be beneficial as a time-release form of glucose in some patients, a dose–response to the starch preparation and careful monitoring of blood glucose levels should be carried out to ensure that treatment is appropriate for individual patients. The authors believe that many patients require an intensive feeding regimen at least until they have stopped growing. This consists of high-starch feedings at intervals of 2–3 hours during the day, continuous nocturnal feeding of a complete, low-lipid-containing (<5% calories) formula, and periodic monitoring to ensure normal blood glucose and lactate levels throughout the day and night. As patients become fully grown and have a relatively lower requirement for glucose,

the uncooked cornstarch regimen may allow discontinuation of the night-time nasogastric feedings. Utilizing modified cornstarch has been shown to ameliorate the metabolic complications [154].

Prognosis

Until the use of nocturnal feedings, the first few years of life were usually marked by frequent hospitalizations for treatment of hypoglycemia and acidosis, with a high rate of death or permanent central nervous system impairment from recurrent and prolonged episodes of hypoglycemia. Patients who survived puberty appeared to have fewer problems than they had when younger. Patients with persistent hyperuricemia had gouty complications during the second and third decades of life, and many patients had complications of hyperlipidemia, with xanthomas, and with higher rates of cardiovascular disease and pancreatitis than those in the general population [155]. Recognition of hepatic adenomas has been relatively recent, and the incidence of complications from benign hepatic adenomas is unclear, although several patients have developed hepatomas [142].

Long-term follow-up of the results of portacaval shunting or nocturnal feedings is not complete. Ten-year follow-up of patients treated with nocturnal feedings indicates that infants so treated have many fewer problems than they had before treatment and that some patients with hepatic adenomas may show resolution after a few years of treatment. Too few patients have been monitored into the third decade of life to permit conclusions, but early observations indicate that, for optimal treatment, the nocturnal feedings are necessary for most young patients, whereas raw cornstarch administration may suffice for older patients. Patients generally have less tendency to hypoglycemia after the age of 20. As long as blood glucose is consistently maintained between 70 and 120 mg/dL, most children appear to lead fairly normal, healthy lives, with normal growth and development [155].

Older patients (>18 years) with suboptimal treatment have a high incidence of progressive renal disease. The affected individuals show progressive glomerular sclerosis with proteinuria as an early manifestation [156]. Renal involvement appears initially with microalbuminuria and hyperfiltration progressing to frank proteinuria and hypertension [157]. Although the cause of the lesion is unclear, it appears that the incidence is lowered by maintenance of good control of blood glucose and other blood abnormalities.

Glycogen storage disease type IB

In 1968, Senior and Loridan described a patient with clinical and laboratory features identical to GSD-I except that no enzyme defect was identified from frozen liver [158]. In addition to the hepatic abnormality, patients have repeated infections because of neutropenia and abnormal leukocyte migration and some show decreased neutrophil phagocytosis-stimulated oxygen consumption, decreased nitroblue tetrazolium reduction, defective bactericidal activity, defective hexose monophosphate shunt activity, and increased incidence of inflammatory bowel disease [159,160]. These patients have been diagnosed as having GSD-IB. There has been little mention of a familial occurrence in the reports of GSD-IB. The number of reported cases is small, however, and the mode of inheritance is presumed to be autosomal recessive.

The reason for the discrepancy between the in vitro and in vivo activity of G6Pase in patients with GSD-IB is not known. Steady-state kinetic measurements led Arion and associates to conclude that the normal microsomal G6Pase is a two-compartment system consisting of a specific glucose-6-phosphate carrier on the outer bilayer of the membrane of the endoplasmic reticulum and a catalytic phosphorylase component located on the inner half of the membrane [159]. Because disruption of isolated microsomes of patients with GSD-IB with cholate or freeze–thawing results in a marked increase in activity, the general assumption has been that the defect in GSD-IB is a deficiency of the translocase or carrier portion of the enzyme system although the putative translocase has never been identified in microsomes from normal liver [160]. Pre-steady-state kinetics have shown that the limiting step in the reaction is not glucose release from the enzyme but the release of phosphate [161]. These findings in normal liver microsomes are similar in the liver of a patient with GSD-IB, although the pre-steady-state kinetics are blunted. These findings question the general concept of a translocase and suggest that patients with GSD-IB may have a configurational abnormality in the enzyme–membrane interaction that can be overcome by alteration of the membrane lipid rather than by an opening of the microsomal vesicle [161].

Molecular basis

Glycogen storage disease type IB is caused by mutation in *SLC37A4*, the gene encoding microsomal glucose-6-phosphate transporter [162]. The gene has been mapped to chromosome 11q23 and is composed of 9 exons spanning a genomic region of 4 kb. The gene is expressed in the liver, kidney, and leukocytes [163]. More than 69 mutations have been described in the gene, resulting in functional deficiency of glucose-6-phosphate transporter, which explains the neutropenia and neutrophil–monocyte dysfunction characteristic of GSD-IB [162,164]. No genotype–phenotype correlations have been described for type IA or IB disorders [165].

Treatment

Treatment of GSD-IB is identical to that of GSD-IA, with the possible exception that prophylactic antibiotics may lessen the tendency for frequent infection [158]. Improvement in neutrophil function with treatment has been reported by some investigators [158]. However, the authors' experience has been that the neutropenia and abnormal migration persists even after 3 months of management that normalized all parameters of disease in the blood, and even after subsequent portacaval shunting [166]. The lack of improvement in neutrophil

function in some of the well-treated patients suggests that the defect in GSD-IB is intrinsic to both the liver and leukocytes. The functional impairment in neutrophils is related to impaired glucose production by neutrophils resulting in endoplasmic stress and increased apoptosis rather than an aberrant neutrophil maturation [167]. Improvement of neutropenia and neutrophil dysfunction occurs in response to granulocyte colony-stimulating factor [168]. Vitamin E supplementation, by decreasing reactive oxygen species, improves mean values of neutrophil counts as well as the frequency and severity of infections, mouth ulcers, and perianal lesions [169].

Glycogen storage disease type III

Amylo-1,6-glucosidase deficiency, GSD-III, first was recognized in 1952, when examination of liver and muscle tissue from a patient revealed atypical structure of glycogen molecules present in excess in both tissues [170]. Short outer chains, as in phosphorylase limit dextrin, were also noted and a deficiency of the debranching enzyme, amylo-1,6-glucosidase, was proposed [171]. Debranching enzyme contains two catalytic activities on a single polypeptide chain. The two activities are oligo-1,4–1,4-glucantransferase and amylo-1,6-glucosidase. The 160 kDa debrancher enzyme has been purified [172]. In 1967, van Hoof and Hers measured debranching enzyme activity by four methods in hepatic and muscle tissue samples from 45 patients known to have the disease [173]. Thirty-four patients exhibited complete absence of enzyme activity in both tissues regardless of the method of measurement; these were designated as having GSD-IIIA. In the remaining patients, residual enzyme activity was apparent in either muscle (GSD-IIIB) or hepatic tissue through at least one method of measurement. These findings have been confirmed by immunoblot analysis of glycogen debranching enzyme in 41 patients with GSD-III [174].

GSD-III also is known as *limit dextrinosis* or *Forbes disease*. Transmission of the disease is autosomal recessive, and it may be diagnosed prenatally [174]. A higher incidence of GSD-III (1 in 5400 births) occurs in non-Ashkenazi Jewish communities of North African descent.

Molecular basis

The human gene encoding for glycogen debranching enzyme, *AGL*, is 85 kb is length and consists of 35 exons [175]. It has been localized to chromosome 1p21 [176]. The cDNA includes a 4545 bp encoding region and 2371 bp 3′-untranslated region. The predicted protein is approximately 172 kDa, consistent with the estimated size of the purified protein [177]. Six mRNA isoforms have been identified [178]. Isoform 1 is expressed in the liver; isoforms 2, 3, and 4 are muscle specific. Isoforms 5 and 6 are minor isoforms. Mutations in the glycogen debranching gene have been described in patients with type IIIa and IIIb. These mutations include missense, nonsense, splicing, and deletion insertion defects [179]. Specific mutations in exon 3 such as 17delAG and Q6x are only seen in type IIIb [180]. The splice mutation IVS32–12A>G was found to cause mild clinical symptoms, whereas mutations 3965delT and 4529insA are associated with a severe phenotype and early onset of clinical symptoms [181]. Gene sequencing has identified 25 novel mutations, further demonstrating the heterogeneity of this disorder [182].

Clinical presentation

The clinical manifestations of GSD-III result directly from its effects on hepatic and muscle tissue, although amylo-1,6-glucosidase deficiency is generalized to all types of cell. Individuals with GSD-III generally tolerate longer periods of fasting without hypoglycemia; therefore, the clinical course of the disease is usually much milder than that of GSD-I.

Symptoms and their severity vary from patient to patient and with age. In infancy and childhood, GSD-III and GSD-I are not readily distinguishable by physical examination alone, primarily because hepatic manifestations predominate in this age group. Growth failure and hepatomegaly may be striking early in life. Hepatic fibrosis may lead to the development of splenomegaly in some children by 4 to 6 years of age. A decrease in liver size, however, has been noted to occur in some patients around puberty [183], and in some adults normal physical examination results have been documented. These patients usually have evidence of hepatic fibrosis but do not necessarily develop cirrhosis and liver failure.

The onset of muscular symptoms usually occurs in adulthood and is manifested primarily as progressive muscle weakness, which may be intensified by brisk walking or climbing, and muscle wasting. Accumulation of glycogen in peripheral nerve axons has been demonstrated in one adult with unsteady gait [184].

Renal enlargement is not seen in GSD-III. Glycogen accumulation in the heart may produce cardiomegaly and non-specific electrocardiographic changes. However, congestive heart failure and arrhythmias have not been reported.

Biochemical and laboratory findings

Laboratory aberrations seen in GSD-III are similar to but less severe than in GSD-I. The onset of fasting-induced hypoglycemia occurs more slowly in most patients with GSD-III. Elevations in lipid levels appear to correlate directly with the tendency toward hypoglycemia; that is, moderately high lipid levels are seen in those patients who develop lower blood glucose levels after fasts of 6–8 hours [183]. Moderate elevations in serum aminotransferase (300–600 IU/L) are seen consistently, with the exception of an occasional patient with more severe enzyme elevations [185]. Lactic acid and uric acid levels are usually normal.

Patients with GSD-III exhibit characteristic responses to the administration of various hormones and nutrients. Galactose and fructose are transformed freely to glucose in these patients, and protein and amino acids cause small but protracted increases in blood glucose levels [183]. Similarly, glucagon and epinephrine administration between 1.5 and

3 hours after a meal raise blood glucose levels. Failure of these hormones to produce increases in blood glucose levels after a prolonged fast seems to provide evidence of available 1,4-glucosyl linkages that can undergo phosphorolysis shortly after a meal [186]. After a prolonged fast, access to 1,4-linkages would be blocked by terminal 1,6-glycosyl linkages, preventing an increase in blood glucose. This has been called the *double glucagon tolerance test*; however, patient response has been inconsistent, possibly because of glucose formation through this pathway. Such testing is, therefore, of little diagnostic value.

Patients with GSD-III have abnormally high hepatic glycogen content. Structurally, hepatic glycogen has been found to have abnormally short outer branch points. These patients also may exhibit alterations in the activity of other enzymes involved in glycogen degradation.

No one test or feature provides information that will differentiate this form of the disease from all others. Therefore, direct measurement of amylo-1,6-glucosidase activity in liver and muscle tissue samples and concomitant examination for abnormal glycogen structure should be relied on to yield a definitive diagnosis. The presence of excess glycogen in muscle and excess plasma creatine kinase also strongly supports the diagnosis.

Treatment

Treatment of this disorder remains investigative. Treatment should be restricted to patients who have obvious muscle involvement, progressive fibrotic changes in the liver, or both. An accurate correlation between the type of glycogen accumulation and progression of liver disease, so that a clear-cut prognosis could be assigned to each patient, would be helpful in showing a positive therapeutic response.

Present investigative efforts combine the technique of nocturnal feedings with the known responses to protein and amino acids [183]. Improved growth and increased muscle strength has been reported for a patient given a high-protein diet during the day and continuous nocturnal intragastric feedings of a high-protein liquid formula (Sustacal) at night [187]. Growth and aminotransferase and blood glucose levels were more positively influenced by a high-starch diet with a standard (recommended dietary allowance) protein intake [188]. This therapy is, therefore, virtually identical to that for GSD-I. A report from France described treatment for a 2-month-old infant with GSD-III and severe cardiomyopathy by combining the use of synthetic ketone bodies (D,L-3-hydroxybutyrate) as an alternative energy source, 2:1 ketogenic diet to reduce glucose intake, and high-protein diet to enhance gluconeogenesis [189]. Two years after the onset of the treatment, echocardiography showed an improvement of cardiomyopathy. Growth and liver size remained normal and no side effects were observed. Blood glucose levels remained within the normal range and insulin levels decreased [189]. This outcome is encouraging, but more extensive follow-up evaluation over a longer period of treatment is needed.

Glucogen storage disease type IV

α-1,4-Glucan-6-glycosyltransferase deficiency, type IV GSD, is a rare form of glycogenosis that was first described clinically and pathologically in 1952 by Anderson [190]. Glycogen possesses abnormally long outer and inner chains of glucose units [191] and there is an absence of branching enzyme activity in this disorder [192]. The few descriptions of the disorder have illustrated its unusual clinical, biochemical, and pathologic aspects.

Type IV GSD also is known as *amylopectinosis* and as *Andersen disease*. The disorder is most likely inherited through autosomal recessive transmission [193]; the possibility of X-linked transmission has not been eliminated, because of the preponderance of males among reported patients [123].

Molecular basis

The human gene, *GBE1*, encoding branching enzyme has been localized to chromosome 3p12 [194]. The human cDNA is 3 kb in length, encoding a protein of 702 amino acid residues [194]. There appears to be a phenotype–genotype correlation, which may explain the clinical variability of the patients [195]. Mutations leading to R515C, F257L, and R524X result in infantile cirrhosis; mutation 873del210 results in infantile myopathy and cardiomyopathy. Mutation giving rise to Y3295/L224P results in non-progressive liver disease [195] while mutation c288delA presents with severe hypotonia [196]. Prenatal diagnosis can be made using polymerase chain reaction-based DNA mutation analysis [197].

Clinical presentation

Clinically, GSD-IV is a heterogeneous disorder with variability that may have congenital, infantile, childhood, or adulthood presentation [198]. The most common form is the classic progressive liver cirrhosis, with onset of symptoms between 3 and 15 months of age. These children usually present with failure to thrive, abdominal distention, hepatosplenomegaly, and other vague gastrointestinal complaints. Later, symptoms associated with progressive liver dysfunction and cirrhosis usually dominate the clinical picture.

Approximately 50% of patients with GSD-IV glycogenosis also experience abnormal neuromuscular development, with abnormal polysaccharide deposition in skeletal muscle [199]. A neuromuscular form of the disease has been described with the usual manifestations of hypotonia, muscular atrophy, decreased or absent tendon reflexes, and evidence that all levels of the neuromuscular axis (i.e. skeletal muscles and the peripheral and central nervous systems) may be affected. A few patients have developed cardiac failure, presumably from myofibrillar damage caused by amylopectin deposition within myocardial cells [123]. In exceptional patients, cardiac and neuromuscular symptoms predominate [200]. A few patients with features suggestive of GSD-IV with amylopectinosis have been reported to have severe progressive cardiomyopathy with and without skeletal myopathy, but normal or near-normal glycogen branching enzyme activity in liver, muscle, and cultured skin fibroblasts [201]. Adults with diffuse central and peripheral nervous systems dysfunction accompanied by accumulation of polyglucosan bodies have been described (adult polyglucosan body disease) [202].

Laboratory findings

Blood electrolytes are usually within normal limits except in patients with renal tubular defects, who have low bicarbonate concentrations. Serum aminotransferase and alkaline phosphatase levels are usually elevated to 3× to 6× normal. Except with malnutrition, late in the disease, serum cholesterol is often slightly elevated. Until liver failure develops, serum albumin, globulin, bilirubin, and ammonia are normal. All liver test results become abnormal as liver failure becomes severe. Glucagon and epinephrine tolerance tests cause a positive glucose response, with increases in blood levels of 15–23 mg/dL, the maximum response occurring about 30 minutes after hormone injection and 2 hours after a meal. Both hormones may allow detection of urinary ketone bodies. Hypoglycemia is not a characteristic feature of the illness until terminal liver failure occurs. Chronic and severe acidosis may occur secondary to a renal tubular defect in hydrogen ion excretion. Oral glucose and fructose tolerance tests show no abnormality, and serum lactate and pyruvate levels are normal.

Biochemical and pathologic features

Individuals with GSD-IV characteristically have hepatic glycogen contents of 3.5 to 5.0%, compared with approximately 6% of wet weight in normal subjects. In one patient, hepatic glycogen content measured 10.7%. The chemical properties of the polysaccharide also differ from those of normal glycogen, because of the abnormal structure of the compound. In GSD-IV, more than 40% of the glucose units are highly susceptible to phosphorylase-induced hydrolysis (normal: about 36%); this could be attributed to its longer outer chain lengths (normal: 8–12 glycosyl units) and fewer branch points (approximately 6%) compared with normal mammalian glycogen (approximately 8%). The polysaccharide is highly chromogenic, with a maximal KI–I_2 absorption band at approximately 525 nm (nl: 460 nm). Leukocytic glycogen also is abnormal, presumably because of the deficiency of branching enzyme in these cells. Skeletal muscle glycogen appears normal. Liver and myocardial glycosyl deposits appear similar histochemically; both are resistant to digestion by α-amylase.

Examination of the liver shows uniform micronodular cirrhosis with broad bands of fibrous tissue extending around and into the lobules. Portal veins, lymphatic channels, and hepatic arteries are normal with slight portal biliary duct proliferation. Liver cell plates are distorted, and, as the disease progresses, the lobules develop prominent sinusoidal channels with fibrous walls coursing between thick liver plates.

Microscopically, liver cell nuclei are frequently eccentric in position. With H&E stain, they appear to be displaced by pale,

(a)

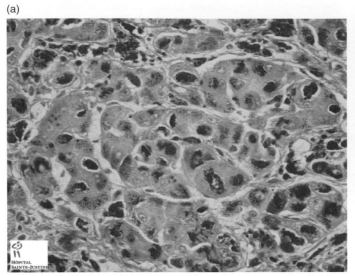

(b)

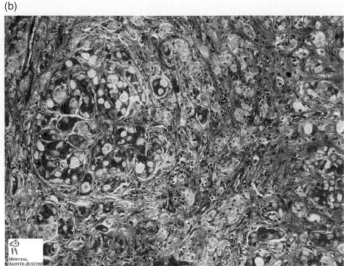

Figure 27.9 Glycogen storage disease type IV. (a) Periodic acid–Schiff-positive inclusions in cytoplasm. (b) Micronodular cirrhosis with hepatocytes containing cytoplasmic inclusions. (Masson trichrome stain; image courtesy of humpath.com.)

slightly eosinophilic, or colorless inclusions deposited in the cytoplasm. This is the most striking and characteristic finding and is generally limited to the periphery of the lobule. The inclusions vary from hyaline to reticulate and are usually sharply demarcated from normal cytoplasm. Clear haloes may surround the contents of the inclusions. In the late stages of the disease, nodular accumulations of a slightly different hyaline, fibrillar material are scattered throughout the hepatic lobules. This material is birefringent, appearing in polarized light as sheaths of crystals that cannot be easily distinguished from deposits that typify α_1-antitrypsin deficiency, except perhaps on the basis of their greater frequency and larger size in GSD-IV. In both conditions, the peripheral lobular deposits are PAS positive and diastase resistant.

Ultrastructural studies show three types of cytoplasmic deposit: glycogen particles, fibrils, and finely granular material. The abnormal glycogen can be detected ultrastructurally or histochemically. Similarly, changes in cytoplasmic deposits are seen in the myocardium, central nervous system, and skeletal muscles. Figure 27.9 shows a liver sample from a patient with GSD-IV, showing massive accumulation of glycogen demonstrated by PAS staining.

Treatment

Three types of treatment, without improvement, were used for one patient. First, a high-protein, low-carbohydrate diet with corn oil added to the milk fat caused no change in weight gain or in the progression of cirrhosis. Second, with progression of the disease, purified α-glucosidase from *Aspergillus niger* was given for 6 days. This treatment resulted in a striking decrease in hepatic glycogen content, from 10 to 2%. Although no unfavorable reaction occurred, liver size did not decrease. Glycogen content was maintained at 3% by a third treatment, intramuscular injection of zinc-glucagon 1 mg three times a day for 24 days. Any positive effect of these treatments remains doubtful but the poor clinical results following the treatments might have been related to the advanced state of cirrhosis before their initiation.

Liver transplantation is the only available option for patients with GSD-IV who progress to liver cirrhosis and failure. Liver transplantation results in resorption of extrahepatic deposits of amylopectin, possibly by systemic microchimerism (i.e. cells of the host organs became mixed with cells with the donor genomes that had migrated from the allograft into the recipient tissues and presumably serve as enzyme carriers) [194]. Predominant neuromuscular and cardiac involvement may preclude liver transplantation.

References

1. Mason HH, Turner ME. Chronic galactosemia. *Am J Dis Child* 1935;**50**:359.

2. Donnell GN, Bergren WR, Cleland RS. Galactosemia. *Pediatr Clin North Am* 1960;**7**:315–332.

3. Gitzelmann R. Hereditary galactokinase deficiency, a newly recognized cause of juvenile cataracts. *Pediatr Res* 1967;**1**:14–23.

4. Gitzelmann R, Steinmann B, Mitchell B, *et al.* Uridine diphosphate galactose-4-epimerase deficiency. IV. Report of eight cases in three families. *Helv Paediatr Acta* 1977;**31**:441–452.

5. Holton JB, Gillett MG, MacFaul R, *et al.* Galactosemia: a new severe variant due to uridine diphosphate galactose-4-epimerase deficiency. *Arch Dis Child* 1981;**56**:885–887.

6. Holton, JB. Galactosaemia: pathogenesis and treatment. *J Inherit Metab Dis* 1996;**19**:3–7.

7. Hopfer U. Membrane transport mechanisms for hexoses and amino acids in the small intestine. In Johnson LR, Christensen J, Jackson MJ (eds.) *Physiology of the Gastrointestinal Tract*,

2nd edn. New York: Raven Press, 1987, pp. 1499–1526.

8. Heinrich MR. The purification and properties of yeast galactokinase. *J Biol Chem* 1964;**239**:50–53.

9. Shin-Buehring YS, Beier T, Tan A, *et al.* Galactokinase and galactose-1-phosphate uridyltransferase (transferase) and galactokinase in human fetal organs. *Pediatr Res* 1977;**11**:1012.

10. Flach JE, Reichardt TKV, Elsas LJ. Sequence of a cDNA encoding human galactose-1-phosphate uridyl transferase. *Mol Biol Med* 1990;**7**: 365–369.

11. Segal S, Blair A. Some observations on the metabolism of d-galactose in normal man. *J Clin Invest* 1961;**40**:2016–2025.

12. Tygstrup N. Determination of the hepatic elimination capacity (LM) of galactose by single injection. *Scand J Clin Lab Invest* 1966;**92**(Suppl 18):118–125.

13. Lemaire HG, Muller-Hill B. Nucleotide sequences of the gal E gene and the gal T gene of *E. coli*. *Nucleic Acids Res* 1986;**14**:7705–7711.

14. Field TL, Reznikoff WS, Frey PA. Galactose-1-phosphate uridylyltransferase: identification of histidine-164 and histidine-166 as critical residues by site-directed mutagenesis. *Biochemistry* 1989;**28**:2094–2099.

15. Reichardt JKV, Woo SLC. Molecular basis of galactosemia: mutations and polymorphisms in the gene encoding human galactose-1-phosphate uridyl transferase. *Proc Natl Acad Sci USA* 1991;**88**:2633–2637.

16. Calderon FR, Pharsalker AR, Crockett DK, *et al.* Mutation database for the galactose-1-phosphate uridyltransferase (*GALT*) gene. *Hum Mutat* 2007;**28**: 939–943.

17. Tyfield L, Reichardt J, Fridovich-Keil J, *et al.* Classical galactosemia and mutations at the galactose-1-phosphate uridyl transferase (*GALT*) gene. *Hum Mutat* 1999;**13**:417–430.

18. Wang BB, Xu YK, Ng WG, *et al.* Molecular and biochemical basis of galactosemia. *Mol Genet Metab* 1998;**63**:263–269.

19. Reichardt JK, Levy HL, Woo SL. Molecular characterization of two galactosemia mutations and one polymorphism: implications for structure–function analysis of human galactose-1-phosphate uridyltransferase. *Biochemistry* 1992;**31**:5430–5433.

20. Belman AL, Moshe SL, Zimmerman RD. Computed tomographic demonstration of cerebral edema in a child with galactosemia. *Pediatrics* 1986;**78**:606–609.

21. Levy HL, Sepe SJ, Shih VE, *et al.* Sepsis due to *Escherichia coli* in neonates with galactosemia. *N Engl J Med* 1977;**297**:823–825.

22. Litchfield WJ, Wells WW. Effects of galactose on free radical reactions of polymorphonuclear leukocytes. *Arch Biochem Biophys* 1978;**188**:26–30.

23. Segal S, Blair A, Roth H. The metabolism of galactose by patients with congenital galactosemia. *Am J Med* 1965;**38**:62–70.

24. Segal S. Disorders of galactose metabolism. In Stanbury JB, Wyngaarden JB, Frederickson DS (eds.) *The Metabolic Basis of Inherited Disease*, 6th edn. New York: McGraw-Hill, 1989, pp. 453–480.

25. Sidbury JB Jr. The role of galactose-1-phosphate in the pathogenesis of galactosemia. In Gardner LE (ed.) *Molecular Genetics and Human Disease*. Springfield, IL: Charles C Thomas, 1960, p. 61.

26. Tada K. Glycogenesis and glycolysis in the liver from congenital galactosemia. *Tohoku J Exp Med* 1964;**82**:168–171.

27. Keppler D, Decker K. Studies on the mechanisms of galactosamine hepatitis: accumulation of galactosamine-1-phosphate and its inhibition of UDP-glucose pyrophosphorylase. *Eur J Biochem* 1969;**10**:219–225.

28. Quan-Ma R, Wells W. The distribution of galactitol in tissues of rats fed galactose. *Biochem Biophys Res Commun* 1965;**20**:486–490.

29. Schwarz V. The value of galactose phosphate determinations in the treatment of galactosemia. *Arch Dis Child* 1960;**35**:428–432.

30. Thier S, Fox M, Rosenberg L, *et al.* Hexose inhibition of amino acid uptake in the rat kidney cortex slice. *Biochim Biophys Acta* 1964;**93**:106–115.

31. Saunders S, Isselbacher KJ. Inhibition of intestinal amino acid transport by hexoses. *Biochim Biophys Acta* 1965;**102**:397–409.

32. van Heyningen R. Formation of polyols by the lens of the rat with "sugar" cataract. *Nature* 1959;**184**: 194–195.

33. Kinoshita JH, Dvornik D, Krami M, *et al.* The effect of aldose reductase inhibitor on the galactose-exposed rabbit lens. *Biochim Biophys Acta* 1968;**158**:472–475.

34. Dische Z, Zelmenis G, Youlous J. Studies on protein and protein synthesis during the development of galactose cataract. *Am J Ophthalmol* 1957;**44**:332–340.

35. Kinoshita JH, Merola LO, Tung B. Changes in cation permeability in the galactose-exposed rabbit lens. *Exp Eye Res* 1968;**7**:80–90.

36. Granett SE, Kozak LP, McIntyre JP, *et al.* Studies on cerebral energy metabolism during the course of galactose neurotoxicity in chicks. *J Neurochem* 1972;**19**:1659–1670.

37. Malone JI, Wells HJ, Segal S. Galactose toxicity in the chick: hyperosmolality. *Science* 1971;**174**:952–954.

38. Knull IIR, Wells WW. Recovery from galactose-induced neurotoxicity in the chick by the administration of glucose. *J Neurochem* 1973;**20**:415–422.

39. Woolley DW, Gommi BW. Serotonin receptors, IV: specific deficiency of receptors in galactose poisoning and its possible relationship to the idiocy of galactosemia. *Proc Natl Acad Sci USA* 1964;**52**:14–19.

40. Sanders RD, Spencer JB, Epstein MP, *et al.* Biomarkers of ovarian function in girls and women with classic galactosemia. *Fertil Steril* 2009;**92**: 344–351.

41. Badik JR, Castaneda U, Gleaso TJ, *et al.* Ovarian function in Duarte galactosemia. *Fert Steril* 2011;**96**: 469–473.

42. Roe TF, Hallat JG, Donnell GN, *et al.* Childbearing by a galactosemic woman. *J Pediatr* 1971;**78**:1026–1030.

43. Robbins SL, Cotran RS. Diseases of infancy and childhood. In Robbins SL, Cotran RS (eds.) *Pathologic Basis of Disease*, 2nd edn. Philadelphia, PA: Saunders, 1979, p. 582.

44. Smetana HF, Olen E. Hereditary galactose disease. *Am J Clin Pathol* 1962;**38**:3–25.

45. Walker FA, Hsia DY, Slatis HM, *et al.* Galactosemia: a study of twenty-seven kindreds in North America. *Ann Hum Genet* 1962;**25**:287–311.

46. Kirkman HN, Bynum E. Enzymic evidence of a galactosemic trait in parents of galactosemic children. *Ann Hum Genet* 1959;**23**:117–126.

47. Mellman WJ, Tedesco TA, Feige P. Estimation of the gene frequency of the Duarte variant of galactose-1-phosphate uridyl transferase. *Ann Hum Genet* 1968;**32**:1.

48. Brandt NJ. Frequency of heterozygotes for hereditary galactosemia in a normal population. *Acta Genet* 1967;**17**:289.

49. Xu YK, Kaufman FR, Donnell GN, *et al.* Radiochemical assay of minute quantities of galactose-1-phosphate uridyl transferase activity in erythrocytes and leukocytes of galactosemia patients. *Clin Chim Acta* 1995;**235**:125–136.

50. Kliegman RM, Sparks JW. Perinatal galactose metabolism. *J Pediatr* 1985;**107**:831–841.

51. Scriver CR. Population screening: report of a workshop. *Prog Clin Biol Res* 1985;**163B**:89–152.

52. Kleijer WJ, Janse HC, van Diggelen OP, *et al.* First-trimester diagnosis of galactosaemia. *Lancet* 1986;**i**:748.

53. Koch R, Donnell GN, Fishler K, *et al.* Galactosemia. In Kelley VC (ed.) *Practice of Pediatrics*. Hagerstown, MD: Harper & Row, 1979, p. 14.

54. Gross KC, Acosta PB. Fruits and vegetables are a source of galactose: implications in planning the diets of patients with galactosaemia. *J Inherit Metab Dis* 1991;**14**:253–258.

55. Walter JH, Collins JE, Leonard JV. Recommendations for the management of galactosaemia. UK Galactosaemia Steering Group. *Arch Dis Child* 1999;**80**:93–96.

56. Manis FR, Cohn LB, McBride-Chang C, *et al.* A longitudinal study of cognitive functioning in patients with classical galactosaemia, including a cohort treated with oral uridine. *J Inherit Metab Dis* 1997;**20**:549–555.

57. Berry GT. The role of polyols in the pathophysiology of hypergalactosemia. *Eur J Pediatr* 1995;**154** (suppl 2): S53–S64.

58. Boxer MB, Shen M, Tanega C, *et al. Toward improved therapy for classic galactosemia. Probe Reports from the NIH Molecular Libraries Program.* Bethesda, MD: National Center for Biotechnology Information, 2010 (updated 3 March 2011).

59. Schweitzer S, Shin Y, Jakobs C, *et al.* Long-term outcome in 134 patients with galactosaemia. *Eur J Pediatr* 1993;**152**:36–43.

60. Hoffmann B, Wendel U, Schweitzer-Krantz S. Cross-sectional analysis of speech and cognitive performance in 32 patients with classic galactosemia. *J Inherit Metab Dis* 2011;**34**:421–427.

61. Renner C, Razeghi S, Uberall MA, *et al.* Hormone replacement therapy in galactosaemic twins with ovarian failure and severe osteoporosis. *J Inherit Metab Dis* 1999;**22**:194–195.

62. Campbell S, Kulin HE. Transient thyroid binding globulin deficiency with classic galactosemia. *J Pediatr* 1984;**105**:335–336.

63. Hennermann JB, Schadewaldt P, Vetter B, *et al.* Features and outcome of galactokinase deficiency in children diagnosed by newborn screening. *J Inherit Metab Dis* 2011;**34**:399–407.

64. Sangiuolo F, Magnani M, Stambolian D, *et al.* Biochemical characterization of two *GALK1* mutations in patients with galactokinase deficiency. *Hum Mutat* 2004;**23**:396.

65. Gitzelmann R, Haigis E. Appearance of active UDP-galactose 4 β-epimerase in cells cultured from epimerase-deficient persons. *J Inherit Metab Dis* 1978;**1**:41.

66. Sachs B, Sternfeld L, Kraus G. Essential fructosuria: its pathophysiology. *Am J Dis Child* 1974;**63**:252.

67. Steinmann B, Gitzelmann R, Van den Berghe G. Disorders of fructose metabolism. In Scriver C, Beaudet A, Sly W, *et al.* (eds.) *The Metabolic and Molecular Bases of Inherited Disease*, vol 1, 8th edn. New York: McGraw-Hill, 2000, pp. 1489–1520.

68. Chalmers RA, Pratt RTC. Idiosyncrasy to fructose. *Lancet* 1956;**ii**:340.

69. Froesch ER, Prader A, Labhart A, *et al.* [Hereditary fructose intolerance, a congenital metabolic disorder unknown until now.] *Schweiz Med Wochenschr* 1957;**87**:1168–1171.

70. Baker L, Winegrad AI. Fasting hypoglycemia and metabolic acidosis associated with deficiency of hepatic fructose-1,6-diphosphatase activity. *Lancet* 1970;**ii**:13–16.

71. Thorens B. Glucose transporters in the regulation of intestinal, renal, and liver glucose fluxes. *Am J Physiol* 1996;**270**: G541–553.

72. Rottmann WH, Tolan DR, Penhoet EE. Complete amino acid sequence for human aldolase B derived from cDNA and genomic clones. *Proc Natl Acad Sci USA* 1984;**81**:2738–2742.

73. Lench NJ, Telford EA, Andersen SE, *et al.* An EST and STS-based YAC contig map of human chromosome 9q22.3. *Genomics* 1996;**38**:199–205.

74. Chambers RA, Pratt RTC. Idiosyncrasy to fructose. *Lancet* 1956;**ii**:340.

75. Froesch VER, Prader A, Labhart A, *et al.* Die hereditare Fructoseintoleranz, eine bisher nicht bekannte kongenitale Stoffwechselstorung. *Schweiz Med Wochenschr* 1957;**87**:1168–1171.

76. Hers HG, Joassin G. Anomaly of hepatic aldolase in intolerance to fructose.] *Enzymol Biol Clin* 1961;**1**: 4–14.

77. Penhoet EE, Kochman M, Rutter WJ. Isolation of fructose diphosphate aldolases A, B and C. *Biochemistry* 1969;**8**:4391–4395.

78. Henry I, Gallano P, Besmond C, *et al.* The structural gene for aldolase B (ALDB) maps to 9q13-32. *Ann Hum Genet* 1985;**49**:173–180.

79. Tolan DR, Penhoet EE. Characterization of the human aldolase B gene. *Mol Biol Med* 1986;**3**:245–264.

80. Cross NC, Tolan DR, Cox TM. Catalytic deficiency of human aldolase B in hereditary fructose intolerance caused by a common missense mutation. *Cell* 1988;**53**:881–885.

81. Cross NC, de Franchis R, Sebastio G, *et al.* Molecular analysis of aldolase B genes in hereditary fructose intolerance. *Lancet* 1990;**335**: 306–309.

82. Sebastio G, de Franchis R, Strisciuglio P, *et al.* Aldolase B mutations in Italian families affected by hereditary fructose intolerance. *J Med Genet* 1991;**28**:241–243.

83. Tolan DR, Brooks CC. Molecular analysis of common aldolase B alleles for hereditary fructose intolerance in North Americans. *Biochem Med Metab Biol* 1992;**48**:19–25.

84. Rellos P, Sygusch J, Cox TM. Expression, purification, and characterization of natural mutants of human aldolase B. Role of quaternary structure in catalysis. *J Biol Chem* 2000;**275**:1145–1151.

85. Coffee EM, Tolan DR. Mutations in the promoter region of the aldolase B gene that cause hereditary fructose intolerance. *J Inherit Metab Dis* 2010;**33**:715–725.

86. Cornblath M, Rosenthal IM, Reisner SH, *et al.* Hereditary fructose intolerance. *N Engl J Med* 1963;**269**:1271–1278.

87. Odievre M, Gentil C, Gautier M, *et al.* Hereditary fructose intolerance in childhood. Diagnosis, management, and course in 55 patients. *Am J Dis Child* 1978;**132**:605–608.

88. Schulte MJ, Widukind L. Fatal sorbitol infusion in a patient with fructose-sorbitol intolerance. *Lancet* 1977;**2**:188.

89. Morris RC, Jun, Ueki I, *et al.* Absence of renal fructose-1-phosphate aldolase activity in hereditary fructose intolerance. *Nature* 1967;**214**:920–921.

90. Perheentupa J, Pitkanen E, Nikkila EA, *et al.* Hereditary fructose intolerance. A clinical study of four cases. *Ann Paediatr Fenn* 1962;**8**:221–235.

91. Gurtler B, Leuthardt F. [Heterogeneity of aldolases.] *Helv Chim Acta*1970;**53**:654–658.

92. Rutter WJ, Richards OC, Woodfin BM. Comparative studies of liver and muscle aldolase. I. Effect of carboxypeptidase on catalytic activity. *J Biol Chem* 1961;**236**:3193–3197.

93. Nordmann Y, Shapira F, Dreyfus JC. A structurally modified aldolase in fructose intolerance: immunologic and kinetic evidence. *Biochem Biophys Res Commun* 1968;**31**:884.

94. Esposito G, Vitagliano L, Santamaria R, *et al.* Structural and functional analysis of aldolase B mutants related to hereditary fructose intolerance. *FEBS J* 2002;**531**:152–156.

95. Froesch ER, Prader A, Wolf HP, *et al.* [Hereditary fructose intolerance.] *Helv Paediatr Acta* 1959;**14**:99 112.

96. Froesch ER. Essential fructosuria, hereditary fructose intolerance, and fructose-1,6-diphosphatase deficiency. In Stanbury JB, Wyngaarden JB, Fredrickson DS (eds.) *The Metabolic Basis of Inherited Disease*, 4th edn. New York: McGraw-Hill, 1978, p. 131.

97. van Den Berg G, Hue L, Hers HG. Effect of administration of fructose on glycolytic action of glucagon. An investigation of the pathogeny of hereditary fructose intolerance. *Biochem J* 1973;**134**:637.

98. Raivio KO, Kekomaki MP, Maenpaa PH. Depletion of liver adenine nucleotides induced by D-fructose. Dose-dependence and specificity of the fructose effect. *Biochem Pharmacol* 1969;**18**:2615–2624.

99. Dormandy TL, Porter RJ. Familial fructose and galactose intolerance. *Lancet* 1961;**i**:1189–1194.

100. Turner RC, Spathis GS, Nabarro JD, *et al.* Familial fructose and galactose intolerance. *Lancet* 1972;**ii**:872.

101. Schwartz R, Gamsu H, Mulligan PB, *et al.* Transient intolerance to exogenous fructose in the newborn. *J Clin Invest* 1964;**43**:333–340.

102. Dubois R, Loeb H, Ooms HA, *et al.* [Study of a case of functional hypoglycemia caused by intolerance to fructose.] *Helv Paediatr Acta* 1961;**16**:90–96.

103. Levin B, Oberholzer VG, Snodgrass GJ, *et al.* Fructosaemia. An inborn error of fructose metabolism. *Arch Dis Child* 1963;**38**:220–230.

104. Lelong M, Alagille D, Gentil C, *et al.* Cirrhose hepatique et tubulopathie par absence congenitale de l'aldolase hepatique: intolerance hereditaire au fructose. *Bull Soc Med Hop* 1962;**113**:58.

105. Nikkila EA, Perheentupa J. Non-esterified fatty acids and fatty liver in hereditary fructose intolerance. *Lancet* 1962;**ii**:1280.

106. Morris RC Jr. An experimental renal acidification defect in patients with hereditary fructose intolerance. II. Its distinction from classic renal tubular acidosis; its resemblance to the renal acidification defect associated with the Fanconi syndrome of children with cystinosis. *J Clin Invest* 1968;**47**:1648–1663.

107. Melancon SB, Khachadurian AK, Nadler HL, *et al.* Metabolic and biochemical studies in fructose 1,6-diphosphatase deficiency. *J Pediatr* 1973;**82**:650–657.

108. Kikawa Y, Shin YS, Inuzuka M, *et al.* Diagnosis of fructose-1,6-bisphosphatase deficiency using cultured lymphocyte fraction: a secure and noninvasive alternative to liver biopsy. *J Inherit Metab Dis* 2002;**25**:41–46.

109. Elpeg ON. The molecular background of glycogen metabolism disorders. *J Pediatr Endocrinol Metab* 1999;**12**:263–379.

110. Hers HG. The control of glycogen metabolism in the liver. *Ann Rev Biochem* 1976;**45**:167–189.

111. von Gierke E. Glykogenspeicherkrankheit der Leber und Nieren [Hepato-nephromegalia glykogenica]. *Beitr Pathol Anat* 1929;**82**:497–513.

112. Cori GT, Cori CF. Glucose-6-phosphatase of the liver in glycogen storage disease. *J Biol Chem* 1952;**199**:661–667.

113. Cori GT. Glycogen structure and enzyme deficiencies in glycogen storage disease. *Harvey Lect* 1953;**48**:145–171.

114. Senior B, Loridan, L. Studies of liver glycogenoses, with particular reference to the metabolism of intravenously administered glycerol. *N Engl J Med* 1968;**279**:958–965.

115. Chen SY, Pan CJ, Nandigama K, *et al.* The glucose-6-phosphate transporter is a phosphate-linked antiporter deficient in glycogen storage disease type Ib and Ic. *FASEB* 2008;**22**:2206–2213.

116. Boyer TD, Manns MP, Sanyal AJ. *Zakim and Boyer's Hepatology*, 6th edn. St. Louis, MO: Saunders-Elsevier, 2011, ch. 66.

117. Shelly LL, Lei KJ, Pan CJ, *et al.* Isolation of the gene for murine glucose-6-phosphatase, the enzyme deficient in glycogen storage disease type 1A. *J Biol Chem* 1993;**268**:21482–21485.

118. Lei KJ, Pan CJ, Shelly LL, *et al.* Identification of mutations in the gene for glucose-6-phosphatase, the enzyme deficient in glycogen storage disease type 1a. *J Clin Invest* 1994;**93**:1994–1999.

119. Chou JY and Masfield B. Mutations in the glucose 6 phosphate (G6PC) gene that cause type 1a glycogen storage disease. *Hum Mutat* 2008;**29**:921–930.

120. Stroppiano M, Regis S, DiRocco M, *et al.* Mutations in the glucose-6-phosphatase gene of 53 Italian patients

with glycogen storage disease type Ia. *J Inherit Metab Dis* 1999;**22**:43–49.

121. Melis D, Pivonello R, Parenti G, et al. The growth hormone-insulin-like growth factor axis in glycogen storage disease type 1: evidence of different growth patterns and insulin-like growth factor levels in patients with glycogen storage disease type 1a and 1b. *J Pediatr* 2010;**156**;663–670.

122. Hers H, Van Hoof F, de Barsy T. glycogen storage disease. In Stanbury JB, Wyngaarden JB, Frederickson DS (eds.) *The Metabolic Basis of Inherited Disease*, 6th edn. New York: McGraw-Hill, 1989, pp. 425–452.

123. Ghishan FK, Greene HL. Inborn errors of metabolism that cause permanent injury to the liver. In Zakim D, Boyer T (eds.) *Hepatology: A Textbook of Liver Disease*, 2nd edn, vol 49. Philadelphia, PA: Saunders, 1990, pp. 1300–1348.

124. Fernandes J, Berger R, Smit GPA. Lactate as a cerebral metabolic fuel for glucose-6-phosphatase deficient children. *Pediatr Res* 1984;**18**:335–339.

125. Coire CI, Qizilbash AH, Castelli MF. Hepatic adenomata in type Ia glycogen storage disease. *Arch Pathol Lab Med* 1987;**111**:166–169.

126. Chen Y-T, Coleman RA, Sheinman JI, et al. Renal disease in type I glycogen storage disease. *N Engl J Med* 1988;**318**:7–11.

127. Slonim AE, Lacy WW, Terry A, et al. Nocturnal intragastric therapy in type I glycogen storage disease: effect on hormonal and amino acid metabolism. *Metabolism* 1979;**28**:707–715.

128. Havel RJ, Balasse EO, Williams HE, et al. Splanchnic metabolism in von Gierke's disease (glycogenesis type I). *Trans Assoc Am Phys* 1969;**82**:305–323.

129. Schwenk WF, Haymond MW. Optimal rate of enteral glucose administration in children with glycogen storage disease type I. *N Engl J Med* 1986;**314**:682–685.

130. Sadeghi-Nejad A, Presente E, Binkiewicz A, et al. Studies in type I glycogenesis of the liver. The genesis and disposition of lactate. *J Pediatr* 1974;**85**:49–54.

131. Jakovcic S, Khachadurian AK, Hsia DY. The hyperlipidemia in glycogen storage disease. *J Lab Clin Med* 1966;**68**:769–779.

132. Forget PP, Fernandes J, Begemann PH. Triglyceride clearing in glycogen storage disease. *Pediatr Res* 1974;**8**:114–119.

133. Fine RN, Strauss J, Donnell GN. Hyperuricemia in glycogen-storage disease type 1. *Am J Dis Child* 1966;**112**:572–576.

134. Jakovcic S, Sorensen LB. Studies of uric acid metabolism in glycogen storage disease associated with gouty arthritis. *Arthritis Rheum* 1967;**10**:129–134.

135. Greene ML, Seegmiller JE. Elevated erythrocyte phosphoribosylpyrophosphate in X-linked uric aciduria: importance of PRPP concentration in regulation of human purine biosynthesis. *J Clin Invest* 1969;**48**:**32a**.

136. Brosh S, Boer P, Kupfer B, et al. De novo synthesis of purine nucleotides in human peripheral blood leukocytes. Excessive activity of the pathway in hypoxanthine-guanine phosphoribosyltransferase deficiency. *J Clin Invest* 1976;**58**:289–297.

137. Holmes EW, McDonald JA, McCord JM, et al. Human glutamine phosphoribosylpyrophosphate amidotransferase. Kinetic and regulatory properties. *J Biol Chem* 1973;**248**:144–150.

138. Greene HL, Wilson FA, Hefferan P, et al. ATP depletion, a possible role in the pathogenesis of hyperuricemia in glycogen storage disease type I. *J Clin Invest* 1978;**62**:321–328.

139. Roe TF, Kogut MD. The pathogenesis of hyperuricemia in glycogen storage disease, type I. *Pediatr Res* 1977;**11**:664–669.

140. Corby DG, Putnam CW, Greene HL. Impaired platelet function in glucose-6-phosphatase deficiency. *J Pediatr* 1974;**85**:71–76.

141. Cooper RA. Abnormalities of cell-membrane fluidity in the pathogenesis of disease. *N Engl J Med* 1977;**297**:371–377.

142. Roe TF, Kogut MD, Buckingham BA, et al. Hepatic tumors in glycogen-storage disease type I. *Pediatr Res* 1979;**13**:931.

143. Parker PH, Burr I, Slonim AE, et al. Regression of hepatic adenomas in type Ia glycogen storage disease with dietary therapy. *Gastroenterology* 1987;**81**:534–536.

144. Wang DQ, Fiske LM, Carreras CT et al. Natural history of hepatocellular adenoma formation in glycogen storage disease type 1. *J Pediatr* 2011;**159**:442–446.

145. Bannasch P, Hacker HJ, Klimek F, et al. Hepatocellular glycogenosis and related pattern of enzymatic changes during hepatocarcinogenesis. *Adv Enzyme Regul* 1984;**22**:97–121.

146. Kishnani PS, Chuang TP, Bali D, et al. Chromosomal and genetic alterations in human hepatocellular adenomas associated with type Ia glycogen storage disease. *Hum Mol Genet* 2009;**18**:4781–4790.

147. McAdams AJ, Hug G, Bove KE. Glycogen storage disease, types I to X: criteria for morphologic diagnosis. *Hum Pathol* 1974;**5**:463–487.

148. Folkman J, Philippart A, Tze WJ, et al. Portacaval shunt for glycogen storage disease: value of prolonged intravenous hyperalimentation before surgery. *Surgery* 1972;**72**:306–314.

149. Riddell AG, Davies RP, Clark AD. Portacaval transposition in the treatment of glycogen-storage disease. *Lancet* 1966;**ii**:1146–1148.

150. Burr IM, O'Neill JA, Karzon DT, et al. Comparison of the effects of total parenteral nutrition, continuous intragastric feeding, and portacaval shunt on a patient with type I glycogen storage disease. *J Pediatr* 1974;**85**:792–795.

151. Greene HL, Slonim AE, Burr IM. Type I glycogen storage disease: a metabolic basis for advances in treatment. *Adv Pediatr* 1979;**26**:63–92.

152. Chen YT, Cornblath M, Sidbury JB. Cornstarch therapy in type I glycogen-storage disease. *N Engl J Med* 1984;**310**:171–175.

153. Collins JE, Leonard JV. The dietary management of inborn errors of metabolism. *Hum Nutr Appl Nutr* 1985;**39**:255–272.

154. Bahttacharya K, Orton RC, Qi X, et al. A novel starch for the treatment of glycogen storage disease. *J Inherit Med Dis* 2007;**30**:350–357.

155. Greene HL, Slonim AE, Burr IM, et al. Type I glycogen storage disease: five years of management with nocturnal intragastric feeding. *J Pediatr* 1980;**96**:590–595.

156. Chen YT, Coleman RA, Scheinman JI, et al. Renal disease in type I glycogen

storage disease. *N Engl J Med* 1988;**318**:7–11.

157. Baker L, Dahlem S, Goldfarb S, *et al.* Hyperfiltration and renal disease in glycogen storage disease, type I. *Kidney Int* 1989;**35**:1345–1350.

158. Senior B, Loridan L. Studies of liver glycogenoses, with particular reference to the metabolism of intravenously administered glycerol. *N Engl J Med* 1968;**279**:958–965.

159. Arion WJ, Wallin BK, Lange AJ, *et al.* On the involvement of a glucose 6-phosphate transport system in the function of microsomal glucose 6-phosphatase. *Mol Cell Biochem* 1975;**6**:75–83.

160. Skaug WA, Warford LL, Figueroa JM, *et al.* Glycogenesis type IB: possible membrane transport defect. *South Med J* 1981;**74**:761–764.

161. Zakim D, Edmondson DE. The role of the membrane in the regulation of activity of microsomal glucose-6-phosphatase. *J Biol Chem* 1982;**257**:1145–1148.

162. Hiraiwa H, Pan CJ, Lin B, *et al.* Inactivation of the glucose 6-phosphate transporter causes glycogen storage disease type 1b. *J Biol Chem* 1999;**274**:5532–5536.

163. Annabi B, Hiraiwa H, Mansfield BC, *et al.* The gene for glycogen-storage disease type 1b maps to chromosome 11q23. *Am J Hum Genet* 1998;**62**: 400–405.

164. Chen LY, Pan CJ, Shieh JJ, *et al.* Structure–function analysis of the glucose-6-phosphate transporter deficient in glycogen storage disease type Ib. *Hum Mol Genet* 2002;**11**: 3199–3207.

165. Elpeleg ON. The molecular background of glycogen metabolism disorders. *J Pediatr Endocrinol Metab* 1999;**12**:363–379.

166. Corbeel L, Hue L, Lederer B, *et al.* Clinical and biochemical findings before and after portacaval shunt in a girl with type Ib glycogen storage disease. *Pediatr Res* 1981;**15**:58–61.

167. Visser G, de Jager W, Verhagen LP, *et al.* Survival but not maturation is affected in neutrophil progenitors from GSD-1b patients. *J Inherit Metab Dis* 2012;**35**:287–300.

168. Ishiguro A, Nakahata T, Shimbo T, *et al.* Improvement of neutropenia and neutrophil dysfunction by granulocyte colony-stimulating factor in a patient with glycogen storage disease type Ib. *Eur J Pediatr* 1993;**152**:18–20.

169. Melis D, Della casa R, Parini R, *et al.* Vitamin E supplementation improves neutropenia and reduces the frequency of infections in patients with glycogen storage disease type 1b. *Eur J Pediatr* 2009;**168**:1069–1074.

170. Forbes GB. Glycogen storage disease: report of a case with abnormal glycogen structure in liver and skeletal muscle. *J Pediatr* 1953;**42**:645–653.

171. Illingworth B, Cori GT. Structure of glycogens and amylopectins: III. Normal and abnormal human glycogen. *J Biol Chem* 1952;**199**: 653–660.

172. Chen Y-T, He J-K, Ding J-H, *et al.* Glycogen debranching enzyme: purification, antibody characterization, and immunoblot analyses of type III glycogen storage disease. *Am J Hum Genet* 1987;**41**:1002–1015.

173. van Hoof F, Hers HG. The subgroups of type III glycogenosis. *Eur J Biochem* 1967;**2**:265–270.

174. Ding J-H, de Barsy T, Brown BI, *et al.* Immunoblot analyses of glycogen debranching enzyme in different subtypes of glycogen storage disease type III. *J Pediatr* 1990;**116**:95–100.

175. Bao Y, Dawson TL, Jr, Chen YT. Human glycogen debranching enzyme gene (*AGL*): complete structural organization and characterization of the 5′ flanking region. *Genomics* 1996;**38**:155–165.

176. Yang-Feng TL, Zheng K, Yu J, *et al.* Assignment of the human glycogen debrancher gene to chromosome 1p21. *Genomics* 1992;**13**:931–934.

177. Yang BZ, Ding JH, Enghild JJ, *et al.* Molecular cloning and nucleotide sequence of cDNA encoding human muscle glycogen debranching enzyme. *J Biol Chem* 1992;**267**:9294–9299.

178. Bao Y, Yang BZ, Dawson TL Jr., *et al.* Isolation and nucleotide sequence of human liver glycogen debranching enzyme mRNA: identification of multiple tissue-specific isoforms. *Gene* 1997;**197**:389–398.

179. Okubo M, Kanda F, Horinishi A, *et al.* Glycogen storage disease type IIIa: first report of a causative missense mutation (G1448R) of the glycogen debranching enzyme gene found in a homozygous patient. *Hum Mutat* 1999;**14**:542–543.

180. Shen J, Bao Y, Liu HM, *et al.* Mutations in exon 3 of the glycogen debranching enzyme gene are associated with glycogen storage disease type III that is differentially expressed in liver and muscle. *J Clin Invest* 1996;**98**: 352–357.

181. Shen JJ, Chen YT. Molecular characterization of glycogen storage disease type III. *Curr Mol Med* 2002;**2**:167–175.

182. Goldstein JL, Austin SL, Boyette K, *et al.* Molecular analysis of the *AGL* gene: identification of 25 novel mutations and evidence of genetic heterogeneity in patients with glycogen storage disease type III. *Genet med* 2010;**12**:424–430.

183. van Creveld S, Huijing F. Glycogen storage disease: biochemical and clinical data in sixteen cases. *Am J Med* 1965;**38**:554–561.

184. Ugawa Y, Inoue K, Takemura T, *et al.* Accumulation of glycogen in peripheral nerve axons in adult-onset Type III glycogenosis. *Ann Neurol* 1986;**19**: 294–297.

185. Alagille D, Odievre M. Inborn errors of metabolism. In Alagille D, Odievre M (eds.) *Liver and Biliary Tract Disease in Children.* New York: Wiley, 1979, pp. 196–242.

186. Hug G, Krill CE Jr, Perrin EV, *et al.* Cori's disease (amylo-1,6-glucosidase deficiency): report of a case in a Negro child. *N Engl J Med* 1963;**268**:113–120.

187. Slonim AE, Terry AB, Moran R, *et al.* Differing food consumption for nocturnal intragastric therapy in types I and III glycogen storage disease. *Pediatr Res* 1978;**12**:512–894.

188. Borowitz SM, Greene HL. Cornstarch therapy in a patient with type III glycogen storage disease. *J Pediatr Gastroenterol Nutr* 1987;**6**:631–634.

189. Valayannopoulos V, Bajolle F, Arnoux JB, *et al.* Successful treatment of severe cardiomyopathy in glycogen storage disease type III with DL-3-hydroxybutyrate, ketogenic and high protein diet. *Pediatr Res* 2011;**70**: 638–641.

190. Anderson DH. Studies on glycogen disease with report of a case in which the glycogen was abnormal. In Ajjar VA (ed.) *Carbohydrate Metabolism.*

Baltimore, MD: Johns Hopkins University Press, 1952, p. 28.

191. Illingworth B, Cori GT. Structure of glycogens and amylopectins. III. Normal and abnormal human glycogen. *J Biol Chem* 1952;**199**: 653–660.

192. Brown BI, Brown DH. Lack of an alpha-1,4-glucan: alpha-1,4-glucan 6-glycosyl transferase in a case of type IV glycogenosis. *Proc Natl Acad Sci USA* 1966;**56**:725–729.

193. Andersen DH. Familial cirrhosis of the liver with storage of abnormal glycogen. *Lab Invest* 1956;**5**:11–20.

194. Thon VJ, Khalil M, Cannon JF. Isolation of human glycogen branching enzyme cDNAs by screening complementation in yeast. *J Biol Chem* 1993;**268**:7509–7513.

195. Bao Y, Kishnani P, Wu J-Y, *et al.* Hepatic and neuromuscular forms of glycogen storage disease type IV caused by mutations in the same glycogen-branching enzyme gene. *J Clin Invest* 1996;**97**:941–948.

196. Li SC, Hwu WL, Lin JL, *et al.* Association of the congenital neuromuscular form of glycogen storage disease type IV with a large deletion and recurrent frameshift mutation. *J Child Neurol* 2012;**27**: 204–208.

197. Shen J, Liu HM, McConkie-Rosell A, *et al.* Prenatal diagnosis of glycogen storage disease type IV using PCR-based DNA mutation analysis. *Prenat Diagn* 1999;**9**:837–839.

198. Maruyama K, *et al.* Congenital form of glycogen storage disease type IV: a case report and a review of the literature. *Pediatr Int* 2004:**46**:474–477.

199. Schochet SS, McCormick WF, Zellweger H. Type IV glycogenosis (amylopectinosis): light and electron microscopic observations. *Arch Pathol* 1970;**90**:354–363.

200. Ferguson IT, Mahon M, Cumming WJK. An adult case of Andersen's disease: type IV glycogenosis. *J Neurol Sci* 1983;**60**:337–351.

201. Das BB, *et al.* Amylopectinosis disease isolated to the heart with normal glycogen branching enzyme activity and gene sequence. *Pediatr Transplant* 2005:**9**:261–265.

202. Bruno C, Servidei S, Shanske G, *et al.* Glycogen branching enzyme deficiency in adult polyglucosan body disease. *Ann Neurol* 1993;**33**:88–93.

Copper metabolism and copper storage disorders

28

Ronald J. Sokol

Introduction

The accumulation of excess copper in the liver is toxic in humans and other mammals and may lead to hepatitis, fulminant hepatic failure, cirrhosis, and death. Of the several human copper storage diseases that have been described, the molecular basis of only Wilson disease is understood with the discovery of the Wilson disease gene (*ATP7B*) in 1993. The therapeutic success using oral copper-chelating agents and zinc therapy make Wilson disease one of the few treatable genetic metabolic liver diseases. In a fulminant presentation or advanced disease at diagnosis, copper chelation is ineffective and liver transplantation is life-saving. Indian Childhood Cirrhosis (ICC) has been defined as a copper-storage disorder affecting children primarily of Indian descent and evolving to cirrhosis and death before age 3 to 4 years without treatment. Children from North America, Asia, Austria, Germany, and other countries have been described with a similar condition, which has been termed *idiopathic copper toxicosis* (ICT). This chapter reviews copper physiology and mechanisms of copper

hepatotoxicity, followed by descriptions of the major copper-storage diseases of childhood.

Copper absorption and metabolism

The normal adult Western diet contains 2–5 mg per day of copper. The efficiency of copper absorption in adults ranges from 40 to 60% [1], with higher absorption at lower intakes. (Figure 28.1) [2]. Foods containing high amounts of copper include unprocessed wheat, dried beans, peas, shellfish (particularly oysters), chocolate, liver, and kidney. The estimated daily copper requirement for adults is approximately 0.9–1.7 mg [1]. Dietary and chemical factors may impair copper absorption. For example, excess intake of zinc, cadmium, and ascorbic acid can interfere with copper bioavailability because of the formation of insoluble copper salts at an alkaline pH [3]. A vegetarian diet, as well as ingested raw meat, have been associated with decreased copper absorption. Gastrointestinal secretions (e.g. saliva, gastric juice, duodenal secretions) form low-molecular-weight soluble complexes that aid in the

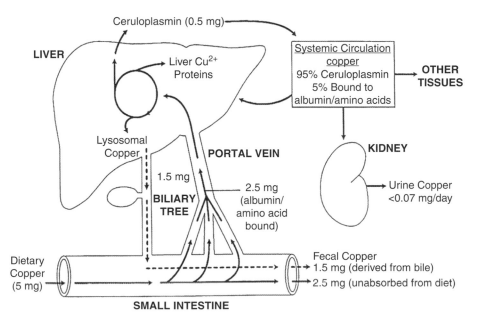

Figure 28.1 Copper balance in humans. Relative amounts of copper arising from 5 mg of daily dietary intake in adult. (Adapted from Sokol, 1992 [2].)

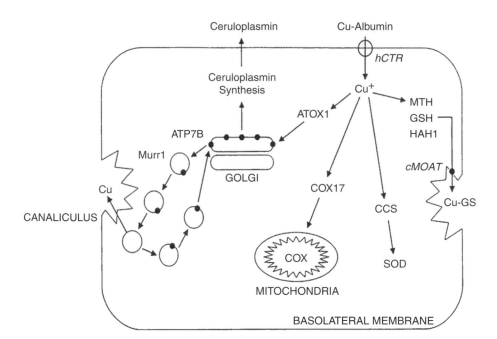

Figure 28.2 Copper metabolism in the hepatocyte. MTH, metallothionein; CCS, Copper chaperone of SOD antibody; SOD, superoxide dismutase; COX, cytochrome *c* oxidase; GSH, glutathione; cMOAT, canalicular multiple organic anion transporter (MRP2). (Adapted from Bacon and Schilsky, 1999 [4].)

absorption of copper by preventing the precipitation of copper salts [3], and certain digestive products (e.g. L-amino acids) facilitate copper absorption. It is the balance between these exogenous and endogenous factors that regulate intestinal absorption of copper. Because dietary intake and absorption generally exceed metabolic needs, a large amount of ingested copper is eventually excreted in bile (see below).

Within the small intestine epithelial cells, absorbed copper is bound to the protein metallothionein or is complexed to amino acids and transported into the portal venous circulation by the copper-transporting ATPase ATP7A. Although enterocyte metallothionein also binds zinc and cadmium, copper is bound most avidly. Because zinc stimulates metallothionein synthesis, it has been shown that increased dietary zinc may impair copper absorption by causing retention of copper in the enterocyte, which is then excreted in the feces following desquamation of the enterocyte. This mechanism forms the basis for oral zinc therapy in Wilson disease (see below).

Once absorbed into the portal venous blood, copper is complexed to albumin and amino acids in equilibrium with a very small fraction of free ionic copper. Copper is then transported into hepatocytes by a specific membrane transport system for albumin-bound copper, the human copper transporter 1 (HCTR1) (Figure 28.2) [1,4]. Among the amino acids present in blood, the binding affinities for copper in decreasing order are histidine, threonine, glutamine, and asparagine. This amino acid-bound copper is most likely the form in which copper is transported to various tissues other than the liver. Within 3 hours of absorption, 60–90% of copper has been transported to and taken up by hepatocytes where copper initially interacts with low-molecular-weight ligands, such as cytosolic metallothionein, glutathione, and HAH1 [5]. The

function of these proteins is to store copper for subsequent metabolic needs of the hepatocyte, to bind and detoxify excess copper, and to provide copper to chaperones that assist in incorporating it into essential proteins that are secreted (e.g. ceruloplasmin) or assist in copper excretion in bile (P-type ATPase). Important hepatic copper metalloenzymes include superoxide dismutase (32 kDa), mitochondrial monoamine oxidase (195 kDa), cytochrome *c* oxidase (290 kDa), and ceruloplasmin. In other tissues, copper is incorporated into tyrosinase and lysyl oxidase.

The *ATP7B* gene (80 kb) is located on chromosome 13, contains 21 exons, and is highly expressed in liver and kidney with lower levels of expression in lung, placenta, and other tissues. Splicing variants of the gene may be present in brain. The encoded protein, ATP7B, is a P-type cation-transporting ATPase, homologous to the Menkes disease gene product (ATP7A) and the copper-transporting ATPase (copA) in copper-resistant *Enterococcus hirae*. The protein structure (Figure 28.3) includes domains for copper binding (six sites), ATP-binding, a phosphorylation region, a transmembrane cation channel, and a transduction domain. Within one membrane-spanning domain is a sequence of amino acids (cysteine–proline–cysteine) that is characteristic of all metal-transporting ATPases. ATP7B is located in the trans-Golgi complex of the hepatocyte and appears necessary for transport of copper into vesicles bound for lysosomes and eventual excretion into the bile canaliculus (Figure 28.2). This process represents the main homeostatic mechanism for copper metabolism in humans. Copper conjugated to glutathione is a minor pathway of copper excretion into bile. ATP7B also makes copper available for the synthesis of ceruloplasmin, possibly within the Golgi apparatus as well. When ATP7B is mutated in Wilson disease, both copper secretion into bile and

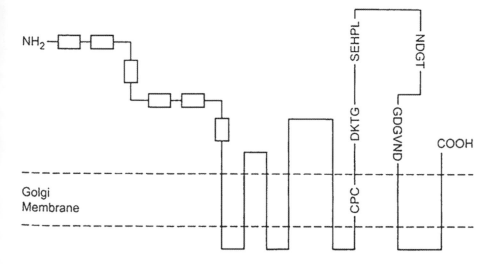

Figure 28.3 Structural features of *ATP7B*, the Wilson disease gene, include six cysteine-rich metal-binding regions (open boxes) near the N-terminus in the cytosol of the cell; eight transmembrane domains, one of which includes the cysteine–proline–cysteine (CPC) sequence common to other metal transporters; DKTG phosphatase and phosphorylation domain; NDGT ATP-binding domain; and the hinge region (GDGVND). (Adapted from Bacon and Schilsky, 1999 [4] and Petrukhin *et al.*, 1994 [6].)

copper incorporation into ceruloplasmin are impaired, resulting in copper accumulation within the hepatocyte.

Metallochaperones play an essential key role in copper homeostasis in mammalian (and yeast) cells. These proteins control delivery of copper to specific intracellular targets, in which copper is incorporated into synthesis of critical enzymes and proteins [7]. Three mammalian copper chaperones (Figure 28.2) have been well characterized: human CCS (homologous to yeast Lys7p), which delivers copper to copper/zinc superoxide dismutase in cytosol; human COX17 (homologous to yeast Cox17p), which delivers copper to cytochrome *c* oxidase in mitochondria [8]; and human ATOX1/HAH1 (homologous to yeast Atx1p), which delivers copper to the secretory pathway for incorporation into the copper transport protein ATP7B (homologous to yeast Ccc2p) in the Golgi compartment [9]. ATX1P has also been found to function as an antioxidant.

Ceruloplasmin, a blue-colored copper-containing α$_2$-globulin (134 kDa), is synthesized mainly by hepatocytes and secreted into the systemic circulation [10]. Its major role as a ferroxidase is to promote iron mobilization from tissues by oxidizing ferrous iron for transfer into transferrin. Consequently, patients homozygous for mutations in *CP*, the gene encoding ceruloplasmin gene (aceruloplasminemia), do not have copper storage but rather develop iron overload in the liver, pancreas, and brain [11]. Ceruloplasmin may also transport copper to other tissues and act as an oxidase toward aromatic amines (e.g. epinephrine, 5-hydroxytryptamine, and dopamine), phenols, cystine, ferrous ion, and ascorbic acid; or as an antioxidant [12]. The normal plasma concentration of ceruloplasmin in older children and adults, measured by the oxidase enzymatic assay, is 20–45 mg/dL and copper is 70–150 μg/dL. In the human newborn, plasma ceruloplasmin is 1.8–13.1 mg/dL and copper varies between 12 and 26 μg/dL [13], increasing to adult levels by age 2 years. This is in contrast to the parturient mother, whose levels are 40–89 mg/dL and 118–302 μg/dL, respectively [13]. Non-ceruloplasmin-bound

copper does not differ between newborn and mother and ranges between 5 and 15 μg/dL. It should be noted that the classic assays for ceruloplasmin were based on its oxidase activity in vitro and, hence, depended on the presence of copper in the molecule [14]. More recent immunoassays detect apoceruloplasmin (which does not contain copper) as well as holoceruloplasmin (which contains copper) and may, therefore, give higher serum values of ceruloplasmin in patients with Wilson disease than does the oxidase method, which only detects holoceruloplasmin [14]. As a result, many patients with Wilson disease may now have low normal plasma concentrations of ceruloplasmin measured by the immunoassays. This may affect the predictive value of ceruloplasmin levels in diagnosing Wilson disease.

Copper bound to albumin and amino acids, not including that contained in ceruloplasmin, is called "non-ceruloplasmin-bound copper" or "free copper," which normally totals about 10% of total plasma copper, with the remainder being accounted for by non-exchangeable copper bound to ceruloplasmin [15]. When copper accumulates in the liver in Wilson disease, or if severe liver injury occurs, copper is released into the circulation and increases the fraction of "free copper" relative to the copper bound to ceruloplasmin. This copper becomes available for renal excretion causing the cupriuria that is characteristic of Wilson disease and patients with other liver injuries, but to a lesser extent.

More than 80% of absorbed copper is excreted in bile (Figure 28.1), totaling approximately 1.2–1.7 mg daily [16]. Exocystosis of lysosomal copper across the canalicular membrane is the major source of biliary copper, which is then complexed to large proteins (e.g. metallothionein) that prevent reabsorption by the small intestine. Recent identification of a new gene in the Bedlington terrier [17] suggests that the gene product MURR1 is required for vesicular copper (ATP7B) movement and excretion (Figure 28.2). Human *MURR1* (*COMMD1*) has been mapped to chromosome region 2p13-16 [18]. Human *MURR1* has been excluded as the gene causing non-Wilson disease hepatic copper toxicosis syndromes. The protein product interacts with the copper-binding N-terminus of ATP7B, providing biochemical evidence in support of the proposed role of MURR1 in hepatic copper toxicosis [19]. However, several more recent studies showed that *MURR1* is not involved in Wilson disease or other causes of human toxicosis.

Metallothionein-bound copper does not account for all of biliary copper. An additional pathway for copper secretion into bile may involve glutathione-conjugated copper secreted into the canaliculus by the canalicular multispecific organic anion transporter (cMOAT; also known as the multidrug resistance-associated protein 2 (MRP2)) (Figure 28.2). There is minimal enterohepatic circulation of copper. Urine, sweat, and menstrual blood are minor pathways for copper excretion. Urine copper ($<100\,\mu g$ daily) is neither indicative of dietary intake nor important in copper homeostasis under normal circumstances. Pathologic processes that interfere with biliary excretion of copper, such as intrahepatic and extrahepatic hepatobiliary cholestatic disorders, produce copper retention in the liver, generally in the lysosomal fraction of hepatocytes, and are associated with elevated plasma copper and ceruloplasmin levels. In fact, hepatic concentrations of copper in intrahepatic cholestatic disorders of childhood and primary biliary cirrhosis in adults may equal or exceed levels found in Wilson disease. Whether or not excess hepatic copper in cholestasis is hepatotoxic remains under debate.

The organ distribution of the 80–100 mg of copper in an adult includes 15% in the liver, with lesser amounts in brain, heart, and kidneys in decreasing order. Althought 50% of the body's copper is stored in muscle and bone, the concentration is low in these tissues. In fetal liver, copper concentration is several-fold higher than that present in older children and adults, most of which is bound to metallothionein in hepatocyte lysosomes [20]. During fetal life, the amount of copper present in the liver declines from over 90% of total body copper during early development to approximately 50–60% at birth. After birth, hepatic copper content falls rapidly, reaching adult levels by 3 months of age. Because of delayed maturation of ceruloplasmin synthesis in the infant's liver, plasma levels of both ceruloplasmin and copper remain low during the first 6 to 12 months of life. Increased blood levels of thyroxine, estrogens, and testosterone [20] are associated with increased plasma ceruloplasmin and copper, making laboratory values difficult to interpret. Insufficiency of corticosteroids decreases biliary copper excretion resulting in elevated plasma copper and ceruloplasmin levels.

Mechanisms of copper toxicity

High levels of orally or parenterally administered copper accumulate in the liver in most mammalian species. Excess hepatic copper has been shown to cause liver injury in rodents, chickens, ruminants, sheep, Bedlington terriers, and humans [15]. Endogenous copper detoxification mechanisms, such as sequestration with metallothionein, export via copper-translocating ATPases, and biliary secretion, have allowed certain animal species (such as the normal dog, Dominican toad, and mute swan) to tolerate higher hepatic copper content. The newborn human has the capacity to tolerate 5- to 100-fold the hepatic copper content of normal adults [21]. Hepatic lysosomal sequestration of excess copper is also an effective mechanism to render non-toxic enormous concentrations of intracellular copper. However, in some species, natural accumulation of dietary copper leads to severe liver injury and death, as observed in sheep and the Bedlington terrier [22].

The precise intracellular target for the toxic action of copper is uncertain. Many cytosolic enzymes that contain sulfhydryl groups may be inhibited in vitro by copper [23]. Copper inhibits polymerization of tubulin, the chief protein of microtubules, possibly perturbing intracellular trafficking of proteins and mitotic spindle formation. Copper also functions as a pro-oxidant, catalyzing the transformation of hydrogen peroxide to the hydroxyl free radical, which, in turn, may react with and damage polyunsaturated fatty acid residues of cell membranes, thiol-rich proteins, and nucleic acids [23]; it may also activate intrinsic apoptotic cell death pathways. These effects may lead to disturbances in plasma membrane function, mitochondrial oxidative phosphorylation, nuclear control of cell processes, protein synthesis by endoplasmic reticulum, and leakage of lysosomal enzymes into the cytosol. In addition, by-products of lipid peroxidation, such as malondialdehyde and 4-hydroxynonenal, have been shown to stimulate collagen gene expression in hepatic stellate cells and promote fibrogenesis [24], as well as stimulate nuclear factor NF-κB and cytokine gene expression [25].

There is considerable evidence that oxidative injury is a key factor in copper toxicity. Lipid peroxidation has been documented in both hepatic lysosomes and mitochondria isolated from copper-overloaded rats [26]. Moreover, hepatic mitochondria isolated from copper-overloaded rats have abnormal respiration and diminished mitochondrial activity of cytochrome *c* oxidase in conjunction with increased lipid peroxidation [26]. Elevated hepatic mitochondrial copper concentrations in patients with Wilson disease and copper-overloaded Bedlington terriers have been associated with excessive lipid peroxidation of these organelles [22] and in patients with Wilson disease with oxidative modification of mitochondrial DNA [23]. Furthermore, the ultrastructurally abnormal mitochondria in hepatocytes of Wilson disease [1] and ICC support the hepatic mitochondrion being one of the target organelles in copper toxicity. Metallothionein has been shown to function as an antioxidant; therefore, it may not only chelate excess copper but may also play a role in reducing oxidative stress stimulated by copper. Interestingly, high intracellular copper levels lead to a conformational change in the antiapoptotic protein X-linked inhibitor of apoptosis that increases its degradation, thereby decreasing its ability to inhibit caspase-3 and leading to a lower apoptotic threshold

Table 28.1 Clinical presentation in 802 patients of all ages with Wilson disease

Series	No.	Symptoms (No. (%))				
		Hepatic (%)	Neuropsychiatric (%)	Hematologic (%)	Endocrine (%)	Asymptomatic (%)
Walshe [31]	217	101 (47)	90 (42)			28 (13)
Scheinberg and Sternlieb [32]	151	68 (45)	85 (56)	19 (13)	4 (3)	
Saito [33]	140	82 (59)	58 (41)			
Giagheddu et al. [34]	68	30 (40)	23 (34)			15 (22)
Dobyns et al. [24]	53	25 (47)	28 (53)			
Stremmel et al. [25]	51	34 (67)	31 (61)	5 (10)		
Aksoy and Erdem [35]	49	14 (29)	31 (63)			4 (8)
Oder et al. [36]	45	27 (60)	12 (27)			6 (13)
Park et al. [37]	28	12 (43)	10 (36)			6 (21)
Total	802	393 (49)	368 (46)	24 (3)	4 (<1)	59 (7)

and cell death [27]. Other studies are consistent with hepatocyte apoptosis being the primary mode of cell death in copper toxicity [28], possibly explaining the characteristic mild elevation of serum aminotransferases associated with Wilson disease. In addition, oxidative modification of mitochondria DNA may result in impaired oxidative phosphorylation and amplification of oxidative stress.

Wilson disease (hepatolenticular degeneration)

History

In 1912, Kinnear Wilson, an American neurologist, described the degenerative disease of the central nervous system associated with cirrhosis that now bears his name [29]. He proposed the term "progressive lenticular degeneration" for this rare, familial, invariably fatal disease of young people that was characterized by softening of the lenticular nuclei and hepatic cirrhosis. In 1921, Hall further characterized hepatic involvement and introduced the term "hepatolenticular degeneration" [15]. It was not until 1948 that Cumings proposed that copper toxicity caused the tissue injury and suggested the novel use of 2,3-dimercaptopropanol (British AntiLewisite) to increase urinary copper excretion and thus treat the disorder. In 1952, Scheinberg and Gitlin discovered that low circulating ceruloplasmin levels was a practical diagnostic test for the disorder; in 1956, Walshe reported the successful use of the oral copper chelator penicillamine for treatment of the condition, and in 1968 Sternlieb and Scheinberg showed that penicillamine could prevent neurologic and hepatic injury in asymptomatic affected siblings [15]. Walshe showed in 1982 that triethylene tetramine (trientine) was effective with less toxicity than penicillamine. The role of liver transplantation as a treatment option under certain circumstances has been defined. In the 1990s, the search for the gene involved in Wilson disease localized it within 13q14-q21 on chromosome 13. Using positional cloning techniques, three groups independently reported the identification of the gene responsible for Wilson disease, designated *ATP7B* [15,30].

Epidemiology

It has long been known that Wilson disease was transmitted by autosomal recessive inheritance, and so consanguinity is relatively common in affected families. Wilson disease is ubiquitous with a worldwide prevalence of approximately 1 in 30 000, and the heterozygote carrier state has a prevalence of approximately 1 in 90 [1]. There are isolated communities in Japan, Sardinia, and Israel with a higher prevalence. Patients present with a variety of clinical manifestations, including hepatic presentations common in childhood and a later-onset predominately neurologic form. Although there are often similarities in the age of onset and clinical findings of Wilson disease in affected siblings, there may be marked differences in organ system involvement and biochemical findings, suggesting that polygenic or environmental factors may play a role in expression of the disease. The disease has been described as late as the eighth decade of life and rarely before 3 years of age [8]. Presentation in 40–60% of patients is with primary features in the second decade of life [31]. The remainder of patients comes to clinical attention during the third and fourth decades with a primarily neurologic (34%) or psychiatric (10%) presentation [31] (Table 28.1). Other presenting features include hematologic and endocrine abnormalities (e.g. amenorrhea) in 12% and renal symptoms in 1% of patients [38]. All patients have liver involvement, although it may be asymptomatic and well compensated. Although symptoms attributable to Wilson disease may start in childhood, the diagnosis may not be made for several years or even decades because of a low index of suspicion by the clinician. Not infrequently, this delay results in advanced hepatic or neurologic manifestations at the time of diagnosis that potentially could have been prevented.

Genetics

Genetic linkage of Wilson disease to the locus of the gene for the red blood cell esterase D indicated that the Wilson disease gene was on the long arm of chromosome 13, which was further mapped to a smaller region, 13q14-q21. The identification of the gene for Menkes disease prompted the search for that in Wilson disease. Menkes disease is a rare autosomal recessive inherited copper deficiency disorder caused by impaired copper absorption at the intestinal level. Because the disease gene, *ATP7A*, was a putative cation-transporting P-type ATPase involved in copper transport, the search began for a homologous gene located in the Wilson disease locus of chromosome 13. The gene was isolated and identified as *ATP7B* (Figure 28.3), with mutations unique to patients with Wilson disease. The database maintained by the University of Alberta lists over 300 distinct mutations identified from patients with Wilson disease (http://www.wilsondisease.med.ualberta.ca/database.asp). Most of these are small deletions or missense mutations, the latter requiring confirmation that they are not merely polymorphisms. Missense mutations are associated with a predominance of neurologic symptoms and a later clinical presentation. Deletions and other mutations causing premature stop codons are associated with an earlier clinical presentation predominated by symptoms of liver disease. Specific mutations appear to be more common among certain ethnic groups. The most common mutation in descendents from northern Europe, leading to H1069Q, may be present in 35–45% of cases, while in Asian populations a mutation resulting in R778L occurs in 57% of affected Asians under 18 years of age. However over half of all mutations occur rarely in any population. This degree of heterogeneity suggests most affected individuals are compound heterozygotes. Because of the wide variety of mutations, genetic techniques to establish the diagnosis of Wilson disease have significant limitations. A battery of mutations common to a given ethnic group can be screened; however, the absence of one of these mutations does not exclude the diagnosis. Therefore, complete *ATP7B* gene sequencing, which is clinically available, is frequently necessary. Haplotype analysis (microsatellite markers) may be particularly helpful in evaluating relatives of a known case in which microsatellite markers are informative.

Pathogenesis

Mutations in *ATP7B* cause impaired biliary copper excretion that leads to progressive accumulation of copper in the liver followed by subsequent deposition in other organs, causing the varied clinicopathologic features of Wilson disease. The initial accumulation of copper in the liver begins in the first few years of life and can be substantial. It has been proposed that there is also failure to clear the high hepatic copper burden that is usually well tolerated in the neonate. By the end of the first or into the second decade of life, the hepatic burden of copper is exceeded, causing release of free copper into the circulation that penetrates other tissues. During this time, hepatic copper may actually decrease in concentration, while brain, kidney, and ocular copper increase [31].

It is clear that mutations in *ATP7B* cause both decreased biliary excretion of copper [1] and defective hepatocyte incorporation of copper into ceruloplasmin [1]. Serum ceruloplasmin levels are low in Wilson disease because of decreased synthesis of holoceruloplasmin and rapid clearance of apoceruloplasmin, which is still secreted by the liver in Wilson disease. The gene *CP*, encoding ceruloplasmin, on chromosome 3 is normal in patients with Wilson disease. Aceruloplasminemia, a congenital deficiency of ceruloplasmin caused by lack of synthesis of apopoceruloplasmin because of homozygous mutations in its gene, causes iron deposition (not copper) in liver, brain and spleen, retinal degeneration, diabetes and dementia. Heterozygotes for Wilson disease may have low ceruloplasmin levels yet no pathologic accumulation of copper in tissues. Conversely, 5–30% of patients with Wilson disease have normal plasma ceruloplasmin levels [1]. The normal ceruloplasmin levels in Wilson disease result from ceruloplasmin being an acute phase reactant that can elevate in the face of acute liver injury, as well as the fact that circulating apoceruloplasmin may be detected by newer immunologic assays for serum ceruloplasmin. Although a very useful biomarker for this disease, the impairment in ceruloplasmin synthesis appears to be a result of, rather than responsible for, the disturbance of copper metabolism in Wilson disease, and it does not, in itself, appear related to any of the manifestations of Wilson disease.

ATP7B is localized in hepatocytes to the trans-Golgi part of the late secretory pathway. With increasing intracellular copper concentrations, the ATPase traffics to a cytoplasmic vesicular compartment that distributes near the canaliculus where it participates in copper excretion into bile. Once the ATP7B sequestration of copper in vesicles reduces the cytoplasmic copper content, ATP7B is recycled back to the trans-Golgi network (Figure 28.2).

The role of ATP7B in the incorporation of copper into ceruloplasmin has been investigated in yeast. The ATP7B orthologue Ccc2 transports copper to Fet3, which is analogous to apoceruloplasmin in mammalian tissues. In yeast lacking Ccc2, ATP7B replaced this activity while mutant ATP7B did not. Mutations in the metal-binding sites closest to the transmembrane domain 1 are more important for this copper transporting activity than sites closer to the N-terminus. Therefore, copper incorporation into ceruloplasmin is dependent on the copper-transport function of ATP7B. Mutations in *ATP7B* result in failure to incorporate copper in ceruloplasmin and the secretion of apocerulosplasmin which is rapidly removed from the circulation.

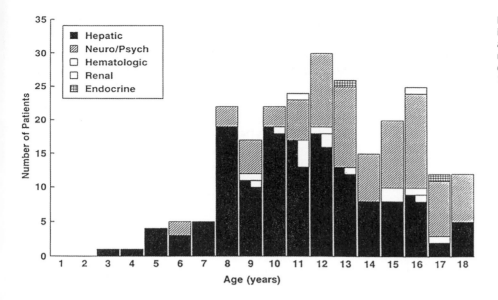

Figure 28.4 Histogram of age distribution of initial mode of clinical presentation in children and adolescents with Wilson disease. Split vertical bars represent combined clinical presentation. (Based on combined data from Scheinberg and Sternlieb, 1984 [32] and Walshe, 1982 [31].)

Clinical features

Wilson disease has a multitude of clinical presentations that can present at almost any age. Although the failure to excrete biliary copper is present from birth, clinical manifestations of Wilson disease are rarely apparent prior to age 3–5 years [32]. Clinical symptoms typically develop sequentially based on the pathophysiologic disturbance of copper metabolism in Wilson disease. Copper silently accumulates in the liver during childhood. After the liver storage capacity for copper becomes saturated, circulating non-ceruloplasmin-bound "free copper" levels rise and copper is then redistributed systemically, accumulating in the nervous system, cornea, kidneys, and other organs and tissues. This change in organ distribution of copper over time is paralleled by the clinical presentations of Wilson disease. Based on the combined large patient series of Walshe [31] and Scheinberg and Sternlieb [32], 83% of patients presented with hepatic symptoms and 17% with neuropsychiatric manifestations prior to age 10 years; 52% presented with hepatic and 48% with neuropsychiatric symptoms at 10–18 years; and 24% presented with hepatic and 74% with neuropsychiatric symptoms after age 18 years (Figure 28.4). Considering patients of all ages using data derived from nine combined series, approximately 49% of patients present with hepatic and 46% with neuropsychiatric symptoms (Table 28.1). The median delay in establishing the diagnosis of Wilson disease in those with neuropsychiatric symptoms was 18 months, which is considerably longer than those with hepatic presentation (median 6 months). During the phase of copper redistribution, other organ systems become involved, with renal, endocrine, and hematologic manifestations appearing after age 10 years (Figure 28.4). A combination of liver dysfunction and other organ system involvement, at any age, should suggest Wilson disease.

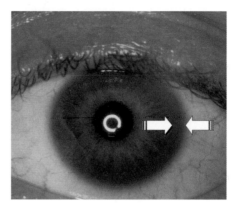

Figure 28.5 Kayser–Fleischer ring (arrows) in 30-year-old male with Wilson disease. (With permission from Sokol, 1992 [2].)

After hepatic saturation, copper accumulating in the ocular cornea may cause the characteristic *Kayser–Fleischer (K-F) ring* (Figure 28.5), a greenish-brown ring at the periphery of the cornea on its posterior surface in Descemet's membrane [32]. This is best detected by slit-lamp examination by an ophthalmologist, although a prominent K-F ring can be seen easily if the iris is of light pigmentation. The color of the ring results from scattering and reflection of light by layers of copper granules. The K-F ring initially appears at the superior poles of the cornea, with subsequent involvement of inferior poles followed by circumferential involvement. Treatment with copper chelators results in gradual resolution of K-F rings over 3 to 5 years in reverse order of appearance, occasionally leading to complete disappearance. This pattern of copper deposition has been said to result from a relative stagnation of solvent flow in the superior poles of the cornea, allowing the precipitation of copper to occur. Analysis by X-ray energy spectroscopy has shown that the K-F ring consists of granules that are rich not only in copper but also in sulfur. This suggests that metallothionein-bound copper in Descemet's membrane is essential for the visual appearance characteristic of K-F rings. The K-F ring does not interfere with visual function. The K-F ring is virtually always present at the time when neurologic or psychiatric symptoms develop, although there are rare exceptions (5% of patients with neurologic symptoms) [1]. Importantly, the K-F ring is frequently absent in children without neurologic involvement but who present with hepatic symptoms. The K-F ring is not pathognomonic for Wilson disease and has also been reported in patients with prolonged cholestatic liver disease, such as chronic hepatitis, chronic intrahepatic and neonatal cholestasis, cryptogenic cirrhosis, and primary biliary cirrhosis [1]. This is a result of diminished biliary excretion and secondary copper overload.

Another characteristic, but less common, ophthalmologic feature of Wilson disease is the grayish-brown "sunflower cataract" that may develop because of deposits of copper in the anterior and posterior lens capsule. Visualizing these cataracts requires an ophthalmoscopic examination; they rarely interfere with vision and resolve with therapy. The other circumstance in which these cataracts may develop is from a copper-containing foreign body lodged intraocularly (chalcosis). Because of these characteristic ocular findings, all patients in whom Wilson disease is suspect should undergo a thorough ophthalmologic examination.

Hepatic presentations

The liver is both the major site of the biochemical defect in Wilson disease and the initial target of copper toxicity. Clinical symptoms of liver disease are very rare prior to age 3–5 years; however, asymptomatic mild elevation of serum aminotransferase levels has been reported and a rare patient has developed fulminant liver failure before age 5 years. Thereafter, symptoms of acute or chronic liver disease may interrupt a presymptomatic period at any time in the first two decades of life. Hepatic presentations include:

- acute hepatitis
- acute liver failure
- chronic hepatitis
- steatohepatitis
- portal hypertension
- cirrhosis
- asymptomatic elevation of serum aminotransferases
- gallstones
- hepatocellular carcinoma.

Elevated aminotransferase levels may be detected in completely asymptomatic patients for whom a chemistry panel is drawn for unrelated reasons, such as seizure medication monitoring or trauma. Exclusion of more common causes of abnormal liver blood tests should lead to consideration of Wilson disease if the tests do not normalize. It is essential that the clinician maintain a high level of suspicion and thoroughly investigate the child with persisting asymptomatic elevation of aminotransferase levels to facilitate diagnosis and initiation of treatment early in the course of Wilson disease.

Acute hepatitis

Acute hepatitis is the mode of presentation in approximately 25% of patients. Clinical signs of jaundice, anorexia, nausea, malaise, pale stools, and dark urine mimic acute infectious hepatitis. Laboratory investigation reveals a conjugated hyperbilirubinemia associated with elevated aminotransferases but normal serum albumin and prothrombin time/international normalized ratio (INR). Although serologic testing for viral hepatitis types A, B, and C and for Epstein–Barr virus is negative, this presentation can be confused with acute viral hepatitis, particularly if the patient makes a complete, although temporary, recovery.

Acute liver failure

Acute liver failure (fulminant Wilson disease) is the presentation in up to 12% of patients, usually occurring in adolescence as an acute icteric hepatitis that rapidly evolves over a few days to several weeks [1,32]. Symptoms progress to fatigue, hepatic insufficiency, extreme jaundice (because of the accompanying hemolysis), severe coagulopathy, ascites, hepatic encephalopathy, renal failure, and death if liver transplantation is not performed [1]. This presentation may be similar to that of acute fulminant viral hepatitis or following ingestion of a hepatotoxin. However, non-immune hemolysis and rapid onset of renal failure with low serum alkaline phosphatase in a female adolescent are characteristic of the Wilson disease presentation.

A similar, and unfortunate, fulminant presentation has been described in patients who had been successfully treated for up to 20 years with copper chelators or zinc therapy but who discontinued therapy or became non-compliant for as little as 8 months [1]. This rapid development of fatal hepatic disease suggests that the therapeutic action of copper chelation may be through formation of non-toxic copper–chelator or copper–protein complexes (e.g. copper–metallothionein) rather than the generally accepted action of chelators in removing excess copper from the patient. The abrupt discontinuation of D-penicillamine or trientine may expose the liver to a large load of free toxic copper released by dissociation of this complex. Similar presentations have occurred after the discontinuation of zinc therapy. For this reason, patients with Wilson disease must be repeatedly and frequently reminded (especially when they feel healthy) that copper chelation or zinc maintenance therapy is lifelong and discontinuation could be fatal.

Chronic hepatitis

Chronic hepatitis is a more common presentation in 10–30% of patients with Wilson disease during adolescence or young adulthood. Cirrhosis is frequently present at time of this diagnosis [1,32]. Malaise, anorexia, fatigue, abdominal pain, and nausea may precede the onset of jaundice and hepatic dysfunction. Amenorrhea, delayed puberty, polyarthralgias, edema, gynecomastia, ascites, clubbing, or spider angiomata, when present, indicate the chronic nature and likelihood of hepatic fibrosis or cirrhosis. Tender hepatomegaly and splenomegaly are typically found on examination; K-F rings may be absent in up to 50%. Neurologic or psychiatric symptoms, or a family history of Wilson disease, should raise suspicion. Laboratory tests show raised serum aminotransferases, low albumin, elevated gammaglobulin, and a variably abnormal prothrombin time/INR. Except for lower serum aminotransferases, patients with Wilsonian chronic hepatitis appear clinically no different than other patients and may even have positive autoantibodies (anti-nuclear antibodies, anti-smooth muscle antibody), except that liver biopsy in Wilson disease may reveal steatohepatitis. With the rising frequency of adolescent obesity, one can expect up to 30% of patients with Wilson disease to be obese, leading to an incorrect diagnosis of non-alcoholic fatty liver disease when steatohepatitis is found on liver biopsy. Unless appropriate diagnostic studies are performed, the patient may well carry a misdiagnosis of autoimmune, viral, alcoholic, or non-alcoholic steatohepatitis or idiopathic chronic hepatitis until neurologic symptoms develop or the liver is examined at transplantation or autopsy. *Therefore, it is imperative that biochemical screening for Wilson disease be undertaken in all patients with chronic hepatitis without a clear defined diagnosis.* The response to copper chelation therapy is generally excellent even if cirrhosis is present. In a series of 20 patients with chronic hepatitis, Schilsky *et al.* [39] described long-term survival in 90% of cirrhotic patients who were compliant with copper chelation therapy. This compares favorably to survival rates of 55–80% in patients with chronic hepatitis and cirrhosis caused by hepatitis B virus, autoimmune hepatitis, or other causes.

Cirrhosis

The cirrhotic presentation of Wilson disease may be insidious with cutaneous signs of chronic liver disease or splenomegaly being the only clues. Alternatively, anorexia, fatigue, abdominal pain, weight loss, jaundice, ascites, gastrointestinal hemorrhage, hypersplenism, coagulopathy, spontaneous bacterial peritonitis, encephalopathy, poor school function, or hepatorenal syndrome may signal the onset [32]. Indeed, none of these features is specific to Wilsonian cirrhosis, so, sadly, patients may be misdiagnosed as having postnecrotic, steatohepatitis or cryptogenic cirrhosis, or as with alcoholic cirrhosis in adults. Although cirrhosis and its complications are relatively common presenting features of Wilson disease in childhood, it may remain silent and asymptomatic well into adulthood, when patients present with neurologic, psychiatric, endocrine or other symptoms.

Cholelithiasis

Cholelithiasis is relatively common in adolescents with Wilson disease, resulting from ongoing hemolysis in the presence of cirrhosis. Abdominal pain in a patient with Wilson disease should prompt ultrasonographic evaluation for gallstones. Analysis of gallstones showed twice the level of cholesterol as

Table 28.2 Neurologic and psychiatric symptoms associated with Wilson disease

Neurologic	Psychiatric
Tremor (resting, intention)	Organic dementia
Drooling, hypersalivation, dysarthria	Neuroses, anxiety, depression, obsessive/compulsive disorder
Coordination defects, clumsiness	Schizophrenia
Dystonia	Bipolar disorder
Writing difficulties	Antisocial behavior
Choreiform movements	Alcoholism
Ataxic gait	
Fixed grin	
Headache	
Seizures	

found in gallstones from children with hemolytic disease, but <30% of that measured in typical cholesterol gallstones. Interestingly, the copper content of gallstones removed from patients with Wilson disease (5.2–85.4 µg/g) was significantly lower than that in pigment gallstones found in non-Wilsonian patients (571.7–1951.8 µg/g) [31], a consequence of impaired biliary excretion of copper.

A retrospective evaluation of 363 patients with Wilson disease in the UK and Sweden demonstrated intra-abdominal malignancies (primarily hepatomas, cholangiocarcinomas, and poorly differentiated adenocarcinomas) in 4.2–5.3% of patients followed for 10–29 years, and 15% for those followed for 30–39 years [40]. Hepatocellular carcinoma may develop in adults but is exceedingly rare in affected children and adolescents.

Neuropsychiatric presentation

In 40 to 45% of patients with Wilson disease, neurologic or psychiatric signs are the first indication of illness (Table 28.1). Neurologic onset has been recorded in children as young as 6 years [39] and in adults as old as 72 years [1]. Neurologic symptomatology is generally limited to motor manifestations of extrapyramidal or cerebellar dysfunction [1,39]. Psychiatric symptomatology can take many forms (Table 28.2). Neurologic symptoms most commonly present during the second and third decade of life with the insidious appearance of a single symptom, followed by gradual worsening of the symptom with development of other motor abnormalities. Recently, neurologic and psychiatric symptoms have been correlated with MRI of the brain. The first subgroup is that of patients with bradykinesia, cognitive impairment, cogwill rigidity, and an organic mood syndrome, termed "pseudoparkinsonian." This presentation was associated with dilatation of the third ventricle. The second subgroup, termed "pseudosclerosis," is manifested by ataxia, tremor, and reduced functional capacity, and is characterized by focal thalamic lesions. Tremors may be of the resting, intention, or postural forms and can become incapacitating. The third subgroup, termed "dyskinesia," includes patients who exhibit dyskinesia, dysarthria, and organic personality syndrome and correlates with focal lesions in the putamen and globus pallidus. Extrapyramidal symptoms include facial grimaces, stereotypic gestures, drooling, a fixed grin, dysphagia, and finally contractures of the jaw or extremities. Titubation, dysmetria, scanning speech, illegible handwriting, and rarely choreiform and athetoid movements also occur. The nature of these abnormalities may lead to misdiagnoses of multiple sclerosis, Parkinson disease, Friedreich ataxia, and so on. Because intelligence is unaffected, patients generally becomes frustrated and depressed.

The neurologic basis for these motor abnormalities is involvement of the basal ganglia and cerebellum. The corticospinal and corticobulbar pathways are also affected to some extent. There appears to be a critical threshold of brain copper deposition above which neurologic injury and symptomatology ensue (40 μg/g wet weight).

Sensory function and intelligence in patients with Wilson disease remain normal; however, there may be mild memory impairment. Lower scores reported on various intelligence tests are most likely the result of impaired ability to perform motor tasks. Other symptoms that may develop include migraine headaches, grand mal, focal motor or partial complex seizures, and various gait disturbances caused by both the tremor and dystonia. Seizures are unusual, with a prevalence rate of 6.2%, and are rarely present initially, but may develop within weeks or months of starting copper chelation therapy. It has, therefore, been proposed that sudden mobilization of large quantities of copper by chelating agents may be responsible for these seizures. Neurologic presentations of Wilson disease are summarized in Table 28.2.

At some time during the course of their life, many patients will suffer from organic dementia, neurotic behavior, bipolar or schizophrenic psychosis, or behavioral abnormalities that may be antisocial in nature. Aggressive behavioral outbursts, deterioration in school performance or hand-writing, or a major change in affect or personality may be the initial symptoms in an adolescent or college student. Therefore, psychiatric evaluation and ongoing psychotherapy in addition to chelation therapy are important elements in the total care of these patients.

In approximately 10–25% of patients with Wilson disease, a psychiatric disturbance is the initial clinical presentation, even before the appearance of any movement disorder. If the diagnosis of Wilson disease is not made, the development of a movement disorder during therapy with drugs for the psychiatric disorder may be attributed to a medication side effect rather than to the possibility of undiagnosed Wilson disease [32]. Psychiatrists must, therefore, maintain a high index of suspicion of Wilson disease and should measure plasma ceruloplasmin and obtain a slit-lamp examination in patients with psychiatric disorders (even if chronic in nature). This is of particular importance if there is a history of liver disease, a family history of a psychiatric disorder or Wilson disease, if the patient is under age 50 years, or if the patient is not responding satisfactorily to conventional psychiatric treatment [32].

Other presentations

Renal manifestations

Renal disturbances may occur in patients with Wilson disease [32]; however, renal disease as a presenting symptom is rare. Copper has been shown to accumulate in the kidneys of patients with Wilson disease, with up to 100 times the normal concentration being observed. Proximal renal tubular dysfunction, decreased glomerular filtration rate, and decreased renal plasma flow characterize the resulting renal dysfunction. The renal tubular dysfunction is manifested by proteinuria, glucosuria, phosphaturia, uricosuria, generalized aminoaciduria, and microscopic hematuria. Distal renal tubular acidosis contributes to an increased tendency for formation of renal stones. In one series, 7 of 45 patients (16%) developed renal stones. Patients with the acute fulminant presentation of Wilson disease and those with end-stage liver disease may develop severe acute kidney injury, requiring temporary renal dialysis. Finally, isosthenuria has been reported. Many of the renal abnormalities improve during copper chelation therapy; however, severe proteinuria and the nephrotic syndrome [32] or a Goodpasture-like syndrome are more likely to occur as a consequence of penicillamine administration rather than of copper toxicity.

Hematologic manifestations

A variety of hematologic manifestations have been reported in Wilson disease. Intravascular hemolysis is frequent and may be the presenting abnormality in approximately 15% of patients. Hemolysis may be transient and occur when there are no associated neurologic or hepatic clinical manifestations. Therefore, Wilson disease should be considered in all children and adolescents with Coombs-negative hemolytic anemia. When associated with the acute fulminant hepatic presentation, hemolysis is a poor prognostic factor, contributing to renal failure by excess hemoglobinuria. Hemolysis is considered secondary to sudden release of copper from the liver, initiating an oxidant stress capable of peroxidizing red cell membrane lipids. If hepatic involvement is advanced, circulating hepatic-derived coagulation factor levels may be low, platelets may have impaired function, and portal hypertension may cause splenomegaly and resultant thrombocytopenia and leukopenia.

Cardiac involvement

Cardiac involvement has been recognized in Wilson disease. Electrocardiographic abnormalities were present in 18 of 53 patients (34%), with a mean age of 21 years, including left ventricular hypertrophy, ST wave depression, and T-wave inversion [41]. Arrhythmias were present in 13% and 19%

had orthostatic hypotension (although asymptomatic) indicating autonomic dysfunction. Histological findings at autopsy have included cardiac hypertrophy, interstitial fibrosis, intramyocardial small vessel sclerosis, and focal inflammation [41]. Sudden death could be caused by arrhythmias in patients with Wilson disease [41].

Skeletal manifestations

Skeletal manifestations of Wilson disease are not uncommon and may even be the first clinical symptoms of the disease. Bone demineralization is the most common feature, possibly caused by the hypercalciuria and hyperphosphaturia resulting from renal tubular dysfunction. Other radiologic changes include rickets and osteomalacia, osteoporosis, spontaneous fractures, bone fragmentation near joints, osteochondritis desiccans, chondromalacia patellae, premature osteoarthrosis, and premature degenerative arthritis of the knees and wrists. Stiffness of larger joints is a complaint of many patients.

Skin manifestations

Skin pigmentation may be increased, particularly on the anterior aspect of the lower legs, through deposition of melanin, and acanthosis nigrans may be present. Blue lunulae of the fingernails have also been reported. Other associated dermatologic findings may be caused by cirrhosis and portal hypertension.

Hormonal imbalance

Hormonal imbalance secondary to chronic liver disease has been thought to lead to amenorrhea in women and gynecomastia in boys. However, more recent studies suggest that primary ovarian dysfunction may be present and that increased androgen levels and abnormalities in the hypothalamic–pituitary–testicular axis in males are probably not a result of liver dysfunction. Additional infrequent associations with Wilson disease include diabetes mellitus, exocrine pancreatic insufficiency, and hypoparathyroidism.

Laboratory findings

Patients with Wilson disease may present with almost any combination of abnormalities in liver blood tests, or even no abnormality at all. Serum aminotransferase levels are characteristically only mild to moderately elevated with aspartate aminotransferase (AST) more than alanine aminotransferase (ALT), even in patients with the acute liver failure presentation. Serum alkaline phosphatase is usually in the low range, particularly when acute liver failure is present. In patients with acute liver failure, the combination of an AST:ALT ratio >2.2 and an alkaline phosphatase:total bilirubin ratio <4 has almost a 100% diagnostic accuracy for Wilson disease as the cause [38].

Serum copper is usually low in Wilson disease; however, during the fulminant presentation, serum copper is actually elevated because of the massive copper release from the necrosing liver and can be helpful in establishing this diagnosis. This released copper also contributes to the hemolytic anemia, hemoglobinuria, and renal failure that are common during this presentation. The non-ceruloplasmin bound copper (serum "free copper") is generally elevated in untreated patients (>25 μg/dL; normal <15 μg/dL), and can be estimated by the serum copper (μg/dL) minus 3× plasma ceruloplasmin (mg/dL). Serum free copper may also be elevated in other causes of acute liver failure and in chronic cholestasis and copper ingestion/poisoning. This calculation depends on accurate serum copper and ceruloplasmin measurements, the latter being subject to variation with the newer immunologic assays currently in use. Consequently, the non-ceruloplasmin-bound copper should not be used to establish the diagnosis of Wilson disease but may be useful in monitoring patients during chelation or zinc therapy. Serum phosphate and uric acid may be low because of renal tubular losses. Recent studies suggest that uric acid may also be oxidized as a result of oxidative stress. A complete Fanconi syndrome, including aminoaciduria and glycosuria, may be evident. Changes on radiologic evaluation of the skeleton may include osteoporosis, rickets, osteomalacia, localized demineralization, osteoarthritis, and other lesions. MRI and CT imaging of the brain may detect changes in the basal ganglia, pons or thalamus. Copper cannot be detected or quantified by standard imaging techniques.

Diagnosis

Establishing the diagnosis of Wilson disease is sometimes straight forward but commonly challenging. However, it is absolutely essential if copper chelation therapy is to be instituted as early as possible in the course of the disease (Table 28.3). For example, if the patient has oliguric renal failure, it is not possible to quantify urinary copper excretion. Alternatively, plasma ceruloplasmin values in Wilson disease may be elevated into the low normal range during acute hepatitis or estrogen therapy, or may be low in patients with other causes of hepatic failure or other sources of protein loss. Severe coagulopathy may prevent percutaneous liver biopsy. Therefore, the specific criteria used to establish the diagnosis of Wilson disease must be tailored to the patient's clinical presentation. No single laboratory test result can establish this diagnosis without confirmatory clinical and laboratory data, with the possible exception of genetic testing. An international group has developed a scoring system to assist with the diagnosis of Wilson disease [42]. The following sections discuss diagnostic criteria in classical and problematic clinical presentations.

Hepatic presentations

In a patient with liver dysfunction, the finding of a plasma or serum ceruloplasmin <20 mg/dL suggests the diagnosis of Wilson disease [1]; however, confirmatory studies are necessary because a number of disease states can also yield low

Table 28.3 Diagnostic studies used in evaluation for Wilson disease

Diagnostic test	Diagnostic values	Causes of false positive	Causes of false negative
Plasma ceruloplasmin	<20 mg/dL	Kwashiorkor, nutritional copper deficiency, protein-losing state, fulminant hepatitis, hepatic failure, hereditary hypoceruloplasminemia or aceruloplasminemia, Wilson disease heterozygote, Menkes syndrome, normal neonate	Acute inflammation (hepatitis), malignancy, pregnancy or estrogen therapy in Wilson disease (5% of patients), immunoassays of apoceruloplasmin
Hepatic copper concentration	>250 µg/g dry weight	Primary biliary cirrhosis, Indian childhood cirrhosis, chronic cholestatic liver disease, primary sclerosing cholangitis, Alagille syndrome, liver tumors, newborn liver	Copper chelation therapy in Wilson disease
Urine copper excretion	>100 µg/24 h	Copper chelation therapy, chronic active hepatitis, chronic cholestatic liver diseases, primary sclerosing cholangitis, hepatic failure, nephrotic syndrome	Copper chelation therapy in Wilson disease
Kayser–Fleischer rings	Present	Chronic cholestatic liver diseases, primary biliary cirrhosis, neonatal cholestasis	Early Wilson disease
Incorporation of ^{64}Cu into ceruloplasmin	Low	Ceruloplasmin <20 mg/dL, Wilson disease heterozygote	Pregnancy, estrogens, inflammation or malignancy in Wilson disease
Genotyping	Identification of two disease-causing mutations in ATP7B	Laboratory error	Mutation not identified but present
Haplotype analysis (microsatellite markers)	Presence of informative markers on both chromosomes	Laboratory error	Absence of informative microsatellite markers in family

Source: adapted from Scheinberg and Sternlieb, 1984 [32].

ceruloplasmin values. For example, low serum ceruloplasmin may also occur with massive protein loss, kwashiorkor, severe copper deficiency, severe hepatic insufficiency, hereditary hypoceruloplasminemia or aceruloplasminemia, acute liver failure, the normal neonate, Menkes syndrome, and 10% of heterozygotes for Wilson disease (Table 28.3). Therefore, the diagnosis of Wilson disease must be confirmed by an elevated urine 24-hour copper excretion (>100 µg; normal <40 µg/24 h), an elevated urine copper during a penicillamine challenge (see below), the presence of a K-F ring (and the absence of other cholestatic liver disorders), elevated hepatic copper content (>250 µg/g dry weight) with consistent liver histology, or the finding of two pathologic *ATP7B* mutations on genetic testing. Plasma ceruloplasmin <5 mg/dL is very suggestive of Wilson disease in the absence of the above confounding conditions. It should also be stressed that a ceruloplasmin concentration between 20 and 35 mg/dL does not conclusively exclude this diagnosis, so if there is reasonable suspicion, further testing should be undertaken as below.

Urine must be collected in copper-free containers to avoid contamination. Additionally, determining if the collection was a full 24-hour collection should be confirmed by measuring total urinary creatinine excretion (normal 10–20 mg/kg in 24 hours). False positive results of a 24-hour urine copper excretion (i.e. >100 µg) may be seen if the patient is receiving any type of copper chelation therapy, if the collection is contaminated by exogenous copper, or if the patient has chronic hepatitis, cholestatic cirrhosis, or nephrotic syndrome. In children and young adults with autoimmune chronic active hepatitis, acute hepatitis, primary sclerosing cholangitis, acute liver failure, or primary biliary cirrhosis, there can be significant overlap in values with Wilson disease. Recent studies indicate that basal 24-hour urinary copper excretion may be even <100 µg at presentation in 16–23% of patients [1], leading some to recommend a threshold of 40 µg in 24 hours for diagnosis [1]. Using this threshold would certainly increase the number of false positive urinary coppers in patients with other liver diseases. To improve the diagnostic accuracy of urine copper, the King's College Hospital group [43] have demonstrated good discrimination between Wilson disease and other liver disorders when 24-hour urine copper excretion was measured *after* a penicillamine challenge (500 mg given orally immediately before and repeated 12 hours into the urine collection); values >25 µmol/24 h (1575 µg) indicated Wilson disease. However, the same group has subsequently reported similar post-penicillamine challenge copper excretion in three children with acute persistent hepatitis A virus infection, cautioning against the use of this test as sole criteria for diagnosing

Wilson disease. Moreover, this test showed poor sensitivity for excluding the diagnosis in asymptomatic siblings.

If plasma ceruloplasmin concentration is >20 but <35 mg/dL, the diagnosis of Wilson disease is not totally excluded if clinical circumstances are suggestive, because 5–30% of patients will have ceruloplasmin in this normal range. Steindl *et al.* [44] reported that 10 of 25 patients (40%) presenting with liver disease had ceruloplasmin values in the normal range, with several exceeding 30 mg/dL. In this study, ceruloplasmin was measured by radial immunodiffusion, an immunologic technique that recognizes both the oxidase-active holoprotein that contains six copper atoms per molecule and the enzymatically inactive apoceruloplasmin. Therefore, such immunologic techniques may yield higher values than those obtained by the older "gold standard" oxidase reaction, confusing the diagnosis. Most commercial laboratories have adopted the more convenient immunoassay, making low ceruloplasmin concentration less valuable as a diagnostic pillar for Wilson disease. If ceruloplasmin is normal but there is a high index of suspicion, then a 24-hour urine copper excretion, slit lamp examination, and liver biopsy should be performed to confirm or exclude the diagnosis. Genetic testing can also be considered.

A percutaneous liver biopsy should be obtained for light microscopy, electron microscopy, and quantitative copper analysis if coagulation studies allow it to be performed safely. Transjugular liver biopsy can be performed if a significant coagulopathy is present. Characteristic histologic findings of Wilson disease (fatty change, periportal glycogenated nuclei) or of other liver disorders (e.g. primary biliary cirrhosis) aid in the diagnosis. Ultrastructural mitochondrial changes of Wilson disease are also valuable. Measuring a quantitative hepatic copper concentration is absolutely essential. Normal hepatic copper content is <50 μg/g dry weight of liver. Assuming an adequate sample has been obtained, it is virtually always >250 μg/g dry weight in Wilson disease, and may reach 3000 μg/g tissue. Recent studies have suggested that the 250 μg/g dry weight is too high a threshold and that some patients may have liver copper as low as 70 μg/g dry weight [1]. Therefore, if liver copper is between 70 and 250 μg/g dry weight, further testing will be indicated [1]. In affected asymptomatic siblings of patients with Wilson disease, liver copper content may be borderline elevated. Although a normal hepatic copper content excludes the diagnosis of Wilson disease, a false positive result can occur in the proper clinical setting. Other conditions associated with elevated hepatic copper values must be excluded by specific diagnostic studies as the clinical circumstances dictate (Table 28.3). The disorders that arise most commonly are autoimmune or infectious chronic hepatitis. The presence of autoimmune markers, plasma ceruloplasmin >30 mg/dL, and 24-hour urine copper excretion (with or without penicillamine challenge) below the threshold will generally exclude Wilson disease.

If the diagnosis remains uncertain despite the testing already described, or if liver biopsy is contraindicated, the rate of incorporation of radiolabeled copper into ceruloplasmin has been used in the past as a diagnostic study [1]. A dose of 2.0 mg cupric acetate containing 0.3–0.5 mCi copper-64 is administered orally in 100–150 mL of fruit juice following an 8-hour fast. The concentration of copper-64 in serum is determined serially (at +1, 2, 4, 24 and 48 hours) over 48 hours. Normally, the radiocopper rises at 1 and 2 hours, falls thereafter with a secondary rise over the ensuing 24 or 48 hours representing incorporation of the radiolabeled copper into newly synthesized ceruloplasmin. In Wilson disease, the secondary rise in serum copper that normally occurs after 4 hours is absent. The pattern is intermediate in Wilson disease heterozygotes. Although this test has performed in the past on occasion, it is now rarely used because of the difficulty in obtaining the isotope.

Molecular genetic testing is now widely available and may yield valuable diagnostic information, particularly if the diagnosis remains in doubt despite the testing already discussed. Haplotype testing may establish the diagnosis if another family member (proband) has Wilson disease. Evaluation of DNA haplotype markers (microsatellite markers) that flank *ATP7B* on chromosome 13 is available in a number of commercial laboratories. Prenatal diagnosis is also possible using this approach, although this has limited application since early postnatal diagnosis allows appropriate timing for treatment. Alternatively, direct genotyping of *ATP7B* can be performed. Because of a multitude of mutations of *ATP7B*, genetic mutation analysis generally employs either a panel of likely mutations for a given ethnic population or sequencing of the entire gene. Some specific ethnic groups who have a single predominant mutation and for whom genotyping may be particularly useful include Sardinian, Icelandic, Korean, Japanese, and Canary Island populations. It is absolutely essential that an experienced geneticist be available to interpret the results of genotyping, inasmuch as non-pathologic variants are common and should not be overinterpreted as disease causing. A challenge with genotyping is the finding of one disease-causing mutation in a suspected patient, raising the question of an unidentified second mutation in the promoter region or introns. Genotype–phenotype correlations are hampered by the high prevalence of compound heterozygotes in *ATP7B*.

Tests that appear to be of no value in establishing the diagnosis of Wilson disease include CT and MRI of the liver, since liver copper content cannot currently be detected or quantified by these modalities. Although advocated by some experts as useful, the non-ceruloplasmin bound serum copper fraction ("free copper") may be elevated in a variety of liver diseases as well as Wilson disease, so its value in establishing the diagnosis is questionable. It is of more value in monitoring treatment.

Figure 28.6 illustrates a suggested approach to diagnosing Wilson disease in patients with a hepatic presentation. Plasma ceruloplasmin, a 24-hour urine collection for copper analysis, and an ophthalmology examination for a K-F ring should be obtained. A liver biopsy should be obtained if any of these are

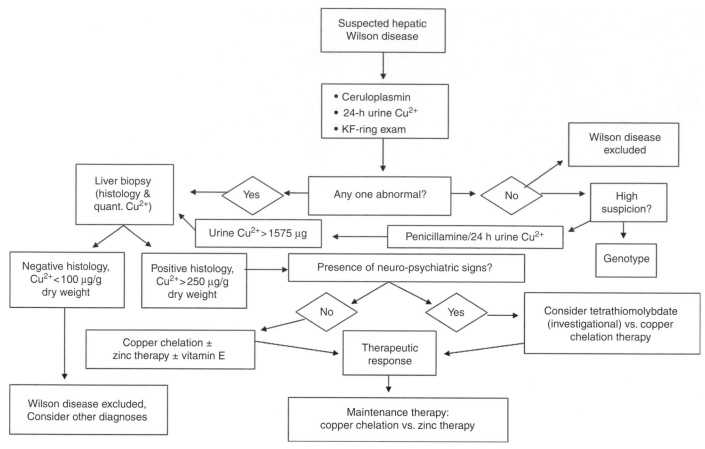

Figure 28.6 Approach to evaluation and treatment of pediatric patient with suspected Wilson disease because of presentation with liver disease.

abnormal or if there is a high suspicion for Wilson disease and the ceruloplasmin is 20–30 µg/dL or if it was measured by an immunologic method and is in the normal range. In addition to routine histology, electron microscopy and quantitative copper analysis should be obtained. If quantitative hepatic copper is >250 µg/g dry weight and other diagnoses are excluded by histology and other appropriate laboratory tests, then the diagnosis of Wilson disease is established. Some may substitute molecular testing to avoid the liver biopsy. Mutation analysis of DNA can be performed for a defined *ATP7B* mutation, common mutations in the appropriate ethnic population, or full sequencing can be performed; haplotype (microsatellite) marker analysis can be performed if a first-degree relative has Wilson disease.

Histopathology of the liver

Although the diagnosis of Wilson disease may not be evident from a single liver biopsy, the sequential changes observed over several years are characteristic. Therefore, a high index of suspicion and an understanding of the characteristic pathology are required to suggest the diagnosis on a single liver biopsy. Earliest histologic findings that may be present in asymptomatic children include periportal glycogen-filled, swollen nuclei [1,32] and hepatic steatosis, initially microvesicular that evolves into macrovesicular fat (Figure 28.7). Soon

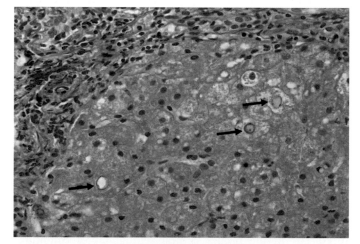

Figure 28.7 Liver histology of Wilson disease in a 3-year-old asymptomatic boy diagnosed because his sister presented with fulminant liver failure caused by Wilson disease. Portal tract mononuclear infiltrate and prominent periportal glycogenated hepatocyte nuclei (arrows) are present. Early evidence of portal fibrosis is also present. (Hematoxylin & eosin, magnification x400.)

thereafter mononuclear cell infiltrates of portal tracts become evident with increasing periportal fibrosis, hyperplasia of Kupffer cells, and pericentral venular fibrosis. In adolescents and adults, the macrovesicular steatosis might mistakenly suggest alcohol-induced liver disease or non-alcoholic

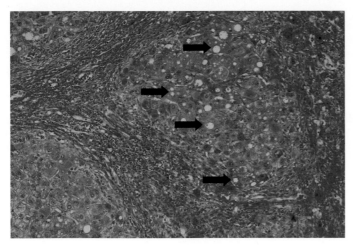

Figure 28.8 Liver histology of Wilson disease in a 16-year-old girl presenting with fulminant liver failure. Macrovesicular steatosis (arrows), mononuclear cell portal tract inflammatory infiltrate, and bridging fibrosis and micronodular cirrhosis. (Masson trichrome stain, magnification ×200.)

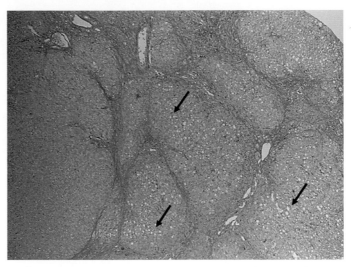

Figure 28.9 Liver histology of Wilson disease in 13-year-old girl. Bridging fibrosis and both mild micro- and macrovesicular hepatocytic steatosis (arrows) are present, with less inflammatory infiltrate than seen in Figure 28.8. (Hematoxylin & eosin, magnification ×100.)

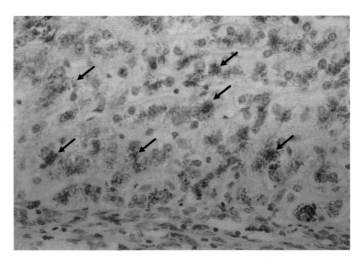

Figure 28.10 Copper staining of liver removed at time of liver transplant from a 16-year-old girl with fulminant hepatic failure caused by Wilson disease (see Figure 28.8). Strongly positive staining of copper-associated proteins in multiple hepatocytes (arrows) by rhodanine histochemical stain (magnification ×1000).

steatohepatitis. During the acute hepatitis phase of Wilson disease, hepatocyte swelling and individual hepatocyte necrosis, mild cholestasis and lymphocytic infiltration are present [32]. The chronic hepatitis lesion exhibits ballooning of hepatocytes, focal hepatocyte necrosis with interface hepatitis, glycogenated nuclei, erosion of the periportal limiting plate, lymphocytic and plasma cell inflammatory infiltrates in portal tracts, periportal fibrosis, and, when advanced, combined micronodular and macronodular cirrhosis (Figures 28.8 and 28.9). This appearance may be indistinguishable from that of autoimmune or chronic infectious hepatitis. The fulminant hepatitis lesion is characterized by microvesicular fat, coagulative cell necrosis, pigment-laden Kupffer cells, collapse of stoma with drop out of hepatocytes, Mallory's hyaline present in cytoplasm, and occasional multinucleated giant cells and bile duct proliferation in a background of cirrhosis [32].

Cirrhosis develops invariably in untreated patients and is characterized by fibrous bands separating regenerative nodules of either a macronodular or mixed micromacronodular pattern (Figure 28.8) [32]. Pericentral venular fibrosis and a pseudo-acinar pattern may be observed. Periportal steatosis and glycogenated nuclei may still be present and are characteristic although non-specific. Mallory's hyaline may be present in hepatocytes at the periphery of regenerative nodules, leading to confusion with Laennec's cirrhosis. Dark pigment representing either lipofuscin, copper-associated protein, or occasionally iron may also be observed in individual hepatocytes. Hepatocellular carcinoma is rarely found in cirrhotic livers from patients with Wilson disease.

Histochemical stains for copper or copper-associated proteins, such as rhodamine, rubeanic acid, orcein, or Timm's silver sulfide, provide qualitative evidence of increased liver copper. However, despite elevated hepatic copper content, these stains are frequently negative in patients with Wilson disease [1,32] and may be very misleading. Although a positive

stain for copper is helpful (Figure 28.10), a negative histochemical stain for copper on a liver biopsy never rules out the diagnosis of Wilson disease. These stains are invariably positive in other conditions causing elevated hepatic copper levels, such as cholestatic liver disorders and ICC; however, in Wilson disease there is no correlation between histochemical staining of copper and quantitative copper measurements on biopsy samples. There are several possible reasons for the absence of stainable copper in Wilson disease: copper is not present in hepatocytes of regenerating nodules that have had insufficient time to accumulate copper, copper has been released because of cell injury, or cytosolic copper is more difficult to identify by histochemistry than the granular

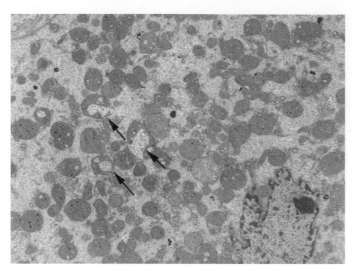

Figure 28.11 Electron microscopy of liver in 10-year-old boy with Wilson disease and liver failure. Pleomorphic mitochondria with dilated and cystic cristae are abundant (arrows) (magnification ×14 000).

appearance of lysosomal copper present in other conditions [32]. *For theses reasons, quantitative measurement of copper in liver biopsies is mandatory.* Liver biopsies must be performed with steel biopsy needles and at least 5 mg, if not 10–15 mg, used for determination of quantitative copper by a reputable laboratory.

Electron microscopy may be helpful in establishing the diagnosis because Wilson disease is one of the few liver diseases with characteristic ultrastructural lesions [32,45]. In the early stages of Wilson disease, hepatocellular mitochondria are pleomorphic and abnormally large, show widened intracristal spaces, increased matrix density, large granules and sometimes crystalline, vacuolated or dense inclusions in the mitochondrial matrix (Figure 28.11). This constellation of mitochondrial changes in a liver with fatty changes is characteristic Wilson disease [45]; however, similar changes may be observed in non-alcoholic steatohepatitis. During penicillamine therapy, these mitochondrial changes regress or disappear [45]. These mitochondrial changes also disappear during progression of the lesion toward cirrhosis [45]. Peroxisomes may become enlarged and granular or flocculent. In the later stages of cirrhosis, these ultrastructural lesions are absent; however, excess copper-rich lipofuscin granules are present [45].

In the central nervous system, lesions include degeneration of the putamen and globus pallidus, and atrophy of the caudate. Degeneration of the cerebral cortex, cerebellum, and white matter in the region of the dentate nucleus has also been described [32].

Neuropsychiatric presentation

If a patient presents with neurologic or psychiatric symptomatology, the absence of a K-F ring makes the diagnosis of Wilson disease unlikely, although up to 5–10% of those with neurologic presentations have recently been found to not have a K-F ring [1]. Thorough examinations for a K-F ring must be carried out by slit lamp examination by an experienced ophthalmologist. However, copper might also be deposited in the cornea in chronic cholestatic liver disease, such as primary biliary cirrhosis or familial cholestatic syndromes, and even in neonates with cholestasis. Consequently, hepatic histology and other blood tests are necessary to exclude other forms of liver disease. Plasma ceruloplasmin is generally very low in those with this presentation but, for the reasons discussed above, there may be false positive and false negative results. Consequently, there is no single test that can be used to diagnose Wilson disease in all circumstances; it is the constellation of clinical history, family history, physical examination, and key laboratory tests that establish the diagnosis.

Brain CT shows that cerebral injury is not limited to the lenticular nuclei in Wilson disease. Williams and Walshe [46] evaluated 60 patients and found a surprisingly high frequency of CT abnormalities: 73% with ventricular dilation, 63% cortical atrophy, 55% brainstem atrophy, 45% hypodense areas in basal ganglia and 10% posterior fossa atrophy. This combination of findings appeared specific for Wilson disease, although the findings alone are observed in a variety of clinical conditions. Only 2 of 40 patients with neurologic symptoms had normal CT scans. Interestingly 75% of those with hepatic presentation and 50% of presymptomatic patients had abnormal scans. Penicillamine therapy resulted in improvement in basal ganglia hypodensities in 10 of 14 patients, as well as clinical improvement [46]. Despite striking abnormalities on brain CT, patients may still respond well to chelation treatment. Therefore, CT examination may be valuable in diagnosis and management of patients with neurologic involvement, even though it is of little prognostic value.

Magnetic resonance imaging has been used to better characterize and follow central nervous system lesions during copper chelation therapy. The most common abnormalities noted by MRI are lesions in the basal ganglia, ventricular dilatation, and generalized atrophy. Not unexpectedly, MRI has identified abnormalities in patients with normal CT scans. Prolongation of T_1-weighted images or darker areas on these images corresponds to necrosis, cystic change, or edema while a shorten T_1, which produces a lighter image, represents increased copper content. On MRI, 10 of 22 patients (46%) had lesions in the caudate, 9 (41%) in putamen, 8 (36%) brain atrophy, 6 (27%) midbrain lesions, 5 (23%) subcortical white matter lesions, 5 (23%) pons lesions, and 2 (10%) in thalamus, vermis, dentate or globus pallidus. Dystonia and bradykinesia correlated with putamen lesions and dysarthria with both putamen and caudate lesions. Using a more sensitive ultra-low-field MRI technique with computerized image processing, a gradual return toward normality was demonstrated in brain lesions of a 13-year-old boy with Wilson disease concomitant with clinical improvement during copper chelation therapy [47]. More recently, positron emission tomography has been used to evaluate brain lesions in Wilson disease. Glucose consumption was reduced in the cerebellum, striatum, cortex, and thalamus, and there was a significant reduction in dopa-decarboxylase, which indicates impaired function of the striatal dopaminergic pathway.

A variety of electrophysiologic and imaging techniques have been used to evaluate patients with Wilson disease and the response to chelation therapy. Auditory evoked potentials showed increased wave latencies in those with central nervous system involvement, were normal in neurologic symptom-free patients, and improved during copper chelation therapy. Visual evoked potentials revealed abnormally prolonged latency in three of eight symptomatic patients tested. Likewise, somatosensory evoked potentials showed central conduction delay in symptomatic patients, were normal in symptom-free patients, and improved during therapy. These findings suggest involvement of sensory pathways as they course through the brainstem, although hearing, vision, and sensory function are unimpaired.

Specific clinical circumstances

Acute hepatitis

Acute hepatitis in Wilson disease is most often confused with acute viral hepatitis, particularly if the patient makes a complete recovery. Serologic markers for hepatitis A, B, and C viruses as well as Epstein–Barr virus, cytomegalovirus and other hepatotrophic viruses are negative. Additionally, markers for toxin-induced hepatitis and autoimmune hepatitis are negative. Some key findings that should alert the clinician to the diagnosis of Wilson disease, include a mild hemolytic anemia or a depressed serum uric acid level (from renal tubular losses), or low alkaline phosphatase. In the absence of positive serologies, patients with acute non-specific hepatitis should be screened for evidence of Wilson disease and autoimmune hepatitis.

Acute liver failure (fulminant hepatitis)

Establishing the diagnosis of Wilson disease in the patient with acute liver failure may be particularly difficult. Liver biopsy may not be possible because of coagulopathy; renal failure may preclude collection of urine; ceruloplasmin may be low because of the liver failure itself; and K-F rings are often absent because of the young age of the patients. This presentation may appear similar to acute fulminant viral, autoimmune, or toxin induced hepatitis, although several clues should suggest Wilson disease. A Coombs-negative hemolytic anemia, with elevated reticulocyte count, caused by rapid release of massive amounts of copper from the necrosing liver is characteristic of Wilson disease, causes an extremely high serum bilirubin (reaching 60–80 mg/dL), and makes this the most likely diagnosis [1]. Occasionally hepatitis A virus triggers hemolysis in patients with glucose-6-phosphate dehydrogenase deficiency or thalassemia trait; however, hepatitis A virus infection can quickly be excluded serologically. Other findings that should suggest Wilson disease include relatively low serum aminotransferase for fulminant hepatic failure of 2–10× upper limit of normal and an abnormally low serum alkaline phosphatase

level for patient age. This latter finding is not caused by interference of copper or bilirubin with the alkaline phosphatase assay, nor is it caused by abnormalities in zinc metabolism. In addition, the serum AST is significantly more elevated than the ALT. In one study of patients in this clinical setting, a ratio of alkaline phosphatase (IU/L) to total serum bilirubin (mg/dL) of <4 combined with an AST:ALT ratio of >2.2, appeared to be diagnostic of Wilson disease [38]. In this presentation, serum copper levels are very elevated, rather than depressed, because of the hepatocyte copper release with hepatic necrosis; however, elevated serum copper could not differentiate Wilsonian patients from other causes of acute liver failure. If present, K-F rings seen on slit-lamp examination will confirm the diagnosis of Wilson disease, although they are commonly absent in the typical adolescent female with Wilson disease and acute liver failure in whom neuropsychiatric symptoms have not yet developed. Results of genotyping are unlikely to be available when decisions surrounding liver transplantation have to be made urgently.

Transjugular liver biopsy can allow tissue to be obtained even if a significant coagulopathy is present provided the patient is stable enough to be moved to the radiology suite. Characteristic histologic findings of Wilson disease, such as fatty change, periportal glycogenated nuclei, and an elevated hepatic copper content, aid in the diagnosis. Ultrastructural mitochondrial changes of Wilson disease are also valuable. If the patient undergoes liver transplant and Wilson disease cannot be diagnosed or excluded based on the histology, electron microscopy, or quantitative copper content of the removed recipient liver, then DNA mutation analysis should be performed.

If the diagnosis of Wilson disease escapes detection, all patients with acute liver failure will die of hepatic or renal failure. Even when appropriately diagnosed, these patients virtually never recover despite copper chelation therapy, plasmapheresis, or postdilution hemofiltration and require urgent liver transplantation. In many patients, it will be obvious that liver transplantation will be required regardless of the underlying diagnosis. Prompt referral to a liver transplantation center for emergency liver transplantation evaluation is essential to save the patient's life.

Chronic hepatitis and cirrhosis

Other than finding a mild hemolytic anemia, there is little to distinguish Wilson disease as a cause of cirrhosis from other causes. A high degree of suspicion is necessary to pursue slit-lamp examination for a K-F ring, investigate for a positive family history, or recognize neuropsychiatric symptoms. For this reason, all children age 3–4 years or older with cirrhosis should undergo evaluation for Wilson disease as described. Referral for a liver transplantation evaluation should be considered if at diagnosis there is an irreversible coagulopathy, encephalopathy, or renal insufficiency, or if hepatic decompensation develops despite the initiation of copper chelation therapy.

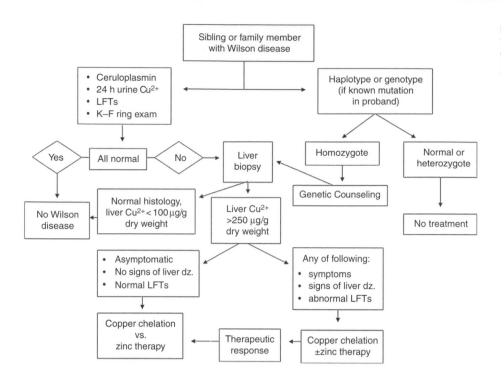

Figure 28.12 Approach to evaluation and treatment of asymptomatic siblings (or other first-degree relative) of patient with Wilson disease. Illustrated are both a "phenotype" and a "genotype" approach to evaluation. dz, disease.

Chronically elevated aminotransferases

All children and adults who have unexplained chronically elevated serum aminotransferases require a plasma ceruloplasmin, slit-lamp examination, 24-hour urine copper excretion, and, most likely, a liver biopsy to establish the underlying diagnosis. Attributing elevated aminotransferases as being caused by non-alcoholic fatty liver disease in obese or overweight patients has the potential of overlooking Wilson disease in a significant number of patients. Institution of copper chelation at this stage of Wilson disease assuredly will prevent serious hepatic or neurologic sequelae if cirrhosis has not yet developed.

Asymptomatic patients with Kayser–Fleischer rings

In an asymptomatic patient for whom a K-F ring is found on routine ophthalmologic examination, plasma ceruloplasmin should be assessed. If it is low, or there is high suspicion and it is normal, a 24-hour urine copper excretion should be performed and consideration given for a liver biopsy or genotyping. Elevated urine copper excretion, low plasma ceruloplasmin, and a K-F ring establish the diagnosis. However, if liver or spleen is enlarged, or liver blood tests are abnormal, a liver biopsy should be considered.

Asymptomatic siblings of patients with Wilson disease

Asymptomatic siblings and other first-degree relatives of a Wilson disease patient should be screened for the disease after 2 years of age, unless hepatomegaly or abnormal aminotransferase levels are found earlier. A thorough history and physical examination, slit-lamp examination, and laboratory analysis

should be performed (Figure 28.12). If all tests are normal, it is very unlikely that the relative has Wilson disease. However, if any of those tests are abnormal, a liver biopsy should be performed for histology, electron microscopy, and quantitative copper analysis. An alternative, less invasive approach is to evaluate the known patient, the sibling, and the parents for DNA haplotype (microsatellite markers) to determine if the sibling in question has inherited the gene for Wilson disease. Haplotype analysis is informative in over 90–95% of cases. Another approach is to genotype the affected relative, and if *ATP7B* mutations are identified, to test the sibling in question for these mutations. Finding two disease-causing mutations or informative microsatellite markers will establish the diagnosis of Wilson disease and preclude the need for liver biopsy, unless there are signs or symptoms of chronic liver disease.

Treatment

Without treatment, Wilson disease is uniformly fatal. The hallmark of medical management in Wilson disease is reducing or chelating the stored copper and preventing copper from reaccumulating. This is accomplished by instituting therapy with one of several copper-chelating agents, a low copper diet, oral zinc, and, possibly, antioxidants (Table 28.4). Stringent dietary restriction of copper-containing foods is impractical, although it is recommended that patients avoid foods with very high copper content, such as chocolate, nuts, legumes, mushrooms, shellfish, and liver. Domestic water softeners should *not* be used because they may increase copper concentrations in drinking water substantially.

Table 28.4 Medications used in treatment of Wilson disease

Medication	Action	Dose	Comments
D-Penicillamine	Copper chelator	*Initial*: 20 mg/kg daily (up to 1.5–2.0 g/day maximum), 3 doses per day, between meals *Maintenance*: 10–20 mg/kg daily (up to 0.75–1.0 g/day) *Oral pyridoxine*: 25–50 mg daily	Initial and maintenance therapy
Trientine	Copper chelator	Same dose as penicillamine	Same as above
Zinc acetate	Inhibits copper absorption, stimulates hepatic metallothionein	25–50 mg 3 times a day between meals	Slower action than copper chelators; useful for maintenance and during pregnancy
Ammonium tetrathiomolybdate	Inhibits copper absorption, copper chelator	120–200 mg/day	Investigational drug used for limited (6–8 weeks) periods of time
Vitamin E	Antioxidant	400–1200 IU/day (2–3 doses per day with meals)	Adjunctive therapy

Copper chelation therapy

Until the 1950s, little effective therapy was available for Wilson disease. British AntiLewisite was then introduced and shown to effectively chelate copper but the need for daily intramuscular injections limited its usefulness. There are currently three commercially available anticopper agents and a fourth agent that is being used under an Investigational New Drug application to the US Food and Drug Administration. These are D-penicillamine (β,β-dimethylcysteine), trientine, zinc, and the investigational drug ammonium tetrathiomolybdate. There is only one recently published randomized trial comparing two of these therapies [48]. Published data include primarily single center experience and combined center reviews. The most published experience is with D-penicillamine because it was the first orally effective drug developed for the treatment of Wilson disease.

D-Penicillamine

The paramount work of Walshe clearly demonstrated the benefits of D-penicillamine in Wilson disease [18]. D-Penicillamine is a sulfhydryl-containing metabolite of penicillin that is absorbed well from the gastrointestinal tract, effectively chelates copper, and is then excreted in the urine. The pharmaceutical form is D-penicillamine (referrred to as D-penicillamine or penicillamine), as L-penicillamine is toxic. The actual mechanism on how this drug works is not known. The major action of penicillamine was originally thought to be a "decoppering effect," although there are conflicting data as to whether it actually reduces total copper content of the liver and other organs. Alternatively, a "detoxification" effect has been proposed in which copper is directly complexed to the drug and induction of metallothionein synthesis occurs. Thus, unbound or "toxic" copper will not be available to injure the liver and central nervous system.

It is recommended to begin penicillamine therapy with 250–500 mg/day and increase by 250 mg increments every 4–7 days to a maximum dose of 1000–1500 mg/day in two to four divided doses in an adult, given ideally at least 30 minutes before or 2 or more hours after meals as food inhibits its absorption [1]. Maintenance dosing is 750–1000 mg/day in two divided doses. In children, the target dose is 20 mg/kg daily, rounded to the nearest multiple of 250 mg and given ideally in three divided doses. After stabilization, the dose can be divided into two or three daily doses not to be given with meals. Penicillamine may have an antipyroxidine effect; therefore, *all treated patients should also receive 25–50 mg pyridoxine daily* [1].

During the first month of penicillamine therapy, the patient should be monitored weekly for fever or rash. A complete blood count and platelet count, urinalysis, renal and liver blood tests should be obtained each 1 to 2 weeks. If the patient responds appropriately with resolution of symptoms and normalization of liver blood tests, monitoring is performed every 1 to 3 months for the first year, and every 6 to 12 months thereafter. Abnormalities in liver blood tests may persist for at least a year of treatment; however, the trend should be toward improvement within the first 6 months of therapy. An annual 24-hour urinary copper excretion is helpful in monitoring chronic penicillamine therapy. Initially, up to several grams of copper may be excreted in 24 hours; however, after months to years of chelation, as little as 200 to 500 µg of copper should be excreted per day [1]. If urinary copper excretion is <200 µg/24 h, poor adherence with chelation therapy should be suspected or overtreatment and excess copper removal. In those with non-adherence, non-ceruloplasmin-bound copper is elevated (>15 µg/dL) and in those with overtreatment, values are low (<5 µg/dL). If copper excretion increases suddenly, this suggests a lapse in adherence, followed by resumption of penicillamine a few days prior to the urine collection. Non-ceruloplasmin-bound copper should normalize with effective therapy. Values should be 5–15 µg/dL during effective therapy. Non-compliance is suspected if, during chronic therapy, the non-ceruloplasmin-bound copper is >20 µg/dL. Values <5 µg/dL should be repeated, and if confirmed, may indicate copper deficiency and the dose of penicillamine should be gradually reduced by 25% and the patient monitored closely. For patients in whom K-F rings had been initially detected, serial ophthalmologic examination is helpful in documenting disappearance or significant reduction of these lesions with adequate copper chelation [1]. Serial ophthalmologic examination may also be useful in patients without K-F rings, as the development of rings would also indicate poor compliance. For patients that require higher doses of penicillamine, the dose can be reduced to 750 to 1000 mg/day once clinical symptoms have resolved [1]. If compliant, penicillamine therapy will maintain the asymptomatic patient in good health. Uninterrupted lifelong therapy is mandatory. A yearly discussion with the patient and family should reinforce the importance of compliance. Patients should be reminded of the essential need to take the penicillamine without fail, and the possible fatal consequences of discontinuing this therapy suddenly. In one series, 8 of 11 patients who discontinued therapy died of fulminant liver failure within 2.6 years.

In 10–50% of patients, neurologic symptoms worsened shortly after penicillamine therapy was started [19]. Continued or reduced dose penicillamine therapy generally resulted in reversal of this worsening, although irreversible neurologic abnormalities have been reported [19]. Therefore, it is recommended that the penicillamine dose be reduced to 250 mg/day if neurologic symptoms worsen and gradually increased every 4–7 days by 250 mg/day until urinary copper excretion exceeds 2000 µg/day. The cause of this neurologic worsening is not known. Some propose that there is a transient brain exposure to increased blood copper as the penicillamine mobilizes hepatic copper stores, or that penicillamine may form a complex with intracellular copper that is more toxic. Although this type of neurologic exacerbation is more common with penicillamine it does not appear to be specific to this agent. Worsening neurologic function has also been reported, although less frequently, following initiation of treatment with trientine, thiomolybdates, and zinc. A seriously neurologically handicapped patient may respond poorly to penicillamine therapy alone and require combined therapy with British AntiLewisite. Recent data suggest that the investigational drug ammonium tetrathiomolybdate may be a better alternative in patients with neurologic symptoms [48] but this drug has not been approved for use.

The effect of penicillamine therapy on psychiatric disturbances is difficult to predict, although improved school performance is commonly observed in treated children. Liver dysfunction generally improves rapidly (by 2–6 months) with penicillamine therapy but if overt fibrosis and cirrhosis are present, the signs of portal hypertension show little response although histology may gradually improve. Hepatic copper content generally decreases but may remain quite elevated despite years of therapy and clinical improvement. Patients with psychiatric disturbances require not only copper chelation therapy but also psychotherapy and appropriate psychotropic medications.

Penicillamine may produce both allergic and toxic side effects in up to 30% of patients, which has limited its use in recent years. Early side effects of penicillamine include a hypersensitivity reaction manifested as fever, skin rash, lymphadenopathy, and pancytopenia [1]. After the first year of therapy, late toxic reactions include proteinuria, nephrotic syndrome, drug-associated systemic lupus erythematosus, Goodpasture syndrome, optic neuritis, agranulocytosis, thrombocytopenia, myasthenia gravis, low serum IgA levels, loss of taste, and anaphylactic reactions [32]. The most common late reactions with penicillamine are observed in the skin because of the interference with cross-linking of collagen and elastin. These include a dermatopathy (cutis laxa) associated with weakening of subcutaneous tissue, elastosis perforans serpiginosa, lichen planus, aphthous stomatitis, systemic sclerosis-like lesions, and pemphigoid lesions in mouth, vagina, and skin. Rarely, hepatotoxicity, hair loss, or dysgeusia have been reported. For treatment of these reactions, penicillamine should be temporarily discontinued until the lesions resolve, and 2 or 3 days before restarting therapy, 0.5 mg/kg prednisone daily should be started. Penicillamine could then be reintroduced at a lower dose and increased gradually with weaning of prednisone when the final dose is reached and tolerated [32]. Alternatively, trientine therapy should be substituted for penicillamine with any significant toxic reaction. If bone marrow toxicity is observed, penicillamine should be immediately withdrawn and trientine substituted. Overall, trientine appears to be associated with a lower frequency of side effects and is recommended by some authorities as a safer initial chelator for Wilson disease.

Penicillamine therapy is ineffective in patients with fulminant Wilson disease (acute liver failure), in patients who develop hepatic failure after penicillamine therapy has been discontinued, and those with advanced cirrhosis [32]. These patients will rarely survive unless liver transplant is performed. As in other patients with acute liver failure, survival is dependent on rapid referral to a liver transplant center, intensive care therapy, and a rapid evaluation for liver transplantation.

Triethylene tetramine dihydrochloride (trientine)

In 1985, trientine was approved by the US Food and Drug Administration for patients who are intolerant to penicillamine [49]. It does not contain sulfhydryl groups but chelates copper by forming a stable complex with copper through its four nitrogen atoms in a planar ring. It is very effective and many advocate it the preferential first-line copper-chelating drug [49], primarily because of its better safety profile. The initial dosage for adolescents and adults and is 750–1500 mg/day in two to three divided doses 30–60 minutes prior to meals or 2 hours after meals. Maintenance therapy is typically 750–1000 mg/day. In children, the dosage is 20 mg/kg daily rounded off to the nearest 250 mg in two or three divided doses. The drug is less toxic than penicillamine. Toxicity includes bone marrow suppression (a sideroblastic anemia), nephrotoxicity, and skin and mucosal lesions [1]. Females may become iron deficient and require iron supplementation. Initiation of therapy requires a clinical and laboratory assessment and adjustment of doses in a similar manner to that for penicillamine. Patients are monitored with 24-hour urinary coppers and other laboratory tests as they are for penicillamine (see above). There appears to be no cross-reactivity in toxicity in those patients who have toxic reactions to penicillamine.

Ammonium tetrathiomolybdate

Brewer *et al.* proposed an alternative approach to the treatment of Wilson disease that is based on whether the patient presents with neurologic or hepatic symptoms [19,48]. Because up to 50% of patients in this series who had neurologic disease showed worsening of their symptoms with penicillamine therapy, they proposed using an alternative drug, ammonium tetrathiomolybdate, for initial therapy in neurologically affected patients [19,48]. This investigational compound acts by forming a stable three-way complex with protein and copper. Given with food, it complexes with dietary copper, preventing its absorption; when taken between meals it is absorbed and complexes with copper and albumin in blood, preventing cellular uptake and resulting in decreased intracellular copper stores. This drug may exhibit a higher affinity for copper than metallothionein in vitro, providing a rationale for its proposed ability to remove copper from cells. An initial study of 33 neurologically affected patients treated for 8 weeks as initial therapy reported that there was no worsening of neurological symptoms. The drug was given for a total of 8 weeks, as 20 mg with meals and snacks and between-meal dose ranging from 20 to 80 mg, three times a day. After 8 weeks, the drug was stopped and patients were maintained on oral zinc acetate 50 mg three times a day. In a follow-up study with 22 additional patients, the incidence of side effects was slightly higher. Of the 22 patients, three dropped out of the study, two developed neurologic deterioration and five had bone marrow suppression. There are concerns over possible bone marrow suppression and other toxicities of this drug.

Recently, a randomized comparison of tetrathiomolybdate and trientine as initial treatment was conducted in 48 patients with Wilson disease presenting with neurologic symptoms [48]. Six in the trientine arm and one in the tetrathiomolybdate arm showed neurologic progression during therapy ($p < 0.05$). Seven receiving tetrathiomolybdate had an adverse event (none serious, four with elevations of aminotransferases) while only one receiving trientine did so. These data suggest a possible benefit of tetrathiomolybdate short term for neurologically affected patients. Continued ongoing prospective evaluation of this potential treatment will hopefully yield useful guidelines for its use and more information about possible side effects. This drug has not been approved for use in patients with Wilson disease.

Zinc therapy

Zinc has been proposed as maintenance or adjunctive therapy for Wilson disease [50,51]. Zinc inhibits intestinal absorption of copper and, possibly, increases metallothionein binding of copper in the liver. The dose of zinc acetate, given between meals, currently advocated is 50 mg elemental zinc in adolescents and adults three times daily or zinc sulfate 150–220 mg given three times daily. Common side effects include headache and gastrointestinal upset, perhaps less with zinc acetate, and iron deficiency. Because of its slower onset of action, zinc therapy is generally not used as initial therapy in symptomatic patients in most, but not all, countries. It is not known whether zinc therapy is beneficial for patients receiving a copper chelator or whether it binds to the chelator and prevents its action, so it is not recommended as combined therapy. Since chelators bind zinc, giving them together to a patient may interfere with the action of both. Zinc therapy may play a role in presymptomatic patients or siblings identified very early in their disease course. Some authorities suggest that since these children have normal liver blood tests, normal or mildly increased urinary copper excretion, and mild to moderate elevation of hepatic copper, they should not be exposed to the possible side effects of copper chelators. Since these children have not yet accumulated a toxic burden of copper, it is proposed that sole treatment with zinc (1 mg/kg elemental zinc dose three times a day between meals) is effective in inhibiting intestinal copper absorption and lowering the copper burden, and zinc is less toxic. Prospective long-term follow-up of such children under various forms of treatment is needed to establish the safest and most effective manner of treating this enlarging group of patients. Although there are a number of reports of successful maintenance therapy with zinc [50], it should be used cautiously as a sole agent and patients monitored very closely [51]. A recent report from Germany suggests that zinc monotherapy was associated with more hepatic treatment failures and worse actuarial survival than with chelating agents [51]. It should also be stressed that patients have deteriorated and developed fulminant liver failure after the discontinuation of zinc therapy.

Antioxidant therapy

The role of antioxidants as adjunctive therapy in Wilson disease has not been thoroughly explored. The basis for this type of therapy is the demonstrated oxidative damage to the hepatocyte in rats with copper overload, Bedlington terriers, and patients with Wilson disease [22,26]. In addition, α-tocopherol (vitamin E) has been shown to protect isolated rat hepatocytes from the toxicity of in vivo copper loading. Hepatic concentrations of antioxidants, such as glutathione and vitamin E [22], are depressed and circulating vitamin E levels are lower in patients with Wilson disease compared with controls. There are several anecdotal reports of patients with liver failure being "rescued" by adjuvunct vitamin E therapy in addition to aggressive copper chelation therapy. Vitamin E, 400–1200 IU/day, can be safely given orally in divided doses with meals.

Table 28.5 Prognostic index in fulminant Wilson disease

Test	Normal	Score				
		0	1	2	3	4
Serum bilirubin (μmol/L (mg/dL))	3–20 (0.2–1.2)	<100 (<5.9)	100–150 (5.9–8.8)	151–200 (8.9–11.8)	201–300 (11.9–17.5)	>300 (>17.5)
Serum aspartate aminotransferase (IU/L)	7–20	<100	100–150	151–200	201–300	>300
Prolongation of prothrombin time (s)		<4	4–8	9–12	13–20	>20

A prognostic total score of 7 or more indicates the need for liver transplantation.
Source: adapted from Nazer *et al.*, 1986 [54] and published by permission of BMJ Publishing Group.

Since high-dose vitamin E may interfere with vitamin K-dependent clotting factor synthesis, the prothrombin time should be monitored and vitamin K supplementation used if necessary. Other antioxidants are not currently recommended until further testing is performed.

Liver transplantation

Orthotopic liver transplantation is well established as a life-saving therapy in patients with Wilson disease and acute fulminant hepatic failure, fulminant hepatic failure after inadvisably discontinuing copper chelation therapy, and patients with decompensated cirrhosis unresponsive to medical therapy. A survey of 57 transplant recipients showed survival of 44 (77%) at a mean of 2.7 years after transplant, a poorer outcome in patients with neurologic disease, and disappearance of K-F rings in 18 out of 20 patients examined [52]. Neurologic symptoms improve in survivors of liver transplantation. In another series of 45 transplant recipients, survival at 5 years was 73% (33), with poorer outcome in those with fulminant hepatic failure [53]. Living-related transplantation from heterozygote parent donors has also been shown to be successful. Liver engraftment appears to cure the underlying biochemical defect making further copper chelation therapy unnecessary.

To better determine criteria for referral for liver transplantation, Nazer *et al.* [54] have developed a prognostic index based on grading from 1 to 4 points the serum bilirubin concentration, serum AST, and prolongation of prothrombin time (Table 28.5). Patients with 7 or more out of a possible 12 points at presentation had fatal courses or required transplantation, and those with 6 points or less survived with medical therapy alone. Dhawan *et al.* [55] evaluated the validity of this scoring system for pediatric patients by retrospectively reviewing the data from 74 patients who either died or survived on medical management. Using 7 points as the cut-off number for death without transplantation, five children with a score >7 survived on chelation therapy. Importantly four children who had a score <7 died on medical management. This translates into a sensitivity of 87% and a specificity of 90%. The authors developed a new index based on serum bilirubin, INR, AST, albumin, and white cell count at presentation. A score of >11, out of a possible 20, was predictive for

death with a 93% sensitivity, 98% specificity, and a positive predictive value of 88% [55]. The new index was then prospectively evaluated in 14 patients. Four patients were predicted to need transplantation, while no patient with a score of <11 died on medical management [55]. One patient with a score of 11 survived on medical management. This index appears to be more sensitive and specific in predicting mortality without transplantation. If further prospective evaluation of this index proves its validity, it may help to facilitate selection of patients for potential liver transplantation. Currently, there does not appear to be a role for gene transfer therapy in Wilson disease because of the availability of other effective treatments and the uncertainties of gene therapy.

Special circumstances
Pregnancy

During pregnancy it is advisable to continue penicillamine therapy at a dose of 750–1000 mg/day [1], although one authority advises discontinuation during the first 12 weeks of gestation, if possible. Several patients who have discontinued therapy for longer periods during pregnancy have had episodes of acute hemolysis or worsening of liver disease [1], including fulminant hepatic failure. Penicillamine has been administered to over 150 pregnant patients with Wilson disease [1,56] and there have been two cases of neonatal transient cutis laxa. However, one infant developed a connective tissue defect, although the mother was being treated with penicillamine for cystinuria. The overall risk of miscarriage and fetal abnormalities in infants whose mothers were maintained on penicillamine during pregnancy (750–1000 mg/day for first two trimesters, and 500 mg/day for last trimester) appear to be the same (144 normal neonates in 153 pregnancies) as for those whose mothers received trientine therapy (19 normal neonates in 22 pregnancies), and for those whose mothers received zinc therapy (24 normal neonates in 26 pregnancies) [56]. Therefore, trientine and zinc therapy are probably equivalent to penicillamine therapy as far as safety during pregnancy [56]. All children fathered by patients with Wilson disease have been normal. Although infants may be at a small risk for a connective tissue or skin abnormality during penicillamine therapy, the risk to mother and infant of discontinuing copper chelation therapy appears to be greater [56]. If cesarean section is anticipated, some authorities recommend reducing the dose of penicillamine to 250 mg/day 6 weeks prior to delivery to reduce the risk for impaired wound healing. Women taking penicillamine should not breast-feed because it is secreted in breast milk and could potentially be harmful to the infant [1].

Surgery

Penicillamine has inhibitory effects on collagen cross-linking. Therefore, in order to prevent interference with wound healing, it is recommended that, when patients with Wilson disease undergo surgery, the dose of penicillamine should be reduced, but not stopped, for 10–14 days postoperatively.

Indian childhood cirrhosis and idiopathic copper toxicosis

There are several additional disorders of hepatic copper toxicosis in childhood. Indian childhood cirrhosis has been a significant cause of mortality in the preschool age child in India and neighboring countries. The cause of this toxicosis has been attributed to excess copper exposure from ingestion of contaminated milk or water sources. Liver biopsies of these patients show extraordinarily high levels of hepatic copper, suggesting that copper may be involved in the pathogenesis of this condition [57]. Clusters of children living in the Austrian province of Tyrol and in northern Germany and isolated cases from North America and other countries have been described in which the clinical course, hepatic histology, and hepatic copper levels are similar to the classic cases from India. These entities have been called endemic Tyrolean infantile cirrhosis and idiopathic copper toxicosis, respectively. They may represent several distinct diseases or the same disease in different populations. Although dietary copper restriction has markedly reduced the number of cases, it is unclear whether excessive intake of copper alone is enough to cause disease. This suggests that there is a second factor contributing to these disorders. Two mechanisms have been suggested for the etiologic role of copper in the development of childhood hepatic toxicosis: (1) copper may act in synergy with a hepatoxin, or (2) patients may have a genetic predisposition to copper-associated liver damage (a so-called ecogenetic disease) [58]. Treatment with copper chelation is promising; without treatment, these diseases are invariably fatal. Both diseases have decreased in frequency with the recognition of the relation to copper contamination of the diet. Both ICC and ICT of childhood will be discussed.

Indian childhood cirrhosis

Epidemiology and genetics

Classically, ICC occurs in children 1–3 years of age, but it has occurred up to age 10 years [57]. There is a positive family history in 30% but the genetics have not been well established.

In India, ICC has been one of the leading causes of cirrhosis in children, and was said to be the fourth most common cause of death in pediatric centers in that country prior to changes in feeding practices that were associated with excessive copper intake. Boys outnumber girls 3:1 without discrimination by social class. A striking epidemiologic association discovered in the 1980s was the observation that boiled animal milk stored in brass utensils, which was the common practice in India, has a very high copper concentration, and that this copper is bound to casein [59]. Compared with control infants who did not develop ICC, children with ICC who lived in small rural communities were less likely to be exclusively breast-fed, received animal milk earlier, and stopped breast-feeding at a younger age. Patients with ICC seemed to have an earlier and larger exposure to milk contaminated with copper leached from brass utensils. Asymptomatic siblings have also been found to have mild to moderate accumulation of copper but no evidence of liver dysfunction. Consequently, it has been proposed that there might be a genetic predisposition to the liver injury in ICC that requires excessive copper intake to lead to disease expression [57]. Indeed, family data from a series of cases from Pune, India showed that 26% of cases were from consanguineous parents, higher than the 13% in children with other liver disorders. The gene causing Wilson disease, *ATP7B*, has been excluded in non-Wilsonian syndromes. A defect in metallothionein synthesis was shown in an American child with an ICC-like illness, however, this defect was not found in three patients with ICC or in two other patients with ICT. Additionally, *MURR1*, responsible for the Bedlington terrier copper toxicosis, has been excluded as the gene causing non-Wilsonian syndromes.

Clinical features

The clinical presentation of ICC has been divided into three stages [57]. In the early stage, anorexia, irritability, and low-grade fever develop, and abdominal distension from an enlarged, smooth liver with a sharp firm edge is found. During the intermediate stage, jaundice and signs of portal hypertension such as splenomegaly and ascites appear, associated with an increased susceptibility to infection. Progression to cirrhosis takes from 1 to 8 months. The late stage is characterized by decompensated cirrhosis with jaundice, a shrinking liver, gastrointestinal bleeding, repeated infections, edema, and, finally, hepatic encephalopathy and death.

Serum aminotransferase, bilirubin, and albumin, and coagulation studies follow the expected changes for the various stages of ICC. Renal tubular dysfunction reveals a generalized amino aciduria and the presence of reducing substances. Other characteristic findings include elevated serum immunoglobulin levels, positive anti-smooth muscle antibodies in up to 45% of cases, elevated serum α-fetoprotein, and low complement levels. Serum ceruloplasmin and copper levels are normal to elevated, distinguishing this disease from Wilson disease.

The course of decompensation from cirrhosis in untreated patients is rapid. Within 4 weeks of presentation, there is 45%

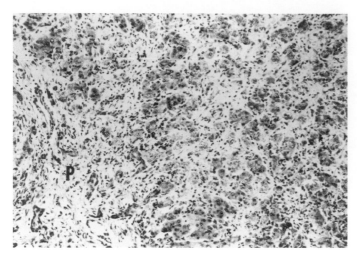

Figure 28.13 Histology of liver in Indian childhood cirrhosis. Low-power view of liver of American child, showing extensive fibrosis throughout hepatic lobules, entrapment of clusters of hepatocytes, and parenchymal inflammation that includes neutrophils and lymphocytes. P, portal tract. (Hematoxylin & eosin, magnification ×150.) (With permission from Sokol, 1992 [2].)

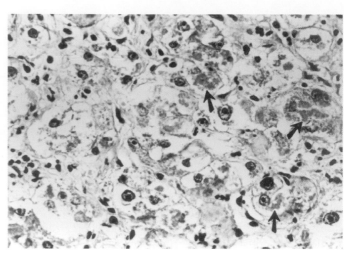

Figure 28.14 Histology of liver in Indian childhood cirrhosis. Hepatocytes are diffusely ballooned and many contain Mallory bodies (arrows). Note the infiltrate of neutrophils and lymphocytes surrounding the hepatocytes. (Hematoxylin & eosin, magnification ×600.) (With permission from Sokol, 1992 [2].)

mortality, and 86% die within 6 months [60]. Occasional children survive longer untreated; however, it is possible that these children suffer from a separate entity. Copper chelation therapy has dramatically changed the natural course of ICC and changes in storage of milk in India have led to a welcome reduction in the number of cases.

Histopathology

The hepatic histology in ICC shows several distinguishing characteristics: (1) hepatocellular necrosis with prominent Mallory's hyaline, (2) marked pericellular fibrosis throughout the hepatic lobule (micro-micronodular cirrhosis), (3) a lack of regenerative nodules, and (4) coarse brown aggregates of copper-associated protein in the hepatocytes (Figures 28.13–28.15). The early histologic lesion consists of ballooned hepatocytes, reflecting hepatocellular injury, with focal inflammatory cell infiltrates near necrotic hepatocytes. For the most part, portal tracts remain uninflamed. Mallory's hyaline affects approximately 15% of the hepatocytes but it may be more prominent in rapidly progressive and fatal cases. Hepatic steatosis is characteristically absent. Creeping intercellular fibrosis creates the characteristic micro-micronodular cirrhosis that eventually develops as small islands of hepatocytes are segregated from the rest of the hepatic lobule by fibrosis. Hepatocyte regenerative changes and regenerative nodules are conspicuously absent. Inflammatory infiltrates in the parenchyma and portal tracts are composed mostly of mononuclear cells and some neutrophils around degenerating hepatocytes. Bile ductular proliferation is a constant feature, with variable degrees of hepatocellular and canalicular cholestasis.

Increased amounts of hepatocellular copper and copper-associated protein are indicated by appropriate histochemical staining, such as the rhodamine and Orcein stains,

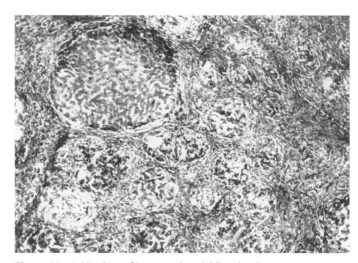

Figure 28.15 Histology of liver in Indian childhood cirrhosis. Low-power micrograph demonstrates its "micro-micronodular" nature. Majority of modules are much smaller than normal hepatic lobule. (Masson trichrome stain, magnification ×60.) (With permission from Sokol, 1992 [2].)

respectively. Glycogen depletion and multinucleated giant cells are characteristic of the advanced cirrhotic lesion. Kupffer cells contain iron and lipofuscin.

Electron microscopy reveals Mallory's hyaline, indistinct mitochondria, and dilated rough endoplasmic reticulum. Lysosomal copper is also evident.

Pathogenesis

Many factors have been considered in the pathogenesis of ICC. Although many etiologic agents may lead to liver failure in children in India, infectious agents have only rarely been associated with ICC. The hepatitis viruses do not play a role in ICC. Aflatoxin, a hepatotoxin produced by the fungus *Aspergillus flavus* has been implicated because this fungus commonly contaminates grain, nuts, and animal feed in India and appears in milk of cows. In addition, cirrhosis in children has been linked to ingestion of peanuts contaminated by aflatoxin. It has been proposed that in addition to copper in milk, ingestion of a second contaminant, such as aflatoxin, might compound the copper toxicity leading to cirrhosis, however there are little data to support its role.

It has also been proposed that synergistic toxicity of pyrrolizidine alkaloids secreted in milk of lactating cows or buffalo may produce liver injury in human infants if the milk is subsequently contaminated with copper. Such a synergy has been demonstrated in sheep and suckling rats, with severe liver damage caused by the combination of agents. Although these alkaloids have been more commonly associated with venoocclusive disease of the liver in the West Indies, when administered with excess copper they increase copper accumulation and toxicity in animals. Although this is an interesting hypothesis, currently few human data support a role of pyrrolizidine alkaloids in ICC.

A nutritional etiology has not been supported since the liver in ICC lacks the steatosis that is common in nutritional liver disease. The immunologic abnormalities of hypergammaglobulinemia, reduced complement levels, depressed delayed type hypersensitivity, and reduced T-cell numbers present in ICC probably reflect hepatocellular damage and malnutrition rather than an autoimmune component. The role of chronic ingestion of copper in this disorder compared with unaffected children is supported by both the high incidence and the earlier introduction of animal milk feedings from brass utensils used to heat and store milk [57], and the documented increase of milk copper concentration from 11.5 to 625 µg/dL when milk is heated and stored in this fashion.

The liver in ICC has the highest copper levels of any human condition. The average hepatic copper content is approximately 1400 µg/g dry weight liver, with values reported up to 4788 µg/g liver [57]. Furthermore, the intracellular distribution of copper includes diffuse hepatocyte cytoplasmic staining for copper, and copper-laden hepatocytes show evidence of severe damage, suggesting that this copper is toxic and involved in the pathogenesis of liver injury [57]. It has been proposed that the excessive copper interferes with assembly of microtubes leading to the accumulation of intermediate filaments that constitute the Mallory's hyaline characteristic of ICC and interfering with intracellular transport of secretory proteins, causing ballooning of hepatocytes.

Compelling evidence that copper is the cause of liver injury in ICC is derived from studies of both treatment and prevention of ICC. Treatment with penicillamine early in the course of disease reduces mortality [61], improves liver histology and reverses cirrhosis, and leads to long-term survival. In fact, penicillamine therapy has been discontinued in a number of children, after a mean of 3–5 years of therapy, without recurrence of disease or relapse. Moreover, the recurrence rate of ICC in children born subsequently to families with an index case was significantly reduced in families who received dietary advice to avoid boiling and storing animal milk in brass utensils compared with those not receiving such advice [57]. Therefore, most experts believe copper is the primary factor in the pathogenesis of liver injury in ICC; however, a genetic defect in copper metabolism or excretion has not been excluded as being a predisposing factor.

Diagnosis and treatment

The diagnosis of ICC is established based on the age of the patient, rapid onset and progression of severe liver disease, absence of other common causes of liver disease, negative serologies for hepatitis viruses, histologic findings on liver biopsy, normal serum ceruloplasmin, and markedly elevated hepatic copper concentration. In a well-conducted controlled trial, copper chelation therapy with penicillamine in 15 patients with advanced cirrhosis showed no benefit compared with untreated cases. In 20 children with less advanced disease (i.e. no ascites or jaundice), treatment with penicillamine 20 mg/kg daily reduced mortality from 93% to 53% during a treatment period of 1–1.5 years. Copper concentration in hepatic biopsies decreased dramatically during therapy. Addition of prednisolone therapy did not seem to improve survival beyond penicillamine therapy alone. Inasmuch as penicillamine may have other effects besides copper chelation, it is not certain that the copper chelation was the precise means by which the hepatic disease was stabilized or improved, but this seems to be very likely. In another trial of penicillamine, histologic evidence of disease regressed and correlated with clinical recovery. Long-term survival after penicillamine therapy (>5 years) was associated with normal growth and development, absence of neurologic abnormalities, reduction of hepatosplenomegaly, and normalization of liver function tests. Liver histology continued to improve and normalized in a number of treated patients. These data support the role of copper in the pathogenesis of ICC and indicate that penicillamine chelation therapy should be instituted in patients in the preicteric phase before end-stage liver disease is present. In patients with decompensated cirrhosis, or those unresponsive to penicillamine, liver transplant should be considered. The use of trientine or other copper chelators, or zinc therapy, in ICC has not been reported to date. Because copper initiates generation of oxygen free radicals, it is possible that adjuvunct antioxidant therapy might be of benefit during copper chelation therapy, although this has not been investigated in ICC.

An important study has validated that prevention of ICC may be possible by the institution of public health measures designed to reduce copper ingestion by infants and young children in India [57]. In this study, decreased use of brass utensils for storage of milk in the Pune District of India, as a result of a public health interventional program, resulted in a dramatic fall of ICC recurrences in families (1 of 86) compared with older siblings (12 of 125) when no dietary advice was given. In an adjacent district without the public education campaign, the prevalence of ICC was unchanged during the study period. Based on these data, it is clear that children in India and nearby countries should not be fed milk that is boiled or stored in copper-containing vessels, such as brass, particularly if there is a family history of ICC. In non-Indian children with hepatic lesions that resemble ICC, copper metabolism should be investigated, drinking water tested for copper contamination, and therapy instituted with copper chelation therapy. If unresponsive end-stage liver disease ensues, liver transplantation should be performed.

Idiopathic copper toxicosis

A growing number of cases of an ICC-like illness have been described in non-Indian infants and young children in Europe, North America, Asia, and the Middle East. The clinical course, liver histology and hepatic copper content of these children most closely resembles that of ICC and clearly differs from that of Wilson disease. This disorder, or group of disorders, has variably been labeled as ICT, copper-associated childhood cirrhosis, copper-associated liver disease, non-Indian childhood cirrhosis and may be identical to endemic Tyrolean infantile cirrhosis [58]. Over a number of years, approximately 30 cases have been reported from a variety of countries, a cluster of 138 cases from the Tyrol area of western Austria [58], and a recent cluster of eight cases from the Emsland area of northern Germany. In general, these patients demonstrate onset of clinical liver disease in the first 2 years of life, with a relatively rapidly progressive course to cirrhosis and liver failure. The liver histology is similar to ICC with cytoplasmic Mallory's hyaline and a markedly elevated hepatic copper content of $>400\,\mu g/g$ dry weight. In addition, these patients have a normal or elevated serum ceruloplasmin concentration.

Clinical features

The age of onset of reported cases of ICT ranges from 2 months to 10 years. Most have onset in first 2 years of life but several patients have not been identified until 5 years of age, with one patient presenting at age 10 years. Clinical features include a distended abdomen and hepatosplenomegaly. Occasionally patients have fever, lethargy, anemia, malaise, and ascites. Jaundice is rare as an initial symptom. Within several weeks to 1 year, complications of cirrhosis and portal hypertension progress rather rapidly to death, suggesting the presence of compensated cirrhosis prior to clinical presentation. Patients with ICT come to clinical recognition at an earlier age range than patients with Wilson disease. These children can be confused with other metabolic liver diseases that present at this age with cirrhosis, such as α_1-antitrypsin deficiency and hereditary tyrosinemia.

Diagnostic testing

The diagnosis of ICT requires high index of suspicion. A family history of infantile liver disease, use of brass utensils to store milk, use of well water or water supply through old copper plumbing might be clinical clues to this diagnosis; however, these factors are frequently not present. Liver function tests are abnormal, consistent with the extent of liver injury and hepatic failure. Serum ceruloplasmin must be normal. Urinary copper excretion is raised. Other causes of cholestatic liver disease that can also lead to copper accumulation must be excluded. These include α_1-antitrypsin deficiency, paucity of intralobular bile ducts, progressive familial intrahepatic cholestasis, and autoimmune hepatitis. In some older children, it may be necessary to perform DNA mutation analysis of *ATP7B* to exclude common mutations for Wilson disease. Finally, copper incorporation into ceruloplasmin using copper-65 was normal in one patient [62], unlike that found in Wilson disease and is not useful in establishing a diagnosis of ICT.

Histopathology

Careful examination of the liver reveals the characteristic lesion of ICC. There is micro-micronodular cirrhosis, Mallory's hyaline, pericellular fibrosis, a mixed inflammatory infiltrate, and on histochemical stain granular copper or copper-associated protein. Early in the clinical course, the liver lesion may be less florid and Mallory's hyaline may be absent. Most importantly, the tissue must be preserved appropriately at the time of biopsy for quantitative copper analysis in an experienced laboratory. Hepatic copper content has usually been $>1000\,\mu g/g$ dry weight, but occasionally in the 400 to $1000\,\mu g/g$ range.

Etiopathogenesis

There is evidence for both a genetic and an environmental component in the etiology of ICT. In cases in the Tyrol [58] and northern Germany, there were both familial clustering and consanguinity, suggesting an autosomal recessive inheritance. However, expression of ICT in the Tyrolean patients was linked closely to the early introduction of copper-contaminated milk from copper or brass vessels, analogous to the suspected etiology of true ICC. Importantly, the Tyrolean endemic cirrhosis disappeared after 1974, when traditional copper cooking utensils were replaced by stainless steel, thus eliminating the excessive copper exposure to infants. Two patients with ICT have also been treated successfully with penicillamine [62]. These data, coupled with the extraordinary high hepatic copper levels, leave little doubt that copper toxicity is the major factor causing the liver injury and cirrhosis in ICT. The burning question is whether this is merely an environmental exposure or a genetic predisposition requiring an additional environmental exposure, a so-called ecogenetic disease [58]. As with ICC, both mutations in *ATP7B*, the Wilson's gene, and *MURR1*, the Bedlington terrier gene, have been eliminated as causes of ICT. A review of a number of ICT cases that have been associated with excess copper intake from a domestic water supply suggested copper toxicity as the sole etiologic factor [58]. However, Scheinberg and Sternlieb reviewed deaths from liver disease in children under 6 years of age in three Massachusetts towns with elevated drinking water copper concentrations of 8.5–8.8 mg/L and showed no deaths from liver disease over a 23-year period, representing 64 124 child-years [63]. They concluded that chronic excess copper intake alone was unlikely the etiology of ICT. In six published cases of ICT, the excess copper intake was attributed to the ingestion of drinking water containing up to 6.8 mg/L. The Tyrolean and northern Germany cases, as well as other reported cases with a suggested hereditary influence, strongly suggest a genetic defect exacerbated by a high copper intake during infancy, as the etiology of ICT. The candidate gene for ICT has yet to be identified but the continued discovery of new proteins involved in cellular copper homeostasis and new genetic techniques, such as homozygosity mapping, should lead to identification of any genetic etiology for ICT.

Treatment

Current treatment of ICT involves establishing an early diagnosis, eliminating excess copper intake, and instituting copper chelation therapy. Evaluation for liver transplantation is indicated if standard criteria for transplantation are met. The water supply of patients should be evaluated for copper content, or substituted by bottled distilled drinking water. Brass and copper utensils should not be used to store or administer infant formula, milk, or water. Some advocate dietary elimination of foods high in copper, such as liver, chocolate, nuts, mushrooms, and shellfish. Consideration should be given to therapy with vitamin E to reduce ongoing oxidant damage until hepatic copper levels are reduced by chelation therapy. Siblings should be screened by liver blood tests, physical examination, and, possibly, urinary copper excretion. To assist with identification of the genetic defect in this rare illness, caretakers of newly identified patients should contact current investigators in this field.

Acknowledgements

The author thanks Drs. Jay Lefkowitch and Bruce Beckwith for providing the photomicrographs.

References

1. Roberts EA, Schilsky ML. Diagnosis and treatment of Wilson disease: an update. *Hepatology*; 2008;**47**:2089–2111.

2. Sokol RJ. Copper storage diseases. In Kaplowitz N (ed.) *Liver and Biliary Disease*. Philadelphia, PA: Williams & Wilkins, 1992, pp. 322–333.

3. Gollan JL. Studies on the nature of complexes formed by copper with human alimentary secretions and their influence on copper absorption in the rat. *Clin Sci Mol Med* 1975;**49**:237.

4. Bacon BR, Schilsky ML. New knowledge of genetic pathogenesis of hemochromatosis and Wilson's disease. *Adv Int Med* 1999;**44**:91–116.

5. Klomp LW, Liu SJ, Yuan DS, *et al.* Identification and functional expression of HAH1, a novel human gene involved in copper homeostasis. *J Biol Chem* 1997;**272**:9221–9226.

6. Petrukhin K, Lutsenko S, Chernov I, *et al.* Characterization of the Wilson disease gene encoding a P-type copper transporting ATPase: genomic organization, alternative splicing, and structure/function predictions. *Hum Mol Genet* 1994;**3**:1647–1656.

7. Harrison MD, Jones CE, Dameron CT. Copper chaperones: function, structure and copper-binding properties. *J Biol Inorg Chem* 1999;**4**:105–115.

8. Wilson DC, Phillips MJ, Cox DW, Roberts EA. Severe hepatic Wilson's disease in preschool-aged children. *J Pediatr* 2000;**137**:719–722.

9. Portnoy ME, Rosenzweig AC, Roe T, *et al.* Structure-function analyses of the ATX1 metallochaperone. *J Biol Chem* 1999;**274**:15041–15045.

10. Sternlieb I, Morell AG, Tucker WD, *et al.* The incorporation of copper into ceruloplasmin in vivo: Studies with copper 64 and copper 67. *J Clin Invest* 1961;**40**:1834.

11. Miyajima H. Aceruloplasminemia, an iron metabolic disorder. *Neuropathology* 2003;**23**:345–350.

12. Frieden E, Hsieh HS. The biological role of ceruloplasmin and its oxidase activity. *Adv Exp Med Biol* 1976;**74**:505.

13. Scheinberg IH, Cook CD, Murphy JA. The concentration of copper and ceruloplasmin in maternal and infant plasma at delivery. *J Clin Invest* 1954;**33**:963.

14. Schilsky ML, Sternlieb I. Overcoming obstacles to the diagnosis of Wilson's disease. *Gastroenterology* 1997;**113**: 350–353.

15. Rosencrantz R, Schilsky M. Wilson disease: pathogenesis and clinical considerations in diagnosis and treatment. *Sem Liver Disease* 2011;**31**:245–259.

16. Frommer DJ. Defective biliary excretion of copper in Wilson's disease. *Gut* 1974;**15**:125.

17. Mueller T, Van de Sluis B, Zhernakova A, *et al.* The canine copper toxicosis gene *MURR1* does not cause non-Wilsonian hepatic copper toxicosis. *J Hepatol* 2003;**38**:164–168.

18. Walshe JM. Penicillamine, a new oral therapy for Wilson's disease. *Am J Med* 1956;**21**:487–495.

19. Brewer GJ, Terry CA, Aisen AM, Hill GM. Worsening of neurologic syndrome in patients with Wilson's disease with initial penicillamine therapy. *Arch Neurol* 1987;**44**:490–493.

20. Evans GW. Copper homeostasis in the mammalian system. *Physiol Rev* 1973;**53**:535.

21. Reed GB, Butt EM, Landing BH. Copper in childhood liver disease. A histologic, histochemical and chemical survey. *Arch Pathol* 1972;**93**:249.

22. Sokol RJ, Twedt D, McKim JM Jr, *et al.* Oxidant injury to hepatic mitochondria in patients with Wilson's disease and Bedlington terriers with copper toxicosis. *Gastroenterology* 1994;**107**:1788–1798.

23. Valko M, Morris H, Cronin MT. Metals, toxicity and oxidative stress. *Curr Med Chem* 2005;**12**: 1161–1208.

24. Dobyns, WB, Goldstein NP, Gordon H. Clinical spectrum of Wilson's disease (hepatolenticular degeneration). *Mayo Clin Proc* 1979;**54**:35–42.

25. Stremmel W, Meyerrose KW, Niederau C, *et al.* Wilson's disease: clinical presentation, treatment and survival. *Ann Intern Med* 1991;**115**:720–726.

26. Sokol RJ. Abnormal hepatic mitochondrial respiration and cytochrome *c* oxidase activity in rats with copper overload. *Gastroenterology* 1993;**105**:178–187.

27. Mufti AR, Burstein E, Csomos RA, *et al.* XIAP Is a copper binding protein deregulated in Wilson's disease and other copper toxicosis disorders. *Mol Cell* 2006;**21**:775–785.

28. Mansouri A, Gaou I, Fromenty B, *et al.* Premature oxidative aging of hepatic mitochondrial DNA in Wilson's disease. *Gastroenterology* 1997;**113**: 599–605.

29. Wilson AK. Progressive lenticular degeneration: a familial nervous disease associated with cirrhosis of the liver. *Brain* 1912;–**34**:295.

30. Bull PC, Thomas GR, Rommens JM, *et al.* The Wilson's disease gene is a putative copper transporting P-type ATPase similar to the Menkes' gene. *Nat Genet* 1993;**5**:327–337.

31. Walshe JM. The liver in Wilson's disease (hepatolenticular degeneration). In Schiff L, Schiff ER (eds.) *Diseases of the Liver*. Philadelphia: Lippincott, 1982, pp. 1037–1050.

32. Scheinberg IH, Sternlieb I (eds.) *Wilson's Disease*. Philadelphia, PA: Saunders, 1984.

33. Saito T. Presenting symptoms and natural history of Wilson's disease. *Eur J Pediatr* 1987;**146**:261–265.

34. Giagheddu A, Demelia L, Puggioni G, *et al.* Epidemiologic study of hepatolenticular degeneration (Wilson's disease) in Sardinia (1902–1983). *Acta Neurol Scand* 1985;**72**:43–55.

35. Aksoy M, Erdem S. Wilson's disease in Turkey, a review of 49 cases in 41 families. *New Istanbul Contrib Clin Sci* 1975;**11**:92–97.

36. Oder W, Grimm G, Kollegger H, *et al.* Neurological and Neuropsychiatric spectrum of Wilson's disease: a prospective study of 45 cases. *J Neurol* 1991;**238**:281–287.

37. Park RHR, McCabe P, Fell GS, *et al.* Wilson's disease in Scotland. *Gut* 1991;**32**:1541–1545.

38. Korman JD, Volenberg I, Balko J, *et al.* Pediatric and Adult Acute Liver Failure Study Groups. Screening for Wilson disease in acute liver failure: a comparison of currently available diagnostic tests. *Hepatology* 2008;**48**:1168–1174.

39. Schilsky ML, Scheinberg IH, Sternlieb I. Prognosis of Wilsonian chronic active hepatitis. *Gastroenterology* 1991;**100**:762–767.

40. Walshe JM, Waldenstrom E, Sams V, Nordlinder H, Westermark K. Abdominal malignancies in patients with Wilson's disease. *Q J Med* 2003;**96**:657–662.

41. Factor SM, Cho S, Sternlieb I, *et al.* The cardiomyopathy of Wilson's disease. Myocardial alterations in nine cases. *Virchows Arch A* 1982;**397**:301–311.

42. Ferenci P, Caca K, Loudianos G, *et al.* Diagnosis and phenotypic classification of Wilson disease. *Liver Int* 2003;**23**:139–142.

43. DaCosta CM, Baldwin D, Portmann B, *et al.* Value of urinary copper excretion after penicillamine challenge in the diagnosis of Wilson's disease. *Hepatology* 1992;**15**:609–615.

44. Steindl P, Ferenci P, Dienes HP, *et al.* Wilson's disease in patients presenting with liver disease: a diagnostic challenge. *Gastroenterology* 1997;**113**:212–218.

45. Sternlieb I. Mitochondrial and fatty changes in hepatocytes of patients with Wilson's disease. *Gastroenterology* 1968;**55**:354.

46. Williams FJB, Walshe JM. Wilson's disease. An analysis of the cranial computerized tomographic appearances found in 60 patients and the changes in response to treatment with chelating agents. *Brain* 1981;**104**:735–752.

47. Linne T, Agartz I, Saaf J, *et al.* Cerebral abnormalities in Wilson's disease as evaluated by ultra-low-field magnetic resonance imaging and computerized image processing. *Magn Reson Imaging* 1990;**8**:819–824.

48. Brewer GJ, Askari F, Lorincz MT, *et al.* Treatment of Wilson disease with ammonium tetrathiomolybdate: IV. Comparison of tetrathiomolybdate and trientine in a double-blind study of treatment of the neurologic presentation of Wilson disease. *Arch Neurol* 2006;**63**:521–527.

49. Dubois RS, Rodgerson DO, Hambidge KM. Treatment of Wilson's disease with triethylene tetramine hydrochloride (trientine). *J Pediatr Gastroenterol Nutr* 1990;**10**:77–81.

50. Schilsky M. Zinc treatment for symptomatic Wilson disease: moving forward by looking back. *Hepatology* 2009;**50**:1341–1343.

51. Weiss KH, Gotthardt DN, Klemm D, *et al.* Zinc monotherapy is not as effective as chelating agents in treatment of Wilson disease. *Gastroenterology* 2011;**140**:1189–1198.

52. Schilsky ML, Scheinberg IH, Sternlieb I. Liver transplantation for Wilson's disease: indications and outcome. *Hepatology* 1994;–**19**:583.

53. Eghtesad B, Nezakatgoo N, Geraci LC, *et al.* Liver transplantation for Wilson's disease: a single-center experience. *Liver Transplant Surg* 1999;**5**:467–474.

54. Nazer H, Ede RJ, Mowat AP, *et al.* Wilson's disease: clinical presentation and use of prognostic index. *Gut* 1986;**27**:1377–1381.

55. Dhawan A, Taylor RM, Cheeseman P, De Silva P, *et al.* Wilson's disease in children: 37-year experience and revised King's score for liver transplantation. *Liver Transplant* 2005;**11**:441–448.

56. Sternlieb I. Wilson's disease and pregnancy. *Hepatology* 2000;**31**:531–532.

57. Tanner MS. Role of copper in Indian childhood cirrhosis. *Am J Clin Nutr* 1998;**67**(Suppl):1074–1081.

58. Müller T, Feichtinger H, Berger H, *et al.* Endemic Tyrolean infantile cirrhosis: an ecogenetic disorder. *Lancet* 1996;**347**:877–880.

59. O'Neill NC, Tanner MS. Uptake of copper from brass vessels by bovine milk and its relevance to Indian childhood cirrhosis. *J Pediatr Gastroenterol Nutr* 1989;**9**:167–172.

60. Bhave SA, Pandit AN, Pradhan AM, *et al.* Liver disease in India. *Arch Dis Child* 1982;**57**:922.

61. Tanner MS, Bhave SA, Pradham AM, *et al.* Clinical trials of penicillamine in Indian childhood cirrhosis. *Arch Dis Child* 1987;**62**:1118–1124.

62. Horslen SP, Tanner MS, Lyon TDB, *et al.* Copper associated childhood cirrhosis. *Gut* 1994;**35**:1497–1500.

63. Scheinberg IH, Sternlieb I. Is non-Indian childhood cirrhosis caused by excess dietary copper. *Lancet* 1994;**344**:1002–1004.

Iron storage disorders

Michael R. Narkewicz and Peter F. Whittington

Iron overload disorders

Iron overload states can be classified as primary or secondary. There are many disorders that can lead to iron overload (Table 29.1) [1]. This chapter focuses on hereditary hemochromatosis (HHC), juvenile hemochromatosis (JHC), and secondary iron overload (primarily transfusion associated) in the

Table 29.1 Classification of iron overload states

Type	Disorders
Primary	Hereditary hemochromatosis, *HFE*-associated
	C282Y homozygotes
	C282Y/H63D compound heterozygotes
	Hereditary hemochromatosis, non–*HFE*-associated
	Hereditary hemochromatosis, *TFR2*-associated
	Juvenile hemochromatosis (hemojuvelin-associated (HJV), hepcidin-associated (HAMP))
	Ferroportin-associated hemochromatosis (*FPN* autosomal dominant)
	Heavy-chain ferritin disease
	Neonatal hemochromatosis
	Autosomal dominant hemochromatosis (Solomon Islands)
	Aceruloplasminemia
	Atransferrinemia
	Fiedreich ataxia
	Divalent metal transporter 1 deficiency
Secondary	Iatrogenic (transfusional iron overload)
	Anemias (sideroblastic anemia, hereditary spherocytosis, β-thalassemia)
	Dietary or medicinal iron overload
	Long-term hemodialysis
	Chronic liver disease (hepatitis B and C, alcoholic liver disease, non-alcoholic steatohepatitis, post-portocaval shunt)
	Porphyria cutanea tarda
	Cystic fibrosis
	Tyrosinemia
	Zellweger syndrome

Adapted from Pietrangelo *et al.*, 2011 [1] with permission.

pediatric patient and in neonatal hemochromatosis (NH). For a discussion of the rarer entities, the reader is referred to a recent review [1].

Physiology and pathophysiology of iron overload

Iron is one of the more tightly regulated nutrients in the body. Humans have no significant excretory pathway for iron. Therefore, body iron stores are normally controlled at the level of absorption, matching absorption to physiologic requirements. Under normal circumstances, only about 1 mg of elemental iron is absorbed each day (Figure 29.1), in balance with gastrointestinal losses. Intestinal iron absorption is increased by low body iron stores (storage regulation), increased erythropoiesis (erythropoietic regulation), anemias associated with ineffective erythropoiesis (thalassemias, congenital dyserythropoietic anemias, and sideroblastic anemia), and acute hypoxia. Both dietary iron intake (dietary regulation) and systemic inflammation can temporarily decrease iron absorption and availability, even in the presence of iron deficiency [2].

Duodenal crypt cells sense body iron status and are programmed for iron absorption as they mature. Duodenal and proximal jejunal enterocytes are responsible for iron absorption. Low gastric pH helps to dissolve iron, which is then enzymatically reduced to the ferrous form by ferrireductase. Divalent metal transporter 1 transfers iron to the enterocyte, where it is either stored as ferritin or moved across the basolateral membrane to reach the plasma, where it is rapidly oxidized to the ferric form by hephaestin and bound to transferrin. Divalent metal transporter 1 levels are altered in response to body iron stores [2].

The central regulatory mechanisms for iron status hinges on hepcidin and ferroportin. Hepcidin is produced in the liver, and its expression and secretion in iron sufficiency is elevated. Hepcidin acts to downregulate the cell surface expression of ferroportin, a transmembrane iron transporter that acts to transfer iron out of intestinal epithelial cells and macrophages [3,4]. During times of low iron status, hepcidin is low and

Liver Disease in Children, Fourth Edition, ed. Frederick J. Suchy, Ronald J. Sokol, and William F. Balistreri. Published by Cambridge University Press. © Cambridge University Press 2014.

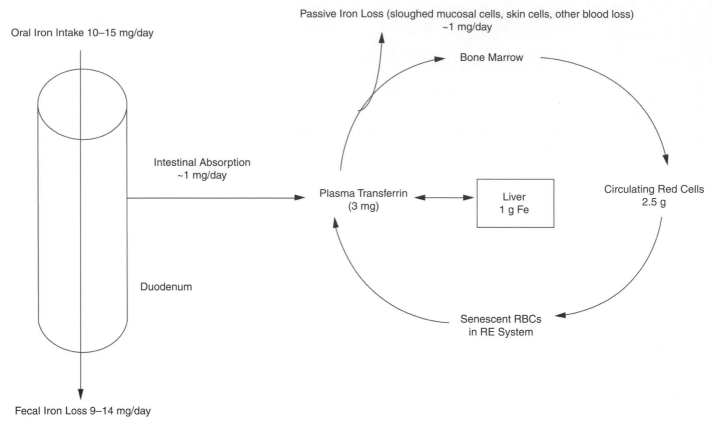

Figure 29.1 Physiology of normal iron metabolism in humans. RE, reticuloendothelial; RBCs, red blood cells; Fe, iron.

ferroportin expression on the basolateral membrane of the enterocyte is maintained. As a consequence, intestinal epithelial cells transport more dietary iron across their basolateral membranes, leading to increased iron absorption. Mutations in the genes for both hepcidin (JHC) and ferroportin (autosomal dominant hemochromatosis) have been described [1]. Hepcidin expression is regulated by the HFE protein (mutated in HHC type 1), transferrin receptor 2 (TFR2; see below), and hemojuvelin (mutated in JHC). This regulation has provided insight into the mechanism of iron overload in the various forms of hemochromatosis (Figure 29.2). In animal models and in humans with hemochromatosis, the normal increase in hepcidin expression with iron loading is lost, leading to lower hepcidin levels and continued iron absorption in the face of iron overload [5].

In humans, iron in the circulation is tightly bound to transferrin. Transferrin can bind up to two molecules of ferric iron, with about 30% of the binding sites on transferrin normally occupied by ferric iron. Diferric transferrin binds to the transferrin receptor 1 (TFR1) on the cellular plasma membrane. This complex is then endocytosed into the cell, where iron is released by the acid environment of the endocytic vesicle. The iron is then transported across the endosomal membrane to the cytoplasm. Therefore, in the setting of a highly saturated transferrin (e.g. HHC), more of the transferrin is in the diferric state, or the more readily absorbable state.

The uptake of iron is primarily regulated by the expression of TFR1 on the cell surface. In iron deficiency, iron regulatory proteins are increased and bind to the TFR1 iron-responsive elements in the $3'$-untranslated region of the TFR1 mRNA. This stabilizes the TFR1 transcript, leading to increased TFR1 expression on the cell surface, increasing iron uptake. Simultaneously, these same iron regulatory proteins bind to the $5'$-untranslated region of ferritin (the iron storage and intracellular sequestration molecule), decreasing its synthesis. In states of iron repletion or excess, there is a reduced level of iron-binding proteins, leading to less TFR1 production and an increase in ferritin and hepcidin synthesis. In the intestine and at other sites, iron is also transported by at least one transporter that is independent of transferrin and TFR1. An active transporter for divalent cations, including iron, called the divalent cation transporter 1, has been reported. Its mRNA is strongly expressed in the enterocytes at the villous tips and is increased in states of iron deficiency.

The second receptor TFR2 binds holotransferrin/diferric transferrin and mediates the uptake of transferrin-bound iron. This protein is predominately expressed in the liver, where, in contrast to TFR1, it is not downregulated by dietary iron overload nor is it in the mouse model for HHC. Hepatic TFR2 provides an explanation for the continued hepatic iron uptake in HHC despite the downregulation of TFR1. Hepcidin synthesis in the liver is also regulated by TFR2.

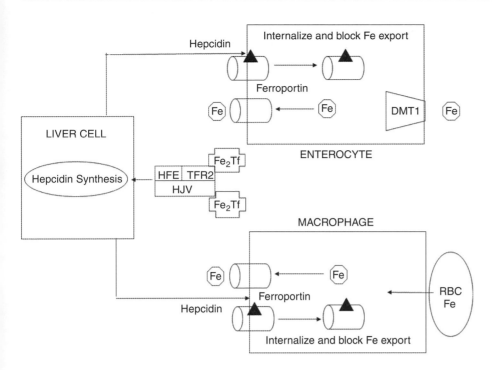

Figure 29.2 Proposed roles of hepcidin, HFE, transferrin receptor 2 (TFR2), and ferroportin in iron absorption. In states of high iron stores and inflammation, hepatic hepcidin synthesis is increased with signaling from HFE, TFR2, and hemojuvelin (HJV). Hepcidin results in phosphorylation and internalization of ferroportin in both enterocytes and macrophages, reducing transport of iron. (Adapted from Vaulont et al., 2005 [4].)

In HHC and JHC, net iron absorption is increased above endogenous losses. In addition, in both disorders, there is loss of the normal downregulation of iron absorption as iron accumulates in the body. This is directly related to inhibition hepatic hepcidin expression by mutations affecting the hepcidin regulatory proteins responsible for HHC and JHC [5,6]. The result is a net gradual increase in total body iron. In HHC, the net increase in total body iron has been estimated at 4–7 mg/day. The increased iron absorption in HHC is the result of inappropriate transfer of iron at the basolateral surface of the enterocyte because of suppression of hepatic hepcidin secretion [6]. In JHC, iron accumulates more rapidly than in HHC, in part because of the more significant role of hemojuvelin in the regulation of hepcidin [7]. Excessive iron intake in the diet can accelerate the accumulation of iron in both HHC and JHC. In a similar manner, increased iron losses (most commonly in menstruating females) can retard the accumulation of iron. In secondary iron overload caused by the hemoglobinopathies, overload is related to both the anemia and increased iron absorption and the excess iron provided by transfusions. In contrast, in aplastic anemias, iron overload is primarily related to transfusion.

Hereditary hemochromatosis (OMIM 235200)

Genetics

Hereditary hemochromatosis has long been recognized as an autosomal recessive disorder. In 1976, it was linked to the human leukocyte antigen (HLA) region of the short arm of chromosome 6. In 1996, using positional cloning in a defined cohort of patients with HHC, the candidate gene for HHC, called *HFE*, was discovered [8]. *HFE* encodes a novel major histocompatibility (MHC) class I-like molecule. Two principal missense mutations of *HFE* have been identified. One results in a change from a cysteine to tyrosine at position 282 (C282Y). A second mutation results in a change from a histidine to aspartate at position 63 (H63D). Upward of 85–90% of patients with classic HHC are homozygous for C282Y, and another 5% are compound heterozygotes (C282Y/H63D). The H63D mutant is quite common (15–20% heterozygote state in the general population), but H63D homozygotes generally do not have significant iron loading. It is also important to note that, in the majority of studies, 10–15% of patients with a clinical syndrome of typical HHC do not have either the C282Y or H63D mutation. However, 55% of patients initially felt to have HHC who carried neither mutation were found to have previously unrecognized causes for secondary iron overload. There remains a subgroup of mutation-negative iron-overloaded patients with typical HHC. Some of these patients have mutations in other hepcidin regulatory proteins. Several new mutations in *HFE* have been described in patients with iron overload, suggesting that other *HFE* mutations may be found in "wild-type" HHC.

The formation of a heterodimer between HFE and β_2-microglobulin (β_2m) is essential for correct intracellular trafficking and transport of HFE to the plasma membrane and cell surface expression of an HFE–β_2m complex. The C282Y mutant protein does not associate with β_2m, resulting in a reduction in cell surface expression of HFE–β_2m in transfected cells. The C282Y mutant protein fails to undergo late Golgi processing and is retained in the endoplasmic reticulum, undergoing accelerated degradation. In contrast, the H63D mutation has no effect on the binding of β_2m or cell surface expression of HFE. Further work has demonstrated that HFE associates with TFR1 on the cell surface, decreasing the affinity of TFR1 for diferric transferrin. The C282Y HFE mutant does not arrive at the cell surface and so does not associate with TFR1. The H63D mutant does associate with TFR1. The affinity of the TFR1 for diferric transferrin decreases less with binding to the H63D mutant than with binding to wild-type HFE.

HFE is widely expressed throughout the body; the highest levels are found in the liver and small intestine. *HFE* is prominently expressed in the deep crypt cells of the duodenum. It now seems clear that HFE is involved in an as yet unknown complex regulation of hepcidin secretion, with subsequent lack of hepcidin mRNA expression and hepcidin secretion in the face of excessive total body iron stores. There are several proposed mechanisms by which this may occur (reviewed by Babitt and Lin [9]).

Further evidence for the role of HFE in iron metabolism comes from several recently studied animal models. Studies in the β_2m knockout mouse have shown that these mice accumulate iron in a pattern similar to that of HHC. The murine *HFE* homologue has been disrupted. The phenotype of this mouse is very similar to HHC, with an elevated transferrin saturation and iron accumulation in the parenchymal cells of the liver and abnormal regulation of hepcidin. Liver-specific HFE disruption leads to a phenotype similar to a complete knockout. There is emerging evidence for a role of HFE in the bone morphogenic protein–ASMAD signaling in the regulation of hepcidin and interplay with TFR1 and TFR2 [9].

Epidemiology

Hereditary hemochromatosis is one of the most common genetic diseases in the white population, with a prevalence of the C282Y homozygous state of 1 in 200–400 [10]. The disease is most common in individuals of northern European descent. The frequency of the C282Y mutation is highest in subjects from northwest Europe (10–20%), less frequent in southern and eastern European populations (2–4%), and rare in natives of Africa, Central or South America, Eastern Asia, and the Pacific Islands [11]. The H63D mutant has a distribution similar to that of C282Y, but it is more common in European groups (15–40%). In a large population-based study of 3011 unrelated white adults in Brusselton, Australia, 14.1% were heterozygous for C282Y and 0.5% were homozygous [11]. It is very unusual to find HHC in African-American or Asian patients [10]. Indeed, no instances of C282Y/C282Y have been found in African patients with iron overload. There also have been reports of non-C282Y/C282Y iron overload in Italian patients.

Overall estimates are that about 6.8% of the US white population is heterozygous for C282Y and 0.5% are homozygous. This is fairly similar to the incidence estimates of 1 in 200 for iron overload in the worldwide white population [12]. Both HHC and the C282Y mutation are uncommon in African-Americans or Asian-Americans [11], the prevalence of clinically diagnosed HHC in African-Americans being about 1 in 1000 [10].

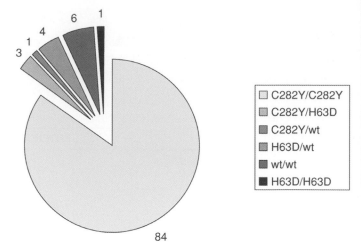

Figure 29.3 Distribution of genotypes in patients with hemochromatosis. Combination of 19 studies encompassing 1618 patients. wt, wildtype. (Adapted from Ramrakhiani S, Bacon R. Hemochromatosis: advances in molecular genetics and clinical diagnosis. *J Clin Gastroenterol* 1998;27:41–6 with permission.)

Therefore, although HHC is a disease with worldwide distribution, it remains predominately a disease of individuals of northern European descent. The distribution of genotypes in this population is shown in Figure 29.3 [13]. Although mutation analysis has assisted in defining the prevalence of the disease in this population, it has not proved useful in other selected populations. Nevertheless, HHC remains one of the more common, if not the most common, inherited disorder in humans.

Clinical features

In adults, HHC may present with the clinical syndrome of diabetes, cirrhosis, and increased skin pigmentation, as initially described in 1865. Although the genetic defect is present at birth, years of increased iron absorption and tissue accumulation (usually >5 g of excess total body iron) are required for the development of clinical symptoms (Figure 29.4). As such, clinical symptoms are rare before adulthood. Before the discovery of the gene for HHC, most adults were diagnosed with clinical symptoms that included liver disease (fibrosis or cirrhosis), diabetes, skin pigmentation, heart failure, arthritis, and endocrinologic disturbances. Screening of asymptomatic adults was restricted to first-degree relatives of affected adults. Consequently, the true prevalence of symptoms was uncertain. Since the discovery of *HFE*, it is recognized that many adults who are homozygous for C282Y mutation are asymptomatic [11]. The disorder is classified into four stages: (1) a genetic predisposition with no abnormality other than possibly an elevated serum transferrin saturation, (2) iron overload (2–5 g) without symptoms, (3) iron overload with early symptoms (lethargy, arthralgia), and (4) iron overload with organ damage. For further data on the clinical manifestations in adults, the reader is referred to a recent review [14].

Table 29.2 Organ involvement in hereditary hemochromatosis

Organ	Histology
Liver	Periportal iron deposition, fibrosis, cirrhosis
Pancreas	Fibrosis with normal exocrine and beta-cell function; abnormal beta-cell function.
Skin	Bronzing secondary to increased melanin
Heart	Dilated and restrictive cardiomyopathy
Joints	Hip, shoulder, knee, metacarpophalangeal joint involvement, chondrocalcinosis
Pituitary	Fibrosis leading to hypogonadotropic hypogonadism

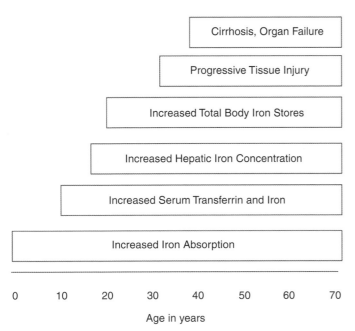

Figure 29.4 Typical progression of iron accumulation and pathology in hereditary hemochromatosis.

As iron accumulates in the tissues, there is progressive fibrosis and injury. As organ failure results, the classic clinical consequences of hemochromatosis are recognized. The organs involved and pathologic findings are listed in Table 29.2.

Disease expression is dependent not only on the mutation but on other genetic and environmental factors, such as sex, age, dietary iron, and other factors affecting iron balance. For example, males with HHC typically present earlier than females, presumably because of the ongoing iron losses in menstruating females. In addition, the association of symptoms with the mutations is quite variable and less common than previously thought.

Most children and adolescents with HHC are asymptomatic. Although most will have abnormal transferrin saturation, a normal ferritin is the rule. Reports of elevated ferritin and death from congestive heart failure in children have not been confirmed by genotype analysis and may represent JHC, a

truly distinct disorder [15]. A study screening the children of 179 homozygotes found that even at a mean age of 37 years, most affected children of parents with HHC were asymptomatic [16].

Several studies in heterozygotes have shown that heterozygotes do not have clinically important iron overload unless another illness is present. Heterozygotes do have slightly higher transferrin saturations than those in normal individuals (men 38% versus 30%; women 32% versus 29%). This suggests that the heterozygote state may be protective for iron deficiency in women.

Diagnosis and screening

Prior to the discovery of *HFE*, the diagnosis of HHC required the documentation of iron overload or HLA linkage to an affected individual. Criteria for iron overload consistent with HHC include (1) grade 3 or 4 stainable iron on liver biopsy, (2) hepatic iron concentration >4500 µg/g dry weight (80 µmol/g), (3) a hepatic iron index (iron concentration in micromoles per gram liver dry weight divided by age in years) of >1.9, or (4) evidence of iron overload of >5 g. These criteria are rarely encountered in children because in the absence of confounding factors (high dietary intake, hepatitis C viral infection, etc.), children typically have not developed this degree of iron overload. Indeed, these criteria are probably not acceptable for individuals identified by family screening, who may be early in the course of iron overload. Some investigators have suggested that any individual with an abnormal hepatic iron concentration (>30 µmol/g (1500 µg/g) dry weight) who has no other reason for iron overload should be suspected of having HHC. A variety of disorders can lead to hepatic iron overload, including chronic liver diseases such as alcoholic liver disease, non-alcoholic steatohepatitis, chronic viral hepatitis, cystic fibrosis, and porphyria cutanea tarda. There is no association with an increased prevalence of *HFE* mutations in either alcoholic liver disease or viral hepatitis [17]. However, in both non-alcoholic steatohepatitis and porphyria cutanea tarda, a higher frequency of the C282Y mutation has been observed [18].

In adults, the transferrin saturation is used to screen individuals, with the threshold for further investigation being 45% in men and 42% in premenopausal women. Abnormal transferrin saturation has been reported in children as young as 2 years. However, fasting transferrin saturation and ferritin level in affected children can be normal, even in known homozygous subjects [19]. Indeed, as many as 30% of women with HHC who are under 30 years of age have normal transferrin saturation [19]. Therefore, transferrin saturation is helpful in phenotypic screening in children when it is abnormal but does not exclude HHC when normal. In contrast, ferritin may be elevated in many inflammatory liver diseases such as chronic viral hepatitis and non-alcoholic steatohepatitis in the absence of HHC and is less helpful in phenotypic screening for HHC in children and adults.

Liver biopsy has been primarily studied in adults. Increased hepatic iron can be demonstrated by Prussian blue staining. Hepatic iron quantification with the determination of the hepatic iron index (micromoles of iron per gram dry weight liver divided by age in years) has been considered one of the more sensitive and specific tests for HHC. Several studies have demonstrated that a hepatic iron index >1.9 in the absence of secondary iron overload is indicative of HHC. However, 10–15% of patients with HCC identified by genetic testing will have a hepatic iron index <1.9, calling into question the use of this test for diagnosis in children [20]. In children with HHC, an abnormal hepatic iron index has been reported in those as young as 7 years. Liver biopsy has given way to MRI quantification of hepatic iron content. Liver biopsy is now reserved for assessment of hepatic fibrosis in HHC [20].

Genetic testing is available on a commercial basis. The distribution of genotypes in patients with hemochromatosis is shown in Figure 29.3. In 150 family members of 61 white American probands, 34 family members had an HHC phenotype. Among the family members, 92% of the C282Y homozygotes and 34% of the C282Y/H63D compound heterozygotes had the HHC phenotype. None of the H63D homozygotes had an HHC phenotype. A few individuals were heterozygous for one mutation and had iron overload. Therefore, testing for *HFE* mutations should include those leading to both C282Y and the H63D. Heterozygosity may contribute to iron overload with an associated condition, but it should not be considered the sole cause of iron overload. Only C282Y/C282Y and compound heterozygosity (C282Y/H63D) should be considered indicative of HHC. However, not all compound heterozygotes will develop HHC. In most cases, these individuals will not require liver biopsy for confirmation of the diagnosis. However, C282Y homozygotes with evidence of liver disease (elevated aminotransferases or hepatomegaly) or with serum ferritin >1000 µg/L should undergo a liver biopsy to assess the degree of liver injury and the possible contribution of other liver disorders to the clinical picture. Liver biopsy is also recommended in suspected iron overload in non-C282Y homozygotes (C282Y heterozygotes, C282Y/H63D, or no mutations).

Approach to the child with a parent with hereditary hemochromatosis

The preferred clinical assessment of a child whose parent has HHC is open to debate. Because symptomatic end-stage organ disease from HHC is easily preventable with early therapy, screening of potentially affected children has been advocated. However, the majority of patients present with clinical disease after the age of 20 years. Biochemical screening (phenotypic strategy, Figure 29.5) may require sequential transferrin saturation and ferritin determinations and MRI for hepatic iron content or liver biopsy. With the advent of genetic mutation testing, Adams *et al.* [16] have shown that it is cost-effective to screen the spouse of the affected parent with mutation analysis (genetic strategy, Figure 29.6). If the unaffected parent is either

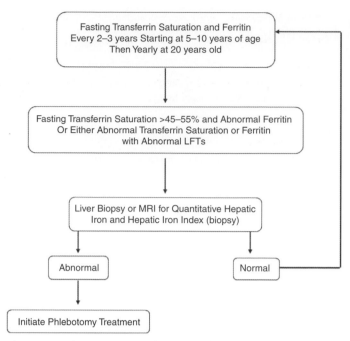

Figure 29.5 Phenotypic strategy for screening for iron overload in a child with a parent with hemochromatosis when the affected parent has no detectable mutation in HFE. LFTs, liver function tests.

heterozygous or homozygous for C282Y, the potentially affected children are then screened with mutation analysis following appropriate counseling and consent [16]. Subsequently, at-risk children are followed with fasting transferrin saturation, ferritin, and liver blood tests. This strategy was found to be more cost-effective when compared with the phenotypic strategy [21]. When the serum ferritin is >200 µg/L or aminotransferases increase, consideration could be given to MRI hepatic iron quantification or direct initiation of phlebotomy therapy.

Iron overload in children with liver dysfunction

In children, iron overload should be considered in the differential diagnosis of liver disease and testing for transferrin saturation and ferritin should be considered in the evaluation of hepatic dysfunction (Figure 29.7). If liver biopsy is performed as part of the evaluation, staining for iron should be done and quantitative hepatic iron determination should be considered. There are older reports of children presenting as young as 5 years with iron overload and presumed HHC, which may have been JHC as these reports predate *HFE* testing. White children with evidence of iron overload (elevated transferrin saturation of >50%, elevated ferritin, increased stainable iron or hepatic iron concentration) would be candidates for possible *HFE* mutation analysis. The yield of *HFE* analysis in African-American and Asian-American children would be expected to be quite low. *HFE* mutation analysis also may be helpful in patients with other diseases that can lead to iron overload (non-alcoholic steatohepatitis, porphyria cutanea tarda).

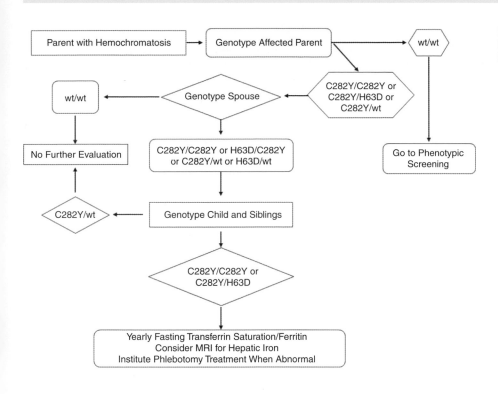

Figure 29.6 Genotypic strategy for screening for hereditary hemochromatosis in a child with a parent with hemochromatosis.

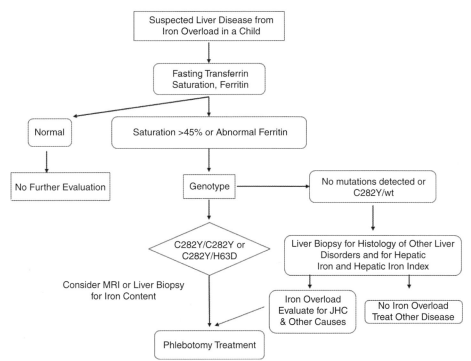

Figure 29.7 Phenotypic strategy for screening for iron overload in a child with liver disease and suspected iron overload.

The role of liver biopsy has not been studied in children. Data from one large adult study have shown that 50% of patients with HCC with a serum ferritin >1000 μg/L, abnormal aspartate aminotransferase, or hepatomegaly had significant fibrosis on liver biopsy [22]. In contrast, none of the patients with HCC without those factors had significant fibrosis [22]. Even before genotyping was available, it was shown that patients diagnosed in the precirrhotic stage who were treated with venisection had a normal life expectancy. Therefore, in patients homozygous for the C282Y mutation, these non-invasive measures may be used to avoid liver biopsy.

Because HHC is a common genetic disorder whose effects can be prevented by presymptomatic intervention, screening of the general population has been considered. Until the cost of the testing is reduced and the implications for insurability and management are clarified, newborn testing has not been

Box 29.1 Standard adult treatment schedule

1. Remove excess iron:
   - phlebotomy: 1–2 times/week, 500 mL (250 mg iron/ 500 mL blood); will remove 12–35 g iron in 1 year
   - check hemoglobin every week
   - check serum iron, transferrin saturation, and ferritin every 2 months
   - check serum ferritin more frequently when <100 mg/dL
   - document iron depletion by liver biopsy or MRI
2. Prevent reaccumulation of iron:
   - phlebotomy every 2–3 months
   - check serum iron, transferrin saturation, and ferritin every year
   - screen for hepatocellular carcinoma if cirrhosis is present

Source: adapted with permission from Niederau *et al.*, 1999 [24].

recommended [23]. In adults, screening strategies have been suggested using a combination of transferrin saturation and confirmation with *HFE* testing.

Treatment

The goals of treatment are to reduce total body iron overload and prevent reaccumulation of iron. When instituted before end-organ injury, successful treatment would ideally prevent the development of cirrhosis and other end-organ disease and reduce the incidence of hepatocellular carcinoma. A standard adult treatment schedule is shown in Box 29.1 [24]. Current recommendations are that venisection is indicated if serum ferritin is >300 µg/L in males or 200 µg/L in females [25]. The goals of therapy are to maintain a ferritin level <50 µg/L. There are few published data on phlebotomy therapy in children as most children with HHC do not meet the preceding criteria. Initial therapy in symptomatic children should include phlebotomy of 5–8 mL/kg weekly or every other week until the ferritin has decreased to <300 µg/L. Thereafter, two to four sessions per year will probably be required. In our experience, therapeutic phlebotomy may need to be less frequent in children with HHC who have asymptomatic iron overload, probably because of their lower total body iron load. Careful attention to the development of iron deficiency is required when treating children. Once identified, children with HHC should be counseled to maintain a low-iron diet and avoid ascorbic acid and vitamin supplements containing iron.

Juvenile hemochromatosis (OMIM 602390)

Juvenile hemochromatosis, or hemochromatosis type 2, is a rare iron-loading disorder that leads to severe iron loading and organ failure, typically before 30 years of age [15]. It is characterized by autosomal recessive inheritance and a pattern of iron distribution and tissue injury similar to that of HHC. However, JHC is not associated with mutations in *HFE* and

does not show linkage to chromosome 6p. In contrast to HHC, males and females are equally affected, and hypogonadism and cardiac dysfunction are the most common symptoms at presentation. The disorder has been reported in several ethnic groups. Most patients present in the second and third decades of life, which may be partly the result of a higher rate of iron accumulation in JHC than in HHC. As such, the phlebotomy requirements to maintain normal iron balance are significantly higher in JHC than in HHC. The JHC locus was initially localized to chromosome 1q. Further study demonstrated that the gene *HJV* at this site encodes hemojuvelin, a key regulatory protein for hepcidin, and accounts for about 90% of the cases reported to date [15]. The most frequent mutation gives rise to G320V in the protein, which was reported to account for 60% of the mutations in the original description and all individuals identified in a French Canadian study. However, many mutations have now been reported (reviewed by Pietrangel *et al.* [1]). *HAMP*, which encodes hepcidin and is located on chromosome 19, accounts for only 10% of the reported cases [26]. Combined mutations in *HFE* and *TFR2* may also present with a phenotype of JHC without mutations in either *HJV* or *HAMP* [1,15].

As a consequence, this disorder should be considered when children and adolescents present with clinically significant liver disease and iron overload. Significant iron overload and clinical liver disease is more likely to be caused by JHC in children and adolescents, even though the disorder is rare. A family history of iron overload and hypogonadism in the absence of *HFE* mutations should raise the clinical suspicion for JHC. It is likely that some of the earlier reports of children with clinically apparent liver disease and iron overload dealt with this disorder and not HHC. With the identification of candidate genes involved in JHC, genetic diagnosis is available for *HJV*, *HAMP*, and the *HFE/TFR2* combination. These offer the opportunity for presymptomatic diagnosis in children from affected families. However, the overall incidence of this disorder must be small in comparison with classic HHC as, in the Australian population study, only 0.5% of the adults with the wild-type/wild-type hemochromatosis genotype had an elevated (>45%) fasting transferrin saturation.

Secondary iron overload

Secondary iron overload is a common problem for children with transfusion-dependent diseases such as the thalassemias, sickle cell disease, and aplastic anemias. This has been referred to as hemosiderosis, primarily because the accumulation of iron begins in the reticuloendothelial cells in the liver. The pathophysiology of secondary iron overload is related to the provision of parenteral iron that bypasses the normal intestinal regulation of iron absorption. In addition, the anemias of ineffective erythropoiesis (thalassemias, congenital dyserythropoietic anemias, and sideroblastic anemias) stimulate iron absorption, resulting in an additional 2–5 g of iron absorbed from the diet per year. With inadequate chelation therapy, clinical symptoms of iron overload typically are not manifest until the second decade of life. However, tissue iron overloading of parenchymal cells is apparent after only 1 year of transfusion therapy. In patients who are receiving transfusions without chelation therapy, symptomatic heart disease has been reported within 10 years [27]. Iron-induced liver disease is a common cause of death in older patients, often aggravated by hepatitis C infection. Fibrosis is present as early as 2 years after starting transfusions, with cirrhosis reported in the first decade of life. With improved survival with iron chelation, iron loading of the anterior pituitary and associated disturbed sexual maturation are quite common.

Although the amount of excess iron that has been provided in the form of transfused iron can be calculated from the volume of red blood cells administered, the biochemical markers of iron overload may be unreliable. Some researchers advocate following ferritin levels for signs of iron overload. Under normal conditions, 1 µg/L ferritin is equivalent to 8–10 mg storage iron. Therefore, a ferritin of 1000 µg/L is equal to about 10 000 mg of storage iron. However, above 4000 µg/L ferritin, there is no longer a correlation between ferritin and iron stores. In addition, ferritin may be increased with hepatic inflammation, which may be related to other factors such as hepatitis C infection. This has led others to suggest that ferritin concentrations are not an accurate reflection of tissue iron accumulation [28]. More accurate estimations of tissue iron burden are obtained by liver or cardiac biopsy and iron quantification by MRI [29] or by investigative SQUID (superconducting quantum interference device) biomagnetometry, which may be better at assessing high tissue iron concentrations.

Treatment

Standard treatment of transfusional iron overload centers on chelation therapy or, when possible, exchange transfusion. Deferoxamine is generally given by continuous subcutaneous administration and is capable of inducing negative iron balance. In general, ferritin should begin to decrease by the end of 1 year of treatment. Generally, the goal is to maintain a ferritin level of <1000 µg/L on treatment. Deferoxamine prevents early cardiac death, arrests the progression to cirrhosis, and stabilizes or reduces total body iron load [30]. The major risks of deferoxamine are growth failure, hearing impairment, and bone abnormalities. These are more common in patients with low iron loads. Direct dose-related toxicities involve the kidneys, lungs, and visual loss. Iron chelation is generally successful at reducing liver and early cardiac toxicity. The early use of deferoxamine in an amount proportional to the transfusional iron overload reduces iron burden and the risk of the development of diabetes mellitus, cardiac disease, and early death in patients with thalassemia major [30]. However, alternative strategies have been applied for serious iron overload. When possible, such as in some cases of sickle cell disease, exchange transfusion can reduce the iron burden from transfusions [31]. Other strategies include intravenous deferoxamine, which can rapidly reduce tissue iron burden in situations of severe iron overload (Figure 29.8). Newer oral chelation agents have recently become available. Deferiprone has been used in Europe and was approved for use in the USA [32]. Deferiprone seems to be more effective at removal of cardiac iron load than deferoxamine and similar in efficacy or slightly less effective for hepatic iron reduction. The major side effects of deferiprone are bone marrow suppression, arthropathy, gastrointestinal symptoms, and zinc deficiency. Deferasirox is another oral chelation therapy approved for use in the USA and several other countries. There has been a large clinical trials experience with deferasirox which suggest that it is very efficient in liver and cardiac iron removal in adults and children. Side effects include gastrointestinal disease. Recent reports suggest a small but increased risk of renal or hepatic failure and gastrointestinal hemorrhage. Combination treatment with deferoxamine and deferiprone or other

(a)

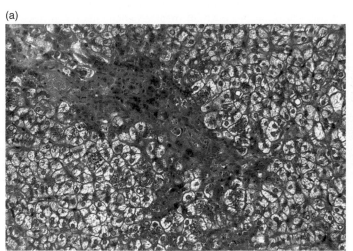

(b)

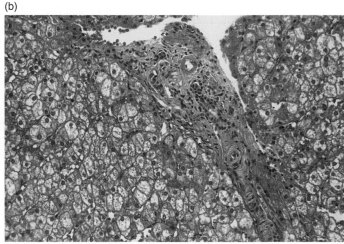

Figure 29.8 Effects of intravenous deferoxamine treatment. (a) Liver biopsy from a 16-year-old girl with β-thalassemia. Increased stainable iron shown on Prussian blue stain. Quantitative hepatic iron of 15 483 µg/g dry weight. (b) Repeat liver biopsy with Prussian blue stain in the same patient following 1 year of daily intravenous deferoxamine (hepatic iron 669 µg/g dry weight). Note the dramatic reduction in stainable iron.

oral chelators, such as deferasirox, suggest an additive effect in the presence of adequate renal function [33].

In the past, researchers have recommended serial liver biopsy to follow iron overload in transfusion-dependent patients. We have found that liver biopsy is helpful in determining the contribution from hepatitis C and iron overload and in guiding the use of more aggressive therapies, such as intravenous deferoxamine. At present, MRI is the test of choice to quantify hepatic iron overload and for longitudinal determinations [29]. Liver biopsy should be reserved for assessment of hepatic injury and fibrosis and for the assessment of the relative contribution of non-iron-related disorders to the process.

Neonatal hemochromatosis

Neonatal hemochromatosis (NH) is a form of secondary iron overload in which fetal liver disease leads to extrahepatic siderosis in a distribution similar to that seen in HHC. The phenotype of severe neonatal liver disease and extrahepatic siderosis (or iron overload) defines NH clinically and has resulted in its many synonyms, emphasizing the iron both in diagnosis and pathogenesis of liver disease: neonatal iron storage disease, perinatal hemochromatosis, perinatal iron storage disease, and congenital hemochromatosis. Its description as a "metabolic disease," mainly because of its recurrence in siblings, resulted in it being classified among the HHC disorders (OMIM 231100), where it most certainly does not belong. Current understanding is that severe liver disease in the fetus, for which there are several causes, leads to disordered fetal iron metabolism and the signature extrahepatic siderosis. Iron appears to have no role in the pathogenesis of the liver disease, which is primary. To emphasize, there is no evidence that NH is anyway related to the family of diseases that fall under the classification of HHC.

Etiology and pathogenesis

Etiology of fetal liver disease leading to the neonatal hemochromatosis phenotype

A hemochromatosis-like disease in a newborn was first described by Cottier in 1957, and a similar disease was described in siblings by Laurende and colleagues in 1961, setting the stage for NH being considered a hereditary disorder of iron metabolism [34]. However, the NH phenotype was found to be associated with cirrhosis in the newborn and questions arose as to whether it resulted from fetal liver disease, although no etiology for such fetal liver disease could be identified until more recently. The fact that NH recurred in sibships led to intense search for a genetic causation, but no gene locus could be identified [35]. Further, the recurrence pattern defied genetic explanation. After the index case in a maternal sibship there is an approximately 90% probability that each subsequent baby born to that mother will be affected [36]. A woman may have unaffected offspring before having the

first child with NH, but thereafter most pregnancies terminate in either a fetal loss or a child born with NH. There are several documented instances of a woman giving birth to affected babies with different male parentage, but not vice versa. It has never been recorded that female siblings of women having a baby with NH themselves have had an affected baby. Consequently, NH appears to be congenital and familial, but not hereditary. This pattern of recurrence is much like that of known maternofetal alloimmune diseases.

Gestational alloimmune liver disease

Gestational alloimmune liver disease (GALD) is the cause of almost all NH [37,38]. While several mechanistic aspects of how alloimmunity against fetal liver develops remain to be elucidated and to date the fetal liver target antigen has not been identified, it is clear that IgG-initiated, complement-mediated hepatocyte injury is the central mechanism leading to GALD-associated fetal liver disease [38]. All gestational alloimmune diseases have the same basic underpinnings [39]. A woman is exposed to a fetal antigen that she does not recognize as self (i.e. has no immune tolerance to) and develops an adaptive immune response. That response can affect the sensitizing fetus or a subsequent fetus expressing the same sensitizing antigen. Since IgG is the only component of adaptive immunity that can effectively bridge the placental interface, it is the effector molecule in gestational alloimmune disease. Specific alloreactive IgG molecules cross the placenta chaperoned by FcRn along with the large repertoire of IgG antibodies that provides protective immunity to the fetus. The movement of IgG across the placenta begins at 12–14 weeks of gestation coincident with the expression of FcRn. Therefore, one component of the necessary package for fetal injury is in place very early in gestation. The next component, the expression on fetal cells and tissues of the sensitizing antigen, may evolve earlier or later. Once bound to the fetal antigen, the IgG can have one or more effects. The one necessary for cell lysis and active tissue injury involves the binding and activation of complement. The final piece to fall in place is adequate synthesis of complement by the fetus (since all fetal complement is synthesized by the fetus) to exact injury. This occurs somewhere between 12 and 20 weeks of gestation. Therefore, by midgestation the table is set for gestational alloimmune disease to adversely affect the fetus. The liver form, GALD, results from classical pathway activation of the terminal complement cascade on the surface of fetal hepatocytes and is the only known immune liver disease to have this singular mechanism of injury [38].

Perinatal liver diseases other than GALD have been associated with the NH phenotype, although in sum they constitute less than 2% of reported NH cases. Reports of clear association include Down syndrome (in particular with myelodysplasia), the bile acid synthetic defect δ-4-oxosteroid reductase deficiency, and the mitochondrial DNA depletion syndrome resulting from mutations in *DGUOK*, encoding deoxyguanosine kinase. Not so clear association has been made to maternal diseases including hepatitis B virus infection and systemic lupus erythematosis. No association has ever been made to maternal *HFE*-associated hemochromatosis or other iron overload conditions.

Regulation of fetal iron stores and its poor regulation in neonatal hemochromatosis associated with gestational alloimmune disease

The fetus regulates placental iron transport to insure adequate iron for the growth and oxygen-carrying capacity needs of the fetus and newborn. The placenta acts as an active interface between the mother's huge iron pool and the highly controlled and relatively small fetal iron pool, assuring adequate iron supply to the fetus and protecting against potentially toxic iron overload. Many of the control mechanisms that function after birth to control accrual of dietary iron also function during fetal life, with the placental trophoblast functioning in analogy to the duodenal mucosa (reviewed by Whitington and Kelly [36]). Ferroportin is highly expressed and colocalizes with HFE in placental trophoblast cells. Ferroportin expression increases with gestational age in parallel with increasing iron needs of the fetus. Fetal hepcidin evidently regulates fetal iron stores: transgenic hepcidin-overexpressing mice are born profoundly anemic and iron deficient. In cases of GALD-associated NH, expression of liver *HAMP*, the gene encoding hepcidin, markedly reduced, from <1% to 10% of normal fetus and newborn liver. This would be expected to limit the capacity for regulating placental iron flux and result in fetal iron overload. Moreover, expression of the gene for transferrin is similarly reduced, and the iron-binding capacity in NH is uniformly low. This results in high iron saturation and probably excess circulating non-transferrin-bound iron for uptake into tissues. This combination of liver injury-related defects is the probable cause of fetal iron overload and tissue siderosis in NH.

Pathology

The liver histopathology in NH typically has the appearance of severe chronic or subacute liver disease (Figure 29.9), which most certainly had its beginnings well before birth and has been described as "congenital cirrhosis" [34]. Loss of hepatocytes is profound: hepatocyte volume density is usually less than 10% of normal newborn liver [40]. In many instances almost no hepatocytes remain. Residual hepatocytes appear damaged and may exhibit giant cell or pseudoacinar transformation. They often show coarsely granular siderosis and hepatocanalicular cholestasis. Parenchymal collapse and fibrosis are pronounced. Up to 50% of patients show regenerative nodules. Portal triads are left intact, although hepatocyte loss and parenchymal collapse lead to their being crowded together.

While the histology of NH as widely described in the literature almost certainly was that of GALD-associated NH, the identification of a precise marker for GALD has led to discovery of some interesting variant histopathology. Patients with GALD can be shown to have complement-mediated hepatocyte injury by immunohistochemical demonstration of C5b-9 complex (the neoantigen created in the formation of membrane attack complex) in more than 75% of residual hepatocytes [38]. As shown in Figure 29.9, GALD produces the subacute/chronic liver disease that typifies NH. However, GALD may produce acute liver failure and fetal demise with or without siderosis of the liver or extrahepatic tissues [41]. These patients show histology of acute liver failure with global hepatocyte injury/death, but with hepatocyte dropout and no parenchymal collapse or fibrosis (Figure 29.9). The parenchyma in NH has been described as "inflamed" or showing acute and chronic inflammation [42]. However, careful studies of patients with GALD show no acute (neutrophils) or chronic (T- and B-cells) inflammation. The hypercellular appearance in these patients comes from the presence of large numbers of oval cells, presumably from attempted regeneration, and in some cases macrophages. The immune liver injury in GALD involves the interaction of the maternal adaptive immune system with the fetal innate immune system. Maternal IgG binding to fetal hepatocytes activates fetal complement, with hepatocyte injury resulting from membrane attack complex. Also part of the fetus' innate immune armamentarium, macrophages, can be recruited by C3a and C5a released during the terminal complement cascade assembly of the membrane attack complex. Their presence and the absence of other acute and chronic inflammation indicate that adaptive cellular immunity plays no role in GALD-related liver injury, as it does in other immune liver diseases such as autoimmune hepatitis.

One of the defining features of NH is extrahepatic siderosis in the pattern of HHC. At autopsy, the most consistently affected tissues and the ones that should be most carefully examined with Perl Prussian blue staining are the exocrine pancreas, the thyroid follicles, the adrenal cortex, and the myocardium. Others in which siderosis can be found include epithelia of renal tubules, gastric and Brunner glands, parathyroid glands, and the thymus (Hassall corpuscles), as well as pancreatic islets, the adenohypophysis, and chondrocytes in hyaline cartilage. The spleen, lymph nodes, bone marrow, and other reticuloendothelial elements contain little or no stainable iron. In living patients, oral mucosal biopsy provides a mechanism of demonstrating extrahepatic siderosis, which can be found in the minor salivary glands. Hepatocytes show siderosis in the majority of patients with NH, as they do in many neonatal liver diseases. Since GALD-related injury is limited to the liver, it seems that the hepatic siderosis may be caused by liver injury, whereas the extrahepatic siderosis results secondarily from iron overload.

Infants with NH sometimes exhibit renal failure caused by dysgenesis of proximal tubules. Correlation with the process of normal renal development dates arrested tubulogenesis to about 24-weeks of gestation. The liver is the source of angiotensinogen, which is required for development of proximal renal tubules. In NH, reduced angiotensinogen synthesis can be correlated with reduced hepatocyte mass, and both with the degree proximal tubular dysgenesis [40]. Therefore, it appears

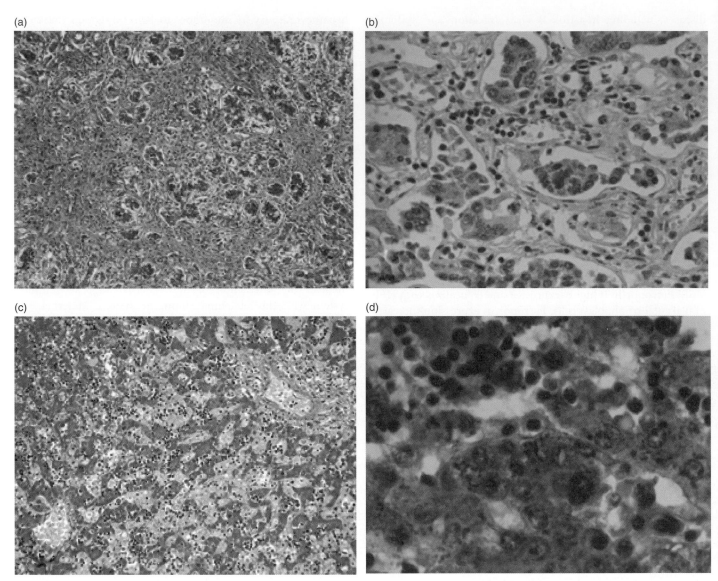

Figure 29.9 Hepatic histology in gestational alloimmune liver disease (GALD). (a) Typical GALD-associated neonatal hemochromatosis showing extreme loss of hepatocytes with parenchymal collapse and fibrosis. Residual hepatocytes take the form of pseudorosettes and multinucleate cells (trichrome stain, original magnification ×100). (b) In typical GALD-associated neonatal hemochromatosis, residual hepatocytes contain C5b-9 complex in dense aggregates and coarse granules (immunohistochemistry for C5b-9 complex, original magnification ×400). (c) GALD in a fetus that died at 32 weeks of gestation. The parenchymal architecture is well preserved with no fibrosis or collapse. The individual hepatocytes are condensed leaving large spaces between cords, which are filled with blood elements (trichrome stain, original magnification ×100). (d) In a similar still birth at 32 weeks of gestation, hepatocytes contain C5b-9 complex in coarse and fine granules (immunohistochemistry for C5b-9 complex, original magnification ×400).

that this extrahepatic manifestation of NH is the result of the profound liver injury and dysfunction that typifies the disease.

Diagnosis

Infants who manifest liver disease antenatally or very shortly after birth should have NH within the differential diagnosis. It should also be suspected in unexplained stillbirth. Demonstration of extrahepatic siderosis is currently necessary to prove the diagnosis. No other disease of the newborn demonstrates the combination of severe liver disease and extrahepatic siderosis, and thus the combination of findings is absolutely diagnostic. Caution should be exercised in

evaluating hepatocyte siderosis for the purpose of diagnosing NH. Finding siderosis in the liver is not diagnostic. The normal newborn liver contains sufficient stainable iron to be confused with pathologic siderosis, although they are qualitatively different to the eyes of experienced pathologists. Furthermore, pathologic hepatic siderosis has been described in several neonatal liver diseases. The absence of stainable iron in the liver does not exclude the diagnosis of NH since in many cases few if any hepatocytes remain, and hepatic siderosis in NH involves hepatocytes exclusively. Often, NH is diagnosed at autopsy, where siderosis of many tissues can be demonstrated if looked for. Proper stains for iron should be performed on the tissues typically involved (see Pathology) when autopsy is performed on any baby with liver failure or suspected liver disease and in unexplained stillbirths.

It should be remembered that NH is a phenotypic expression of several fetal and perinatal liver diseases, with GALD being the most common. The gestational history of the mother is particularly important in the diagnosis of GALD. A mother who has had recurrent stillbirths is highly suspicious because women who have a baby with NH have had, on average, one in eight of their pregnancies ending in stillbirth. Also an important historical finding is one or more maternal siblings with early neonatal liver disease or death. The death need not be recorded as caused by liver failure since many of these cases are misdiagnosed as "sepsis" or carry non-specific diagnoses such as anasarca, hydrops, and bleeding diathesis. Other perinatal liver diseases associated with NH (see Etiology and pathogenesis) are familial and thus could produce recurrent NH; however, this has never been recorded.

Clinical diagnosis can be difficult and NH should be suspected in any neonate with evidence of cirrhosis or liver failure, as it is by far the most common cause of neonatal liver failure. Bear in mind, however, that there is a spectrum of disease presentation. In some cases, the liver disease takes a prolonged course and is manifest days to weeks after birth. Some "affected" babies have no clinical disease. Twins may have disparate clinical findings, with one severely affected and the other minimally so [43]. Most affected live-born babies show evidence of fetal insult (i.e. intrauterine growth restriction and oligohydramnios), and premature birth is common. Hypoglycemia, marked coagulopathy, hypoalbuminemia, edema with or without ascites, and oliguria are prominent features. Jaundice develops during the first few days after birth. Most infants exhibit significant elevations of both conjugated and non-conjugated bilirubin, with total bilirubin levels often exceeding 30 mg/dL. Serum aminotransferase concentrations are disproportionately low for the degree of hepatic injury, whereas circulating concentrations of α-fetoprotein are characteristically very high, usually 100–600 µg/mL (normal newborn values <80 µg/mL). Studies of iron status often show hypersaturation of available transferrin, with hypotransferrinemia and hyperferritinemia (values >0.8 µg/mL). Nearly all patients with NH will exhibit elevated ferritin levels; however, this finding is non-specific in liver disease of the newborn infant. Furthermore, the degree of elevated ferritin does not discriminate NH from other liver diseases, as levels >15 µg/mL have been observed in both. Also characteristic of NH is persistent patency of the ductus venosus, which can be demonstrated by sonography, the cause of which is unclear.

The differential diagnosis of infants with liver failure is limited and GALD-associated NH is first on the list. Mitochondrial hepatopathy is a consideration. Infants with GALD-associated NH do not show evidence of mitochondrial dysfunction, such as pronounced elevation of blood lactate. If such signs are present, evaluation of mitochondrial disease should be undertaken, in particular gene analysis for *DGUOK* mutations. Bile acid synthetic defects also should be considered.

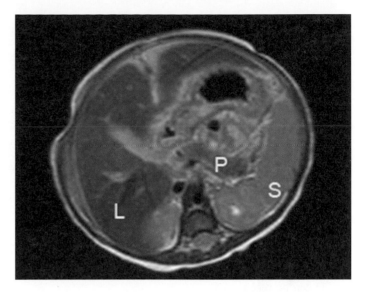

Figure 29.10 Gestational alloimmune liver disease (GALD)-associated neonatal hemochromatosis in a term infant with liver failure at birth. The MRI T$_2$ sequence shows attenuation of signal in liver (L) and pancreas (P), which appear black relative to spleen (S). This indicates excess iron in liver and pancreas. This child fully recovered with medical treatment (double volume exchange transfusion and intravenous immunoglobulin). Autopsy remains of a previous stillborn maternal sibling were used to demonstrate alloimmune liver injury and prove the diagnosis of GALD.

The results of urine mass spectroscopy (see Chapter 21) do not show the findings characteristic of synthetic defects and usually show elevated levels of normal bile acids. Patients may receive the erroneous diagnosis of tyrosinemia based upon elevated serum tyrosine levels, which are reflective of failed hepatic metabolic function. However, succinylacetone is absent in the urine. Viral infections such as herpes simplex virus and echovirus must be excluded by appropriate examinations. Hemophagocytic lymphohistiocytosis also appears as a cause of neonatal liver failure.

Demonstration of extrahepatic siderosis in living babies can be by tissue biopsy or by MRI (Figure 29.10). Biopsy of the oral mucosa is a clinically useful approach to obtain glandular tissue in which to demonstrate siderosis [44]. Differences in magnetic susceptibility between iron-laden and normal tissues on T$_2$-weighted MRI can document siderosis of various tissues, particularly the pancreas and liver [45]. The diagnostic utility of these approaches has never been formally evaluated. Experience suggests that oral mucosal biopsy and MRI each have a diagnostic sensitivity of about 60% relative to autopsy in proven cases of NH. The two examinations are not always positive in the same patient, however, and together they have a sensitivity approaching 80%. Therefore, the diagnostic approach should be to perform one test and, if negative, do the other. The choice of which to start with is often determined by the ease with which it can be performed in the individual patient setting. Oral mucosal biopsy often fails because of an inadequate specimen not containing submucosal glands is obtained. Therefore, the surgeon should be instructed to take as deep and generous a specimen as possible. MRI has not been useful in identifying extrahepatic hemochromatotic siderosis in utero.

Although GALD may be diagnosed in the absence of extrahepatic siderosis, it does not always produce the NH phenotype [41]. Examination of liver specimens for alloimmune injury involves immunohistochemistry for C5b-9 complex in hepatocytes [38]. This test is performed on paraffin-embedded archival tissue and so can be applied to autopsy materials from maternal siblings in order to achieve a diagnosis of a current patient. Even autopsy materials from fetal products of late intrauterine demise, where autolysis and maceration prevented diagnosis of NH-associated liver disease and no siderosis was detectable, have been used to make a diagnosis of GALD. Liver biopsy with examination for C5b-9 complex in hepatocytes has been used to make a diagnosis of GALD in neonates with severe liver disease and negative studies for extrahepatic siderosis. This test is at present only performed in one laboratory and is not commercially available. Clearly, better diagnostic tests and/or criteria are needed before the full spectrum of GALD can be recognized.

Treatment and outcome
Medical therapy

A cocktail containing both antioxidants and an iron chelator has been used to treat NH but with limited success [46]. This therapy was based on the hypothesis that oxidative injury caused by iron overload was central to disease pathogenesis, which appears not to be the case. Treatment for alloimmune liver injury with double-volume exchange transfusion and intravenous immunoglobulin has been shown to improve outcome over conventional medical therapy and liver transplant in an uncontrolled trial involving 16 infants with severe NH [47]. Ongoing data collection from nearly 40 infants treated in this way shows an approximate 80% survival (PF Whitington, unpublished data). While this approach appears to be a clear advance, it is fraught with difficulty. Infants with GALD-associated NH have severe advanced liver disease. The therapy can only ease ongoing alloimmune injury and permit recovery, which can take weeks to months. The infant must be supported in an intensive care setting with intravenous glucose infusions, blood products, and other therapies to prop up an ailing liver in order for recovery to occur. Sepsis and other catastrophic events may intervene and are the major reasons for the 20% failure rate of this therapy. Of the elements of the chelation–antioxidant cocktail that might be retained in this therapy, only N-acetylcysteine and vitamin E have potential value outweighing negligible risk. Desferrioxamine should be avoided since it is toxic to neutrophils and its use incurs sepsis risk.

With double-volume exchange transfusion and intravenous immunoglobulin therapy, recovery from liver failure to the point at which the infant can be discharged to home has varied from 1 to 4 months. However, it takes 2–4 years for full recovery from liver disease to occur. The liver in infants with NH appears to be plastic, with the ability to remodel completely. Two such babies who are siblings underwent liver biopsy as neonates and again after 2–4 years [48]. The initial biopsies demonstrated typical histology of severe NH with a pathologic diagnosis of cirrhosis, while the repeat biopsies demonstrated normal histology with no pathologic findings.

Liver transplantation

In the first 3 months of life, NH is a frequent indication for liver transplantation [49,50]. When performed for NH, the difficulties attendant to transplantation in newborns are frequently compounded by prematurity, small size for gestational age, and multiorgan failure [51]. Taking all the major published series of liver transplantation for treatment of NH into consideration, the overall survival rate with transplantation appears to be somewhat less than 40%, even though some centers report a high success rate in a small number of patients. With the apparent clear superiority in the results of medical treatment over those of transplantation for the indication of NH [47], it seems that transplantation might be totally abandoned as a therapeutic option. However, the question is asked as to whether the two approaches might be included in a therapeutic strategy. That appears to be difficult. When it becomes clear that medical therapy has failed, usually in association with a catastrophic event, transplantation is no longer an option. Conversely, if transplant is performed, the potential for recovery with medical therapy is eliminated.

Preventive thrapy

Recurrence of severe GALD-associated NH can be prevented by treatment during gestation [36]. The current recommended treatment consists of intravenous immunoglobulin 1 g/kg body weight administered at 14 weeks, 16 weeks, and then weekly for a total of 20 doses. Women who have had a gestation affected with proven NH should be treated in lieu of any other marker for high risk of recurrence. At the time of writing, this therapy has been administered in 100 pregnancies at risk for recurrence of NH. One pregnancy was lost at 21 weeks after starting intravenous immunoglobulin at 18 weeks: the baby had proven GALD. All other treatments have resulted in babies who survived. No intrauterine growth restriction, fetal liver disease, or other evidence of fetal distress has been detected in 98 infants. One infant in distress for unknown cause was born at 26 weeks of gestation and survived. Five babies born after gestational treatment had significant clinical liver disease and all survived. However, biochemical evidence suggests that about 80% of babies were affected: elevated serum α-fetoprotein (observed range 100–700 µg/mL) and/or elevated serum ferritin (observed range 0.8–16 µg/mL). This growing experience suggests that treatment with high-dose intravenous immunoglobulin during gestation can modify GALD so that it is not lethal to the fetus or the newborn.

Acknowledgements

Michael Narkewicz thanks Dr. Sarah Mengshol for providing the photomicrographs. This work was supported in part by grant M01 R00069 from the General Clinical Research Centers Program of the National Center for Research Resources,

National Institutes of Health and the Hewit–Andrews Endowed Chair in Pediatric Liver Disease. The contribution by Peter Whitington was supported in part by the Sally Burnett Searle Endowed Professorship in Pediatrics and Transplantation, the Siragusa Foundation (Chicago, IL), and the Liver Foundation for Kids (Lemont, IL).

References

1. Pietrangelo A, Caleffi A, Corradini E. Non-HFE hepatic iron overload. *Semin Liver Dis* 2011;**31**:302–318.

2. Evstatiev R, Gasche C. Iron sensing and signalling. *Gut* 2012;**61**:933–952.

3. Donovan A, Lima CA, Pinkus JL, *et al.* The iron exporter ferroportin/Slc40a1 is essential for iron homeostasis. *Cell Metab* 2005;**1**:191–200.

4. Vaulont S, Lou DQ, Viatte L, Kahn A. Of mice and men: the iron age. *J Clin Invest* 2005;**115**:2079–2082.

5. De Domenico I, Ward DM, Kaplan J. Hepcidin and ferroportin: the new players in iron metabolism. *Semin Liver Dis* 2011;**31**:272–279.

6. Pietrangelo A. Hepcidin in human iron disorders: therapeutic implications. *J Hepatol* 2011;**54**:173–181.

7. Huang FW, Pinkus JL, Pinkus GS, Fleming MD, Andrews NC. A mouse model of juvenile hemochromatosis. *J Clin Invest* 2005;**115**:2187–2191.

8. Feder JN, Gnirke A, Thomas W, *et al.* A novel MHC class I-like gene is mutated in patients with hereditary haemochromatosis. *Nat Genet* 1996;**13**:399–408.

9. Babitt JL, Lin HY. The molecular pathogenesis of hereditary hemochromatosis. *Semin Liver Dis* 2011;**31**:280–292.

10. Phatak PD, Sham RL, Raubertas RF, *et al.* Prevalence of hereditary hemochromatosis in 16031 primary care patients. *Ann Intern Med* 1998;**129**:954–961.

11. Olynyk JK, Cullen DJ, Aquilia S, *et al.* A population-based study of the clinical expression of the hemochromatosis gene. *N Engl J Med* 1999;**341**:718–724.

12. Edwards CQ, Griffen LM, Goldgar D, *et al.* Prevalence of hemochromatosis among 11,065 presumably healthy blood donors. *N Engl J Med* 1988;**318**:1355–1362.

13. Ramrakhiani S, Bacon R. Hemochromatosis: advances in molecular genetics and clinical diagnosis. *J Clin Gastroenterol* 1998;**27**:41–46.

14. Pietrangelo A. Hereditary hemochromatosis: pathogenesis, diagnosis, and treatment. *Gastroenterology* 2010;**139**: 393–408, e1–2.

15. Pietrangelo A. Juvenile hemochromatosis. *J Hepatol* 2006;**45**:892–894.

16. Adams PC, Kertesz AE, Valberg LS. Screening for hemochromatosis in children of homozygotes: prevalence and cost-effectiveness. *Hepatology* 1995;**22**:1720–1727.

17. Grove J, Daly AK, Burt AD, *et al.* Heterozygotes for *HFE* mutations have no increased risk of advanced alcoholic liver disease. *Gut* 1998;**43**:262–266.

18. Bonkovsky HL, Jawaid Q, Tortorelli K, *et al.* Non-alcoholic steatohepatitis and iron: increased prevalence of mutations of the *HFE* gene in non-alcoholic steatohepatitis. *J Hepatol* 1999;**31**: 421–429.

19. Kowdley KV, Trainer TD, Saltzman JR, *et al.* Utility of hepatic iron index in American patients with hereditary hemochromatosis: a multicenter study. *Gastroenterology* 1997;**113**:1270–1277.

20. Martin DR, Semelka RC. Magnetic resonance imaging of the liver: review of techniques and approach to common diseases. *Semin Ultrasound CT MR* 2005;**26**:116–131.

21. Adams PC. Implications of genotyping of spouses to limit investigation of children in genetic hemochromatosis. *Clin Genet* 1998;**53**:176–178.

22. Guyader D, Jacquelinet C, Moirand R, *et al.* Noninvasive prediction of fibrosis in C282Y homozygous hemochromatosis. *Gastroenterology* 1998;**115**:929–936.

23. Whitlock EP, Garlitz BA, Harris EL, Beil TL, Smith PR. Screening for hereditary hemochromatosis: a systematic review for the US Preventive Services Task Force. *Ann Intern Med* 2006;**145**:209–223.

24. Niederau C, Erhardt A, Haussinger D, *et al.* Haemochromatosis and the liver. *J Hepatol* 1999;**30**(Suppl 1):6–11.

25. EASL. Clinical practice guidelines for HFE hemochromatosis. *J Hepatol* 2010;**53**:3–22.

26. Gehrke SG, Pietrangelo A, Kascak M, *et al. HJV* gene mutations in European patients with juvenile hemochromatosis. *Clin Genet* 2005;**67**:425–428.

27. Wolfe L, Olivieri N, Sallan D, *et al.* Prevention of cardiac disease by subcutaneous deferoxamine in patients with thalassemia major. *N Engl J Med* 1985;**312**:1600–1603.

28. Nielsen P, Fischer R, Engelhardt R, *et al.* Liver iron stores in patients with secondary haemosiderosis under iron chelation therapy with deferoxamine or deferiprone. *Br J Haematol* 1995;**91**:827–833.

29. Carneiro AA, Fernandes JP, de Araujo DB, *et al.* Liver iron concentration evaluated by two magnetic methods: magnetic resonance imaging and magnetic susceptometry. *Magn Reson Med* 2005;**54**:122–128.

30. Brittenham GM, Griffith PM, Nienhuis AW, *et al.* Efficacy of deferoxamine in preventing complications of iron overload in patients with thalassemia major. *N Engl J Med* 1994;**331**:567–573.

31. Cabibbo S, Fidone C, Garozzo G, *et al.* Chronic red blood cell exchange to prevent clinical complications in sickle cell disease. *Transfus Apher Sci* 2005;**32**:315–321.

32. Piga A, Roggero S, Vinciguerra T, *et al.* Deferiprone: new insight. *Ann N Y Acad Sci* 2005;**1054**:169–174.

33. Cappellini MD, Musallam KM, Taher AT. Overview of iron chelation therapy with desferrioxamine and deferiprone. *Hemoglobin* 2009;**33**(Suppl 1):S58–S69.

34. Knisely AS, Mieli-Vergani G, Whitington PF. Neonatal hemochromatosis. *Gastroenterol Clin North Am* 2003;**32**:877–89, vi–vii.

35. Kelly AL, Lunt PW, Rodrigues F, *et al.* Classification and genetic features of neonatal haemochromatosis: a study of 27 affected pedigrees and molecular analysis of genes implicated in iron metabolism. *J Med Genet* 2001;**38**: 599–610.

36. Whitington PF, Kelly S. Outcome of pregnancies at risk for neonatal hemochromatosis is improved by treatment with high-dose intravenous

immunoglobulin. *Pediatrics* 2008;**121**: e1615–e1621.

37. Whitington PF. Neonatal hemochromatosis: a congenital alloimmune hepatitis. *Semin Liver Dis* 2007;**27**:243–250.

38. Pan X, Kelly S, Melin-Aldana H, Malladi P, Whitington PF. Novel mechanism of fetal hepatocyte injury in congenital alloimmune hepatitis involves the terminal complement cascade. *Hepatology* 2010;**51**: 2061–2068.

39. Hoftman AC, Hernandez MI, Lee KW, Stiehm ER. Newborn illnesses caused by transplacental antibodies. *Adv Pediatr* 2008;**55**:271–304.

40. Bonilla SF, Melin-Aldana H, Whitington PF. Relationship of proximal renal tubular dysgenesis and fetal liver injury in neonatal hemochromatosis. *Pediatr Res* 2010;**67**:188–193.

41. Whitington PF, Pan X, Kelly S, Melin-Aldana H, Malladi P. Gestational alloimmune liver disease in cases of fetal death. *J Pediatr* 2011;**159**:612–616.

42. Silver MM, Beverley DW, Valberg LS, *et al*. Perinatal hemochromatosis. Clinical, morphologic, and quantitative iron studies. *Am J Pathol* 1987;**128**: 538–554.

43. Ekong UD, Kelly S, Whitington PF. Disparate clinical presentation of neonatal hemochromatosis in twins. *Pediatrics* 2005;**116**:e880–e884.

44. Knisely AS, O'Shea PA, Stocks JF, Dimmick JE. Oropharyngeal and upper respiratory tract mucosal-gland siderosis in neonatal hemochromatosis: an approach to biopsy diagnosis. *J Pediatr* 1988;**113**:871–874.

45. Udell IW, Barshes NR, Voloyiannis T, *et al*. Neonatal hemochromatosis: radiographical and histological signs. *Liver Transplant* 2005;**11**:998–1000.

46. Leonis MA, Balistreri WF. Neonatal hemochromatosis: it's OK to say "NO" to antioxidant-chelator therapy. *Liver Transplant* 2005;**11**:1323–1325.

47. Rand EB, Karpen SJ, Kelly S, *et al*. Treatment of neonatal hemochromatosis with exchange transfusion and intravenous immunoglobulin. *J Pediatr* 2009;**155**:566–571.

48. Ekong UD, Melin-Aldana H, Whitington PF. Regression of severe fibrotic liver disease in 2 children with neonatal hemochromatosis. *J Pediatr Gastroenterol Nutr* 2008;**46**: 329–333.

49. Grabhorn E, Richter A, Burdelski M, Rogiers X, Ganschow R. Neonatal hemochromatosis: long-term experience with favorable outcome. *Pediatrics* 2006;**118**:2060–2065.

50. Rodrigues F, Kallas M, Nash R, *et al*. Neonatal hemochromatosis: medical treatment vs. transplantation: the king's experience. *Liver Transplant* 2005;**11**:1417–1424.

51. Sundaram SS, Alonso EM, Whitington PF. Liver transplantation in neonates. *Liver Transplant* 2003;**9**:783–788.

Chapter 30

Heme biosynthesis and the porphyrias

Robert J. Desnick, Manisha Balwani, and Karl E. Anderson

Introduction

The porphyrias are metabolic disorders each resulting from the deficiency of a specific enzyme in the heme biosynthetic pathway (Figure 30.1 and Table 30.1) [1–5]. These enzyme deficiencies are inherited as autosomal dominant X-linked, recessive, traits, with the exception of porphyria cutanea tarda (PCT), which usually is sporadic. The porphyrias are classified as either *hepatic* or *erythropoietic* depending on the primary site of overproduction and accumulation of porphyrin precursors or porphyrins (Table 30.2) although some have overlapping features. The hepatic porphyrias are characterized by overproduction and initial accumulation of porphyrin precursors and/or porphyrins primarily in the liver, whereas in the erythropoietic porphyrias, overproduction and initial accumulation of the pathway intermediates occur primarily in bone marrow erythroid cells.

The major manifestations of the acute hepatic porphyrias, which typically present after puberty, are neurologic, including neuropathic abdominal pain, neuropathy, and mental disturbances. The neurologic involvement appears to be the result of hepatic production of a neurotoxic substance, as liver transplantation has prevented further occurrences in several patients who had frequent attacks of acute intermittent porphyria (AIP) [6,7]. Steroid hormones, drugs, and nutrition influence the hepatic production of porphyrin precursors and porphyrins, thereby precipitating or increasing the severity of some hepatic porphyrias. Rare homozygous variants of the autosomal dominant hepatic porphyrias have been identified and usually manifest clinically before puberty. The symptoms in these patients are usually more severe and occur earlier than those of patients with the respective autosomal dominant porphyria (see below) [1].

The erythropoietic porphyrias usually present with cutaneous photosensitivity at birth or in early childhood, or in the case of congenital erythropoietic porphyria (CEP), even in utero as non-immune hydrops fetalis [1,8]. Cutaneous sensitivity to sunlight results from excitation of excess porphyrins in the skin by long-wave ultraviolet light, leading to cell damage, scarring, and deformation. Therefore, the porphyrias

are metabolic disorders in which environmental, physiologic, and genetic factors interact to cause disease.

Because many symptoms of the porphyrias are non-specific, diagnosis is often delayed [2]. First-line diagnostic testing involves the determination of the porphyrin precursors and/or porphyrins in urine, plasma, or erythrocytes (see below). A definitive diagnosis is based on demonstration of the specific enzyme deficiency and/or gene mutation(s). The isolation and characterization of the genes encoding the heme biosynthetic enzymes have permitted identification of the mutations causing each porphyria. Molecular genetic analyses now make it possible to provide precise heterozygote or homozygote identification and prenatal diagnoses in families with known mutations.

Recent reviews of the porphyrias are available [1–5]. Informative and up-to-date websites are sponsored by the American Porphyria Foundation (www.porphyriafoundation.com) and the European Porphyria Initiative (www.porphyriaeurope.org). An extensive list of unsafe and safe drugs for individuals with porphyria is given at the Drug Database for Acute Porphyrias (www.drugs-porphyria.com).

Heme biosynthesis

Heme biosynthesis involves eight enzymatic steps in the conversion of glycine and succinyl-coenzyme A (CoA) to heme (Figure 30.1 and Table 30.1) [1]. These eight enzymes are encoded by nine genes, as the first enzyme in the pathway, $5'$-aminolevulinate synthase (ALA synthase), has two genes that encode unique housekeeping and erythroid-specific isozymes. The first and the last three enzymes in the pathway are located in the mitochondrion, whereas the other four are in the cytosol. Heme is required for a variety of hemoproteins, such as hemoglobin, myoglobin, respiratory cytochromes, and the cytochrome P450 enzymes (CYPs). Hemoglobin synthesis in erythroid precursor cells accounts for approximately 85% of daily heme synthesis in humans. Hepatocytes account for most of the rest, primarily for synthesis of CYPs, which are particularly abundant in the liver endoplasmic reticulum and turn over more rapidly

Liver Disease in Children, Fourth Edition, ed. Frederick J. Suchy, Ronald J. Sokol, and William F. Balistreri. Published by Cambridge University Press. © Cambridge University Press 2014.

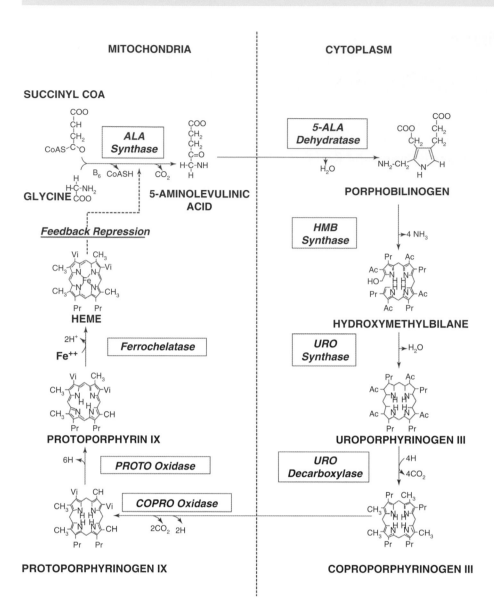

Figure 30.1 The human heme biosynthetic pathway.

than many other hemoproteins, such as the mitochondrial respiratory cytochromes. As shown in Figure 30.1, pathway intermediates are the porphyrin precursors, 5'-ALA and porphobilinogen (PBG), and porphyrins (mostly in their reduced forms, known as porphyrinogens). At least in humans, these intermediates do not accumulate in significant amounts under normal conditions or have important physiologic functions.

The first enzyme, ALA synthase, catalyzes the condensation of glycine, activated by pyridoxal phosphate and succinyl-CoA, to form ALA. In the liver, this rate-limiting enzyme can be induced by a variety of drugs, steroids, and other chemicals. The distinct non-erythroid (i.e. housekeeping) and erythroid-specific forms of ALA synthase are encoded by separate genes located on chromosomes 3p21.1 (*ALAS1* encoding ALA synthase 1 (ALAS1)) and Xp11.2 (*ALAS2* encoding ALA synthase 2 (ALAS2)). Loss-of-function mutations in the erythroid gene *ALAS2* cause X-linked sideroblastic anemia [1], while gain-of-function mutations in the last exon of *ALAS2* cause X-linked protoporphyria (XLP) [9].

The second enzyme, ALA dehydratase, catalyzes the condensation of two molecules of ALA to form PBG. Four molecules of PBG condense to form the tetrapyrrole uroporphyrinogen (URO) III by a two-step process catalyzed by the third enzyme, hydroxymethylbilane (HMB) synthase (also known as PBG deaminase), and the fourth enzyme, URO III synthase (URO synthase). The third step, catalyzed by HMB synthase, is the head-to-tail condensation of four PBG molecules by a series of deaminations to form the linear tetrapyrrole HMB. The fourth enzyme, URO synthase, catalyzes the rearrangement and rapid cyclization of HMB to form URO III, the asymmetric, physiologic URO isomer required for heme synthesis.

Table 30.1 Human heme biosynthetic enzymes and genes

Enzyme	Gene symbol	Chromosomal location	cDNA (bp)	Gene Size (kb)	Exons[a]	Protein (aa)	Subcellular location	Known mutations[b]	3D structure[c]
5'-Aminolevulinate synthase									
Housekeeping	ALAS1	3p21.1	2199	17	11	640	M	–	
Erythroid-specific	ALAS2	Xp11.2	1937	22	11	587	M	64	–
5'-Aminolevulinate dehydratase									
Housekeeping	ALAD	9q32	1149	15.9	12 (1A + 2–12)	330	C	12	Y
Erythroid-specific	ALAD	9q32	1154	15.9	12 (1B + 2–12)	330	C	–	
Hydroxymethylbilane synthase									
Housekeeping	HMBS	11q23.3	1086	11	15 (1 + 3–15)	361	C	376	E
Erythroid-specific	HMBS	11q23.3	1035	11	15 (2–15)	344	C		
Uroporphyrinogen III synthase									
Housekeeping	UROS	10q26.2	1296	34	10 (1 + 2B–10)	265	C	35	H
Erythroid-specific	UROS	10q26.2	1216	34	10 (2A+ 2B–10)	265	C	4	
Uroporphyrinogen decarboxylase	UROD	1p34.1	1104	3	10	367	C	109	H
Coproporphyrinogen oxidase	CPOX	3q12.1	1062	14	7	354	M	64	H
Protoporphyrinogen oxidase	PPOX	1q23.3	1431	5.5	13	477	M	166	–
Ferrochelatase	FECH	18q21.31	1269	45	11	423	M	138	B

3D, three-dimensional; aa, amino acid residues; C, cytoplasm; M, mitochondria.
[a] Number of exons and those encoding separate housekeeping and erythroid-specific forms indicated in parentheses.
[b] Number of known mutations from the Human Gene Mutation Database (www.hgmd.org) as of January 3, 2012.
[c] Crystallized from human (H), murine (M), *Escherichia coli* (E), *Bacillus subtilis* (B), or yeast (Y) purified enzyme; references in Protein Data Bank (www.rcsb.org).
Source: from Anderson *et al.* [1].

The fifth enzyme in the pathway, URO decarboxylase, catalyzes the sequential removal of the four carboxyl groups from the acetic acid side-chains of URO III to form coproporphyrinogen (COPRO) III, a tetracarboxylate porphyrinogen. This then enters the mitochondrion, where COPRO oxidase, the sixth enzyme, catalyzes the decarboxylation of two of the four propionic acid groups to form the two vinyl groups of protoporphyrinogen (PROTO) IX, a dicarboxylate porphyrinogen. Next, PROTO oxidase, the seventh enzyme, oxidizes PROTO IX to protoporphyrin IX by the removal of six hydrogen atoms. The product of the reaction is a porphyrin (oxidized form), in contrast to the preceding tetrapyrrole intermediates, which are porphyrinogens (reduced forms). Finally, ferrous iron is inserted into protoporphyrin IX to form heme, a reaction catalyzed by the eighth enzyme in the pathway, ferrochelatase (FECH; also known as heme synthetase or protoheme ferrolyase).

Regulation of heme biosynthesis

Regulation of heme synthesis differs in the two major heme-forming tissues, the liver and erythron. In the liver, "free" heme regulates the synthesis and mitochondrial translocation of the housekeeping form of ALAS1 [10]. Heme represses the synthesis of the *ALAS1* mRNA and interferes with the transport of the enzyme from the cytosol into mitochondria. Hepatic ALAS1 is increased by many of the same chemicals that induce CYPs in the endoplasmic reticulum of the liver. Because most of the heme in the liver is used for the synthesis of CYPs, hepatic ALAS1 and CYPs are regulated in a coordinated fashion, and many drugs that induce hepatic ALAS1 also induce CYPs. The other hepatic heme biosynthetic enzymes are presumably synthesized at constant levels, although their relative activities and kinetic properties differ. For example, normal individuals have

Table 30.2 Human porphyrias: major clinical and laboratory features

Porphyria	Deficient enzyme	Inheritance	Principal symptoms	Enzyme activity (% normal)	Increased porphyrin precursors and/or porphyrins[a]		
					Erythrocytes	Urine	Stool
Hepatic							
5-ALA dehydratase-deficient porphyria	ALA dehydratase	AR	NV	~5	Zn-protoporphyrin	ALA, coproporphyrin III	–
Acute intermittent porphyria	HMB synthase	AD	NV	~50	–	ALA, PBG, uroporphyrin	–
Porphyria cutanea tarda	URO decarboxylase	AD	CP	~20	–	Uroporphyrin, 7-carboxylporphyrin	Isocoproporphyrin
Hereditary coproporphyria	COPRO oxidase	AD	NV & CP	~50	–	ALA, PBG, coproporphyrin III	Coproporphyrin III
Variegate porphyria	PROTO oxidase	AD	NV & CP	~50	–	ALA, PBG, coproporphyrin III	Coproporphyrin III, protoporphyrin
Erythropoietic							
Congenital erythropoietic porphyria	URO synthase	AR	CP	1–5	Uroporphyrin I, coproporphyrin I	Uroporphyrin I, coproporphyrin I	Coproporphyrin I
Erythropoietic protoporphyria	Ferrochelatase	AR[b]	CP	~20–30	Protoporphyrin	–	Protoporphyrin
X-linked protoporphyria	ALA synthase 2	XL	CP	~100[c]	Protoporphyrin	–	Protoporphyrin

AD, autosomal dominant; ALA, 5′-aminolevulinate; AR, autosomal recessive; COPRO, coproporphyrinogen; CP, cutaneous photosensitivity; HMB, hydroxymethylbilane; NV, neurovisceral; PROTO, protoporphyrinogen; URO, uroporphyrinogen; XL, X-linked.
[a] Increases that may be important for diagnosis.
[b] A polymorphism in intron 3 of the wild-type allele affects the level of enzyme activity and clinical expression.
[c] Increased activity from "gain-of-function" mutations in *ALAS2* exon 11.

much higher activities of ALA dehydratase than HMB synthase, the latter being the second rate-limiting step in the pathway [1].

In the erythron, novel regulatory mechanisms allow for the production of the very large amounts of heme needed for hemoglobin synthesis. The response to stimuli for hemoglobin synthesis occurs during cell differentiation, leading to an increase in cell number. The erythroid-specific *ALAS2* is expressed at higher levels than the hepatic form, and an erythroid-specific control mechanism regulates iron transport into erythroid cells. During erythroid differentiation, the activities of other heme biosynthetic enzymes may be increased. Separate erythroid-specific and non-erythroid or "housekeeping" transcripts are known for the first four enzymes in the pathway. As noted above, ALAS1 and ALAS2 are encoded by genes on different chromosomes, but for each of the next three genes in the pathway, both erythroid and non-erythroid transcripts are transcribed by alternative promoters from their single respective genes.

Classification of the porphyrias

The porphyrias can be classified as either hepatic or erythropoietic, depending on whether the heme biosynthetic intermediates that accumulate arise initially from the liver or the developing erythrocytes, or as *acute* or *cutaneous*, based on their clinical manifestations. Table 30.2 lists the porphyrias, their principal symptoms, and major biochemical abnormalities. Of the five hepatic porphyrias, AIP, hereditary coproporphyria (HCP), variegate porphyria (VP), and ALA dehydratase-deficient porphyria (ADP), present with acute attacks of neurologic manifestations and elevated levels of one or both of the porphyrin precursors ALA and PBG; they are, therefore, classified as acute porphyrias. Symptoms of neuropathic abdominal pain, peripheral neuropathy, and mental disturbances typically develop during adult life [1,6,7]. The fifth hepatic porphyria, PCT, usually presents in adults with blistering skin lesions and not acute attacks. Both HCP and VP may cause cutaneous manifestations similar to those of PCT in addition to acute neurologic symptoms.

The erythropoietic porphyrias CEP and erythropoietic protoporphyria (EPP), including the recently described X-linked form, XLP, are characterized by elevations of porphyrins in bone marrow and erythrocytes and usually present in infancy with cutaneous photosensitivity [9]. The skin lesions in CEP resemble those of PCT but are usually much more severe, whereas EPP and XLP cause a more immediate, painful, non-blistering type of photosensitivity. Presentation of symptoms before puberty is most common with EPP and XLP. Around 20% of patients with EPP (and presumably XLP) develop minor abnormalities of liver function, and up to 5% develop more severe hepatic complications that may be life threatening.

Diagnosis of porphyrias

A few specific and sensitive first-line laboratory tests should be used whenever symptoms or signs suggest the diagnosis of porphyria [5]. If a first-line test is significantly abnormal, more comprehensive testing should follow to establish the type of porphyria.

Acute porphyrias

An acute porphyria should be suspected in patients with neurovisceral symptoms after puberty, such as abdominal pain, when the initial clinical evaluation does not suggest another cause, and the urinary porphyrin precursors (ALA and PBG) should be measured. Urinary PBG is virtually always increased during acute attacks of AIP, HCP, and VP and is not substantially increased in any other medical condition. Therefore, this measurement is both sensitive and specific. A method for rapid, in-house testing for urinary PBG, such as the Trace PBG kit (Thermo-Fisher Scientific, Waltham, MA, USA), should be available. Results from spot (single-void) urine specimens are highly informative because very substantial increases in PBG are expected during acute attacks of porphyria. A 24-hour collection may unnecessarily delay diagnosis. The same spot urine specimen should be saved for quantitative determination of ALA and PBG to confirm the qualitative PBG result and also to detect elevations of ALA in rare patients with ADP. Urinary porphyrins may remain increased longer than porphyrin precursors in HCP and VP. Therefore, it is useful to measure total urinary porphyrins in the same sample, keeping in mind that urinary porphyrin increases are often non-specific. Measurement of urinary porphyrins alone should be avoided for screening because these may be increased in disorders other than porphyrias, such as chronic liver disease, and misdiagnoses of porphyria may result from minimal increases in urinary porphyrins that have no diagnostic significance. Measurement of erythrocyte HMB synthase is not useful as a first-line test in the acute setting because it does not differentiate latent from active AIP. Moreover, the enzyme activity is not decreased in all patients with AIP and is never deficient in other acute porphyrias. Once a biochemical diagnosis is established, mutation analysis for the appropriate heme biosynthetic genes should be undertaken. Molecular diagnostic studies are also useful to identify at-risk family members once the specific mutation is known in the index case.

Cutaneous porphyrias

Blistering skin lesions caused by porphyria are virtually always accompanied by increases in total plasma porphyrins. A fluorometric method is preferred because the porphyrins in plasma in VP are mostly covalently linked to plasma proteins and may be less readily detected by high-performance liquid chromatography. The normal range for plasma porphyrins is somewhat increased in patients with end-stage renal disease. Although a total plasma porphyrin determination will usually detect EPP and XLP, which have symptoms of non-blistering photosensitivity, an erythrocyte protoporphyrin determination is more sensitive. However, because increases in erythrocyte protoporphyrin occur in many other conditions, the diagnosis of EPP must be confirmed by showing a predominant increase in free protoporphyrin rather than zinc protoporphyrin. In XLP, both free and zinc protoporphyrin are markedly increased, the zinc protoporphyrin being 15–50% of the total erythrocyte porphyrins [9].

More extensive testing is justified when an initial test is positive [5]. A substantial increase in PBG may be caused by AIP, HCP, or VP. These acute porphyrias can be distinguished by measuring erythrocyte HMB synthase, urinary porphyrins (using the same spot urine sample), fecal porphyrins, and plasma porphyrins. Enzymatic assays for COPRO oxidase and PROTO oxidase are not widely available. The various porphyrias that cause blistering skin lesions are differentiated by measuring porphyrins in urine, feces, and plasma. Confirmation at the DNA level by the demonstration of the causative mutation(s) is important after the diagnosis is established by biochemical testing and also permits family studies. Further details are provided in the following sections on each type of porphyria.

Testing for subclinical porphyria

It is often difficult to diagnose or "rule out" porphyria in patients who had suggestive symptoms months or years in the past, and in relatives of patients with acute porphyrias, because porphyrin precursors and porphyrins may be normal. More extensive testing and consultation with a specialist laboratory and physician may be needed. Before evaluating relatives, the diagnosis of porphyria should be firmly established in an index case and the laboratory results reviewed to guide the choice of tests for the family members. The index case or another family member with confirmed porphyria should be retested if necessary. Identification of a disease-causing mutation in an index case greatly facilitates detection of additional gene carriers.

The hepatic porphyrias

The major manifestations of the hepatic porphyrias, which typically present after puberty, are neurologic, although some also have cutaneous symptoms.

5′-Aminolevulinate dehydratase-deficient porphyria

Severe deficiency of ALA dehydratase activity gives rise to a rare autosomal recessive acute hepatic porphyria [1,6]. To date, there are only a few documented cases, including five in children or adolescents, in which specific gene mutations have been identified [1,11,12]. These affected homozygotes had less than 10% of normal ALA dehydratase activity in erythrocytes, but their clinically asymptomatic parents and heterozygous relatives had about half-normal levels of enzyme activity and did not excrete increased levels of ALA. The frequency of ALA dehydratase-deficient porphyria is not known, but the frequency of heterozygous individuals with less than 50% normal ALA dehydratase activity was approximately 2% in a population screening study in Sweden. Because there are multiple causes for deficient ALA dehydratase activity, it is important to confirm the diagnosis of ALA dehydratase-deficient porphyria by mutation analysis.

Clinical features

The clinical presentation is variable, presumably depending on the amount of residual ALA dehydratase activity. All patients had significantly elevated levels of plasma and urinary ALA and markedly decreased ALA dehydratase activity. Four of the reported patients were male adolescents with symptoms resembling those of AIP, including abdominal pain and neuropathy [11]. One patient was an infant with more severe disease, including failure to thrive beginning at birth. Earlier onset and more severe manifestations in this patient reflected a more significant deficiency of ALA dehydratase activity [11]. Another patient was essentially normal until age 63, when he developed an acute motor polyneuropathy that was associated with a myeloproliferative disorder. This patient was heterozygous for an ALA dehydratase mutation that presumably was present in erythroblasts that underwent clonal expansion because of the bone marrow malignancy.

Diagnosis

Patients have increased urinary levels of ALA and COPRO III. Urinary PBG is normal or slightly increased. In erythrocytes, ALA dehydratase activity is less than 10% of normal. Hereditary tyrosinemia type I (fumarylacetoacetase deficiency) and lead intoxication should be considered in the differential diagnosis because either succinylacetone (which accumulates in hereditary tyrosinemia type I and is structurally similar to ALA) or lead can inhibit ALA dehydratase, increase urinary excretion of ALA, and cause manifestations that resemble those of the acute porphyrias. Heterozygotes are clinically asymptomatic and do not excrete increased levels of ALA but can be detected by demonstration of intermediate levels of erythrocyte ALA dehydratase activity or a specific mutation in the gene for ALA dehydratase. To date, molecular studies of patients with ALA dehydratase-deficient porphyria have identified nine missense/nonsense and two splice-site mutations, as well as a two-base deletion in *ALAD*, encoding ALA dehydratase (Human Gene Mutation Database, www. hgmd.org) [12]. The parents in each case were not cosanguineous, and the index cases had inherited a different *ALAD* mutation from each parent. Prenatal diagnosis of this disorder should be possible by determination of the ALA dehydratase activity and/or gene mutation in cultured chorionic villi or amniocytes. Of note, a common polymorphism (K59N) has been identified that alters zinc binding but retains normal activity [13].

Treatment

The treatment of acute attacks in the four males who developed symptoms during adolescence was similar to that of AIP (see below) and included decreased symptoms from intravenous hemin treatment. The severely affected patient who did not survive infancy was supported by hyperalimentation and periodic blood transfusions, but did not respond biochemically or clinically to hemin or liver transplantation.

Acute intermittent porphyria

Acute intermittent porphyria is an autosomal dominant condition resulting from the half-normal level of HMB synthase activity. The disease is widespread but may be more common in Scandinavia and Great Britain. In most heterozygous individuals, clinical expression is highly variable. Activation of the disease is often related to environmental or hormonal factors, such as drugs, diet, and steroid hormones. Attacks can often be prevented by avoiding known precipitating factors. Rare homozygous dominant AIP also has been described in children (see below).

Clinical features

Induction of the rate-limiting hepatic enzyme ALAS1 is thought to underlie acute attacks in AIP and the other acute porphyrias. In the great majority of heterozygous carriers of *HMBS* mutations, AIP remains latent (or asymptomatic), and this is almost always the case before puberty. In patients with no history of acute symptoms, porphyrin precursor excretion is usually normal, suggesting that half-normal hepatic HMB synthase activity is sufficient for normal hepatic heme synthesis, and ALAS1 activity is not increased. When heme synthesis is increased in the liver, half-normal HMB synthase activity may become limiting and ALA, PBG, and other heme pathway intermediates may accumulate. Common precipitating factors include endogenous and exogenous gonadal steroids, porphyrinogenic drugs, alcohol ingestion, and low-calorie diets, usually instituted for weight loss.

The fact that AIP is almost always latent before puberty suggests that adult levels of steroid hormones are important for clinical expression. Symptoms are more common in women, which suggest a role for female hormones. Premenstrual attacks are probably the result of endogenous progesterone. Acute porphyrias are sometimes exacerbated by exogenous steroids, including oral contraceptive preparations containing progestins. Surprisingly, pregnancy is usually well tolerated, suggesting that beneficial metabolic changes may ameliorate the effects of high levels of progesterone. Table 30.3 is a partial list of the major drugs that are harmful in AIP (and also in HCP, VP, and probably ALA dehydratase-deficient porphyria). An extensive list of unsafe and safe drugs for individuals with porphyria is given at the Drug Database for Acute Porphyrias (www.drugs-porphyria.com). Reduced intake of calories and carbohydrates, as may occur with illness or attempts to lose weight, may also increase porphyrin precursor excretion and induce attacks of porphyria. Increased carbohydrates may ameliorate attacks. Recent findings indicate that hepatic ALAS1 is regulated by the peroxisome proliferator-activated receptor-γ coactivator 1α (PGC-1α), which may represent an important link between nutritional status and the acute porphyrias [14]. Attacks also may be provoked by infections, surgery, and ethanol. Some patients have repeated attacks without identifiable precipitants.

Because the neurovisceral symptoms are often non-specific, a high index of suspicion is required to make the diagnosis. The disease is rarely fatal if diagnosed promptly. Abdominal pain, the most common symptom, is usually steady and poorly localized but may be cramping. Constipation, abdominal distension, and decreased bowel sounds are common. Increased bowel sounds and diarrhea are less common. Because inflammation is absent, abdominal tenderness, fever, and leukocytosis are usually not prominent. Additional common manifestations include nausea; vomiting; tachycardia; hypertension; mental symptoms; extremity, neck, or chest pain; headache; muscle weakness; sensory loss; tremors; sweating; dysuria; and bladder distension.

The peripheral neuropathy is the result of axonal degeneration (rather than demyelination) and primarily affects motor neurons. Findings such as tachycardia, hypertension, sweating, and tremors may be the result of sympathetic overactivity. Motor neuropathy affects the proximal muscles initially, more often in the shoulders and arms. Muscle weakness may progress to respiratory and bulbar paralysis and death, particularly when diagnosis and treatment are delayed. Sudden death occurs occasionally, perhaps from sympathetic overactivity or cardiac arrhythmia.

Mental symptoms are often prominent during attacks and may include insomnia, agitation, disorientation, hallucinations, and depression. Seizures may be a neurologic manifestation of the disease or may be the result of hyponatremia. The latter results from inappropriate vasopressin secretion or electrolyte depletion. Abdominal pain may resolve within hours and paresis within days. However, severe motor neuropathy

Table 30.3 Some major drugs considered unsafe and safe in acute porphyrias[a]

Unsafe	Safe
Alcohol	Acetaminophen
Barbiturates[b]	Aspirin
Carbamazepine[b]	Atropine
Carisoprodol[b]	Bromides
Clonazepam (high doses)	Cimetidine
Danazol[b]	Erythropoietin[b,c]
Diclofenac and possibly other	Gabapentin
Non-steroidal anti-inflammatory drugs[b]	Glucocorticoids
Ergots	Insulin
Estrogens[c,d]	Narcotic analgesics
Ethchlorvynol[c]	Penicillin and derivatives
Glutethimide[b]	Phenothiazines
Griseofulvin[b]	Ranitidine[b,c]
Mephenytoin	Streptomycin
Meprobamate[b] (also mebutamate,[b] tybutamate[b])	
Methyprylon	
Metoclopramide[b]	
Phenytoin[b]	
Primidone[b]	
Progesterone and synthetic progestins[b]	
Pyrazinamide[b]	
Pyrazolones (aminopyrine, antipyrine)	
Rifampin[b]	
Succinimides (ethosuximide, methsuximide)	
Sulfonamide antibiotics[b]	
Valproic acid[b]	

[a] A more extensive list of drugs and their status is available in Anderson et al. [1] and at the following websites: www.porphyriafoundation.com, www.porphyria-europe.com and www.drugs-porphyria.com.

[b] Porphyria is listed as a contraindication, warning, precaution, or adverse effect in US labeling for these drugs. For drugs listed as unsafe, absence of such cautionary statements in US labeling does not imply lower risk.

[c] Although porphyria is listed as a precaution in US labeling, these drugs are regarded as safe by other sources.

[d] Estrogens have been regarded as harmful, mostly from experience with estrogen–progestin combinations and because they can exacerbate porphyria cutanea tarda. Although evidence that they exacerbate acute porphyrias is weak, they should be used with caution. Low doses of estrogen (e.g. transdermal) have been used safely to prevent side effects of gonadotropin-releasing hormone analogues in women with cyclic attacks.

Table 30.4 Homozygous forms of porphyria

| Porphyria | Deficient enzyme | Clinical onset | Principal symptoms | | Other symptoms |
			Neurovisceral	Cutaneous photosensitivity	
Hepatic					
Homozygous dominant acute intermittent porphyria	HMB synthase	Infancy & childhood	+	–	Absence of acute attacks, development delay
Hepatoerythropoietic porphyria	URO decarboxylase	Childhood	–	+	Rare anemia
Homozygous dominant coproporphyria	COPRO oxidase	Childhood	+	+	Growth retardation
Harderoporphyria	COPRO oxidase	Infancy & childhood	–	+	Neonatal hemolytic jaundice & anemia
Homozygous dominant variegate porphyria	PROTO oxidase	Infancy & childhood	+	+	Absence of acute attacks, mental retardation, hand deformities
Erythropoietic					
Homozygous erythropoietic protoporphyria	Ferrochelatase	Childhood	–	+	
Congenital erythropoietic porphyria	URO synthase	Infancy, childhood and later onset	–	+	Anemia

COPRO, coproporphyrinogen; HMB, hydroxymethylbilane; PROTO, protoporphyrinogen; URO, uroporphyrinogen.
Source: modified from Elder, 1997 [5].

may continue to improve over several years. Long-term risks for hypertension, impaired renal function, and hepatocellular carcinoma are increased.

Diagnosis

Both ALA and PBG levels are increased in plasma and urine during acute attacks [1,2]. Although the diagnosis of an acute attack is based on clinical findings and not the absolute level of these porphyrin precursors, the increase is expected to be substantial. Excretion of PBG is usually 50–200 mg/24 h (220–880 mmol/24 h; normal, 0–4 mg/24 h (0–18 mmol/24 h)), and urinary ALA excretion is 20–100 mg/24 h (150–760 mmol/24 h; normal, 1–7 mg/24 h (8–53 mmol/24 h)). Levels of these porphyrin precursors decrease after an attack but usually remain elevated, except with prolonged remissions. Decreases after hemin infusions are dramatic but usually transient (see below). A normal urinary PBG level effectively excludes AIP as a cause for current symptoms. Fecal and plasma porphyrins are normal or minimally increased in AIP, in contrast to HCP and VP. Most asymptomatic ("latent") heterozygotes with HMB synthase deficiency, particularly those who have never had symptoms, have normal urinary excretion of ALA and PBG. The enzyme deficiency is detectable in erythrocytes from most AIP heterozygotes (Table 30.4).

However, the activity is higher in young erythrocytes, and a concurrent condition that increases erythropoiesis may increase the enzyme into the normal range in a patient with AIP. Therefore, the detection of the family's HMB synthase mutation is important for diagnostic confirmation of symptomatic patients and for identification of asymptomatic family members with this enzyme deficiency.

Of note, the erythroid and housekeeping forms of HMB synthase are encoded by a single gene (*HMBS*) with two promoters; some mutations, usually found within exon 1, particularly in the initiation of translation codon, affect only the non-erythroid enzyme, and the erythroid enzyme is transcribed normally. Therefore, patients with the rare erythroid form of AIP (erythroid, or variant, AIP) have normal enzyme levels in erythrocytes and deficient activity in non-erythroid tissues [1].

More than 375 mutations in *HMBS* have been identified in AIP, including missense, nonsense, and splicing mutations and insertions and deletions, with most mutations found in only one or a few families (Human Gene Mutation Database; www.hgmd.org) [12]. Identification of the gene in an index case enables detection of latent family members and prenatal diagnosis of an at-risk fetus using cultured amniotic cells or chorionic villi. However, this is seldom done because the prognosis of individuals with *HMBS* mutations is generally favorable.

Treatment

During acute attacks, narcotic analgesics are usually required for abdominal pain, and phenothiazines are effective for nausea, vomiting, anxiety, and restlessness. Insomnia and restlessness are treated with chloral hydrate or low doses of short-acting benzodiazepines. Carbohydrate loading, usually with intravenous glucose (at least 300 mg/day), may be effective in milder acute attacks of porphyria (without paresis, hyponatremia, etc.). Because intravenous hemin is more effective and the response slower if treatment is delayed, it is no longer recommended that hemin therapy for a moderate to severe attack be started only after an unsuccessful trial of intravenous glucose for several days. Hemin should be used initially for moderate to severe attacks and for mild attacks that do not respond to carbohydrate loading within 1–2 days. The standard regimen is 3–4 mg heme in the form of lyophilized hematin (Recordati Rare Diseases, Milan, Italy), heme albumin (hematin reconstituted with human albumin), or heme arginate (Orphan Europe, Paris, France), infused daily for 4 days [5]. Heme arginate and heme albumin are chemically stable and are less likely than hematin to produce phlebitis or an anticoagulant effect. Recovery depends on the degree of neuronal damage and is usually rapid if therapy is started early, but patients with severe motor neuropathy may require months or years. Inciting factors are usually multiple, and removal of one or more hastens recovery and helps to prevent future attacks. Frequent attacks that occur during the luteal phase of the menstrual cycle may be prevented with a gonadotropin-releasing hormone analogue, which prevents ovulation and progesterone production.

The long-term risk of hypertension and chronic renal disease is increased in AIP; a number of patients have undergone successful renal transplantation. Chronic, low-grade abnormalities in liver function tests are common, and the risk of hepatocellular carcinoma is increased. Such tumors in patients with AIP have not been associated with increases in serum α-fetoprotein. Therefore, hepatic imaging is recommended at least yearly for early detection of these tumors.

An allogeneic liver transplantation was first performed on a 19-year-old female AIP heterozygote who had 37 acute attacks in the 29 months before transplantation [2]. Post-transplantation, her elevated urinary ALA and PBG levels returned to normal in 24 hours and she did not experience acute neurologic attacks for more than 3 years post-transplant. Two patients with AIP had combined liver and kidney transplants secondary to uncontrolled acute porphyria attacks, chronic peripheral neuropathy, and renal failure requiring dialysis. Both patients had a marked improvement with no attacks and normal urinary PBG levels post-transplant, as well as improvement of their neuropathic manifestations [3]. To date, a number of women with AIP have had successful liver transplants for severe recurrent neurologic attacks and secondary organ damage, with amelioration of their neurologic attacks and normalization of their heme precursors [2,3].

However, liver transplantation is a high-risk procedure and should be considered as a last resort in patients with severe recurrent attacks [15]. Recently, liver-directed gene therapy has been successful in the prevention of drug-induced biochemical attacks in a murine model of human AIP [16]. Liver transplantation is a high-risk procedure and should not be considered an established treatment for acute porphyrias.

Homozygous dominant acute intermittent porphyria

Homozygous dominant AIP is a rare form of porphyria presenting in infancy in which patients inherit HMB synthase mutations from each of their heterozygous parents and, therefore, have very low (<2%) enzyme activity (Table 30.4). The disease has been described in a Dutch girl, two young British siblings, and a Spanish boy [17,18]. In these homozygous affected patients, disease manifestations included failure to thrive, developmental delay, bilateral cataracts, and/or hepatosplenomegaly. Acute attacks did not occur. Urinary ALA and PBG were markedly elevated. Interestingly, the HMB synthase mutations (R167W, R167Q, and R172Q) in these patients were in exon 10 within five bases of each other. Brain MRI of children with homozygous AIP have suggested damage primarily in white matter that was myelinated postnatally, whereas tracks that myelinated prenatally were normal [18]. These findings suggest that a neurotoxic endogenous product such as ALA or PBG present in large amounts postnatally, rather than heme deficiency, caused nervous tissue damage. Prenatally, excess amounts of ALA and PBG would cross the placenta and be excreted in the mother's urine. Most children with homozygous AIP die at an early age.

Porphyria cutanea tarda

Porphyria cutanea tarda, the most common of the porphyrias, may be either sporadic (type 1) or familial (types 2 and 3) and may also develop after exposure to halogenated aromatic hydrocarbons. Hepatic URO decarboxylase is deficient in all types of PCT, and for clinical symptoms to manifest, this enzyme deficiency must be substantial (~20% of normal activity or less). Generation of a URO decarboxylase inhibitor, specifically in the liver in the presence of iron and under conditions of oxidative stress, is suspected to cause this decrease, although this inhibitor remains to be isolated and characterized [19].

The majority of patients with PCT (~80%) have no URO decarboxylase mutations and are said to have type 1 (sporadic) disease, or type 3 if relatives are affected. Patients with PCT who are heterozygous for URO decarboxylase mutations have familial (type 2) PCT. In these patients, inheritance of a URO decarboxylase mutation from one parent results in half-normal enzyme activity in liver and all other tissues, which is a significant predisposing factor but is insufficient by itself to cause symptomatic PCT. As discussed below, other genetic and environmental factors contribute to susceptibility to all types of PCT. For this reason, penetrance of this genetic trait is low,

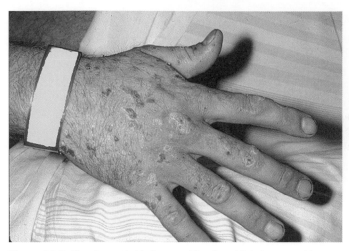

Figure 30.2 Chronic, crusted lesions resulting from blistering caused by photosensitivity on the dorsum of the hand of a patient with porphyria cutanea tarda. (Reproduced with permission from Anderson *et al.*, 2001 [1].)

and many patients who present with type 2 PCT have no family history of the disease and may appear to have sporadic disease. Homozygous type 2 PCT is termed hepatoerythropoietic porphyria (HEP), which usually presents with clinical symptoms in childhood (see below).

Deficient hepatic URO decarboxylase and a porphyrin pattern resembling PCT can be produced in rodents by a number of halogenated aromatic hydrocarbons, such as hexachlorobenzene and 2,3,7,8-tetrachlorodibenzo-*p*-dioxin (TCDD, dioxin). Outbreaks and isolated cases of PCT have been reported in humans exposed to these chemicals. Most notably, PCT affected thousands of children and adults in eastern Turkey during a period of food shortage, when seed wheat treated with hexachlorobenzene as a fungicide was consumed rather than planted [19].

Clinical features

Blistering skin lesions that appear most commonly on the backs of the hands are the major clinical feature (Figure 30.2). These rupture and crust over, leaving areas of atrophy and scarring. Lesions may also occur on the forearms, face, legs, and feet. Skin friability and small white papules termed *milia* are common, particularly on the backs of the hands and fingers. Hypertrichosis and hyperpigmentation, particularly on the face, are particularly troublesome in women. Occasionally, the skin over sun-exposed areas becomes severely thickened, with scarring and calcification that resembles systemic sclerosis. Neurologic features are absent.

A number of susceptibility factors in addition to inherited mutations in *UROD*, encoding URO decarboxylase, in type 2 PCT can be recognized clinically and may affect management. The importance of excess hepatic iron is underscored by the increased prevalence of the common hemochromatosis-causing mutations, C282Y and H63D in the HFE protein, in

patients with types 1 and 2 PCT [20]. There is also a strong association of PCT with hepatitis C virus in southern Europe and the USA. For example, in a series from the USA, this viral infection was found in 29 of 39 patients with PCT (74%), often in association with other risk factors [21]. Excess alcohol is a long-recognized contributor, as is estrogen use in women. Infection with HIV is probably an independent but less common risk factor, which, like hepatitis C virus, does not occur in isolation. Multiple susceptibility factors that appear to act synergistically can be identified in the individual patient with PCT [20].

Patients with PCT characteristically have evidence of chronic liver disease, such as persistently abnormal liver function tests, even when the disease occurs in the absence of susceptibility factors that cause liver damage, such as hepatitis C infection and excess ethanol use. Cirrhosis or hepatocellular carcinoma may develop in the long term [3].

Diagnosis

Porphyrins are increased in the liver, plasma, urine, and stool [1]. The urinary ALA may be slightly increased, but PBG is normal. Urinary porphyrins consist mostly of uroporphyrin and heptacarboxylate porphyrin, which is a diagnostic pattern for PCT and HEP, with lesser amounts of coproporphyrin and hexa- and pentacarboxylate porphyrins. Plasma porphyrins are also increased, which is useful for screening. Fluorometric scanning of diluted plasma at neutral pH can rapidly distinguish VP and PCT. There is an increase in isocoproporphyrins, particularly in feces, which is diagnostic for URO decarboxylase deficiency. These tetracarboxylate porphyrins result from a normally minor pathway that is accentuated by URO decarboxylase deficiency, whereby pentacarboxylate porphyrinogen is metabolized to iso-COPRO by COPRO oxidase, the enzyme that follows in the pathway.

In erythrocytes, URO decarboxylase activity is generally about half normal in type 2 PCT and normal in types 1 and 3. A genetic basis for type 3 PCT, which would clearly distinguish it from type 1, has not been established. Because most patients with familial (type 2) PCT have no family history of the disease, the finding of half-normal URO decarboxylase activity in erythrocytes is useful for identifying this predisposing genetic trait, although DNA analysis to identify a specific mutation is more reliable. More than 105 mutations have been identified in the *UROD* in type 2 PCT and HEP (Human Gene Mutation Database; www.hgmd.org) [12]. Of the mutations listed in the Human Gene Mutation Database, approximately 65% are missense/nonsense, and approximately 10% are splice-site mutations; most have been identified in only one or two families.

Treatment

Discontinuing risk factors such as alcohol, estrogens, and iron supplements is recommended but may not result in timely improvement. A complete response can almost always be achieved by the standard therapy, which at most centers is repeated phlebotomy to reduce hepatic iron [6]. A unit (450 mL) of blood can be removed approximately every 2 weeks. The aim is to gradually reduce iron until the serum ferritin reaches the lower limits of normal [19]. Hemoglobin levels or the hematocrit should be followed closely to prevent anemia. Because iron overload is not marked in most cases, the target ferritin level can often be achieved after only five or six phlebotomies; however, patients with PCT with hemochromatosis may require many more phlebotomies. To document improvement in PCT, it is most convenient to follow the total plasma porphyrin concentration, which becomes normal some time after the target ferritin level is reached. After remission, continued phlebotomy may not be needed. Plasma porphyrin levels are followed at intervals of 6–12 months for early detection of recurrences, which occur in a minority of patients and may be treated again by phlebotomy.

A low-dose regimen of chloroquine or hydroxychloroquine, which in some manner mobilizes excess porphyrins from the liver and promotes their excretion, is a useful alternative to phlebotomy, particularly when phlebotomy is contraindicated or poorly tolerated. Small doses (e.g. 125 mg chloroquine phosphate twice weekly) should be given because standard doses may induce the rapid release of stored hepatic porphyrins, transient marked increases in photosensitivity, and hepatocellular damage. Hepatic imaging can detect or exclude complicating hepatocellular carcinoma. Treatment of PCT in patients with end-stage renal disease is facilitated by administration of erythropoietin.

Hepatoerythropoietic porphyria

The homozygous form of familial (type 2) PCT, HEP, resembles CEP clinically (see below). Most patients have inherited different mutations from unrelated parents. In HEP, URO decarboxylase activity is markedly deficient, with levels typically 3–10% of normal. Mutations associated with HEP are generally associated with expression of some residual enzyme activity. Excess porphyrins originate mostly from liver, with a pattern consistent with severe URO decarboxylase deficiency (see above).

There also is a substantial increase in erythrocyte zinc protoporphyrin in HEP, as in other homozygous dominant forms of the acute porphyrias, ALA dehydratase-deficient porphyria, and some cases of CEP. Apparently, porphyrinogens accumulate in the marrow while hemoglobin synthesis is most active and are metabolized to protoporphyrin (and chelated with zinc by FECH) after hemoglobin synthesis is complete.

Like CEP, HEP usually presents with blistering skin lesions, hypertrichosis, scarring, and red urine in infancy or childhood. Sclerodermoid skin changes are sometimes prominent. Unusually mild cases have been described. Concurrent conditions that affect liver function may alter disease severity. For example, hepatitis A virus caused the disease to become manifest in a 2-year-old child and then improved with recovery from this viral infection.

Hepatoerythropoietic porphyria is readily distinguished from CEP by increases in both uroporphyrin and heptacarboxyl porphyrin in urine and in isocoproporphyrins in stool. In most cases of CEP, the excess erythrocyte porphyrins are predominantly uroporphyrin I and coproporphyrin I rather than zinc protoporphyrin. Erythropoietic protoporphyria and XLP are readily distinguished by their non-blistering photosensitivity and normal urine porphyrins and by demonstrating that the excess erythrocyte protoporphyrin is mostly free or, for XLP, may be complexed with zinc for 15–50% of total protoporphyrin levels. As in CEP, avoidance of sunlight is most important in managing this disease. The outlook depends on the severity of the enzyme deficiency and may be favorable if sunlight can be avoided. Phlebotomy has shown little or no benefit.

Hereditary coproporphyria

Hereditary coproporphyria is an autosomal dominant hepatic porphyria that results from the half normal activity of COPRO oxidase. The disease usually presents with acute attacks, as in AIP. However, cutaneous photosensitivity also may occur, but much less commonly than in VP. In two studies of more than 100 patients with HCP, over 80% had abdominal pain but only 5–29% had cutaneous symptoms [22,23]. The disorder is less common than AIP or VP [24]. Homozygous dominant HCP and harderoporphyria, a biochemically distinguishable variant of HCP, present with clinical symptoms in children (see below).

Clinical features

Hereditary coproporphyria is influenced by the same factors that cause attacks in AIP. The disease is latent before puberty, and neurovisceral symptoms, which are virtually identical to those of AIP, are more common in women. In general, HCP is less severe than AIP, although severe and fatal motor neuropathy may occur. Blistering skin lesions are identical to those in PCT and VP and begin in childhood in rare homozygous cases.

Diagnosis

Coproporphyrin III is markedly increased in the urine and feces in symptomatic patients and often persists, particularly in feces, when there are no symptoms [1,2]. Urinary ALA and PBG levels may be less increased during acute attacks and, with recovery from an attack, may revert to normal more quickly than in AIP [6]. Plasma porphyrins are usually normal or only slightly increased but may be higher in patients with skin lesions. The diagnosis of HCP is readily confirmed by increased fecal porphyrins, consisting almost entirely of coproporphyrin III, which distinguishes it from other porphyrias. An increase in the fecal coproporphyrin III/COPRO I ratio is useful for detecting latent disease.

Although the diagnosis can be confirmed by measuring COPRO oxidase activity, assays for this mitochondrial enzyme are not widely available and require cells other than erythrocytes. Since the gene *CPOX*, encoding COPRO, oxidase was cloned, more than 60 mutations, two-thirds of which are missense, have been identified in unrelated patients (Human Gene Mutation Database; www.hgmd.org) [12].

Treatment

Neurologic symptoms are treated as in AIP (see above). Phlebotomy and chloroquine are ineffective for the cutaneous manifestations.

Homozygous dominant hereditary coproporphyria and harderoporphyria

Individuals with mutations in both their *COPOX* alleles have been described. Several had homozygous dominant HCP and five had a variant form called harderoporphyria. One patient with homozygous HCP was a young girl, the daughter of consanguineous parents, who at the age of 4 years had symptoms of growth retardation, hypertrichosis, and skin hyperpigmentation. In her 20s, she had acute porphyric attacks. She had markedly increased fecal coproporphyrin III, approximately 10% of normal COPRO oxidase activity, and was homozygous for the missense mutation R331W [25].

Individuals with harderoporphyria, which is a biochemical and clinical variant form of HCP in which hemolysis and erythropoietic features are prominent, usually present in early childhood with jaundice, hemolytic anemia, hepatosplenomegaly, and skin photosensitivity [1]. However, the symptoms may be variable; one patient had only jaundice in childhood but developed mild anemia and skin lesions in adulthood, whereas two other patients had both neonatal anemia and skin photosensitivity. Urinary coproporphyrin III, fecal porphyrins (66–90% harderoporphyrin), and erythrocyte zinc protoporphyrin are increased.

Most patients with harderoporphyria reported to date are either homoallelic or heteroallelic for the K404E missense mutation. Studies of the crystallized COPRO oxidase protein and hydrophobic cluster analysis have shown that the amino acids at residues 400–404 are involved in the second step of the conversion of COPRO III to PROTO IX, and mutations affecting any one of these amino acid residues may result in the release and accumulation of the reaction intermediate, harderoporphyrinogen [26,27]. Occasionally, heterozygotes for mutations in this region may develop typical HCP [28]. Recently, a Turkish infant with the harderoporphyria phenotype and probable acute neurologic attacks was described who was homoallelic for the *CPOX* missense mutation resulting in H327R [29]. Structural studies predicted that H327R interacts with residue W399 in the active site, thereby accounting for the harderoporphyria phenotype [29].

Variegate porphyria

Variegate porphyria is an autosomal dominant hepatic porphyria that results from deficient activity of PROTO oxidase, the seventh enzyme in the heme pathway, and may present with neurologic symptoms, photosensitivity, or both. It is particularly common in South Africa, where 3 of every 1000 whites have the disorder. Most are descendants of a couple who emigrated from Holland to South Africa in 1688 [30]. In other countries, VP is less common than AIP. Homozygous dominant VP is rare and presents early in childhood.

Clinical features

Acute attacks identical to those in AIP and often precipitated by drugs, hormones, or diet develop in a minority of heterozygotes for PROTO oxidase deficiency. Blistering skin manifestations are identical to those in PCT but are more difficult to treat and usually of longer duration. Attacks are generally milder than in AIP and less often fatal. In two large studies of patients with VP, approximately 60% had only skin lesions, 20% had only acute attacks, and approximately 20% had both [30].

Diagnosis

Urinary excretion of ALA and PBG is increased during acute attacks but may be less increased and return to normal more quickly than in AIP. Increases in fecal protoporphyrin and coproporphyrin III and in urinary coproporphyrin III are more persistent. Plasma porphyrin levels also are increased, particularly when there are cutaneous lesions, but are increased in latent disease more commonly than fecal porphyrins. The fluorescence emission spectrum of porphyrins in plasma at neutral pH in VP is distinctive and can rapidly distinguish VP from all other porphyrias, particularly PCT, which is much more common [31].

Assays of PROTO oxidase activity in cells such as lymphocytes for confirming the diagnosis are not widely available, and identifying the specific *PPOX* mutation is preferred once a diagnosis has been established in an index case. More than 130 mutations have been identified in the *PPOX* from unrelated patients with VP (Human Gene Mutation Database; www.hgmd.org) [12]. The missense mutation R59W is the common mutant in most South Africans with VP of Dutch descent [32].

Treatment

Acute attacks are treated as in AIP, and hemin should be started early in most cases. Other than avoiding sun exposure and wearing protective clothing, there are few effective measures for treating the skin lesions. Beta-carotene, phlebotomy, and chloroquine are not helpful.

Homozygous dominant variegate porphyria

Affected individuals with homozygous dominant VP have mutations affecting both *PPOX* alleles, resulting in very low enzyme activity levels. These patients generally develop cutaneous symptoms, including photosensitivity and hypertrichosis, before the age of 2 years. Scarring and deformities of the face and digits may be prominent. Most patients do not have acute attacks. Neurologic symptoms in some patients include mental retardation, convulsions, growth retardation, and nystagmus. A patient with homozygous dominant VP followed for over 20 years developed mild sensory neuropathy and an unexplained immunoglobulin A nephropathy besides having severe cutaneous problems. Laboratory findings include elevated erythrocyte zinc protoporphyrin levels, as in other homozygous dominant porphyrias. Missense and/or splice-site mutations have been identified in most homozygous patients with VP. Expression studies have indicated that these mutations have residual activity.

Erythropoietic porphyrias

In the erythropoietic porphyrias, excess porphyrins from bone marrow erythrocyte precursors are transported in plasma to the skin and lead to cutaneous photosensitivity. The most common of these, EPP, may be complicated by severe, life-threatening liver disease.

Congenital erythropoietic porphyria

Congenital erythropoietic porphyria is an autosomal recessive disorder, also known as Günther disease, that is the result of the markedly deficient, but not absent, activity of URO synthase and the resultant accumulation of uroporphyrin I and coproporphyrin I isomers. Uroporphyrinogen I, which is derived from the non-enzymatic cyclization of the substrate HMB, is metabolized by URO decarboxylase to COPRO I, but the latter is not a substrate for COPRO oxidase. Congenital erythropoietic porphyria is associated with hemolytic anemia and severe cutaneous photosensitivity. Excess porphyrins are also deposited in teeth and bones.

Clinical features

Severe cutaneous photosensitivity begins in early infancy in most patients [8]. The disease may be recognized in utero as a cause of non-immune hydrops fetalis. The skin over light-exposed areas is friable, and bullae and vesicles are prone to rupture and infection. Skin thickening, focal hypo- and hyperpigmentation, and hypertrichosis of the face and extremities are characteristic. Secondary infection and bone resorption may lead to disfigurement of the face and hands. The teeth are reddish brown and fluoresce on exposure to long-wave ultraviolet light. Hemolysis is probably the result of the marked increase in erythrocyte porphyrins and leads to splenomegaly. A milder form of the disease in adults is a complication of a myeloproliferative or myelodysplastic disorder.

Diagnosis

Uroporphyrin and coproporphyrin (mostly type I isomers) accumulate in the bone marrow and are also found in circulating erythrocytes, plasma, urine, and feces. The predominant porphyrin in feces is coproporphyrin I. The diagnosis can be confirmed by demonstration of markedly deficient URO synthase activity or the identification of specific mutations in *UROS*. The disease can be detected in utero by measuring porphyrins in amniotic fluid and URO synthase activity in cultured amniotic cells or chorionic villi or by the detection of the family's specific gene mutations. Molecular analyses of the mutant alleles from unrelated patients have revealed the presence of over 35 mutations in *UROS*, including four in its erythroid-specific promoter [8,33]. More recently, CEP caused by a mutation in *GATA1*, an X-linked transcription factor common to globin genes and heme biosynthetic enzymes in erythrocytes, has been reported [34].

Treatment

Severe CEP often requires chronic transfusions for anemia, which can be started in utero. Chronic transfusions sufficient to suppress erythropoiesis are effective in reducing porphyrin production, but result in iron overload and other complications [35]. Splenectomy may reduce hemolysis and decrease transfusion requirements. Protection from sunlight is essential, and minor skin trauma should be avoided. Complicating bacterial infections should be treated promptly. Bone marrow and cord blood transplantation have proved effective in several transfusion-dependent children [e.g. 36], providing the rationale for stem-cell gene therapy [8].

Erythropoietic protoporphyria

Erythropoietic protoporphyria is an inherited disorder resulting from the partially deficient activity of FECH, the last enzyme in the heme biosynthetic pathway. It is not only the most common erythropoietic porphyria but is also the most common porphyria in children and the second most common in adults [1]. Patients with EPP have FECH activity as low as 15–25% in lymphocytes and cultured fibroblasts. Protoporphyrin accumulates primarily in bone marrow reticulocytes during hemoglobin synthesis, and then appears in plasma, is taken up in the liver, and is excreted in bile and feces. Protoporphyrin transported to the skin causes photosensitivity. In most symptomatic patients (~90%) with this autosomal recessive disorder, a mutation in one *FECH* allele is inherited with a relatively common (~10% in European Caucasians) mutation, IVS3–48T>C, that results in the low expression of the normal enzyme. In about 5–10% of EPP families, two *FECH* loss-of-function mutations have been found [21,24,37]. Recently, an X-linked form of EPP, XLP, has been found to result from gain-of-function mutations in exon 11 of *ALAS2* [9] and is clinically indistinguishable from EPP. The *ALAS2* mutations alter the C-terminal amino acid sequence and result in increased ALAS2 activity and the accumulation of protoporphyrin. X-linked protoporphyria accounts for less than 5% of patients with the EPP phenotype [37].

Clinical features

Skin photosensitivity, which differs from that in other porphyrias, usually begins in childhood and consists of pain, redness, and itching occurring within minutes of sunlight exposure. This occurs only in patients with substantial elevations in erythrocyte protoporphyrin and a genotype that results in FECH activity below approximately 35% of normal. Vesicular lesions are uncommon. The burning pain developing shortly after sun exposure can be excruciating, and not relieved by narcotic analgesics. Subsequently, the exposed area becomes red and swollen. Symptoms may seem out of proportion to the visible skin lesions. Vesicles and bullae are sparse and occur in only about 10% of patients. Chronic skin changes may include lichenification, leathery pseudovesicles, labial grooving, and nail changes. Severe scarring is rare, as are pigment changes, friability, and hirsutism. Unless hepatic or other complications develop, protoporphyrin levels and symptoms of photosensitivity remain remarkably stable over many years in most patients. Factors that exacerbate hepatic porphyrias play little or no role in EPP or XLP.

The primary source of excess protoporphyrin is the bone marrow reticulocyte. Erythrocyte protoporphyrin is almost all free (not complexed with zinc) and is mostly bound to hemoglobin. In XLP, free and zinc protoporphyrin are both increased in erythrocytes [9]. In plasma, protoporphyrin is bound to albumin. Hemolysis and anemia are usually absent or mild.

Although EPP and XLP are erythropoietic porphyrias, up to 20% of patients with EPP may have minor abnormalities of liver function; in about 5% of patients, the accumulation of protoporphyrin causes liver disease, which may be chronic but sometimes develops rapidly and may progress to liver failure and death. Protoporphyrin is insoluble, and excess amounts form crystalline structures in liver cells and can decrease hepatic bile flow in bile fistula in rats. Studies in a mouse model of EPP suggest that excess protoporphyrin alters bile composition in a manner that is toxic to bile duct epithelium, leading to ductular proliferation and fibrosis [38]. Rapidly progressive liver disease in human EPP is associated with increasing protoporphyrin levels in liver, plasma, and erythrocytes and increased photosensitivity. Protoporphyric liver disease may cause severe abdominal pain, particularly in the right upper quadrant, and back pain. Gallstones composed at least in part of protoporphyrin may be symptomatic in patients with EPP and need to be excluded as a cause of biliary obstruction in patients with hepatic decompensation. Hepatic complications appear to be higher in autosomal recessive EPP caused by two *FECH* mutations and in XLP [39].

Diagnosis

A substantial increase in erythrocyte protoporphyrin, which is predominantly free and not complexed with zinc, is the hallmark of EPP, while erythrocyte free and zinc protoporphyrin accumulate in XLP. Protoporphyrin levels are also variably increased in bone marrow, plasma, bile, and feces. Plasma and fecal porphyrins are increased less than in most other cutaneous porphyrias and are sometimes normal. Therefore, measuring erythrocyte protoporphyrin is important for their diagnosis. Although erythrocyte protoporphyrin concentrations are increased in other conditions, such as lead poisoning,

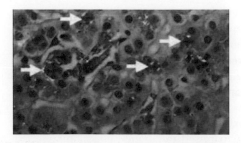

Figure 30.3 Polarization microscopy of a liver biopsy specimen from a patient with erythropoietic protoporphyria shows that the pigment deposits are birefringent because of the presence of protoporphyrin crystals (arrows). The crystal on the left is in the form of a centrally located dark Maltese cross. (Reproduced with permission from McGuire *et al.*, 2005 [40].)

iron deficiency, various hemolytic disorders, and all homozygous forms of porphyria, and are sometimes somewhat increased, even in acute porphyrias, in all these conditions, in contrast to EPP (but not XLP), protoporphyrin is complexed with zinc. Therefore, after an increase in erythrocyte protoporphyrin is found in a patient with suspected EPP, it is important to confirm the diagnosis by an assay that distinguishes free and zinc-complexed protoporphyrin, and then to perform mutation analyses of *FECH* and *ALAS2*.

Erythrocytes in EPP and XLP exhibit red fluorescence when examined by fluorescence microscopy at 620 nm (Figure 30.3). Urinary levels of porphyrins and porphyrin precursors are normal. Activity of FECH in cultured lymphocytes or fibroblasts is decreased in EPP, but such assays are not widely available. Mutation analysis of *FECH* is recommended to detect the causative mutation and, in most affected families, the presence of the IVS3–48T>C low-activity allele. To date, more than 135 loss-of-function mutations have been identified in *FECH*, many of which result in an unstable or absent enzyme protein [12]. Studies suggest that patients with EPP with a null allele *in cis* and the IVS3–48T>C low-expression allele *in trans* have a greater risk for developing severe liver complications than do those with mutations that encode some enzyme activity [39]. In XLP, the erythrocyte protoporphyrin levels appear to be higher than other forms of EPP, and the proportions of free and zinc protoporphyrins are approximately equivalent. To-date, several *ALAS2* exon 11 gain-of-function mutations have been described, which markedly increase ALAS2 activity and cause XLP [9].

Treatment

Avoiding sunlight exposure and wearing clothing designed to provide protection for conditions with chronic photosensitivity are essential. Oral beta-carotene (120–180 mg/dL) may improve tolerance to sunlight if the dose is adjusted to maintain serum carotene levels in the range 10–15 μmol/L (600–800 μg/dL), causing mild skin discoloration through to carotenemia. The beneficial effects of beta-carotene may involve quenching of singlet oxygen or free radicals. Recently, clinical studies have shown that treatment with an alpha-melanocyte-stimulating hormone analogue, which darkens the skin, can increase the amount of patient exposure to sunlight without pain [41].

Treatment of hepatic complications, which may be accompanied by motor neuropathy, is difficult. Colestyramine and other porphyrin absorbents, such as activated charcoal, may interrupt the enterohepatic circulation of protoporphyrin and promote its fecal excretion, leading to some improvement. Splenectomy may be helpful if the disease is accompanied by hemolysis and significant splenomegaly. Plasmapheresis and intravenous hemin are sometimes beneficial. However, liver transplant is sometimes necessary and is often successful in the short term (reviewed by McGuire *et al.* [40]). Liver disease often recurs eventually in the transplanted liver because of continued bone marrow production of excess protoporphyrin. In a retrospective study of 17 patients with EPP who had received a liver transplant, 11 (65%) had recurrent EPP liver disease [40]. Post-transplantation treatment with hemin and plasmapheresis may help to prevent recurrence of this complication. However, bone marrow transplantation, which has been successful in human EPP and prevented liver disease in a mouse model [42], should be considered along with or after liver transplantation.

Dual porphyria

Patients with porphyria and deficiencies of two heme biosynthetic enzymes have been described, but few are documented by molecular studies. These patients are said to have dual porphyria but have diverse combinations of enzyme deficiencies and differing clinical presentations. Families with individuals having both VP and familial PCT have been described. Combined deficiencies of both HMB synthase and URO decarboxylase may lead to symptoms of AIP, PCT, or both. An infant with severe porphyria inherited a COPRO oxidase deficiency from one parent and URO synthase deficiency from both. Dual deficiencies of URO synthase and URO decarboxylase were described in a patient with features of an erythropoietic porphyria. Molecular studies of a patient initially thought to have both VP and AIP revealed a *PPOX* mutation, but no *HMBS* mutation. A patient with both sporadic PCT and HCP due to an inherited *CPOX* mutation was identified based on a urinary porphyrin pattern consistent with PCT. Recently, mutations in two different heme biosynthetic pathway genes were documented in two individuals with biochemical data consistent with a dual porphyria. One patient, diagnosed after an acute porphyric attack, had a missense mutation in one *CPOX* allele and a missense mutation in one *ALAD* allele [43]. His urinary porphyria pattern suggested HCP except for higher-than-expected ALA levels, which suggested ALA dehydratase-deficient porphyria. The second patient had a splice-site mutation in one *HMBS* allele and a novel two-base insertion in one *UROD* allele [28]. The 25-year-old woman presented with a bullous rash in sun-exposed areas after starting on birth control pills. Her PBG was elevated, and the initial diagnosis was VP; however, studies of her urinary and plasma porphyrins did not support that diagnosis and indicated a dual porphyria.

Animal models of porphyrias

Animal models of the human porphyrias are extremely valuable in studying the pathophysiology and possible treatments of the porphyrias. Earlier models of acute hepatic porphyrias include rodents treated with chemicals such as allylisopropylacetamide and 1,4-dihydro-3,5-dicarbethoxycollidine (DDC). Rodents and hepatocytes treated with hexachlorobenzene and other halogenated polycyclic aromatic hydrocarbons have been useful models for PCT and produce URO decarboxylase deficiency confined to the liver, as in human type 1 PCT. Mouse models produced by gene targeting technology have been generated for AIP, CEP, PCT, VP, and EPP. In general, knockout mice that are homozygous for a null mutation have been fetal lethals. However, knockin mice, which have residual activity expressed by the targeted gene, survive and have the biochemical and/or clinical features of their human counterparts [44–46]. In addition, an EPP mouse model has been generated by ethylnitrosourea-induced mutagenesis, resulting in a point mutation in *Fech*, which is expressed as a recessive trait [47].

An AIP mouse model with HMB synthase deficiency, produced by gene targeting, when treated with a barbiturate had impaired motor function, ataxia, increased levels of ALA in brain and plasma, and decreased heme saturation of liver tryptophan pyrrolase. A motor neuropathy resembling that seen in AIP may develop in these mice, with normal or only slightly increased plasma or urinary ALA, suggesting a role for heme deficiency in nervous tissue [48].

Two mouse models of CEP using knockin techniques have been reported in which the mice have low URO synthase, hepatosplenomegaly, and hemolytic anemia [45,46]; one model also had the characteristic light-induced cutaneous involvement.

A knockout mouse heterozygous for *Urod*, with only approximately 50% of normal activity in all tissues, did not show symptoms of PCT unless injected with iron dextran or given oral ALA [49]. These treatments decreased URO decarboxylase activity to around 20% of normal. When the heterozygous $Urod^{+/-}$ mice were bred to $Hfe^{-/-}$ mice, the combined $Urod^{+/-}/Hfe^{-/-}$ mice became uroporphyric without exogenous chemical treatment [49]. Of interest, knockin mice homozygous for the *Hfe* C282Y mutation also developed symptoms of PCT if given 10% ethanol in their drinking water. A mouse model of VP with the common South African R59W mutation in the gene for PROTO oxidase had biochemical findings similar to those of VP [50]. The heterozygous knockout mouse for EPP had skin photosensitivity but no liver disease, whereas the EPP mouse model generated by ethylnitrosourea-induced mutagenesis, when homozygous for the induced point mutation, has approximately 5% of normal Fech activity, skin lesions, jaundice, and severe hepatic dysfunction with massive protoporphyrin deposits [46].

Acknowledgements

This work was supported in part by grants from the NIH Rare Disease Clinical Research Network for the Porphyrias Consortium (U54 DK083909), National Institutes of Health, including a research grant (5 R01 DK026824); the General Clinical Research Center Programs at the Mount Sinai School of Medicine (5 M01 RR00071) and the University of Texas Medical Branch (5 M01-RR0073) from the National Center for Research Resources; the US Food and Drug Administration (FD-R-002604); and the American Porphyria Foundation. MB is the recepient of an NIH Career Development award (K23 DK095940).

References

1. Anderson KE, Sassa S, Bishop DF, *et al.* Disorders of heme biosynthesis: X-linked sideroblastic anemias and the porphyrias, In Scriver CR, Beaudet AL, Sly WS, *et al.* (eds.) *The Metabolic and Molecular Basis of Inherited Disease.* New York: McGraw-Hill, 2001, pp. 2991–3062.

2. Anderson KE, Bloomer JE, Bonkovsky HL, *et al.* Recommendations for the diagnosis and treatment of the acute porphyrias. *Ann Intern Med* 2005;**142**:439–512.

3. Desnick RJ, Anderson KE, Astrin KH. Inherited porphyrias. In Rimoin DL, Conner JM, Pyeritz RE, *et al.* (eds.) *Emery and Rimoin's Principles and Practice of Medical Genetics*, 5th edn. Edinburgh: Churchill-Livingstone, 2007, pp. 2331–2358.

4. Puy H, Gouya L, Deybach JC. Porphyrias. *Lancet* 2010;**375**:924–937.

5. Elder GH. Hepatic porphyrias in children. *J Inherit Metab Dis* 1997;**20**:237–246.

6. Soonawalla ZF, Orug T, Badminton MN, *et al.* Liver transplantation as a cure for acute intermittent porphyria. *Lancet* 2004;**363**:705–706.

7. Wahlin S, Harper P, Sardh E, *et al.* Combined liver and kidney transplantation in acute intermittent porphyria. *Transplant Int* 2010;**23**: 18–21.

8. Desnick RJ, Astrin KH. Congenital erythropoietic porphyria: advances in pathogenesis and treatment. *Br J Haematol* 2002;**117**:779–795.

9. Whatley SD, Ducamp S, Gouya L, *et al.* C-terminal deletions in the alas2 gene lead to gain of function and cause x-linked dominant protoporphyria without anemia or iron overload. *Am J Hum Genet* 2008;**83**:408–414.

10. May BK, Dogra SC, Sadlon TJ, *et al.* Molecular regulation of heme biosynthesis in higher vertebrates. *Prog Nucleic Acid Res Mol Biol* 1995;**51**:1–51.

11. Akagi R, Kato N, Inoue R, *et al.* Delta-aminolevulinate dehydratase (ALAD) porphyria: the first case in North America with two novel *ALAD* mutations. *Mol Genet Metab* 2006;**87**:329–336.

12. Stenson PD, Ball EV, Mort M, *et al.* Human Gene Mutation Database (HGMD): 2003 update. *Hum Mutat* 2003;**21**:577–581.

13. Astrin KH, Bishop DF, Wetmur JG, *et al.* Delta-aminolevulinic acid dehydratase isozymes and lead toxicity. *Ann N Y Acad Sci* 1987;**514**:23–29.

14. Handschin C, Lin J, Rhee J, *et al.* Nutritional regulation of hepatic heme biosynthesis and porphyria through PGC-1alpha. *Cell* 2005;**122**:505–515.

15. Dowman JK, Gunson BK, Mirza DF, *et al.* Liver transplantation for acute intermittent porphyria is complicated by a high rate of hepatic artery thrombosis. *Liver Transplant* 2012;**18**:195–200.

16. Yasuda M, Bishop DF, Fowkes M, *et al.* AAV8-mediated gene therapy prevents induced biochemical attacks of acute intermittent porphyria and improves neuromotor function. *Mol Ther* 2010;**18**:17–22.

17. Llewellyn DH, Smyth SJ, Elder GH, *et al.* Homozygous acute intermittent porphyria: compound heterozygosity for adjacent base transitions in the same codon of the porphobilinogen deaminase gene. *Hum Genet* 1992;**89**:97–98.

18. Solis C, Martinez-Bermejo A, Naidich TP, *et al.* Acute intermittent porphyria: studies of the severe homozygous dominant disease provides insights into the neurologic attacks in acute porphyrias. *Arch Neurol* 2004;**61**: 1764–1770.

19. Phillips JD, Bergonia HA, Reilly CA, *et al.* A porphomethane inhibitor of uroporphyrinogen decarboxylase causes porphyria cutanea tarda. *Proc Natl Acad Sci USA* 2007;**104**: 5079–5084.

20. Egger NG, Goeger DE, Payne DA, *et al.* Porphyria cutanea tarda: multiplicity of risk factors including *HFE* mutations, hepatitis C, and inherited uroporphyrinogen decarboxylase deficiency. *Dig Dis Sci* 2002;**47**:419–426.

21. Kuhnel A, Gross U, Doss MO. Hereditary coproporphyria in Germany: clinical-biochemical studies in 53 patients. *Clin Biochem* 2000;**33**:465–473.

22. Martasek P. Hereditary coproporphyria. *Semin Liver Dis* 1998;**18**:25–32.

23. Martasek P, Nordmann Y, Grandchamp B. Homozygous hereditary coproporphyria caused by an arginine to tryptophane substitution in coproporphyrinogen oxidase and common intragenic polymorphisms. *Hum Mol Genet* 1994;**3**:477–480.

24. Lee DS, Flachsova E, Bodnarova M, *et al.* Structural basis of hereditary coproporphyria. *Proc Natl Acad Sci USA* 2005;**102**:14232–14237.

25. Schmitt C, Gouya L, Malonova E, *et al.* Mutations in human *CPO* gene predict clinical expression of either hepatic hereditary coproporphyria or erythropoietic harderoporphyria. *Hum Mol Genet* 2005;**14**:3089–3098.

26. Hasanoglu A, Balwani M, Kasapkara CS, *et al.* Harderoporphyria due to homozygosity for coproporphyrinogen oxidase missense mutation H327R. *J Inherit Metab Dis* 2011;**34**:225–231.

27. Meissner P, Hift RJ, Corrigall A. Variegate porphyria. In Kadish KM, Smith K, Guilard R (eds.) *Porphyrin Handbook*, part II. San Diego, CA: Academic Press, 2003, pp. 93–120.

28. Poh-Fitzpatrick MB. A plasma porphyrin fluorescence marker for variegate porphyria. *Arch Dermatol* 1980;**116**:543–547.

29. Meissner PN, Dailey TA, Hift RJ, *et al.* A R59W mutation in human protoporphyrinogen oxidase results in decreased enzyme activity and is

prevalent in South Africans with variegate porphyria. *Nat Genet* 1996;**13**:95–97.

30. Solis C, Aizencang GI, Astrin KH, *et al.* Uroporphyrinogen III synthase erythroid promoter mutations in adjacent *GATA1* and *CP2* elements cause congenital erythropoietic porphyria. *J Clin Invest* 2001;**107**:753–762.

31. Phillips JD, Steensma DP, Pulsipher MA, Spangrude GJ, Kushner JP. Congenital erythropoietic porphyria due to a mutation in *GATA1*: the first trans-acting mutation causative for a human porphyria. *Blood* 2007;**109**:2618–2621.

32. Piomelli S, Poh-Fitzpatrick MB, Seaman C, *et al.* Complete suppression of the symptoms of congenital erythropoietic porphyria by long-term treatment with high-level transfusions. *N Engl J Med* 1986;**314**:1029–1031.

33. Dupuis-Girod S, Akkari V, Ged C, *et al.* Successful match-unrelated donor bone marrow transplantation for congenital erythropoietic porphyria (Günther disease). *Eur J Pediatr* 2005;**164**: 104–107.

34. Gouya L, Martin-Schmitt C, Robreau AM, *et al.* Contribution of a common single-nucleotide polymorphism to the genetic predisposition for erythropoietic protoporphyria. *Am J Hum Genet* 2006;**78**:2–14.

35. Whatley SD, Mason NG, Holme SA, *et al.* Molecular epidemiology of erythropoietic protoporphyria in the United Kingdom. *Br J Dermatol* 2010;**162**:642–646.

36. Wahlin S, Floderus Y, Stål P, Harper P. Erythropoietic protoporphyria in Sweden: demographic, clinical, biochemical and genetic characteristics. *J Intern Med* 2011;**269**:278–288.

37. Meerman L, Koopen NR, Bloks V, *et al.* Biliary fibrosis associated with altered bile composition in a mouse model of erythropoietic protoporphyria. *Gastroenterology* 1999;**117**:696–705.

38. Minder EI, Gouya L, Schneider-Yin X, *et al.* A genotype–phenotype correlation between null-allele mutations in the ferrochelatase gene and liver complication in patients with erythropoietic protoporphyria. *Cell Mol Biol* 2002;**48**:91–96.

39. McGuire BM, Bonkovsky HL, Carithers RL Jr, *et al.* Liver transplantation for erythropoietic protoporphyria liver disease. *Liver Transplant* 2005;**11**: 1590–1596.

40. Harms J, Lautenschlager S, Minder CE, Minder EI. An alpha-melanocyte-stimulating hormone analogue in erythropoietic protoporphyria. *N Engl J Med* 2009;**360**:306–307.

41. Fontanellas A, Mazurier F, Landry M, *et al.* Reversion of hepatobiliary alterations by bone marrow transplantation in a murine model of erythropoietic protoporphyria. *Hepatology* 2000;**32**:73–81.

42. Akagi R, Inoue R, Muranaka S, *et al.* Dual gene defects involving delta-aminolaevulinate dehydratase and coproporphyrinogen oxidase in a porphyria patient. *Br J Haematol* 2006;**132**:237–243.

43. Harraway JR, Florkowski CM, Sies C, *et al.* Dual porphyria with mutations in both the *UROD* and *HMBS* genes. *Ann Clin Biochem* 2006;**43**:80–82.

44. Lindberg RL, Porcher C, Grandchamp B, *et al.* Porphobilinogen deaminase deficiency in mice causes a neuropathy resembling that of human hepatic porphyria. *Nat Genet* 1996;**12**: 195–199.

45. Bishop DF, Johansson A, Phelps R, *et al.* Uroporphyrinogen III synthase knock-in mice have the human congenital erythropoietic porphyria phenotype, including the characteristic light-induced cutaneous lesions. *Am J Hum Genet* 2006;**78**:645–658.

46. Bishop DF, Clavero S, Mohandas N, Desnick RJ. Congenital erythropoietic porphyria: characterization of murine models of the severe common (C73R/ C73R) and later-onset genotypes. *Mol Med* 2011;**17**:748–756.

47. Tutois S, Montagutelli X, Dasilva V, *et al.* Erythropoietic protoporphyria in the house mouse: a recessive inherited ferrochelatase deficiency with anemia, photosensitivity, and liver disease. *J Clin Invest* 1991;**88**:1730–1736.

48. Lindberg RL, Martini R, Baumgartner M, *et al.* Motor neuropathy in porphobilinogen deaminase-deficient mice imitates the peripheral neuropathy of human acute porphyria. *J Clin Invest* 1999;**103**:1127–1134.

49. Phillips JD, Jackson LK, Bunting M, *et al.* A mouse model of familial porphyria cutanea tarda. *Proc Natl Acad Sci USA* 2001;**98**:259–264.

50. Medlock AE, Meissner PN, Davidson BP, *et al.* A mouse model for South African (R59W) variegate porphyria: construction and initial characterization. *Cell Mol Biol* 2002;**48**:71–78.

Tyrosinema

31

Grant Mitchell, Pierre A. Russo, Josée Dubois, and Fernando Alvarez

Introduction

Hepatorenal tyrosinemia is a fascinating inborn error of metabolism that can affect numerous organs, particularly the liver, kidneys, and peripheral nerves. (For simplicity, this chapter uses the generic term tyrosinemia to refer to hepatorenal tyrosinemia (also known as fumarylacetoacetate hydrolase deficiency, tyrosinemia type I or congenital tyrosinosis; MIM 27670). Other forms of hypertyrosinemia are referred to by their specific names.) The first report of a patient with elevated blood tyrosine was in 1932 [1]. Patients with a more typical clinical and biochemical picture of tyrosinemia were then described in the late 1950s [2]. Since then, more than 500 patients have been reported in the literature or enrolled in the International NTBC Trial (of 2-(2-nitro-4-trifluoromethyl benzoyl)-1,3-cyclohexanedione (nitisinone)). Previously, almost all patients died in infancy and early childhood, and only isolated case reports described affected adults. In the 50 years since the description of tyrosinemia, the course of the disease has been improved successively by the introduction of diet therapy, neonatal screening, and hepatic transplantation. The advent of liver and kidney transplantation as a definitive treatment revolutionized the outcome [3]. Recently, the availability of nitisinone, a chemical commercialized as Orfadin (Swedish Orphan International, Stockholm, Sweden), has provided hope for a non-surgical solution for some patients [4]. On a fundamental level, tyrosinemia raises questions in hepatology, biochemical and population genetics, cell biology, oncology, and public health.

Pathophysiology

Tyrosinemia is caused by a deficiency of fumarylacetoacetate hydrolase (FAH; EC 3.7.1.2), the last enzyme of tyrosine degradation (Figure 31.1a). The site of the primary metabolic block in tyrosinemia was elegantly deduced by Lindblad et al. in 1977 [5] and subsequently confirmed enzymatically by others [6]. The enzyme is a 419 amino acid residue cytosolic homodimer present in the liver and to some extent in the kidney, lymphocytes, erythrocytes, fibroblasts, and chorionic

villi [7]. Human liver FAH cDNAs (GenBank NM000137) and the human gene *FAH* have been cloned and sequenced and the human gene mapped to chromosome 15q23-q25 [8]. Early studies of tyrosinemia showed that other enzymes of tyrosine degradation, particularly 4-hydroxyphenylpyruvate dioxygenase (4HPPD), are reduced in tyrosinemic liver. These changes have subsequently been shown to be secondary to the deficiency of FAH.

The mechanism of the hepatic and renal symptoms of tyrosinemia is largely conjectural, although much circumstantial evidence favors a toxic effect of the final compounds of tyrosine metabolism. Tyrosine and its early metabolites (4-hydroxyphenylpyruvate and homogentisate; Figure 31.1a) are present at high levels in other hereditary diseases that have no hepatic or renal symptoms and so these compounds are unlikely to cause the hepatorenal manifestations of tyrosinemia. In contrast, the compound immediately upstream from the FAH reaction, fumarylacetoacetate and its derivatives succinylacetoacetate and succinylacetone, have potent biologic activity. For example, fumarylacetoacetate and its precursor, maleylacetoacetate, resemble maleic acid, a well-known toxin that can induce renal Fanconi syndrome [9], and the histologic changes of maleic acid-induced Fanconi syndrome mimic the renal changes of tyrosinemia (see Pathology). Maleylacetoacetate and fumarylacetoacetate are reactive unstable compounds. The latter can form glutathione adducts [5], and free glutathione concentration is somewhat reduced in tyrosinemic liver samples [10]. The significance of this observation is unknown, but free sulfhydryl groups are known to be important for protection against free radicals and other toxic compounds.

In tyrosinemic livers, discrete nodules with normal FAH activity can be identified and can be shown to result from somatic mutations in one *FAH* allele that restored a normal sequence [11]. Revertant nodules are frequent in tyrosinemic livers and may be large, presumably reflecting the highly mutagenic environment of the tyrosinemic hepatocyte and a selective growth advantage of revertant cells. Of note, fumarylacetoacetate is a mutagen [11]. In 25 tyrosinemic livers from French Canadian patients, 20 (80%) had revertant nodules that

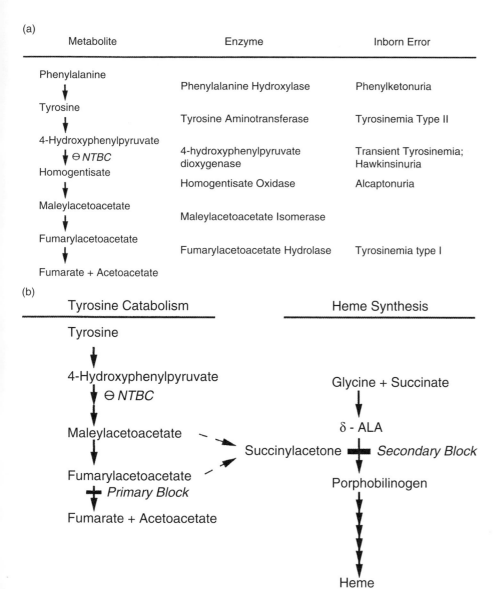

(a)

Metabolite	Enzyme	Inborn Error
Phenylalanine		
↓	Phenylalanine Hydroxylase	Phenylketonuria
Tyrosine		
↓	Tyrosine Aminotransferase	Tyrosinemia Type II
4-Hydroxyphenylpyruvate		
↓ ⊖ NTBC	4-hydroxyphenylpyruvate dioxygenase	Transient Tyrosinemia; Hawkinsinuria
Homogentisate		
↓	Homogentisate Oxidase	Alcaptonuria
Maleylacetoacetate		
↓	Maleylacetoacetate Isomerase	
Fumarylacetoacetate		
↓	Fumarylacetoacetate Hydrolase	Tyrosinemia type I
Fumarate + Acetoacetate		

(b)

Tyrosine Catabolism

Tyrosine
↓
4-Hydroxyphenylpyruvate
↓ ⊖ NTBC
Maleylacetoacetate
↓
Fumarylacetoacetate
＋ *Primary Block*
↓
Fumarate + Acetoacetate

Heme Synthesis

Glycine + Succinate
↓
δ - ALA
↓
Succinylacetone ＋ *Secondary Block*
↓
Porphobilinogen
↓
Heme

Figure 31.1 Tyrosine metabolism. (a) Degradation of the aromatic amino acids. The metabolic intermediates, the degradative enzymes, and the inborn errors associated with dysfunction of these enzymes are indicated. Quantitatively, minor pathways of tyrosine metabolism are not shown but are of physiologic significance. These pathways include synthesis of catecholamines and the synthesis of melanin pigments and are felt to be normal in tyrosinemia. (b) Inter-relationship of tyrosine catabolism in tyrosinemia and of heme biosynthesis. Succinylacetone is derived from the intermediates that accumulate upstream from the primary enzyme block. It inhibits the synthesis of porphobilinogen from δ-aminolevulinic acid (δ-ALA). The resulting δ-ALA accumulation is thought to cause the clinical signs of neurologic crises. Each solid arrow represents a single enzymatic step. The hatched arrows reflect the uncertainty regarding the mechanism by which succinylacetone arises from related compounds in the pathway of tyrosine degradation. The site of action of nitisinone (2-(2-nitro-4-trifluoromethylbenzoyl)-1,3-cyclohexanedione (NTBC)) is indicated.

occupied up to 36% of the surface studied; interestingly, the extent of replacement by revertant nodules correlated inversely with the patients' clinical severity.

Mouse models of FAH deficiency have hepatic and renal symptoms resembling those of tyrosinemic patients but a more fulminant course, resulting in neonatal death [12]. Nitisinone treatment can permit growth to adulthood, but mice rapidly develop hepatic failure if nitisinone is withdrawn [13]. Also, following challenge with homogentisic acid, a tyrosine metabolite downstream from the nitisinone-induced block (Figure 31.1b), hepatocytes undergo apoptosis [14]. Mice deficient in FAH are useful for studies of the pathophysiology of tyrosinemia. However, mouse liver and nutrition have numerous differences from those of humans, such as a marked propensity to develop hepatocellular carcinoma, probably by mechanisms different from those in humans, and it is generally agreed that results from mouse models cannot be extrapolated directly to humans.

The most clearly established pathophysiologic mechanism in tyrosinemia is the role of succinylacetone in neurologic crises (Figure 31.1b). Succinylacetone is a potent inhibitor of the porphyrin synthetic enzyme δ-aminolevulinic acid dehydratase, and caused a marked accumulation of δ-aminolevulinic acid in children with tyrosinemia [15]. δ-Aminolevulinic acid toxicity has been shown to be associated with neurotoxicity in acute intermittent porphyria, hereditary deficiency of δ-aminolevulinic acid dehydratase, and lead poisoning [15]. Available clinical, biochemical, and pathologic evidence suggests that the neurologic crisis of tyrosinemia results from δ-aminolevulinic acid toxicity and that it represents the most severe porphyria-like condition known in humans.

Genetics and screening

Tyrosinemia is an autosomal recessive trait [16]. It is important that couples with an affected child be aware that they have a 25% risk of having another affected child in each subsequent pregnancy. Heterozygotes for hepatorenal tyrosinemia are asymptomatic and have normal levels of tyrosine-related metabolites.

Large numbers of patients with tyrosinemia have been reported in two regions: the province of Quebec, Canada, and northern Europe, particularly Scandinavia. In Quebec, tyrosinemia is common because of a well-documented but complex founder effect [16]. Tyrosinemia is particularly frequent in the Saguenay-Lac St-Jean area of northern Quebec, where the carrier rate for tyrosinemia is 1 in 20 and where 1 in 1846 live births results in an affected child. Overall, the birth rate of affected children in Quebec is 1 in 16 786, compared with an estimated 1 in 100 000–20 000 elsewhere, including Scandinavia [7]. Tyrosinemia has been reported in many ethnic groups, and lack of French Canadian or Scandinavian ancestry does not exclude the diagnosis.

Many mutations in *FAH* have been described in patients with tyrosinemia [17]. The IVS12+5ga allele accounts for about 90% of mutant *FAH* alleles in the Saguenay-Lac St-Jean area of Quebec [17]. Both IVS12+5ga and IVS6–1gt are frequent in patients of diverse ethnic origins [18]. In addition, W262X is prevalent in Finns [17] and Q64H (192GT) in Pakistanis. R341W causes pseudodeficiency (see Diagnosis). In view of the protean manifestations of tyrosinemia, it will be interesting to search for genotype–phenotype correlations. However, affected subjects from the same family may have different clinical presentations [17]. We know of one family with three affected children, two of whom died in infancy: one from a hepatic crisis, another from a paralytic neurologic crisis. The surviving sibling is now a young adult with renal tubulopathy and modest liver disease. Clearly, environmental and genetic factors unrelated to *FAH* play a major role in determining the clinical severity of tyrosinemia. Mild tyrosinemia type I disease may be caused by an Ala35Thr mutation and presents atypically without increase of the diagnostically important toxic metabolites succinylacetone and succinylacetoacetate [19].

Diagnosis

Tyrosinemia should be suspected in any infant or child with evidence of hepatocellular necrosis, cirrhosis, or decreased hepatic synthetic function (particularly perturbed coagulation studies) of unknown cause. If the diagnosis is considered clinically, the most discriminating test is assay of succinylacetone in urine (or blood). Elevated levels of succinylacetone occur only in hepatorenal tyrosinemia and clear elevations are present in the vast majority of tyrosinemic patients who are not treated with nitisinone. Minute amounts of succinylacetone in fact occur in normal individuals, but most laboratories establish a threshold for reporting above this level and typically succinylacetone is reported as absent in normal individuals [20].

Other clinical signs may suggest the diagnosis. Rarely, patients may present with coagulopathy in the absence of overt liver disease [21]. Rickets or characteristic renal or neurologic findings, particularly if associated with abnormal hepatic function, also suggest this diagnosis [7].

Elevated plasma tyrosine levels are a non-specific finding, in contrast to succinylacetone, which is specific for tyrosinemia. Plasma tyrosine levels are initially elevated to a variable degree in almost all symptomatic patients, although older patients with a chronic course and patients treated with low-protein diets often do not show hypertyrosinemia [7]. Furthermore, hypertyrosinemia is a non-specific finding. Blood tyrosine is elevated after meals. Therefore, hypertyrosinemia should be diagnosed only in fasting samples. Hypertyrosinemia may be associated with all forms of liver failure as well as with a diverse group of conditions involving the pathway of tyrosine catabolism (Figure 31.1). The same is true of plasma methionine levels, which may be markedly elevated in tyrosinemia, and of phenylalanine levels, which are often initially somewhat elevated at diagnosis as well. The demonstration of elevated levels of succinylacetone on dried filter paper blood samples, in plasma or in urine, is pathognomonic for tyrosinemia [22]. We have never observed a tyrosinemic patient who did not have elevated levels of succinylacetone in blood and urine. Rare case reports exist of patients with normal tyrosine levels and with undetectable levels of succinylacetone. We have encountered a small number of patients in whom blood succinylacetone levels are very low and in which it is more convenient to demonstrate the presence of succinylacetone in urine samples.

An assay for FAH is not widely used for the diagnosis of affected or carrier individuals. False positive and negative results are possible. In selected patients, it is useful to perform FAH assays. It can be assayed in lymphocytes and erythrocytes as well as in liver tissue [6,23]. Even in liver, the level of FAH activity can be falsely high, for example in revertant nodules of patient samples, or falsely low, in the case of pseudodeficiency. Pseudodeficiency occurs when an enzyme that functions adequately in vivo yields low values under the in vitro conditions used in the enzyme assay. Carrier detection by these techniques is imperfect; some heterozygotes for the deficiency may have high levels of residual FAH activity. Conversely, a pseudodeficient *FAH* allele is common in certain populations. This allele is not associated with clinical symptoms but has a very low activity when assayed in vitro. Enzyme assay results, therefore, need to be interpreted in light of the patients' clinical and biochemical findings. For the above reasons, carrier detection by enzymatic means is not recommended as a screening technique.

In patients with an established diagnosis of tyrosinemia, molecular diagnosis is useful because it permits the detection of heterozygotes among family members who desire specific genetic counseling and because it is useful for prenatal diagnosis in subsequent pregnancies of the couple [12]. In at-risk populations, molecular testing for common alleles is an appropriate first step. Complete sequencing of *FAH* exons and deletion-duplication analysis are also available clinically and are useful in patients who are not at risk for common alleles. Even in regions with a strong founder effect, some rare mutant alleles exist. A negative molecular screening test does not completely eliminate carrier status in patients from such regions. In at-risk populations, carrier screening is possible by molecular testing for common alleles but a negative molecular screening test does not completely eliminate carrier status.

Prenatal diagnosis of tyrosinemia is possible by the measurement of succinylacetone in the amniotic fluid and by FAH assay using cultured amniocytes or chorionic villus cells [23]. Molecular diagnosis can be offered to families in which the causal mutation is known. Prenatal diagnosis should be supervised by an experienced genetician.

Neonatal screening for tyrosinemia has been undertaken in Quebec since 1970 using blood samples dried on filter paper. Currently, succinylacetone is used as a marker for screening. Screening using blood tyrosine as a marker leads to many false positive results in children with transient tyrosinemia (Figure 31.1a), in those with other hereditary tyrosinemias (Figure 31.1a), and occasionally in children with hepatic problems other than hepatorenal tyrosinemia. More importantly, false negative results may be obtained in children affected with hepatorenal tyrosinemia, particularly in this era of low neonatal protein intake (breast-feeding, humanized formulae) and early hospital discharge, two factors that reduce the levels of blood tyrosine in predischarge samples. Succinylacetone, in contrast, is elevated in childhood (and also prenatally as a marker for diagnosis in amniotic fluid).

Differential diagnosis

In practice, for tyrosinemic children presenting to the hepatologist in the first year of life, the differential diagnosis is that of diseases causing hepatic failure [24]. In older children and young adults, the differential diagnosis includes other diseases leading to cirrhosis.

At any age, the presence of a suggestive family history or of typical neurologic crises in a patient with signs of liver dysfunction is strongly suggestive of tyrosinemia, and the demonstration of elevated succinylacetone in blood or urine establishes the diagnosis. Renal tubular dysfunction in patients with hepatocellular failure is suggestive of tyrosinemia but is also seen in other hereditary metabolic diseases, such as galactosemia, hereditary fructose intolerance, Wilson disease, certain lactic acidoses, and glycogen storage disease type I [24]. Elevation of serum α-fetoprotein (AFP) is consistent with tyrosinemia, although it is not specific. In patients not treated with nitisinone, the level of AFP is consistently elevated in young acutely ill patients and in most other patients but may be normal in some young adults with an indolent course of disease.

Other forms of hypertyrosinemia

Biochemically, many patients have hypertyrosinemia secondary to hepatic failure, and the pattern of plasma amino acids is not particularly helpful in diagnosis. A practical consideration is that tyrosine can be elevated in plasma in non-fasting subjects, along with several other amino acids. Experienced interpretation and repeated plasma amino acid chromatography are necessary before initiating investigations if the clinical symptomatology does not suggest tyrosinemia.

Several inborn errors of metabolism and some acquired conditions may result in isolated hypertyrosinemia [7]. Transient tyrosinemia of the newborn is felt to be the result of an immaturity of the enzyme 4HPPD, which causes a transient deficiency of the enzyme. It is found most frequently in newborns who are premature, who receive large amounts of protein (such as are found in cow's milk), or who are deficient in vitamin C, the cofactor for 4HPPD. Transient tyrosinemia is generally felt to be a benign trait, unnoticed unless plasma amino acids are studied. It disappears spontaneously within days to weeks, although mild developmental delay has been reported [25]. Biochemical normalization also may be hastened by the administration of vitamin C (50–100 mg/day) or by dietary restriction of phenylalanine and tyrosine.

Hawkinsinuria is a rare autosomal dominant trait in which affected infants may develop acidosis and hypertyrosinemia. Clinical manifestations arise at the time of weaning from breast milk. Hawkinsinuria is hypothesized to be the result of an abnormal function of 4HPPD and is diagnosed by the presence of an unusual organic compound (hawkinsin) in the urine of symptomatic patients. The prognosis seems to be excellent, and hepatic function was not markedly perturbed in the reported cases.

Patients with tyrosinemia type III have primary 4HPPD deficiency [26]. Presentations vary from asymptomatic to mental retardation and neurologic signs. It is not formally proven that this represents a true clinical phenotype and it may, in fact, reflect an ascertainment bias (i.e. a fortuitous discovery in patients in whom amino acid chromatography was performed for mental retardation caused by unrelated factors). Conversely, because of the suspicion of neurologic risk, treatment with a phenylalanine and tyrosine-restricted diet is recommended to lower circulating tyrosine concentrations.

Tyrosinemia type II (oculocutaneous tyrosinemia) is also clinically distinct from tyrosinemia and is caused by the autosomal recessively inherited deficiency of tyrosine aminotransferase [26]. Patients with tyrosinemia type II develop hyperkeratosis of the palms and soles and painful lesions of the ocular cornea that resemble ocular herpes infection. Patients affected by tyrosinemia type II develop hyperkeratosis of the palms and soles and corneal thickening, and they may have developmental delay, but hepatic and renal functions remain intact.

Interestingly, the other inborn errors of aromatic amino acid catabolism shown in Figure 31.1 are associated with neither hypertyrosinemia nor signs of liver disease. Phenylketonuria is usually revealed by high blood levels of phenylalanine at neonatal screening, and its major manifestation, mental retardation, can be prevented by dietary phenylalanine restriction. The signs of alcaptonuria are arthritis in middle age, a darkening of urine when exposed to air, and excessive urinary excretion of homogentisic acid.

Clinical findings in non-nitisinone-treated patients

This section describes the natural history of tyrosinemia and the impact of diet therapy and neonatal screening. Our experience with nitisinone, which radically improves the clinical course, is described later (see Treatment). Patients with tyrosinemia have traditionally been divided into having acute and chronic forms based on the clinical picture. This distinction is not always clear because some children have a stormy course in the first year of life typical of the acute form but then have an indolent course compatible with the chronic form. Moreover, children over 2 years of age defined as having chronic tyrosinemia remain at risk for acute life-threatening liver and neurologic crises. The liver, kidneys, and peripheral nerves are the main organs affected by tyrosinemia [26].

Liver crises

Liver crises typically present before 2 years of age and decrease in frequency and severity thereafter. In Quebec, where, because of neonatal screening, diet therapy is introduced before 1 month of age, the severity of episodes of liver decompensation in infants appears to be decreased; however, these episodes may occur, and in our experience, patients treated early with diet alone all eventually develop cirrhosis [7,26]. Acute episodes are often heralded by an intercurrent viral infection, with anorexia, irritability, and vomiting. Infants with liver decompensation typically emit an odor resembling that of boiled cabbage. Within a few hours to days, overt liver disease may develop, with a rapid increase in liver size, ascites, anasarca, and marked coagulopathy. Jaundice is usually a terminal event and is not a feature of most patients. Historically, over 80% of all patients with tyrosinemia died before 2 years of age from an acute liver crisis, some infants presenting with 6–10 episodes in the first year of life [7,27].

The first laboratory indication of an impending liver crisis is disproportionate prolongation of the coagulation time [27], and a bleeding diathesis without other symptoms of liver disease may be the mode of presentation. Prothrombin and partial thromboplastin times may be alarmingly prolonged despite normal or near normal serum aminotransferases. These abnormalities also may be seen in clinically stable infants and are unresponsive to oral or parenteral vitamin K supplementation. Infusions of fresh frozen plasma are effective at restoring near normal coagulation in most instances. Interestingly, factor V levels, frequently used in other liver diseases as a marker of liver synthetic function, may be within or close to the normal range in tyrosinemic infants at the beginning of a crisis. In contrast, factors XI and XII, as well as vitamin K-dependent factors II, VII, IX, and X, may be exceedingly low (<15%), with normal factor VIII levels.

During a liver crisis, serum aminotransferases are initially only mildly elevated (<2× normal values), if at all, in contrast to the pathologic coagulation profile [7]. Serum amino acids, particularly tyrosine, methionine, and phenylalanine, are elevated and may be accompanied by generalized aminoaciduria in patients who have renal dysfunction. Serum AFP may be extremely high (up to 400 μg/mL), declining over several weeks to months after the crisis.

Chronic liver disease

A chronic course was seen in less than 40% of Quebec patients but may have been more prevalent in northern Europe [7,27]. With the systematic newborn screening program in Quebec, dietary management is instituted by 3–4 weeks of age. Despite early dietary intervention, in our experience, all non-nitisinone-treated children eventually develop cirrhosis, although at highly variable rates. During the first 2 years of life, the child is particularly at risk for liver and neurologic crises. Thereafter, the dominant liver problem is the risk of hepatocarcinoma [28].

Clinical examination reveals hepatosplenomegaly in approximately 70% and rarely other signs of liver dysfunction, such as spider hemangiomas or clubbing. Rickets may be apparent in those with moderate or severe renal disease.

In Quebec, 40% of our population with a chronic course has abnormal coagulation parameters but no overt bleeding [29]. Serum AFP is elevated in virtually all patients, ranging from 100 to 400 000 ng/mL (normal, <10 ng/mL), with exacerbations during hepatic crises. At birth, AFP levels are extremely high and decrease to a variable extent with dietary therapy. This reduction of AFP with diet therapy alone should be remembered when evaluating results of nitisinone therapy. Serum aminotransferase concentrations are usually normal or mildly elevated, with normal albumin and bilirubin in the majority. The serum gamma-glutamyltransferase level is usually slightly elevated and may reflect renal involvement, although this has not been carefully evaluated.

Risk of hepatocarcinoma

The incidence of hepatocarcinoma in tyrosinemia is difficult to estimate because systematic autopsies have not been performed in all children dying of the disease; even in autopsied patients, livers have not always been examined in detail.

Although the mechanism(s) underlying the mutagenic activity of fumarylacetoacetate and other metabolites remains to be identified, glutathione depletion by fumarylacetoacetate may play an important role in mutagenicity. Moreover, hepatic stress in hereditary tyrosinemia type I activates the AKT survival pathway in the *Fah*[−/−] knockout mice model and inhibits intrinsic apoptosis to confer cell death resistance in vivo, thus favoring hepatocarcinogenesis [30]. This continual production of proliferative and stress-related survival signals, coupled with the mutagenicity of fumarylacetoacetate, may instigate a mutator phenotype that could end in tumorigenesis and/or mutation reversion [31].

At Hôpital Sainte-Justine, 31 tyrosinemic livers have been studied at autopsy or transplantation since 1986 (Table 31.1). In 23 of 31 livers (74%), nodules were identified by either ultrasonography or CT. Four livers (13%) showed one or more foci of hepatocarcinoma, and four had evidence of high-grade dysplasia. The frequency of carcinoma is lower than the widely cited figure of 37% by Weinberg *et al.* [32], who reviewed all 42 cases of tyrosinemia published before 1976 and added their personal experience with one patient. Fourteen of their patients, from older literature, had a presumed diagnosis of tyrosinemia not always documented pathologically. The incidence of hepatocarcinoma may be less than initially reported, and this may have implications when considering the urgency of liver transplantation for children with clinically stable disease and no evidence of nodules on imaging. However, there is no question that the risk of hepatocarcinoma is high, even in infants. Hepatocarcinoma can occur before 2 years of age [3].

As in other liver disease, serial serum AFP levels do not reliably predict the presence of carcinoma. They may increase greatly following acute liver crises and do not accurately discriminate regenerating or fatty nodules from hepatocarcinoma (Figure 31.2). Hepatocarcinoma may occur in tyrosinemia in the presence of normal or low AFP levels [29]. Nevertheless, a high degree of suspicion should be maintained if there is a significant increase in AFP levels from the usual baseline in a clinically stable patient with no evidence of an acute exacerbation such as a liver crisis, because this may indicate the development of hepatocarcinoma. If a nodule is visualized radiologically or by ultrasonography, imaging characteristics cannot reliably rule out malignancy (see below, Imaging in tyrosinemia). Hepatoblastoma has also been reported [33].

Table 31.1 Children with tyrosinemia undergoing liver transplantation who had not received previous nitisinone treatment

Patient	Age at OLT (years)	Nodules/HCC or dysplasia*	Outcome
1	1⅔	−/Dysplasia grade 1	Death, primary non-function
2	8	−/−	A&W
3	9	−/−	A&W
4	3½	+/HCC and dysplasia grade 3	A&W
5	2	+/Dysplasia grade 3	A&W
6	10	+/−	A&W
7	1½	+/Dysplasia grade 1	A&W
8	12	+/−	A&W
9	1½	−/Dysplasia grade 1	A&W
10	17	−/−	Liver/kidney, A&W
11	6	+/Dysplasia grade 2	A&W
12	3	−/Dysplasia grade 2	A&W
13	2	−/Dysplasia grade 1	A&W
14	⅓	+/Dysplasia grade 2	Death, primary non-function
15	9½	+/Dysplasia grade 3	A&W
16	1	+/Dysplasia grade 3	A&W
17	2½	+/Dysplasia grade 1	A&W
18	2½	+/Dysplasia grade 1	A&W
19	11	+/HCC and dysplasia grade 3	A&W
20	½	+/Dysplasia grade 2	A&W
21	3	+/Dysplasia grade 1	A&W
22	11/12	+/Dysplasia grade 3	A&W
23	2	+/Dysplasia grade 2	A&W

A&W, alive and well; OLT, orthotopic liver transplantation; HCC, hepatocarcinoma; nitisinone (NTBC: 2-(2-nitro-4-trifluoromethyl benzoyl)-1,3-cyclohexanedione); −, absent; +, present.

Neurologic crises

Neurologic crises are a hallmark of non-nitisinone-treated tyrosinemia. The crises have two phases: first, an active period of painful paresthesias, autonomic signs such as hypertension [15], tachycardia, and sometimes progressive paralysis; second, a period of recuperation, seen in crises with weakness or paralysis. In our series of 48 French Canadian patients, 20 (42%) had crises, higher than in previous series [15]. Crises may truly be less frequent in other populations, or perhaps crises were under-reported or not identified in earlier series.

Painful crises are the most frequent. During the prodrome, which often occurs following a minor infection, the child is irritable and less active than usual. The child then develops severe pain, often in the legs. Patients frequently adopt a position of extreme hyperextension of the trunk and neck, which can be mistaken for opisthotonus or meningismus. Older patients have claimed that this alleviates the pain somewhat. This hypertonia may be mistaken for tonic convulsions, but in fact the patients are conscious. True convulsions also may be observed, often in association with severe hyponatremia.

About one-third of crises in our series were associated with weakness or paralysis, and in 8 of 104 crises, mechanical ventilation was necessary because of respiratory weakness, in one child for more than 3 months. Electrophysiologically, there was evidence of axonal degeneration, with nerve conduction studies showing normal velocity but decreased wave amplitude and an increased threshold of stimulation, progressing to absence of peripheral nerve function. Recuperation from paralytic crises is possible, although patients with repeated severe crises may have chronic weakness. Patients in whom oral anesthesia develops as part of a crisis may seriously

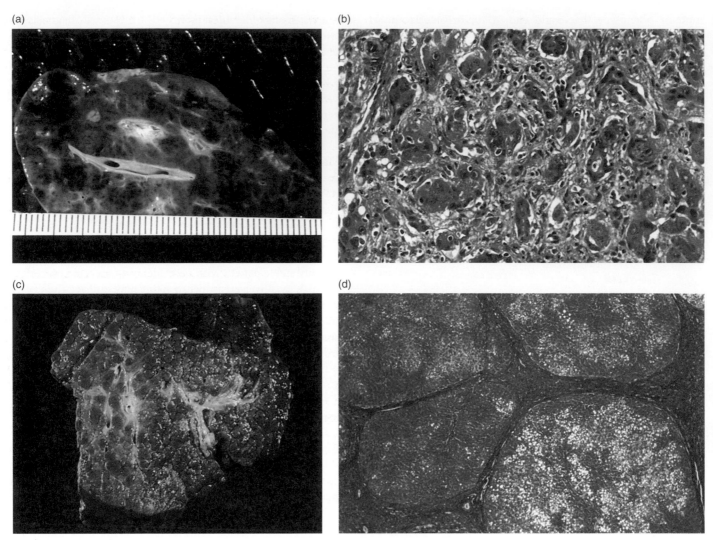

Figure 31.2 Liver pathology in tyrosinemia of acute and chronic courses. (a,b) A 3-month-old girl with the acute form of tyrosinemia. (a) Microscopic appearance of liver, which was firm, shrunken, and vaguely nodular. (b) Histologic examination of the liver revealed massive parenchymal collapse and fibrosis. There is cholangiolar proliferation, and surviving hepatocytes are frequently arranged in a pseudoglandular pattern. There is intracellular cholestasis and hemosiderin deposition as well as a mild, non-specific chronic inflammatory infiltrate (original magnification ×125). (c,d) A 2-year-old boy with a chronic form of the disease. (c) Enlarged, cirrhotic liver with a coarsely nodular external and cut surface. (d) Low-power histologic examination reveals a mixed macro- and micronodular cirrhosis. The nodules appear histologically heterogeneous because of a variable degree of fat content in the hepatocytes. (HPS stain, original magnification 30×.) (b,d) Hematoxylin–phloxine–saffron stain. See color section.

lacerate their tongue, develop severe bruxism, and dislodge teeth. Hypertension and sustained tachycardia are common during the initial phase of crises, as are electrolytic imbalances, particularly in children with tubulopathy. Vomiting and ileus occur frequently and may complicate nutritional management. It is important to note that the mental development of children with tyrosinemia is normal and that during crises their level of consciousness is not diminished. The active phase of crises usually lasts for 1–7 days.

Of note, the neurologic crises of tyrosinemia are not usually associated with deterioration of standard liver tests. Plasma aminotransferases, prothrombin times, and bilirubin are unchanged from periods between crises. There was no readily apparent difference between succinylacetone levels during crises when compared with values observed between

crises. Urinary levels of δ-aminolevulinic acid tend to be higher during crises than between crises, but in our retrospective series this had little diagnostic or predictive value for a given episode. Results of routine cerebrospinal fluid analyses are normal during neurologic crises [15]. In some cases, catecholamine excretion is increased.

Neurologic crises are a major cause of distress in non-nitisinone-treated patients with tyrosinemia. There is an appreciable risk of death, particularly in paralytic crises. In our series of 20 children who had experienced at least one crisis, 11 of 14 deaths occurred during crises, and all 11 were associated with the complications of respiratory insufficiency [15]. All tyrosinemic children who are ill and who are not receiving nitisinone therapy should be observed closely for the signs of neurologic decompensation, particularly respiratory insufficiency, because it may develop rapidly; consequently, children with signs suggestive of an impending neurologic crisis should be hospitalized.

Coma is *not* a feature of isolated neurologic crises. The development of coma in a tyrosinemic patient should not be attributed to a neurologic crisis without first excluding other causes requiring treatment, including liver failure with encephalopathy and a false diagnosis of coma in a patient with paralysis.

The dramatic nature of painful neurologic crises is described in the following paragraph written by the mother of one of our patients, reproduced here from the first edition [34].

> For 2 or 3 days before the crisis, P would sleep fitfully with increasing crankiness. No position seemed comfortable, and he became more unsteady on his feet. His face was drawn and pale. His appetite was poor, and he was always nauseous. His belly became bloated. He lost interest in playing and was very sensitive to the slightest touch. This was followed by periods of intense pain for about 3 days, which decreased in frequency over the next few days. When he felt the pain coming, he would place his forearms under his chin, and would tense up and tremble. He would screw up his face and wring his hands to the point of causing bruises. He would arch his back until his head touched his heels, tear out his hair, pull out his teeth, and bite his cheeks and lips despite all the bandages we had placed to prevent him from hurting himself. He would shriek a lot but was drowsy most of the time. He would throw up a lot, and he usually had some fever. He would lose about 2–3 pounds with every crisis. It would take 2–3 weeks for him to get back to his usual state. When I asked him what the pain felt like, he would say there were two types: one was like he had large needles in his muscles and bones everywhere and the other as if he were being squeezed in a vice.

Renal disease

Renal involvement is almost always present in children with tyrosinemia, and it is as varied as that of the liver [7]. Symptoms range from no evidence of renal disease to overt renal failure. Even those with no evidence of renal disease, including an intact glomerular filtration rate (GFR), may show some degree of fibrosis on biopsy (see Pathology). Both renal tubular dysfunction and glomerular involvement may occur in tyrosinemia. The severity of dysfunction is variable to some extent with the clinical state of the patient, increasing during periods of decompensation. Generalized aminoaciduria and glycosuria are sometimes seen, but rickets is the principal clinical manifestation of renal tubular dysfunction in tyrosinemia and figured prominently in its initial clinical descriptions [2]. In some patients, it is the main medical problem.

Some clinical evidence of proximal tubular dysfunction was present in only 10 of 37 patients evaluated at Hôpital Sainte-Justine. However, at the time of study all these patients were on a phenylalanine and tyrosine-restricted diet and some were receiving nitisinone, both of which can partially reverse Fanconi syndrome in tyrosinemia. Conversely, in an adult in whom chronic tubular and glomerular dysfunction was present, we have observed that tubular dysfunction may persist even after prolonged nitisinone treatment, suggesting that permanent tubular abnormalities may occur. Over 80% of the children evaluated at Hôpital Sainte-Justine have some degree of nephromegaly on ultrasonography, and 33% have evidence of mild to moderate nephrocalcinosis (Table 31.2).

Chronic renal failure may occur in adolescents and young adults. In the Hôpital Sainte-Justine series, GFRs, as assessed by diethylenetriamine pentaacetic acid clearance, were generally decreased but over a wide range of severity (Table 31.2).

Other clinical manifestations

Some infants have episodes of hypoglycemia that in our experience may be refractory to treatment. In rare patients, hypoglycemic episodes occur even during chronic nitisinone treatment or after hepatic transplantation (personal observations). Although hypertrophy of the islets of Langerhans is frequent in tyrosinemia (see Pathology) and hyperinsulinism has occasionally been documented [35], in others it is clearly ruled out. Therefore, hypoglycemia in a tyrosinemic patient requires a complete evaluation as for non-tyrosinemic patients. One tyrosinemic child has been reported to have diabetes mellitus type 1, although the relationship of this condition to tyrosinemia is uncertain, and the pancreatic histology in this patient was normal.

Clinically significant hypertrophic cardiomyopathy has been reported in tyrosinemia and has even been reported to be frequent and to respond to nitisinone treatment [36]. We have not observed this despite systematic focused evaluations, but physicians should be alert to this possibility.

Imaging in tyrosinemia
Liver

This section describes our experience before the availability of nitisinone and during the first 5 years of the Quebec NTBC protocol. It is important to note that not all nodules are detectable by imaging. In cirrhotic livers examined after transplantation or at autopsy, only a minority of the nodules were detected in previous ultrasonograms or scans.

In our series of 30 patients evaluated before nitisinone treatment, ultrasonography was more sensitive than CT in the evaluation of liver changes in tyrosinemia [37]. However, the sensitivity is highly dependent on the experience of the ultrasonographer, and ultrasonographic examination is more difficult to standardize than CT. The earliest ultrasonographic change, which may be subtle, is an inhomogeneity of the liver parenchyma without the presence of distinct nodules. Inhomogeneity is often the first sign of micronodular cirrhosis but also may be a transient finding. We speculate that transient ultrasonographic inhomogeneity may reflect the presence of multiple small foci of fatty change, which we have observed in some biopsy samples. Subsequently, in the development of cirrhosis, hypoechogenic micronodules (<5 mm) appear and

Table 31.2 Evaluation of renal disease in 37 patients with tyrosinemia

Patient	Age (years)	Nephromegaly	Nephrocalcinosis	GFR pretransplantation (mL/min per 1.73/m^2)[a]
1	0.7	+	+	40
2	8	+	−	69
3	9	+	−	137
4	3.5	+	+	142
5	1.5	+	−	105
6	9.7	+	−	47
7	1.5	+	−	64
8	18	+	+	34
9	8	+	+	36
10	12	+	−	83
11	2.0	+	−	108
12	18	+	+	27
13	6	+	−	52
14	2.0	−	−	173
15	2.5	−	−	73
16	2.8	+	−	ND
17	3.5	+	−	ND
18	1.9	−	−	ND
19	8	+	+	ND
20	1.8	+	−	ND
21	9	+	+	117
22	0.3	+	−	82
23	4	+	+	93
24	6	+	+	65
25	2.0	+	−	86
26	0.7	+	−	182
27	0.9	+	+	155
28	2.0	−	−	147
29	2.0	+	+	125
30	0.5	−	−	141
31	2.0	+	−	107
32	9	−	−	124
33	2.0	+	+	90
34	2.5	−	−	116
35	4	+	−	128
36	1.0	−	+	120
37	3.0	−	−	128

GFR, glomerular filtration rate; ND, not determined; −, absent; +, present.
[a] Clearance of diethylene triamine pentaacetic acid.

then macronodules (≥ 5 mm), which may be either hyper- or hypoechogenic. In our pre-nitisinone series [37], the echodensity of nodules was not predictive of the presence of dysplasia or malignancy. If portal hypertension is suspected, Doppler ultrasonography should be performed.

Use of CT reveal most macronodules. Of technical note, some nodules are obscured by contrast studies whereas the detection of others is enhanced. We routinely perform both examinations. Our experience with MRI is limited, but this technique merits further study in tyrosinemia, particularly in children old enough to remain motionless to undergo the examination without sedation.

Our experience with MRI of tyrosinemic nodules is limited because our patients now rarely develop cirrhotic changes. MRI can provide useful information about regenerative, dysplastic, or hepatocarcinomatous nodules. Sensitivity of detection is increased when a paramagnetic contrast agent such as mangafodipir is used. This liver-specific contrast agent is taken up by hepatocytes and excreted into bile. Nodules of functioning hepatocytes, such as in regenerative nodules, show homogeneous enhancement, whereas some hepatocellular carcinomas show reduced enhancement with this agent. This technique has been applied to one reported tyrosinemic patient who had multiple hepatic nodules and in whom the hepatic nodularity regressed and AFP levels reduced when adequate nitisinone treatment was instituted [38]. The nodules enhanced normally and were felt to be benign. The positive predictive value of this method has not been estimated. Diffusion-weighted imaging has been reported to be more sensitive than T_2-weighted imaging for the detection of hepatocarcinoma, but no imaging method can eliminate hepatocarcinoma with certainty [39]. Our clinical approach to hepatic nodules in tyrosinemia is discussed below (see Chronic liver disease, under Pathology).

Kidney

In our pre-nitisinone series [37], ultrasonography revealed nephromegaly in about half the patients, cortical hyperechogenicity in one-third, and nephrocalcinosis in one-fourth. Abdominal CT also can detect the nephromegaly. Nephrocalcinosis is best detected in scans performed without contrast. In some contrast studies, a delayed nephrogram is apparent, possibly reflecting diminished function.

Pancreas

Most patients have normal pancreatic imaging studies. Rarely, hyperechogenicity has been reported.

Pathology

Liver

Fulminant liver disease

In fulminant liver disease, morphologic alterations are variable, although the liver is generally slightly to moderately enlarged, frequently pale, and often nodular; in other patients,

the liver may be shrunken and firm, with a brownish discoloration [9]. Histologic examination usually reveals micronodular cirrhosis and, often, marked bile duct proliferation within portal tracts and fibrotic septa (Figure 31.2). The hepatocytes are characterized by varying degrees of steatosis, and their usual regular trabecular arrangement is replaced by pseudo-acinar or pseudoglandular formations around a central canaliculus, often containing prominent bile plugs. A significant accumulation of iron pigment may be seen within Kupffer cells and hepatocytes. Giant cell transformation is also occasionally observed. These changes reflect the non-specific nature of the early insult, are shared by a wide variety of infantile hepatopathies, and may include a neonatal hepatitis-like picture [40]. In the infant, neonatal hepatitis is a non-specific response of the liver to a wide variety of metabolic and infectious insults and is not characteristic of any single entity.

Chronic liver disease

In chronic liver disease, the liver is characteristically coarsely nodular and frequently enlarged as a result of usually well-established mixed micro- and macronodular cirrhosis [9,41]. There is steatosis, varying in extent between the various nodules or even within a single nodule. Fibrous septa vary in width and frequently contain a mild lymphoplasmacytic infiltrate. Ductular proliferation usually is minimal. Intralobular cholestasis or inflammation is usually insignificant, which correlates with the usually normal bilirubin levels of these children. Most ominous in the older child is the development of hepatic carcinoma. Sometimes, but not always, this is apparent by gross examination. In one of our patients, a single large hemorrhagic nodule was noted in the autopsy specimen. In a second patient, a hepatectomy specimen was obtained at transplantation, and a large grayish white nodule of hepatoma could be easily distinguished from the surrounding nodules in the cirrhotic liver (Figure 31.3). However, numerous sections through the rest of the liver revealed multiple microscopic foci of hepatocellular carcinoma as well as multiple areas of nuclear atypia and hyperchromatism qualifying as hepatocellular dysplasia.

Liver cell dysplasia, of large cell or small cell type, has been reported in hereditary tyrosinemia in the absence of, as well as in association with, hepatocellular carcinoma [41]. Liver cell dysplasia, particularly the small cell type, is widely accepted as a premalignant condition and underlines the need for early transplantation in these patients. The occurrence of dysplasia and the high incidence of hepatocellular carcinoma in hereditary tyrosinemia, far greater than the incidence of hepatocellular carcinoma in adults with cirrhosis resulting from hepatitis, are highly suggestive of a powerful underlying carcinogenic influence, presumably related to abnormal metabolites [10]. Ultrastructurally, morphologic changes in the liver are quite non-specific and characterized by the presence of fat droplets in the hepatocytes, usually without displacement of the nucleus. Mild dilatation of the endoplasmic reticulum, as well as non-specific minor changes in the mitochondria, has

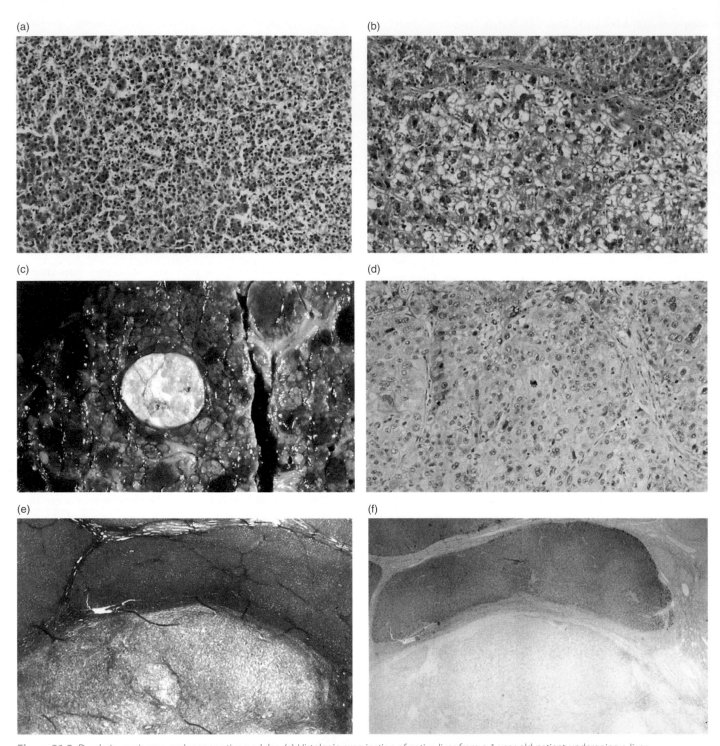

Figure 31.3 Dysplasia, carcinoma, and regenerative nodules. (a) Histologic examination of native liver from a 1-year-old patient undergoing a liver transplantation revealed multiple foci of dysplasia. This microphotograph shows the small cell variant, composed of fetal hepatocyte-like cells with increased nucleocytoplasmic ratio and hyperchromatic nuclei. (Hematoxylin–phloxine–saffron (HPS) stain, original magnification ×200.) (b) Foci of large cell dysplasia are shown in the liver from the same patient, characterized by irregular hyperchromatic nuclei and an increased nucleocytoplasmic ratio. Distinction from a microscopic hepatocellular carcinoma may be very difficult. (HPS stain, original magnification ×200.) (c) Native liver from a 4-year-old hepatic transplant recipient showing cirrhosis and one nodule that clearly stood out from the rest of the parenchyma. (d) Histologic examination of the nodule in (c) revealed hepatocellular carcinoma with extensive nuclear irregularity and many mitoses. (HPS stain, original magnification ×200.) (e) Native liver from an 11-year-old liver transplant recipient with extensive macronodular cirrhosis; one large focus of hepatocellular carcinoma was noted (pale staining nodule, lower portion of figure). (HPS stain, original magnification ×20.) (f) Immunostaining with an antibody to fumarylacetoacetate hydrolase revealed a positive reaction in many of the regenerating nodules, indicating reacquisition of the missing enzyme by the regenerating hepatocytes, suggesting reversion of the mutation. Note that the carcinomatous nodule remains negative, indicating absence of reversion. (Avidin–biotin–peroxidase technique with hematoxylin counterstaining; original magnification ×20.) See color section.

been noted. In dysplastic liver cells, irregular nuclear profiles with large nucleoli and reduction of cytoplasmic organelles are characteristic ultrastructural features [42].

At least one case of hepatoblastoma has been documented in a 15-month-old tyrosinemic child [32]. Because the treatment of hepatoblastoma differs from that of hepatocarcinoma, it is important to consider this rare possibility in the evaluation of liver masses in tyrosinemia.

Kidneys

Renal tubular dysfunction, characterized by Fanconi syndrome and hypophosphatemic rickets, may be a major clinical manifestation of tyrosinemia [27]. Renal failure, when present, has been reported in patients with long-standing disease. Although non-specific, the characteristic morphologic change noted, particularly in young patients with the fulminant form of the disease, has been nephromegaly, characterized by an increase in kidney weight with microscopically irregular dilatations of the proximal tubules and vacuolization of tubular epithelial cells. Glycogen accumulation in collecting tubules has been reported. Nephrocalcinosis, sometimes extensive and visualized by clinical imaging, is present in most samples. Ultrastructural examination reveals simplification of the epithelial cells, with loss of the brush border, and cytoplasmic vacuolization, particularly in the periapical area. Although non-specific, these changes are strongly reminiscent of those encountered in experimental Fanconi syndrome induced by maleic acid.

An unusual finding was the report of hyperplasia of the juxtaglomerular apparatus in one infant. This appears to be unique: this finding has not been reported since and was absent from our series of kidney biopsies despite a careful search. The inference that this represents a secondary change is strengthened by the profound electrolytic disturbances in that patient, which, as the author discussed, may have induced a change in the juxtaglomerular apparatus. Although liver transplantation may correct the metabolic derangement in many patients, some biochemical anomalies of renal tubular function may persist [43].

In 9 of 24 patients with tyrosinemia where renal tissue was examined at the Hôpital Sainte-Justine, there was a mild to moderate degree of glomerulosclerosis and interstitial fibrosis – mild glomerulosclerosis being defined as the occurrence of sclerosis in at least 10% of glomeruli accompanied by interstitial changes [9]. Significant glomerular changes have been reported infrequently in hereditary tyrosinemia. In two patients, renal failure accompanied the glomerular changes, the latter attributed to the metabolic disease rather than a consequence of pyelonephritis or an unrelated glomerulopathy [44]. Eight of the nine patients in our series were older than 2 years, and in four the findings were noted in renal biopsies obtained either shortly before or at the time of liver transplantation. Immunofluorescence studies usually did not reveal any significant immune deposits in the glomeruli, although the occasional presence of immunoglobulin A, a non-specific

finding related to chronic liver disease, was noted. No renal malignancies were observed in our series nor have any been reported to our knowledge.

Pancreas

Hyperplasia and hypertrophy of the islets of Langerhans have been reported in a large number of patients [27] and have rarely been associated with chronic hypoglycemia, although most patients have normal blood glucose levels. However, the variability and inconsistency of these changes are likely related both to difficulties in the accurate assessment of the relative volume of pancreatic islet cells, particularly in the infant where there is a relatively high proportion of islet tissue, and to probable differences in the amount of islet tissue present in different areas of the pancreas. Hyalinization of the islets also has been reported in some patients, but whether this change may result in diabetes is purely conjectural; one patient was described in whom diabetes was associated with tyrosinemia but the islets were seen to be normal [45].

Heart

Myocardial hypertrophy has been associated with ultrastructural changes characterized principally by increased numbers of mitochondria in the myocytes [36]; these patients had a significant incidence of cardiomyopathy as detected by echocardiography but a low incidence of clinical heart disease. By comparison, an obstructive cardiomyopathy has been described in two symptomatic patients [36]. We have not observed these changes in any of our cases.

Peripheral nerves

Three peripheral nerve specimens have been analyzed during the period of recuperation, 2–6 weeks following paralytic crises [15]. All three samples revealed axonal degeneration and secondary demyelination, similar to the changes seen in acute intermittent porphyria.

Management

Nitisinone treatment for tyrosinemia

Treatment protocols

Nitisinone is started at a daily dosage of 1–2 mg/kg. Nitisinone has a long half-life (>50 hours) and is provided in one or two daily doses. The prescription is adjusted to maintain (1) an absence of detectable urinary and blood succinylacetone and (2) plasma nitisinone at >50 µmol/L. In non-screened patients who present acutely with symptoms suggestive of tyrosinemia, an initial dose of 2 mg/kg daily is prescribed after adequate diagnostic samples have been obtained (the administration of nitisinone rapidly reduces the levels of succinylacetone in urine and blood, and pretreatment samples are critical for precise diagnosis). The dose is then adjusted as above when the acute phase has subsided.

In the Quebec NTBC protocol, the goal for plasma tyrosine level is 250–400 μmol/L maintained by dietary phenylalanine and tyrosine restriction, which requires specialized dietary supervision and supplementation with special formulae providing the remaining nutrients for growth. Of note, whereas plasma tyrosine is a non-specific and imprecise reflection of metabolic control in non-nitisinone-treated patients, it is an accurate measure in those receiving nitisinone because the pharmacologic block in metabolism is close to tyrosine (Figure 31.1). Plasma tyrosine is used to adjust dietary prescriptions in nitisinone-treated patients. A tandem mass spectrometry-based assay for simultaneous determination of nitisinone, succinylacetone, tyrosine, phenylalanine, and methionine levels on a dried blood spot has been reported [46].

The above recommendations for nitisinone, succinylacetone, and tyrosine levels are reasonable based upon current knowledge but have not been formally shown to be optimal. More experience will be required to formulate evidence-based recommendations.

The monitoring protocol during nitisinone treatment involves the collection of pretreatment baseline specimens of blood and urine, close observation for immediate adverse effects after initiating nitisinone administration (none has been detected to date), and metabolic monitoring for 1 week in hospital and with decreasing frequency until 6 months, at which time metabolic testing is performed at 3-month intervals (with closer surveillance if clinically indicated). Metabolites (plasma tyrosine and phenylalanine, urinary δ-aminolevulinic acid and urine succinylacetone, every 3 months), markers of liver function (plasma levels of AFP, aminotransferases, and gamma-glutamyltransferase, every 3 months), and coagulation tests (every 6 months) are followed. Dietary records for 72 hours are used to calculate phenylalanine plus tyrosine intake every 3 months. Imaging currently includes abdominal ultrasonography every 6 months and abdominal MRI annually, and isotopic GFR every 4 years. Baseline ophthalmologic assessment (see Complications) is done before or soon after beginning treatment and slit lamp assessments are repeated if ocular symptoms develop.

Results

The results of the first 15 years of the Quebec protocol have recently been analyzed [47]. Patients were divided into those that received nitisinone before 1 month of age ("early" treatment group, 24 patients) and those who received their first dose after 1 month ("late" group, 26 patients) and a historical control group born in the previous decade who never received nitisinone before receiving a transplant or death (28 patients). There were striking differences among these three groups with respect both to acute complications (hospitalizations for tyrosinemia-related reasons and neurologic crises) and to chronic outcomes (transplantation, death). Acute complications stopped with the onset of treatment. For example, no hospitalizations for acute complications were observed in over 5700 patient-months of nitisinone treatment, compared with 184 hospitalizations in 1312 patient-months without nitisinone treatment (p < 0.001).

Liver transplantation was performed in 20 of the non-treated patients (71%) at a median age of 26 months, versus seven late-treated patients (26%; p < 0.001) and no early-treated patient (p < 0.001). Ten deaths occurred in non-nitisinone-treated patients versus two in treated patients (p < 0.01). The two deaths in treated patients were caused by complications related to liver transplantation not to tyrosinemia-related complications. It is impossible to conclude whether the development of nodules in late-treated patients represents only the expected repair and regeneration in response to severe pretreatment liver damage or whether there was also a component of true progression of the disease during nitisinone treatment. However, data from the early-treated patients hint at a near-complete suppression of hepatic disease in compliant patients who receive nitisinone. Inclusion of patients for analysis in the early treatment group was restricted to patients with over 5 years of follow-up, in order to assure a follow-up time over twice the median age for liver transplantation of untreated patients. Patients who began nitisinone treatment more recently than that have similar results but were not analyzed because of their shorter follow-up time. None of the early-treated patients had detectable liver disease by repeated ultrasound and abdominal MRI imaging, and none had biochemical evidence of coagulopathy or liver disease.

It is important to guard against overconfidence. Nitisinone was propelled from an unlikely origin (an agricultural chemical) to the status of a therapeutic agent without passing through typical phase II and III trials. The long-term effects of nitisinone administration are unknown. Vigilance, meticulous follow-up of individual patients, and ongoing compilation of the world experience with nitisinone treatment will be required to obtain adequate data collection.

The efficacy of nitisinone treatment has kindled debate about the optimal management paradigm for tyrosinemic patients (Figure 31.4). Should regions other than those at high risk perform neonatal screening for tyrosinemia? Most of the world's tyrosinemic patients are born outside Quebec and northern Europe, in areas where newborn screening with succinylacetone is not currently practiced. The technical obstacles to incorporating succinylacetone determination into expanded neonatal screening are being overcome [48]. Efficient neonatal screening combined with early nitisinone treatment, often makes the difference between presymptomatic initiation of an effective and possibly curative medical treatment and the situation with late detection, often when liver failure or irreversible liver damage has occurred.

Complications

To date, in our series, the only complication attributable to nitisinone has been ocular. One nitisinone-treated patient developed corneal crystals, presumably representing tyrosine precipitation, which disappeared within 24 hours of initiating

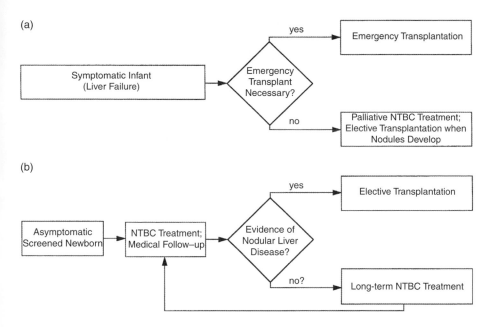

Figure 31.4 Management paradigms for hepatorenal tyrosinemia. (a) Without neonatal screening. (b) Efficient neonatal screening plus nitisinone (2-(2-nitro-4-trifluoromethylbenzoyl)-1,3-cyclohexanedione (NTBC)) treatment. The question mark reflects the unknown course of tyrosinemia with long-term nitisinone treatment.

a strict low-phenylalanine and tyrosine diet. Similar lesions have occurred in other nitisinone-treated patients and occur in rats following tyrosine loading or nitisinone treatment [13,49,50]. Photophobia and ocular inflammation in a nitisinone-treated patient are considered to be indications for emergency ophthalmologic examination to eliminate the presence of corneal crystals.

The risk of hepatocellular carcinoma in early-treated patients is a major unknown. Hepatocarcinoma can develop in FAH-deficient mice despite nitisinone treatment [13]. However, it would be inappropriate to extrapolate directly to humans, in whom (1) tyrosinemia evolves more slowly than in mice, (2) the turnover of tyrosine and phenylalanine (milligrams/kilogram daily) is about ten-fold less than in mice, (3) nitisinone intake can be more reliably assured than has been the case for mice, and (4) the mechanisms of hepatocellular carcinogenesis show major differences from those in rodents [28]. However, this observation should encourage physicians to perform close, well-controlled follow-ups of tyrosinemic patients treated with nitisinone and to share their results in the context of multicenter trials so that non-anecdotal data can be accumulated.

It is also noteworthy that mental retardation is common in hereditary hypertyrosinemias because of deficiencies of tyrosine aminotransferase (tyrosinemia type II; Figure 31.1a) and 4HPPD, the enzyme inhibited by nitisinone (tyrosinemia type III). To some extent, particularly for tyrosinemia type III, this may reflect ascertainment bias (i.e. a fortuitous discovery on amino acid chromatography performed for unrelated neurologic abnormalities). Although our cohort of nitisinone-treated patients is developing well, this observation is striking enough to recommend strict dietary control to maintain low levels of circulating tyrosine and ongoing surveillance of school performance and development.

Sometimes irreversible changes are present before nitisinone therapy. However, even in patients where permanent damage has occurred, such as one instance in our series of an established renal tubulopathy, or where cirrhosis is established, nitisinone is predicted to prevent or greatly slow further deterioration.

Diet therapy

In nitisinone-treated patients, the principles of diet therapy are the provision of an adequate intake of phenylalanine plus tyrosine to enable adequate growth while avoiding excess intake that results in hypertyrosinemia. Adequate amounts of other nutrients including other amino acids must be provided. Diet should be managed by an experienced team including a dietician and a physician familiar with the principles of management of hereditary metabolic diseases.

Apart from dietary intake of tyrosine and phenylalanine, the principle variable in the control of tyrosine degradation is metabolic state. Under catabolic stresses such as infections, fasting, surgery, or burns, muscle and other organs can liberate large amounts of amino acids. This release of endogenous phenylalanine and tyrosine can exceed the body's tolerance and result in hypertyrosinemia in nitisinone-treated patients. In non-nitisinone-treated patients, increased tyrosine catabolism during acute stress can precipitate crises. A major goal of therapy in this situation is to provide sufficient calories to encourage anabolism and treating the underlying acute condition.

In non-nitisinone-treated patients, the effect of dietary restriction of phenylalanine and tyrosine on the long-term outcome of tyrosinemia, while conceptually evident, has not been documented in detail. Available evidence suggests that dietary therapy can improve renal tubular function and slows but does not prevent the progression of liver disease. Cirrhosis and hepatocellular carcinoma may develop in tyrosinemic patients complying with a strict diet. Readers are referred to the first edition of this chapter and to other sources [29] for further discussion of dietary therapy in non-nitisinone-treated patients.

In infants diagnosed clinically, we eliminate all tyrosine and phenylalanine from the diet for 24–48 hours while providing adequate amounts of other amino acids, vitamins, and minerals by the use of energy-rich formulae containing no phenylalanine or tyrosine. After that, depending on the state of the child, tyrosine and phenylalanine are gradually reintroduced in the form of humanized milk formulae or breast milk.

Methionine levels usually normalize with other liver functions in the days and weeks following diagnosis and therapy [27]. We have not specifically restricted methionine intake, but in patients in whom prolonged hypermethioninemia was observed, some investigators have restricted dietary methionine. Of note, hypermethioninemia is apparently not toxic in itself, being well tolerated in other hereditary states such as methionine adenosyltransferase deficiency.

After the acute phase, the intake of phenylalanine plus tyrosine is titrated according to the child's growth and, the plasma phenylalanine and tyrosine levels. As a starting approximation, a minimum of about 90 mg/kg daily of phenylalanine plus tyrosine is sufficient for normal growth in infants, and 700–900 mg daily is sufficient for older children. Slightly more than half of this amount is provided as phenylalanine. Treatment must be individualized according to the child's metabolic state and individual requirements for tyrosine and phenylalanine by maintaining normal growth and ensuring that plasma tyrosine is maintained within the target range.

Acute liver crises

In our experience, acute liver crises do not occur in nitisinone-treated patients. Urgent administration of nitisinone in addition to the following measures is the treatment of choice. Infections and other precipitants of liver crises should be treated aggressively. Observation in hospital; provision of sufficient energy intake, often with gavages or parenteral nutrition; and medical treatment for the accompanying complications, such as ascites, are important. A reduction or cessation of phenylalanine and tyrosine intake for 24–48 hours is usually indicated. Oral or nasogastric feeding is preferred over intravenous administration because it permits greater energy intake. In acutely ill tyrosinemic children, supplemental intravenous glucose is useful in our experience to prevent catabolism and to reduce the risk of a neurologic crisis. Most acute crises resolve within days to weeks, but fulminant liver failure may develop in non-nitisinone-treated patients, necessitating urgent liver transplantation. After the first 2 years of life, episodes of liver decompensation become less frequent. The physician should remain vigilant to this possibility at all ages.

Chronic liver disease and liver transplantation

Liver transplantation cures tyrosinemic liver disease (Table 31.1). The optimal timing for liver transplantation in the patient with chronic stable liver disease requires individual decision making. In the United Network for Organ Sharing database, 125 patients have required liver transplantation secondary to hereditary tyrosinemia type I [51]. The mean age at transplant was 2.5 years (SD, 3.6). Overall, 1- and 5-year patient survival was 90.4% and 90.4%, respectively. Some children with nodules found at transplantation to be hepatocarcinoma have died with recurrence of carcinoma after transplantation [3] but some children are nodule-free with normal growth. Even before nitisinone therapy, we often delayed transplantation for such patients by several years. In practice, we follow patients without liver nodules who have stable renal and liver function, clinically and with serial imaging.

Some groups have advocated early liver transplantation for all patients with tyrosinemia as being both curative of the disease and preventive of the complications from neurologic crisis and liver failure. Although small infants survive transplantation more frequently than they did previously and the reduced liver technique has allowed for greater availability of livers, children with a stable course probably would benefit from waiting until they reach at least 10 kg. This is especially true because nitisinone treatment has eliminated or greatly reduced the risk of acute decompensation [4].

Before nitisinone was available, we considered a single neurologic crisis to be an indication for transplantation, given the high incidence of relapse and mortality; also, a history of hepatic crises was a relative indication. In nitisinone-treated patients, neither is an indication for transplantation because recurrence of these complications is prevented by nitisinone treatment.

Patients with ultrasonographic evidence of micronodular cirrhosis are followed closely by imaging for the development of distinct nodules. The presence of a single persistent nodule is considered an indication for transplantation. In some situations where the nodule is accessible, biopsy may be an option. However, in our experience, macronodules arise only in cirrhotic livers that, in fact, have many other nodules not detectable by imaging. Although the lack of dysplasia or carcinoma in a biopsied nodule may reduce the urgency of transplantation, in our experience, the presence of cirrhosis would not eliminate the need for transplantation.

We have not encountered the situation of an increasing AFP level in a patient without a detectable nodule. This would place the clinician in the uncomfortable position of deciding between transplantation based on a (non-specific) laboratory result and ongoing surveillance of a presumably localized, poorly differentiated population of hepatocytes. A liver biopsy to establish the presence or absence of cirrhosis would be performed in such circumstances. The presence of cirrhosis would be important in the decision regarding transplantation. Causes unrelated to tyrosinemia would be considered before accepting an isolated biochemical anomaly as an indication for transplantation. More sensitive and specific tests for hepatocellular carcinomas are required for optimum medical surveillance. Hopefully in the future, new imaging methods and serial images will permit the reliable discrimination of hepatocellular cancer from regenerative nodules based upon the characteristics and temporal course of individual lesions.

After transplantation, we permit a normal diet and we do not continue treatment with nitisinone. Some investigators raise the possibility that the disease may progress in other organs despite liver transplantation, and recommend continued nitisinone and diet therapy. In patients receiving transplants since the mid-1980s, we have found no clinical evidence of disease progression in our patients after liver transplantation and do not have sufficient grounds to continue to impose this added burden on patients.

Liver tumors in tyrosinemia

The treatment of hepatocellular carcinomas is similar in children with and without tyrosinemia, and readers are referred to the pertinent chapters in this book for further information. Tyrosinemia arguably confers the strongest known predisposition to the development of hepatocarcinoma. Nonetheless, a concerted study of the biology of tyrosinemic hepatocarcinoma has not been performed. It will be pertinent to pursue whether the biology of tyrosinemic hepatocarcinomas is similar to that of hepatocarcinomas that arise in other diseases.

Importantly, at least one case of hepatoblastoma has been documented, in a 15-month-old tyrosinemic child [32]. Because the treatment of hepatoblastoma differs from that of hepatocarcinoma, hepatoblastoma is an important consideration in the evaluation of liver masses in tyrosinemic children [33].

Neurologic crises

The most important treatment principles are supportive care with surveillance of respiratory status and rapid nitisinone administration. Paralysis and respiratory failure can develop rapidly and may be overlooked in patients in pain, to whom analgesics and sedation are often prescribed. Nitisinone produces a striking decrease in the excretion of δ-aminolevulinic acid (see Pathophysiology) within 12 hours [47], suggesting that the risk of crisis is reduced almost immediately. The recurrence of neurological crises has not been observed in compliant patients receiving nitisinone.

During the acute phase, analgesia is provided for the severe pain, using narcotic analgesics if necessary. A high level of carbohydrate is critically important because glucose inhibits δ-aminolevulinate synthase, reducing the production of δ-aminolevulinic acid. Hypertension, hyponatremia, hypokalemia, and hypophosphatemia are treated symptomatically if present. Extreme hyponatremia has caused convulsions in several cases. Dental consultation and use of a protective oral prosthesis are necessary in bruxism, tongue biting, and oral anesthesia. Crises are not expected to intensify after this point,

but recovery in patients with paralysis will reflect the time course of axonal regeneration. Ventilatory support including mechanical ventilation may be necessary for several weeks during convalescence. It is important that the patient, family, and hospital personnel be aware that recuperation is possible and that an optimistic attitude be adopted during this period. In patients with tyrosinemia, we avoid the use of medications that can aggravate porphyria, such as barbiturates (see Pathophysiology), before and for at least 1 week following nitisinone treatment.

Hematin, which inhibits δ-aminolevulinic acid synthetase, has been proposed as a therapeutic option in neurologic crises. In one child, a relationship was reported between hematin administration and motor improvement [52], but the child nonetheless remained intubated for 2 months. The use of hematin carries a risk of coagulopathy. The availability of nitisinone should render the use of hematin unnecessary in tyrosinemia.

Following liver transplantation, no patient has had neurologic crisis.

Renal involvement

Renal tubular dysfunction in tyrosinemia usually responds to some extent to dietary therapy [49]. Rickets is the main clinical sign of tubular dysfunction in tyrosinemia. At least three mechanisms may be implicated in its pathogenesis: urinary phosphate loss, impaired hepatic hydroxylation of vitamin D, and impaired renal hydroxylation of vitamin D. Rachitic patients with tyrosinemia should be evaluated individually and treatment tailored according to the patient's needs. The need for treatment should be reassessed after several weeks of nitisinone treatment. The relationship of treatment of rickets to other complications, such as nephrocalcinosis, is unclear.

It has been suggested that the damage in both liver and kidney is the result of decreased sulfhydryl compounds in these tissues and the use of N-acetylcysteine has been advocated to bring about repletion of tissue glutathione content [27]. Results of reported acute trials with oral or intravenous N-acetylcysteine, however, were not encouraging and we have seen neurologic crises and liver progression in patients receiving this therapy orally. Whether the long-term use of N-acetylcysteine is of some benefit in tyrosinemia remains unproved.

Careful attention to the degree of renal involvement is required at the time of transplant evaluation (Table 31.2). This includes evaluation of tubular and glomerular functions, including phosphate reabsorption, aminoaciduria, glycosuria, and GFR by creatinine or radioisotope clearance. It would be prudent to assess the extent to which the dysfunction is reversible with nitisinone treatment.

Kidney transplantation alone was performed in an adult with tyrosinemia and renal failure who had little clinical evidence of liver involvement, although micronodular cirrhosis was present at the time of transplantation [44]. The patient subsequently required dialysis because of chronic rejection, but liver function apparently remained normal until death 3 years after transplantation. It seems unlikely that kidney transplantation alone would significantly alter the risk of hepatocarcinoma.

Results with combined transplantation have been promising in tyrosinemia and in other hereditary diseases. Despite the fact that no cross-match (aside from ABO blood group compatibility) has been performed in our combined transplantations for tyrosinemia or other liver–kidney diseases (oxalosis type 1 and Alagille syndrome), the kidneys have not shown evidence of rejection. In fact, in combined transplantations, the liver may have fewer episodes of rejection, both in our experience and in that of others (D. Freese, personal communication).

The choice between liver alone or combined liver–kidney transplantation can be a dilemma in a patient with moderate non-reversible renal disease. Currently used immunosuppressive agents such as cyclosporine and tacrolimus are nephrotoxic and could further reduce the function of an already compromised kidney. The calcineurin inhibitors cause a significant decrease in GFR in children who undergo liver transplantation, regardless of the underlying liver disease. This effect must be considered when evaluating a child with tyrosinemia for transplantation.

At our institution, 29 tyrosinemic children have undergone transplantation with livers alone, with follow-up of more than 15 years. In our series, the long-term course of GFR after hepatic transplantation was similar in tyrosinemic patients and patients transplanted for other reasons, suggesting that tyrosinemic patients are not more sensitive than other patients to the nephrotoxic effects of immunosuppressants [53]. Some other tyrosinemic children with affected glomerular function before liver transplantation alone have improved their GFR after transplantation, but most have decreased their GFR despite low cyclosporine levels (100–120 ng/mL). Observations that the rate of decrease is similar in tyrosinemic patients and in children undergoing transplantation for other diseases suggest that liver transplantation may slow or stop the kidney disease of tyrosinemia. This is anecdotal, however, and more data are needed. Perhaps the use of three daily doses of cyclosporine may have reduced the incidence of nephrotoxicity. Alternatively, it cannot be excluded that the long-term concomitant use of calcium channel blockers may have played a beneficial role. Following hepatic transplantation, there is a marked reduction but not a complete normalization of succinylacetone excretion, the source of the succinylacetone presumably being the kidney itself or other extrahepatic tissues and the significance of which is unknown.

In practice, until less nephrotoxic immunosuppressive agents become available, we consider combined liver–kidney transplantation when the pretransplantation GFR is low enough (<40 mL/min per 1.73 m^2) for the predicted decrease in the post-transplantation GFR to affect growth. Longer follow-up of renal function in tyrosinemic patients who have undergone hepatic transplantation may allow us to further refine our approach to the renal disease of tyrosinemia.

Gene therapy or hepatocyte transplantation in tyrosinemia

Tyrosinemia is potentially an attractive candidate disease for gene therapy or hepatocyte replacement. Correction of FAH in hepatocytes would offer similar benefits to those of transplantation and presumably would correct clinically detectable risks of tyrosinemia. Cells with normal FAH activity have a growth advantage over FAH-deficient hepatocytes and may overgrow and repopulate the liver. Mice with FAH deficiency have an aggressive liver disease that resembles human tyrosinemia and provides an interesting model system for preclinical testing. Fundamental research is exploring several variants of this theme, including viral transformation and gene replacement of FAH-deficient cells in vivo or ex vivo. These approaches are intuitively appealing, easy to understand, and, if successful, would offer a cure without the risks of transplant and immunosuppression. Parents, therefore, often spontaneously ask about them, sometimes even assuming that they are available and efficient.

Although gene therapy and hepatocyte transplantation currently are not treatment options, they have received considerable publicity and are producing interesting results in tyrosinemic and other mice [54]. Gene replacement therapy is theoretically more difficult in tyrosinemia than in certain other inborn errors because the toxic intermediates in tyrosinemia are felt to be capable of inducing hepatocarcinoma and possibly kidney disease, even in the presence of normal circulating tyrosine levels. Therefore, for treatment of tyrosinemia, it would not suffice to simply produce a sufficient number of cells to normalize plasma tyrosine: all hepatocytes would have to express normal FAH to avoid the risk of progression to cancer. Biologically, cells with a functional *FAH* would have a selective advantage and might overgrow FAH-deficient cells, particularly in mice [54]. However, it is not clear how nodules that would arise from this process could be reliably distinguished from neoplastic nodules. Adeno-associated virus gene repair appears to have been successful in correcting a mouse model of hereditary tyrosinemia in vivo. As predicted, in this model, repaired hepatocytes had a selective growth advantage and were thus able to proliferate to efficiently repopulate mutant livers and cure the underlying metabolic disease [55].

At a clinical level, it is not clear how nodules that would arise from this process could be reliably distinguished from neoplastic nodules. If major improvements occur in gene transfer technology, in vivo cell selection, and detection of hepatocellular carcinoma, they could have an important impact on the feasibility of gene therapy or hepatocyte transplantation in tyrosinemia. Hepatocyte transplantation would also require lifelong immunosuppression.

Liver disease-specific induced pluripotent stem cells offer great promise to model and potentially treat metabolic liver disease. These cells have already been produced from skin fibroblasts derived from tyrosinemic patients as a proof of principle [56,57]. In the murine model of tyrosinemia type I fibroblast-derived $FAH^{-/-}$-induced pluripotent stem cells were used as targets for gene correction in combination with the tetraploid embryo complementation method. The gene correction was validated functionally by the long-term survival and expansion of FAH-positive cells in these mice after withdrawal of rescuing therapy with nitisinone [58]. Producing such autologous cell therapies would avoid immune suppression and enable correction of the gene defect prior to cell transplantation. Practical considerations prevent immediate application of these exciting fundamental developments.

Future clinical challenges

The disease paradigm of tyrosinemia has been transformed by nitisinone treatment. Patients and their families previously lived in fear of the frequent and often fatal acute hepatic and neurologic crises. The chronic anxiety of parents over the risk of cirrhosis, liver cancer, rickets, and chronic renal failure was sustained by the occurrence of these signs in the patient him or herself, or in other patients who belonged to the patient association. In Quebec, a generation of patients who have received nitisinone treatment since the newborn period and who have never experienced the complications of tyrosinemia is reaching adolescence. The repeated explications of physicians about the potential complications of tyrosinemia are discordant with the daily experience of these families, for whom the child has always enjoyed normal health.

Compliance with treatment and monitoring are major concerns. Although most families have integrated nitisinone and the dietary restrictions into their daily routine, some question their pertinence for their child, as well as the need for repeated standardized medical evaluation. For these families, the sentiment that the disease is "cured" is reinforced by the lack of symptoms despite suboptimal drug or dietary compliance. We have observed neurologic crises in patients who have neglected to take nitisinone as prescribed (as reflected by extremely low plasma nitisinone levels and/or high succinylacetone concentrations) and corneal ulcers in other patients with high plasma tyrosine levels. Non-compliant patients must be considered to be at increased risk for the development of the chronic complications of tyrosinemia.

Pregnancy in women with tyrosinemia is controversial. For the foreseeable future, it will be difficult to provide confident recommendations to tyrosinemic women considering pregnancy. Prenatal exposure to nitisinone and its accompanying prenatal hypertyrosinemia pose potential but as-yet theoretical risks to the fetus. From the experience with maternal phenylketonuria, in which the normal fetus of affected mothers can be severely mentally handicapped if the disease is poorly controlled in the mother during early pregnancy, these considerations must be taken seriously. At the time of writing, only three nitisinone-treated pregnancies are known to the authors. From these pregnancies, children without gross malformations or neurologic problems were born. These children are still very young and the long-term outcome of the babies is unknown.

The subject of pregnancy should be discussed openly with patients as well as the limits of current knowledge. Women with tyrosinemia wishing to avoid pregnancy should be counseled about contraception; oral contraceptives with high estrogen content are avoided because of the associated low risk of hepatic adenomas. Other options of family planning include adoption. If a tyrosinemic woman elects to become pregnant, the following general considerations would apply. It would be prudent to continue nitisinone during the pregnancy because of the clear risk to the mother and the fetus if a tyrosinemic crisis occurs during pregnancy. Regarding diet, in the absence of adequate clinical experience, we would recommend stringent control before pregnancy with frequent monitoring of plasma phenylalanine and tyrosine, and strict dietary surveillance before and throughout pregnancy, analogous to the recommendations for the dietary treatment of phenylketonuria during the pregnancy of an affected mother. Close dietary follow-up would be necessary to avoid dietary deficiencies, particularly given the rapid changes that occur in nutritional requirements during pregnancy. The outcome and course of each pregnancy of nitisinone-treated tyrosinemic children should be reported, because it provides a substantial contribution to current knowledge.

It is important to avoid complacency. Early treatment with nitisinone has been extremely successful to date but outcomes beyond adolescence are unknown, for liver and kidney function, for psychomotor performance, and for ocular complications. The special diet provides patients with a greater choice than ever before but increasing the variety and palatability of low-tyrosine foods is a major goal in normalizing lifestyle for patients. The optimal levels of tyrosine, phenylalanine, and nitisinone are not established and to determine this may require large collaborative series. It is still not possible to distinguish malignancy in hepatic nodules non-invasively with certainty. Meticulous clinical monitoring and high vigilance for the development of complications are important for the long-term follow-up of tyrosinemic patients.

Conclusions

The outcome of tyrosinemia has completely changed since its description over 60 years ago, most recently with the discovery of nitisinone. Nitisinone treatment has had a profound impact on the quality of life and the outcome of tyrosinemic patients, by eliminating the occurrence of acute liver and neurologic crises that previously were a daily threat. The combination of neonatal screening and early nitisinone treatment is undoubtedly the medical treatment of choice for tyrosinemia. It delays and may prevent the long-term complications of tyrosinemia, although longer follow-up is necessary prior to concluding on this point. Physicians and families must remain alert for the development of complications resulting from the disease or its treatment. If major improvements occur in gene transfer technology, in vivo cell selection, and detection of hepatocellular carcinoma, they could improve the feasibility of gene therapy or hepatocyte transplantation in tyrosinemia. The potential advantages to the patient of such new therapies will have to be weighed against the excellent results currently obtained with neonatal screening and early nitisinone and diet therapy.

Acknowledgements

We wish to acknowledge the participation of numerous people involved in the many facets of patient care for tyrosinemic children, including Jean Larochelle, Marie Lambert, Andrée Rasquin-Weber, Ernest Seidman, Louis Dallaire, Yolande Lefèvre, Martyne Gosselin, Danièlle Régimbald, Manon Bouchard, Khazal Paradis, Claude Roy, Sean O'Regan, C. Ronald Scott, and our other colleagues in the Quebec NTBC Study. This work was supported in part by the Canadian Liver Foundation, the Garrod Association of Canada, and the US Food and Drug Administration, and André Imbeau.

References

1. Medes G. A new error of tyrosine metabolism: tyrosinosis. The intermediary metabolism of tyrosine and phenylalanine. *Biochem J* 1932;**26**:917–940.

2. Baber MD. A case of congenital cirrhosis of the liver with renal tubular defects akin to those in the Fanconi syndrome. *Arch Dis Child* 1956;**31**(159):335–339.

3. Mieles LA, Esquivel CO, Van Thiel DH, *et al.* Liver transplantation for tyrosinemia. A review of 10 cases from the University of Pittsburgh. *Dig Dis Sci* 1990;**35**:153–157.

4. McKiernan PJ. Nitisinone in the treatment of hereditary tyrosinaemia type 1. *Drugs*. 2006;**66**:743–750.

5. Lindblad B, Lindstedt S, Steen G. On the enzymic defects in hereditary tyrosinemia. *Proc Natl Acad Sci USA* 1977;**74**:4641–4645.

6. Kvittingen EA, Jellum E, Stokke O. Assay of fumarylacetoacetate fumarylhydrolase in human liver-deficient activity in a case of hereditary tyrosinemia. *Clin Chim Acta* 1981;**115**:311–319.

7. Kvittingen EA. Hereditary tyrosinemia type I: an overview. *Scand J Clin Lab Invest Suppl* 1986;**184**:27–34.

8. Phaneuf D, Labelle Y, Berube D, *et al.* Cloning and expression of the cDNA encoding human fumarylacetoacetate hydrolase, the enzyme deficient in hereditary tyrosinemia: assignment of the gene to chromosome 15. *Am J Hum Genet* 1991;**48**:525–535.

9. Russo P, O'Regan S. Visceral pathology of hereditary tyrosinemia type I. *Am J Hum Genet* 1990;**47**:317–324.

10. Jorquera R, Tanguay RM. The mutagenicity of the tyrosine metabolite, fumarylacetoacetate, is enhanced by glutathione depletion. *Biochem Biophys Res Commun* 1997;**232**:42–48.

11. Kvittingen EA, Rootwelt H, Brandtzaeg P, Bergan A, Berger R. Hereditary tyrosinemia type I. Self-induced correction of the fumarylacetoacetase defect. *J Clin Invest* 1993;**91**:1816–1821.

12. Grompe M, al-Dhalimy M, Finegold M, *et al.* Loss of fumarylacetoacetate hydrolase is responsible for the neonatal hepatic dysfunction phenotype of lethal albino mice. *Genes Dev* 1993;**7**:2298–2307.

13. Al-Dhalimy M, Overturf K, Finegold M, Grompe M. Long-term therapy with NTBC and tyrosine-restricted diet in a murine model of hereditary tyrosinemia type I. *Mol Genet Metab* 2002;**75**:38–45.

14. Kubo S, Sun M, Miyahara M, *et al.* Hepatocyte injury in tyrosinemia type 1 is induced by fumarylacetoacetate and is inhibited by caspase inhibitors. *Proc Natl Acad Sci USA* 1998;**95**:9552–9557.

15. Mitchell G, Larochelle J, Lambert M, *et al.* Neurologic crises in hereditary tyrosinemia. *N Engl J Med* 1990;**322**:432–437.

16. De Braekeleer M, Larochelle J. Genetic epidemiology of hereditary tyrosinemia in Quebec and in Saguenay-Lac-St-Jean. *Am J Hum Genet* 1990;**47**:302–307.

17. Rootwelt H, Hoie K, Berger R, Kvittingen EA. Fumarylacetoacetase mutations in tyrosinaemia type I. *Hum Mutat* 1996;**7**:239–243.

18. Ploos van Amstel JK, Bergman AJ, van Beurden EA, *et al.* Hereditary tyrosinemia type 1: novel missense, nonsense and splice consensus mutations in the human fumarylacetoacetate hydrolase gene; variability of the genotype–phenotype relationship. *Hum Genet* 1996;**97**:51–59.

19. Cassiman D, Zeevaert R, Holme E, Kvittingen EA, Jaeken J. A novel mutation causing mild, atypical fumarylacetoacetase deficiency (tyrosinemia type I): a case report. *Orphanet J Rare Dis* 2009;**4**:28.

20. Jakobs C, Dorland L, Wikkerink B, *et al.* Stable isotope dilution analysis of succinylacetone using electron capture negative ion mass fragmentography: an accurate approach to the pre- and neonatal diagnosis of hereditary tyrosinemia type I. *Clin Chim Acta* 1988;**171**:223–231.

21. Croffie JM, Gupta SK, Chong SK, Fitzgerald JF. Tyrosinemia type 1 should be suspected in infants with severe coagulopathy even in the absence of other signs of liver failure. *Pediatrics* 1999;**103**:675–678.

22. Magera MJ, Gunawardena ND, Hahn SH, *et al.* Quantitative determination of succinylacetone in dried blood spots for newborn screening of tyrosinemia type I. *Mol Genet Metab* 2006;**88**:16–21.

23. Kvittingen EA, Brodtkorb E. The pre- and post-natal diagnosis of tyrosinemia type I and the detection of the carrier state by assay of fumarylacetoacetase. *Scand J Clin Lab Invest Suppl* 1986;**184**:35–40.

24. Shanmugam NP, Bansal S, Greenough A, Verma A, Dhawan A. Neonatal liver failure: aetiologies and management: state of the art. *Eur J Pediatr* 2011;**170**:573–581.

25. Rice DN, Houston IB, Lyon IC, *et al.* Transient neonatal tyrosinaemia. *J Inherit Metab Dis* 1989;**12**:13–22.

26. Scott CR. The genetic tyrosinemias. *Am J Med Genet C* 2006;**142**:121–126.

27. Larochelle J, Prive L, Belanger M, *et al.* [Hereditary tyrosinemia. I. Clinical and biological study of 62 cases.] *Pediatrie* 1973;**28**:5–18.

28. Castilloux J, Laberge AM, Martin SR, Lallier M, Marchand V. "Silent" tyrosinemia presenting as hepatocellular carcinoma in a 10-year-old girl. *J Pediatr Gastroenterol Nutr* 2007;**44**:375–377.

29. Paradis K, Weber A, Seidman EG, *et al.* Liver transplantation for hereditary tyrosinemia: the Quebec experience. *Am J Hum Genet* 1990;**47**:338–342.

30. Orejuela D, Jorquera R, Bergeron A, Finegold MJ, Tanguay RM. Hepatic stress in hereditary tyrosinemia type 1 (HT1) activates the AKT survival pathway in the fah$^{-/-}$ knockout mice model. *J Hepatol* 2008;**48**:308–317.

31. van Dyk E, Pretorius PJ. Point mutation instability (PIN) mutator phenotype as model for true back mutations seen in hereditary tyrosinemia type 1: a hypothesis. *J Inherit Metab Dis* 2012;**35**:407–411.

32. Weinberg AG, Mize CE, Worthen HG. The occurrence of hepatoma in the chronic form of hereditary tyrosinemia. *J Pediatr* 1976;**88**:434–438.

33. Nobili V, Jenkner A, Francalanci P, *et al.* Tyrosinemia type 1: metastatic hepatoblastoma with a favorable outcome. *Pediatrics* 2010;**126**: e235–e238.

34. Paradis K, Mitchell GA, Russo, P. Tyrosinemia. In Suchy FJ (ed.) *Liver Disease in Children.* St. Louis, MO: Mosby, 1994, p. 203.

35. Baumann U, Preece MA, Green A, Kelly DA, McKiernan PJ. Hyperinsulinism in tyrosinaemia type I. *J Inherit Metab Dis* 2005;**28**:131–135.

36. Edwards MA, Green A, Colli A, Rylance G. Tyrosinaemia type I and hypertrophic obstructive cardiomyopathy. *Lancet* 1987;**i**: 1437–1438.

37. Dubois J, Garel L, Patriquin H, *et al.* Imaging features of type 1 hereditary tyrosinemia: a review of 30 patients. *Pediatr Radiol* 1996;**26**:845–851.

38. Crone J, Moslinger D, Bodamer OA, *et al.* Reversibility of cirrhotic regenerative liver nodules upon NTBC treatment in a child with tyrosinaemia type I. *Acta Paediatr* 2003;**92**:625–628.

39. Parikh T, Drew SJ, Lee VS, *et al.* Focal liver lesion detection and characterization with diffusion-weighted MR imaging: comparison with standard breath-hold T$_2$-weighted imaging. *Radiology* 2008;**246**:812–822.

40. Yu JS, Walker-Smith JA, Burnard ED. Neonatal hepatitis in premature infants simulating hereditary tyrosinosis. *Arch Dis Child* 1971;**46**:306–309.

41. Dehner LP, Snover DC, Sharp HL, *et al.* Hereditary tyrosinemia type I (chronic form): pathologic findings in the liver. *Hum Pathol* 1989;**20**:149–158.

42. Tremblay M, Belanger L, Larochelle J, Prive L, Gagnon PM. [Hereditary tyrosinemia: examination of the liver by electron microscopy of hepatic biopsies: observation of 7 cases]. *L'union Med Can* 1977;**106**:1014–1016.

43. Tuchman M, Freese DK, Sharp HL, *et al.* Contribution of extrahepatic tissues to biochemical abnormalities in hereditary tyrosinemia type I: study of three patients after liver transplantation. *J Pediatr* 1987;**110**:399–403.

44. Kvittingen EA, Talseth T, Halvorsen S, *et al.* Renal failure in adult patients with hereditary tyrosinaemia type I. *J Inherit Metab Dis* 1991;**14**:53–62.

45. Lindberg T, Nilsson KO, Jeppsson JO. Hereditary tyrosinaemia and diabetes mellitus. *Acta Paediatr Scand* 1979;**68**:619–620.

46. la Marca G, Malvagia S, Materazzi S, *et al.* LC-MS/MS method for simultaneous determination on a dried blood spot of multiple analytes relevant for treatment monitoring in patients with tyrosinemia type I. *Anal Chem* 2012;**84**:1184–1188.

47. Larochelle J, Alvarez F, Bussieres JF, *et al.* Effect of nitisinone (NTBC) treatment on the clinical course of hepatorenal tyrosinemia in Quebec. *Mol Genet Metab* 2012;**107**:49–54.

48. la Marca G, Malvagia S, Pasquini E, *et al.* The inclusion of succinylacetone as marker for tyrosinemia type I in expanded newborn screening programs. *Rapid Commun Mass Spect* 2008;**22**:812–818.

49. Lock EA, Gaskin P, Ellis MK, *et al.* Tissue distribution of 2-(2-nitro-4-trifluoromethylbenzoyl)cyclohexane-1-3-dione (NTBC): effect on enzymes involved in tyrosine catabolism and relevance to ocular toxicity in the rat. *Toxicol Appl Pharmacol* 1996;**141**: 439–447.

50. Ahmad S, Teckman JH, Lueder GT. Corneal opacities associated with NTBC treatment. *Am J Ophthalmol* 2002;**134**:266–268.

51. Arnon R, Annunziato R, Miloh T, *et al.* Liver transplantation for hereditary tyrosinemia type I: analysis of the UNOS database. *Pediatr Transplant* 2011;**15**:400–405.

52. Rank JM, Pascual-Leone A, Payne W, *et al.* Hematin therapy for the neurologic crisis of tyrosinemia. *J Pediatr* 1991;**118**:136–139.

53. Herzog D, Martin S, Turpin S, Alvarez F. Normal glomerular filtration rate in long-term follow-up of children after orthotopic liver transplantation. *Transplantation* 2006;**81**:672–677.

54. Grompe M. Therapeutic liver repopulation for the treatment of metabolic liver diseases. *Hum Cell* 1999;**12**:171–180.

55. Paulk NK, Wursthorn K, Wang Z, *et al.* Adeno-associated virus gene repair corrects a mouse model of hereditary tyrosinemia in vivo. *Hepatology* 2010;**51**:1200–1208.

56. Ghodsizadeh A, Taei A, Totonchi M, *et al.* Generation of liver disease-specific induced pluripotent stem cells along with efficient differentiation to functional hepatocyte-like cells. *Stem Cell Rev* 2010;**6**:622–632.

57. Asgari S, Pournasr B, Salekdeh GH, *et al.* Induced pluripotent stem cells: a new era for hepatology. *J Hepatol* 2010;**53**:738–751.

58. Wu G, Liu N, Rittelmeyer I, *et al.* Generation of healthy mice from gene-corrected disease-specific induced pluripotent stem cells. *PLOS Biol* 2011;**9**:e1001099.

Lysosomal storage disorders

32

T. Andrew Burrow and Gregory A. Grabowski

Introduction

Lysosomes are membrane bound cellular organelles that contain multiple hydrolases needed for the digestion of various macromolecules including mucopolysaccharides, glycosphingolipids and oligosaccharides. The lysosomal storage diseases are a group of over 40 diseases that are characterized by defective lysosomal function, leading to an accumulation of specific substrates within the lysosomes and eventual impairment of cellular function. A schematic of the lysosomal system enzyme trafficking and substrate accumulation is shown in Figure 32.1.

These diseases are classified by the nature of the stored material that results from the defects in selected lysosomal enzymes, their cofactors, and/or enzyme or substrate transport (Table 32.1). The lysosomal storage diseases are heterogeneous, progressive, multisystem diseases that have a spectrum of ages of onset, severity, rate of progression, and organ involvement. Lysosomal storage diseases have significant morbidity and mortality in the absence of effective treatment. The majority of these diseases are autosomal recessive and, although individually rare, the combined birth prevalence is approximately 1 in 7 000 live births [2]. The diseases are traditionally diagnosed biochemically, but in many cases may also be confirmed molecularly by the identification of pathogenic mutations in one or both copies (X-linked conditions or autosomal recessive, respectively) of the specific genes.

The liver is nearly always involved in lysosomal storage diseases; this can be seen at the light or electron microscopic level. The degree of clinical involvement depends upon the disorder. In many cases, mild abnormalities in liver enzymes and/or hepatomegaly are the only manifestations. However, significant hepatic injury may be present, resulting in considerable morbidity. For each of the diseases, the nature of the organ involvement will depend on the tissue-specific lysosomal enzyme content, substrate composition and turnover, and the rate of cell turnover/replacement. The resultant pathophysiologies are poorly understood but likely are the consequence of numerous proinflammatory and inflammatory events initiated by excess substrate and/or deficient products and their

consequent disruption of lysosomal membrane integrity and/or other components of the autophagocytic and endosomal systems.

Traditionally, these conditions were treated utilizing symptom-based management. Over the past several decades, safe and effective treatments for many of these conditions have been developed, with variable degrees of success. The potential for effective treatment of these conditions prior to the onset of irreversible damage has led to proposals for the addition of lysosomal storage diseases to newborn screen panels. The benefits and limitations of newborn screening for the lysosomal storage diseases have been debated, and further studies aimed at determining the utility of such testing are indicated.

The objective of this chapter is to provide clinicians with a broad overview of the lysosomal storage diseases that significantly affect the liver.

Sphingolipidoses

Mutations in the structures of the primary enzyme or their essential cofactors – that is, sphingolipid activator proteins (saposins) – lead to defective or absent hydrolysis of specific sphingolipids and their abnormal accumulation within lysosomes. Sphingolipids are critical structural components of cell membranes that also function in protein sorting and in cell signaling and recognition. Among the sphingolipidoses, Gaucher disease variants, Niemann–Pick types A and B (NPA and NPB), Farber disease, and G_{M1}-gangliosidosis are discussed here because of their specific effects on the liver.

Gaucher disease

Gaucher disease, a common lysosomal storage disease, is inherited in an autosomal recessive manner. The phenotypes result from defective cleavage of glucosylceramide and its deacylated analogue, glucosylsphingosine, by acid β-glucosidase in all nucleated cells [3]. Over 430 mutations in *GBA1*, the gene that encodes the lysosomal enzyme acid β-glucosidase, have been discovered in affected patients. Gaucher disease has a frequency of approximately 1 in 57 000 in the general

Liver Disease in Children, Fourth Edition, ed. Frederick J. Suchy, Ronald J. Sokol, and William F. Balistreri. Published by Cambridge University Press. © Cambridge University Press 2014.

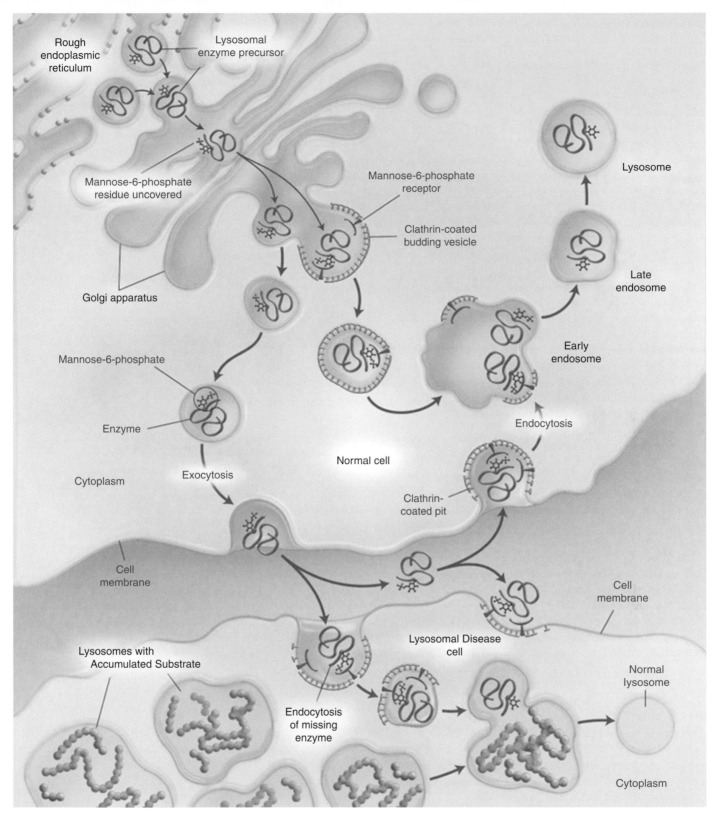

Figure 32.1 The lysosomal system in normal (upper) and lysosomal disease (lower) cells. Lysosomal enzymes are synthesized on the rough endoplasmic reticulum, transported through the Golgi apparatus, and delivered to the lysosomes. In the rough endoplasmic reticulum, oligosaccharide chains are cotranslationally added to the nascent polypeptide. Sequential glycosidic modifications occur in the Golgi apparatus to trim terminal α-glucosidic and α-mannosidic residues, and specific glycosyltransferases add N-acetylglucosamine, β-galactose, and sialic acid. On selected high mannose chains, mannose-6-phosphates are exposed and used to target soluble lysosomal hydrolases to the lysosomes. Membrane-bound lysosomal proteins are targeted to lysosomes by specific peptides within the protein sequence. The glycosidic, proteolytic, and macromolecular processing of the lysosomal proteins occurs vectorially from *cis*- to *trans*-Golgi. The fully mature proteins and cofactors are delivered to the lysosomes after transit through the *trans*-Golgi network and endosomal system. Some lysosomal enzymes are lost from the cells by exocytosis into the surrounding intercellular milieu. Such enzymes, either exogenously supplied or available by secretion, can be internalized by receptor-mediated endocytosis using the mannose-6-phosphate receptor or other receptor (e.g. macrophage mannose receptor) system. The intralysosomal deficiency of specific hydrolases or cofactors leads to an inability to cleave macromolecules (glycosaminoglycans, glycosphingolipids, oligosaccharides, etc.) and their resultant accumulation within distended lysosomes. The degree and rate of accumulation of such specific substrates will depend on the endogenous synthesis and/or exogenous delivery of substrates to particular cells and/or tissues. In the lysosomal storage diseases, the accumulated substrates elicit cellular reactions (proinflammatory, transcriptional, etc.) by mechanisms that remain undetermined. (Adapted from Muenzer and Fisher, 2004 [1].)

Table 32.1 Lysosomal storage disorders involving the liver

Disease	Protein defect	Storage material	Degree of liver involvement	Established therapy
Sphingolipidoses				
Gaucher disease	Acid β-glucosidase	Glucosylceramide	+→++	+
Niemann–Pick disease type A	Sphingomyelinase	Sphingomyelin	++–+++	–
Niemann–Pick disease type B	Sphingomyelinase	Sphingomyelin	++–+++	+
Farber disease	Acid ceramidase	Ceramide	+–+++	–
G_{M1}-gangliosidosis	β-Galactosidase	G_{M1} ganglioside	+–+++	–
Cholesterol transport defect				
Niemann–Pick disease type C	NPC1 or NPC2	Unesterified cholesterol/ sphingolipids	+–+++	–
Glycoprotein storage diseases				
Fucosidosis	α-L-Fucosidase	Fucose-rich oligosaccharides, glycolipids, and glycoproteins	+	–
α-Mannosidosis	α-Mannosidase	Mannose-rich oligosaccharides	+	–
Sialidosis	Lysosomal neuraminidase	Sialic acid-rich oligosaccharides, glycolipids, and glycoproteins	+	–
Galactosialidosis	Protective protein/ cathepsin A	Gangliosides and sialic acid-rich oligosaccharides and glycoproteins	+–+++	–
Glycogen storage disease				
Pompe disease	Acid α-glucosidase	Glycogen	+	+
Cholesteryl ester storage disorders				
Wolman disease	Lysosomal acid lipase	Cholesteryl esters, triglycerides	+→+++	–
Cholesteryl ester storage disease	Lysosomal acid lipase	Cholesteryl esters, triglycerides	+→+++	Phase III trials
Mucopolysaccharidoses				
Type I (Hurler, Scheie, Hurler–Scheie)	α-L-Iduronidase	Dermatan sulfate, heparan sulfate	+	+
Type II (Hunter) (attenuated and severe)	Iduronate sulfatase	Dermatan sulfate, heparan sulfate	+	+
Type IIIA (Sanfilippo A)	Heparan *N*-sulfatase	Heparan sulfate	+	–
Type IIIB (Sanfilippo B)	α-*N*-Acetylglucosaminidase	Heparan sulfate	+	-
Type IIIC (Sanfilippo C)	Acetyl-CoA: α-glucosaminide *N*-acetyltransferase	Heparan sulfate	+	–
Type IIID (Sanfilippo D)	*N*-acetylglucosamine 6-sulfatase	Heparan sulfate	+	–
Type IV (Morquio A)	Galactose 6-sulfatase	Keratan sulfate, chondroitin 6-sulfate	+	Phase III trials
Type IV (Morquio-B)	β-Galactosidase	Keratan sulfate	+	–
Type VI (Maroteaux-Lamy)	Arylsulfatase B	Dermatan sulfate	+	+
Type VII (Sly)	β-Glucuronidase	Dermatan sulfate, heparan sulfate, chondroitin 4-, 6-sulfates	+	–
Type IX	Hyaluronidase	Hyaluronic acid	+	–

Table 32.1 (*cont.*)

Disease	Protein defect	Storage material	Degree of liver involvement	Established therapy
Disorder of enzyme transport				
Mucolipidosis type II (I-cell disease)	Phosphotransferase	Oligosaccharides, glycosaminoglycans, lipids	+–++	–
Mucolipidosis type III (pseudo-Hurler)	Phosphotransferase	Oligosaccharides, glycosaminoglycans, lipids	+–++	–
Miscellaneous disorder				
Multiple sulfatase deficiency	FGly-generating enzyme	Sulfated glycosaminoglycans, glycolipids, glycopeptides, and hydroxysteroids	+	–

CoA, coenzyme A; +, ++, +++, or – refer to progressively severe involvement from absent (–) to (→) very severe (+++).

population and approximately 1 in 855 in the Ashkenazi Jewish population.

In visceral tissues, cells of macrophage lineage are primarily involved, whereas a variety of CNS neurons may be affected in some variants. These engorged macrophages, Gaucher cells, are 20–100 µm in diameter, with tubular inclusions resembling wrinkled tissue paper (Figure 32.2). Gaucher cells are abundant in liver, spleen, lung, bone marrow, and lymph nodes, and can lead to hepatosplenomegaly, anemia, thrombocytopenia, pulmonary disease, lymphadenopathy, and destructive bone disease.

Three clinical variants of Gaucher disease have been described, based upon the absence or presence and severity of neuronopathic disease.

Gaucher disease type 1. This is the non-neuronopathic variant and accounts for approximately 90% of cases of the disease in Europe and the USA. The associated phenotypes are restricted to visceral organs. The onset of disease is highly variable and occurs from childhood to adulthood. Survival is frequently reduced, but many patients live into adulthood. A significant number of patients are discovered serendipitously in the sixth to eighth decades of life. This variant is prevalent among those of Ashkenazi Jewish heritage.

Gaucher disease types 2 and 3. These variants are neuronopathic variants that are distinguished by the age of onset of neurologic signs and symptoms and their severity. Although relatively rare in the European and North American populations, these neuronopathic variants are most frequent in Asia, Africa, and South and Central America [3]. Gaucher disease type 2 can have onset in utero to 6 months of life, with rapidly progressing neurologic deterioration and visceral disease. Death occurs at a mean age of 9 months. Gaucher disease type 3 has less fulminant neuronopathic involvement. Indeed, horizontal supranuclear gaze palsy may present early without

progression and with concomitant variable degrees of visceral disease. Survival is usually less than 40 years [3]. The demarcation between types 2 and 3 is blurred and these variants represent a continuum of CNS disease.

Hepatomegaly is nearly universal in patients with Gaucher disease, and there is great variation in the degree of enlargement. Massive enlargement of the liver, up to 10-fold normal volume, can occur, and the largest livers are noted in the youngest and splenectomized patients [3]. Typically, the liver is enlarged 1.5- to 2.5-fold. Clinically, elevations of serum aminotransferase and alkaline phosphatase levels are frequent. Liver dysfunction, including hepatic failure occurs, but is infrequent [3]. The most significant clinical and histological liver disease is observed in patients who have had splenectomy.

Portal hypertension, with associated complications of esophageal varices, severe fibrosis and cirrhosis, and hepatic failure, has been reported [4] but is unusual and generally associated with concomitant viral infection (i.e. hepatitis C virus). Hepatocellular carcinoma is an unusual complication of Gaucher disease but has not been reported in children. This complication may be associated with secondary, known carcinogenic processes such as hepatitis B infection, but in a minority of patients there were no known risk factors other than Gaucher disease.

Grossly, the liver may appear yellow-brown in the presence of severe Gaucher cell replacement, grayish red with white streaks in Gaucher cell infiltration, or dark-red to purple in areas of extramedullary hematopoiesis [3]. In more severely affected patients, the liver may have micronodules or larger nodules (Figure 32.2).

Examination of liver biopsies from patients with Gaucher disease types 1, 2, and 3 reveals a broad spectrum of histopathological features [4]. Little difference is found in the pathological findings among patients with any of the three disease variants. However, cirrhosis was only observed in patients with Gaucher disease type 1 [4].

(a)

(b)

(c)

(d)

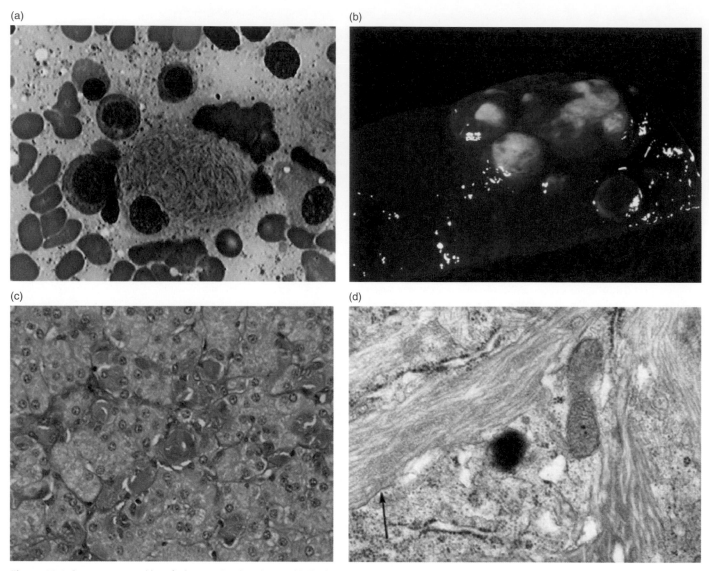

Figure 32.2 Bone marrow and liver findings in Gaucher disease. (a) The bone marrow macrophage is typical of the storage cells, that is, Gaucher cells. The typical "crinkled paper" cytoplasmic inclusions are evident. (b) Liver slice showing nodules (white/yellow) made up almost entirely of Gaucher cells. (c) By light microscopy, only Kuppfer cells contain visible storage material, glucosylceramide, whereas the hepatocytes do not. Periodic acid–Schiff staining is negative in Kuppfer cells. (d) Electron micrograph showing characteristic tubular storage material of Gaucher disease cellular inclusions (magnification ×20 000). (Courtesy of D. Witte.)

Gaucher cell accumulation and fibrosis are the most common pathological features of untreated disease. The degree of involvement varies from scattered aggregates of Gaucher cells in sinusoids with few other abnormalities to more severe manifestations. Pericellular fibrosis is commonly in a diffuse pattern, but severely atrophic and diminished numbers of hepatocytes is unusual. Central zonal (zone 3) distribution of Gaucher cells is common. The central veins are frequently compressed and obscured. Storage cell accumulation is occasionally noted in the portal zones, periportal regions, and mid-zones, but rarely to the degree observed in the central zones. Hepatocytes close to the storage cells may show degenerative changes and atrophy. Pericellular fibrosis is frequently observed and is characterized by thick fibrous septa surrounding

the central vein with replacement of the normal hepatic parenchyma in some cases. Fibrotic linkage of adjacent central zones by fibrous bands, with involvement of the portal triads, consistent with micronodular cirrhosis, as well as regenerative activity, has also been reported. Additionally, extramedullary hematopoiesis has been noted in a few patients. Cholestasis is not usually identified in pathological specimens [4].

Severe liver involvement in Gaucher disease type 1 manifests with enlarged, nodular livers with extensive central, acellular fibrosis, surrounded by parenchymal nodules, frequently incorporating portal tracts. The fibrous tissue may involve the portal tracts with focal ductal proliferation and surround small parenchymal nodules, some of which exhibit canalicular cholestasis. Gaucher cells are most often found at the fibrotic margins.

One study documented severe, early-onset liver dysfunction in a child with Gaucher disease type 2 [5]. The child presented at 7 days of age with cholestasis and hepatosplenomegaly. The clinical course was complicated by progressive portal hypertension, worsening degree of hepatosplenomegaly, but improvement in cholestasis. Liver histology showed progressive fibrosis, without inflammatory cell infiltrates, and Gaucher cells around the periportal space and surrounding the central hepatic veins. The child died of uncontrollable upper gastrointestinal bleeding at 4.5 months [5].

The diagnosis of Gaucher disease is made by demonstration of abnormally low acid β-glucosidase activity in nucleated cells, most commonly peripheral blood leukocytes or cultured skin fibroblasts. The enzyme is not normally present in erythrocytes or plasma/serum. It may also be diagnosed by the identification of pathogenic mutations in both copies of *GBA1*. Mutational analyses provide guidance for prognostication and the risk of CNS or non-CNS involvement, and overall disease severity [3]. These genotype–phenotype correlations are based on associations and are not definitive. Counseling based on risk factors is rapidly evolving and should be conducted by healthcare professionals with expertise in this area.

Treatment for the variants of Gaucher disease is based on the multisystem involvement and the need for coordinated care management plans. Although enzyme therapy (see below) has become the standard of care, treatment of patients with Gaucher disease involves supportive management for the complications of Gaucher disease, including appropriate orthopedic procedures and management of hematologic and CNS signs and symptoms. Bone marrow transplantation can prove curative; however, it carries a significant risk of complications and has limited use since the advent of enzyme therapy.

Enzyme therapy for the variants of Gaucher disease is the standard of care for the control and reversal of visceral manifestations. Intravenous enzyme therapy has not been proven to have direct beneficial effects on the CNS involvement but plays a supportive/palliative role for type 2, and can be lifesaving in type 3 disease. Enzyme therapy is provided by regular intravenous infusions of recombinant human acid β-glucosidase that has been modified for preferential uptake into macrophages. Therapeutic goals and expected outcomes have been developed and are frequently updated.

Three enzyme therapy products are currently approved for use in the treatment of Gaucher disease: imiglucerase (Cerezyme, Genzyme Corporation, Cambridge, MA, USA; approved by the US Food and Drug Administration in 1991), velaglucerase (VPRIV, Shire Human Genetic Therapies, Cambridge, MA, USA; approved in 2010), and taliglucerase alfa (Elelyso, Pfizer, New York, USA approved for adults in 2012). The products differ in their manufacturing processes, glycosylation patterns, and at amino acid residue 495.

In a study of 1028 patients with Gaucher disease type 1 treated with imiglucerase, a 20–30% decrease in liver volumes within 1–2 years was achieved after initiation of treatment. Additional reductions to near normal were achieved by 5 years.

In patients with massive livers, the rate of decrease was slower, but overall gains were substantial. These findings were concomitant with improvements in anemia and thrombocytopenia [6]. The dose dependency of these responses provides guidance for the use of these drugs. While enzyme therapy can stabilize existent advanced liver disease, irreversible damage may never respond. The safety profile of imiglucerase has been extensively reviewed and shows that the drug is generally safe and well tolerated. Although long-term data are not available for velaglucerase or taliglucerase alfa, phase II and III studies demonstrate similar safety and efficacy to imiglucerase.

Orthotopic liver transplantation has been successful in patients with end-stage liver disease. Regardless, primary therapies for the disease (enzyme therapy or substrate reduction therapy) remain an important component of treatment for these individuals, particularly to address the extrahepatic organ involvement.

A secondary therapy has been approved for use in patients in whom enzyme therapy cannot be used for medical reasons. The approach inhibits the synthetic pathway for glucosylceramide, glucosylceramide synthase. The overall concept is to allow the residual mutant enzyme present in all patients with Gaucher disease to degrade a smaller inflow of the substrate and thereby reduce storage. This approach might fill a void for patients who develop sensitivity to enzyme therapy or have additional complications that may not respond to enzyme treatments.

Miglustat (*N*-butyldeoxynojirimycin (Zavesca), Actelion Pharmaceuticals, South San Francisco, CA, USA), a substrate reduction agent, is licensed for use in the USA, Europe, and Israel in adults with mild to moderate Gaucher disease type 1 for whom enzyme replacement therapy is unavailable or contraindicated.

Clinical trials of miglustat have shown some effect on liver and splenic volumes, but hematologic status was only improved slightly. Miglustat may also help to reduce the incidence of bone pain and improve bone mineral density in affected patients. However, it has also become evident that miglustat monotherapy might not be sufficient to maintain the same adequate disease control in all patients. The drug also has several common side effects, including diarrhea and peripheral neuropathy, which may be unacceptable for some patients.

Phase I and II clinical trials of eliglustat tartrate, a second substrate reduction therapeutic agent, have been completed [7], and phase III clinical trials are currently underway. In the phase II study, 20 patients completed a total of 2 years of therapy. In these patients, statistically significant percentage improvements from baseline were observed for platelet count, hemoglobin level, spleen volume, liver volume, and bone mineral density of the lumbar spine. Greatest improvements in hemoglobin and organ-volume reductions were observed in individuals with more extensive baseline disease manifestations. In general, eliglustat tartrate is well tolerated at therapeutic doses. Indeed, most adverse events were mild to moderate in intensity, and many of the side effects noted for miglustat, especially diarrhea, were not experienced [7].

Neither enzyme replacement therapy nor substrate reduction therapy has demonstrated effectiveness in preventing or improving neurologic dysfunction in patients with Gaucher disease types 2 and 3.

Acid sphingomyelinase deficiency: Niemann–Pick types A and B

Acid sphingomyelinase deficiencies are heterogeneous, autosomal recessive lysosomal disorders characterized by an accumulation of undegraded sphingomyelin and other lipids in the lysosomes of multiple cell types, particularly those of macrophage/monocyte lineage, which are termed Niemann–Pick cells. The gene *SMPD1* encodes sphingomyelin phosphodiesterase-1 (acid sphingomyelinase) and maps to chromosome 11p15.4-p15.1. More than 50 mutations have been found in *SMPD1* of affected patients.

The two forms, NPA and NPB, are phenotypes within a continuum of disease that vary by age of onset, absence or presence of neurological disease, severity of features, and survival. Visceral features may include growth retardation; hepatomegaly, often without liver dysfunction; splenomegaly; gastrointestinal disturbances; hyperlipidemia; pulmonary disease; osteoporosis; lymphadenopathy; pancytopenia; and ocular abnormalities, particularly cherry red maculae. The incidence of NPA and NPB has not been well studied, and varies depending upon the specific population. However, the combined frequency of NPA and NPB was estimated at approximately 1 in 248 000 in Australia [8].

Niemann–Pick type A. This is the most severe phenotype and displays progressive neurovisceral disease within the first several months of life. Survival depends upon supportive care, but usually does not extend beyond age 2–3 years. Prolonged neonatal jaundice, hepatosplenomegaly, usually without liver dysfunction, and failure to thrive are among the earliest features [9]. Affected individuals experience progressive hypotonia, muscle weakness, intellectual decline, and loss of milestones that transforms to spasticity and rigidity at the end stages of the disease. It is particularly prevalent in the Ashkenazi Jewish population in which approximately 1 in 80 is a carrier [9].

Niemann–Pick type B. This is a heterogeneous, non-neuronopathic form with the visceral features described above. It is frequently diagnosed in childhood to adolescence with survival into adulthood. Hepatosplenomegaly is most prevalent during childhood but tends to become less conspicuous with age [9]. Within a subpopulation of patients with this subtype of disease, pulmonary disease is a significant source of morbidity. The disease is pan-ethnic in nature, with highest incidence in individuals of Turkish, Arabic, and North African descent, and less frequently among those of Ashkenazi Jewish heritage.

Intermediate variants of acid sphingomyelinase deficiency are common and are seen in over 60% of affected individuals in central Europe. These intermediate variants are defined by a cluster of visceral features and a protracted neuronopathic course. A rapidly progressive, early fatal, visceral variant without major CNS involvement has also been described.

Hepatomegaly is a common finding in acid sphingomyelinase deficiency. In 29 patients with NPB, the mean liver volume was 1.91-fold increased. Mild, stable elevations of serum aminotransferase and bilirubin were common in patients in this study [10]. Although not common in acid sphingomyelinase deficiency, hepatic fibrosis, cirrhosis, portal hypertension, and liver failure have been reported in adults and children, typically resulting in a poor outcome [11]. However, in a minority of patients, other comorbidities, such as hepatitis B virus, may have contributed to liver dysfunction. Orthotopic liver transplantation has been successfully performed in a number of individuals with NPB.

The liver in patients with NPB is often smooth, firm, and yellow to orange in coloration [11]. Hepatocytes and Kupffer cells contain vacuolated storage material within the cytoplasm, imparting a foamy appearance (Figure 32.3). Their distribution may initially be spotty, but may become generalized in later stages of the disease. Niemann–Pick cells are approximately 25 to 75 μm in size and stain negative with periodic acid–Schiff (PAS) stain, but positive for lipid with Sudan black B and Oil red O. During the disease course, Niemann–Pick cells initially accumulate in the sinusoids but later extend to involvement of the portal areas [9]. These cells can accumulate

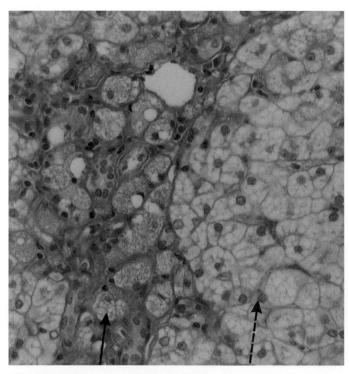

Figure 32.3 Photomicrograph of a liver section from a 6-year old girl with Neumann–Pick type B. Obvious "foamy" Kupffer cells are present (hyphenated arrow). Storage in hepatocytes is also clearly observed (sold arrow). The storage material is Periodic acid–Schiff–diastase negative (magnification ×400). (Courtesy of M. Collins.)

to such a degree within the sinusoids that intrahepatic obstruction can result. Ultrastructurally, the storage material resembles parallel membranes or concentrically laminated structures. Increasing degrees of fibrosis are observed and progressed to cirrhosis in advanced disease [11].

The diagnosis of NPB and NPA is established by the deficiency of acid sphingomyelinase in nucleated cells. The type and severity of disease does not correlate well to the amount of residual enzyme activity. The enzyme is not present in significant amounts in erythrocytes or plasma/serum. The diseases may also be diagnosed by the identification of pathogenic mutations in both copies of *SMPD1*.

Current management of NPB and NPA is symptomatic. Bone marrow transplantation (BMT) has been performed in multiple individuals with NPA and NPB, but despite evidence of engraftment, the patients exhibited progression of their CNS disease [12]. Enzyme replacement therapy has been developed and a phase I study evaluating the safety of the product in adults with NPB began in 2006.

Farber disease

Farber disease is a rare, progressive, autosomal recessively inherited lysosomal storage disorder resulting from mutations in *ASAH*, the gene encoding the lysosomal enzyme acid ceramidase. The diagnosis is established by detection of markedly deficient acid ceramidase activity in plasma, leukocytes, and cultured skin fibroblasts, or by molecular evaluation. The level of in vitro residual enzyme activity does not correlate with disease severity. *ASAH* is located at chromosome 8p21.3-p22. Many types of mutation result in Farber disease; however, genotype–phenotype correlations are not solid because of the rarity of the disease.

Several subtypes of Farber disease are recognized, varying by phenotypic features, severity and survival. Variable degrees of pulmonary, cardiac, hepatic, splenic, reticuloendothelial, and nervous system involvement may also be present [13].

Classic Farber disease. This is the most common subtype and is characterized by the classic triad of laryngeal, subcutaneous, and joint involvement that develops within the first months of life. Affected individuals experience failure to thrive. Swallowing dysfunction and pulmonary compromise develop as a result of granulomas in the epiglottis and larynx, requiring gastrostomy tube feedings and tracheostomies in the most severe cases [13]. These granulomatous lesions also occur in connective tissue, the heart, spleen, reticuloendothelial system, liver, bone, and the nervous system, contributing to the disease process [13]. Hepatomegaly is observed in approximately 40% of affected individuals, but liver dysfunction is uncommon [13]. Death occurs in the first few years of life, often from pulmonary disease [13]. An attenuated variant displays similar, albeit milder, features of the classical disease. The age of onset is later in childhood and survival is frequently into adulthood [13].

Neonatal-visceral subtype. This severe form has neonatal or early infantile onset and is characterized by liver dysfunction, with death occurring in early infancy, often before the development of classical features of Farber disease [13]. In the most severe cases, it may present as hydrops fetalis.

Progressive neurologic subtype. This is manifested by progressive, generalized, neurologic deterioration and seizures within the first few years of life, followed by death in early childhood. Although subcutaneous nodules and joint disease have been described in these patients, those features do not predominate and the visceral organs are not typically affected.

Pathologic features include an accumulation of storage material within macrophages or histiocytes, termed foam cells. Granulomas can be present and contain a central core of foam cells surrounded by macrophages, lymphocytes, and multinucleated cells, as well as fibrosis in older nodules [13]. Ultrastructurally, the foam cells contain distended lysosomes filled with curvilinear tubular structures, Farber bodies [13].

The liver can be firm, nodular in texture, and yellow in coloration [14]. The variable liver histopathology is a spectrum from microscopic normal to minimal fatty infiltration. In more severe disease, granulomatous lesions are present [14]. The liver in neonatal-visceral Farber disease can exhibit sinusoidal fibrosis, with weakly eosinophilic, vacuolated storage cells filling the sinusoids [14]. Mild intracellular and canalicular cholestasis can be present. Mild biliary ductal proliferation has been noted in the expanded portal zones [14].

Symptomatic management has been the therapy for the disease. Several individuals with classic Farber disease, including neurologic dysfunction, have received BMT. A significant improvement was observed in their visceral features, but neurological deterioration continued until death [15]. Recently, BMT in two patients with the attenuated phenotypes of Farber disease and normal neurological function led to significant reductions in the disease features and improvement in their quality of life [16].

G_{M1}-gangliosidosis

G_{M1}-gangliosidosis is a heterogeneous, progressive neurovisceral disorder that results from a deficiency of β-galactosidase with resultant G_{M1}-ganglioside, asialo-G_{M1}-ganglioside, oligosaccharides, and keratin sulfate accumulation in a variety of tissues. The disease is autosomal recessive and caused by mutations in *GLB1*, encoding the β-galactosidase. *GLB1* maps to chromosome 3p21.33. It has been well characterized and dozens of disease-causing mutations have been identified, including missense, nonsense, duplication, insertion, and splice defect mutations.

The disorder has three variants (types 1, 2, and 3), based upon age of onset, severity of neurological involvement,

Table 32.2 G_{M1} gangliosidosis variants

Parameter sign	Type 1	Type 2	Type 3
Age at onset	0–6 months	0.5–3 years	Childhood/adulthood
Hepatosplenomegaly	++→++++	++→+++	+/−
CNS progression	++++	+++	+++
Cherry-red spot	+++	+/−	Rare
Dysmorphic facies	+++	+	+
Skeletal dysplasia	+++	+	+/−
Death	1–2 years	5 years	Adulthood

The symbols +, ++, +++, ++++ or − refer to progressively severe involvement from absent (−) to (→) very severe (++++) of different clinical manifestations.

presence or absence of visceral disease, and survival (Table 32.2). The prevalence is approximately 1 in 384 000 individuals. The disease is allelic to another condition, Morquio type B disease (a mucopolysaccharidosis lacking neurologic or hepatic features), but only G_{M1}-gangliosidosis is discussed here. The condition has a similar phenotype to galactosialidosis, as β-galactosidase exists as a multienzyme complex with N-acetylgalactosamine-6-sulfate sulfatase and protective protein/cathepsin A and defects of the last (as seen in galactosialidosis) result in secondary deficiencies of β-galactosidase and N-acetylgalactosamine-6-sulfate sulfatase.

Early infantile-onset (type 1) G_{M1}-gangliosidosis. This presents within the first 6 months of life with significant neurodegenerative changes, feeding difficulties and failure to thrive, coarse features, cherry-red maculae, and dysostosis multiplex. Hepatomegaly is usually present at or shortly after birth, and is often associated with other features including generalized peripheral edema, ascites, or abnormalities in liver studies; the last may occur independently of hepatomegaly. Hydrops fetalis may be observed. Overt liver dysfunction is not usually present.

Late infantile/juvenile-onset (type 2) G_{M1}-gangliosidosis. This presents from around 6 months to 3 years of age and is associated with neurodegenerative disease. The patients may or may not exhibit coarse facies, cherry-red maculae, and hepatosplenomegaly [17]. Death frequently occurs by 5 years of age.

Adult-onset/chronic (type 3) G_{M1}-gangliosidosis. This is a slowly progressive CNS disease. Dementia, ataxia, speech disturbances, dystonia, and parkinsonism are common neurological features in this subtype. Hepatosplenomegaly may or may not be observed.

In hepatocytes, neurons, glomerular cells, and myocytes, storage material accumulates, stains pink with hematoxylin and eosin and is PAS positive [17]. Cells of monocyte/macrophage lineage, including Kupffer cells, also accumulate storage materials within affected organs [17]. Ultrastructurally,

affected cells exhibit numerous, pleomorphic storage material-laden lysosomes that appear empty or contain fibrillar and granular material. The liver can appear normal under microscopic examination, particularly in individuals with later onset disease [17].

G_{M1}-gangliosidosis is diagnosed by demonstrating severely decreased acid β-galactosidase activity in lymphocytes, fibroblasts, or plasma. The disease can be confirmed molecularly by the detection of *GLB1* mutations. Well-defined genotype–phenotype correlations have not been recognized; therefore, mutation analysis cannot be used to predict the clinical phenotype. Although the disease phenotype does not correlate well with the level of residual enzyme activity, individuals with greater degrees of residual enzyme activity have generally been noted to have later onset and milder disease [17]. The detection of complex carbohydrates in the urine, including keratin sulfate, adds further support to the diagnosis, but is not diagnostic.

The treatment for this disease is symptomatic management. Bone marrow transplantation is generally unsuccessful in stabilizing/reversing the neurological deterioration in individuals with G_{M1}-gangliosidosis.

Niemann–Pick disease type C

Although originally classified with NPA and NPB variants as an acid sphingomyelinase deficiency, the two forms of NPC (NPC1 and NPC2) result from lipid-trafficking defects that are not primarily related to *SMPD1* mutations. The NPC1 and NPC2 phenotypes are essentially identical [18,19]. However, the NPC nomenclature is engrained in the literature and will be used here. The prevalence of NPC has been estimated to be approximately 1 in 120 000–150 000 in Western Europe; however, it is pan-ethnic in nature [18,20]. Based on age of onset, CNS features, and survival, three clinical forms have been delineated: neonatal/infantile, childhood, and adolescent/adult [21].

NPC1 and NPC2 are autosomal recessive neurovisceral diseases with highly variable ages of onset, pathological features, and survival [19,20]. Defective lipid trafficking, storage of lipids (unesterified cholesterol, phospholipids, sphingomyelin, and glycolipids) in lysosomes of affected cells, and secondary sphingomyelinase deficiency results in progressive neurocognitive dysfunction with visceral disease, particularly hepatic and splenic involvement [20]. Although the onset and degree of progression is variable among the phenotypes, visceral disease (when present) may occur before or after the development of neurological symptoms [19]. However, the visceral findings may be absent or minimal, particularly in adult-onset disease, particularly at the time of diagnosis [19].

The neonatal/infantile subtype accounts for around 20–30% of NPC. The disease is a rapidly progressive neurovisceral disease, presenting within the first few months of life as developmental delay. Severe hepatic dysfunction can manifest perinatally, as ascites or hydrops fetalis. In early infancy, liver disease/dysfunction (i.e. infantile cholestatic disease or idiopathic neonatal hepatitis) often develops, frequently in association with progressive hepatosplenomegaly [19,22]. In approximately 10% of such patients, hepatic failure develops and death occurs [22]. Those surviving show resolution by the second to fourth months of life. Hepatosplenomegaly may remain, but splenomegaly is usually predominant [22]. However, survivors may "grow into their organs" such that hepatosplenomegaly may not be detected later in childhood [21].

Of those who recover from the liver dysfunction, some immediately demonstrate neurological symptoms whereas others have resolution of symptoms only to present at a later age with progressive neurodegenerative disease, including hypotonia, developmental delay, loss of acquired skills, spasticity, dystonia, dysphagia, seizures, and pyramidal signs [20,21].

Vertical supranuclear gaze palsy is classically observed in individuals with NPC but is not as common in those with neonatal/infantile presentations as in other subtypes [20]. Generalized failure to thrive and growth retardation occur.

In some infants, particularly those with mutations of *NPC2*, a significant infiltrative pulmonary disease may also occur as a primary feature or accompanying hepatic involvement, which may act as a significant source of morbidity and mortality [21]. Death usually occurs by 5 years of age.

The childhood NPC1 variant accounts for about 50–70% of affected individuals. Children with this variant may initially have normal development, but by early to late childhood, they exhibit neurocognitive deterioration, initially presenting as clumsiness, behavioral problems, and poor school performance [20]. Psychiatric disturbances, including psychosis, may develop around the time of puberty. Other signs of neurodegenerative disease gradually appear, including ataxia, vertical supranuclear gaze palsy, dystonia, seizures, cataplexy, dysarthria, and dysphagia [20]. Dysphagia is progressive and eventually makes oral feeding impossible. The individuals eventually become dependent on caregivers for all of their needs. Survival into teenage years and adulthood can occur, and death is usually the result of pulmonary disease [20]. Significant liver dysfunction is unusual.

The adolescent/adult-onset NPC2 variant accounts for around 5–10% of cases and presents with psychiatric and/or neurological symptoms. Indeed, these findings frequently overshadow the visceral findings of the disease [20]. The psychiatric symptoms often mimic depression or schizophrenia and can be quite debilitating. Dementia often occurs, but there is a slower rate of progression than in other subtypes of the disease. Vertical supranuclear gaze palsy may be subtle and difficult to recognize. Hepatomegaly and splenomegaly are observed in approximately 13% and 50% of patients, respectively [20].

Histopathologically, NPC exhibits accumulation of free cholesterol and sphingolipids within cells of monocyte/macrophage origin, in the visceral organs (i.e. hepatocytes), and

neurons and glial cells of the nervous system [20]. The storage cells exhibit a foamy appearance and stain positively with PAS and filipin. Because of their microscopic appearance, storage cells of monocyte/macrophage origin are often referred to as "foam cells." Ultrastructurally, these lipid-laden cells contain numerous, pleomorphic membrane-bound lipid inclusions with structures varying from crystalline to electron-dense laminated inclusions [22].

At autopsy, the liver is enlarged and firm, with a surface that is pale yellow to green in appearance [23]. The neonatal liver disease may resemble idiopathic neonatal hepatitis with severe giant cell transformation of the hepatic cells and/or cholestasis [22,24]. Liver biopsies from 25 individuals with a history of neonatal liver disease showed cellular and canalicular cholestasis with biliary rosette formation with variable degrees of parenchymal damage, little hepatocellular necrosis, but evidence of previous cell loss in the form of reticulin collapse. The last was severe enough to produce bridging collapse and/or prominent fibrosis-induced fragmentation of the specimen core in half of the individuals. In addition to lobular inflammation, four patients had hematopoietic activity and multinucleated giant hepatocytes. Portal edema and ductal proliferation were also observed. In early biopsy specimens, the identification of storage cells was difficult because of the presence of activated Kupffer cells loaded with ceroid and bile pigment [22].

Liver biopsy specimens of 15 patients with a history of mild, persistent liver disease 1 to 8 years after resolution of symptoms showed that inflammation and cholestasis had vanished (12 of 15), but variable degrees of inactive, postnecrotic fibrosis remained, with progression to cirrhosis in five. Storage material was noted in some hepatocytes and storage cells were identified in the parenchyma and to a lesser extent within portal and fibrous areas [22]. In patients without a history of liver dysfunction, normal hepatic architecture was present, but there was obvious storage material in hepatocytes and Kupffer cells [22].

Mutations of two genes, *NPC1* and *NPC2*, are present in NPC. The *NPC1* and *NPC2* genes map to chromosomes 18q11-q12 and 14q24.3, respectively. The *NPC1* gene product functions as an integral membrane transport protein in the lysosomal/late endosomal system for cholesterol, glycolipids, and other materials [18,20]. The *NPC2* gene product is a soluble lysosomal cholesterol transporter. Abnormal function of the NPC1 and NPC2 proteins leads to accumulation of free cholesterol and glycolipids within the lysosomes as well as a secondary sphingomyelinase deficiency. Additionally, delayed low density lipoprotein-mediated regulatory responses appear to contribute to the disease process [18,20]. *NPC1* mutations account for approximately 95% of NPC; *NPC2* mutations account for the remaining 5%. Although mutations in both genes result in remarkably similar phenotypes, severe pulmonary disease is a unique complication in patients with *NPC2* mutations and is a cause of early demise.

Because of the variability in phenotypes within this disease, NPC is not always initially suspected. The diagnosis is often delayed because of the absence of hepatosplenomegaly or storage cells in the bone marrow at initial presentation. However, NPC should be considered in all patients with idiopathic neonatal hepatitis [24]. A biochemical diagnosis can be made by the demonstration of impaired cholesterol esterification and positive filipin staining in cultured fibroblasts. Despite accumulation of sphingolipids in the lysosomes of affected cells, sphingomyelinase activity is normal. Molecular studies may also be employed for diagnosis but this method is often somewhat challenging, as many disease-causing mutations are private.

The treatment of patients with NPC relies upon symptom management, particularly the neurologic and psychiatric symptoms. Although BMT has been studied, this had no impact on the neurologic dysfunction and ultimate disease course. Likewise, liver transplantation improved hepatic function but did not appear to ameliorate CNS disease progression.

Various pharmacologic agents have also been studied as potential disease-specific therapies for NPC, including cholesterol-lowering therapies, sterol-binding agents, and neurosteroids, with varying degrees of success. Recently miglustat has been studied as a treatment for the neurologic manifestations observed in NPC. Miglustat is an *N*-alkylated imino sugar that functions as a competitive inhibitor of glucosylceramide synthase. Preclinical studies showed that miglustat is capable of crossing the blood–brain barrier and reducing excess storage of neurotoxic glycolipids, which are thought to contribute to the neurologic manifestations in NPC [25]. Clinical trials of miglustat in children and adolescents/adults indicated that the agent might have some efficacy at stabilizing the neurologic manifestations of NPC [26]. Indeed, based upon these studies, miglustat was approved by the European Union in 2009 for the treatment of neurologic manifestations in adults and children with NPC. However, a recent study of miglustat in a mouse model of Sandhoff disease (a lysosomal storage disease with CNS and visceral manifestations) showed unanticipated elevations in glycosphingolipids in the CNS despite delayed loss of motor function and coordination and extended lifespan [27]. This finding is contradictory to the expected finding of diminished levels of glycosphingolipids in the CNS. The significance of this finding is unclear, but it warrants further investigation to ensure the long-term safety of this agent, with particular emphasis on CNS disease, in patients with similar conditions.

Miglustat has not been demonstrated to have an effect on the visceral manifestations of the disease. Additionally, certain side effects, including gastrointestinal signs (e.g. osmotic diarrhea, weight loss, bloating, and belching), and neurological signs (e.g. tremor and peripheral neuropathy) are frequently reported in patients taking miglustat, similar to patients with Gaucher disease treated with miglustat (see above).

Additionally, cyclodextrin has been explored as a potential therapeutic agent for NPC1.

Disorders of glycoprotein degradation

Fucosidosis, α-mannosidosis, sialidosis, and galactosialidosis are lysosomal storage diseases resulting from defects in glycoprotein degradation. Deficiencies of specific exoglycosidases result in an inability to remove terminal sugar moieties from glycoproteins and oligosaccharides, and in the subsequent accumulation of excessive amounts of undigested substrates in the lysosomes of affected cells. All are inherited as autosomal recessive traits.

Fucosidosis

Fucosidosis is caused by a deficiency in the lysosomal enzyme α-L-fucosidase, which cleaves fucose moieties from the non-reducing end of a variety of oligosaccharides, glycoproteins, and glycolipids [28]. A deficiency in this enzyme results in cellular accumulation and urinary excretion of fucose-containing macromolecules, including oligosaccharides, glycoproteins, and glycolipids in the lysosomes of affected cells [28,29]. The gene for α-L-fucosidase (*FUCA1*) has been mapped to chromosome 1p34-1p36, and many types of mutations have been shown to result in fucosidosis, including point mutations, deletions, duplications, and insertions.

The clinical features include varying degrees of hearing loss, ocular abnormalities, coarse facial appearance, skeletal dysplasia, hepatosplenomegaly, frequent infections, growth retardation, skin abnormalities (including angiokeratoma and telangiectasia), and progressive neurologic deterioration and mental retardation [29]. Variability in disease severity may be seen even in individuals with similar phenotypes, including members of the same family [29]. The disease is pan-ethnic with about 100 cases being described worldwide. A relatively high number of patients have Italian and the Mexican-Native American (Colorado and New Mexico) backgrounds [29].

The two variants (types I and II), are probably more appropriately viewed as a continuum of severities [29]. In the more severe type I presentations, patients experience neurologic dysfunction within the first year of life, often progressing to a vegetative, decorticate state, with death occurring prior to 6 years of age [28]. Conversely, individuals with type II disease are distinguished by a less severe and slower rate of progression of phenotypic features, usually beginning between 1 and 2 years of life, and longer survival (~3 decades) [28,29]. Angiokeratoma and telangiectasia develop with age. The other phenotypic features of fucosidosis are relatively consistent among individuals displaying both phenotypes.

The hepatic findings are mild and characterized by non-progressive hepatomegaly and/or elevation in liver function studies. In one study, 40% of those affected with fucosidosis exhibited hepatomegaly and 25% had elevations in their liver enzymes, independent of liver volume [29]. Liver dysfunction does not occur and liver failure has not been described in patients with fucosidosis [29].

By light microscopy, affected cells have a foamy appearance. Ultrastructurally, the storage material is heterogeneous in appearance (light and reticular, electron dense, or lamellar) a consequence of the many types of fucose-containing macromolecules stored in this disease [28–30].

Detailed and electron microscopic examination of liver biopsy tissue from a boy aged 3½ years with fucosidosis revealed well-preserved architecture and no signs of an inflammatory process or fibrosis. Many cell types, including Kupffer cells, hepatocytes, bile duct epithelial cells, and blood vessel endothelial cells, were packed with storage-material-laden vacuoles [30]. Foam cells were regularly seen in the portal areas. The sinusoids were frequently obscured by storage material-laden Kupffer cells, and isolated necrotic periportal cells were occasionally observed. Ultrastructurally, the storage material was heterogeneous in appearance.

Fucosidosis is often suspected upon recognition of the classical pattern of phenotypic features. Evidence of excessive urinary excretion of fucose-containing oligosaccharides and glycoproteins by thin layer chromatography further supports the diagnosis. Diagnosis of fucosidosis requires the demonstration of severely diminished α-L-fucosidase activity (<5%) in cultured fibroblasts and white blood cells or by mutation analysis. However, enzymatic diagnosis must be made cautiously because 10% of the normal population carries a polymorphism that reduces the enzyme activity to 10–30% of control [29].

Treatment for this disorder relies mostly upon symptomatic management. An 8-month-old boy received BMT because of early neurological involvement by fucosidosis. Despite evidence of mild neurodevelopmental delay, the procedure was considered a success as he exhibited a less severe phenotype than his sibling who did not receive a transplant [31]. Gene and enzyme therapies are not available for this disorder.

α-Mannosidosis

α-Mannosidosis is an autosomal recessive disorder caused by a deficiency of the lysosomal enzyme α-mannosidase, resulting in an accumulation of mannose-rich macromolecules in affected cells. α-Mannosidase cleaves terminal mannose moieties from oligosaccharides and glycoproteins. The deficiency of α-mannosidase leads to an accumulation of α-mannosyl-terminated compounds in lysosomes of cells and in urine. The gene for α-mannosidase (MANB) has been mapped to chromosome 19p13-q12. α-Mannosidosis results from a variety of disease-causing mutations of MANB, including splice site, missense, nonsense, insertions, and deletions. Because of the rarity of the condition, genotype–phenotype correlations are not well described.

The variable phenotypic features include progressive mental deterioration, coarse facial appearance, deafness, ocular abnormalities, skeletal dysplasia, recurrent infections, hernias, and hepatosplenomegaly [28]. The disease has a prevalence of approximately 1 in 500 000 [7].

Two variants (types I and II) are have been classically described based on age of onset and severity of disease.

Individuals exhibiting type I α-mannosidosis present in infancy with severe, rapidly progressive mental deterioration and clinical features, and death often occurs within the first decade of life [28]. Type II α-mannosidosis has a more slowly progressive phenotype with normal early development, but mental deterioration, hearing loss and other clinical features become apparent by childhood or adolescence [28]. Hepatomegaly is present, particularly in type I, but hepatic dysfunction does not occur.

Through further characterization of the condition, significant phenotypic variability has been identified (even among individuals with similar phenotypes, i.e. affected relatives) such that it may be more appropriate to consider α-mannosidosis as a continuum of disease presentations. Considering this, an alternative classification scheme, consisting of three variants has been described: type 1 is a "mild" variant with slowly progressive neurologic deterioration, myopathy, absence of skeletal abnormalities, and recognition at >10 years of age; type 2 is a moderate variant with skeletal abnormalities, myopathy, slowly progressive neurologic deterioration, and recognition in the first decade of life; and type 3 is a severe, early-onset (prenatal or early infancy) phenotype with skeletal abnormalities and rapidly progressive neurologic involvement, leading to death at an early age.

Liver biopsies show well-preserved architecture with no signs of inflammation. Fibrosis can be present in the portal areas and around Kupffer cells. Hepatocytes, bile duct epithelial cells, Kupffer cells, and blood vessel endothelial cells are engorged with storage-material-laden vacuoles. Foam cells are consistently found in the portal areas. The sinusoids can be obscured by engorged Kupffer cells. The storage material is heterogeneous by electron microscopy [32].

Definitive diagnosis of the disorder requires the demonstration of low levels of α-mannosidase activity in cultured fibroblasts or white blood cells or the presence of disease causing mutations in both MANB alleles [28].

Symptomatic management is the mainstay of treatment but BMT in affected children (<2 years of age) may lead to resolution of the sinopulmonary disease and organomegaly, improvement in the skeletal disease, and variable effects on neurocognitive function. However, there may also be significant morbidity/morality from the procedure.

Recent studies evaluating enzyme replacement and gene therapies in animal α-mannosidosis models have provided optimism that disease-specific treatment for this condition may be available in the future.

Sialidosis

Sialidosis is an autosomal recessive disorder caused by a deficiency of the lysosomal enzyme α-neuraminidase, resulting in accumulation of sialic acid-rich molecules in the lysosomes and excretion in the urine. The disease is rare, approximately 1 in 4 000 000 live births.

Its clinical features vary according to age of onset, organ involvement, and severity of symptoms. The two variants of sialidosis (types I and II) vary in age of onset and progression, but share progressive CNS disease and cherry-red spots.

Sialidosis type I. This milder, adult-onset phenotype is characterized by progressive ophthalmological disease (visual impairment and development of cherry-red spots) and neurologic disease (myoclonus, ataxia, seizures, and nystagmus). For this reason, the condition is also frequently referred to as "cherry-red spot-myoclonus syndrome." The visceral findings (including liver involvement) are generally absent in individuals with this variant [28].

Sialidosis type II. This most severe form of the condition is an early-onset (occasionally congenital), mucopolysaccharidosis-like phenotype, with progressive neurological and visceral disease [28]. Hepatosplenomegaly is universal but liver dysfunction does not occur. Many patients with type II disease are stillborn; however, some individuals may survive into the second decade of life [28].

The gene for lysosomal neuraminidase (*NEU1*) has been mapped to chromosome 6p21.3, and mutations in this gene are responsible for both subtypes of sialidosis. The enzyme exists as a multienzyme complex with β-galactosidase and protective protein cathepsin A. The last is critical for lysosomal transport and proper function of lysosomal neuraminidase [33,34].

Neuraminidase catalyzes the cleavage of terminal α2,3- and α2,6-linked sialic acid residues from numerous sialic acid-rich oligosaccharides and glycoproteins [34]. A deficiency in this enzyme results in cellular accumulation of sialic acid-containing glycopeptides and oligosaccharides in the urine and lysosomes of affected cells.

The liver histology in type II disease shows well-preserved architecture and membrane-bound vacuoles containing heterogeneous material in the hepatocytes, Kupffer cells, and vascular endothelial cells. The sinusoids can be widened and occluded by Kupffer cells and free foamy material. There was no evidence of necrosis, fibrosis, or inflammatory infiltration in several studies [30]. Hepatomegaly is not a feature of type I disease, but storage material can be observed by light microscopy [28].

Sialidosis is often suspected when the phenotypic features described above are observed. Definitive diagnosis of the disorder requires the demonstration of low levels of lysosomal neuraminidase activity in cultured fibroblasts or identification of two pathogenic mutations in *NEU1* [28]. Galactosialidosis, a similar disorder with defective β-galactosidase and neuraminidase activities, can confuse the diagnosis. The presence of large amounts of mannose-containing oligosaccharides and glycopeptides in the urine support the diagnosis. Therapy is symptomatic.

Galactosialidosis

Galactosialidosis is an autosomal recessively inherited, heterogeneous disorder caused by a defect in the protein protective protein/cathepsin A; the gene has been mapped to chromosome 20q13.1. Protective protein/cathepsin A forms a multienzyme complex with β-galactosidase and lysosomal α-neuraminidase and is required for proper intracellular transport and function of both enzymes [33,34]. Additionally, it has separate enzymatic functions. Consequently, defects in this enzyme results in defective β-galactosidase and lysosomal neuraminidase activity, with a resultant accumulation of sialic acid-rich oligosaccharides and glycoproteins and gangliosides in affected cells, and excretion of sialic acid-rich oligosaccharides in the urine [33]. Galactosialidosis has a prevalence of approximately 1 in 2.5 million in the Netherlands [2].

Because the disorder is partially a result of lysosomal neuraminidase deficiency, many of its phenotypic characteristics are similar to sialidosis, including coarse facies, cherry-red spots, and dysostosis multiplex. Galactosialidosis is classified into three subtypes based on age of onset, organ involvement, and severity of disease: early infantile, late infantile, and juvenile/adult onset [33].

Early infantile phenotype. In addition to the features described above, those with the early infantile phenotype demonstrate fetal hydrops, edema, ascites, kidney disease, neurodegeneration, and early death (mean, ~7 months) [33]. Hepatosplenomegaly develops early and the liver can reach volumes greater than two times normal. Elevations in liver enzymes may be observed, but overt liver dysfunction does not occur.

Late infantile phenotype. The presentation is characterized by growth retardation, cardiac involvement, and, less frequently, neurologic involvement. This phenotype is compatible with prolonged survival.

Juvenile/adult-onset phenotype. This is particularly associated with neurologic signs/symptoms and angiokeratoma, with a similar distribution and appearance as in fucosidosis and Fabry disease. This phenotype is also compatible with prolonged survival [33].

Hepatosplenomegaly of lesser degrees than seen in the early infantile presentation may be observed in the later onset presentations, but liver dysfunction does not occur. On microscopic examination, hepatocytes, Kupffer cells, and epithelial cells contain numerous storage material-containing vacuoles. Ultrastructurally, the storage material is quite heterogeneous in appearance.

A diagnosis of galactosialidosis requires the demonstration of decreased β-galactosidase, lysosomal neuraminidase, and cathepsin A enzyme activity in white blood cells or cultured skin fibroblasts or mutation analysis. Determination of cathepsin A activity, solely, is not advisable as one could theoretically fail to identify a patient with a defect in the protective rather than the catalytic function of the enzyme [33]. Therapy relies upon symptom management. However, mouse studies have suggested a potential benefit of bone marrow transplantation.

Glycogen storage disease type II (Pompe disease)

Glycogen storage disease type II (Pompe disease) is an autosomal recessive disorder caused by a deficiency in the lysosomal enzyme acid α-glucosidase, which results in an abnormal accumulation of glycogen in lysosomes of cells. The gene *GAA* maps to chromosome 17q25.2-q25.3.

The three phenotypes vary by age of onset and severity and progression of symptoms: infantile, childhood/juvenile, and adult onset. The disease is rare with a frequency of 1 in 14 000–300 000 depending on the geographic area or ethnic group [35].

The clinical phenotypes have classically been considered to result from glycogen accumulation in cardiac, skeletal, and smooth muscles. However, many other cells contain excessive glycogen, including neurons. Although their role in the disease process is not clear, evidence suggest that involvement of the CNS and the peripheral nervous system is a significant contributor to the clinical phenotype.

The "classic" infantile phenotype of glycogen storage disease type II is a severe, progressive disease that presents within the first few months of life with feeding problems, poor weight gain, cardiac disease, respiratory difficulties, macroglossia, and generalized myopathy [35,36]. Despite the presence of a severe myopathic disease, skeletal muscles are often firm and hypertrophic in appearance [35]. Cardiomegaly results from a progressive hypertrophic cardiomyopathy that affects the walls of both ventricles and the interventricular septum, with diminished volume of the ventricular chambers [35] (Figure 32.4). Moderate hepatomegaly without liver dysfunction is noted in up to 90% of patients [36]. Feeding difficulties are almost universal in this patient population, and patients often require enteral sources of nutritional support. Impairment of the respiratory muscles results in respiratory difficulties and many also require assisted ventilation. Cognition is considered grossly normal [35]; however, neuromuscular disease results in obvious neurologic abnormalities and associated fine and gross motor skill delays. The disease is rapidly progressive and death occurs with a median age of 9 months [35]. Residual

(a) (b)

(c)

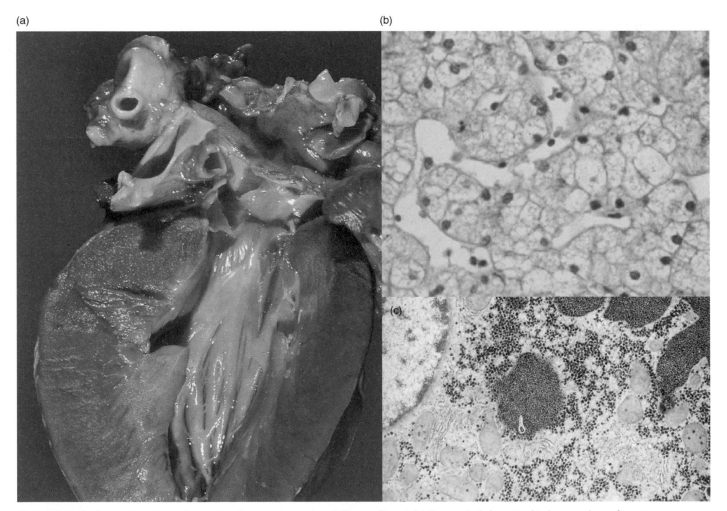

Figure 32.4 Cardiac and hepatic involvement in glycogen storage type II (Pompe disease). (a) The massively hypertrophied myocardium of a patient younger than 1 year with infantile Pompe disease. (b) Photomicrograph showing massive glycogen accumulation in hepatocytes and Kupffer cells (hemotoxylin & eosin staining.) (c) Ultrastructure showing lysosomal and free cytoplasmic glycogen particles (magnification ×200 000). (Courtesy of K. Bove.)

tissue acid α-glucosidase levels are less than 1% of normal in affected patients.

A less common phenotype with early onset has been described with less severe cardiac disease. Such patients show progressive muscle weakness and hypotonia within the first few months of life. Pseudohypertrophy of the calf muscles and Gower sign may cause this variant to resemble Duchenne muscular dystrophy [37]. Ventilatory insufficiency, frequently requiring ventilatory assistance, is a significant source of morbidity and mortality for this population. Indeed, ventilatory failure is a frequent cause of death, which often occurs in early childhood [37].

The childhood/juvenile-onset phenotype is primarily a neuromuscular variant with onset in the first decade. Cardiac disease is uncommon [35]. Typically, delayed motor milestones, progressive proximal muscle weakness, and involvement of the respiratory muscles are present [35]. Pulmonary compromise can lead to the need for ventilatory assistance, particularly during sleep. Many individuals become wheelchair bound. Moderate hepatomegaly without liver dysfunction is observed in up to 30% of affected patients. The levels of residual enzyme activity in tissue is frequently less than 10% of normal. Death usually results from respiratory failure [35].

The adult onset phenotype is a neuromuscular variant with slowly progressive proximal myopathy with respiratory insufficiency in about 30% and onset in the third to sixth decades [35]. However, many patients recall symptoms from childhood. The lower extremities are often more significantly involved than the upper extremities, and regional variation in muscle involvement occurs [35]. Cardiac complications are not common and moderate hepatomegaly without liver dysfunction is observed in around 30% [38]. Serum aminotransferases may be elevated in this population, but this may represent enzyme release from muscle tissues. Individuals with adult-onset disease have higher levels of residual enzyme activity (possibly 40% of normal) than those with infantile- or childhood/juvenile-onset disease. Like the juvenile-onset phenotype, many individuals are eventually wheelchair bound, and impairment of the respiratory muscles frequently results in respiratory difficulties, often requiring ventilatory support, particularly during sleep [35,39]. Death usually occurs from respiratory failure.

Pompe disease results from the accumulation of glycogen of normal structure within lysosomes and cytoplasm of affected cells, including liver, heart, smooth and skeletal muscle, and nervous system [35]. The storage material stains positively with PAS. Within the liver, glycogen is abundant and is in the form of scattered cytoplasmic rosettes and smaller β- and α-particles in the lysosomes (Figure 32.4) [35]. The liver architecture remains intact.

Pompe disease is suspected in infants with massive cardiomegaly and hypotonia/muscle weakness. The diagnosis may be more elusive in individuals with muscle weakness and lack of severe cardiac involvement (i.e. those with atypical phenotypes or later-onset disease). Diagnosis requires the detection of markedly diminished acid α-glucosidase activity in cultured fibroblasts and/or muscle tissue. However, the levels of residual acid α-glucosidase in adults can approach levels observed in unaffected carriers and the lower end values found in normal individuals, confusing the diagnosis [35]. The diagnosis can be confirmed by the discovery of disease-causing mutations in both alleles of GAA. In general, mutations that lead to the least amounts of residual enzyme activity are associated with infantile-onset disease and those that result in greater amounts of enzyme activity cause juvenile- and adult-onset disease [35].

Althought BMT has been performed, it was unsuccessful. Enzyme therapy with recombinant algucosidase alfa is the standard of care for the treatment of Pompe disease. Myozyme (alglucosidase alfa, Genzyme, Cambridge, MA, USA) is approved for use in infantile Pompe disease, whereas Lumizyme (alglucosidase alfa, Genzyme) is approved for the treatment of patients 8 years and older with non-infantile variants of Pompe disease. Both preparations are administered by intravenous infusions at doses of 20–40 mg/kg every 2 weeks.

In clinical trials of alglucosidase alfa, significant improvement in overall survival, survival free of ventilatory support, and improvement in cardiac structure and function were noted compared with untreated patients. Progress in motor development was more variable but the results suggested that patients who begin enzyme replacement therapy at an early age (i.e. <6 months) experience greater improvement in motor function than those who begin receiving therapy at later ages [40]. Similarly, clinical trials of Lumizyme in individuals with later-onset disease have shown stabilization of motor and pulmonary function in treated patients. Some individuals may develop IgE antibodies, which may be associated with anaphylactic reactions. Furthermore, some patients may develop IgG antibodies to the recombinant enzyme, diminishing its effectiveness. Enzyme replacement therapy is not expected to cross the blood–brain barrier and, therefore, is not expected to have a therapeutic effect on the neurologic manifestations.

Supportive therapy is an important component in the treatment of this disease and can improve the quality of life and minimize complications. However, it does not alter the disease course.

Lysosomal acid lipase deficiency: Wolman disease and cholesteryl ester storage disease

Deficiency of lysosomal acid lipase leads to the accumulation of cholesteryl esters, triglycerides, and other lipids within the lysosomes. Two major phenotypes include Wolman disease and cholesteryl ester storage disease (CESD).

The gene LIPA encodes lysosomal acid lipase and maps to chromosome 10q23.2-q23.3. Both diseases result from mutations in LIPA with nearly complete deficiency of lysosomal acid lipase activity in Wolman disease and significant residual enzyme activity in CESD.

Wolman disease presents in the neonatal period with feeding difficulties, persistent forceful vomiting, profuse watery diarrhea, abdominal distension, progressive hepatomegaly, and failure to thrive because of malabsorption. The malabsorption syndrome does not improve with medical interventions or changes in diet and may necessitate parenteral nutrition. Generalized lymphadenopathy and splenomegaly are also present. Neurologic development is not normal, but specific signs related to CNS dysfunction are uncommon and may relate to malnutrition and severe disability [41].

Radiographic evaluation reveals enlarged adrenal glands with punctuate calcifications. Laboratory studies reveal progressive anemia, vacuolization of the lymphocytes, and elevated serum aminotransferases indicative of hepatic involvement. Plasma cholesterol and triglycerides levels are usually normal. Death occurs within the first year. Wolman disease is rare and has an incidence of approximately 1 in 500 000 [7].

Cholesteryl ester storage disease is a heterogeneous disorder that can present between infancy to adulthood. Hepatomegaly is the primary and sometimes sole finding in this phenotype. Hepatic involvement is often progressive with pathologic features of non-alcoholic steatosis and fibrosis with progression to cirrhosis. Some patients affected with CESD can have a more severe course with symptoms much like those in Wolman disease, including vomiting and watery diarrhea, failure to thrive, adrenal calcification, and liver dysfunction. Laboratory studies often reveal hyperlipidemia, particularly type IIb hyperlipoproteinemia, and elevated serum aminotransferases.

Progressive, premature atherosclerosis occurs and may result in vascular compromise. Age of death is variable and depends on severity of hepatic and atherosclerotic disease, but survival into adulthood is common. The incidence of homozygotes for the most common mutation in CESD (an exon 8 splice junction mutation leading to E8SJM,) was estimated to be approximately 1 in 170 000 in Germany [42].

Cholesteryl esters and triglycerides accumulate in the liver and other affected organs but not the CNS. This storage material stains positively with Oil red O and Sudan black, and cholesterol crystals are observed under polarized light in frozen sections. In fixed tissues, clefts or voids can be visualized, representing lipid that was dissolved during tissue fixation. This storage material has an equally heterogeneous appearance under the electron microscope [41].

The liver of patients with Wolman disease is markedly enlarged (often greater than two times the normal size), firm in consistency, and yellow in coloration, with a cut surface that is greasy. Hepatic architecture may be preserved early in the course, but may become quite distorted [43]. Hepatocytes and Kupffer cells are engorged with lipid laden vacuoles (Figure 32.5). Foam cells are present in the portal and periportal areas and tend to cluster between parenchymal cells. Infiltration with inflammatory cells occurs. Portal and periportal fibrosis may be observed, and often progress to micronodular

cirrhosis. Ultrastructural examination reveals lipid accumulation, particularly in the lysosomes, with a heterogeneous globular to crystalline appearance [44].

The gross appearance of the liver in CESD is similar to that in individuals with Wolman disease but is often more orange than yellow in coloration. Fatty infiltration of hepatocytes can be profound and may mimic non-alcoholic steatosis. Kupffer cells and foam cells are involved similarly to those in Wolman disease. Periportal accumulation of lymphocytes and plasma cells may be dramatic. Fibrosis eventually develops and can develop into micronodular cirrhosis [41].

Both diseases result from defects in lysosomal acid lipase. This enzyme catalyzes the breakdown of cholesteryl esters and triglycerides that are delivered to liposomes by low density lipoprotein receptor-mediated endocytosis [41]. Cleavage of these substrates leads to liberation of free cholesterol and fatty acids, which are transported out of the lysosomes and into the cytoplasm. Disruption of this major pathway for neutral lipid metabolism leads to a dysregulation of the negative and positive feedback mechanisms that normally ensure intracellular cholesterol homeostasis.

Wolman disease should be suspected in infants with a combination of gastrointestinal symptoms, hepatomegaly, and bilateral adrenal cortical calcifications [41]. Likewise, CESD should be suspected in individuals with hyperlipidemia and unexplained hepatomegaly with or without dysfunction. Diagnosis can be made by the detection of significantly diminished lysosomal acid lipase activity in leukocytes or cultured skin fibroblasts and the demonstration of disease-causing mutations in both copies of LIPA.

There are no approved specific therapies for Wolman disease and CESD. Treatment primarily involves symptomatic management, particularly to prevent malnutrition and vitamin deficiencies. While BMT has been performed in patients with Wolman disease, mortality may depend on the initial status of the patient. A surviving individual exhibited improvement in clinical status and normalization of lysosomal acid lipase levels in peripheral blood cells [44]. Orthotopic liver transplantation may be beneficial for treatment of hepatic manifestations. Studies to determine the efficacy of 3-hydroxy-3-methylglutarate-CoA (HMG-CoA) reductase inhibitors in treating CESD have been performed, with mixed results; further research is necessary to determine the efficacy of this treatment. The major benefit appears to be a decrease in serum cholesterol levels. The results from enzyme replacement and gene therapy studies in mice have been encouraging and enzyme therapy is being used in clinical trials.

Mucopolysaccharidoses

The mucopolysaccharidoses (MPSs) are a group of seven lysosomal storage diseases characterized by a deficiency of various lysosomal enzymes that catalyze the degradation of glycosaminoglycans (previously called mucopolysaccharides). All are autosomal recessive in nature, except for Hunter disease

(a)

(b)

(c)

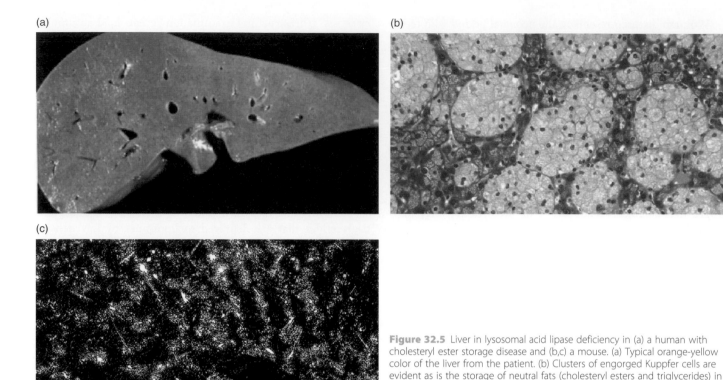

Figure 32.5 Liver in lysosomal acid lipase deficiency in (a) a human with cholesteryl ester storage disease and (b,c) a mouse. (a) Typical orange-yellow color of the liver from the patient. (b) Clusters of engorged Kuppfer cells are evident as is the storage of neutral fats (cholesteryl esters and triglycerides) in hepatocytes (magnification ×200). (c) Polarized light micrograph of lysosomal acid lipase-deficient mouse liver section. Cholesterol crystals are evident as are numerous other befringence bodies. (Courtesy of H. Du.) Livers in patients with Wolman disease and cholesteryl ester storage disease are similar.

(MPS II), which is X-linked. Depending on the enzyme affected, a single or combinations of glycosaminoglycans accumulate in cells and appear in urine.

The mucopolysaccharidoses are variable in age of onset, organ involvement, severity, and survival (Table 32.3). Many features are shared, including progressive course, coarse facial appearance, hearing loss, hepatosplenomegaly, obstructive airway disease, skeletal abnormalities, joint stiffness, and cardiac disease, with variable degrees of severity. Mental retardation and neurologic deterioration are variable between and among the types of MPSs. The combined frequency of MPS was approximately 1 in 22 500 in an Australian population, accounting for 35% of all lysosomal storage diseases [7].

Hepatosplenomegaly is observed in many patients with MPS, and may be massive, but hepatic dysfunction is usually not a feature associated with the MPS.

Variable cytoplasmic vacuolization from deposition of incompletely degraded glycosaminoglycans is present in most organs, including the liver, although this varies among individuals and types of MPS. Within the liver, storage material accumulates within the hepatocytes and Kupffer cells. There is an abundance of sinusoidal Kupffer cells, contributing to an obliteration of the sinusoids [46]. Ultrastructurally, these vacuoles contain heterogeneous storage material [46]. Significant fibrosis extending from portal to portal space and encircling the lobules with areas of hepatocyte disintegration can be present in patients with MPS I, II, and III [46].

The diagnosis of an MPS is suggested by the presenting phenotypic features. The observation of characteristic patterns of glycosaminoglycans in urine aids in the diagnosis and helps to pinpoint the enzyme deficiency. Definitive diagnosis requires the observation of deficient enzyme activity in serum, lymphocytes, or cultured fibroblasts, but residual enzyme activity is not a valid predictor of disease outcome. Molecular techniques may also be employed to diagnose these disorders, but requires identification of unusual or private mutations.

Bone marrow transplant has been performed in patients with various forms of the MPS. Success in stabilizing or improving clinical features has varied with the MPS variant. The CNS dysfunction in MPS I can be ameliorated or stabilized if BMT occurs early in the disease (<24 months). Successful BMT outcomes for CNS function have been controversial in other MPS diseases.

Enzyme therapy has been approved for MPS I, II, and VI. Despite evidence for the efficacy of enzyme replacement therapy in these conditions, significant limitations exist. The limited capacity to treat the CNS manifestations of these diseases was noted above. Clinical trials evaluating the safety and efficacy of intrathecally administered enzyme therapy in individuals with MPS I and II demonstrating CNS disease are ongoing. In addition, the skeletal manifestations of mucopolysaccharidoses respond poorly to enzyme therapy. Indeed, even patients receiving chronic infusions of enzyme replacement therapy since

Table 32.3 The mucopolysaccharidoses

Type	Enzyme defect	Glycosaminoglycan stored	Clinical features
MPS I-H, severe (Hurler)	α-L-Iduronidase	Dermatan sulfate, heparan sulfate	Mental retardation, corneal clouding, hepatosplenomegaly, severe dysostosis multiplex, joint stiffness, growth retardation, death in childhood
MPS I-H/S, moderate (Hurler–Scheie)	α-L-Iduronidase	Dermatan sulfate, heparan sulfate	Normal intelligence, corneal clouding, hepatosplenomegaly, moderate dysostosis multiplex, joint stiffness, growth retardation, survival into adulthood
MPS I-S, attenuated (Scheie)	α-L-Iduronidase	Dermatan sulfate, heparan sulfate	Normal intelligence to mild mental retardation, corneal clouding, hepatosplenomegaly, mild dysostosis multiplex, joint stiffness, normal stature, survival into adulthood
MPS II, attenuated (Hunter)	Iduronate 2-sulfatase	Dermatan sulfate, heparan sulfate	Normal intelligence, hepatosplenomegaly, moderate dysostosis multiplex, stiff joints, growth retardation, survival into adulthood
MPS II, severe (Hunter)	Iduronate 2-sulfatase	Dermatan sulfate, heparan sulfate	Mental retardation, retinal degeneration, hepatosplenomegaly, moderate dysostosis multiplex, stiff joints, survival into teens
MPS IIIA (Sanfilippo A)	Heparan N-sulfatase (sulfamidase)	Heparan sulfate	Neurologic deterioration, mental retardation, behavioral problems, hepatosplenomegaly, mild dysostosis multiplex, stiff joints
MPS IIIB (Sanfilippo B)	α-N-Acetylglucosaminidase	Heparan sulfate	Similar to MPS IIIA
MPS IIIC (Sanfilippo C)	Acetyl-CoA: α-glucosaminide N-acetyltransferase	Heparan sulfate	Similar to MPS IIIA
MPS IIID (Sanfilippo D)	N-Acetylglucosamine 6-sulfatase	Heparan sulfate	Similar to MPS IIIA
MPS IVA (Morquio A)	Galactose 6-sulfatase (N-acetylgalactosamine 6-sulfatase)	Keratan sulfate, chondroitin 6-sulfate	Normal intelligence, corneal clouding, hepatosplenomegaly, severe dysostosis multiplex, survival into adulthood
MPS IVB (Morquio B)	β-Galactosidase	Keratan sulfate	Normal intelligence, corneal clouding, hepatosplenomegaly, severe dysostosis multiplex, survival into adulthood
MPS VI (Maroteaux–Lamy)	N-Acetylgalactosamine 4-sulfatase (arylsulfatase B)	Dermatan sulfate	Mental retardation, corneal clouding, hepatosplenomegaly, severe dysostosis multiplex, variable survival
MPS VII (Sly)	β-Glucuronidase	Dermatan sulfate, heparan sulfate, chondroitin 4-, 6-sulfates	Mental retardation, no corneal opacities, hepatosplenomegaly, severe dysostosis multiplex, growth retardation, variable survival
MPS IX	Hyaluronidase	Hyaluronic acid	Short stature, periarticular soft tissue masses

MPS, mucopolysaccharidosis.
Source: adapted from Valle *et al.*, 2006 [45].

early childhood may expect a great likelihood of significant skeletal complications from their disease.

Mucolipidosis types II and III

Mucolipidosis types II and IIIα/β and IIIγ are progressive, autosomal recessively inherited lysosomal storage diseases that result from deficient activity of uridine diphosphate-N-acetylglucosamine-lysosomal enzyme N-acetylglucosaminyl-1-phosphotransferase (referred to as phosphotransferase).

Phosphotransferase contributes to the addition of a mannose 6-phosphate recognition marker on lysosomal enzymes. This recognition marker is critical for the transport of lysosomal enzymes from the Golgi apparatus to lysosomes in mesenchymal cells, and in its absence, lysosomal enzymes are secreted out of cells. The result is a deficiency of multiple lysosomal enzymes, and in many, but not all, cell types accumulations of undigested substrates occur within the lysosomes of affected cells [47]. In comparison, hepatocytes, Kupffer cells, and leukocytes demonstrate nearly normal levels of intracellular lysosomal enzyme activity, suggesting that alternative lysosomal enzyme transportation pathways are active within these cell types, and this provides a possible explanation for the diminished severity of pathological features observed in these cells [47].

Phosphotransferase is composed of three subunits, α_2, β_2, and γ_2 [47]. Evidence suggests that the α- and β-subunits serve as the catalytic components of the enzyme and the γ-subunit serves in substrate recognition [47]. The genes for the α- and β-subunits (*GNPTAB*) and γ-subunit (*GNPTG*) are mapped at chromosomes 12p and 16p, respectively. Mucolipidosis type II results from mutations in *GNPTA*, whereas, mucolipidosis type III types α/β and γ result from mutations in *GNPTAB* and *GNPTAG*, respectively.

Mucolipidosis type II is a rare pan-ethnic condition for which estimates of prevalence vary from 1 in 123 5000 to 1 in 625 000 [2,48]. However, a large cohort of affected individuals has been identified in the French Canadian population. Mucolipidosis IIIα/β is also pan-ethnic condition. Although data regarding the prevalence are not available, the prevalence may be similar to that of mucolipidosis type II. Mucolipidosis IIIγ is a rare condition, for which data regarding prevalence are not available. However, many reported patients are from the Middle East.

Mucolipidosis type II is often referred to as I-cell disease because of characteristic intracellular inclusions in cultured fibroblasts. The progressive phenotype presents from the neonatal period to the first year with features suggestive of MPS I, including neurological deterioration and visceral disease, with failure to thrive, growth retardation, facial coarsening, skin thickening, corneal clouding, cardiac disease, abdominal distension, hepatosplenomegaly, skeletal dysplasia and anomalies, and joint contractures [47]. However, unlike MPS I, the onset of disease is earlier and features are often more severe. Hydrops fetalis has also been reported. Death usually occurs in the first decade of life from cardiopulmonary disease [47].

In patients with mucolipidosis II, hepatomegaly presents in the neonatal period or shortly after and may be associated with elevated liver enzymes, but overt hepatic dysfunction is rarely observed. One infant with mucolipidosis type II presented with cholestasis, and biochemical and histological evidence of liver dysfunction. The cholestasis improved with ursodeoxycholic acid therapy.

Previously grouped into a single classification, mucolipidosis type III has recently been separated into α/β and γ subtypes. However, given the relatively small number of cases reported with the γ subtype, it is unclear how these two variants differ. In general, mucolipidosis type III is a less severe and more slowly progressive phenotype of mucolipidosis that presents in childhood with variable degrees of growth retardation, coarse facial appearance, corneal clouding, cardiac

valvular abnormalities, restrictive lung disease, skin thickening, skeletal dysplasia, joint contractures and destruction, and carpal tunnel syndrome [47]. Developmental delay or learning disability occurs in approximately 50% of patients, but is not as severe as in type II [49]. Hepatosplenomegaly is not common and is not associated with liver dysfunction. Mucolipidosis type III is compatible with survival into adulthood [47].

Intermediate phenotypes (i.e. physical features similar to but milder than the type II phenotype) with clinical courses more like that of patients with type III disease have also been described [50]. In such patients, the demarcation between types II and III is blurred, suggesting that it may be more appropriate to consider these diseases as a continuum of disease severity.

The hepatic architecture remains intact, but storage material is noted in portal mononuclear cells, and sinusoidal Kupffer cells, but to lesser degrees in hepatocytes [51]. Ultrastructurally, these inclusions are membrane bound and heterogeneous in appearance, appearing fibrillogranular, globular, and membranous [47,51].

The diagnosis of mucolipidosis types II and III is made by finding deficient activity of multiple lysosomal enzymes in cultured fibroblasts and massive elevations of multiple lysosomal enzymes in fibroblast culture medium or serum. Additionally, phosphotransferase activity can be directly measured in white blood cells or in cultured fibroblasts. Mucolipidosis types II and III cannot be differentiated on the basis of residual enzyme activity or localization because these are similar in both disorders [47]. Mutation analysis may also be employed to identify disease causing mutations in *GNPTAB* or *GNPTG*. An additional benefit of molecular diagnosis is identification of potential genotype–phenotype correlations. Mucolipidosis type II is associated with *GNPTAB* mutations predicting near-total absence of phosphotransferase activity; whereas mucolipidosis type IIIα/β is associated with *GNTAB* mutations predicting retention of low levels of phosphotransferase activity. Because of limited numbers of patients with mucolipidosis type IIIγ, no genotype–phenotype data are available.

There are no specific treatments for these forms of mucolipidosis, and therapy relies upon symptom management. Physical therapy may diminish the progression of joint immobility in those with type III disease [47]. Limited experience with BMT suggests some potential benefits.

Multiple sulfatase deficiency

Multiple sulfatase deficiency is an autosomal recessive disorder characterized by impaired activity of all known cellular sulfatases caused by deficiency of an enzyme essential for post-translational modification of an active site cysteine common to all members of the sulfatase family [52]. The phenotype is heterogeneous and combines features of the individual sulfatase deficiency disorders: metachromatic leukodystrophy, multiple mucopolysaccharidoses, X-linked ichthyosis, and chondrodysplasia punctata [52]. It is a rare disease, with an incidence of approximately 1 in 1.4 million [7].

The disorder presents in early infancy with varying degrees of progressive neurological dysfunction, developmental delays, growth retardation, facial coarsening, corneal clouding, hepatosplenomegaly, cardiac disease, ichthyosis, skeletal abnormalities, and stiff joints. Detailed histology on liver involvement is not available, but hepatomegaly and mild elevations in liver enzymes occur.

Multiple sulfatase deficiency is diagnosed biochemically based upon the characteristic pattern of deficient multiple sulfatase activities in leukocytes, plasma, and cultured fibroblasts. Excess mucopolysaccharides and sulfatides are usually identified in tissue samples and urine, further supporting the diagnosis. Sequencing of *SUM1* may also be used for diagnosing. Genotype–phenotype correlations are not well described because of the rarity of the condition; however, mutations resulting in very low residual enzyme activity may be associated with more severe phenotypes than those allowing higher residual enzyme activity. There is no known treatment for multiple sulfatase deficiency and therapy relies on symptomatic management, but studies into therapies for individual sulfatase deficiencies are ongoing.

References

1. Muenzer J, Fisher A. Advances in the treatment of mucopolysaccharidosis type I. *N Engl J Med* 2004;**350**: 1932–1934.

2. Poorthuis BJ, Wevers RA, Kleijer WJ, *et al.* The frequency of lysosomal storage diseases in the Netherlands. *Hum Genet* 1999;**105**(1–2):151–156.

3. Grabowski GA, Petsko GA, Kolodny EH. Gaucher disease. In Valle D, Beaudet AL, Vogelstein B, *et al.* (eds.) *The Online Metabolic & Molecular Bases of Inherited Disease.* (http://www.ommbid.com, accessed 22 July 2013).

4. James SP, Stromeyer FW, Chang C, Barranger JA. Liver abnormalities in patients with Gaucher's disease. *Gastroenterology* 1981;**80**:126–133.

5. Barbier C, Devisme L, Dobbelaere D, *et al.* Neonatal cholestasis and infantile Gaucher disease: a case report. *Acta Paediatr* 2002;**91**:1399–1401.

6. Weinreb NJ, Charrow J, Andersson HC, *et al.* Effectiveness of enzyme replacement therapy in 1028 patients with type 1 Gaucher disease after 2 to 5 years of treatment: a report from the Gaucher Registry. *Am J Med* 2002;**113**:112–119.

7. Lukina E, Watman N, Arreguin EA, *et al.* Improvement in hematological, visceral, and skeletal manifestations of Gaucher disease type 1 with oral eliglustat tartrate (Genz-112638) treatment: 2-year results of a phase 2 study. *Blood* 2010;**116**:4095–4098.

8. Meikle PJ, Hopwood JJ, Clague AE, Carey WF. Prevalence of lysosomal storage disorders. *JAMA* 1999;**281**: 249–254.

9. Schuchman EH, Desnick RJ. Niemann–Pick disease types A and B: acid sphingomyelinase deficiencies. In Valle D, Beaudet AL, Vogelstein B, *et al.* (eds.) *The Online Metabolic & Molecular Bases of Inherited Disease.* (http://www.ommbid.com, accessed 22 July 2013).

10. Wasserstein MP, Desnick RJ, Schuchman EH, *et al.* The natural history of type B Niemann–Pick disease: results from a 10-year longitudinal study. *Pediatrics* 2004;**114**: e672–e677.

11. Takahashi T, Akiyama K, Tomihara M, *et al.* Heterogeneity of liver disorder in type B Niemann–Pick disease. *Hum Pathol* 1997;**28**:385–388.

12. Victor S, Coulter JB, Besley GT, *et al.* Niemann–Pick disease: sixteen-year follow-up of allogeneic bone marrow transplantation in a type B variant. *J Inherit Metab Dis* 2003;**26**:775–785.

13. Levade T, Sandhoff K, Schulze H, Medin JA. Acid Ceramidase Deficiency: Farber Lipogranulomatosis. In Valle D, Beaudet AL, Vogelstein B, *et al.* (eds.) *The Online Metabolic & Molecular Bases of Inherited Disease.* (http://www.ommbid.com, accessed 22 July 2013).

14. Kattner E, Schafer A, Harzer K. Hydrops fetalis: manifestation in lysosomal storage diseases including Farber disease. *Eur J Pediatr* 1997;**156**:292–295.

15. Yeager AM, Uhas KA, Coles CD, *et al.* Bone marrow transplantation for infantile ceramidase deficiency (Farber disease). *Bone Marrow Transplant* 2000;**26**:357–363.

16. Vormoor J, Ehlert K, Groll AH, *et al.* Successful hematopoietic stem cell transplantation in Farber disease. *J Pediatr* 2004;**144**:132–134.

17. Suzuki Y, Nanba E, Matsuda J, Higaki K, Oshima A. B-Galactosidase deficiency (B-galactosidosis): GM1 gangliosidosis and morquio B disease. In Valle D, Beaudet AL, Vogelstein B, *et al.* (eds.) *The Online Metabolic & Molecular Bases of Inherited Disease.* (http://www.ommbid.com, accessed 22 July 2013).

18. Vanier MT, Millat G. Niemann–Pick disease type C. *Clin Genet* 2003;**64**: 269–281.

19. Vanier MT. Niemann–Pick disease type C. *Orphanet J Rare Dis* 2010;**5**:16.

20. Patterson MC, Vanier MT, Suzuki K, *et al.* Niemann–Pick disease Type C: A lipid trafficking disorder. In Valle D, Beaudet AL, Vogelstein B, *et al.* (eds.) *The Online Metabolic & Molecular Bases of Inherited Disease.* (http://www.ommbid.com, accessed 22 July 2013).

21. Patterson M. Niemann–Pick disease type C. In Pagon RA, Bird TD, Dolan CR, Stephens K (eds.) *GeneReviews.* Seattle, WA: University of Washington, Seattle, 1993– (website, updated July 2008; accessed March 13, 2012).

22. Kelly DA, Portmann B, Mowat AP, Sherlock S, Lake BD. Niemann–Pick disease type C: diagnosis and outcome in children, with particular reference to liver disease. *J Pediatr* 1993;**123**: 242–247.

23. Gilbert EF, Callahan J, Viseskul C, Opitz JM. Niemann–Pick disease type C. Pathological, histochemical, ultrastructural and biochemical studies. *Eur J Pediatr* 1981;**136**:263–274.

24. Yerushalmi B, Sokol RJ, Narkewicz MR, *et al.* Niemann–Pick disease type C in neonatal cholestasis at a North American Center. *J Pediatr Gastroenterol Nutr* 2002;**35**:44–50.

25. Zervas M, Somers KL, Thrall MA, Walkley SU. Critical role for glycosphingolipids in Niemann–Pick

disease type C. *Curr Biol* 2001;**11**: 1283–1287.

26. Wraith JE, Vecchio D, Jacklin E, *et al.* Miglustat in adult and juvenile patients with Niemann–Pick disease type C: long-term data from a clinical trial. *Mol Genet Metab* 2010;**99**:351–357.

27. Ashe KM, Bangari D, Li L, *et al.* Iminosugar-based inhibitors of glucosylceramide synthase increase brain glycosphingolipids and survival in a mouse model of Sandhoff disease. *PLOS One* 2011;**6**: e21758.

28. Thomas GH. Disorders of glycoprotein degradation: α-mannosidosis, B-mannosidosis, fucosidosis, and sialidosis. In Valle D, Beaudet AL, Vogelstein B, *et al.* (eds.) *The Online Metabolic & Molecular Bases of Inherited Disease.* (http://www.ommbid.com, accessed 22 July 2013).

29. Willems PJ, Gatti R, Darby JK, *et al.* Fucosidosis revisited: a review of 77 patients. *Am J Med Genet* 1991;**38**: 111–131.

30. Freitag F, Blumcke S, Spranger J. Hepatic ultrastructure in mucolipidosis I (lipomucopolysaccharidosis). *Virchows Arch B Cell Pathol* 1971;**7**:189–204.

31. Vellodi A, Cragg H, Winchester B, *et al.* Allogeneic bone marrow transplantation for fucosidosis. *Bone Marrow Transplant* 1995;**15**:153–158.

32. Monus Z, Konyar E, Szabo L. Histomorphologic and histochemical investigations in mannosidosis. A light and electron microscopic study. *Virchows Arch B Cell Pathol* 1977;**26**:159–173.

33. d'Azzo A, Andria G, Strisciuglio P, Galjaard H. Galactosialidosis. In Valle D, Beaudet AL, Vogelstein B, *et al.* (eds.) *The Online Metabolic & Molecular Bases of Inherited Disease.* (http://www.ommbid.com, accessed 22 July 2013).

34. van der Spoel A, Bonten E, d'Azzo A. Transport of human lysosomal neuraminidase to mature lysosomes requires protective protein/cathepsin A. *EMBO J* 1998;**17**:1588–1597.

35. Hirschhorn R, Reuser AJJ. Glycogen storage disease type II: acid α-glucosidase (acid maltase) deficiency. In Valle D, Beaudet AL, Vogelstein B, *et al.* (eds.) *The Online Metabolic & Molecular Bases of Inherited Disease* (http://www.ommbid.com, accessed 22 July 2013).

36. van den Hout HM, Hop W, van Diggelen OP, *et al.* The natural course of infantile Pompe's disease: 20 original cases compared with 133 cases from the literature. *Pediatrics* 2003;**112**:332–340.

37. Leslie N, Tinkle B. Glycogen storage disease type II (Pompe disease). In Pagon RA, Bird TD, Dolan CR, Stephens K (eds.) *GeneReviews*. Seattle, WA: University of Washington, Seattle, 1993– (website, updated August 2010).

38. Kishnani PS, Howell RR. Pompe disease in infants and children. *J Pediatr* 2004;**144**(5 Suppl):S35–43.

39. Hagemans ML, Winkel LP, Van Doorn PA, *et al.* Clinical manifestation and natural course of late-onset Pompe's disease in 54 Dutch patients. *Brain.* 2005;**128**(Pt 3):671–677.

40. Kishnani PS, Corzo D, Leslie ND, *et al.* Early treatment with alglucosidase alpha prolongs long-term survival of infants with Pompe disease. *Pediatr Res* 2009;**66**:329–335.

41. Assmann G, Seedorf U. Acid Lipase deficiency: Wolman disease and cholesteryl ester storage disease. In Valle D, Beaudet AL, Vogelstein B, *et al.* (eds.) *The Online Metabolic & Molecular Bases of Inherited Disease.* (http://www.ommbid.com, accessed 22 July 2013).

42. Muntoni S, Wiebusch H, Jansen-Rust M, *et al.* Prevalence of cholesteryl ester storage disease. *Arterioscler Thromb Vasc Biol* 2007;**27**:1866–1868.

43. Grabowski G, Bove K, Du H. Lysosomal acid lipase deficiencies: Wolman disease and cholesteryl ester storage disease. In Walker WA, Goulet OJ, Kleinman RE (eds.) *Pediatric Gastrointestinal Disease:* *Pathophysiology, Diagnosis and Management.* Hamilton, Ontario: Decker, 2004, pp. 1429–1439.

44. Krivit W, Freese D, Chan KW, Kulkarni R. Wolman's disease: a review of treatment with bone marrow transplantation and considerations for the future. *Bone Marrow Transplant* 1992;**10**(Suppl 1):97–101.

45. Valle D, Beaudet AL, Vogelstein B, *et al.* (eds.). *Online Metabolic and Molecular Bases of Inherited Disease,* 2006 (http://www.ommbid.com, updated March 2011, accessed 10 November 2013).

46. Parfrey NA, Hutchins GM. Hepatic fibrosis in the mucopolysaccharidoses. *Am J Med* 1986;**81**:825–829.

47. Kornfeld S, Sly WS. I-cell disease and pseudo-Hurler polydystrophy: disorders of lysosomal enzyme phosphorylation and localization. In Valle D, Beaudet AL, Vogelstein B, *et al.* (eds.) *The Online Metabolic & Molecular Bases of Inherited Disease.* (http://www.ommbid.com, accessed 22 July 2013).

48. Pinto R, Caseiro C, Lemos M, *et al.* Prevalence of lysosomal storage diseases in Portugal. *Eur J Hum Genet* 2004;**12**:87–92.

49. Kelly TE, Thomas GH, Taylor HA, Jr., *et al.* Mucolipidosis III (pseudo-Hurler polydystrophy): Clinical and laboratory studies in a series of 12 patients. *Johns Hopkins Med J* 1975;**137**:156–175.

50. Cathey SS, Leroy JG, Wood T, *et al.* Phenotype and genotype in mucolipidoses II and III alpha/beta: a study of 61 probands. *J Med Genet* 2010;**47**:38–48.

51. Kenyon KR, Sensenbrenner JA, Wyllie RG. Hepatic ultrastructure and histochemistry in mucolipidosis II (I-cell disease). *Pediatr Res* 1973;**7**:560–568.

52. Hopwood JJ, Ballabio A. Multiple sulfatase deficiency and the nature of the sulfatase family. In Valle D, Beaudet AL, Vogelstein B, *et al.* (eds.) *The Online Metabolic & Molecular Bases of Inherited Disease.* (http://www.ommbid.com, accessed 22 July 2013).

Disorders of bile acid synthesis and metabolism

33

Kenneth D. R. Setchell

Introduction

The importance of bile acid synthesis and metabolism to normal physiology and their role in pathophysiological states is well recognized. For such small and relatively simple molecules, bile acids have amazingly diverse properties and functions. To the lipidologist, bile acid biosynthesis represents one of the major pathways for regulating cholesterol homeostasis – each day approximately 0.5 g cholesterol is metabolized to bile acids. To the hepatologist, these molecules are seen as essential for providing the major driving force for the promotion and secretion of bile and, therefore, are key elements in the development and maintenance of an efficient enterohepatic circulation. The gastroenterologist recognizes the importance of bile acids in facilitating the solubilization and absorption of fats and fat-soluble vitamins from the small bowel, although in the large bowel these molecules if in excess are potentially harmful in that they are carthartic, membrane damaging, and promoters of colonic disease. More recently, bile acids have become of interest to the endocrinologist because of their hormone-like actions of relevance to obesity and glucose and insulin regulation, where they are now regarded as important molecules that signal through orphan receptors to regulate metabolism. This chapter will, therefore, provide an overview of the pathways of bile acid synthesis and metabolism and will focus on specific inborn errors in bile acid synthesis and metabolism that are now regarded as a cause of progressive cholestatic liver disease and of syndromes of fat-soluble vitamin malabsorption or neurological disease.

Pathways of bile acid synthesis from cholesterol

Structurally, bile acids possess a cyclopentanoperhydrophenanthrene (ABCD-ring) nucleus and, therefore, belong to the chemical class of steroids [1]. They differ from steroid hormones and neutral sterols, such as cholesterol in having a five-carbon atom side-chain with a terminal carboxylic acid (Figure 33.1). Bile acids are synthesized in the liver from cholesterol by a complex series of chemical reactions catalyzed

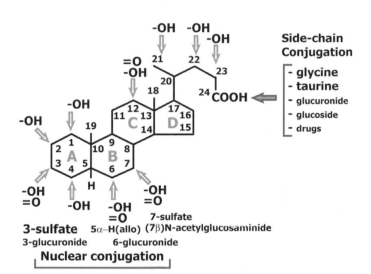

Figure 33.1 The 5β-cholanoic acid nucleus that is the basic structure of C_{24}-bile acids of mammalian species. Indicated are the ABCD rings, the numbering system for the carbon atoms, and the metabolic sites of substitution of functional groups occurring under normal and pathophysiologic conditions. Unsaturation can also occur in the nucleus (mainly at positions Δ^4, Δ^5), and in the side-chain. The smaller font size signifies the relative quantitative importance of the conjugation reactions.

by 17 different hepatic enzymes located in the endoplasmic reticulum, mitochondria, cytoplasm, and peroxisomes; consequently, there is considerable trafficking of intermediates between these subcellular compartments. Several of the enzymes are also found in extrahepatic tissues. The enzymes involved in bile acid biosynthesis have all been isolated and well characterized in pioneering work performed in the late 1960s and 1970s, and more recently the role that each enzyme plays in the regulation of bile acid synthesis has been elucidated from studies of gene knockout animal models and humans with genetic defects in bile acid synthesis. Complimentary DNAs have now been described for these enzymes, including the rate-limiting enzyme in the bile acid biosynthetic pathway, the cytochrome P450 liver-specific enzyme *cholesterol 7α-hydroxylase* (CYP7A1), and these have provided important tools to examine the regulation of bile acid synthesis and to confirm genetic defects in bile acid synthesis.

Liver Disease in Children, Fourth Edition, ed. Frederick J. Suchy, Ronald J. Sokol, and William F. Balistreri. Published by Cambridge University Press. © Cambridge University Press 2014.

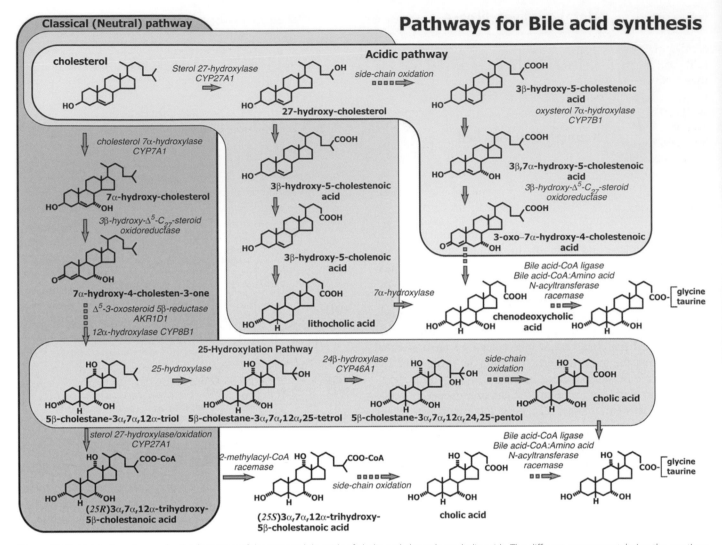

Figure 33.2 Metabolic pathways for the formation of the primary bile acids of cholic and chenodeoxycholic acids. The different enzymes catalyzing the reactions are indicated in italics. The broken arrows indicate multiple steps in the conversion. Shown by the shaded areas are the classical (neutral) pathway, the acidic pathway, and several alternative pathways leading to bile acid synthesis for bile acid synthesis.

Conjugated (glycine and taurine) cholic and chenodeoxy-cholic acids are the two primary bile acids synthesized in humans but there is considerable variability in the qualitative pattern of bile acid synthesis among animal species. Rodents, synthesize mostly cholic and the 6β-hydroxylated bile acid β-muricholic (3α,6β,7β-trihydroxy-5β-cholanoic acid) and these are predominantly taurine conjugated, while pigs synthesize a 6α-hydroxylated bile acid, hyodeoxycholic (3α,6α-dihydroxy-5β-cholanoic acid) and 6-oxo-lithocholic acid.

Although there is a tendency to illustrate the reactions in the bile acid synthetic pathway to occur in a linear fashion (Figure 33.2), moving from initiation of changes to the steroid nucleus through modification of the side-chain, in reality there is considerable substrate promiscuity for the 17 enzymes catalyzing the various reactions, which results in a vast number of different bile acids and intermediates being synthesized. This is particularly evident during early development, a period of physiological cholestasis, and in pathological conditions that interfere with the integrity of the enterohepatic circulation. Furthermore, intestinal bacterial modifications, resulting in the formation of "secondary" bile acids, add a further level of complexity to the bile acid composition of biological fluids.

There are two main pathways leading to primary bile acid synthesis. These are termed the "neutral" and "acidic" pathways, the former being the classical one that is initiated by CYP7A1 leading to cholic acid synthesis, and the latter being initiated by the action of cholesterol 27-hydroxylase (CYP27A1) on the side-chain to yield chenodeoxycholic acid [2]. This acidic pathway leads to the formation of 3β-hydroxy-5-cholenoic and lithocholic acids, as intermediates to cheno-deoxycholic acid and these markedly hepatotoxic monohydroxy-bile acids are increased in early life and in cholestatic liver diseases. 27-Hydroxylation occurs in the liver and in many other tissues, including brain, alveolar macro-phages, vascular endothelia, and fibroblasts; its extrahepatic role appears related to the cellular regulation of cholesterol homeostasis by its ability to generate oxysterols that are potent repressors of cholesterol synthesis. It is now accepted that the "acidic" pathway contributes significantly to overall total bile acid synthesis, and particularly to chenodeoxycholic acid synthesis. Normal levels of bile acids are synthesized in mice even when the gene encoding CYP7A1 is knocked-out, and bile acid synthesis is sustained in rats when CYP7A1 is inhibited. However, $Cyp7A1^{-/-}$ mice die within the first few weeks of life from liver failure and the consequences of fat-soluble vitamin malabsorption unless fat-soluble vitamins and cholic acid are fed to these animals immediately after birth. Despite being deficient in CYP7A1, primary bile acid synthesis occurs in this model via the developmental expression of an oxysterol 7α-hydroxylase (CYP7B1) specific to the acidic pathway. This enzyme is essential in protecting the liver from hepatotoxic monohydroxy-bile acids that are formed as intermediates in this pathway [3]. The above examples show that primary bile acid synthesis is not exclusively dependent on CYP7A1, and under certain conditions, alternative pathways are induced. For some time it was evident that there were a number of different 7α-hydroxylases; this was confirmed following the isolation and characterization of CYP7B1 and CYP39A1 [2]. CYP7B1 has high activity in human liver and is also found in brain, kidney, and prostate, but its regulation is not fully understood. It has broad substrate specificity, being active on the oxysterols, 27- and 25-hydroxycholesterol, on the bile acids 3β-hydroxy-5-cholenoic and 3β-hydroxy-5-cholestenoic acids, and also on C_{19} steroids. *CYP7B1* is localized to chromosome 8q21.3 and in close proximity to *CYP7A1*. Genetically engineered $Cyp7B1^{-/-}$ mice lacking this enzyme have elevated levels of 27- and 25-hydroxycholesterol, but not 24-hydroxycholesterol [4]. Similarly, extremely high levels of 27-hydroxycholesterol and hepatotoxic monohydroxy bile acids, 3β-hydroxy-5-cholenoic and 3β-hydroxy-5-cholestenoic acids, were found in an infant with a genetic defect in *CYP7B1* [3]. A mutation in *CYP7B1* will cause a phenotype of progressive and fatal liver disease [3,5,6] and indicates the quantitative importance of the "acidic" pathway in early human life.

Following the synthesis of 7α-hydroxycholesterol, modifications to the steroid nucleus take place that result in oxido-reduction and C-12 hydroxylation, consequently preparing the sterol intermediates for direction into either the *cholic acid* (3α,7α,12α-trihydroxy-5β-cholan-24-oic), or *chenodeoxycholic acid* (3α,7α-dihydroxy-5β-cholan-24-oic) pathways. According to convention, 7α-hydroxycholesterol is converted to 7α-hydroxy-4-cholesten-3-one, a reaction catalyzed by a microsomal NAD-dependent 3β-hydroxy-Δ^5-C_{27}-steroid oxidoreductase (C_{27}3β-HSD), formerly referred to as a 3β-hydroxy-Δ^5-C_{27}-steroid dehydrogenase/isomerase. This enzyme shows substrate specificity toward 7α-hydroxylated sterols and bile acids possessing a 3β-hydroxy-Δ^5 nucleus and is inactive on 7β-hydroxylated analogues. Comparable reactions occur in steroid hormone synthesis; however, the enzyme active on bile acid intermediates is a distinct single enzyme that shows absolute specificity toward C_{27} sterols, differing from

the isozymes active on C_{19} and C_{21} neutral steroids. Expression of the gene for C_{27}3β-HSD is not exclusive to the liver but is also seen in fibroblasts, which enables its activity to be determined in patients with a genetic defect in this enzyme [7]. Mutations in the gene encoding this enzyme are associated with progressive intrahepatic cholestasis [8,9] and this is often the cause of late-onset chronic cholestasis.

12α-Hydroxylation of the product of the above reaction will direct the Δ^4-3-oxo intermediate into the cholic acid pathway. This reaction is catalyzed by a liver-specific microsomal cytochrome P450 12α-hydroxylase (CYP8B1), which is highly expressed in rabbit and human liver, two species where deoxycholic acid is quantitatively important. When the gene encoding this enzyme is knocked out in mice, there is loss of cholic acid and reduced cholesterol absorption [2]. The primary structures of the rabbit, mouse, and human enzymes have been established by molecular cloning of their cDNAs. The activity of CYP8B1 determines the relative proportion and synthetic rate of cholic relative to chenodeoxycholic acids and appears in humans to be upregulated by interruption of the enterohepatic circulation, and in animals by starvation. It is possible that in utero there may be reduced activity of this enzyme because fetal bile has a predominance of chenodeoxycholic acid [10]. In contrast, the ratio of cholic acid to chenodeoxycholic acid is very high in neonatal bile compared with adult bile. The neonatal period is associated with a phase of physiological cholestasis, which may lead to upregulation in CYP8B1 activity with a consequent increase in cholic acid synthesis.

7α-Hydroxy-4-cholesten-3-one and 7α,12α-dihydroxy-4-cholesten-3-one both undergo reduction with formation of a 3-oxo-5β(H)-structure and this generates the basic *trans*-configuration of the A/B-rings of the steroid nucleus that is common to the majority of bile acids in most mammalian species. Allo(5α-*H*)-bile acids are often major bile acid species of lower vertebrates but are found in small proportions in biological fluids from humans. These are formed by an analogous reaction but catalyzed by a hepatic 5α-reductase. The K_m of 5α-reductase is high and consequently under normal conditions 5β-reduction is favored. The Δ^4-3-oxosteroid 5β-reductase (AKR1D1), a cytosolic aldo-keto reductase, is a protein of approximately 38 kDa comprising 326 amino acid residues that differs significantly in structure from the 5α-reductase and has broad substrate specificity. Its crystal structure and the effect of a number of point mutations on the substrate-binding sites and enzyme activity were recently reported [11,12]. Although under normal conditions, this enzyme does not appear to be of regulatory importance for bile acid synthesis, its activity parallels the activity of CYP7A1 and therefore measurement of the plasma concentration of 7α-hydroxy-4-cholesten-3-one can be used as an indirect assessment of hepatic CYP7A1 activity. The finding of elevated proportions 3-oxo-Δ^4-bile acids in biological fluids during early life and in advanced cholestatic liver disease suggests that under pathological conditions it is this enzyme that becomes rate-limiting for bile acid synthesis rather than CYP7A1. Mutations in *AKR1D1*, the gene encoding AKR1D1, are clinically manifest as progressive intrahepatic cholestasis and biochemically by the production of large amounts of C_{24}-3-oxo-Δ^4-bile acids and allo-bile acids [12–14].

The enzyme catalyzing the conversion of the 3-oxo-5β(H)-sterols to the corresponding 3α-hydroxy-5β(*H*) intermediates is a soluble 3α-hydroxysteroid dehydrogenase (AKR1C4). This enzyme catalyzes the oxido-reduction of a number of substrates, and several cDNA clones with sequence similarity to other aldo-keto reductases have been described suggesting the existence of multiple isozymes. This final step in modification of the steroid nucleus results in the formation of the key intermediates 5β-cholestane-3α,7α-diol and 5β-cholestane-3α,7α,12α-triol (bile alcohols), which then undergo a sequence of reactions leading to side-chain oxidation and consequent shortening by three carbon atoms (Figure 33.2).

The initial step in side-chain oxidation of the bile alcohols involves hydroxylation of the C-27 carbon atom, a reaction that is catalyzed by mitochondrial CYP27A1 and leads to the formation of 5β-cholestane-3α,7α,12α,27-tetrol. CYP27A1 is also responsible for the complete oxidation reaction that yields directly 3α,7α,12α-trihydroxy-5β-cholestanoic acid. 5β-Cholestane-3α,7α,12α,27-tetrol may also undergo oxidation by the combined actions of soluble or mitochondrial alcohol and aldehyde dehydrogenases, but the relative importance of these reactions compared with the complete CYP27A1-catalyzed reaction is not known. Complementary DNAs encoding the rat, rabbit, and human sterol 27-hydroxylase have been isolated. This enzyme is expressed in many extrahepatic tissues and its function appears to be important in facilitating the removal of cellular cholesterol. It shows substrate specificity toward many sterols, including cholesterol and vitamin D and is the same enzyme that catalyzes the formation of 27-hydroxycholesterol, the first step in the "acidic" pathway. When the gene *CYP27A1* encoding sterol 27-hydroxylase is disrupted in the mouse, bile acid synthesis is markedly reduced; however, mutations in this gene, which cause the rare lipid storage disease of cerebrotendinous xanthomatosis (CTX), have only a modest effect on bile acid synthesis, partly because alternative pathways for bile acid synthesis support the production of compensatory levels of cholic acid [15].

Using radiolabeled precursors, it was shown that 5β-cholestane-3α,7α,12α-triol can be first 25-hydroxylated in the microsomal fraction, then 24β-hydroxylated and finally oxidized to cholic acid. This pathway is specific for cholic acid since little or no hydroxylation of 5β-cholestane-3α,7α-diol has been demonstrated. Based on studies of patients with CTX, it was proposed that the C-25 hydroxylation pathway may be a major pathway for cholic acid synthesis in humans. The C-25 hydroxylation pathway accounts for less than 5% of the total bile acids synthesized in healthy adults and less than 2% in adult rats. Hydroxylation of cholesterol also occurs at the C-24 and C-25 positions in addition to the aforementioned cholesterol 27-hydroxylation to yield oxysterols, which are potent

repressors of cholesterol synthesis. Cholesterol 24-hydroxylase (CYP46A1) is expressed in the brain to a greater extent than in the liver, where it is considered to play a role in cholesterol secretion. In gene knockout mouse models of cholesterol 24- and 25-hydroxylases, bile acid synthesis is unaffected [2].

The cholestanoic acids are next converted to CoA esters by the action of a bile acid-CoA ligase (synthetase) of which two forms have been identified; one that activates newly synthesized C_{27} cholestanoic acids, the other activates cholanoic acids formed as secondary bile acids returning to the liver for reconjugation. The product of this reaction is the formation of the CoA esters of (25R)-3α,7α-dihydroxycholestanoic and (25R)-3α,7α,12α-trihydroxycholestanoic acids. The (25R)-diastereoisomers must be racemized to their (25S)-forms in order to penetrate the peroxisome for subsequent oxidation. This reaction is catalyzed by a 2-methylacyl coenzyme A racemase that is also active on branched-chain fatty acids such as phytanic acids. A mutation in the gene encoding this enzyme leads to the accumulation of (25R)-cholestanoic acids and phytanic acids and presents with neurologic and liver disease [16].

The final stage in modification of the side-chain involves the beta-oxidation of the cholestanoic acids, which occurs by a multiple-step reaction within peroxisomes. The sequence of these reactions is analogous to the beta-oxidation of fatty acids. The CoA esters of the cholestanoic acid are acted on by a specific peroxisomal acyl-CoA oxidase (ACOX2). This reaction is rate limiting and the enzyme has been partially purified from rat liver and found to differ from the analogous acyl-CoA oxidase (ACOX1) utilizing fatty acids as substrates. The situation in humans is somewhat different in that a single peroxisomal oxidase acts on both branched-chain fatty acids and the bile acid intermediates. Formation of a C-24 hydroxylated derivative occurs by the action of a bifunctional enoyl-CoA hydratase/β-hydroxyacyl-CoA dehydrogenase, a reaction that goes through a Δ^2-4-intermediate. Photoaffinity labeling experiments have shown that this enzyme is the same one that is involved in the peroxisomal beta-oxidation of fatty acids. The dehydrogenase activity of the bifunctional enzyme yields a 24-oxo derivative that, following thiolytic cleavage by peroxisomal thiolase 2, releases three carbon atoms in the form of propionic acid. This results in the formation of the C_{24} bile acid CoA end-product. With the exception of the acyl-CoA oxidase, defects in any of the other enzymes responsible for the beta-oxidation of very-long-chain fatty acids exhibit abnormalities in primary bile acid biosynthesis [2].

Some mention of allo(5α-reduced) bile acids is warranted even though under physiological conditions these account for relatively small proportion of the total bile acids in biological fluids of humans. In humans, 5α-reduced bile acids are usually formed by the action of intestinal microflora on 3-oxo-5β-bile acids during their enterohepatic circulation and consequently are found in significant amounts in feces. In rodents, these can be formed in the liver from 5α-cholestanol. This pathway begins with 7α-hydroxylation of 5α-cholestanol and the product is then converted to 5α-cholestane-3α,7α-diol via the intermediate 7α-hydroxy-5α-cholestan-3-one. Hepatic 12α-hydroxylation of 5α-sterols is very efficient in the rat and readily leads to the formation of allo-cholic acid. A further pathway for allo-bile acid formation involves the hepatic 5α-reduction of 7α-hydroxy- and 7α,12α-dihydroxy-3-oxo-4-cholen-24-oic acids, a reaction catalyzed by a Δ^4-3-oxosteroid 5α-reductase. The finding of large proportions of allo-bile acids in infants with severe cholestatic liver disease caused by AKR1D1 deficiency indicates these to be primary bile acids of hepatic origin in humans [16]. Both 5α-reductase isozymes are expressed in the liver beginning from birth [2].

A striking feature of bile acid synthesis and metabolism during early life is the relatively large proportion of polyhydroxylated, unsaturated, and oxo-bile acids that are synthesized; these are not found in the bile of healthy adults [10]. Although frequently referred to as "atypical," this is a misnomer since they are, in fact, typical of the developmental phase of hepatic metabolism. Interestingly, the qualitative and quantitative bile acid composition of biological fluids in early life closely resembles that of adults with severe cholestatic liver disease, suggesting that in the diseased liver there is a reversion to more primitive pathways of synthesis and metabolism [10]. The most notable distinction in ontogeny is the prevalence of cytochrome P450 hydroxylation pathways, which rapidly decline in importance over the first year of life. The most important hydroxylation reactions are 1β-, 4β-, and 6α-hydroxylations that are of hepatic origin [17]. The concentrations of several of the metabolites, in particular hyocholic (3α,6α,7α-trihydroxy-5β-cholanoic) and 3α,4β,7α-trihydroxy-5β-cholanoic acids, exceed that of cholic acid in fetal bile [10]. The role of these hydroxylation pathways is uncertain, but additional hydroxylation of the bile acid nucleus will increase the polarity of the bile acid and facilitate its renal clearance, while also decreasing its membrane-damaging potential. In early life, and particularly in the fetus, an immaturity in canalicular and ileal bile acid transport processes leads to a sluggish enterohepatic circulation and hydroxylation serves as a hepatoprotective mechanism.

Bile acid conjugation

Irrespective of the pathway by which cholic and chenodeoxycholic acids are synthesized, the CoA thioesters of these primary bile acids are ultimately conjugated to the amino acids glycine and taurine. This two-step reaction is catalyzed by a rate-limiting bile acid-CoA ligase enzyme followed by a bile acid CoA:amino acid N-acyltransferase (EC 2.3.1.65) [18]. The genes encoding both enzymes, SLC27A5 and BAAT, have been cloned. The conjugation reaction was originally believed to take place in the cytosol, but the highest activity of the conjugating enzymes was found to be in peroxisomes.

Genetic defects in the bile acid amidation have been associated with fat-soluble vitamin malabsorption states with variable degrees of liver disease [19]. Bile acid CoA:amino acid N-acyltransferase utilizes glycine, taurine, and,

interestingly, β-fluoroalanine but not alanine, as substrates. It will also conjugate very-long-chain fatty acids to glycine. The specificity of the enzyme has been examined in detail and found to be influenced by the length of the side-chain of the bile acid; bile acids having a C_4 side-chain, that is nor(C_{23})-bile acids and homo(C_{25})-bile acids, are poor substrates for amidation [18]. However cholestanoic (C_{27}) acids are predominantly taurine conjugated. Significant species differences in substrate specificity are observed, which should be considered when working with animal models. Human bile acid-CoA:amino acid N-acyltransferase conjugates cholic acid with both glycine and taurine, whereas the mouse enzyme showed selectivity toward taurine. This is consistent with the mouse being an obligate taurine conjugator of bile acids, as is the rat and the dog.

In humans, the final products of this complex multistep pathway are the two conjugated primary bile acids of cholic and chenodeoxycholic acids, and these are then secreted in canalicular bile and stored in gallbladder bile. In humans, glycine conjugation predominates with a ratio of glycine to taurine conjugates of 3.1:1 for normal adults. In early human life, >80% of the bile acids in bile are taurine conjugated because of the abundance of hepatic stores of taurine [10].

Although the principal bile acids in humans and most mammalian species are amidated, other conjugates occur naturally, including sulfates, glucuronide ethers and esters, glucosides, N-acetylglucosaminides, and conjugates of some drugs. These conjugates account for a relatively large proportion of the total urinary bile acids. Conjugation significantly alters the physicochemical characteristics of the bile acid and serves an important function in increasing the polarity of the molecule, thereby facilitating its renal excretion and minimizing the membrane-damaging potential of the more hydrophobic unconjugated species. Under physiological conditions, these alternative conjugation pathways are quantitatively less important. However, in cholestatic liver disease, or when the liver is subjected to a bile acid load, as during treatment with ursodeoxycholic acid (UDCA), the concentrations of these conjugates in biological fluids may change. Detailed knowledge of these metabolic pathways is limited but it is evident that there is significant localization of bile acid conjugating enzymes in the kidneys.

Sulfation of bile acids, most commonly at the C-3 position but also at C-7, is catalyzed by a bile acid sulfotransferase, an enzyme that in the rat, but not human, exhibits sex-dependent differences in activity. Although much has been written about the potential importance of sulfation in early life, it is evident from the finding of a relatively small proportion of bile acid sulfates in fetal bile that hepatic sulfation is negligible in the fetus and neonate [10]. Indeed, it is most probable that urinary bile acid sulfates originate mainly by renal sulfation; 60–80% of urinary bile acids are sulfated and their excretion increases in cholestasis. Only traces of bile acid sulfates are found in bile despite efficient canalicular transport of perfused bile acid sulfates.

A number of glucuronosyltransferases catalyze the formation of glucuronide ethers and esters. The enzymes show substrate selectivity in that bile acids possessing a 6α-hydroxyl group are preferentially conjugated at the C-6 position forming 6-O-ether glucuronides, while short-chain bile acids form mainly glucuronides. Purification of the hyodeoxycholic acid-specific human UDP-glucuronosyltransferase and subsequent cloning of a cDNA indicate that this enzyme is highly specific toward hyodeoxycholic (3α,6α-dihydroxy-5β-cholanoic) acid; no glucuronidation of hyocholic (3α,6α,7α-trihydroxy-5β-cholanoic) acid could be detected. It is probable that there is a family of isozymes that catalyze the glucuronidation of different bile acids.

Glucosides and N-acetylglucosaminides of non-amidated and amidated bile acids have been identified in normal human urine with quantitative excretion comparable to that of glucuronide conjugates. A microsomal glucosyltransferase has been isolated and purified from human liver but is also present in extrahepatic tissues. The enzyme responsible for N-acetylglucosaminide formation exhibits remarkable substrate specificity in that it preferentially catalyzes the conjugation of bile acids having a 7β-hydroxyl group; consequently, these conjugates account for >20% of the urinary metabolites of patients administered UDCA. Finally, the full extent to which drugs may compete for the conjugating enzymes is not known, however bile acid conjugates of 5-fluorouracil have been identified.

Formation of secondary bile acids

Intestinal microflora play an important role in bile acid synthesis and metabolism. Bacterial enzymes metabolize primary bile acids, altering significantly their physicochemical characteristics and influencing their physiological actions during enterohepatic recycling. The result is the formation of a spectrum of secondary bile acids that are mainly excreted in feces. Deconjugation of conjugated bile acids followed by 7α-dehydroxylation are quantitatively the most important reactions, but bacterial oxido-reduction and epimerization at various positions of the bile acid nucleus also take place along the intestinal tract. This is evident from bile acid profiles along the entire length of the human intestine obtained at autopsy, which show relatively high proportions of secondary bile acids in the proximal jejunum, mid-small bowel, ileum, and cecum [20]. The enzymes that catalyze these reactions are found in a variety of organisms, such as *Escherichia coli* and *Bacteroides*, *Clostridia*, and *Bifidobacteria* spp., and some of these reactions occur in the proximal small intestine. Deconjugation precedes 7α-dehydroxylation, and the bacterial peptidases responsible for this reaction exhibit remarkable substrate specificity in that the length of the side-chain is a crucial factor influencing the reaction. 7α-Dehydroxylation of cholic and chenodeoxycholic acids, a reaction that proceeds via a 3-oxo-Δ^4-intermediate, results in the formation of deoxycholic and lithocholic acids, respectively, and these secondary bile acids make up the largest

proportion of total fecal bile acids. Lithocholic and deoxycholic acids are relatively insoluble and consequently poorly absorbed. However, both bile acids are returned to the liver and can regulate bile acid synthesis. It should be noted that, in rats, deoxycholic acid is efficiently 7α-hydroxylated in the liver and converted back to cholic acid, but this reaction does not take place in humans. Serum concentrations of deoxycholic acid, therefore, could provide a useful means of assessing the extent of impairment of the enterohepatic circulation in cholestatic liver diseases.

Regulation of bile acid synthesis

The major factor influencing bile acid synthesis is negative feedback by bile acids returning to the liver via the portal vein during their enterohepatic recycling. There are marked differences in the ability of different bile acids to regulate CYP7A1. For example, while the primary bile acids cholic and chenodeoxycholic acids downregulate synthesis, bile acids possessing a 7β-hydroxy group, such as UDCA, do not, and UDCA may actually increase synthesis rates. This observation has relevance to the treatment of inborn errors of bile acid synthesis. Interruption of the enterohepatic circulation, by biliary diversion or the feeding of anion exchange resins that bind bile acids in the intestinal lumen, results in an upregulation of CYP7A1 activity. In general, factors that influence CYP7A1 activity cause concomitant changes in the activity of HMG-CoA reductase, the rate-limiting enzyme for cholesterol synthesis and this serves to regulate cholesterol synthesis and maintain a constant cholesterol pool size. Interestingly, CYP7A1 exhibits a diurnal rhythm that is synchronous with the activity of HMG-CoA reductase and is reflected by diurnal changes in bile acid synthesis rates. A significant nocturnal rise in bile acid synthesis takes place that may be regulated by glucocorticoids because this regulation can be abolished by adrenalectomy, or hypophysectomy.

The mechanism involved in regulating CYP7A1 activity and, therefore, bile acid synthesis is complex and mediated through an ever-increasing number of nuclear receptors and transcription factors that have specificity for bile acids and oxysterols [2,21]. Bile acids have been shown to enter the nucleus of the hepatocyte and nuclear concentrations increase with bile acid feeding. These nuclear receptors include the farnesoid X receptor (FXR (NHR1H4)), short heterodimer partner, liver receptor homologue 1, hepatocyte nuclear factor-4α, liver X receptor-α, pregnane X receptor, constitutive androgen receptor, and fibroblast growth factor 19 and its receptor, and the G protein-coupled bile salt receptor TGR5. Much has been learned about the regulation of cholesterol and bile acid synthesis from gene knockout models of these nuclear receptors. New bile acid molecules have been recently synthesized as specific agonists for these receptors in order to devise ways of regulating cholesterol homeostasis and glucose metabolism and these are in clinical trials. In addition to influencing the transcriptional regulation of CYP7A1 in the liver, these

3β-Hydroxy-Δ⁵-C₂₇-steroid oxidoreductase

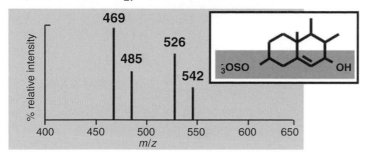

2-Methylacyl-CoA racemase

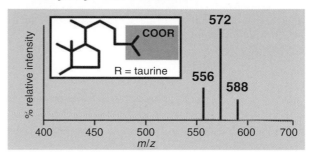

Δ⁴-3-Oxosteroid 5β-reductase

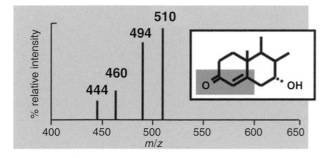

Sterol 27-hydroxylase

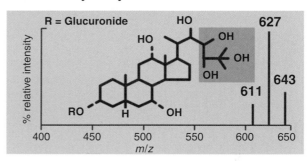

Oxysterol 7α-hydroxylase

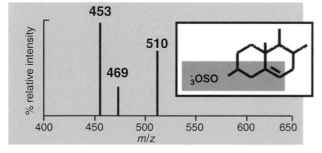

Conjugation (amidation) deficiency

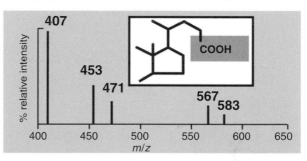

Figure 33.3 Reconstructed negative ion mass spectra generated from fast atom bombardment–mass spectrometry analysis of urine extracts typically observed in patients with six different genetic defects in bile acid synthesis. For simplicity, only the dominant and key diagnostic ions are shown for the specific metabolites formed in each genetic defect and the depiction of the chemical structure that characterize these diagnostic ions in the spectra.

receptors also induce transcription of the ileal bile acid-binding protein that is involved in the ileal uptake and conservation of the bile acid pool.

Defects in bile acid synthesis causing metabolic liver disease and syndromes of fat-soluble vitamin malabsorption

Defects in bile acid synthesis have profound effects on hepatic and gastrointestinal function and on cholesterol homeostasis, particularly when the cause is a genetic mutation encoding the enzymes responsible for primary bile acid synthesis. Such defects lead to an overproduction of hepatotoxic bile acids, which are synthesized from intermediates accumulating in the pathway proximal to the inactive enzyme, and a progressive cholestasis exacerbated by the lack of primary bile acids that are critical for promoting bile flow. Marked alterations in

urinary, serum, and biliary bile acids are found in all infants and children with liver disease and it can be difficult to determine whether such changes are primary or secondary to the liver dysfunction.

The first bile acid synthetic defect causing liver disease was discovered as a result of applying the liquid secondary ionization mass spectrometry (LSIMS) technique of fast atom bombardment ionization mass spectrometry (FAB-MS) [22]. This permitted the direct analysis of bile acids from a small drop of urine. While FAB-MS is still a definitive technique for diagnosing bile acid synthetic defects, newer mass spectrometric approaches have since been used, including electrospray ionization tandem mass spectrometry (ESI-MS) [23] and also gene sequencing techniques. However, mass spectrometry continues to offer the fastest and most accurate method of screening for these disorders because the mass spectra generated (Figure 33.3) permit accurate identification

Table 33.1 Genetic defects in bile acid synthesis causing liver disease, fat-soluble vitamin malabsorption, or neurological disease

Bile acid disorder	Gene and location
Steroid ring disorders	
Cholesterol 7α-hydroxylase (CYP7A1)	*CYP71A* (8q11-q12)
Oxysterol 7α-hydroxylase (CYP7B1)	CYP7B1 (8q21.3)
12α-Hydroxylase (CYP8B1)*	*CYP8B* (3p21.3-p22)
3β-Hydroxy-Δ^5-C$_{27}$-steroid oxidoreductase	*HSD3B7* (16p11.2-p12)
Δ^4-3-Oxosteroid 5β-reductase deficiency (AKR1D1)	*AKR1C4* (7q32-q33)
Side-chain modifications	
Sterol 27-hydroxylase (CYP27A1)	*CYP27A1* (2p23.3-p24.1)
2-Methylacyl-CoA racemase (AMACR)	*AMACR* (5p13.2-q11.1)
Sterol 25-hydroxylase	*CH25H* (10q23.31)
Bile acid-CoA ligase (BACL)	*BACL* (19q13.43)
Bile acid-CoA:N-acyl amino acid transferase (BAAT)	*BAAT* (9q22.3)
Secondary bile acid synthetic defects	
Peroxisomal biogenesis disorders (PEX defects)	multiple *PEX* genes
L-bifunctional protein	*EHHADH* (3q26.3-q28)
Δ^7-Dehydrocholesterol reductase (Smith–Lemli–Opitz)	*DHCR7* (11q13.4)

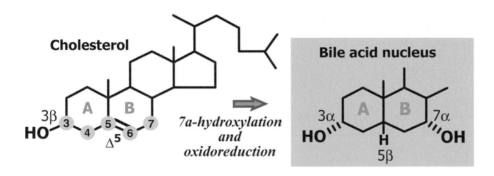

Figure 33.4 Sites of metabolic reactions on the AB-rings of cholesterol leading to the synthesis of the key intermediates in bile acid synthesis.

of the lack of primary bile acids and presence of atypical bile acids specific to each defect [22]. To date, eight well defined defects in bile acid synthesis have been described [3,13,15,16,19,24,25]; all have a highly variable phenotypic expression of familial and progressive infantile or late-onset cholestasis, of syndromes of fat-soluble vitamin malabsorption, and of variable degrees of neurologic involvement (Table 33.1). Based on experience from an international screening program at Cincinnati Children's Hospital Medical Center, bile acid synthesis defects have been identified in 2% of approximately 11 000 screened cases of idiopathic cholestatic liver disease in infants and children. Broadly, these defects can be categorized as deficiencies in the activity of enzymes responsible for catalyzing reactions to the steroid nucleus or to the side-chain.

Defects involving reactions to the steroid nucleus

Four defects have been identified involving enzymes catalyzing reactions that modify the AB-rings of the steroid nucleus (Figure 33.4). The clinical presentations of C$_{27}$3β-HSD (*HSD3B7*), Δ^5-3-oxosteroid 5β-reductase (*AKR1D1*), and CYP7B1 deficiencies are of progressive cholestatic liver disease. Typical biochemical abnormalities include elevations in serum liver enzymes, conjugated hyperbilirubinemia, and evidence of fat-soluble vitamin malabsorption. A normal serum gamma-glutamyltransferase is highly associated with, although not an exclusive feature of, all of the bile acid synthetic defects. Serum cholesterol concentrations are generally normal. The early clinical history of these patients often shows fat-soluble vitamin malabsorption, and in some cases rickets that precedes any evidence of liver dysfunction [26]. These abnormalities are usually responsive to oral vitamin supplementation, but these patients eventually present later in life with hepatosplenomegaly and elevated serum liver enzymes. The $C_{27}3\beta$-HSD deficiency is the most common of the bile acid synthetic defects, frequently accounting for cases of late-onset chronic cholestasis [27].

Cholesterol 7α-hydroxylase (CYP7A1) deficiency

Although not presenting as cholestatic liver disease, a deficiency in CYP7A1 was found to be responsible for hypertriglyceridemia and gallstone disease in three related adults [25]. This finding followed screening of *CYP7A1* for mutations in patients presenting with elevated low density lipoprotein (LDL)-cholesterol who were resistant to HMG-CoA reductase inhibitors. A 2 bp deletion (1302–1303delTT) was observed in exon 6 of the gene, resulting in a frameshift mutation and causing a Leu to Arg substitution that when transfected into HEK 293 cells led to an inactive protein product. All three patients were homozygous for this mutation and had serum cholesterol concentrations >300 mg/dL, LDL-cholesterol >180 mg/dL, and elevated triglycerides [25]. The heterozygous relatives of the two patients described also had elevated cholesterol. There was no evidence for cholestasis, fibrosis, or inflammation but fatty changes in the liver were reported following biopsy. Fecal bile acid analysis revealed markedly reduced total bile acid output (6% of normal) and a high (chenodeoxycholic + lithocholic)/(cholic + deoxycholic) acid ratio, consistent with preferential synthesis of chenodeoxycholic acid via the "acidic pathway" for bile acid synthesis. This clinical phenotype differs from that of the $Cyp7a1^{-/-}$ mouse knockout, which has normal cholesterol levels.

Oxysterol 7α-hydroxylase (CYP7B1) deficiency

The discovery of a genetic defect in *CYP7B1* [3] emphasizes the quantitative importance of the "acidic" pathway for bile acid synthesis in early life. Unlike the mouse, where the enzyme appears to be developmentally regulated, or the rat where it is induced when there is suppression of CYP7A1 activity, it would appear that in the neonatal period of humans CYP7B1 is more important than CYP7A1 for bile acid synthesis. This genetic defect presents as severe progressive cholestatic liver disease. It was first described in a 10-week-old boy of parents who were first cousins [3,5,6]. The index patient had severe cholestasis, cirrhosis, and liver synthetic failure from early infancy. He became progressively jaundiced by 8 weeks of age, had hepatosplenomegaly and markedly elevated serum amintransferases, but a normal serum gamma-glutamyltransferase. The liver biopsy revealed cholestasis, bridging fibrosis, extensive giant-cell transformation, and bile duct proliferation. A similar clinical picture and liver histology was reported for a 5-month-old Taiwanese infant [5], and a 6-month-old Japanese infant [6]. Oral UDCA therapy proved ineffective or led to a deterioration in liver function

tests in all of these patients. Oral cholic acid therapy was also ineffective in the index case; that patient underwent liver transplantation at 4 months of age. The Taiwanese infant died at 11 months of age before transplant could be performed, but the infant from Japan underwent living donor transplantation with a graft from the mother who had a compound heterozygous mutation (R112X/R417C) in *CYP7B1* and the child was reportedly still alive 2 years after transplantation [6]. These examples highlight the severity of this bile acid synthetic defect. It is possible that this cause of idiopathic liver disease may go unrecognized because of its rapid downhill course in the early months of life. The therapeutic strategy for patients with this defect should, in the future, target downregulation of sterol 27-hydroxylase.

Diagnosis of all three cases was by mass spectrometry: FAB-MS analysis of the urine from the index case revealed an absence of primary bile acids and in their place large concentrations of unsaturated monohydroxy-C_{24} bile acids as sulfate (*m/z* 453) and glyco-sulfate (*m/z* 510) conjugates (Figure 33.3). Use of gas chromatography (GC)-MS confirmed that these atypical bile acids were the unsaturated monohydroxy-bile acids, 3β-hydroxy-5-cholenoic and 3β-hydroxy-5-cholestenoic acids, which accounted for 97% and 86%, respectively, of the total serum and urinary bile acids. Additionally, 27-hydroxycholesterol concentrations in serum and urine were >4500 times normal and no 7α-hydroxylated sterols were detected [3]. Similar GC-MS profiles were reported for the two Asian infants [5,6]. The formation of 3β-hydroxy-5-cholenoic and 3β-hydroxy-5-cholestenoic acids occurs exclusively via the acidic pathway and the mass spectrometry findings definitively establish a CYP7B1 deficiency while illustrating how important the acidic pathway is for bile acid synthesis in early life. Monohydroxy-bile acids with the 3β-hydroxy-Δ^5 structure and oxysterols are good ligands for FXR, which would suppress CYP7A1, preventing bile acids being synthesized by the classical pathway [3]. Furthermore, these unsaturated bile acids are extremely cholestatic and the hepatotoxicity in these patients would be exacerbated by the lack of primary bile acids necessary to maintain bile flow. Active CYP7B1 is essential for protecting the liver from hepatotoxic and cholestatic 3β-hydroxy-Δ^5-monohydroxy bile acids that otherwise would accumulate in the acidic pathway (Figure 33.5).

Molecular studies on liver tissue from the first patient showed no CYP7B1 activity, or mRNA, and gene sequencing revealed a C388T transition mutation in exon 5, providing unambiguous confirmation of the genetic defect in *CYP7B1* [3]. This patient was homozygous for this nonsense mutation, while both parents were heterozygous. When cells were transfected with the cDNA having the R388* mutation, there was no detectable CYP7B1 activity. Immunoblot analysis confirmed that the mutated gene encoded a truncated protein unable to catalyze 7α-hydroxylation [3]. In the Taiwanese infant, a single substitution C538T in exon 3 of *CYP7B1* caused an amino acid transition from arginine to a stop codon at position 112 (R112→Stop) [5]. The Japanese infant

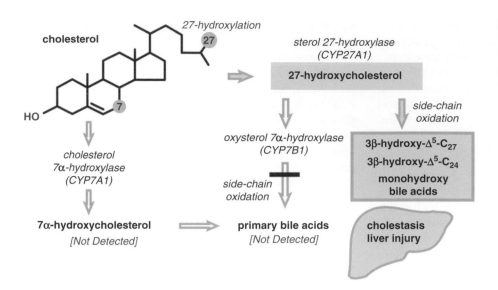

Figure 33.5 The metabolic pathways for primary bile acid synthesis from cholesterol depicting the biochemical presentation in patients with a deficiency of oxysterol 7α-hydroxylase (CYP7B1) activity causing severe neonatal cholestatic liver disease.

had a compound heterozygous mutation (R112X/R417C) in exons 3 and 6 of *CYP7B1* [6]. In all cases, the patients were homozygous for their respective mutations and the parents heterozygous.

3β-Hydroxy-Δ^5-C$_{27}$-steroid oxidoreductase deficiency

The most common of the disorders of bile acid synthesis involves the second step in the pathway – the conversion of 7α-hydroxycholesterol into 7α-hydroxy-4-cholesten-3-one, a reaction catalyzed by microsomal C$_{27}$3β-HSD [2]. Deficiency of this sterol-specific enzyme [24] results in the accumulation of 7α-hydroxycholesterol within the hepatocyte. The other enzymes involved in bile acid synthesis catalyze the remaining transformations, including side-chain oxidation, so that in place of the normal primary bile acids, C$_{24}$-bile acids are synthesized retaining the 3β-hydroxy-Δ^5 structure characteristic of the substrate for the enzyme (Figure 33.6).

This defect was first described in a Saudi Arabian patient, the third infant of five to be affected by progressive idiopathic neonatal cholestasis; the two previous infants had died following a similar clinical history and were products of a consanguineous marriage [24]. All of the affected infants had progressive jaundice, elevated serum aminotransferases, and a conjugated hyperbilirubinemia. This generalized clinical presentation is common to all recognized cases so far [28–30]. Upon clinical examination, patients with C$_{27}$3β-HSD deficiency usually present with hepatomegaly, fat-soluble vitamin malabsorption, and mild steatorrhea. Pruritus is usually not a symptom. This inborn error is highly associated with elevated serum bilirubin and aminotransferases and a normal serum gamma-glutamyltransferase, and this biochemical picture is a useful clinical marker for a suspected defect. Furthermore, serum bile acid concentrations, if measured by enzymatic or immunoassay methods, can be normal and seemingly incompatible with the extent of cholestasis. Therefore, the inclusion

of serum bile acid determination in the clinical evaluation may provide a further clue to this defect. Histological examination of the liver of these patients shows the presence of giant cells and is consistent with cholestasis as evidenced by canalicular plugs, bile stasis, and inflammatory changes [24,28,30,31].

As with most of the inborn errors involving the reactions responsible for nuclear modification, the C$_{27}$3β-HSD deficiency is progressive and familial in nature and may be fatal if untreated. Age at onset and diagnosis is variable, ranging from 3 months into the adult years. Recently it was diagnosed in a 24-year-old woman with cirrhosis of unknown etiology; remarkable was the finding that her sister and a first cousin had died of cirrhosis at ages 19 and 6 years, respectively, and another 32-year-old first cousin was also affected [27]. Homozygosity mapping was used to identify a mutation in *HSD3B7*, which established the diagnosis of a C$_{27}$3β-HSD deficiency as the cause of liver failure. This was subsequently confirmed by FAB-MS analysis of the serum from the living 32-year-old woman and deceased family members [27]. These cases indicate that a bile acid synthetic defect should be considered in late-onset chronic cholestasis [22]. Indeed the majority of these patients are now being diagnosed outside of the neonatal period.

Multiple 3β-hydroxy-Δ^5-hydroxysteroid oxidoreductases exist that catalyze analogous reactions in steroid hormone metabolism but the lack of endocrine abnormalities in these patients is consistent with the specificity of this enzyme toward C$_{27}$-sterols.

Diagnosis of C$_{27}$3β-HSD deficiency is definitively established by FAB-MS or ESI-MS analysis of urine [22,23], which reveals an absence of the normal glycine- and taurine-conjugated primary bile and the presence of the sulfate and glycosulfate conjugates 3β,7α-dihydroxy- and 3β,7α,12α-trihydroxy-5-cholenoic acids. These atypical bile acids are recognized by their respective negative ions of *m/z* 469, 485, 526, and 542 [22]. Some differences are observed between FAB-MS and ESI-MS spectra as evident from a report of a 26-year-old

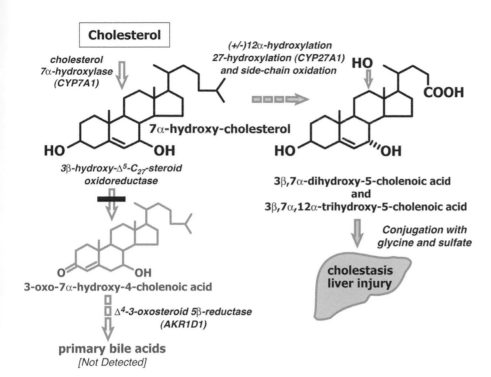

Figure 33.6 The metabolic pathways for primary bile acid synthesis from cholesterol depicting the biochemical presentation in patients with a deficiency of 3β-hydroxy-Δ^5-C_{27}-steroid dehydrogenase/isomerase activity presenting as early- or late-onset chronic cholestasis.

patient with a genetically confirmed mutation in *HSD3B7* who showed (in the urine) a single dominant ion at m/z 462 by ESI-MS, and an absence of the ions typically observed with FAB-MS [29]. When the same urine sample was later analyzed by FAB-MS, this ion was of minor intensity and the characteristic ions at m/z 469, 485, 526, and 542 served to identify this defect (KDR Setchell; unpublished observation). These differences in ionization between the techniques require consideration in order to avoid misdiagnosis. Tetrahydroxy- and pentahydroxy-bile alcohols with a $3\beta,7\alpha$-dihydroxy-Δ^5 and $3\beta,7\alpha,12\alpha$-trihydroxy-Δ^5 nuclei are also found in greatly increased amounts in the urine, plasma, and bile [32]. These bile alcohols are mainly sulfated, in contrast to the glucuronide conjugates of saturated bile alcohols observed in CTX [22]. Although primary bile acids are not detectable in the urine, the bile may contain small proportions of cholic acid resulting from intestinal bacterial metabolism of the 3β-hydroxy-Δ^5-bile acids during enterohepatic recycling. This may facilitate bile secretion to explain the delay in onset of cholestasis and longer survival of these patients.

Fibroblasts also contain $C_{27}3\beta$-HSD, which means its activity can be measured in cultured fibroblasts using 7α-hydroxy-cholesterol as substrate. In contrast to healthy controls, patients with this defect have no detectable enzyme activity in fibroblasts [7,23]. Their parents have a low but measurable activity consistent with a heterozygous phenotype. Sequencing of *HSD3B7*, localized to chromosome 16p11.2-12, has failed to find a common mutation for this disorder. In 16 patients, 12 different mutations were identified, including, point mutations, small insertions, and deletions [9]. A 2 bp deletion in exon 6 accounted for the inactivity of this enzyme in the index case with this bile acid defect [8]. In four patients, mutations were compound heterozygous while the majority were inherited in homozygous form. When several of the identified mutations were expressed in HEK 293 cells, impaired synthesis of the normal protein could be demonstrated and this lacked enzyme activity [9].

The mechanism of liver injury is considered to be by the accumulation of atypical bile acids concomitant with a lack of primary bile acids. In animal models, 3β-hydroxy-5-cholenoic acid produces cholestasis, but this is not the case for $3\beta,7\alpha$-dihydroxy-5-cholenoic acid, which is rapidly metabolized to chenodeoxycholic acid in animals. This conversion does not occur in patients lacking $C_{27}3\beta$-HSD. Studies using rat liver canalicular membrane vesicles have shown *tauro*-$3\beta,7\alpha$-dihydroxy-5-cholenoic acid to be markedly cholestatic [33].

Oral administration of the primary bile acid, cholic acid (5–15 mg/kg body weight daily), the therapeutic approach for these patients, is expected to resolve the biochemical and histological abnormalities and to improve growth [22,30]. Chenodeoxycholic acid has also been effective [34] but is more cathartic and may cause loose stools or diarrhea in young infants. In some cases, patients have been maintained temporarily on UDCA [30], which is choleretic but does not inhibit bile acid synthesis, or a combination of UDCA and chenodeoxycholic acid [34]. Cholic acid is a ligand for FXR, which downregulates hepatic CYP7A1 activity to limit production of hepatotoxic 3β-hydroxy-Δ^5-bile acids, while additionally providing the stimulus for bile flow. Concomitant with the disappearance of 3β-hydroxy-Δ^5-bile acids after initiating therapy, there are clinical and biochemical improvements with a normalization of liver function tests and resolution of jaundice in virtually all treated patients [22,28]. Furthermore, oral primary bile acid therapy in these patients avoids the need for liver transplantation, which is the only alternative therapy.

Δ^4-3-Oxosteroid 5β-reductase (AKR1D1) deficiency:

A deficiency of cytosolic AKR1D1 responsible for the catalytic conversion of 7α-hydroxy- and 7α,12α-dihydroxy-4-cholesten-3-one into the corresponding 3-oxo-5β(H) analogues was first described in monochorionic twins born with a marked and progressive cholestasis [13]. A previous sibling with neonatal hepatitis had died of liver failure following a similar clinical course. Evaluation revealed elevated serum aminotransferases, marked hyperbilirubinemia, and coagulopathy. Unlike C_{27}3β-HSD deficiency, serum gamma-glutamyltransferase concentrations are generally elevated. Liver biopsies showed marked lobular disarray as a result of giant-cell and pseudoacinar transformation of hepatocytes, hepatocellular and canalicular bile stasis, and extramedullary hematopoiesis. Electron micrographs showed small bile canaliculi that were slit-like in appearance, lacking the usual microvilli and containing variable amounts of electron-dense material [13,28,31,35]. Deficiency of AKR1D1 was identified in both twins by urinary FAB-MS analysis, which indicated an elevated bile acid excretion and a predominance of bile acid conjugates with molecular weights consistent with unsaturated oxo-hydroxy- and oxo-dihydroxy-cholenoic acids (Figure 33.3). Confirmation that these were 3-oxo-7α-hydroxy-4-cholenoic and 3-oxo-7α,12α-dihydroxy-4-cholenoic acids was established after extraction, hydrolysis, and derivatization of bile acids and GC-MS analysis [13]. Small proportions of allo(5α-H)-isomers of cholic and chenodeoxycholic acids were also present and there was a lack of primary bile acids. These atypical bile acids accounted for up to 90% of the total urinary bile acids. There was a high concentration of allo-chenodeoxycholic, allo-cholic, and Δ^4-3-oxo-bile acids in serum. Only trace amounts (<2 μmol/L) of bile acids were detected in bile. Studies using rat canalicular membrane vesicles showed that Δ^4-3-oxo-bile acids are poor substrates for the canalicular bile acid transporters [33], presumably because of their poor solubility or low affinity for the transporters. The presence of appreciable levels of allo-bile acids, normally minor metabolites, is explained by the accumulated substrates exceeding the K_m and V_{max} for the hepatic steroid 5α-reductase in the absence of AKR1D1 activity. Interestingly, steroid hormone studies of one patient with a C662T missense mutation in AKR1D1 deficiency found an almost total absence of 5β-reduced steroid hormone metabolites and a dominance of 5α-reduced metabolites, yet the patient had no obvious endocrine abnormalities [36].

As *AKR1D1* is not expressed in fibroblasts, further evidence for a primary enzyme defect was established by immunoblot analysis of the cytosolic fraction from the liver using a monoclonal antibody raised against rat AKR1D1. This monoclonal antibody recognized the 38 kDa protein in the liver from patients with liver disease of other etiologies, but not from the patients with AKR1D1 deficiency. The cDNA for human *AKR1D1* (*SRD5B*) was reported and studies of three patients with high levels of Δ^4-3-oxo-bile acids in urine and low or absent primary bile acids, revealed three different mutations in this gene, consistent with a primary enzyme defect in each case [14]. Two patients were homozygous for missense mutations C662T in one patient and C385T in another; a third patient was homozygous for a single base deletion (511 delT) in exon 5, leading to a premature stop codon. The liver biopsies of all three patients were characterized by giant-cell transformation, a common feature of many of the inborn errors in bile acid synthesis [28,31]. Since these early reports, additional different mutations have been linked to a deficiency in AKR1D1 activity in infants [12,30]. In a patient from Japan who met biochemical criteria for a deficiency in this enzyme, sequence analysis revealed a single silent mutation in the coding region of the gene, but immunoblot analysis of the liver homogenate using a monoclonal antibody revealed expression of the normal protein, thus excluding a primary genetic defect. Increased production of Δ^4-3-oxo-bile acids is not uncommon in patients with severe liver disease and is a feature of immaturity in hepatic bile acid synthesis in infants during the first few weeks of life. Several infants presenting with neonatal hemochromatosis were reported to have an AKR1D1 deficiency [37]. Since primary bile acids are involved in the canalicular transport of iron, the question of whether the iron-storage defect may be secondary to the bile acid synthetic defect, or vice versa, has been raised. In suspected AKR1D1 deficiency, it is important to perform a repeat analysis of urine because, on some occasions, resolution of the liver disease occurs and these atypical bile acids spontaneously disappear. Furthermore the findings ideally should be supported by confirmation of a mutation in the gene.

The liver injury in this defect is the consequence of diminished primary bile acid synthesis and the hepatotoxicity of the accumulated Δ^4-3-oxo-bile acids. The unique morphologic findings on electron microscopy of the liver of the first patients described suggest that maturation of the canalicular membrane and the transport system for bile acid secretion may require a threshold concentration of primary bile acids in early development [35]. Primary bile acid therapy resulted in a normalization of the immature-appearing bile canalicular structures with a disappearance of the electron-dense material seen in and around the canaliculi.

Treatment of this disorder with oral cholic acid (5–15 mg/kg body weight daily) has in most patients resulted in clinical and biochemical improvement, resolution of jaundice, and normalization in liver function tests, provided that therapy was initiated before significant liver damage occurred [30,35]. Use of UDCA was reported not to be ineffective, but it has been used in combination with cholic or chenodeoxycholic acids in some patients [30,38]. In theory, cholic acid is best administered as a divided dose to optimize downregulation in bile acid

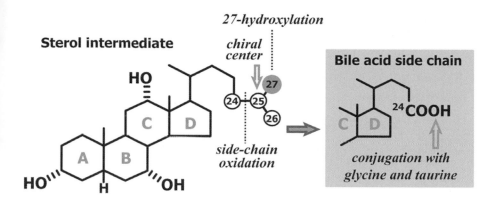

Figure 33.7 Sites of metabolic reactions on the sterol side-chain leading to the synthesis of the key intermediates in bile acid synthesis.

synthesis. The presence of the Δ^4-3-oxo-bile acids in urine should be monitored and the dose titrated according to biochemical and clinical responses [22]. In a few patients, cholic acid has failed to reverse the liver injury; this was likely because the diagnosis was established at an advanced stage when there was cirrhosis and end-stage liver disease.

Defects involving reactions leading to side-chain modification

Defects in the reactions involved in side-chain hydroxylation and oxidation generally present as neurological disturbances and/or syndromes of fat-soluble vitamin malabsorption. These manifestations emphasize the crucial role that bile acids play in the intestinal absorption of lipids. The structural position of these defects is indicated in Figure 33.7. Liver disease is generally mild and may not necessarily be the primary clinical presentation, because low levels of primary bile acids are often made via alternative pathways of synthesis. Cerebrotendinous xanthomatosis was the first defect in bile acid synthesis to be described [15,39] and has been shown conclusively to be caused by mutations in the gene for sterol 27-hydroxylase. More recently, defects in bile acid conjugation and a specific single enzyme defect in peroxisomal beta-oxidation have been described. Generalized disorders in peroxisomal structure and function, distinct from single-enzyme defects in the fatty acid oxidation system, ultimately lead to progressive liver disease, but this is secondary to the underlying genetic disease.

Sterol 27-hydroxylase deficiency (CYP27A1): cerebrotendinous xanthomatosis

Cerebrotendinous xanthomatosis is a rare autosomal recessive lipid-storage disease has an estimated prevalence of 1 in 70 000. The disease is usually not diagnosed until the second or third decade of life when it becomes symptomatic, but it has been detected in a few children. The clinical presentation includes symptoms of progressive neurologic dysfunction, dementia, ataxia, cataracts and the presence of xanthomas in the brain and tendons. It has been suggested that the presence of bilateral juvenile cataracts and a history of chronic diarrhea, although not specific for CTX, may represent an early clinical

manifestation of the disease. More recently, it has been associated with a transient increase in serum liver enzymes in several infants, suggesting the earliest clinical picture may be that of mild cholestasis that ultimately resolves over the first few months of life [40]. In one case report, it was associated with fatal cholestasis in infancy [41]. The main biochemical features of this disease are a significantly reduced synthesis of primary bile acids; elevated biliary, urinary, and fecal excretion of bile alcohol glucuronides; a normal or low plasma cholesterol concentration with excessive deposition of cholesterol and cholestanol in tissues; and a markedly elevated plasma cholestanol concentration.

In the 1970s, Salen and coworkers demonstrated that the basic defect in this disorder was an impairment in side-chain oxidation [39]. Chenodeoxycholic acid synthesis was affected to a greater extent than cholic acid synthesis. Conclusive evidence that the primary defect in CTX is a defect in sterol 27-hydroxylase (Figure 33.8) finally came from molecular studies, facilitated by the cloning of the human sterol 27-hydroxylase cDNA [15]. Since these original findings, over 40 different mutations have been identified in *CYP27A1*, which have included insertion, deletion, and point mutations [15]. Interestingly, the mitochondrial sterol 27-hydroxylase also catalyzes hepatic 25-hydroxylation of vitamin D, yet despite this, 25-hydroxyvitamin D levels are not usually altered in patients with CTX.

A striking feature of this disease is the accumulation of 5α-cholestan-3β-ol (cholestanol) in the nervous system and the markedly elevated concentrations of this sterol, but not cholesterol, in the plasma [15]. The cholestanol:cholesterol ratio in plasma may be of diagnostic value, although an elevation of this ratio, and an increased urinary excretion of bile alcohol glucuronides, is often seen in patients with cholestatic liver diseases. The most plausible explanation is that the high cholestanol levels arise from sterol intermediates that accumulate in the absence of sterol 27-hydroxylase activity. A pathway has been proposed involving 7α-hydroxylation of cholesterol, and conversion to 7α-hydroxy-4-cholesten-3-one, followed by 7α-dehydroxylation that is hepatic rather than intestinal and yields cholest-4,6-dien-3-one as an intermediate. Radiolabeling studies confirmed this pathway, and patients with CTX have

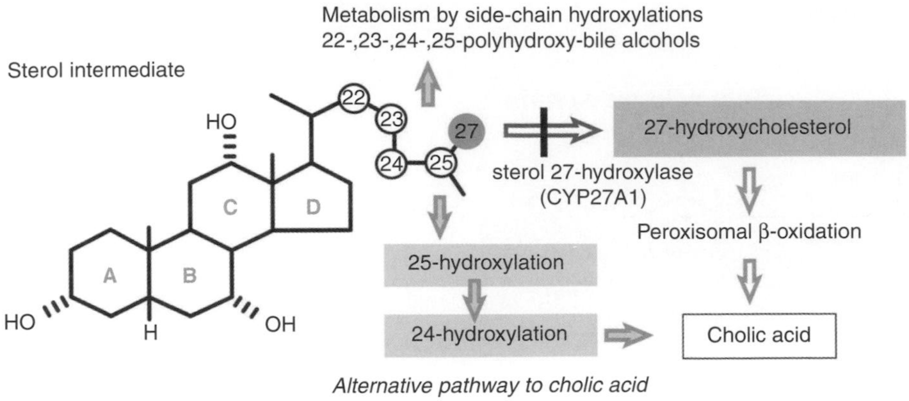

Figure 33.8 The metabolic pathways for primary bile acid synthesis from cholesterol depicting the biochemical presentation in patients with a sterol 27-hydroxylase deficiency (CYP27A1) causing cerebrotendinous xanthomatosis, leading to diminished primary bile acid synthesis and excessive production of bile alcohols. Note, cholic acid is synthesized by the alternative 25-hydroxylation pathway (see also Figure 33.2).

elevated plasma 7α-hydroxy-4-cholesten-3-one and cholest-4,6-dien-3-one levels [15]. Furthermore, colestyramine administration, which increases CYP7A1 activity, leads to increased plasma cholestanol concentrations, while chenodeoxycholic acid administration has the opposite effect.

Diagnosis of CTX at an early age is essential to limit neurologic and cardiovascular complications resulting from the chronic and irreversible deposition of cholesterol and cholestanol in tissues. Diagnosis is generally based on a greatly increased plasma cholestanol:cholesterol ratio, although in some cases this is not entirely reliable, and/or an elevated excretion of bile alcohols in urine [22]. These analyses are highly specialized, time consuming, complex, and outside the scope of routine clinical laboratories. However, using MS it is possible to rapidly and definitively diagnose CTX from an analysis of urine, which reveals the presence of increased levels of bile alcohol glucuronides [22]. The typical FAB-MS negative ion spectrum from a patient with CTX reveals [M-H]$^-$ characteristic of bile alcohol glucuronides (Figure 33.3). In health, bile acid conjugates and bile alcohol glucuronides are excreted in such low levels that these compounds are barely detectable. In CTX, the ions at m/z 611, 627, and 643 become dominant in the spectrum and these represent tetrahydroxy-, pentahydroxy- and hexahydroxy-bile alcohol glucuronides, respectively. Further confirmation of CTX can be achieved by complementing the MS analysis with DNA sequencing of *CYP27A1* and identification of the specific mutation.

Effective treatment of CTX has been achieved by oral bile acid administration [42]. Chenodeoxycholic acid (750 mg/day) normalizes plasma cholestanol with a concomitant decrease in the excretion of urinary bile alcohol glucuronides, consistent with downregulation in endogenous CYP7A1 activity. These biochemical changes are accompanied by an improvement in clinical symptoms, particularly the neurological disturbances and are most effective when initiated prior to the onset of significant symptomology. Cholic and deoxycholic acids also decrease plasma cholestanol and in infants may be preferable, but UDCA is ineffective. Bile acid therapy may be more effective in CTX if combined with an HMG-CoA reductase inhibitor, which additionally inhibits endogenous cholesterol synthesis and reduces plasma cholestanol concentrations.

2-Methylacyl-CoA racemase deficiency

2-Methylacyl-CoA racemase deficiency was reported in a 3-week-old female infant presenting with mildly elevated liver enzymes and low serum 25-hydroxyvitamin D and vitamin E concentrations [16]. Identification of this defect was based on MS analysis of the urine and serum, complemented by molecular studies. Molecular analysis of the gene encoding the enzyme showed a missense mutation yielding an inactive protein (S52P) in this patient. Interestingly, the same mutation was reported in two of three patients with an adult-onset sensory neuropathy characterized by elevated serum phytanic and pristanic acids, but neither fat-soluble vitamin malabsorption nor liver disease were features of the three adult cases. 2-Methylacyl Co-A racemase catalyzes the racemization of the (25R)-diastereoisomers of di- and trihydroxycholestanoic acids to their (25S)-isomers; this reaction is a prerequisite for the initiation of peroxisomal beta-oxidation of the side-chain of these C$_{27}$ bile acid intermediates. It is also responsible for the racemization of (2R)-pristanoyl Co-A to its (2S)-diastereoisomer prior to peroxisomal beta-oxidative degradation, and this broad substrate specificity explains why in this genetic disease very-long-chain fatty acids are normal while pristanic acid, a branch-chained fatty acid, is elevated (Figure 33.9). The urinary FAB-MS analysis from one patient gave a spectrum (Figure 33.3) identical to that observed in Zellweger syndrome; however, plasma very-long-chain fatty acids and other peroxisomal enzyme markers were all normal. Use of high-performance liquid chromatography (HPLC) with ESI-MS was used to separate the diastereoisomers of di- and trihydroxycholestanoic acids and to confirm the presence of exclusively the (25R)-forms in the serum and bile of the patient [16].

This patient responded successfully to fat-soluble vitamin supplementation and cholic acid therapy (15 mg/kg daily), with normalization of liver function tests; she was neurologically and developmentally normal at age 3.5 years. The clinical history is remarkable for a previous sibling who was initially healthy until 5.5 months of age but died suddenly following an intracranial bleed that was secondary to vitamin K deficiency. The liver of this sibling, apparently having the same bile acid synthetic defect, was transplanted, and the recipient was alive

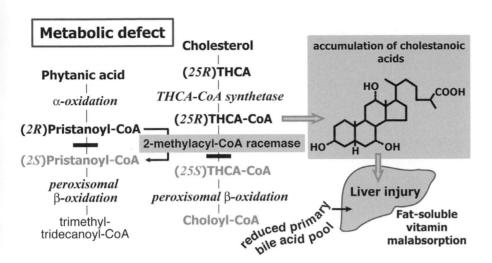

Figure 33.9 Biochemical defect clinical presentation of a deficiency in the activity of 2-methylacyl-CoA racemase. The metabolic pathways for primary bile acid synthesis and branched-chain fatty acid synthesis utilize the same 2-methylacyl-CoA racemase enzyme. THCA, trihydroxycholestanoic acid.

5 years later but receiving oral bile acid therapy [16]. Dietary restriction of phytanic acid should be implemented in this disorder to prevent longer-term neurological damage caused by the accumulation of branched-chain fatty acids. A 2-methyl-acyl-CoA racemase knockout mouse model confirms the importance of phytol restriction in preventing neurological and hepatic manifestations [43]. Since the primary presentation in this infant and her deceased sibling was fat-soluble vitamin malabsorption, this discovery makes a strong case for the screening for bile acid synthetic defects in unexplained fat-soluble vitamin malabsorption or rickets to permit therapeutic intervention with primary bile acids.

Side-chain oxidation defect in the 25-hydroxylation pathway

A defect in side-chain oxidation in the 25-hydroxylation pathway was proposed by Clayton *et al.* for a 9-week-old infant presenting with familial giant-cell hepatitis and severe intrahepatic cholestasis [44]. The diagnosis was based upon the findings of reduced cholic and chenodeoxycholic acid concentrations, and elevated serum concentrations of bile alcohol glucuronides, specifically 5β-cholestane-3β,7α,12α,24-tetrol, 5β-cholest-24-ene-3β,7α,12α,24-tetrol, and 5β-cholestane-3β,7α,12α,25-tetrol. These bile alcohols are not normally found in the plasma of infants with liver disease. Bile alcohol glucuronides were major metabolites in the urine [44]. Although this profile resembled that of patients with CTX, it was concluded on the basis of the liver disease, which at that time had not been previously described as a feature of CTX, that this represented an oxidation defect downstream of the 25-hydroxylation step in this minor pathway for bile acid synthesis. The implications of the findings are that the 25-hydroxylation pathway, considered of negligible importance in adults, may be important in infants. The patient was treated with chenodeoxycholic and cholic acids, which led to normalization in serum aminotransferases and suppression of bile alcohol production.

Peroxisomal disorders

Disorders involving peroxisomal assembly and function have a significant impact upon bile acid synthesis. This is perhaps not surprising since the peroxisome packages at least 40 enzymes, including those required for the beta-oxidation of fatty acids and bile acids, as well as the enzymes catalyzing bile acid conjugation. Most of the disorders in bile acid synthesis in peroxisomopathies are secondary to the primary defect of organelle dysfunction. A review of the clinical and biochemical abnormalities appears in Chapter 37; consequently, this section will highlight only the features pertinent to bile acid metabolism. The early diagnosis of a peroxisomopathy is interestingly often the result of referral of the patient to a gastroenterologist for evaluation of abnormal liver biochemistries.

Many of the peroxisomal disorders show similarities and overlap in clinical and biochemical presentation. Conditions in which there is a generalized impairment in peroxisomal function exhibit abnormalities in bile acid synthesis and metabolism, and these patients often have significant liver disease. Pin-pointing the exact nature of the peroxisomopathy can be challenging and requires a battery of tests to examine the entire beta-oxidation pathway of bile acids and very-long-chain fatty acids, complemented by immunoblotting techniques to identify the presence and activity of other peroxisomal enzymes and genetic screening to sequence the *PEX* gene exons for peroxisomal biogenesis disorders.

Mass spectrometry, both LSIMS (FAB-MS or ESI-MS) and GC-MS, of the urine and plasma/serum permits accurate identification of abnormalities in peroxisomal beta-oxidation of bile acids [22], particularly when there is evidence of progressive liver disease. A typical FAB-MS of the urine reveals the presence of [M-H]⁻ corresponding to unconjugated trihydroxycholestanoic acid (m/z 449), taurine-conjugated trihydroxycholestanoic acid (m/z 556), and taurine-conjugated tetrahydroxylated cholestanoic acids (m/z 572), which tends to be dominant (Figure 33.3). Elevated levels of di- and trihydroxycholestanoic acids and a C_{29}-dicarboxylic bile acid in biological fluids are a consistent feature of patients with Zellweger syndrome, neonatal adrenoleukodystrophy, infantile Refsum disease and pseudo-Zellweger syndrome [45], and peroxisomal biogenesis disorders [46,47]. Of the single enzyme defects, X-linked adrenoleukodystrophy and pseudo-neonatal adrenoleukodystrophy both show normal bile acid synthesis with no accumulation of cholestanoic acids. Dihydroxycholestanoic acid concentrations are in general much lower than trihydroxycholestanoic acid, particularly in younger patients, and this is explained by its preferential conversion to trihydroxycholestanoic acid by 12α-hydroxylation. The origin of a C_{29}-dicarboxylic acid found in serum of many patients with Zellweger synrome is presumed to be from side-chain elongation in the endoplasmic reticulum. Although bile acid synthetic rates are low in patients with Zellweger syndrome, increased serum concentrations of primary bile acids are frequently found and are probably a consequence of impaired hepatic function. Additional metabolism of trihydroxycholestanoic acid by microsomal hydroxylation in the side-chain (to produce C-24 hydroxylated, varanic acid isomers), and in the nucleus (to produce C-1 and C-6 tetrahydroxycholestanoic acids) gives rise to many tetrahydroxylated cholestanoic acids that are excreted in urine and present in plasma, and these are of diagnostic value [45]. The urine from the parents of patients with Zellweger syndrome, who are heterozygous for this most severe form of peroxisomal defect, will have normal urinary bile acid excretion with negligible or no detectable cholestanoic acids [45]. In genetic counseling of affected families, prenatal diagnosis is possible by specific detection of elevated concentrations of di- and trihydroxycholestanoic acids in amniotic fluid.

While the diagnosis of Zellweger syndrome is often straightforward, characterizing and differentiating patients with less severe phenotypes and with single enzyme defects involving peroxisomal enzymes is more difficult. There have been several case reports of presumed trihydroxycholestanoic acid-CoA oxidase deficiencies, and phytanic and pristanic acids, when measured, have been elevated in these patients. All presented with ataxia, and unlike patients with 2-methylacyl-CoA racemase deficiency, who share a similar biochemical profile [16], there was no evidence for any neurological disorder. With the more recent recognition of the complexity of peroxisomal biogenesis disorders, it is possible that some of these previously reported cases could have been caused by mutations in *PEX* genes, of which there are 12 known.

Treatment of the peroxisomopathies is difficult because of the multiorgan pathophysiology of the diseases and is to a large extent restricted to managing the symptoms. Dietary restriction of very-long-chain fatty acids and phytanic acid, and administration of oleic acid, have provided minimal to no benefit in the full-blown Zellweger syndrome. Clofibrate, which has been shown in rats to induce peroxisomal proliferation, has proven to be of no therapeutic value. In general, the

prognosis in most peroxisomal disorders is poor, and patients with Zellweger syndrome generally succumb to respiratory failure. The progressive liver disease that commonly develops in peroxisomal disorders may in part result from increased synthesis and accumulation of C_{27}-bile acids and reduced primary bile acid synthesis. Infusion of *tauro*-trihydroxycholestanoic acid in rats induces red-cell hemolysis and produces a hepatic lesion showing mitochondrial disruption similar to that found in patients with Zellweger syndrome. In an attempt to limit the severity of liver injury in a patient with Zellweger syndrome, primary bile acids were given orally and resulted in a marked improvement in biochemical markers of liver injury and histology, most notably a decrease in the extent of bile duct proliferation and inflammation [45]. This improvement was concomitant with a decrease in the urinary and serum concentrations of cholestanoic acids. A striking and sustained increase in growth and significant improvement in neurologic symptoms were also noted. Based upon this observation and following the successful treatment of patients with primary enzyme defects in bile acid synthesis, cholic acid therapy has now been used in a number of patients with peroxisomal disorders, with variable outcomes [22]. In a study of patients with a variety of peroxisomopathies, including Refsum disease, neonatal adrenoleukodystrophy, and Zellweger syndrome, treatment with cholic acid (10–15 mg/kg daily) for periods ranging from 4.7 to 11 years in duration had variable outcomes. Not surprisingly, the treatment failures mostly included those patients with the more severe Zellweger syndrome, while those patients with single enzyme defects in peroxisomal function causing abnormal bile acid synthesis showed greater responsiveness and may benefit from oral cholic acid therapy [22]. Patients with the peroxisomal biogenesis defects may benefit, as evidenced from the successful treatment of a patient with a PEX10 defect, who so far has been receiving oral cholic acid for more than 14 years [47].

Bile acid-CoA conjugation defects

Hepatic conjugation of bile acids in humans is extremely efficient and as a result negligible amounts of unconjugated bile acids (<2%) typically appear in bile under normal and most cholestatic conditions and even after therapeutic doses of the unconjugated bile acid UDCA are administered. As detailed above, two enzymes catalyze the reactions leading to bile acid amidation. A CoA thioester is first formed by the rate-limiting bile acid-CoA ligase, and then the amino acids, glycine or taurine, are coupled in a reaction catalyzed by a cytosolic bile acid-CoA:amino acid *N*-acyltransferase. The genes encoding both these enzymes have been cloned, thus allowing identification of mutations to be determined in suspected defects in bile acid conjugation.

A defect in bile acid amidation was first described in 1994 in a 14-year-old boy presenting with fat and fat-soluble vitamin malabsorption. This child was of Laotian descent and in

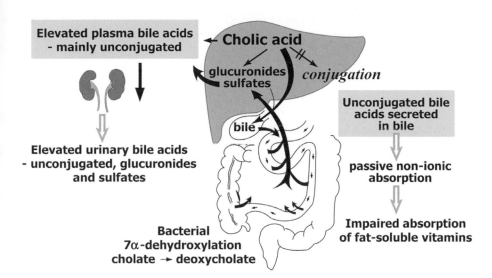

Figure 33.10 Pathophysiological basis for a defect in bile acid conjugation causing fat-soluble vitamin malabsorption.

the first 3 months of life presented with conjugated hyperbilirubinemia, elevated serum aminotransferases, and a normal gamma-glutamyltransferase. Two other patients, a 5-year-old Saudi Arabian boy and his 8-year-old sister, who were products of a consanguineous marriage, were soon after identified with the same bile acid defect, and remarkable was the fact that the boy had undergone a Kasai procedure for a mistakenly diagnosed biliary atresia, while the sister was reportedly asymptomatic at the time of diagnosis. Conjugation defects have since been identified in additional patients with a clinical history of normal or mildly elevated liver function tests but with a severe fat-soluble vitamin malabsorption and rickets [19,48]. All had subnormal levels of vitamin E, vitamin K, 25-hydroxyvitamin D and 1,25-dihydroxyvitamin D. The phenotype of the amidation defect is variable, with severe cholestasis and liver failure requiring liver transplantation in one patient. The clinical presentation and biochemical features of defective amidation (Figure 33.10) closely paralleled the predicted features hypothesized by Hofmann and Strandvik [49]. This conjugation defect was also reported in a number of patients from an Amish kindred and was also associated with mutations in *BAAT*, encoding the bile acid-CoA:amino acid *N*-acyltransferase, and for unexplained reasons also in *TJP2*, encoding tight junction protein 2, in some of these patients [48]. More recently, the first confirmed defect associated with a mutation in *SLC27A5* encoding the bile acid-CoA ligase was reported [19]. The patient, of Pakistani origin born to consanguineous parents, presented with cholestasis, elevated serum bilirubin and aminotransferases levels, normal serum gamma-glutamyltransferase and low fat-soluble vitamins. The liver biopsy showed extensive fibrosis. The patient was found to be homozygous for a missense mutation C1012T in *SLC27A5*, and a second mutation was discovered in BSiEP, encoding the bile salt export pump. No mutations were found in *BAAT*.

Diagnosis of a bile acid amidation defect is readily achieved by MS; FAB-MS and ESI-MS negative ion spectra of the urine, serum, and bile reveal a major ion at *m/z* 407 that corresponds to unconjugated cholic acid (Figure 33.3). In addition, ions characterizing sulfate and glucuronide conjugates of dihydroxy- and trihydroxy-bile acids are usually present. There is a complete lack of the usual glycine- and taurine-conjugated bile acids, and this may be confirmed after chromatographic separation of the individual bile acid conjugate fractions by GC-MS analysis or HPLC with ESI-MS [19]. Serum and urinary bile acids are markedly elevated in these patients and comprise predominantly cholic and deoxycholic acids. Acid *N*-acyltransferase requires the use of molecular techniques to sequence *SLC27A5* and *BAAT* for mutations or immunostaining of a liver biopsy for the presence of bile acid-CoA ligase or bile acid-CoA:amino acid *N*-acyltransferase, because the MS profiles of these two defects are indistinguishable.

While inborn errors in bile acid synthesis usually present as well-defined progressive familial cholestatic liver disease, by contrast, cholestasis is generally not a primary manifestation of a bile acid conjugation defect, presumably because synthesis of high levels of unconjugated cholic acid is sufficient to maintain bile flow (Figure 33.10). The main feature of fat-soluble vitamin malabsorption occurs because of reduced biliary secretion of bile acids and an inability to form mixed micelles owing to rapid passive absorption of unconjugated cholic acid in the proximal small intestine. Although these patients do conjugate bile acids with glucuronic and sulfuric acids, such conjugated bile acids do not promote lipid absorption. Treatment with oral administration of glycocholic acid was effective in resolving the fat-soluble vitamin malabsorption of five patients with the amidation defect caused by mutations in *BAAT*, while UDCA therapy was been used successfully in one patient with a mutation in *SLC27A5* [19]. The recognition that genetic defects in bile acid synthesis are associated with unexplained

Table 33.2 Comparative features of patients with intrahepatic cholestasis from bile acid synthetic defects and Byler syndrome

Feature	Bile acid synthetic defects	PFIC1 and PFIC2[a]
Age at presentation	Variable, late onset	<1 year[b,c]
Prognosis	Excellent	Fatal in first[c] to second[b] decade
Liver	Hepatosplenomegaly	Hepatosplenomegaly[b,c]
Pruritus	Usually absent	Severe[b,c]
Growth failure	Mild	Severe[b,c]
Jaundice	±	Mild/severe[b,c]
Serum aminotransferases	Elevated	Slight[b] to substantial[c] elevations
Serum gamma-glutamyltransferase	Generally normal	Normal[b,c]
Serum cholesterol	Normal or low	Low[b,c]
Fat-soluble vitamins	Malabsorption	Malabsorption[b,c]
Bile acids	No primary bile acids	Primary bile acids[b,c]
Treatment	Bile acid therapy	Transplantation[b,c]

[a] Byler syndrome has recently been separated into progressive familial intrahepatic cholestasis type 1 (Byler syndrome) and type 2 (bile salt export pump defect): PFIC1 is caused by *FIC1* mutations, PFIC2 is caused by *BSEP* mutations.
[b] *FIC1* mutations.
[c] *BSEP* mutations.

fat-soluble vitamin malabsorption warrants a more concerted effort to explore this patient population for these disorders.

Other disorders influencing bile acid synthesis and metabolism

In conditions that alter the integrity of the enterohepatic circulation, significant changes in bile acid synthesis and metabolism will occur. Since serum bile acid concentrations reflect a balance between intestinal input and hepatic extraction, it is evident that pathophysiological changes to the intestinal tract will be reflected by secondary changes in bile acid synthesis and metabolism. Such examples include ileal resection and bacterial overgrowth, while an inborn error in ileal bile acid transport has been shown to cause bile acid malabsorption [50]. Genetic defects in cholesterol synthesis, such as the Smith–Lemli–Opitz syndrome also alter bile acid synthesis because of the reduced availability of cholesterol.

Increased concentrations and alterations in bile acid metabolism can be found in patients with cholestatic diseases, but discerning whether these are primary or secondary to the liver injury can be difficult. Primary bile acid synthetic defects, particularly those involving the steroid nucleus, present as progressive familial intrahepatic cholestasis (PFIC), and represent a distinct entity of the PFIC syndromes separate from those recognized to arise from defects in the canalicular organic anion transporter proteins. A shared feature of Byler disease, designated PFIC type 1 (Byler disease), PFIC type 2 (the bile salt export pump defect), and bile acid synthesis disorders is a consistently low serum gamma-glutamyltransferase, but differential diagnosis can be made based on bile acid analysis. Patients with PFIC types 1 and 2 present with high serum bile acid concentrations, whereas primary bile acids are lacking in patients with the bile acid synthetic defects (Table 33.2).

For bile acid synthetic defects, save the CYP7B1 deficiency, the prognosis is excellent provided oral primary bile acid therapy is initiated before there is significant loss of quantitative liver function, and the need for liver transplantation can be avoided. It is, therefore, important in the clinical evaluation of patients with PFIC to screen for potential defects in bile acid synthesis as early as possible. All of these defects can be recognized by a combination of molecular and analytical studies and bile acid and phospholipid analysis of bile is helpful in the differential diagnosis.

References

1. Hofmann AF, Sjövall J, Kurz G, *et al.* A proposed nomenclature for bile acids. *J Lipid Res* 1992;**33**:599–604.

2. Russell DW. The enzymes, regulation, and genetics of bile acid synthesis. *Annu Rev Biochem* 2003;**72**:137–174.

3. Setchell KDR, Schwarz M, O'Connell NC, *et al.* Identification of a new inborn error in bile acid synthesis: mutation of the oxysterol 7α-hydroxylase gene causes severe neonatal liver disease. *J Clin Invest* 1998;**102**:1690–1703.

4. Li-Hawkins J, Lund EG, Turley SD, Russell DW. Disruption of the oxysterol 7alpha-hydroxylase gene in mice. *J Biol Chem* 2000;**275**:16536–16542.

5. Ueki I, Kimura A, Nishiyori A, *et al.* Neonatal cholestatic liver disease in an Asian patient with a homozygous mutation in the oxysterol 7alpha-hydroxylase gene. *J Pediatr Gastroenterol Nutr* 2008;**46**:465–469.

6. Mizuochi T, Kimura A, Suzuki M, *et al.* Successful heterozygous living donor liver transplantation for an oxysterol 7alpha-hydroxylase deficiency in a Japanese patient. *Liver Transplant* 2011;**17**:1059–1065.

7. Buchmann MS, Kvittingen EA, Nazer H, *et al.* Lack of 3β-hydroxy-Δ5-C27-steroid dehydrogenase/isomerase in fibroblasts from a child with urinary excretion of 3β-hydroxy-Δ5-bile acids. A new inborn error of metabolism. *J Clin Invest* 1990;**86**:2034–2037.

8. Schwarz M, Wright AC, Davis DL, *et al.* The bile acid synthetic gene 3beta-hydroxy-delta(5)-C(27)-steroid oxidoreductase is mutated in progressive intrahepatic cholestasis. *J Clin Invest* 2000;**106**:1175–1184.

9. Cheng JB, Jacquemin E, Gerhardt M, *et al.* Molecular genetics of 3β-hydroxy-Δ5-C27-steroid oxidoreductase deficiency in 16 patients with loss of bile acid synthesis and liver disease. *J Clin Endocrinol Metab* 2003;**88**:1833–1841.

10. Setchell KDR, Dumaswala R, Colombo C, Ronchi M. Hepatic bile acid metabolism during early development revealed from the analysis of human fetal gallbladder bile. *J Biol Chem* 1988;**263**:16637–16644.

11. Di Costanzo L, Drury JE, Penning TM, Christianson DW. Crystal structure of human liver delta4–3-ketosteroid 5beta-reductase (AKR1D1) and implications for substrate binding and catalysis. *J Biol Chem* 2008;**283**:16830–16839.

12. Drury JE, Mindnich R, Penning TM. Characterization of disease-related 5beta-reductase (*AKR1D1*) mutations reveals their potential to cause bile acid deficiency. *J Biol Chem* 2010;**285**:24529–24537.

13. Setchell KDR, Suchy FJ, Welsh MB, *et al.* Δ4-3-oxosteroid 5β-reductase deficiency described in identical twins with neonatal hepatitis. A new inborn error in bile acid synthesis. *J Clin Invest* 1988;**82**:2148–2157.

14. Lemonde HA, Custard EJ, Bouquet J, *et al.* Mutations in *SRD5B1* (*AKR1D1*), the gene encoding Δ4-3-oxosteroid 5β-reductase, in hepatitis and liver failure in infancy. *Gut* 2003;**52**:1494–1499.

15. Bjorkhem I, Hansson M. Cerebrotendinous xanthomatosis: an inborn error in bile acid synthesis with defined mutations but still a challenge.

Biochem Biophys Res Commun 2010;**396**:46–49.

16. Setchell KDR, Heubi JE, Bove KE, *et al.* Liver disease caused by failure to racemize trihydroxycholestanoic acid: gene mutation and effect of bile acid therapy. *Gastroenterology* 2003;**124**:217–232.

17. Dumaswala R, Setchell KDR, Zimmer-Nechemias L, *et al.* Identification of 3α,4β,7α-trihydroxy-5β-cholanoic acid in human bile: reflection of a new pathway in bile acid metabolism in humans. *J Lipid Res* 1989;**30**:847–856.

18. Shonsey EM, Sfakianos M, Johnson M, *et al.* Bile acid coenzyme A: amino acid N-acyltransferase in the amino acid conjugation of bile acids. *Methods Enzymol* 2005;**400**:374–394.

19. Chong CP, Mills PB, McClean P, *et al.* Bile acid-CoA ligase deficiency - a new inborn error of bile acid metabolism. *J Inherit Metab Dis* 2012;**35**:521–530.

20. Hamilton JP, Xie G, Raufman JP, *et al.* Human cecal bile acids: concentration and spectrum. *Am J Physiol Gastrointest Liver Physiol* 2007;**293**:G256–G263.

21. Chiang JY. Bile acids: regulation of synthesis. *J Lipid Res* 2009;**50**:1955–1966.

22. Setchell KDR, Heubi J. Defects in bile acid synthesis: diagnosis and treatment. *J Pediatr Gastroenterol Nutr* 2006;**43** (Suppl 1):S17–S22.

23. Haas D, Gan-Schreier H, Langhans CD, *et al.* Differential diagnosis in patients with suspected bile acid synthesis defects. *World J Gastroenterol* 2012;**18**:1067–1076.

24. Clayton PT, Leonard JV, Lawson AM, *et al.* Familial giant cell hepatitis associated with synthesis of 3β,7α-dihydroxy- and 3β,7α,12α-trihydroxy-5-cholenoic acids. *J Clin Invest* 1987;**79**:1031–1038.

25. Pullinger CR, Eng C, Salen G, *et al.* Human cholesterol 7α-hydroxylase (*CYP7A1*) deficiency has a hypercholesterolemic phenotype. *J Clin Invest* 2002;**110**:109–117.

26. Loomes KM, Setchell KDR, Rheingold SR, Piccoli DA. Bile acid synthetic disorder in a symptomatic patient with normal liver enzymes. *J Pediatr Gastroenterol Nutr* 1998;**26**:579.

27. Molho-Pessach V, Rios JJ, Xing C, *et al.* Homozygosity mapping identifies a bile acid biosynthetic defect in an adult with

cirrhosis of unknown etiology. *Hepatology* 2012;**55**:1139–1145.

28. Bove KE, Heubi JE, Balistreri WF, Setchell KDR. Bile acid synthetic defects and liver disease: a comprehensive review. *Pediatr Dev Pathol* 2004;**7**:315–334.

29. Fischler B, Bodin K, Stjernman H, *et al.* Cholestatic liver disease in adults may be due to an inherited defect in bile acid biosynthesis. *J Intern Med* 2007;**262**:254–262.

30. Gonzales E, Gerhardt MF, Fabre M, *et al.* Oral cholic acid for hereditary defects of primary bile acid synthesis: a safe and effective long-term therapy. *Gastroenterology* 2009;**137**:1310–1320.

31. Bove K, Daugherty CC, Tyson W, *et al.* Bile acid synthetic defects and liver disease. *Pediatr Development Pathol* 2000;**3**:1–16.

32. Ichimiya H, Egestad B, Nazer H, *et al.* Bile acids and bile alcohols in a child with hepatic 3β-hydroxy-Δ5-C27-steroid dehydrogenase deficiency: effects of chenodeoxycholic acid treatment. *J Lipid Res* 1991;**32**:829–841.

33. Stieger B, Zhang J, O'Neill B, Sjovall J, Meier PJ. Differential interaction of bile acids from patients with inborn errors of bile acid synthesis with hepatocellular bile acid transporters. *Eur J Biochem* 1997;**244**:39–44.

34. Riello L, D'Antiga L, Guido M, *et al.* Titration of bile acid supplements in 3beta-hydroxy-delta 5-C27-steroid dehydrogenase/isomerase deficiency. *J Pediatr Gastroenterol Nutr* 2010;**50**:655–660.

35. Daugherty CC, Setchell KDR, Heubi JE, Balistreri WF. Resolution of liver biopsy alterations in three siblings with bile acid treatment of an inborn error of bile acid metabolism (Δ4-3-oxosteroid 5β-reductase deficiency). *Hepatology* 1993;**18**:1096–1101.

36. Palermo M, Marazzi MG, Hughes BA, *et al.* Human delta4-3-oxosteroid 5beta-reductase (AKR1D1) deficiency and steroid metabolism. *Steroids*. 2008;**73**:417–423.

37. Shneider BL, Setchell KD, Whitington PF, Neilson KA, Suchy FJ. Δ4-3-Oxosteroid 5β-reductase deficiency causing neonatal liver failure and hemochromatosis [see comments]. *J Pediatr* 1994;**124**:234–238.

38. Clayton PT, Mills KA, Johnson AW, Barabino A, Marazzi MG. Delta 4-3-oxosteroid 5beta-reductase deficiency: failure of ursodeoxycholic acid treatment and response to chenodeoxycholic acid plus cholic acid. *Gut* 1996;**38**:623–628.

39. Setoguchi T, Salen G, Tint GS, Mosbach EH. A biochemical abnormality in cerebrotendinous xanthomatosis. Impairment of bile acid biosynthesis associated with incomplete degradation of the cholesterol side chain. *J Clin Invest* 1974;**53**:1393–1401.

40. Clayton PT, Verrips A, Sistermans E, *et al.* Mutations in the sterol 27-hydroxylase gene (*CYP27A*) cause hepatitis of infancy as well as cerebrotendinous xanthomatosis. *J Inherit Metab Dis* 2002;**25**:501–513.

41. von Bahr S, Bjorkhem I, Van't Hooft F, *et al.* Mutation in the sterol 27-hydroxylase gene associated with fatal cholestasis in infancy. *J Pediatr Gastroenterol Nutr* 2005;**40**: 481–486.

42. Berginer VM, Salen G, Shefer S. Long-term treatment of cerebrotendinous xanthomatosis with chenodeoxycholic acid. *N Engl J Med* 1984;**311**:1649–1652.

43. Savolainen K, Kotti TJ, Schmitz W, *et al.* A mouse model for alpha-methylacyl-CoA racemase deficiency: adjustment of bile acid synthesis and intolerance to dietary methyl-branched lipids. *Hum Mol Genet* 2004;**13**: 955–965.

44. Clayton PT, Casteels M, Mieli-Vergani G, Lawson AM. Familial giant cell hepatitis with low bile acid concentrations and increased urinary excretion of specific bile alcohols: a new inborn error of bile acid synthesis? *Pediatr Res* 1995;**37**(4 Pt 1):424–431.

45. Setchell KDR, Bragetti P, Zimmer-Nechemias L, *et al.* Oral bile acid treatment and the patient with Zellweger syndrome. *Hepatology* 1992;**15**:198–207.

46. Zeharia A, Ebberink MS, Wanders RJ, *et al.* A novel *PEX12* mutation identified as the cause of a peroxisomal biogenesis disorder with mild clinical phenotype, mild biochemical abnormalities in fibroblasts and a mosaic catalase immunofluorescence pattern, even at 40 degrees C. *J Hum Genet* 2007;**52**:599–606.

47. Steinberg SJ, Snowden A, Braverman NE, *et al.* A PEX10 defect in a patient with no detectable defect in peroxisome assembly or metabolism in cultured fibroblasts. *J Inherit Metab Dis* 2009;**32**:109–119.

48. Carlton VEH, Harris BZ, Puffenberger EG, *et al.* Complex inheritance of familial hypercholanemia with associated mutations in *TJP2* and *BAAT*. *Nat Genet* 2003;**34**:91–96.

49. Hofmann AF, Strandvik B. Defective bile acid amidation: predicted features of a new inborn error of metabolism. *Lancet* 1988;**ii**:311–313.

50. Heubi JE, Balistreri WF, Fondacaro JD, Partin JC, Schubert WK. Primary bile acid malabsorption: defective in vitro ileal active bile acid transport. *Gastroenterology* 1982;**83**:804–811.

34

Inborn errors of fatty acid oxidation

Melanie B. Gillingham and Robert D. Steiner

Introduction

Mitochondrial fatty acid oxidation (FAO) is an essential component of energy production and homeostasis in humans. During periods of limited glucose supply, FAO in the liver provides energy for hepatic function and the acetyl-CoA substrate needed for hepatocytes to synthesize and release ketone bodies into circulation. Ketone bodies provide an alternative energy substrate for peripheral tissues when glucose supply is limited. Other tissues such as skeletal and cardiac muscle rely on FAO for energy production. The oxidation of fatty acids can provide up to 80% of the energy requirements for cardiac and skeletal muscle while sparing glucose for use by the brain and CNS during moderate exercise, fasting, or illness. Disorders in the ability to use fatty acids for energy production manifest during periods of increased energy demands or reduced energy intake.

At least 22 different inherited genetic disorders in the mitochondrial FAO pathway have been described. Most of the disorders have an increasingly broad range of recognized phenotypes from mild to severe. Severe phenotypes typically present in infancy with catastrophic episodes of fasting or illness-induced hypoketotic hypoglycemia. The most common clinical presentation in childhood of FAO disorders generally includes nausea, vomiting, somnolence, and hepatic encephalopathy, similar to what was once known as Reye syndrome, which can progress to coma and death if untreated. Cardiomyopathy can be a life-threatening complication of acute metabolic decompensation in some FAO defects. These defects may also present as sudden unexpected death in infancy; prior to the introduction of expanded newborn screening for these disorders, as many as one-third of the initial episodes were fatal [1]. Alternatively, mild phenotypes of FAO deficiency may not present until adolescence or adulthood and these patients present with exercise intolerance with recurrent episodes of rhabdomyolysis and myoglobinuria. Patients with milder phenotypes who present later in life typically have not reported episodes of hypoketotic hypoglycemia during fasting or illness [1].

The reported combined incidence of FAO disorders across Australia, Germany, and the USA is 1 in 9300 live births [2]. The incidence is lower among Asians. All of the FAO disorders are inherited in an autosomal recessive manner. Specific gene defects have been identified for most of the disorders. Table 34.1 lists the enzymes in the FAO pathway that will be described in this chapter, their corresponding OMIM number, and gene location. This chapter will review the current knowledge in the field of FAO disorders with a specific focus on the liver phenotypes observed.

Regulation of fatty acid oxidation

Most tissues can use a variety of substrates to produce energy: skeletal muscle and liver can use glucose or fatty acids and the CNS can use glucose or ketones. The choice of substrate depends a great deal on substrate availability. During postprandial periods of abundant glucose supply, insulin is released from the pancreatic beta-cell. Insulin increases glucose uptake into muscle and adipose tissue and suppresses free fatty acid release from adipocytes. The predominant substrate available and oxidized is glucose. Glucose oxidation raises the cytosolic concentration of malonyl-CoA, which allosterically inhibits carnitine palmitoyltransferase (CPT)-I, the first and rate-limiting step in FAO [3]. In the fed state, FAO is inhibited and glucose is the primary energy substrate.

During periods of fasting, glucose and insulin concentrations decrease, and free fatty acids are mobilized and released into circulation. Free fatty acids are transported into the cell for oxidation via a variety of cellular fatty acid transporters. Intracellular malonyl-CoA concentrations decrease and release the inhibition on CPT-I. Fatty acids enter the mitochondria via the carnitine transport system and are oxidized to produce ATP. In the liver, acetyl-CoA from FAO is used to produce the ketone bodies, acetoacetate, and β-hydroxybutyrate. In the fasting state, FAO is upregulated and fatty acids and ketones become the primary energy substrate.

Dietary macronutrient composition can also influence flux through the FAO pathway. High-fat diets increase FAO because many fatty acids are ligands for the peroxisome

Table 34.1 Enzymes of the fatty acid oxidation pathway

Enzyme	Deficiency syndrome	OMIM No.	Gene, location
Organic cation transporter 2	Primary carnitine deficiency/carnitine uptake defect	603377	*SLC22A5*, 5q31.1
Carnitine palmityltransferase-IA	Enzyme deficiency	600528	*CPT1A*, 11q13
Carnitine palmityltransferase-IB	Unknown	601987	*CPT1B*, 22qter
Carnitine palmityltransferase-IC	Unknown	608846	*CPT1C*, 19q13.33
Carnitine/acylcarnitine translocase	Enzyme deficiency	212138	*SLC25A20*, 3p21.31
Carnitine palmityltransferase-II	Enzyme deficiency	600650	*CPT2*, 1p32
Very-long-chain acyl-CoA dehydrogenase	Enzyme deficiency	609575	*ACADVL*, 17p13
Long-chain acyl-CoA dehydrogenase	Unknown	201460	*ACADL*, 2q34-q35
Mitochondrial trifunctional protein (TFP)	TFP deficiency, long-chain 3-hydroxyacyl-CoA dehydrogenase deficiency	600890 (α-subunit) 143450 (β-subunit)	*HADHA* and *HADHB*, 2p23
Medium-chain acyl-CoA dehydrogenase	Enzyme deficiency	607008	*ACADM*, 1p31
Medium-chain 3-ketoacyl-CoA thiolase (T1)	Enzyme deficiency	602199	*T1*, 18q.21.1?
Short-chain acyl-CoA dehydrogenase	Enzyme deficiency	201470	*ACADS*, 12q22-qter
Short-chain enoyl-CoA hydratase (crotonase)	Unknown	602292	*ECHS1*, 10q26.2-q26.3
Medium/short-chain 3-hydroxyacyl-CoA dehydrogenase (3-hydroxyacyl-CoA dehydrogenase 1)	Enzyme deficiency	300256	Xp11.2
Short-chain 3-ketoacyl-CoA thiolase (β-ketothiolase, T2)	Enzyme deficiency	607809	*T2*, 11q22.3-q23.1
Electron transfer flavoprotein, α-polypeptide	Multiple acyl-CoA dehydrogenase deficiencies/glutaric aciduria IIA	608053	*ETFA*, 15q24.2-q24.3
Electron transfer flavoprotein, β-polypeptide	Multiple acyl-CoA dehydrogenase deficiencies/glutaric aciduria IIB	130410	*ETFB*, 19q13.41
Electron transfer flavoprotein dehydrogenase	Multiple acyl-CoA dehydrogenase deficiencies/glutaric aciduria IIC	231675	*ETFDH*, 4q32.1

proliferator-activating receptor (PPAR) family of nuclear hormone transcription factors. Dietary fatty acids bind to PPARα and PPARβ and the ligand/transcription factor complex translocates to the nucleus. The PPARs bind nuclear receptor response elements in the promoter region of target genes. PPAR–ligand binding enhances transcription and translation of these genes, including CPT-1 and very-long-chain acyl-CoA dehydrogenase (VLCAD), among others, which stimulates the transport, esterification and oxidation of fatty acids [4].

Exercise can increase FAO by increasing energy demands and mobilizing fatty acids for oxidation. Moderate intensity exercise increases hormones such as adrenaline, glucagon, and adrenocorticotropic hormone, increasing lipolysis of triglycerides in adipose tissue. Increased energy utilization depletes tissue glucose stores and lowers intracellular malonyl-CoA concentrations. Low malonyl-CoA concentrations increase CPT-I activity and entry of fatty acids into the mitochondria for oxidation.

Figure 34.1 is a schematic of FAO pathway. Substrate availability and hormonal regulation acutely regulate the pathway. In addition, cellular energy demands can affect FAO flux. Finally, long-term regulation by hormone transcription factors such as the PPAR family can also alter flux through the FAO pathway.

Fatty acid oxidation

Circulating free fatty acids or fatty acids released from lipoproteins by lipoprotein lipase are taken up into the cell via a variety of cell surface fatty acid transporters. Some of these transporters have endogenous acetyl-CoA synthetase activity and some do not. All fatty acids are rapidly esterified to acyl-CoAs via the transporter itself or by acyl CoA synthetase. From the cytosol, fatty acids must enter the mitochondria for further oxidation. Medium- and short-chain fatty acids can diffuse into the mitochondria but long-chain fatty acids are

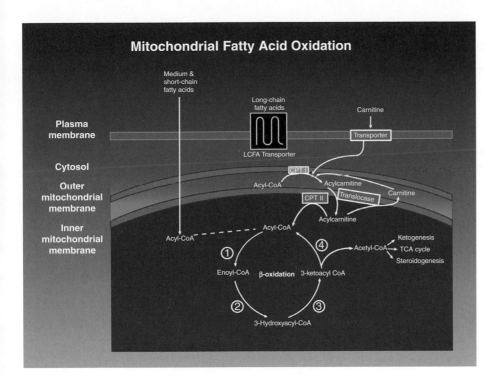

Figure 34.1 Mitochondrial fatty acid beta-oxidation. LCFA, long-chain fatty acid; TCA, tricarboxylic acid. CPT, carnitine palmitoyltransferase.

shuttled into the mitochondria by the CPT system. The first and rate-limiting step of long-chain FAO is CPT-I (Figure 34.2, step 1). This enzyme catalyzes the conversion of a long-chain fatty acyl-CoA to a fatty acylcarnitine. There are three isoforms, which are products of three separate genes: CPT-IA is the isoform expressed in liver, kidney, brain, fibroblasts, and leukocytes; CPT-IB is expressed in muscle and white adipose tissue [5]; and CPT-IC is localized to brain and testes but its function in FAO is unclear. The acylcarnitine conjugates are then transported into the mitochondria by carnitine:acylcarnitine translocase (Figure 34.2; step 2). Once inside the mitochondria, the reaction is reversed by CPT-II and free carnitine and a long-chain fatty acyl-CoA are reformed (Figure 34.2; step 3).

Fatty acyl-CoAs undergo beta-oxidation in a repeating four-enzyme cycle. Each cycle releases one molecule of acetyl-CoA and a chain-shortened fatty acid (Figure 34.2; steps 4–7). At least two and up to four distinct enzymes catalyze each spiral of the FAO pathway (Table 34.1), the enzymes having chain-length specificity and enzymatic activity with substrate specificity for long-chain, medium-chain, or short-chain fatty acids. Long-chain FAO represents the major pathway for ATP synthesis from fatty acids because >95% of dietary fatty acids as well as the majority of endogenous lipid stores are long-chain fatty acids. Oxidation of medium- and short-chain fatty acids is primarily from the successful oxidation of long-chain fats to shorter chain lengths and/or the oxidation of short-chain fatty acids from colonic fermentation. Most diets contain low concentrations of medium- or short-chain fatty acids (<5% of total lipid) unless specifically supplemented with medium-chain triglycerides (MCT).

Acyl-CoA dehydrogenases

The first reaction is performed by one of five acyl-CoA dehydrogenases, the choice of enzyme depending upon the structure and chain length of the fatty acid substrate (Figure 34.2; step 4). The dehydration reaction generates a double bond between the α- and the β-carbon of the acyl-CoA and forms the 2-enoyl-CoA product. All these reactions require riboflavin in the form of flavin adenine dineucleotide (FAD) as a cofactor and produce reducing equivalents (FADH). The FADH is coupled directly to ATP synthesis through electron transfer flavoprotein and electron transfer flavoprotein:coenzyme Q oxidoreductase to coenzyme Q of the electron transport chain.

Very-long-chain acyl-CoA dehydrogenase

Straight chain fatty acids 12–18 carbons in length are metabolized by VLCAD [6]. This enzyme was originally isolated from rat liver mitochondria and differed from the other human acyl-CoA dehydrogenases because it is a homodimer bound to the inner mitochondrial membrane [7]. The *ACADVL* gene contains 20 exons, is about 5.4 kb long, and has been mapped to human chromosome 17p11.13-p11.2 [8,9].

Long-chain acyl-CoA dehydrogenase

Long-chain branched or unsaturated fatty acids are the likely substrates for long-chain acyl-CoA dehydrogenase (LCAD), an enzyme found within the mitochondrial matrix [10]. This is a homotetramer of four identical subunits; each subunit binds one molecule of FAD. Lauric acyl-CoA (C_{12}) is the preferred

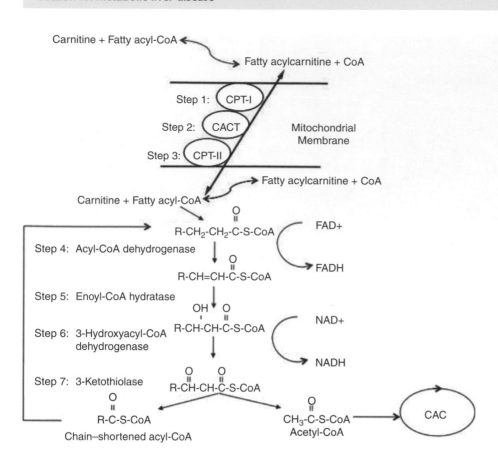

Figure 34.2 Fatty acid oxidation reaction. CAC, carnitine acylcarnitine translocase; CPT, carnitine palmitoyltransferase.

substrate of the recombinant protein [11]. *ACADL* encodes LCAD protein and is mapped to chromosome 2q34-p35 [12]. Expression of *ACADL* is very low in human liver and cardiac and skeletal muscle, which calls into question the physiological importance of this enzyme in humans [13]. Patients previously described with LCAD deficiency have all been subsequently found to have VLCAD deficiency. To date, no deficiency disorder of LCAD has been identified in humans.

Acyl-CoA dehydrogenase 9

Long-chain polyunsaturated fatty acids may also be dehydrogenated by a newly identified enzyme, acyl-CoA dehydrogenase 9 (ACAD9). This enzyme has a substrate preference for polyunsaturated fatty acids and is the primary acyl-CoA dehydrogenase expressed in the CNS [14]. Traditionally, the CNS is believed to be glycolytic and to use only glucose and ketones as energy substrates. However, all of the FAO enzymes are synthesized in the CNS [6]. Two additional ACAD proteins were recently described in human CNS, ACAD11 and ACAD10 [7]. These ACAD enzymes have substrate specificities for long-chain polyunsaturated fatty acids and regional localization in the adult and fetal brain. The expression of multiple ACAD enzymes as well as the other FAO enzymes in the CNS suggests an important role in neuronal function but what role FAO plays in energy metabolism or in other essential CNS processes remains to be elucidated.

Medium-chain acyl-CoA dehydrogenase

Chain shortened fatty acids (C_{6-12}) become the substrate of medium-chain acyl-CoA dehydrogenase (MCAD). The gene encoding this enzyme, *ACADM*, contains 12 exons and maps to chromosome 1p31.1 [15]. The enzyme is a homotetramer located in the mitochondrial matrix, similar to LCAD. MCAD is an important enzyme in humans, and deficiency of MCAD is the most common FAO defect.

Short-chain acyl-CoA dehydrogenase

Short-chain acyl-CoA dehydrogenase (SCAD) catalyzes the initial dehydrogenation of the short-chain fatty acids (C_{4-6}). The gene encoding it, *ACADS*, consists of 10 exons spanning 13 kb of DNA on chromosome 12q [16]. SCAD is also a homotetramer located in the mitochondrial matrix like LCAD and MCAD, suggesting a common ancestral origin. It is controversial whether SCAD deficiency alone is sufficient to cause human disease.

2-Enoyl-CoA hydratases

The second step in FAO is hydration of the 2-enoyl-CoA to form a 3-hydroxyacyl-CoA (Figure 34.2; step 5). There are two separate hydratase enzymes. Long-chain fatty acids are the substrate for the long-chain enoyl-Co hydratase catalyzed by mitochondrial trifunctional protein (TFP). The TFP also

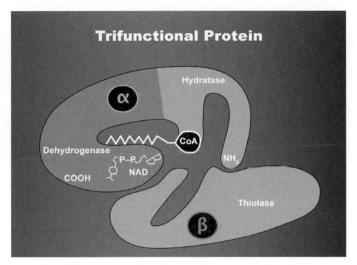

Figure 34.3 The mitochondrial trifunctional protein complex. This is composed of a hetero-octamer of 4α- and 4β-subunits. The α-subunit contains the hydratase and the NAD$^+$-dependent dehydrogenase enzyme activities, and the β-subunit contains the thiolase enzyme activities. COOH, carboxylic acid (functional group).

catalyzes two additional steps of FAO (see below). Medium- and short-chain fatty acids are the substrate for the enzyme short-chain 2,3-enoyl-CoA hydratase (crotonase).

Trifunctional protein

The next three reactions in long-chain FAO are catalyzed by TFP, which is bound to the inner mitochondrial membrane: long-chain enoyl-CoA hydratase, long-chain 3-hydroxyacyl-CoA dehydrogenase, and long-chain ketothiolase activities. Mitochondrial TFP is a hetero-octomer composed of 4α- and 4β-subunits encoded by two different genes, *HADHA* and *HADHB* (Figure 34.3). Both genes are located on chromosome 2p23 in a head-to-head configuration with coordinately regulated expression [17].

The long-chain acylCoA hydratase and the long-chain hydroxyacyl-CoA dehydrogenase activity are encoded in the α-subunit and the long-chain acyl-CoA ketothialase activity is encoded in the β-subunit.

Short-chain enoyl-CoA hydratase

2,3-Enoyl-CoA hydratase is a homohexamer localized in the mitochondrial matrix and encoded by *ECHS1*. The gene is located on chromosome 10q26.2-q26.3 and is highly expressed in human liver, as well as in fibroblasts and muscle [18]. 2,3-Enoyl-CoA hydratase acts on fatty acids of C_4 or longer but activity toward long-chain fatty acids decreases with increasing chain length.

3-Hydroxyacyl-CoA dehydrogenases

The hydroxyl group is dehydrogenated to a keto group at carbon 3 in the third step of FAO (Figure 34.2; step 6). There are two 3-hydroxyacyl-CoA dehydrogenases: LCHAD, which

is part of the TFP (see above), and medium/short-chain 3-hydroxyacyl-CoA dehydrogenase, encoded by *HADH*. Niacin in the form of niacin adenine dinucleotide (NAD) is a required cofactor for both dehydrogenases. Reducing equivalents (NADH) generated in this step are coupled to complex I of the electron transport chain to generate ATP. The medium/short-chain 3-hydroxyacyl-CoA dehydrogenase is a soluble mitochondrial matrix protein with broad activity toward C_4–C_{16} fatty acids. However, its highest activity is toward 3-hydroxydeconyl-CoA (C_{10}) [19]. Conventionally, the enzyme was designated as a short-chain 3-hydroxydeconyl-CoA dehydrogenase, but this was misleading as there is a 3-hydroxydeconyl-CoA dehydrogenase in brain that plays a role in brain development [20]. The protein involved in FAO is now referred to as 3-hydroxyacyl-CoA dehydrogenase or HAD [21].

3-Ketoacyl-CoA thiolases

The final cleavage step is catalyzed by three distinct thiolase enzymes: long-chain 3-ketothiolase within TFP (see above) for long-chain fatty acids, medium-chain 3-ketoacyl-CoA thiolase for medium-chain fatty acids, and short-chain 3-ketoacyl-CoA thiolase (β-ketothiolase) for short-chain fatty acids (Figure 34.2; step 7). The product of this reaction is one molecule of acetyl-CoA and a chain-shortened fatty acid.

Medium-chain ketoacyl-CoA thiolase

The medium-chain ketoacyl-CoA thiolase has also been called mitochondrial 3-oxoacyl-CoA thiolase. The mRNA for this thiolase is highly expressed in human muscle, liver, and fibroblasts. There is some substrate overlap between medium-chain and short-chain 3-ketoacyl-CoA thiolases. The medium-chain thiolase former can cleave C_4 into 2 acetyl-CoA molecules as well as cleave longer fatty ketoacyl-CoA moieties, with highest activity toward C_{10}. It is believed to be the primary thiolase in the medium- and short-chain FAO pathway.

Short-chain 3-ketoacyl-CoA thiolase

The short-chain 3-ketoacyl-CoA thiolase is encoded by *ACAT1* on chromosome 11q22.3-q.23.1, which contains 12 exons and 11 introns. The cDNA is 1.5 kb and encodes a 427 amino acid residue peptide; the enzyme is a homotetramer of four identical 41 kDa subunits. It cleaves C_4 into two molecules of acetyl-CoA and is thought to be primarily involved in ketone body synthesis.

Oxidation of odd-chain fatty acids

Very small amounts of odd chain fatty acid are found in dairy food products, are digested and absorbed into circulation, and must be stored or oxidized [22]. These unique fatty acids are oxidized in the same four-step process as described above to yield multiple acetyl-CoAs and one C_3 intermediate: propionyl-CoA. Propionyl-CoA is converted to succinyl-CoA, a tricarboxylic acid (TCA) cycle intermediate by three

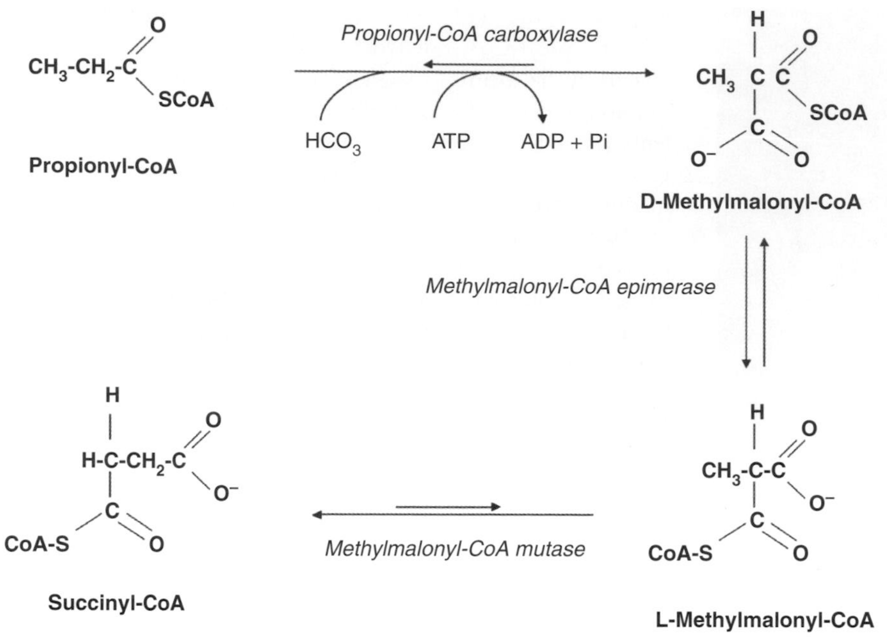

Figure 34.4 Beta-oxidation of odd-carbon fatty acids. The three-carbon propionyl-CoA product of the beta-oxidation of an odd-chain fatty acid is converted to succinyl-CoA by three specialized enzymes. Succinyl-CoA is a tricarboxylic acid cycle intermediate that can enter the cycle.

enzymes (Figure 34.4). First, propionyl-CoA is carboxylated to D-methylmalonyl-CoA by propionyl-CoA carboxylase, a biotin-dependent enzyme. D-Methylmalonyl-CoA is then converted to its L isomer, L-methylmalonyl-CoA, by methylmalonyl-CoA epimerase. L-Methylmalonyl-CoA is converted to succinyl-CoA by methylmalonyl-CoA mutase, a vitamin B_{12}-dependent reaction. The addition of succinyl-CoA to the pool of TCA cycle intermediates via the oxidation of odd-chain fatty acids or branched-chained amino acids is a process termed anaplerosis [23].

Unsaturated fatty acids

Unsaturated fatty acids such as oleic acid (18:1n-9), linoleic (18:2n-6), and linolenic (C18:3n-3) constitute a significant portion (6–8%) of the total energy consumed by humans. Polyunsaturated fatty acids can be used for membrane synthesis and complex lipid structures or oxidized to produce ATP. These fatty acids undergo beta-oxidation as described above until the double bond is reached. The double bonds typically occur every third carbon in a *cis* formation. A double bond between the C_3 and C_4 atoms (*cis*-3-enoyl-CoA) is rearranged to a *trans* double bond by enoyl-CoA isomerase (Figure 34.5). The *trans*-2-enoyl-CoA becomes the substrate for long-chain acyl-CoA hydratase or short-chain enoyl-CoA hydratase depending on the fatty acid chain length and continues through the beta-oxidation cycle. When the double bond is located between the C_2 and C_3 atoms, 2,4-dienoyl-CoA reductase changes the bond into the *trans*-3-enoyl-CoA. Enoyl-CoA isomerase rearranges the bond to form 2-enoyl-CoA and the fatty acid proceeds through the normal beta-oxidation process.

Final products of fatty acid oxidation

The product for each cycle of the FAO system is a chain-shortened fatty acid and one molecule of acetyl-CoA. In the liver and muscle, acetyl-CoA generated through FAO is a substrate for the TCA cycle and the respiratory chain to produce ATP, CO_2, and water. Energy generated through FAO spares glycogen and prevents glucose depletion. Acetyl-CoA generated from FAO is also necessary for the liver to make ketone bodies during periods of fasting. Ketone bodies are released into circulation and provide an alternative fuel for the brain.

Fatty acid oxidation disorders
Carnitine shuttle defects

Defects in the carnitine-dependent transport of long-chain fatty acids into the mitochondria include

- carnitine transport defects (organic cation transporter 2 (OCTN2)
- CPT-IA deficiency
- CPT-II deficiency
- carnitine/acylcarnitine translocase deficiency.

Carnitine transport defects

Carnitine is consumed in the diet from meat, fish, and dairy products but it can also be synthesized from lysine and methionine in the liver. No primary defect in carnitine synthesis has been described but primary/systemic carnitine deficiency refers to a defect in tissue OCTN2. Tissues such as muscle and heart cannot make carnitine and must take up circulating carnitine via the transporter. Defects in OCTN2

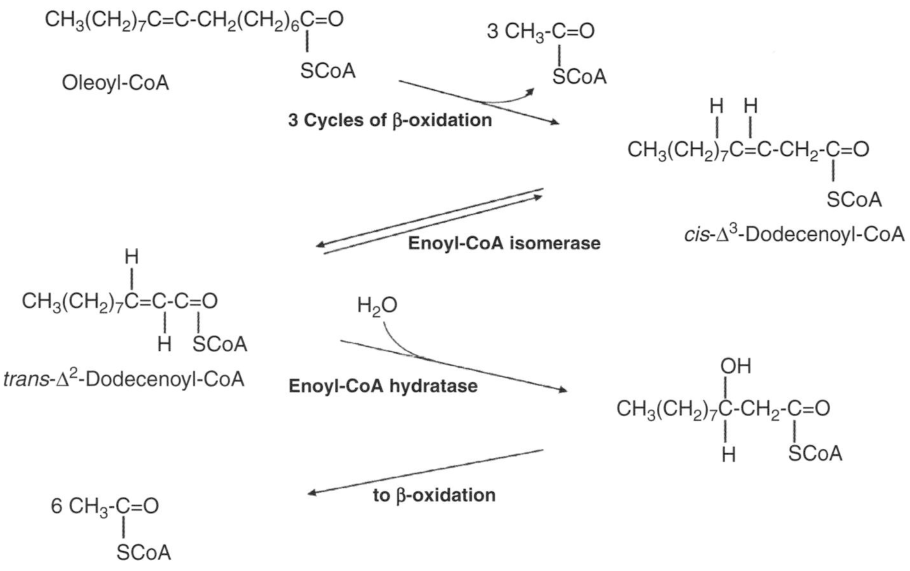

CH₃(CH₂)₇C=C-CH₂(CH₂)₆C=O
|
SCoA

Oleoyl-CoA

3 Cycles of β-oxidation

3 CH₃-C=O
|
SCoA

H H
| |
CH₃(CH₂)₇C=C-CH₂-C=O
|
SCoA

cis-Δ³-Dodecenoyl-CoA

Enoyl-CoA isomerase

H
|
CH₃(CH₂)₇C=C-C=O
| |
H SCoA

trans-Δ²-Dodecenoyl-CoA

H₂O

Enoyl-CoA hydratase

OH
|
CH₃(CH₂)₇C-CH₂-C=O
| |
H SCoA

6 CH₃-C=O
|
SCoA

to β-oxidation

Figure 34.5 Beta-oxidation of unsaturated fatty acids. The beta-oxidation of unsaturated fatty acids is catabolized by two additional mitochondrial enzymes. An isomerase arranges the *cis*-Δ3 double bond to a *trans*-Δ2 double bond, and the subsequent hydration by a hydratase allows the rearranged fatty acid to continue into the normal beta-oxidation pathway.

will lead to muscle and heart carnitine depletion. Muscle depletion of carnitine presents with weakness; cardiac depletion causes cardiomyopathy, and hepatocellular depletion can cause hepatic steatosis or fulminant Reye-like syndrome with hepatic failure, any of which can be precipitated during stress or minor periods of starvation. Sudden unexpected death in infancy, or sudden death in older individuals, has been reported in patients with OCTN2 defects.

Carnitine palmityltransferase-IA

Deficiency of CPT-IA causes symptomatic fasting hypoketotic hypoglycemia and occasionally hepatocellular damage. The heart and muscle are rarely involved because CPT-IA is the liver isoform of the enzyme. We reported one case of CPT-I deficiency with muscle pain and rhabdomyolysis in a previously asymptomatic adult [24]. We also observed hepatic presentation of CPT-I deficiency in one sibling and muscle presentation in another sibling in a family. In CPT-I deficiency, total and free plasma carnitine are characteristically elevated; this observation is unique among all known FAO defects and is otherwise seen only in association with carnitine supplementation or renal insufficiency.

Carnitine palmityltransferase-II

In CPT-II deficiency, an infantile form presents with severe hypoglycemia, myopathy, and cardiomyopathy and often resulting in death [25]. Plasma free carnitine is low with elevated acylcarnitines. A milder form presents with lipid myopathy, recurrent rhabdomyolysis, and myoglobinuria in young adults. Carnitine/acylcarnitine translocase deficiency is clinically similar to infantile CPT-II deficiency. Patients often present in the neonatal or infancy period with severe hypoketotic hypoglycemia; hyperammonemia, probably from liver failure; and elevated acylcarnitines associated with intercurrent illness [26].

Long-chain fatty acid oxidation disorders
Very-long-chain acyl-CoA-dehydrogenase deficiency

Deficiency of VLCAD presents with three main phenotypes: the severe *infantile* presentation with cardiomyopathy, the *childhood/adolescent* form with hypoketotic hypoglycemia and recurrent rhabdomyolysis, and the *adult-onset* form with recurrent rhabdomyolysis. The severe phenotype is characterized by dilated or hypertrophic cardiomyopathy early in life [9]. The cardiomyopathy may be severe and result in early demise. The presentation can also be characterized by hypoketotic hypoglycemia and hepatic steatosis [27]. Cardiomyopathy may resolve with the initiation of treatment with carbohydrates and MCT supplements but this may not always result in a favorable outcome. Carnitine supplementation in the long-chain FAO defects is controversial, because theoretically it could lead to increased concentration of potentially toxic long-chain acylcarnitines. In addition, there is little evidence of the efficacy of carnitine supplementation in these disorders. A reasonable approach would seem to be to use carnitine supplementation judiciously in those with free carnitine levels below normal. Rarely older patients may present with cardiomyopathic complications.

The intermediate phenotype often presents as hypoketotic hypoglycemia in childhood, similar to MCAD deficiency, along with myopathy or rhabdomyolysis. During acute illness, there are characteristic increases in plasma long-chain acylcarnitines including C14:0, C14:1, C16:0, C16:1, C18:0, C18:1 and C18:2 acylcarnitine esters but particularly in C14:1 [28]. Rhabdomyolysis and myoglobinuria are often related to a bout of prolonged exercise, an illness with fever or poor oral intake, cold temperatures, or a combination of these factors. Creatine phosphokinase can be extremely elevated and rhabdomyolysis/myoglobinuria can cause renal failure requiring hemodialysis.

The mild adult-onset form is most often associated with exercise intolerance and myoglobinuria. Adults have presented with a history of recurrent rhabdomyolysis, muscle pain, and weakness that begins in adolescence and may continue intermittently for decades prior to a diagnosis of VLCAD deficiency or with an acute rhabdomyolysis event and no prior history of muscle disease [29]. More than 80 different mutations spanning the gene encoding VLCAD, *ACADVL*, have been reported and no common mutation has been identified [30].

Acyl-CoA dehydrogenase 9

Deficiency of ACAD9 has been described in three patients. The clinical presentation was similar to other FAO disorders including hypoketotic hypoglycemia, fulminant liver failure, and dilated cardiomyopathy. In addition, neurological symptoms such as cerebral stroke were present in all three patients. *ACAD9* is highly expressed in the brain and appears to have a substrate preference for long-chain polyunsaturated fatty acids [7].

Since the initial report, ACAD9 has been implicated as an essential protein for mitochondrial complex 1 assembly and function [31]. Mutations in *ACAD9* have been identified among several patients with mitochondrial disease complex 1 deficiency symptoms suggesting that ACAD9 may play a role in complex assembly and function rather than having a primary role in long-chain FAO. Further research is needed to define the phenotype of subjects with *ACAD9* mutations and the role of ACAD9 in the oxidation of fatty acids.

Long-chain 3-hydroxyacyl-CoA dehydrogenase

Selective loss of the LCHAD activity within TFP and loss of TFP itself (so all three enzymatic functions) have similar presentations and clinical course. Children typically present with hypoketotic hypoglycemia associated with metabolic acidosis, hepatocellular dysfunction, and sometimes cardiomyopathy. Elevated plasma long-chain hydroxyacylcarnitines, including C16:0-OH, C16:1-OH, C18:0-OH, C18:1-OH, C18:2-OH, are diagnostic of LCHAD or TFP deficiency. Pigmentary retinopathy with vision loss during childhood, and progressive peripheral neuropathy are complications specific to LCHAD/TFP deficiency that are not observed in the other FAO disorders [32]. Not all patients experience all complications of the disease. While the underlying etiology of the hypoketotic hypoglycemia appears to be a deficiency of energy from depleted carbohydrate stores, the etiology of the other complications is not completely understood. A depletion of energy or the toxic effects of the accumulation of metabolic products are thought to be causative [33].

Isolated LCHAD deficiency results from the selective loss of LCHAD activity and relative preservation of hydratase and ketothiolase activity of TFP. A common missense mutation, (c.G1528C) accounts for 87% of the alleles in LCHAD deficiency [17]. This common mutation decreases LCHAD activity but does not alter the level of protein expression of either mitochondrial TFP subunit. Other mutations in both the

α- and β-subunits have been shown to result in the loss of all three enzyme activities and TFP deficiency.

There appear to be some clinical differences between LCHAD and TFP deficiencies. Patients who are homozygous for the common LCHAD mutation (c.G1528C) are more likely to develop progressive chorioretinopathy leading to vision impairment than patients who have β-subunit mutations [33]. The infantile form of TFP deficiency appears to be severe, resulting in neonatal death. In our experience, milder forms of TFP deficiency are associated with severe peripheral neuropathy, impairing mobility, more often than isolated LCHAD deficiency. Patients who are heterozygotes for the common LCHAD mutation and a private mutation may develop some aspects of both the chorioretinopathy with vision loss and peripheral neuropathy with impaired mobility.

Medium chain acyl-CoA dehydrogenase deficiency

Deficiency of MCAD is the most common defect in FAO, with an incidence of approximately 1 in 9000 live births [2]. The typical acute clinical presentation includes fasting- or illness-induced hypoketotic hypoglycemia, often associated with metabolic acidosis and hepatocellular dysfunction [34]. Micro- and/or macrovascular steatosis is often observed in symptomatic patients. The most severe manifestation is sudden unexpected death in infancy [35]. Sudden unexpected death has been reported in the first few days after birth almost exclusively in breast-fed infants, presumably because of the relative fasting status in nursing infants. However, some MCAD-deficient individuals may never become symptomatic. The reason some individuals never develop symptoms is not known but is hypothesized to be because these individuals never develop carnitine depletion coincident with sufficient stress to induce a metabolic crisis or because they carry mutations with relatively mild physiologic effects.

In 1990, a common mutation in *ACADM*, a c.A985G point mutation, was identified resulting in a lysine to glutamic acid substitution at position 304 of the mature protein [36]. This missense mutation was subsequently shown to account for a large majority of the alleles in identified patients, although with newborn screening identifying affected individuals, the prevalence of this mutation may change [30]. Other point mutations have been identified in the first 11 of 12 exons but the c.A985G point mutation still accounts for the majority of disease-causing alleles. The c.A985G mutation results in decreased but not absent expression of the mutant protein, activity loss being related to defective protein folding [30].

Symptomatic patients with MCAD deficiency have typically presented in infancy and early childhood (typically 6 months to 6 years of age) but recent reports of adults with MCAD deficiency have challenged the concept that this is exclusively a disorder of childhood [37]. Adults have typically presented to the emergency room with acute neurological deterioration, and subsequent ventricular arrhythmias. These patients were hypoglycemic with lactic acidosis and elevated medium-chain acylcarnitines similar to childhood cases. The initial presenting illness was fatal in 29% of reviewed cases suggesting a potentially lethal and severe presentation is possible in adulthood [37].

Since the advent of newborn screening for MCAD deficiency, many infants have been identified and treated with excellent outcome. The vast majority of affected patients who are treated are completely healthy, although they may need to receive intravenous fluids containing glucose when ill or fasting to prevent metabolic crisis. Some neurological impairment has been noted later in life, rarely, in MCAD-deficient patients, particularly in unscreened populations, but the evidence for neurological impairment in treated patients who have avoided metabolic crisis is scant. Deficits in learning and speech/language communication have been reported in symptomatic individuals prior to newborn screening but further study is needed to determine the prevalence of these complications in screened and early effectively treated populations [38].

Short-chain acyl-CoA dehydrogenase deficiency

Deficiency of SCAD has been associated with failure to thrive, hypoglycemia, hypotonia, developmental delay, and seizures, although it is unclear whether SCAD deficiency causes these symptoms. Deficiency of SCAD with the potential of affecting human health is characterized by increased urinary ethylmalonic acid excretion [39].

Two common sequence variants in *ACADS* have been described (c.C511T and c.G625A) but population studies have found that up to 14% of the general population is homozygous or compound heterozygous for these common missense mutations [39]. This observation combined with new findings that many infants identified with SCAD deficiency by newborn screening remain asymptomatic has led to considerable debate about the clinical relevance of the common mutations and clinical presentation of true SCAD deficiency. A follow-up study of 14 patients who were identified by newborn screening or who presented symptomatically reported that most patients had other medical and neurodevelopmental characteristics that could have been responsible for the symptoms reported [40]. Other rare sequence variants in *ACADS* have been described. Some newborn screening programs are sufficiently confident that SCAD deficiency is a non-disease and they have discontinued testing for this condition. Perhaps a reasonable interpretation is that the sequence variant in *ACADS*, both common and rare, are susceptibility genes, which, together with other environmental factors, may result rarely in symptomatic SCAD deficiency.

3-Hydroxyacyl-CoA dehydrogenase (HAD) deficiency

3-Hydroxyacyl-CoA dehydrogenase deficiency has a similar presentation to other FAO defects including hypoglycemia, hypotonia, and seizures. A small number of patients with this deficiency have been described in the literature so that the phenotype is likely incompletely characterized. What sets this condition apart from other FAO defects is hyperinsulinemia with mild elevations in ammonia associated with postprandial hypoglycemia among subjects with null mutations despite dietary therapy [41]. A leucine-restricted diet may help decrease the hyperinsulinemia. Diagnosis and metabolic status is evaluated using plasma free 3-hydroxy fatty acid profiles because short- and medium-chain 3-hydroxy fatty acids do not readily form acylcarnitine conjugates. The mutations in *HADH* among these patients is heterogeneous.

Medium-chain 3-ketoacyl-CoA thiolase

There has been a single case of deficiency in medium-chain 3-ketoacyl-CoA thiolase described [42]. The patient had lactic acidosis, hepatic dysfunction, and hypoglycemia in the first few days of life. He continued to deteriorate with hyperammonemia, myoglobinuria, respiratory, and renal failure, and he died on day 13 of life. Elevated urine C_{12}-C_{16} dicarboxcylic organic acids were detected along with reduced fibroblast octanoate oxidation and decreased medium-chain 3-ketoacyl-CoA thiolase protein expression. Based on this single case, medium-chain 3-ketoacyl-CoA thiolase deficiency appears to be a severe and lethal condition, but additional patients will need to be identified before the phenotype can be described with confidence.

Glutaric aciduria type II

Glutaric acidemia type II is also known as multiple acyl-CoA dehydrogenation deficiency, an inborn error of fatty acid and amino acid metabolism in which the reoxidation of several mitochondrial dehydrogenases is impaired because of the inability of FAD to transfer electrons to the electron transfer flavoprotein complex caused by a defect in the electron transfer flavoprotein or its dehydrogenase. There is clinical heterogeneity, and generally three groups of patients have been described: those with neonatal onset with congenital abnormalities, those with neonatal onset without abnormalities, and those with a late onset with muscle weakness and carnitine deficiency. Patients with severe neonatal-onset with congenital abnormalities present with hypotonia, macrocephaly, severe hypoglycemia, metabolic acidosis, and enlarged kidneys; it is often associated with prematurity. Many of these patients die in the first week of life or early infancy. Congenital abnormalities include dysmorphic facial features, rocker-bottom feet, muscular and abdominal wall defects, and genital abnormalities. Patients with the neonatal-onset form without congenital abnormalities also present with hypotonia, metabolic acidosis, hypoglycemia, tachypnea, hepatomegaly, and may develop an acrid odor or odor of sweaty feet. Patients typically die in a few months as the result of severe cardiomyopathy.

Patients with the milder, late-onset form present with episodic vomiting, hypoglycemia, and acidosis. Hepatomegaly, carnitine deficiency, and lipid storage myopathy have been described. Glutaric aciduria type II urinary organic acid profiles demonstrate an accumulation of ethylmalonic acid, glutaric acid, and 2-hydroxyglutaric acid. Urinary acylglycine analysis shows accumulation of isovalerylglycine and hexanoylglycine. Plasma acylcarnitine analysis reveals elevated levels of butyrylcarnitine, isovalerylcarnitine, glutarylcarnitine, and medium- and long-chain acylcarnitine species. The biochemical findings can vary, not all affected patients exhibit all these abnormalities on testing. Glutaric acidemia type II is most often caused by mutations in the genes encoding the α- or β-subunit of electron transfer flavoprotein or electron transfer flavoprotein dehydrogenase.

Sudden infant death

The most severe presentation of a FAO disorder is sudden infant death (SID) [9,35]. Retrospective studies of siblings of known cases in autopsy studies of SID suggest about 5% of SID could be caused by FAO disorder. Many cases occur during intercurrent illness or after prolonged fasting. The advent of screening for FAO disorders has decreased the incidence of SID in screened populations [43]. However, no screening program can completely eliminate the possibility of sudden death in affected individuals; some infants die 2–4 days after birth for example, too early for newborn screening to be preventive. Any unexplained death of an infant with a mild illness or after fasting should be investigated for a FAO disorder.

Diagnosis

The advent of expanded newborn screening typically utilizing tandem mass spectrometry has changed the way many patients are being diagnosed. Most patients with a disorder of FAO are currently diagnosed after identification by newborn screening. Each specific FAO defect amenable to identification by newborn screening is associated with a unique newborn screening filter paper blood spot tandem mass spectrometric acylcarnitine profile. All states in the USA and most developed countries include acylcarnitine profiling for FAO defects and organic acid disorders from filter paper blood spots as part of the newborn screening program. Tandem mass spectrometry newborn screening can detect affected children presymptomatically and, with proper dietary and medical treatment, prevent catastrophic illness and death, although no newborn screening program in the world can prevent death in the first 2–4 days of life, which rarely occurs in some FAO defects [2]. For this and other reasons, autopsy screening for FAO defects in unexplained death can be useful and many states in the USA routinely pursue such testing in unexplained childhood or infant deaths. Once a FAO defect has been suggested by newborn screening or in symptomatic patients by initial laboratory testing, further specific tests are usually necessary to confirm the diagnosis. Confirmatory tests may include plasma carnitine levels and acylcarnitine profiles; fibroblast in vitro FAO probe; direct enzymatic assays in peripheral blood lymphocytes, cultured skin fibroblasts from skin biopsy sample, and/or liver biopsy tissue; or mutation analysis typically from blood, saliva, or buccal cells. Table 34.2 lists diagnostic tests and observed abnormalities for each FAO disorder. Some FAO defects, such as MCAD or LCHAD deficiencies, are associated with common disease-causing mutations in the gene in question, making mutation analysis, quick and easy to perform, less expensive than enzymatic testing, and diagnostic if the patient is homozygous for a common mutation. The common mutations associated with these conditions are responsible for most but not all cases, so negative findings on specific mutation analysis does not definitively rule out these disorders. In that case, analysis for additional common mutations or complete gene sequencing can be performed. Some cases may be missed by newborn screening and present symptomatically later in life, making it important to pursue diagnostic testing in patients with suggestive symptoms for FAO defects even in individuals who have had normal newborn screening results. Diagnostic testing for patients presenting symptomatically rather than by newborn screening includes plasma acylcarnitine profiling typically as the first step, and additional confirmatory testing when indicated just as described above for those identified by newborn screening. Defects in FAO should be considered in patients presenting with Reye-like syndrome, myopathy, rhabdomyolysis/myoglobinuria, cardiomyopathy, unexplained liver disease, and/or hypoglycemia (particularly when hypoketotic). Metabolic screening tests often employed when metabolic diseases are suggested that may indicate a defect in FAO include urine organic acids, which may show dicarboxycylic aciduria, urine acylglycine analysis that may yield diagnostic metabolites, and plasma carnitine levels showing free carnitine deficiency or excess and/or abnormal free/acylcarnitine levels depending on specific FAO defect. One exception is medium-/short-chain 3-hydroxyacyl-CoA dehydrogenase deficiency in which acylcarnitine profiles are not diagnostic. Hyperinsulinemia with hypoketotic hypoglycemia is suggestive and a serum fatty acid profile will detect short-chain 3-hydroxyl fatty acids. Low free carnitine concentrations suggest a primary carnitine uptake defect that must be confirmed with uptake studies or mutation analysis. Prenatal diagnostic testing is available routinely for many of the defects in FAO and theoretically available for all of those for which the gene defect has been identified. Most families with children with the treatable FAO defects such as MCAD deficiency do not choose to undergo prenatal diagnostic testing but rather to treat the infant presumptively until postnatal diagnostic testing results are available. Specific diagnostic indicators for each FAO disorder are listed in Table 34.2.

Treatment

The goal of treatment for all FAO defects is to minimize FAO by avoidance of fasting and providing adequate non-fat calories during stresses such as intercurrent illness, either orally or parenterally if needed. Provision of adequate energy and frequent feedings sufficient to avoid fasting should be initiated in infants suspected of having a FAO disorder prior to confirmation of the diagnosis. Additional treatment modalities such as carnitine supplementation, dietary fat restriction, and/or MCT supplementation (for long-chain defects only,

Table 34.2 Metabolic abnormalities detected in fatty acid oxidation disorders

Fatty acid oxidation disorder	Plasma acylcarnitine	Urine organic acids[a]
Carnitine uptake defect	$\downarrow C_0$ (free carnitine), $\downarrow$ long-chain acylcarnitines	Normal or $\uparrow$ dicarboxylic acids
Carnitine palmitoyltransferase-I	$\uparrow C_0$, $\downarrow$ long-chain acylcarnitines	Usually normal
Carnitine palmitoyltransferase-II	$\uparrow C_{16}$, $C_{18:1}$, C_{14}, low C_2	Normal
Carnitine acylcarnitine translocase	$\uparrow C_{16}$, $C_{18:1}$, C_{14}, low C_2	Normal or $\uparrow$ dicarboxylic acids
Very-long-chain acyl-CoA dehydrogenase	$\uparrow C_{14}$, $C_{14:1}/C_{12:1}$	$\uparrow$ Dicarboxylic acids
Long-chain 3-hydroxyacyl-CoA dehydrogenase/mitochondrial trifunctional protein	$\uparrow C_{16}$ OH, $C_{18:1}$ OH, C_{14} OH	$\uparrow$ Dicarboxylic acids, $\uparrow$ hydroxydicarboxylic acids (3-hydroxyadipic acid, 3-hydroxysebacic acid)
Medium-chain ketoacyl-CoA thiolase	Unknown	$\uparrow$ Lactic, 3-hydroxybutyric, saturated and unsaturated C_6–C_{16} dicarboxylic acids
Multiple acyl-CoA dehydrogenase/ glutaric aciduria II	$\uparrow C_4$, C_5, C_5 DC, C_6, C_8, C_{10}, C_{12}, C_{14}	$\uparrow$ Glutaric acid, isobutyrylglycine, ethylmalonic acid, dicarboxylic acids, acylglycines (phenylpropionylglycine), 2-hydroxyglutaric acid
Succinyl-CoA: oxoacid transferase	Normal	Normal
Medium-chain acyl-CoA dehydrogenase	$\uparrow C_8$, C_{10}, $C_{10:1}$	$\uparrow$ Dicarboxylic acids, acylglycines (suberylglycine, hexanoylglycine), 5-hydroxyhexanoic acid, octanedioic acid, decanedioic acid
Medium/short-chain acyl-CoA dehydrogenase	$\uparrow$ 3-OH-C_4	$\uparrow$ Dicarboxylic acids, 2-hydroxyglutaric acid
Short-chain acyl-CoA dehydrogenase	$\uparrow C_4$ (butyrylcarnitine and butyrylglycine)	$\uparrow$ Ethylmalonate, methylsuccinate
Ethylmalonic encephalopathy	$\uparrow C_4$, C_5	$\uparrow$ Lactic acid, ethylmalonate, methylsuccinate
2,4-Dienoyl reductase	Hypocarnitinemia, 2-*trans*, 4-*cis*-decadienoylcarnitine in both urine and blood	Normal
3-Hydroxy-3-methylglutaryl-CoA synthase 2	Normal	Normal
3-Hydroxy-3-methylglutaryl-CoA lyase	$\uparrow C_5$OH	$\uparrow$ 3-Methylglutaric acid, 3-methylglutaconic acid, 3-hydroxy-3-methylglutaric acid, 3-methylcrotonylglycine
β-Ketothiolase	Normal or $\downarrow C_0$	Tiglylglycine, acetoacetic acid, 2-methylacetoacetic acid

[a] Normal urine organic acids usually contain small amounts of various dicarboxylic acids. In addition to disorders of fatty acid oxidation, dicarboxylic aciduria occurs in ketosis, several peroxisomal disorders, and medium-chain triglyceride supplementation.

contraindicated in medium-chain defects) have been incompletely studied. Most treatments are based primarily on anecdotal report and expert opinion; these treatments can vary widely across metabolic centers around the world. Here we will review the evidence or reasoning behind current and potential treatments for FAO disorders.

Avoidance of fasting

Healthy infants and children adapt to fasting by turning on glycogenolysis, increasing hepatic gluconeogenesis, and mobilizing fat stores for ketogenesis (in that order sequentially), in order to maintain adequate blood levels of substrates for systemic energy production. Glycogenolysis can only supply glucose for a matter of hours before glycogen supplies would be depleted, and gluconeogenesis can only prevent hypoglycemia for up to approximately 24 hours in older children and adults, less in infants. Therefore, mobilization of fat stores and FAO for ketogenesis and energy production is the main alternative to glucose oxidation in most infants who are fasting, and older children and adults who fast for prolonged periods. A FAO disorder reduces the capacity to utilize free fatty acids for energy and ketone production. This is compounded by the increased systemic need for glucose resulting from the lack of ketones under fasting conditions, ultimately leading to hypoglycemia. Controlled fasting may rarely be indicated diagnostically in patients suspected of having a disorder of FAO, and also for the development of guidelines for the treatment of patients with a known FAO disorder. Such controlled studies should only be carried out after routine confirmatory testing has been completed, and under supervision of specialists experienced in the treatment of FAO disorders, as fasting individuals with FAO defects may be dangerous.

Multiple fasting studies in patients with deficiency, the most common of the FAO disorders, have been published [34]. Based on an analysis of 35 fasting studies performed on 31 patients with MCAD deficiency, a maximum duration of fasting of 8 hours between 6 months and 1 year of age, 10 hours in the second year of life, and 12 hours thereafter has been recommended [44]. These authors defined a safe duration of fasting as the period during which no clinical symptoms (lethargy, vomiting, sweating, tachycardia) or hypoglycemia (glucose <47 mg/dL) was observed. In 6 out of 35 fasting tests in patients with MCAD deficiency, clinical symptoms were observed before hypoglycemia was noted, consistent with the generally held belief that blood glucose levels are a poor indicator of metabolic status in patients with FAO disorders. Because lethargy, sweating, or tachycardia may precede hypoglycemia, and for the reasons stated above, blood glucose monitoring is usually not helpful in the management of these disorders and may provide a false sense of security to families. Other fasting studies have used abnormal metabolites such as a rise in acylcarnitines as an end-point. Plasma acylcarnitines may rise before plasma glucose falls during these controlled fasts and the effects of elevated plasma acylcarnitines on clinical outcomes are not completely understood.

In general, the results of controlled fasting studies suggest prolonged periods of fasting, defined as fasting >12 hours (shorter in younger children), should be avoided. The usefulness of more specific fasting guidelines is debatable; most healthy children and adults will choose to eat frequently, approximately every 6 to 8 hours during waking hours. However, some metabolic centers use the following guidelines: infants younger than 4 months of age should not exceed 4 hours; between 5 and 12 months, an additional hour can be added for each month. Dietary therapy that includes avoidance of fasting and frequent high-carbohydrate meals for the routine management of all FAO disorders prevents most episodes of metabolic decompensation [1]. It is important to note that controlled fasting studies have been conducted in healthy FAO subjects. The majority of episodes of metabolic decompensation in subjects with FAO disorders occur with intercurrent illness or prolonged exercise. The ability of patients with FAO disorders to tolerate fasting during illness or stress is significantly reduced.

Acute management

Illness increases energy requirements while decreasing appetite and potentially increasing energy and fluid loss from emesis and diarrhea. The result is a negative energy balance

that induces increased FAO to produce ATP. Increasing fluid and carbohydrate intake is essential during illness or stress. Frequent intake of sweetened beverages such as fruit juices can be used to manage an illness at home under the direction of the supervising physician. Most oral rehydration solutions contain insufficient carbohydrates to be used as the major hydration solution for those with FAO disorders. Patients with FAO disorders are often provided with emergency treatment plans outlining the steps to be taken by the family or the emergency department, with contact information for the FAO specialist in the event of illness. Should the patient develop alteration in mental status or hypoglycemia, emergency care should be initiated immediately. Metabolic acidosis is a common complication of metabolic decompensation in FAO disorders and is most often associated with elevated blood lactate concentrations. Acute treatment with glucose-containing intravenous fluids can resolve both the hypoglycemia and lactic acidosis if instituted sufficiently early in the illness. Aggressive treatment for the acidosis is usually unnecessary. Large boluses of concentrated glucose solutions can lead to a hyperinsulinemic response followed by rebound hypoglycemia and are to be avoided, unless this is the only way to provide glucose rapidly, for example in the field by paramedics. However, this treatment needs to be followed up immediately by constant provision of glucose until the patient's condition stabilizes. Emergency resuscitation and critical care should be instituted when necessary as per age-appropriate guidelines for patients without FAO, with the reminder to ensure adequate provision of glucose at all times, and modifications for hepatic and cardiac disease when present, as well as monitoring for cerebral edema.

Preventing night-time hypoglycemia

Night-time hypoglycemia has been reported in some patients with FAO disorders and is a major concern for parents. The risk of night-time hypoglycemia appears to diminish as the child ages, and most affected patients can safely sleep through the night by age 4 years or earlier. Both uncooked cornstarch (1 g/kg) at bedtime or overnight tube feedings have been used to provide a continuous source of carbohydrate throughout the night, although neither are usually indicated in patients with MCAD deficiency. Overnight tube feedings carry their own risks, for example with inadvertent disconnection of the tubing overnight leading to hypoglycemia, so that care, such as alarm systems, needs to be taken to lower the risks.

L-Carnitine supplementation

Carnitine is found in meat and dairy products in the diet or synthesized in vivo from lysine and methionine in the liver. Carnitine deficiency is rare but can occur in liver or kidney disease, malnutrition, vegetarian or vegan diets, and malabsorption in addition to FAO disorders. No primary defect of carnitine synthesis is currently known. Patients with carnitine transport defects (OCTN2 defects) otherwise known as primary/systemic carnitine deficiency will have carnitine deficiency if untreated because of defects in absorption. Patients with FAO disorders can develop secondary carnitine deficiency because of high acylcarnitine excretion in the urine that may exceed synthetic capabilities.

L-Carnitine (typically 50–300 mg/kg daily orally or cautious administration of up to 300 mg/kg daily intravenously) is often prescribed for some disorders of FAO to prevent or treat carnitine deficiency and to enhance urinary excretion of potentially toxic FAO intermediates as carnitine conjugates. However, few controlled trials of carnitine supplementation have been performed to prove its clinical efficacy [45]. Certainly carnitine supplementation is indicated in primary carnitine deficiency and the prescription form of L-carnitine is life saving in such conditions. In patients with MCAD deficiency, carnitine supplementation does increase the excretion of medium-chain acylcarnitine moieties but this has not been shown to improve symptoms precipitated by fasting or acute illness [45]. Carnitine supplementation also impairs the formation of medium-chain glycine conjugates, which is the major pathway of excretion for potentially toxic medium-chain metabolites, suggesting that long-term carnitine supplementation may not be beneficial [45]. Carnitine supplementation in patients with medium-chain defects is controversial, and it may be useful in preventing metabolic crisis even when plasma carnitine levels are normal, and is probably indicated when plasma carnitine levels are low.

Carnitine supplementation in children with long-chain FAO defects is also controversial. Some clinicians are concerned that carnitine supplementation will increase plasma levels of potentially toxic acylcarnitines while others believe carnitine supplementation will improve the excretion of these abnormal metabolites. Two reports of subjects with LCHAD/TFP deficiency concluded that carnitine supplementation was not associated with decreased incidence of metabolic decompensation or lower plasma hydroxylated acylcarnitines but did not cause obvious harm [1,32]. However, carnitine supplementation in children with the infantile form of VLCAD deficiency complicated by severe cardiomyopathy may be life-saving.

Dietary fat restriction

Restricting dietary fat intake in patients with short- or medium-chain defects does not appear to be beneficial. To date, there has been no study examining the effects of a low-fat diet on clinical outcomes in MCAD deficiency. In practice, some metabolic centers recommend that patients with MCAD deficiency consume a diet moderately low in fat (30% of total energy from fat) similar to a heart healthy diet, while others do not recommend a specific restriction in dietary fat. There is no research establishing the clinical benefit or lack thereof of dietary fat restriction among patients with MCAD deficiency,

but instruction on use of a heart healthy diet would be reasonable.

Restricting dietary fat intake decreases the accumulation of potentially toxic metabolites such as acylcarnitines among patients with CPT-II, LCHAD, TFP, or VLCAD deficiency. In addition, supplemental MCT provides an alternative energy source downstream of the enzymatic block and decreases long-chain fatty acid oxidation [32]. (Note that MCT supplementation should not be given to patients with medium- or short-chain FAO defects.) Patients with LCHAD or TFP deficiency consuming 10% of energy from long-chain fatty acid and 10–20% energy from MCT have significantly lower plasma hydroxylated acylcarnitines than subjects consuming more long-chain fatty acid or less MCT. While the relationship between increasing dietary long-chain fat intake and increasing circulating acylcarnitine concentrations is well established, the effects of lowering acylcarnitines on long-term outcomes has not been determined for all long-chain FAO disorders. To date, restricting dietary fat intake and lowering long-chain acylcarnitines in patients with VLCAD or CPT-II deficiency has not been correlated with an improvement in clinical outcomes such as a decreased incidence of rhabdomyolysis. However, lower hydroxyacylcarnitines in subjects with LCHAD or TFP deficiency is associated with improved retinal function and a slower progression of chorioretinopathy of LCHAD [33]. Subjects with LCHAD and TFP deficiency who maintained lower hydroxyacylcarnitines had significantly fewer hospitalizations, better vision, and slower progression of chorioretinopathy over 5 years of follow-up. In contrast, feeding a very high fat can be detrimental and precipitate metabolic decompensation.

Essential fatty acid replacement

Biochemical essential fatty acid deficiency has been diagnosed in treated patients with LCHAD, TFP, and VLCAD deficiency although overt clinical symptoms of deficiency are rarely documented [32]. Patients with long-chain FAO defects on low-fat diets are at high risk for essential fatty acid deficiency, and plasma fatty acid levels should be regularly monitored, preferably by a quantitative method. Providing 4% of energy as linoleic acid and 0.6% as α-linolenic acid normalized plasma levels of essential fatty acids in two children with VLCAD deficiency [46]. Therefore, saturated long-chain fatty acid intake from prepared foods should be minimized and the majority of the long-chain fatty acid intake should be provided by oils rich in essential fatty acids. In addition to preventing essential fatty acid deficiency, consuming more polyunsaturated fatty acids and decreasing consumption of saturated fat may lower plasma acylcarnitine concentrations.

A specific deficiency of docosahexaenoic acid (C22:6n-3) has been noted in some children with LCHAD, TFP, and VLCAD deficiency [32]. Docosahexaenoic acid is an essential component of cell membranes and is necessary for normal retinal and brain function. Whether the cause of the deficiency is related to the low-fat diet or to poor synthesis of docosahexaenoic acid from its precursor α-linolenic acid is not known. Supplementing children with LCHAD, TFP and VLCAD deficiency with preformed docosahexaenoic acid (60 mg/day for infant and toddlers; 100 mg/day for children and teens) will normalize plasma levels and may slow progression of pigmentary retinopathy and peripheral neuropathy in LCHAD/TFP deficiency [33].

Treated children with LCHAD, TFP, and VLCAD deficiency may also be at risk for fat-soluble vitamin deficiency because of the low-fat diet. Adequate vitamin A and D intake is promoted by regular consumption of 2–3 cups of skim milk per day. Dietary intake of skim milk provides a low-fat source of protein, B vitamins, vitamins A, and vitamin D. A daily multivitamin and mineral supplement providing the RDA for vitamins A, D, and E seems prudent for patients with LCHAD, TFP or VLCAD deficiency consuming fat-restricted diet. Vitamin K is not routinely found in multivitamins but no biochemical or clinical deficiencies of this micronutrient have been noted in patients with FAO defects.

Triheptanoate

Energy production in the TCA cycle and the electron transport chain is dependent upon maintaining mitochondrial pools of TCA intermediates. Several investigators have suggested that TCA intermediates may become depleted in subjects with long-chain FAO disorders. Substrates that increase the TCA intermediate pools are termed anaplerotic. Anaplerotic therapy has been suggested as a way to increase energy metabolism in subjects with long-chain FAO disorders. Heptanoate (C7:0), an odd carbon number medium-chain fatty acid, is oxidized by enzymes of the medium-chain FAO pathway to two acetyl-CoA and one proprionyl-CoA. Proprionate is anaplerotic and can be converted to succinate. Observational studies using dietary triheptanoate supplements as an anaplerotic therapy in metabolic disorders compared biochemical and physical outcomes of subjects with a variety of FAO disorders and specifically in CPT-II deficiency before and after treatment with triheptanoate [47]. There was significant improvement in cardiomyopathy and decreased frequency and severity of rhabdomyolysis when subjects were supplemented with triheptanoate. Plasma levels of C_4 and C_5 ketones were higher and disease-specific acylcarnitines were lower on triheptanoate therapy. Further research comparing isocaloric amounts of MCT and triheptanoate are needed to determine the benefit of triheptanoate over traditional MCT oil.

B vitamin supplementation

All of the acyl-CoA dehydrogenase enzymes utilize riboflavin as a cofactor. Outside of SCAD deficiency, which may be a non-disease, there is no evidence that riboflavin is helpful in FAO defects. Niacin is the required cofactor for the LCHAD function of TFP and for 3-hydroxyacyl-CoA dehydrogenase. However, there are no reports of supplemental niacin improving residual enzyme activity or of niacin deficiency in these disorders. Niacin supplementation above normal requirements does not appear to be warranted.

Liver disease in pregnancy

Mothers carrying fetuses affected by certain FAO defects have a greater propensity toward late pregnancy complications including pre-eclampsia, HELLP syndrome (hemolysis, elevated liver enzymes, and low platelets) and AFLP (acute fatty liver of pregnancy) than the general population [48]. The incidence of maternal HELLP and AFLP is particularly high in mothers carrying fetuses with LCHAD/TFP deficiency but it has been documented in pregnancies in which the fetus was subsequently diagnosed with other FAO defects as well. The cause of the toxicity of the affected fetus of the heterozygote mother is not known but it has been suggested that the placenta performs substantial FAO and may produce potentially toxic metabolites that would be filtered into the mother's circulation.

Bezafibrate

Bezafibrates are PPARα agonists that have been used to treat hypertriglyceridemia in humans. In human subjects with CPT-II deficiency, treatment with bezafibrates decreased muscle pain and lethargy and improved biochemical parameters such as acylcarnitine profiles [49]. Bezafibrate treatment is a potential new therapy for long-chain FAO disorders, but is not approved by the US Food and Drug Administration and further studies are needed.

Conclusion

Mitochondrial FAO disorders are a family of disorders characterized by hypoketotic hypoglycemia with fasting. Many of the disorders described in this chapter may have concomitant liver disease with micro- and macrovesicular steatosis, and occasionally with a Reye-like syndrome and frank liver failure. Since the identification of the first FAO disorder in the 1980s, over 22 different disorders have been described. Our ability to diagnose affected infants has greatly improved with the advent of expanded newborn screening. Maternal liver disease during pregnancy results in significant morbidity and mortality in both mother and infant. Treatment of infants and children is based on nutritional interventions designed to decrease FAO and provide adequate energy. Further understanding of the natural history of these disorders and the development of future treatments are areas of ongoing research in the field.

References

1. Saudubray JM, Martin D, de Lonlay P, et al. Recognition and management of fatty acid oxidation defects: a series of 107 patients. *J Inherited Metab Dis* 1999;**22**:488–502.

2. Lindner M, Hoffmann GF, Matern D. Newborn screening for disorders of fatty-acid oxidation: experience and recommendations from an expert meeting. *J Inherit Metab Dis* 2010;**33**:521–526.

3. McGarry JD, Takabayashi Y, Foster DW. The role of malonyl-CoA in the coordination of fatty acid synthesis and oxidation in isolated rat hepatocytes. *J Biol Chem* 1978;**253**:8294–8300.

4. Gulick T, Cresci S, Caira T, Moore DD, Kelly DP. The peroxisome proliferator-activated receptor regulates mitochondrial fatty acid oxidative enzyme gene expression. *Proc Natl Acad Sci USA* 1994;**91**:11012–11016.

5. Bonnefont JP, Demaugre F, Prip-Buus C, et al. Carnitine palmitoyltransferase deficiencies. *Mol Genet Metab* 1999;**68**:424–440.

6. Andresen BS, Bross P, Vianey-Saban C, et al. Cloning and characterization of human very-long-chain acyl-CoA dehydrogenase cDNA, chromosomal assignment of the gene and identification in four patients of nine different mutations within the *VLCAD* gene. *Hum Mol Genet* 1996;**5**:461–472.

7. Strauss AW, Powell CK, Hale DE, et al. Molecular basis of human mitochondrial very-long-chain acyl-CoA dehydrogenase deficiency causing cardiomyopathy and sudden death in childhood. *Proc Natl Acad Sci USA* 1995;**92**:10496–0500.

8. Lea W, Abbas AS, Sprecher H, Vockley J, Schulz H. Long-chain acyl-CoA dehydrogenase is a key enzyme in the mitochondrial beta-oxidation of unsaturated fatty acids. *Biochim Biophys Acta* 2000;**1485**(2–3):121–128.

9. Eder M, Krautle F, Dong Y, et al. Characterization of human and pig kidney long-chain-acyl-CoA dehydrogenases and their role in beta-oxidation. *Eur J Biochem* 1997;**245**:600–607.

10. Indo Y, Coates PM, Hale DE, Tanaka K. Immunochemical characterization of variant long-chain acyl-CoA dehydrogenase in cultured fibroblasts from nine patients with long-chain acyl-CoA dehydrogenase deficiency. *Pediatr Res* 1991;**30**:211–215.

11. Maher AC, Mohsen AW, Vockley J, Tarnopolsky MA. Low expression of long-chain acyl-CoA dehydrogenase in human skeletal muscle. *Mol Genet Metab* 2010;**100**:163–167.

12. Oey NA, Ruiter JP, Ijlst L, et al. Acyl-CoA dehydrogenase 9 (ACAD 9) is the long-chain acyl-CoA dehydrogenase in human embryonic and fetal brain. *Biochem Biophys Res Commun* 2006;**346**:33–37.

13. Reichmann H, Maltese WA, DeVivo DC. Enzymes of fatty acid beta-oxidation in developing brain. *J Neurochem* 1988;**51**:339–344.

14. He M, Rutledge SL, Kelly DR, et al. Identification and characterization of new long chain acyl-CoA dehydrogenases. *Mol Genet Metab* 2011;**102**:418–429.

15. Matsubara Y, Narisawa K, Tada K. Medium-chain acyl-CoA dehydrogenase deficiency: molecular aspects. *Eur J Pediatr* 1992;**151**:154–159.

16. Corydon MJ, Andresen BS, Bross P, et al. Structural organization of the human short-chain acyl-CoA dehydrogenase gene. *Mamm Genome* 1997;**8**:922–926.

17. Ijlst L, Ruiter P, Hoovers JM, Jakobs ME, Wanders RJ. Common missense mutation G1528C in long-chain 3-hydroxyacyl-CoA dehydrogenase deficiency. Characterization and expression of the mutant protein, mutation analysis on genomic DNA and chromosomal localization of the mitochondrial trifunctional protein alpha subunit gene. *J Clin Invest* 1996;**98**:1028–1033.

18. Kanazawa M, Ohtake A, Abe H, et al. Molecular cloning and sequence analysis of the cDNA for human mitochondrial short-chain enoyl-CoA hydratase. *Enzyme Protein* 1993;**47**:9–13.

19. He XY, Yang SY, Schulz H. Assay of L-3-hydroxyacyl-coenzyme A dehydrogenase with substrates of different chain lengths. *Anal Biochem* 1989;**180**:105–109.

20. Yang SY, He XY, Schulz H. Multiple functions of type 10 17beta-hydroxysteroid dehydrogenase. *Trends Endocrinol Metab* 2005;**16**:167–175.

21. Yang SY, He XY, Schulz H. 3-Hydroxyacyl-CoA dehydrogenase and short chain 3-hydroxyacyl-CoA dehydrogenase in human health and disease. *FEBS Lett* 2005;**272**:4874–4883.

22. Stoop WM, Schennink A, Visker MH, et al. Genome-wide scan for bovine milk-fat composition. I. Quantitative trait loci for short- and medium-chain fatty acids. *J Dairy Sci* 2009;**92**:4664–4675.

23. Brunengraber H, Roe CR. Anaplerotic molecules: current and future. *J Inherit Metab Dis* 2006;**29**(2–3):327–331.

24. Brown NF, Mullur RS, Subramanian I, et al. Molecular characterization of L-CPT I deficiency in six patients: insights into function of the native enzyme. *J Lipid Res* 2001;**42**:1134–1142.

25. Brivet M, Boutron A, Slama A, et al. Defects in activation and transport of fatty acids. *J Inherit Metab Dis* 1999;**22**:428–441.

26. Lopriore E, Gemke RJ, Verhoeven NM, et al. Carnitine-acylcarnitine translocase deficiency: phenotype, residual enzyme activity and outcome. *Eur J Pediatr* 2001;**160**:101–104.

27. Pons R, Cavadini P, Baratta S, et al. Clinical and molecular heterogeneity in very-long-chain acyl-coenzyme A dehydrogenase deficiency. *Pediatr Neurol* 2000;**22**:98–105.

28. Vianey-Saban C, Divry P, Brivet M, et al. Mitochondrial very-long-chain acyl-coenzyme A dehydrogenase deficiency: clinical characteristics and diagnostic considerations in 30 patients. *Clin Chim Acta* 1998;**269**:43–62.

29. Hoffman JD, Steiner RD, Paradise L, et al. Rhabdomyolysis in the military: recognizing late-onset very long-chain acyl Co-A dehydrogenase deficiency. *Mil Med* 2006;**171**:657–658.

30. Gregersen N, Andresen BS, Bross P. Prevalent mutations in fatty acid oxidation disorders: diagnostic considerations. *Eur J Pediatr* 2000;**159** (Suppl 3):S213–S218.

31. Haack TB, Danhauser K, Haberberger B, et al. Exome sequencing identifies *ACAD9* mutations as a cause of complex I deficiency. *Nat Genet* 2010;**42**:1131–1134.

32. Gillingham M, van Calcar S, Ney D, Wolff J, Harding C. Dietary management of long-chain 3-hydroxyacyl-CoA dehydrogenase

deficiency (LCHADD). A case report and survey. *J Inherit Metab Dis* 1999;**22**:123–131.

33. Gillingham MB, Weleber RG, Neuringer M, *et al.* Effect of optimal dietary therapy upon visual function in children with long-chain 3-hydroxyacyl CoA dehydrogenase and trifunctional protein deficiency. *Mol Genet Metab* 2005;**86**(1–2):124–133.

34. Stanley CA, Hale DE, Coates PM, *et al.* Medium-chain acyl-CoA dehydrogenase deficiency in children with non-ketotic hypoglycemia and low carnitine levels. *Pediatr Res* 1983;**17**:877–884.

35. Brackett JC, Sims HF, Steiner RD, *et al.* A novel mutation in medium chain acyl-CoA dehydrogenase causes sudden neonatal death. *J Clin Invest* 1994;**94**:1477–1483.

36. Andresen BS, Bross P, Jensen TG, *et al.* A rare disease-associated mutation in the medium-chain acyl-CoA dehydrogenase (MCAD) gene changes a conserved arginine, previously shown to be functionally essential in short-chain acyl-CoA dehydrogenase (SCAD). *Am J Hum Genet* 1993;**53**:730–739.

37. Lang TF. Adult presentations of medium-chain acyl-CoA dehydrogenase deficiency (MCADD). *J Inherit Metab Dis* 2009;**32**:675–683.

38. Joy P, Black C, Rocca A., Haas M, Wilcken B. Neuropsychological functioning in children with medium chain acyl coenzyme a dehydrogenase deficiency (MCADD): the impact of early diagnosis and screening on outcome. *Child Neuropsychol* 2009;**15**:8–20.

39. Pedersen CB, Kolvraa S, Kolvraa A, *et al.* The *ACADS* gene variation spectrum in 114 patients with short-chain acyl-CoA dehydrogenase (SCAD) deficiency is dominated by missense variations leading to protein misfolding at the cellular level. *Hum Genet* 2008;**124**:43–56.

40. Waisbren SE, Levy HL, Noble M, *et al.* Short-chain acyl-CoA dehydrogenase (SCAD) deficiency: an examination of the medical and neurodevelopmental characteristics of 14 cases identified through newborn screening or clinical symptoms. *Mol Genet Metab* 2008; **95**(1–2):39–45.

41. Molven A, Matre GE, Duran M, *et al.* Familial hyperinsulinemic hypoglycemia caused by a defect in the SCHAD enzyme of mitochondrial fatty acid oxidation. *Diabetes* 2004;**53**: 221–227.

42. Kamijo T, Indo Y, Souri M, *et al.* Medium chain 3-ketoacyl-coenzyme A thiolase deficiency: a new disorder of mitochondrial fatty acid beta-oxidation. *Pediatr Res* 1997;**42**:569–576.

43. Goddard P. Newborn screening for medium chain acyl-CoA dehydrogenase deficiency (MCADD) in the UK. *J Fam Health Care* 2004;**14**:90–92.

44. Derks TG, van Spronsen FJ, Rake JP, *et al.* Safe and unsafe duration of fasting for children with MCAD deficiency. *Eur J Pediatr* 2007;**166**:5–11.

45. Rinaldo P, Schmidt-Sommerfeld E, Posca AP, *et al.* Effect of treatment with glycine and L-carnitine in medium-chain acyl-coenzyme A dehydrogenase deficiency. *J Pediatr* 1993;**122**:580–584.

46. Ruiz-Sanz JI, Aldamiz-Echevarria L, Arrizabalaga J, *et al.* Polyunsaturated fatty acid deficiency during dietary treatment of very long-chain acyl-CoA dehydrogenase deficiency. Rescue with soybean oil. *J Inherit Metab Dis* 2001;**24**:493–503.

47. Roe CR, Sweetman L, Roe DS, David F, Brunengraber H. Treatment of cardiomyopathy and rhabdomyolysis in long-chain fat oxidation disorders using an anaplerotic odd-chain triglyceride. *J Clin Invest* 2002;**110**:259–269.

48. Ibdah JA, Bennett MJ, Rinaldo P, *et al.* A fetal fatty-acid oxidation disorder as a cause of liver disease in pregnant women. *N Engl J Med* 1999;**340**: 1723–1731.

49. Bonnefont JP, Bastin J, Laforet P, *et al.* Long-term follow-up of bezafibrate treatment in patients with the myopathic form of carnitine palmitoyltransferase 2 deficiency. *Clin Pharmacol Ther* 2010;**88**:101–108.

Mitochondrial hepatopathies

35

Ronald J. Sokol

Introduction

Alterations of mitochondrial structure and function are now recognized as the etiology of a growing and wide variety of pathologic disorders, including monogenic mitochondrial disorders as well as more common pathologic conditions. Indeed, studying patients with respiratory chain disorders has contributed much to our current knowledge about mitochondrial biology [1]. Genetic defects in the synthesis of mitochondrial proteins, ribosomal RNA, and transfer RNA (tRNA), caused by mutations in 228 nuclear genes and 13 mitochondrial DNA (mtDNA) genes, are the underlying cause of diseases affecting the nervous system, skeletal and cardiac muscle, liver, bone marrow, endocrine and exocrine pancreas, kidney, inner ear, and small and large intestines (Table 35.1) [2]. Resultant perturbations in mitochondrial function yield defective oxidative phosphorylation (OXPHOS) and ATP generation, increased generation of reactive oxygen species, accumulation of hepatocytic lipid, impairment of other mitochondria-based metabolic processes, and activation of apoptotic, autophagic and necrotic cell death pathways [2]. The spectrum and genetic etiologies of inherited mitochondrial hepatic and gastrointestinal disorders continue to expand. In addition, mitochondrial dysfunction may be one of the key targets and determinants for hepatocyte survival in other disorders not directly related to the mitochondrion. Consequently, the concept of primary (or genetic) and secondary (or acquired) mitochondrial hepatopathies has developed. Because mitochondria possess a distinct and unique extranuclear genome, a new class of maternally inherited mitochondrial diseases has also emerged. The tissue-specific accumulation over time of new somatic (non-inherited) mutations of mitochondrial genes may also be involved in several neurodegenerative diseases [3], hepatopathies, and the process of aging itself [4]. This chapter will review continued advances in our understanding of the genetics, structure, and function of the mitochondrion, classification of mitochondrial hepatopathies, the evolving diagnostic approach for these disorders, and treatment modalities including liver transplantation.

Table 35.1 Systemic presentations of mitochondrial disorders

System	Presentation
Cardiac	Hypertrophic cardiomyopathy Heart block, sudden death Barth syndrome (cardiomyopathy, cyclic neutropenia)
Eye	Cataracts, optic atrophy, pigmentary retinopathy
Ear	Sensorineural deafness Aminoglycoside deafness
Renal	Proximal tubular disorder (Fanconi syndrome) Nephritis, nephrotic syndrome
Endocrine	Diabetes mellitus Short stature, and growth hormone deficiency Hypoparathyroidism, hypothyroidism
Hematologic	Pancytopenia, sideroblastic anemia Vacuolization
Gastrointestin	Pancreatic insufficiency, pancreatitis Intestinal villus atrophy Intestinal pseudo-obstruction
Dermatologic	Mottled pigmentation Hypertrichosis, dry brittle hair, alopecia
Metabolic	Lactic acidosis Hyperammonemia

Mitochondrial structure and genetics

The mitochondrion is a double-membrane structure containing a soluble matrix and its own unique genome. The outer membrane serves as a "corset" to hold the highly folded inner membrane in place; as a regulator of efflux of mitochondrial enzymes, cations (including calcium), and substrates into the cytosol; as well as a specific transport site for a variety of mitochondrial substrates that must be taken up from cytosol. The inner mitochondrial membrane contains specialized transport sites for small molecules, the electron transport chain, that accepts electrons generated from the tricarboxylic acid (TCA) cycle, and ATP synthase that carries out OXPHOS and ATP synthesis. The mitochondrial matrix is a concentrated mixture of enzymes that are active in the TCA cycle, fatty acid oxidation (FAO), urea synthesis, and other metabolic pathways. Specific enzyme defects have been described for many of these matriceal enzymes, most coded for by nuclear DNA, leading to familiar, although rare, disorders of FAO, urea synthesis, gluconeogenesis, and so on.

One of the most unique characteristics of mitochondria in mammalian cells is the presence of a separate genome and the enzymes necessary for the replication, transcription, translation, and expression of nucleic acids independently [5]. Virtually all mtDNA in a cell is derived from the unfertilized oocyte (sperm contribute virtually no mitochondria), and hence all characteristics encoded by the mtDNA are maternally inherited. Therefore, affected men do not transmit the genetic defect. In general, deleted molecules are not transmitted from clinically affected women to their children; however, a woman with a heteroplasmic mtDNA point mutation or duplications may transmit a variable amount of mutated DNA to their children [6]. The mitochondrial genome is a double-stranded, circular molecule containing 16 569 bp that has been fully sequenced and shown to encode 37 genes, including 2 ribosomal RNAs, 22 tRNAs for protein synthesis, 13 of the subunits of complex I, III, IV, and V of the respiratory chain (Table 35.2). The mtDNA sequences do not contain introns, as opposed to nuclear genes. Early during development of the female germline, there is a reduction of number of mtDNA molecules within each oocyte followed by amplification to reach approximately 100 000 genomes per mature oocyte. This "genetic bottleneck" influences the variability between oocytes. The mtDNA also depends on nuclear genes for its enzymes of replication, transcription, translation, and repair, and nuclear genes encode all the other proteins of the metabolic pathways located in mitochondria [1]. Net mitochondrial morphology depends on the balance between motility, fission, and fusion of mitochondria. There has been recent progress in characterizing the mammalian mitochondrial proteome, with more than 1100 proteins assigned to this compartment [7]; mutations in genes coding for any of these proteins could potentially cause mitochondrial dysfunction. It should be noted that most subunits of the respiratory chain proteins are encoded by nuclear DNA and imported into the mitochondria after assembly elsewhere in the cell (Table 35.2). Therefore, abnormalities in OXPHOS can be the result of both nuclear and mtDNA mutations.

Each mitochondrion contains 2 to 10 copies of the genome, and since cells can contain hundreds or thousands of mitochondria, thousands of copies of this genome can be present in an individual cell [5]. Usually, all mtDNA is

Table 35.2 Mitochondrial respiratory chain protein complexes: polypeptide subunits

Complex	Total number of subunits	Subunits encoded by nuclear DNA	Subunits encoded by mtDNA
I	41	34	7: ND_1, ND_2, ND_3, ND_4, ND_{4L}, ND_5, ND_6
III	11	10	1: cyt b
IV	13	10	3: cyt. oxidase I, cyt. oxidase II, cyt. oxidase III
V	14	12	2: ATPase 6, ATPase 8

cyt, cytochrome.

identical, called *homoplasmy*; however, normal and mutant mtDNA can coexist in various proportions in a single cell (*heteroplasmy*). The phenotype of the cell is determined by the relative proportion of normal and mutated genomes. Mutations occur in mtDNA 10–20 times as frequently as nuclear DNA, resulting in point mutations, deletions, and duplications. This DNA has neither protective histones nor an effective repair system and it is constantly exposed to reactive oxygen species generated by OXPHOS that can induce DNA damage and mutations. During cell division, mitochondria are randomly partitioned into daughter cells, resulting in non-uniform distribution of mutated mtDNA in progeny cells. The threshold of mutated mitochondrial genome needed to produce a deleterious phenotype varies among people, organ systems, and within individual tissues. The threshold for biochemical expression is about 60% mutant for mtDNA deletions and up to 95% for tRNA mutations [4]. Therefore, there is variable clinical expression among patients with the same genotypic mutations, sometimes with abnormalities in OXPHOS activity detected only in the involved tissues. The degree of organ dysfunction will depend on a tissue's energy requirements, with brain, muscle, and liver most commonly involved. During cell division, the proportion of mutant and wild-type mtDNA may shift, explaining how some patients with mitochondrial disorders may actually shift from one clinical phenotype to another as they age. In addition, mutations in a growing group of nuclear genes interrupt mtDNA replication or stabilization, resulting in generalized depletion of mtDNA. Cell damage in these disorders results from an inadequate supply of energy in metabolically active cells and tissues, increased generation of injurious reactive oxygen species as a consequence of perturbed flow of electrons down the respiratory chain, alterations of cellular ion homeostasis, release of cytochrome *c* and apoptosis-inducing factor into cytoplasm, or other undefined mechanisms.

Functions of mitochondria

The essential functions of mitochondria are related to the multitude of enzyme systems located in the various compartments of this organelle [1]. Mitochondria from different organs exhibit distinct patterns of substrate use, biosynthetic capacities, and even variable ultrastructural features across tissues [1]. While respiratory chain complexes are largely invariant across organs, the protein composition of the mitochondrial ribosome can differ between tissues and there are tissue-specific isoforms of complex IV that should have functional consequences. A major function of mitochondria is to synthesize ATP by the process of OXPHOS, which drives energy-dependent reactions and transport processes in all cells. The transduction of energy by the transfer of electrons from substrates of the TCA cycle (via NADH) and from the FAO cycle (via NADH and FADH$_2$) to oxygen is facilitated by the respiratory chain, a group of five large protein complexes embedded in the inner mitochondrial membrane, plus ubiquinone (coenzyme Q; CoQ) and cytochrome c (Figure 35.1). These include complex I (NADH-CoQ reductase), complex II (succinate-CoQ reductase), complex III (reduced CoQ-cytochrome c reductase), complex IV (cytochrome c oxidase), and complex V (ATP synthase) [8]. The free energy generated from these stepwise redox reactions is converted into a transmembrane proton gradient by the extrusion of protons through the inner membrane at complexes I, III, and IV. At complex V, protons flow back into the mitochondrial matrix and the released energy is used by ATP synthetase to drive ATP synthesis. When ADP and inorganic phosphate are bound to the active site, protons are allowed to move down the concentration gradient and the free energy is enzymatically coupled to the formation of a bond between ADP and phosphate. Three ATP molecules are generated for each molecule of NADH oxidized. Free NAD$^+$ is regenerated for use in the TCA cycle and other integral mitochondrial matrix enzyme pathways. In addition to its role as the final electron receptor in the respiratory chain, 2–3% of the oxygen utilized by mitochondria results in the generation of superoxide by complexes I and III. This superoxide is normally converted to hydrogen peroxide by the manganese-superoxide dismutase present in the matrix or combines with nitric oxide to form peroxynitrite. The hydrogen peroxide may diffuse into cytosol or remain in the mitochondrial matrix, only to be reduced to water by glutathione peroxidases present in both the mitochondria and cell cytoplasm. If the balance of generation and scavenging of these reactive oxygen species is upset, increased oxidative stress may develop within the mitochondria, damaging mitochondrial proteins and mtDNA.

Both primary and secondary defects in function of the respiratory chain have severe consequences for the metabolic homeostasis of the cell [1]. These include a generalized deficiency of high-energy molecules; a substantially increased dependence on glycolysis, with increased lactate production in the cytosol; an increase in the intramitochondrial and

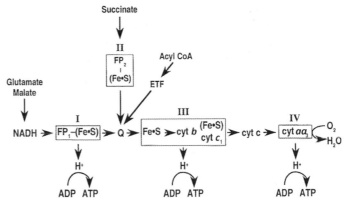

Figure 35.1 The respiratory chain protein complexes and oxidative phosphorylation of the mitochondria. During glycolysis, fatty acid oxidation, and the tricarboxylic acid cycle, reducing equivalents are derived from the sequential metabolism of each metabolic fuel. NADH acts as a carrier of reducing equivalents from glycolysis into the mitochondria matrix, and NADH and FADH$_2$ shuttle reducing equivalents produced by fatty acid oxidation and the TCA cycle. Succinate carries reducing equivalents derived from the TCA cycle. In order to transduce this reducing power into energy, a system of electron carriers (protein complexes I through IV, coenzyme Q and cytochrome c) in the inner mitochondrial membrane convert the reducing equivalents into ATP through the efficient transport of electrons down this chain, resulting in the generation of a transmembrane proton gradient that drives the synthesis of ATP by complex V. FP, flavoprotein, Fe·S, iron–sulfur cluster, cyt, cytochrome.

cytoplasmic concentration of reducing equivalents; the functional impairment of the TCA cycle through this altered redox state (an excess of NADH and lack of NAD); and an increase in the generation of oxygen free radicals with resultant oxidation of lipids in membranes, thiol-containing proteins, and mitochondrial nucleic acids and opening of the mitochondrial permeability pore. The mitochondrial permeability transition releases cytochrome c and apoptosis-inducing factors into the cytosol, triggering the activation of caspases and the irreversible process of cellular apoptosis. In addition, the permeability transition results in loss of mitochondrial membrane potential and interruption of ATP synthesis. Therefore, both metabolic failure and the induction of hepatocyte apoptosis or necrosis could result from impairment of normal electron flow in the respiratory chain.

Another important intermediary metabolic pathway within mitochondria involves the fate of pyruvate. Glucose oxidation via glycolysis in the cytoplasmic compartment results in the formation of two moles of pyruvate from each mole of glucose. Without mitochondrial oxidation, pyruvate is anaerobically reduced to lactate; yielding only 2 of the total 38 moles of potentially available ATP if pyruvate were metabolized via the TCA cycle. Pyruvate can be translocated across the mitochondrial membrane and oxidized to acetyl-coenzyme A (CoA) by the pyruvate dehydrogenase complex; acetyl-CoA then enters the TCA cycle by combining with oxaloacetate to form citrate. The TCA cycle enzymes are located in the mitochondrial matrix and depend on transporters imbedded in the otherwise impermeable inner mitochondrial membrane for the influx of substrates and efflux of generated products.

Table 35.3 Epidemiologic studies of mitochondrial diseases

Study population	Mutations or disease	Disease prevalence/100 000 (95% CI)	Mutation prevalence/ 100 000 (95% CI)
Majamaa et al. (1998) [12], northern Finland (n = 245 201 adults)	Adult point prevalence of A3243G identified in 615 patients	5.71 (4.53–6.89)	16.3 (11.3–21.4)
Chinnery et al. (2000) [13], northern England (n = 1 582 584 adults)	Adult point prevalence of all mtDNA mutations; identified 104 patients and 161 maternal relatives	6.57 (5.30–7.83)	12.48 (10.75–14.23)
Uusimaa et al. (2000) [14], Finland (n = 146 482 children)	All mtDNA mutations in children with respiratory chain disorder; identified 26 children	Unable to calculate from data	Unable to calculate from data
Darin et al. (2001) [15], western Sweden (n = 358 616 children)	Pediatric point prevalence of pediatric mitochondrial encephalomyopathies; identified 32 children	4.76 (2.80–7.60)	Unable to calculate from data

CI, confidence interval; mt, mitochondrial.
Source: with permission from Gillis and Sokol, 2003 [16].

Long-chain FAO is the predominant source of energy for cardiac and skeletal muscle at all times and becomes the major pathway for energy production during fasting in liver, cardiac, and skeletal muscle. With prolonged fasting, fatty acids are converted into ketone bodies in the liver and exported to extrahepatic tissues as an alternative fuel when the supply of glucose is limited, thus sparing glucose utilization for more obligate organ users such as the brain. Fatty acid oxidation leads to the generation of electron-rich substrates for the respiratory chain, $FADH_2$ and NADH. Imbedded in the mitochondrial membrane is the enzyme that catalyzes the conversion of long-chain acyl-CoA esters to acylcarnitines, the transporters of both acyl- and free carnitine across the membrane, and the enzyme which converts acylcarnitines back to acyl-CoAs on the inner side of the inner mitochondrial membrane. In this location are the enzymes of the beta-oxidation cycle, which catalyze the repetitive cleavage of C_2 fragments from the fatty acid chain and the generation of acetyl-CoA. Acetyl-CoA either condenses with oxaloacetate to form citrate and enters the TCA cycle or becomes available for ketogenesis during fasting. Two other mitochondrial matrix enzymes catalyze the synthesis of acetoacetate and its reduction to β-hydroxybutyrate.

Other metabolic pathways partially housed in the mitochondria, include the urea cycle, bile acid synthesis, methylmalonic acid and ethanol metabolism, and fatty acid synthesis. In addition, the mitochondrion plays a key role in intracellular calcium homeostasis. For purposes of this chapter, "mitochondrial diseases" that affect the respiratory chain will be emphasized. These disorders are caused by primary defects or are secondary to other inter-related metabolic defects or drug interactions. With the advent of rapid DNA sequencing technologies in recent years, it has become apparent that many unexplained diseases of infancy and early childhood are caused by genetic disorders of electron transport and OXPHOS. In this chapter, disorders of liver, pancreatic, and intestinal dysfunction in their primary presentation either alone or as part of a more global picture of CNS, muscle, bone marrow, or renal disease will be described, with emphasis on the clinical manifestations, diagnosis, and treatment. Other common manifestations of these disorders are diabetes, cardiomyopathy, deafness, and retinitis pigmentosa. Details of the pathophysiology and molecular biology of these disorders are contained in several excellent reviews [1].

Epidemiology of mitochondrial disorders

Pathogenic mtDNA mutations cause a wide variety of pediatric and adult mitochondrial diseases; in excess of 300 pathogenic point mutations, deletions, insertions, and rearrangements have been identified since the first mitochondrial mutations were reported in 1988 [9,10]. A minimal prevalence of 1 in 7634 live births has been proposed for respiratory chain disorders with onset at any age [11] (Table 35.3). Most estimate that mitochondrial diseases affect 1 in 5000–10 000 in the population, from infancy through adulthood. Approximately 20% of patients with mitochondrial disease have evidence of liver involvement. An estimated 90% of mitochondrial diseases are caused by mutations in nuclear genes, now totaling about 228 genes linked to human diseases [1]. As a general rule, point mutations of mtDNA genes are usually maternally inherited, whereas deletions or rearrangements of mtDNA are either sporadic or inherited in an autosomal recessive manner (caused by mutations in nuclear genes).

Mitochondrial disorders are a challenge for the genetic epidemiologist. Factors that influence the prevalence of mitochondrial disorders include the mutation rate, inheritance pattern, population structure, and the genetic background. Accurate diagnosis may be difficult, and it is not always possible to identify the underlying mitochondrial molecular genetic defect in the blood [17]. Clinical presentations vary considerably and so there may be significant delays in diagnosis. Moreover, transmission of a pathogenic mutation does not necessarily result a clinical phenotype. Most epidemiological studies determined the frequency of a specific mtDNA mutation in patients with a specific clinical presentation, failing to account for phenotypic variability. As the spectrum of mtDNA

Table 35.4 Mitochondrial encephalomyopathies

Syndrome/dysfunction	Features
Leigh syndrome	Subacute necrotizing encephalomyopathy
Kearns–Sayre syndrome	Ophthalmoplegia, retinal degeneration, heart-block
MERRF syndrome	Myoclonus, epilepsy, ragged red fibers
MELAS syndrome	Myopathy, encephalopathy, lactic acidosis and stroke-like episodes
LHON	Leber's hereditary optic neuropathy
NARP	Neuropathy, ataxia and retinitis pigmentosa
MIMyCa	Maternally inherited myopathy and cardiomyopathy
Mitochondrial DNA deletions	Myopathy and multiple deletions of mitochondrial DNA
Mitochondrial DNA depletion syndrome	Generalized depletion
MNGIE	Mitochondrial neurogastrointestinal encephalomyopathy
CHERP	Calcification, hearing loss, hypogonadism, encephalopathy, retinitis pigmentosa
CPEO	Chronic progressive external ophthalmoplegia
OCRL	Ocular cerebrorenal syndrome
Alpers–Huttenlocher disease	Progressive infantile poliodystrophy
Hereditary myopathies	With or without lactic acidosis
Fatty acid oxidation defects	Defects/deficiencies of enzymes of fatty acid oxidation and other carnitine transport and deficiency states
Electron transfer flavoprotein	Electron transfer flavoprotein and its dehydrogenase deficiencies (glutaric acidemia type II)
Possible other disorders	Parkinson disease, Huntington disease, Alzheimer disease

disease continues to rapidly expand, with novel genotypes and phenotypes, epidemiological data will accordingly require future revisions. The population frequency of nuclear gene abnormalities causing mitochondrial diseases has not been accurately estimated.

Neuromuscular mitochondrial disorders

The majority of the diseases initially associated with maternal inheritance and later with mtDNA mutations are neuromuscular in nature (Table 35.4). Many are caused by large deletions or missense mutations of mitochondrial genome involving tRNA genes or subunits of the electron transport chain complexes, or mutations of nuclear genes encoding subunits of these complexes. These disorders include Leber hereditary optic neuropathy, MELAS syndrome (mitochondrial encephalomyopathy, lactic acidosis and stroke-like episodes), MERRF (myoclonic epilepsy with ragged red fibers) syndrome, Kearns–Sayre syndrome, Leigh disease, and others [18,19]. The A3243G mutation in tRNA is the most common single base change and has been associated with MELAS, the G8344A mutation in tRNA being found in MERRF [19]. Many of these mitochondrial encephalomyopathies have their onset in childhood and must be kept in mind by those evaluating children with neurologic and muscular disorders [20]. The number of disorders that can be caused by mitochondrial enzyme defects, abnormal OXPHOS, or other mtDNA mutations has grown at a rapid pace and now includes several gastrointestinal diseases (see below) as well as the mitochondrial hepatopathies. Although most commonly presenting in childhood, many of these mitochondrial hepatopathies can also have delayed onset during adulthood (e.g. Alpers–Huttenlocher syndrome and mitochondrial neurogastrointestinal encephalomyopathy). These disorders can be grouped into the primary (or congenital) and the secondary (or acquired) mitochondrial hepatopathies (Table 35.5).

Classification of mitochondrial hepatopathies

In a variety of hepatic disorders, genetic or acquired defects in either specific biochemical pathways or more general dysfunction of mitochondria have been described. These conditions are frequently, but not universally, associated with morphologic changes of hepatic mitochondrial structure or number or with neuromuscular or other systemic involvement. These disorders (mitochondrial hepatopathies) have undergone classification based on clinical phenotype, as well as more recently by genotype. In the phenotypic classification scheme (Table 35.5), the disorders are divided into *primary hepatopathies*, in which the mitochondrial defect is

Table 35.5 Phenotypic classification of mitochondrial hepatopathies

Type	Hepatopathy
Primary disorders	
Respiratory chain (electron transport) defects)	Neonatal liver failure: Complex I deficiency Complex IV deficiency (*SCO1* mutations) Complex III deficiency (*BCS1L* mutations) Multiple complex deficiencies (*TSFM, EFG1, EFTu* mutations) Mitochondrial DNA depletion syndrome (*DGUOK, MPV17, POLG1, SUCLG1, C10orf2* mutations) Later-onset liver dysfunction or failure Alpers–Huttenlocher syndrome (*POLG1* mutations) Pearson's marrow–pancreas syndrome (mtDNA deletion) Mitochondrial neurogastrointestinal encephalomyopathy (*TYMP* mutations) Chronic diarrhea (villus atrophy) with hepatic involvement (complex III deficiency) Navajo neurohepatopathy (mtDNA depletion; *MPV17* mutations)
Fatty acid oxidation defects	Long-chain hydroxyacyl CoA dehydrogenase (*HADHA*) deficiency Acute fatty liver of pregnancy (*ACADL* mutations) Carnitine palmitoyltransferase I and II deficiencies Carnitine acylcarnitine translocase deficiency
Urea cycle enzyme deficiencies	
Electron transfer flavoprotein deficiencies	Electron transfer flavoprotein and electron transfer flavoprotein dehydrogenase deficiencies
Gluconeogenesis	Phosphoenolpyruvate carboxykinase deficiency (mitochondrial)
Glycine cleavage enzyme deficiency	Non-ketotic hyperglycinemia
Citrin deficiency	Neonatal intrahepatic cholestasis caused by citrin deficiency (*SLC25A13* mutations)
Secondary disorders	
Reye syndrome	
Hepatic copper overload	Wilson disease Indian childhood cirrhosis Idiopathic infantile copper toxicosis Cholestasis
Hepatic iron overload	Hereditary hemochromatosis, juvenile hemochromatosis Neonatal iron storage disease Tyrosinemia, type I Zellweger syndrome
Drugs	Valproic acid, salicylic acid, nucleoside analogues (fialuridine, didanosine, zidovudine), amiodarone, tetracycline, chloramphenicol, quinilones, linezolid, barbiturates, acetaminophen
Toxins	Chemical toxins: iron, ethanol, cyanide, antimycin A, rotenone, others. Bacterial toxins: cerulide (*Bacillus cereus* emetic toxin), Ekiri
Conditions causing mitochondrial lipid peroxidation or microauthophagy	Cholestasis Hydrophobic bile acid toxicity (cholestasis, bile acid synthesis and canalicular transport defects) Non-alcoholic fatty liver disease and steatohepatitis: associated with obesity, insulin resistance, diabetes mellitus, drugs, parenteral nutrition, bacterial contamination of small bowel, jejuno-ileal bypass, or idiopathic α_1-Antitrypsin deficiency
Cirrhosis	

Source: adapted from Treem and Sokol, 1998 [21].

Table 35.6 Molecular classification of primary mitochondrial hepatopathies

Gene	Respiratory chain complex	Protein	Hepatic steatosis	Hepatic fibrosis	Other organs involved
Class 1A: mtDNA genes					
Deletion	Multiple (Pearson)		+	+	K, H, CNS, M
Class 1B: nuclear genes					
Causing mtDNA depletion syndrome					
DGUOK	I, III, IV	Deoxyguanosine kinase, mitochondrial nucleotide salvaging	+	+	K, CNS, M
MPV17	I, III, IV	Mitochondrial inner membrane protein	+	+	CNS, PNS
SUCLG1	I, III, IV	α-Subunit of succinate coenzyme A ligase (SUCL)	+		K, CNS, M
POLG1	I, III, IV	DNA polymerase gamma	+		CNS, M
C10orf2 TWINKLE	I, III, IV	Hexameric mtDNA helicase	+		CNS, M
Nuclear assembly factors: respiratory chain complexes					
SCO1	IV	Copper chaperone of complex IV (cytochrome *c* oxidase)	+	+	M
BCS1L	III (GRACILE)	Assembly protein of complex III (ubiquinol cytochrome *c* reductase)			CNS±, M±
Nuclear transfer factor genes					
TRMU	I, III, IV	tRNA-modifying enzyme	+	+	
EFG1	I, III, IV	Mitochondrial translation elongation factor	+		M
EFTu	I, III, IV	Isoform of α-subunit of elongation factor-1 complex	?		CNS
TSFM	I, IV	EFTs, the mitochondrial translation elongation factors			CNS, K, H

CNS, central nervous system; M, skeletal muscle; K, kidney; PNS, peripheral nervous system; H, heart, GRACILE: growth retardation, aminoaciduria, cholestasis, iron overload, lactic acidosis, early death.
Source: adapted with permission from Leonard and Schapira, 2 000 [23].

the primary cause of the liver disorder, and *secondary hepatopathies,* in which a secondary insult to mitochondria is caused by either a gene defect that affects non-mitochondrial proteins or by an acquired (e.g. exogenous or endogenous toxin) injury to mitochondria. Leonard and Schapira originally divided primary mitochondrial diseases into those caused by mutations affecting mtDNA genes (class 1A) and those caused by mutations in nuclear genes that encode mitochondrial respiratory chain proteins or cofactors (class 1B) [22,23]. This schema has been further expanded into a genotypic classification of mitochondrial hepatopathies (Table 35.6). There has been a virtual explosion in the genetics underlying mitochondrial cytopathies since the 1990s, with over 225 nuclear and 13 mtDNA genes now linked to a human

disorder [1]. Many of the nuclear gene mutations affecting OXPHOS result in primary neuromuscular disease. However, more recently, nuclear genes encoding subunits for respiratory chain complex III (*BCS1L*) and complex IV (*SCO1*) have been shown to lead to significant hepatic involvement in addition to muscle disease (Table 35.6). Mutations in nuclear genes coding for non-respiratory chain mitochondrial proteins may also cause mitochondrial cytopathies. For example, many patients with Leigh syndrome have now been shown to have mutations in the nuclear gene encoding SURF1, a mitochondrial protein involved in cytochrome *c* oxidase assembly. Specifically linked to liver disease are nuclear genes encoding mtDNA replication and assembly, and transfer and elongation factors that stabilize mtDNA. The hepatic disorders and their genes include mitochondrial neurogastrointestinal encephalomyopathy (thymidine phosphorylase, gene *ECGF1*); mtDNA depletion syndrome (MDS), which is linked to a number of defects (deoxyguanosine kinase (DGUOK), thymidine kinase 2 (TK2), DNA polymerase-γ (POLG), mitochondrial inner protein (MPV17), hexameric mtDNA helicase (twinkle), thymidine phosphorylase); and autosomal dominant progressive external ophthalmoplegia (adenine nucleotide translocator 1 (ANT1)). These phenotypically and genotypically heterogeneous disorders appear to share a common mechanism of disturbed mitochondrial nucleoside pools or mtDNA stability [20]. The identification of pathologic mutations in many additional nuclear genes regulating mitochondrial function are the focus of exhaustive research efforts in the field of mitochondrial medicine that will certainly lead to new genetic diseases among the over 1000 nuclear-encoded mitochondrial proteins [1].

Emphasis in this chapter will be placed on those mitochondrial diseases involving the electron transport proteins (respiratory chain) and mtDNA stability in the liver. These usually present as neonatal liver failure (either a single life-threatening event or recurrent episodes); as a gradually progressive liver disease that may suddenly deteriorate in early childhood, frequently associated with neuromuscular symptoms; or as a chronic fibrosing liver disease leading to portal hypertension and its complications. In the secondary disorders, hepatic mitochondria undergo injury or function is impaired secondary to another pathologic process. Among these disorders are diseases of uncertain etiology but clearly involving hepatic mitochondria (e.g. Reye syndrome); conditions caused by mitochondrial toxins, drugs or metals; and other conditions in which mitochondrial lipid peroxidation, microauthophagy, and/or abnormal electron transport have been observed and may be involved in the pathogenesis of liver dysfunction. The remainder of this chapter will focus on prototypic and important mitochondrial hepatopathies, particularly those involving electron transport and OXPHOS. The reader is referred to other chapters for detailed discussions about the deficiencies of other specific mitochondrial enzyme systems.

Primary mitochondrial hepatopathies

The liver and the gastrointestinal tract are among the major target organs in inherited defects of mitochondrial function. Disorders of electron transport and OXPHOS affecting the liver are most severe subgroup of the primary mitochondrial hepatopathies (Table 35.5). Reduced activity of respiratory chain complexes and OXPHOS has been associated with liver disease of varying severity and at different ages, however, neonatal and early childhood presentations predominate [2].

Neonatal liver failure

One of the more common presentations of respiratory chain defects in childhood is that dominated by severe liver failure in the first weeks to months of life. This presentation is characterized by unremitting lactic acidosis, jaundice, conjugated hyperbilirubinemia, serum alanine aminotransferase (ALT) values 2–12 times normal, coagulopathy, ketotic hypoglycemia, and hyperammonemia [24]. Symptoms include lethargy and hypotonia, vomiting and a poor suck from birth, seizures (sometimes subtle), and failure to thrive. In others, in an apparently normal infant, a viral infection or some other undefined inciting event triggers hepatic and, sometimes, neurologic deterioration. The key biochemical features in most of these infants are the markedly elevated plasma lactate concentration, an elevated molar ratio of plasma lactate to pyruvate (>25 and frequently >30 mol/mol), and elevation of β-hydroxybutyrate and the arterial ketone body ratio of β-hydroxybutyrate to acetoacetate (>2.0 mol/mol). The lactic acidosis may worsen during the provision of intravenous glucose, a paradoxical finding that should increase suspicion of a respiratory chain defect. However, normal plasma lactate may be present in some of these conditions (e.g. MPV17 disease) and thus does not exclude respiratory chain defects.

Antenatal manifestations are common in infants affected by respiratory chain disorders. Low birth weight was present in 22.7% of children and 7% had other associated anomalies, including polyhydramnios, hypertrophic cardiomyopathy, cardiac rhythm abnormalities, hydronephrosis, ventricular septal defects, and others in excess of normal newborns. These findings suggest that metabolism is perturbed long before the infant is born.

Liver histology shows predominantly microvesicular (sometimes combined with macrovesicular) steatosis, canalicular cholestasis with bile duct thrombi and bile ductular proliferation, and, in some cases, hepatocellular cholestasis. Inflammation is usually absent or minimal. Periportal and centrilobular fibrosis may be extensive, with loss of broad bands of hepatocytes causing a micronodular cirrhotic appearance. Glycogen depletion is a near constant feature; and iron deposition, usually in hepatocytes, is often observed leading to confusion with neonatal iron storage disease, particularly in DGOUK deficiency. Ultrastructural evidence of mitochondrial injury may be observed as swollen mitochondria, abnormal cristae, paracrystalline arrays, and a fluffy matrix, although normal mitochondrial morphology may be present. Mitochondria density may be increased in each hepatocyte, as commonly observed in muscle of patients with mitochondrial myopathies, presumably as a compensatory mechanism for impaired function of individual mitochondria.

These infants may progress rapidly from onset of symptoms to death from liver failure, aspiration or sepsis in the first months of life despite supportive treatment [24]. Unfortunately, most patients have severe neurologic involvement in infancy with a weak cry, poor suck, hypotonia, recurrent apnea, myoclonic epilepsy, or a combination of these conditions, which should preclude consideration for liver transplantation [19]. However, since the degree of expression of the underlying defect in different tissues is not uniform, a number of affected infants have undergone successful liver transplantation in the absence of detectable extrahepatic manifestations [2]. Others have developed progressive neuromuscular symptoms following liver transplant. We have successfully given a transplant to one such infant with cytochrome *c* oxidase deficiency who has shown no apparent neuromuscular, cardiac, or ocular involvement during 14 years of follow-up. The long-term outcome in these infants will not be known for some time since neuromuscular features in other mitochondrial disorders may not become apparent until adulthood [20]. Other more variable parts of the neonatal presentation include intrauterine growth retardation, hydrops fetalis, neonatal ascites, hypoalbuminemia, elevated α-fetoprotein, and renal tubular dysfunction [24]. The hepatic activity of either isolated or combinations of respiratory chain complex IV, complex I, complex III and occasionally of complex II, has been found to be very low in these infants The implication is that a deficiency of these enzyme complexes, or factors regulating the activity of these enzymes, was the underlying cause of the liver failure. Among these, cytochrome *c* oxidase (complex IV) deficiency is the most common.

Genetics

Although in most cases of cytochrome *c* oxidase deficiency, the disease expression includes developmental delay, progressive myopathy, or subacute necrotizing encephalomyelopathy (Leigh syndrome), which has been observed in patients with mutations in *SURF1* and *SCO2*, there are other patients with cytochrome *c* oxidase deficiency who present with predominantly hepatic failure in infancy. Neonatal liver failure with multivisceral involvement has also been linked to a de novo homoplasmic mutation in the mitochondrial gene for cytochrome *b*. In another affected family, hepatic failure, lactic acidosis, and neurodevelopmental delays were associated with mutations in the cytochrome *c* oxidase assembly gene *SCO*1. The gene product is believed to transfer copper from a chaperone to a subunit of cytochrome *c* oxidase. In other cases, the use of valproic acid to treat myoclonic seizures has seemingly precipitated hepatic failure, even if no prior liver involvement was evident.

Mutations or deletions in mtDNA have not been discovered in most patients with neonatal liver failure. Rather, many appear to have mutations in nuclear genes that code for subunits or assembly factors of single respiratory chain complexes or that cause MDS, the last explaining the decreased activities of complex I, III, and IV in the same patient (see below). Mutations in the nuclear gene *BCS1L* have been reported in infants with hepatic failure, lactic acidosis, renal tubulopathy, and variable degrees of encephalopathy who were found to have deficient activity of complex III of the respiratory chain in liver, fibroblasts, or muscle. Mutations in *BCS1L* have been associated with fatal complex III deficiency, hypotonia, hypoglycemia, lactic acidosis, renal tubular dysfunction, and liver failure in two siblings. Liver histology showed microvesicular steatosis, periportal fibrosis with cholangiolar proliferation, severe cholestasis, hemosiderosis, and pseudoacinar

transformation of hepatocytes. The severest form of mutated *BCS1L* gives rise to the GRACILE syndrome (growth restriction, aminoaciduria, cholestasis, iron overload, lactic acidosis, and early death) [24]. This nuclear gene encodes a chaperone responsible for incorporating the Rieske iron sulfur protein into complex III, and it may be responsible for a substantial portion of infants who present with neonatal liver failure and lactic acidosis.

A neonatal presentation of autosomal recessive DNA polymerase gamma (POLG1) disease has also been described (so-called myocerebrohepatopathy) characterized by lactic acidosis and encephalopathy with or without seizures. If infants survive long enough, typical features of Alpers–Huttenlocher disease may become evident (see below). Neonatal liver failure and early death has been reported in several infants with *TSFM* mutations. This gene encodes for a mitochondrial translation elongation factor S and can present with intrauterine growth retardation, severe lactic acidosis, hypotonia, renal tubulopathy, cholestasis, and liver failure in the first months of life. EFG1, EFTu, and MRPS16 are other translation/elongation factors where mutations are associated with severe neonatal liver presentations. It is likely that additional novel nuclear genes encoding subunits or assembly of respiratory chain complexes and mtDNA translational machinery will be discovered in coming years that will be responsible for other patients with this presentation of neonatal liver failure. In addition, many infants with MDS present with neonatal liver failure.

Mitochondrial DNA depletion syndrome

Mitochondrial DNA depletion syndrome, the underlying cause of many cases of fatal liver failure in infancy, is characterized by a tissue-specific reduction in mtDNA copy number [25]. There are two clinical phenotypes of MDS: a myopathic and a hepatocerebral form. Initial reports stressed the myopathic presentation in infancy or later in childhood. However, phenotypic heterogeneity has been reported, with both myopathic and hepatocerebral presentations of MDS occurring within the same family. For example, mtDNA depletion has been reported to affect the liver alone in one infant with an 88% depletion of mtDNA, and the muscle alone in a second cousin whose liver mtDNA was normal.

Infants with the hepatocerebral form of MDS present generally within the first few weeks or months of life with progressive liver failure; neurological abnormalities, including hypotonia and seizures; hypoglycemia; and unremitting lactic acidosis. It should be noted that, since the underlying molecular basis of MDS has been determined in recent years, several genotypes causing MDS may not be invariably fatal as previously thought. Symptoms include vomiting and severe gastroesophageal reflux, failure to thrive, and developmental delay [19]. Lactic acidemia and hypoglycemia are accompanied by modestly elevated serum aspartate aminotransferase (AST) and ALT, and eventually total and conjugated bilirubin.

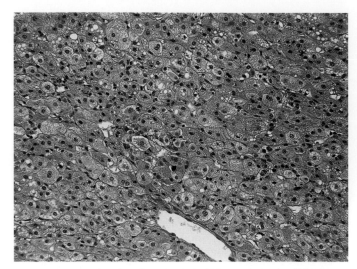

Figure 35.2 Liver histology from 11-week-old boy with mtDNA depletion caused by *POLG* mutations. Biopsy at presentation with diarrhea, weakness, failure to thrive, and elevated aspartate aminotransferase, alanine aminotransferase, international normalized ratio, and plasma lactate. Biopsy shows mild hepatocyte swelling with scattered microvesicular steatosis and cholestasis. Portal tracts are normal and there is no fibrosis. (Hematoxylin & eosin stain, magnification ×200.)

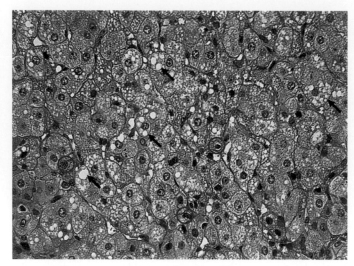

Figure 35.3 Higher power views of liver histology from the patient with mtDNA depletion syndrome in Figure 35.2, showing microvesicular steatosis (arrows) and canalicular cholestasis (circles). (Periodic acid–Schiff–diastase stain, magnification ×800.)

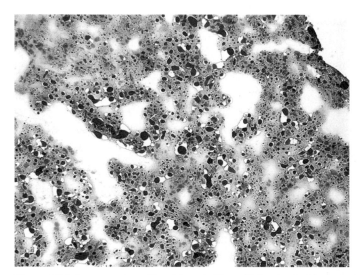

Figure 35.4 Frozen section of liver biopsy in Figure 35.2, stained with Oil-red-O and showing marked microvesicular steatosis in most hepatocytes, despite benign appearance of the biopsy. (Magnification ×100.)

However, evidence of impaired hepatic synthetic function (prolonged prothrombin time/international normalized ratio, low serum albumin, and elevated blood ammonia) may be present even early in the course. In most reported patients, neurologic abnormalities developed prior to death, although the initial hypotonia may have been attributed to the lactic acidosis [25]. In patients without neurologic symptoms, particularly those caused by *DGUOK* mutations, clinical course may be more protracted. Death usually occurs from liver failure, sepsis, bleeding, or aspiration by 1 year of age. Histological findings in MDS liver biopsies include microvesicular steatosis, both cytoplasmic and canalicular cholestasis, an absence of inflammation, and iron deposition in hepatocytes and sinusoidal cells (Figures 35.2–35.4). The lesion may appear quite bland for the degree of hepatic synthetic failure. Eventually loss of hepatocyte mass, cholangiolar proliferation (bile ductular reaction), and portal fibrosis develop. Ultrastructural findings include lipid vacuoles and mitochondria having aspects of "oncocytic transformation," with pleomorphic shape, marked variation in size, dilatation and other abnormalities of the cristae, and changes in matrix density (Figure 35.5). Not uncommonly there is an increased mitochondrial density in hepatocytes. Although the individual histological and ultrastructural findings are non-specific, when taken together in the appropriate clinical context, they are highly suggestive of a respiratory chain disorder [2]. Diagnosis is established by the demonstration of a low ratio of amount of mtDNA to nuclear DNA in affected tissues, generally <10% of normal, with a normal mtDNA sequence [17]. In most patients, there are decreased activities of the electron transport chain complexes for which subunits are coded by mtDNA (I, III, IV, V); however this may only be present in the liver or other affected tissues and not in fibroblasts or circulating mononuclear cells. The severity of mtDNA depletion correlates with the severity of tissue involvement and biochemical defects.

Genetics

Heteroplasmy of mtDNA with differential tissue involvement has suggested that MDS is a mitochondrial disease. However, no convincing cases of mtDNA mutations or maternal transmission have been reported. The consanguineous origin of cases further suggested an autosomal recessive form of inheritance, indicating that a primary nuclear gene defect was most likely the cause of the mtDNA depletion. This hypothesis was supported by experiments in which enucleated fibroblasts

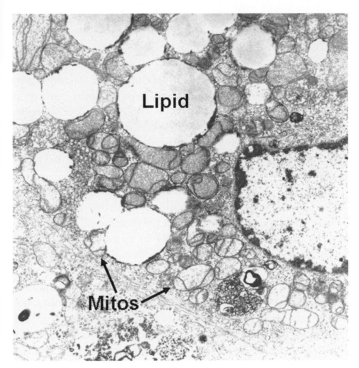

Figure 35.5 Electron microscopy (original magnification ×13 700) of liver in the patient from Figure 35.2 with mtDNA depletion syndrome. Small droplets of neutral lipid are present in hepatocyte. Virtually all mitochondria are abnormal with enlargement and pleomorphic size and shape, unusual cristae, and flocculent matrix.

from a patient with fatal neonatal hepatic failure and mtDNA depletion were fused with a human-derived Rho cell line lacking mtDNA; and the hybrid cells grown in medium lacking pyruvate and uridine to select for the restoration of respiratory chain function. Growth of these cells and the demonstration by Southern blot of normal amounts of mtDNA and normal activity of respiratory chain enzymes in the F1 hybrids confirmed that mtDNA depletion resulted from a defect in a nuclear gene and this led to further investigations of nuclear encoded factors that were responsible for mtDNA maintenance.

The mtDNA processing enzyme activities are dependent on several factors, including deoxyribonucleotide (dNTP) concentrations within the mitochondria, availability of ATP, nuclear translation and elongation factors, and several metal cofactors. Imbalance of any of these cofactors or enzymes could affect mtDNA stability. The mitochondrial pool is maintained by either import of cytosolic dNTPs through dedicated transporters or by salvaging deoxynucleosides within the mitochondria. The mitochondrial deoxynucleoside salvage pathway is regulated by nuclear-encoded enzymes, including DGUOK and TK2. Human DGUOK phosphorylates deoxyguanosine and deoxyadenosine, whereas TK2 phosphorylates deoxythymidine, deoxycytidine, and deoxyuridine. Imbalance of this mitochondrial dNTP pool has been proposed to be responsible for both the hepatocerebral and myopathic forms of MDS.

In 2001, mutations in two genes involved in this pathway were identified in patients with MDS: *DGUOK* in the hepatocerebral form and *TK2* in the myopathic form. The frequency of *DGUOK* mutations in 21 patients with hepatocerebral MDS was 14% in a recent study [26], suggesting that *DGUOK* is not the only gene responsible for mitochondrial depletion in the liver. No genotype–phenotype correlation was demonstrated. Unique characteristics of patients with DGUOK disease include the clinical findings of nystagmus; elevation of ferritin, α-fetoprotein, and transferring saturation mimicking that of neonatal hemochromatosis (gestational alloimmune liver disease); spontaneous survival if there are limited neurologic symptoms; a risk of hepatocellular carcinoma in survivors; reasonably good outcome from liver transplant if no neurologic involvement [25].

More recently, two other nuclear genes have been linked to the hepatocerebral form of MDS. POLG1 is confined to mitochondria but is encoded by a nuclear gene [27]. Mutations have now been described in infants with MDS as well older children with Alpers disease. Most of the presentations of severe disease in infancy or with mtDNA depletion in early childhood are associated with at least one mutation in the linker region of the gene, and one in the polymerase domain. Mutations in *MPV17* have also been found in families affected by the hepatocerebral form of MDS [28], neonatal liver failure, and Navajo neurohepatopathy. This gene encodes an inner mitochondrial membrane protein of still uncertain function, although it may be involved in the metabolism of reactive oxygen species. With the availability of clinical genotyping in commercial laboratories (see http://www.genetests.org), genetic diagnosis of MDS is now feasible. Mitochondrial-toxic anticonvulsants may trigger or worsen a mitochondrial disorder and can precipitate to hepatic failure. Valproic acid has been known to exhibit a deleterious effect in patients with *POLG1* mutations and in patients with myoclonic epilepsy with ragged red fibers (MERF) syndrome [29].

Other genes recently linked to MDS include *SUCLG1*, which encodes the α-subunit of succinate coenzyme A ligase, an enzyme catalyzing the conversion of succinyl CoA and ADP or GDP to succinate and ATP or GTP. SUCLG1 disease involves not only the liver but also the kidney, CNS, and muscle. Twinkle is a hexameric DNA helicase that plays a key role in mtDNA replication and is encoded by *C10orf2*e. Pathologic mutations in this gene have been associated with mtDNA depletion in neonates, with lactic acidosis, hypoglycemia, and severe truncal hypotonia. Hepatic involvement included hepatomegaly, hepatic steatosis, cholestasis, and elevated AST/ALT.

Later-onset progressive liver failure in early childhood (Alpers–Huttenlocher syndrome)

Deficiencies of respiratory chain complex I, complex IV, or combinations of respiratory chain enzymes have been associated with a later onset of recognizable liver disease in infancy and early childhood [2]. The onset of symptoms generally occurs between 3 months and 8 years of life with a second peak between 17 and 24 years of life and is characterized by hepatomegaly and jaundice, with hepatic failure evolving over time. In most of these children, liver failure is preceded by the development of hypotonia, feeding difficulties, symptoms of gastroesophageal reflux or intractable vomiting, failure to thrive, and ataxia followed by the onset of relatively refractory partial motor epilepsy or multifocal myoclonus. The seizure disorder may necessitate the use of multiple anticonvulsants, including valproic acid, which may trigger liver failure in these patients within months through its effects on mitochondrial respiratory chain enzyme activity. On some occasions, monitoring of liver blood tests initiated solely because of the use of anticonvulsants yields the first recognition that there is an abnormality in liver function. In addition to mild to moderate elevation of aminotransferases, evidence of hepatic synthetic failure may be present (low serum albumin, prolonged prothrombin time, depressed clotting factor V or VII). Progressive neurologic deterioration may ensue rapidly. In other children, the neurologic features are less severe or with somewhat later onset. This clinical presentation has also been called the Alpers–Huttenlocher syndrome (Alpers progressive infantile poliodystrophy). Neurological evaluation may reveal elevated blood or cerebrospinal fluid lactate and pyruvate levels, characteristic electroencephalography findings (high-amplitude slow activity with polyspikes, asymmetric abnormal visual evoked responses), and low-density areas or atrophy in the occipital or temporal lobes on CT of the brain [30]. A family history of an affected sibling has been reported in up to 50% of cases. In some patients, NADH oxidoreductase (complex I) deficiency has been found in liver or muscle mitochondria. The generally accepted clinical diagnostic criteria for this syndrome are (1) refractory, mixed type seizures that often include a focal component; (2) psychomotor regression that is often episodic and triggered by intercurrent infections; and (3) hepatopathy with or without acute liver failure [19].

Striking microscopic changes in the brain include spongiosis, neuronal loss, and astrocytosis, which progress down through the cortical layers and involve the basal ganglia, cerebellum, and brainstem [31]. Early in the course of the liver disease, liver pathology may only be notable for microvesicular steatosis, focal hepatocyte degeneration, and portal fibrosis (Figure 35.6). However, hepatic decompensation may ensue rapidly and lead to death in 1–2 months. At autopsy, the liver shows macrovesicular steatosis with accompanying micronodular cirrhosis, massive hepatocyte dropout (probably caused by apoptosis), parenchymal collapse, and bile ductular proliferation within broad bands of fibrous tissue (Figure 35.6b,c). On electron microscopy, there may be an increased number and density of normal-appearing mitochondria in each hepatocyte or mitochondria may be swollen and pleomorphic with a less dense matrix and few cristae (Figure 35.7). Most children die by 3 years of age but some survive into their teenage years. In those who show marked deterioration following the start of therapy for seizures, death has been attributed to hepatotoxicity caused by the valproate; however, treatment with this drug may have only accelerated the natural history of the disease. Gene testing for *POLG* should be considered in any young child who presents with or develops intractable seizures, particularly when there is a history of psychomotor regression [33] and if valproic acid therapy is considered. Occasionally, this disorder is not recognized prior to liver transplantation in a child with acute liver failure; progressive neurologic deterioration commonly follows transplantation despite normal function of the liver allograft.

In recent years it has become apparent that most children with Alpers–Huttenlocher syndrome have two mutations in *POLG*, which encodes the mtDNA polymerase [27]. This association was first described in 2004 in three children, one of whom developed acute liver failure within 3 weeks of initiation of valproic acid for refractory seizures. All three children were homozygous for a E873Stop mutation, which was believed to be causative, and were also heterozygous for the A467T mutation, whose role was not known. Subsequently a number of groups confirmed this association. Mutations of *POLG* were found in 8 of 10 patients referred with Alpers–Huttenlocher syndrome [34], and in 13 of 15 sequential patients (87%) with Alpers–Huttenlocher syndrome [35], suggesting that *POLG* mutations are responsible for the majority of cases. It should be pointed out that *POLG* mutations were first identified in families with autosomal dominant chronic progressive external ophthalmoplegia (PEO), which is associated with accumulation of multiple mtDNA deletions in affected tissues [31], and then were discovered in autosomal recessive progressive external ophthalmoplegia. There is a wide spectrum of disease caused by mutations in this gene, with most affected children under age 7 years demonstrating significant hepatic involvement [36]. In one series, all patients had either A467T or W748S mutations, so that screening for these two mutations was thought to be an effective and sensitive means for confirming the diagnosis of Alpers–Huttenlocher syndrome. However, there are currently over 180 disease-producing mutations of *POLG* that vary in age of onset, mode of inheritance, and clinical features.

Pancreatic insufficiency, bone marrow abnormalities and liver involvement (Pearson syndrome)

Pearson marrow–pancreas syndrome was described in 1979 in four children with neonatal-onset severe macrocytic anemia, variable neutropenia and thrombocytopenia, vacuolization of erythroid and myeloid precursors, and ringed-sideroblasts in the bone marrow [37]. Later in infancy or early childhood, diarrhea and fat malabsorption developed and the patients were found to have pancreatic insufficiency caused by extensive pancreatic fibrosis and acinar atrophy. Partial villous atrophy of the small intestine was noted in a number of patients. Marked hepatomegaly, hepatic steatosis, and cirrhosis has been associated with liver failure and death in some patients before the age of 4 years.

(a)

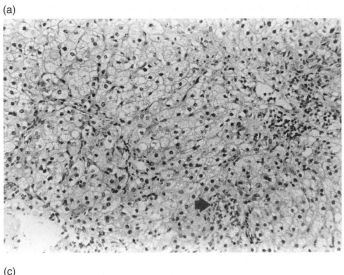

(b)

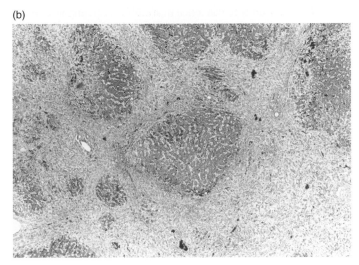

(c)

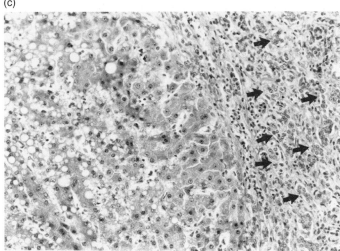

Figure 35.6 Liver histology obtained from girl aged 5 years and 7 months with Alpers–Huttenlocher disease. (a) Biopsy at the time of presentation with liver involvement, showing periportal inflammation (solid arrow), microvesicular steatosis, and mild portal fibrosis. (b) Autopsy liver specimen obtained 2 months later demonstrating micronodular cirrhosis and extensive fibrosis, with prominent regenerative nodules and bile ductular proliferation. (c) Higher power view of edge of a regenerative nodule, demonstrating massive collapse of parenchyma with extensive portal fibrosis and bile ductular proliferation (solid arrows) and microvesicular steatosis in hepatocytes of regenerative nodules. (With permission from Narkewicz *et al.*, 1991 [32].)

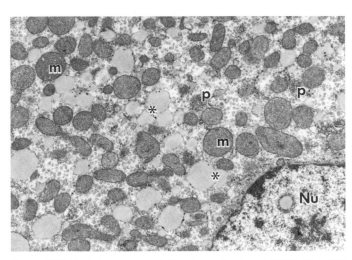

Figure 35.7 Electron microscopy (original magnification ×13 700) of the child in Figure 35.6 with liver in Alpers–Huttenlocher disease. Hepatocyte obtained at onset of liver disease showing microvesicular steatosis (asterisks), normal peroxisomes (p), and morphologically normal mitochondria (m) but increased in number. Nu, nucleus. (With permission from Narkewicz *et al.*, 1991 [32].)

It is now established that mtDNA rearrangements are present in all patients with Pearson syndrome with large (4000–5000 bp) deletions predominating in three-quarters of reported cases [38]. Of the respiratory chain enzymes encoded by mtDNA, complex I is the most severely affected by this deletion; however, it also encompasses genes that encode two subunits of complex V, one subunit of complex IV, and five tRNA genes [24]. While oxidation of NADH is abnormal in lymphocytes from these patients, oxygen consumption and respiratory chain enzyme activities are normal in muscle mitochondria. Southern blotting has shown that a mixed population of normal and deleted mitochondrial genomes is present in all tissues tested (heteroplasmy), but different proportions of deleted mtDNA molecules are noted. In the clinically more severely affected tissues, such as bone marrow, polymorphonuclear leukocytes, lymphocytes, pancreas, and gut, mtDNA deletions are found in 80–90% of cells; but in only 50% of muscle cells. It appears that the phenotypic expression of Pearson syndrome in a given tissue requires a minimum threshold number of mutated mtDNA molecules. The lack of maternal inheritance or positive family histories, and the absence of mtDNA rearrangements in the lymphocytes of parents or siblings of cases, suggests that many are caused by de novo mutations occurring during oogenesis or the early development of fertilized eggs.

Other clinical manifestations of Pearson syndrome include renal tubular disease (Fanconi syndrome), patchy erythematous skin lesions and photosensitivity, diabetes mellitus, adrenal insufficiency, hydrops fetalis, and the late development of visual impairment, tremor, ataxia, proximal muscle weakness, external ophthalmoplegia, and a pigmentary retinopathy. These symptoms are similar to those found in Kearns–Sayre syndrome, a mitochondrial disease also characterized by a large 5 kb mtDNA deletion. The occurrence of Kearns–Sayre syndrome in patients with Pearson syndrome who survive to childhood is another example of the dependence of phenotypic expression on random partitioning of mutated mtDNA during cell division, changes in the proportion of rearranged mtDNA in various tissues over time, and the possible accumulation of other somatic mutations [17]. Supporting this hypothesis is the clinical observation that patients with Pearson syndrome frequently do not require blood transfusions after the age of 2 years. This may be because the number of hematopoietic cells containing a high proportion of deleted mtDNA decreases with time as a result of selection of cells with normal mtDNA. When suspected, Pearson syndrome can generally be diagnosed by analyzing for the characteristic mtDNA deletion [17]. Stem cell transplant corrected hematologic and metabolic abnormalities in one patient who then died of a secondary malignancy.

Chronic diarrhea and intestinal pseudo-obstruction with liver involvement

Severe anorexia, vomiting, chronic diarrhea, and villus atrophy may be the initial manifestations of a rare mtDNA rearrangement syndrome appearing late in the first year or during the second year of life and associated with mild elevations of liver enzymes, hepatomegaly, and steatosis [39]. Diarrhea, vomiting, and lactic acidosis worsens in these patients with high-dextrose intravenous infusions or enteral nutrition. Diarrhea improves and even resolves completely by 5 years of age, in association with normalization of intestinal biopsies. However, retinitis pigmentosa, cerebellar ataxia, sensorineural deafness, and proximal muscle weakness may become evident late in the first decade of life, leading to death soon thereafter. Respiratory chain enzyme assays are normal in circulating lymphocytes but were abnormal in skeletal muscle tissue, revealing a complex III deficiency.

Mitochondrial neurogastrointestinal encephalomyopathy

Mitochondrial neurogastrointestinal encephalomyopathy (MNGIE) is a multisystem syndrome, first described in 1983, that involves skeletal muscle, peripheral and central nervous systems, the intestinal tract, and the liver [40–42].

In 1994, the syndrome was called mitochondrial neurogastrointestinal encephalomyopathy [43]. It is characterized by myopathy with ragged red fibers, peripheral sensorimotor neuropathy, progressive external ophthalmoplegia, ptosis, leukoencephalopathy, and chronic intestinal pseudo-obstruction. The disease onset ranges from 5 months to 43 years of age [44]. Non-specific gastrointestinal signs and symptoms of nausea, vomiting, abdominal pain, borborygmi, diarrhea, constipation, and abdominal distension often lead to a diagnosis of intestinal dysmotility or "pseudo-obstruction." Gastrointestinal symptoms typically have onset in childhood and were the presenting complaint in 45–67% of patients [45]. Sensory neuropathy, hearing loss, or ocular symptoms were the initial manifestations in 42–49% of patients. Thin body habitus and short stature are constant findings, presumably secondary to chronic malnutrition and malabsorption. Small-bowel diverticulosis, presumably secondary to markedly delayed intestinal motility, appears in early adult years in 30–67% of patients. The chronic intestinal pseudo-obstruction has been attributed to a visceral smooth muscle myopathy, with atrophic fibrotic longitudinal smooth muscle in the intestinal wall but normal ganglion cells in some reported patients. In other patients, autopsy has suggested an autonomic neuropathy with fibrosis and vacuolization of autonomic ganglia in the myenteric plexus and decreased nerve fibers innervating intestinal smooth muscle.

MNGIE is an autosomal recessive disease associated with multiple mtDNA deletions and/or depletion in skeletal muscle. In the limited number of patients studied, skeletal muscle respiratory chain defects consisting of complex IV, complex I, or combination defects have been identified. Following the mapping of MNGIE to chromosome 22q13.32-qter in four kindreds, loss-of-function mutations in *TYMP*, encoding thymidine phosphorylase have been identified. Fifty-four different *TYMP* mutations in ethnically diverse MNGIE pedigrees have been found [42]. Thymidine phosphorylase is a multifunctional enzyme that has an important role in the nucleoside salvage pathway, catalyzing the breakdown of thymidine to be reutilized for mtDNA synthesis as deoxythymidine triphosphate (dTTP). Thymidine phosphorylase also produces 2-deoxyribose, which is an endothelial cell chemoattractant in angiogenesis induction. None of the patients with MNGIE have had vascular abnormalities, suggesting that the absence of thymidine phosphorylase activity does not interfere with normal angiogenesis. Impaired thymidine metabolism has been demonstrated by biochemical analysis in patients with MNGIE, with markedly elevated plasma levels of thymidine ($8.6 \pm 3.4\,\mu mol/L$, normal $<0.05\,\mu mol/L$) and deoxyuridine ($14.2 \pm 4.4\,\mu mol/L$, normal $<0.05\,\mu mol/L$) and depletion of the mitochondrial dTTP pool used for DNA synthesis. Recent studies have demonstrated both mtDNA depletion and deletions in smooth muscle from the small intestine of affected patients [46]. The pathogenesis of these findings in MNGIE, like MDS, appears to be related to an imbalance of the mitochondrial nucleoside pool. Allogeneic hematopoietic stem cell transplantation has been recently shown to correct biochemical features of MNGIE; its effect on clinical symptoms and course are under study but experience in individual patients appears to be encouraging [42].

Navajo neurohepatopathy

Navajo neurohepatopathy is a sensorimotor neuropathy with progressive liver disease that is confined to Navajo children [47]. This disorder is manifested by the development of weakness, hypotonia, areflexia, loss of sensation in the extremities, acral mutilation, corneal ulceration, poor growth, short stature, and serious systemic infections. An association of Reye-like syndrome episodes, hepatic dysfunction, and death from liver failure at a young age was seen in three patients. Cerebral MRI further demonstrated the presence of progressive white matter lesions, and peripheral nerve biopsies showed severe loss of myelinated fibers. Multiple investigations of infectious, biochemical, and metabolic causes failed to yield an etiology for this multisystem disorder, yet the inheritance appeared to be autosomal recessive. The hepatic findings were thoroughly characterized in 20 patients [47]: there were three clinical presentations, including an infantile presentation, in which failure to thrive and jaundice progress to hepatic failure and death within the first 2 years of life, with or without neurologic findings; a childhood form, presenting between 1 and 5 years of age with rapid development of liver failure; and the classical form in which progressive neurological findings dominate although liver dysfunction (and even cirrhosis) was present in all patients. Elevation of AST, ALT, alkaline phosphatase, and gamma-glutamyltransferase were present in all patients. Liver histology demonstrated portal fibrosis or micronodular cirrhosis, macro- and microvesicular steatosis, pseudoacinar formation, multinucleated giant cells, cholestasis, and periportal inflammation [2]. Non-specific mitochondrial changes, such as swollen mitochondria and ringed cristae, were seen in several patients. Blood lactate and pyruvate levels were normal in patients tested, and skin fibroblasts had normal respiration from one patient. The liver involvement in this disorder is progressive with liver failure developing within months to years in most patients. Neurologic symptoms have progressed after liver transplant, questioning the value of transplant in this disorder. There has been no effective treatment to date for affected children.

It is now established that Navajo neurohepatopathy is a MDS caused by mutations in *MPV17* [48]. A homozygous R50Q mutation in all affected patients with Navajo neurohepatopathy extends the phenotypic spectrum associated with *MPV17* mutations and establishes a clear founder effect in this disease. This discovery will now allow for the possibility of both prenatal and postnatal genetic diagnosis of Navajo neurohepatopathy, even in presymptomatic patients, with the hope that an effective treatment can now be developed.

Fatty acid oxidation defects and electron transport deficiency

Other inborn errors of metabolism can alter the transfer of electrons and generation of ATP by the respiratory chain by generating toxic metabolites that specifically inhibit one or more of the enzyme complexes or non-specifically perturb the mitochondrial membrane and other electron transport pathways.

Long-chain 3-hydroxyacyl CoA dehydrogenase (LCHAD) deficiency is an autosomal recessively inherited defect in the third enzyme in the intramitochondrial beta-oxidation pathway of FAO, which shares several features with respiratory chain disorders [49]. For example, profound lactic acidemia occurs during episodes of metabolic crisis, in contrast to other FAO disorders. Deficiency of LCHAD has been associated with neonatal liver failure, progressive hepatic fibrosis, and cirrhosis, unlike other FAO defects that usually result in micro- and macrovesicular steatosis without permanent liver damage. It also involves the nervous system, including the inevitable development of retinitis pigmentosa in all patients who survive the neonatal and early childhood period and the appearance of a progressive peripheral neuropathy in some long-term survivors. Several groups have demonstrated that the long-chain fatty acid esters palmityl-CoA and 3-hydroxy-palmityl-CoA, intermediates that would be expected to accumulate within mitochondria in patients with LCHAD deficiency, inhibit respiratory chain driven ATP synthesis in cultured skin fibroblasts from normal humans. This inhibition of ATP synthesis appears to be localized to both the transport of succinate into mitochondria and of electrogenic ADP/ATP carrier on the inner mitochondrial membrane. A patient has been described with complex I deficiency who had clinical and biochemical features of LCHAD deficiency, which included cardiomyopathy, liver failure and the characteristic organic acid pattern in urine [50]. He was treated effectively with carnitine, a low-fat diet with medium-chain triglyceride oil and essential fatty acid supplements, succinate, and ascorbate. This underscores the need to consider respiratory chain disorders in patients who have abnormal urine organic acid patterns that suggest FAO disorders, and that there is an overlap in clinical phenotype in these two types of mitochondrial hepatopathies.

Accumulating CoA esters of long-chain fatty acids found in the livers of patients with Reye syndrome have been shown to uncouple OXPHOS and reduce intramitochondrial ATP formation. These same metabolites have been linked to liver damage in other diseases characterized histologically by intrahepatic microvesicular steatosis including acute fatty liver of pregnancy [51]. Reports of acute fatty liver of pregnancy in LCHAD-deficient heterozygote mothers who are carrying an affected fetus suggest that toxic long-chain fatty acid metabolites from the fetus may enter the maternal circulation and play a role in maternal liver injury during the latter stages of pregnancy in heterozygote women. The expression of this fetomaternal disorder requires the presence of an increased load of toxic metabolites from the fetus and a maternal liver with a limited capacity to degrade these compounds.

Other primary mitochondrial hepatopathies

These disorders include nuclear gene-encoded defects in other specific enzymes or structural proteins affecting mitochondria, including FAO defects, urea cycle enzyme deficiencies, phosphoenolpyruvate carboxykinase deficiency, carnitine acyl-carnitine translocase deficiency (*SLC25A20*), carnitine palmityltransferase I and II deficiency, and others (Table 35.5). The specific clinical manifestations of each disorder depend on the pathophysiological consequences of the individual biochemical pathway that is disrupted and the type of toxic metabolites or precursors that accumulate. The reader is referred to other chapters of this textbook for descriptions of these conditions.

Secondary mitochondrial hepatopathies

Secondary mitochondrial hepatopathies are caused by an injurious metal, drug, toxin, xenobiotic, or endogenous metabolite (Table 35.5). Acquired abnormalities of mitochondrial respiration caused by these factors may be involved in the pathogenesis of these disorders. Several prototypic disorders will be discussed.

Reye syndrome

Reye syndrome is the classic secondary mitochondrial hepatopathy and is caused by the interaction of a viral infection (influenza, varicella, enteroviruses, other viruses) and salicylate, perhaps in combination with an underlying undefined metabolic/genetic predisposition. In past years passed, many cases that were initially labeled as Reye syndrome were undoubtedly undiagnosed genetic metabolic diseases, such as FAO defects, urea cycle disorders, and respiratory chain defects. However, there are several characteristics that lead us to conclude that there still are patients who present with this clinical entity [52]. Liver and brain electron microscopy in patients with Reye syndrome reveals striking abnormalities in mitochondrial structure (Figure 35.8) and mitochondrial function is perturbed, resulting in defective ureagenesis and ketogenesis, hyperammonemia, hypoglycemia, elevated serum free fatty acids, lactate, and dicarboxylic acids. Impairment of beta-oxidation of fatty acids by mitochondria is also present. Salicylates have been shown to impair mitochondrial FAO in vitro, possibly by reversible inhibition of LCHAD activity. Cells from patients with Reye syndrome were found to be more susceptible to inhibition by low concentrations of salicylates than controls.

Most cases of Reye syndrome traditionally occurred in the autumn and winter (influenza season) with the peak age between 5 and 15 years [52]. Symptoms developed several

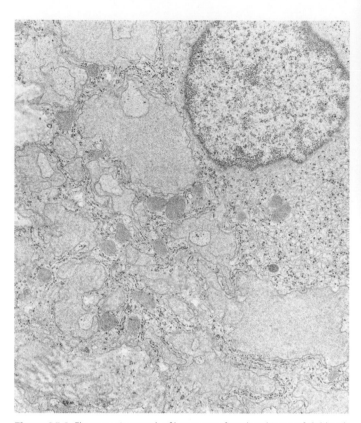

Figure 35.8 Electron micrograph of hepatocyte from liver biopsy of child with Reye syndrome. Peroxisomes are increased in number and size. There is marked reduction of cytoplasmic glycogen. Mitochondrial abnormalities include marked pleomorphism and swelling, with absent dense bodies and a flocculent matrix. (Osmium tetroxide fixation in Millonig phosphate buffer, magnification ×21 000).

days following onset of influenza A or B infections, or varicella. There was a strong association of aspirin use during these illnesses and the development of Reye syndrome. Frequently, the child appeared to be recovering from a viral illness after 3 to 5 days when sudden, unremitting vomiting developed. After several hours of vomiting, and not uncommonly dehydration, variable degrees of encephalopathy developed. Early mild stages of encephalopathy (grades 0–2) were associated with quietness, lethargy, and sleepiness and progressed in many affected patients to stages 3 and 4 with delirium, decorticate and decerebrate posturing, and eventually brainstem herniation caused by cerebral edema and raised intracranial pressure. Liver dysfunction was always present when vomiting developed and was characterized by elevated AST, ALT, and blood ammonia, with mild to moderate prolongation of prothrombin time, variable hypoglycemia, but normal serum bilirubin values. Metabolic support with hypertonic dextrose infusions and control of cerebral edema and intracranial pressure became the most important facets of clinical treatment, until spontaneous recovery occurred or irreversible brain injury developed. Mortality was high when patients presented in deeper stages of coma and correlated with high levels of blood ammonia at presentation.

Abnormal mitochondrial morphology and function characterize this disorder, with involvement of liver, brain, muscle, and kidney. Although patients present with hepatic dysfunction, hyperammonemia, and coma, the encephalopathy may be caused by direct involvement of CNS mitochondria as well as the accumulating metabolic toxins. Liver biopsies are characterized by microvesicular steatosis in the absence of hepatic inflammation or necrosis and characteristic swelling and pleomorphism of mitochondria under electron microscopy [52] (Figure 35.8). The liver makes a full recovery in this disease, despite progressive and sometimes fatal cerebral edema. The mortality of Reye syndrome remains high primarily because most patients nowadays are diagnosed in deeper stages of coma. A detailed discussion of the pathophysiology and treatment of Reye syndrome is found in the first edition of this textbook [52]. In more recent years, many young patients once thought to have Reye syndrome have been found subsequently to have defects in FAO, a form of primary mitochondrial hepatopathy. Since the incidence of Reye syndrome has decreased dramatically in western countries following the public warnings of salicylate use in children with viral infections, it is imperative to thoroughly evaluate all children who are diagnosed with Reye syndrome for FAO defects, particularly those under 5 years of age. Although salicylate use has not been associated with Reye syndrome in some countries, its reduced use in the USA and UK has clearly diminished the frequency of cases of Reye syndrome. Others believe that the increasing ability to diagnose FAO defects and other metabolic diseases over the past two decades also account for the decreased incidence of Reye syndrome.

Wilson disease

Mitochondrial involvement in the pathogenesis of liver injury in Wilson disease has been implicated for many years, since the early observation by Sternlieb of abnormal mitochondrial morphology on electron microscopy of liver biopsies that is so characteristic of this disorder of copper metabolism [53]. Changes in mitochondrial shape, density, and size are common early in the course of Wilson disease, including decreased matriceal density, enlarged intermembranous spaces, dilatation and vacuolization of cristae, crystalline inclusions, and vacuoles in the matrix [53,54]. Recent studies in experimental animals and naturally occurring copper toxicity in dogs and in humans have shown that the mitochondrion is a major intracellular target for copper toxicity. The accumulation of copper in the hepatic mitochondria leads to oxidant stress (increased free radical generation) with subsequent lipid peroxidation and oxidative alterations of thiol-containing proteins. In a rat model of copper overload, a 60% decrease of cytochrome c oxidase activity was demonstrated in hepatic mitochondria in conjunction with significant lipid peroxidation. Similar increased lipid peroxidation has been demonstrated in hepatic mitochondria isolated from copper-overloaded dogs and from patients with Wilson disease

undergoing liver transplantation. Recent studies in an *Atp7b* mouse knockout model of Wilson disease similarly demonstrate abnormal respiratory chain activity and mitochondrial dysfunction. This oxidant damage in hepatic mitochondria also leads to mtDNA deletions in young adults with Wilson disease [55]. These data suggest that perturbed hepatic mitochondrial electron transport may be an important factor in the pathogenesis of liver dysfunction and liver failure in copper overload states. The underlying defect in Wilson disease is caused by mutations in the *ATP7B*, encoding the P-type ATPase, which is present in the *trans*-Golgi and might be transported to hepatic mitochondria. The function of the P-type ATPase in mitochondria and how this may relate to the pathogenesis of Wilson disease has not been determined. In addition to copper chelation therapy, treatment to reduce the oxidative stress (e.g. with antioxidants) in the liver of patients with Wilson disease may help to protect the mitochondria from injury in this disease and in other metal overload conditions.

Drugs and toxins

Acquired abnormalities of mitochondrial respiration may be caused by a number of drugs and toxins (Table 35.5). Some drugs can fragment mtDNA, inhibit its replication, decrease mitochondrial transcripts, and impair mitochondrial protein synthesis [56]. Ion homeostasis or the mitochondrial permeability transition pore can also be disrupted. Severe impairment of OXPHOS decreases hepatic ATP, causing cell dysfunction or necrosis. Beta-oxidation can be secondarily inhibited leading to steatosis [57]. Mitochondria have a central role in programmed death through the release of cytochrome c and other proapoptotic factors, in the loss of transmembrane potential, the disruption/modulation of cellular calcium ions, and the production of reactive oxygen species. The release of mediators, including caspases, calpains, lysosomal proteases, and endonucleases, is the main executioner of cell death, and these mediators often cooperate during the execution stage of apoptosis.

Valproic acid is a C_8 branched-chain fatty acid that can be metabolized into a potential mitochondrial toxin, 4-en-valproic acid, and it may also inhibit beta-oxidation in itself. Individual genetic variation in mitochondrial beta-oxidation may determine the sensitivity of some individuals to a severe toxic reaction with valproic acid, causing a Reye-like syndrome or fulminant hepatic failure. Children with underlying MDS, Alpers–Huttenlocher syndrome (*POLG1* mutations), and respiratory chain defects (complex I deficiency) are more sensitive to valproic acid; its use has precipitated liver failure. It has also been recently shown that harboring a single mutation in *POLG1*, even in adults, predisposes to severe valproic acid-induced acute liver injury. For other drugs, the mechanism causing inhibition of mitochondrial respiration is still unclear. A number of toxins inhibit specific protein complexes of the respiratory chain (e.g. cyanide, antimycin A, rotenone) and lead to reduced ATP production and increased oxidative stress. The emetic toxin of *Bacillus cereus*, cereulide, has been demonstrated to cause inhibition of respiratory chain activity and is a causative agent for fulminant liver failure. Other drugs with potential mitochondrial inhibitory effects include tetracycline, linezolid, chloramphenicol, quinolones, and propofol.

Two important toxins/drugs that cause mitochondrial injury will be discussed in more detail: ethanol and nucleoside analogues.

Ethanol toxicity

Acquired respiratory-chain defects have been implicated in the pathogenesis of the intrahepatic microvesicular steatosis that develops during ethanol hepatotoxicity [58]. Ethanol consumption increases the generation of reactive oxygen species by hepatic mitochondria, decreases the intrahepatic mitochondrial glutathione levels, and increases the susceptibility of hepatic mitochondria to lipid peroxidation. Because mtDNA lacks protective histones and DNA repair enzymes and lies in close proximity to the site of free radical generation, both reactive oxygen species and lipid peroxidation products may damage mtDNA. The majority of alcoholics with microvesicular steatosis had an acquired mtDNA deletion that mimicked the large approximately 5000 bp deletion characteristic of Pearson syndrome in childhood; however, it was present in a much lower percentage of cells. This mtDNA deletion was present in 6 of 10 alcoholics with microvesicular steatosis, 2 of 17 alcoholics with macrovesicular steatosis, 0 of 23 alcoholics with acute alcoholic hepatitis or cirrhosis, and 0 of 62 age-matched non-alcoholic patients with various other liver diseases or normal liver histology. The pathogenesis of the microvesicular steatosis may be related to the excess of reducing equivalents (NADH) produced by ethanol in hepatic mitochondria. As LCHAD is dependent on NAD as a cofactor; the accumulation of intramitochondrial NADH inhibits LCHAD activity thus decreasing beta-oxidation of long-chain fatty acids. In addition, reduced reoxidation of NADH caused by an acquired complex I (mtDNA deletion) defect may also contribute to a reduction in long-chain FAO and the development of microvesicular steatosis. Strategies at improving mitochondrial respiration or reducing the generation of reactive oxygen species may be of potential benefit, and are under study.

Nucleoside analogues and other anti-HIV drugs

Several drugs of the nucleoside analogues (reverse transcriptase inhibitors) type directly inhibit protein complexes of the intramitochondrial respiratory chain or intramitochondrial beta-oxidation enzymes or interfere with mtDNA replication (Table 35.5) and lead to hepatotoxicity and microvesicular steatosis. An example of drug-induced mitochondrial toxicity was the fatal lactic acidosis and liver failure that developed in seven adults with chronic hepatitis B infection who were treated with the experimental antiviral nucleoside analogue fialuridine [59]. Most of these patients presented with fatigue,

nausea, constipation and abdominal pain, coagulopathy, hyperammonemia, and profound lactic acidosis, with only mild jaundice and minimal increases in serum aminotransferase values. Pancreatitis, peripheral neuropathy, and myopathy, reminiscent of inherited mitochondrial disorders of the respiratory chain, also developed in several patients. Liver tissue from the five patients who underwent liver transplantation showed marked microvesicular and macrovesicular steatosis, cholestasis, and swollen dysmorphic mitochondria. The mechanism of fialuridine toxicity is based on its incorporation directly into mtDNA in the place of thymidine, thus interrupting transcription of mtDNA and its gene products. This has a profound effect on mtDNA-encoded proteins, with impaired mitochondrial respiration and FAO that resulted in microvesicular steatosis, morphologic changes in mitochondria, and severe lactic acidosis.

Nucleos(t)ide-reverse transcriptase inhibitors are the main source of antiretroviral therapy-related mitochondrial hepatotoxicity in large part because of their ability to inhibit DNA POLG [60]. Examples of implicated drugs include zidovudine, stavudine, lamivudine, zalcitabine, and emtricitabine. The correlation between mitochondrial hepatotoxicity and potency in inhibiting POLG is not absolute in that zidovudine is more toxic to mitochondria than lamivudine in vitro despite lower potential to inhibit POLG. This suggests that other mechanisms may contribute to mitochondrial hepatotoxicity. There is emerging evidence that HIV protease inhibitors (e.g. ritonavir, indinavir, and nelfinavir) and non-nucleoside reverse transcriptase inhibitors (e.g. efavirenz, nevirapine, and delavirdine), which do not lead to mtDNA depletion, are also toxic to mitochondria, possibly through adverse effects on mitochondrial bioenergetics and induction of cell death pathways.

Hydrophobic bile acid toxicity

Hydrophobic bile acids, which accumulate in the liver in cholestasis (including bile acid transport defects), are toxic to hepatocytes through several mechanisms, including activation of cell death receptor and protein kinase signaling pathways, the induction of the mitochondrial membrane permeability transition, and the generation of oxidative stress [61]. Experimental cholestasis induced by bile duct ligation in the rat is associated with reduced activity of the electron transport chain in hepatic mitochondria, with an increased density of mitochondria per hepatocyte. Moreover, hydrophobic bile acids inhibit complex I and complex III activity in isolated hepatic mitochondria. Pathophysiologic concentrations of hydrophobic bile acids induce the mitochondrial membrane permeability transition and hydroperoxide generation as well as activating of downstream cell death pathways. Therefore, it has been proposed that, during cholestasis and in patients with bile acid synthesis and canalicular transport defects, increased concentrations of hydrophobic bile acids induce generation of reactive oxygen species from the altered electron transport chain of hepatocyte mitochondria, with the resultant opening of the permeability pore and the onset of cellular necrosis or apoptosis. The C_{34}-bile acids, found in some inborn errors of bile acid metabolisms, are even more cytotoxic than mature C_{30}-bile acids. The C_{27}-bile acids are potent inhibitors of OXPHOS and enhance mitochondrial reactive oxygen species production by inhibiting the respiratory chain. The antioxidant vitamin E has provided significant protection against bile acid toxicity in an in vivo rat model. The extent of the role of mitochondrial dysfunction in human cholestatic liver disease and whether this could be targeted for new therapies has not been fully explored and awaits further investigation.

Non-alcoholic steatohepatitis

Another category of secondary mitochondrial hepatopathy is the broad group of disorders now called non-alcoholic fatty liver disease and steatohepatitis. In these disorders micro- or macrovesicular steatosis is accompanied by varying degrees of necroinflammatory change and portal fibrosis, in the absence of significant intake of alcohol but generally in the presence of insulin resistance [62]. There is also ultrastructural evidence of mitochondrial damage in non-alcoholic steatohepatitis, which may be progressive and culminate in cirrhosis and hepatocellular carcinoma. It is commonly associated with obesity, diabetes mellitus type 2, jejuno-ileal bypass surgery, parenteral nutrition, bacterial overgrowth of the small intestine, and various drugs. There is growing evidence that acquired mitochondrial electron transport abnormalities may underlie the oxidant stress generated and contribute to the intracellular accumulation of microvesicular fat. Circulating lipopolysaccharide and tumor necrosis factor-α levels are elevated in several of the associated conditions and may contribute to both the oxidant stress and mitochondrial dysfunction. Use of antioxidant therapy for non-alcoholic steatohepatitis, including vitamin E, is discussed in Chapter 36.

Diagnosis of respiratory chain disorders

General clinical features and diagnostic approach

Diagnosing a mitochondrial respiratory chain defect in patients with liver disease requires a high index of suspicion. Clinical findings that should suggest these disorders include (1) association of neuromuscular symptoms with liver dysfunction; (2) multisystem involvement in a patient with acute or chronic liver disease; (3) a rapidly progressive course of liver disease, particularly in the presence of lactic acidosis, hepatic steatosis, or ketonemia; and (d) onset of liver disease in the first 2 years of life. Although CNS and neuromuscular syndromes have been the predominant findings in many patients, a report of 100 patients with respiratory chain deficiencies at one European center showed that 56% presented with a non-neuromuscular problem, which included liver presentations [63]. A more complete list of presenting clinical symptoms at various ages has been published by Munnich et al. [63] (Table 35.1). Most patients with respiratory chain defects

(involving any tissue) present early in life. In one large series, 36% presented before 1 month of life, 44% between 1 month and 2 years, and 20% after 2 years of age.

With modern advances in next-generation DNA sequencing, the identification of clear mitochondrial disease phenotypic patterns and a large and growing number of genes linked to mitochondrial pathology, the diagnostic approach to these patients is undergoing rapid evolution. Within several years, whole genome or whole exome sequencing will be commercially available and will cost less than single gene sequencing costs today. Therefore, analyzing large panels of nuclear and mtDNA genes causing mitochondrial disorders will be feasible and cost-effective. These panels are currently available from several clinical laboratories in the USA. Interpretation of genotyping results will be critical to making the proper diagnosis. A tiered approach to diagnosing hepatic mitochondrial disorders is recommended, as below, with initial screening tests (tier one), followed by either biochemical assays in affected tissues or genotyping for relatively common causative genes (tier two), followed by further molecular and biochemical evaluations (tier 3).

Screening tests for respiratory chain defects

Laboratory findings which suggest the presence of a respiratory chain defect are listed in Table 35.7 [2,17]. Persistent elevation of plasma lactic acid (>2.5 mmol/L), an elevated molar ratio of plasma lactate to pyruvate (>20:1), and elevation of the ketone body ratio (β-hydroxybutyrate to acetoacetate: >2:1) are highly suggestive of respiratory chain disorders. It should be stressed, however, that lactic acid and these ratios are not elevated in all patients with respiratory chain defects (e.g. Alpers–Huttenlocher syndrome, Navajo neurohepatopathy) [35]. Elevated ratios are indicative of an increase in reducing equivalents (excess of NADH and lack of NAD) caused by impaired transfer of electrons from NADH to oxygen as a result of disrupted OXPHOS. The plasma lactate to pyruvate ratio is a reflection of the NADH to NAD balance in the cytosol, and the ketone body ratio is a reflection of the NADH to NAD ratio within the mitochondrion. The elevated ketone body ratio is a consequence of functional impairment of the TCA cycle, with ketone body synthesis increasing (particularly after meals) through channeling of acetyl CoA away from reacting with oxalate to form citrate and into the ketogenic pathway. After feeding or intravenous dextrose, the exaggerated paradoxical production of ketones is even more evident, as ketone production should normally decrease after meals (or glucose infusion) through the suppressive effect of insulin on ketogenesis. Similarly, the abnormal plasma lactate to pyruvate ratio is particularly apparent in the postprandial period when more NAD is required for adequate oxidation of glycolytic substrates. In the presence of decreased NAD, pyruvate will be diverted by anaerobic metabolism to lactate. Therefore, to fully evaluate the patient, some have recommended that the concentration of these substrates and their molar ratios, as well as

Table 35.7 Screening tests for respiratory chain defects

Test	Result
Initial tests	
Plasma lactate	>2.5 mmol/L (persistently elevated)
Plasma molar lactate:pyruvate ratio	>20–25:1
Arterial molar ketone body ratio	β-Hydroxybutyrate/acetoacetate >2:1
Plasma ketone bodies/lactate after food	Paradoxical ↑ in plasma ketone bodies or lactate after meals or intravenous dextrose
Oral glucose load	2 g/kg load: repeat plasma lactate:pyruvate testing each 15 min for 90 min
Gas chromatography–mass spectroscopy of urine	Lactate, succinate, fumarate, malate, 3-methylglutaconic acid, 3-methylglutaric acid
Other tests	
Creatine kinase, acyl carnitine profile	For fatty acid oxidation disorders
Serum amino acid profiles	Elevated alanine
Plasma thymidine	For MNGIE syndrome (mitochondrial neurogastrointestinal encephalomyopathy)
Coenzyme Q in leukocytes, serum methylmalonic acid	Elevated in succinate-CoA ligase deficiencies (*SUCLA* and *SUCLG1*)
Cerebral spinal fluid lactate and pyruvate	If normal in serum

Source: adapted from Treem and Sokol, 1998 [21].

blood glucose and free fatty acids, should be determined before and 1 hour after meals. Occasionally, it is necessary to load a fasted patient with oral glucose (2 g/kg) in order to provoke lactic acidemia and abnormal ratios if the values are normal under baseline conditions. Substrates and ratios should be measured every 15 minutes for 90 minutes after the load. The lactate to pyruvate molar ratio in cerebrospinal fluid may be helpful when no elevation in plasma lactate is observed, particularly in the patient with CNS involvement. *Pitfalls* in interpretation of these ratios include false positives in patients with systemic hypotension or with impaired ventilation. In addition, pyruvate and acetoacetate are less stable than lactate and β-hydroxybutyrate, and artefacts of sample preparation or delayed processing may result in spuriously increased ratios. Complex II deficiency should theoretically not affect the plasma lactate to pyruvate and ketone body ratios because a block at that level would not affect NADH oxidation. It should be pointed out that patients with the later presentation of liver dysfunction (e.g. Alpers–Huttenlocher syndrome) frequently do not have elevations of plasma lactate or increased plasma lactate to pyruvate and arterial ketone body ratios. Patients with pyruvate dehydrogenase deficiency generally have low plasma lactate to pyruvate ratios (<10). Defects in the TCA cycle may also result in elevated lactate to pyruvate ratios but ketone body ratios should be low (<1). Renal tubular dysfunction can cause lower plasma lactate levels, thus making the lactate to pyruvate ratio less accurate. Diabetes mellitus may impair pyruvate entry into the TCA cycle.

Investigation of urine is also useful. Proximal renal tubular dysfunction may lower plasma lactate and increase urinary lactate. In these cases, gas chromatography–mass spectrometry (GC-MS) can detect elevated urinary lactate, TCA cycle intermediates (succinate, fumarate, and malate), and at times, 3-methyl-glutaconic and 3-methylglutaric acid.

It should be emphasized that these are screening tests and may not be abnormal if the respiratory chain defect is confined to one or two organs. Therefore, searching for dysfunction or abnormal histology/biochemistry of the target organs is also important.

Other useful screening tests may include creatine kinase, acyl carnitine profile (for FAO disorders; measured by tandem mass spectrometry), serum amino acid profiles (searching for elevated alanine), plasma thymidine (if considering MNGIE syndrome), coenzyme Q levels in leukocytes, serum methyl-malonic acid levels (elevated in succinate-CoA ligase deficiencies (*SUCLA* and *SUCLG1*), and cerebral spinal fluid lactate and pyruvate (if normal in the serum).

Definitive diagnostic tests
Measurement of mitochondrial respiration

If freshly obtained affected tissue and the laboratory expertise are available, analysis of oxygen consumption in mitochondrial-enriched fractions of tissues (liver, muscle, lymphocytes, fibroblasts) can be performed by polarographic studies in the presence of a series of respiratory substrates to define the site of the respiratory impairment [2,63]. Patients with complex I deficiency (NADH oxidoreductase) will show impaired respiration (oxygen consumption by mitochondria) with NADH-producing substrates such as glutamate and malate; those with complex II (succinate oxidoreductase) with FADH-producing substrates such as succinate; and those with complex III (ubiquinone-cytochrome *c* oxidoreductase) and complex IV (cytochrome *c* oxidase) with both types of substrates. Complex V (ATP synthetase) deficiency will produce impaired respiration with all substrates, but the addition of agents which uncouple electron transfer from phosphorylation (2,4-dinitrophenol or calcium ions) will return the respiratory rate to normal. Polarographic studies have the advantage of requiring relatively small amounts of tissue (100–200 mg muscle; 10 mL blood for circulating lymphocytes); however, these assays require fresh tissue for immediate isolation and analysis of mitochondria. Therefore, biopsies must be conducted at the center performing these studies. Polarographic testing is available on fresh liver biopsy specimens at very few centers around the world and is impractical for evaluation of most patients.

Enzymatic activity of respiratory chain complexes

Direct measurement of the enzymatic activity of the mitochondrial respiratory chain complexes on frozen tissue is more commonly used to establish deficiency of the respiratory chain [64]. These studies can be performed on frozen samples of small biopsies of liver, muscle, kidney, myocardium, or other tissue since they do not require the isolation of mitochondrial fractions, and can be carried out on tissue homogenates, lymphocytes, or cultured skin fibroblasts. Tissue biopsy samples must be frozen immediately at the bedside or in the operating room and stored at $-80°C$ until analyzed. Measurement of respiratory chain enzyme activities separately or in groups is performed in specialized laboratories spectrophotometrically using specific electron acceptors and donors. In general, the tissues chosen for study should be those which clinically express the disease. It may also be useful to obtain skin fibroblasts and lymphocytes for testing, although a defect may be absent in these cells and confined to the involved organ. In some countries (Australia, Netherlands, USA), micromethods have allowed these analyses to be performed on frozen portions of percutaneous liver and muscle biopsy specimens (10–15 mg tissue). However, in most centers, these analyses usually require surgical liver or muscle biopsies. Pitfalls in these measurements include the following. Normal values may have a wide range, so overlap may be found in affected patients. For this reason, some experts recommend expressing results as ratios of one protein complex activity to another to detect deficiencies of one enzyme that may be in the low to normal range [65]. Normal respiratory activity does not exclude a defect in mtDNA, since heteroplasmy may allow for reasonably normal enzymatic activity in some areas of a given tissue. Molecular analysis of mtDNA should be performed in these instances. Certain cells (e.g. lymphocytes and cultured fibroblasts) are not good for detecting abnormalities in complex I activity.

Finally, blue native polyacrilamide gel electrophoresis of tissue can detect incompletely assembled respiratory chain subunits and may be helpful in establishing the diagnosis.

Histopathological investigations

It is possible to detect deficiencies of subunits of several of the respiratory chain complexes by histochemical examination of biopsy material. Polyclonal and monoclonal antibodies directed against cytochrome *c* oxidase (complex IV) subunits can be used to stain liver and muscle. Tissue specimens must be frozen immediately in liquid nitrogen-cooled isopentane for these studies. Other immunohistochemical techniques for staining NADH tetrazolium reductase and succinate dehydrogenase are also available. Histology and electron microscopy of muscle and liver may also reveal characteristic findings of respiratory chain disorders (e.g. ragged red fibers in muscle).

Magnetic resonance imaging

Magnetic resonance imaging may be useful in diagnosis of mitochondrial disease and in documenting whether the brain is involved if liver transplantation is being considered [66]. Abnormal findings may be non-specific, such as cerebral atrophy. The basal ganglia are particularly vulnerable to a failure of energy metabolism with T_2-weighted hyperintensities commonly seen on MRI in the putamen, globus pallidus, and caudate nuclei. Findings can also be even more characteristic of a given disorder such as stroke-like (MELAS) lesions that do not respect vascular boundaries. Cerebral lactate measurements, the end-product of non-oxidative metabolism (glycolysis), can be done using ^1H magnetic resonance spectroscopy. Elevations of lactic acid in the CNS occurring in the absence of peripheral lactic academia are particularly important. Other features of energy metabolism, as measured with phosphorus-31 spectroscopy, may also have utility in characterizing mitochondrial disease.

Molecular analyses of mtDNA and nuclear DNA

Molecular diagnosis has become very useful as more nuclear genes are identified that cause specific respiratory chain and mtDNA depletion disorders. For nuclear genes, whole blood for isolation of genomic DNA will usually suffice [17]. For mtDNA deletions and mutations, the involved tissue may be necessary for analysis because of heteroplasmy. In addition, the DNA of biopsied tissue (including liver) can be isolated, electrophoresed, blotted, and hybridized with probes for nuclear and mitochondrial genes. Autoradiographic signals after hybridization can be measured and the mtDNA level expressed as the ratio of the signal of the mitochondrial probe to that of the nuclear probe in order to determine if mtDNA depletion is present. Deletions and mutations of mtDNA can be screened by the single-strand conformational polymorphism technique. To detect mtDNA deletions, techniques using digestion of mtDNA with restriction enzymes can demonstrate two populations of mtDNA. For characterization of the nucleotide sequence at the boundaries of the mtDNA deletions, amplification with the polymerase chain reaction is performed followed by automated nucleotide sequencing. Massively parallel sequencing (next-generation sequencing) is now being used as a one-step comprehensive molecular analysis of the whole mitochondrial genome for patients in whom a mitochondrial disease is suspected [67].

Using these molecular techniques, specific mutations or deletions can be sought and even the entire mitochondrial genome can be sequenced. Genetic mutations in mtDNA have not been detected in most infants with neonatal liver failure caused by respiratory chain defects [24]. However, mutations in *SCO1* and *BCS1L* may be identified in infants with neonatal hepatic failure or GRACILE syndrome. In patients with suspected or proven hepatic MDS, *dGUOK*, *POLG*, and *MPV17* should be genotyped initially, and *SUCLG1* and *TWINKLE* then considered [1]. In patients with the clinical presentation of MNGIE syndrome, mutations of *TYMP*, encoding thymidine phosphorylase, should be sought. In patients with the later-onset liver failure presentation characteristic of Alpers–Huttenlocher syndrome, *POLG* (Navajo neurohepatopathy), *MPV17*, and *DGUOK*, *TWINKLE*, and *SUCLG1* should be analyzed [27]. Other genes to consider (Table 35.6) include *TRMU*, *EFG1*, *EFTu*, and *TSFM*, encoding nuclear translation factors. Pearson marrow–pancreas syndrome requires mtDNA analysis to detect the common mtDNA deletion (4997 bp). In addition, multiple mtDNA duplications have been reported in Pearson syndrome. Molecular DNA analysis is now becoming a useful tool in the diagnosis of patients with primary respiratory chain defects and may replace the need to obtain tissue for respiratory chain enzyme activity analysis and mtDNA depletion studies, as the genetic tests become less expensive and available from approved clinical laboratories (see http://www.genetests.org). As stated, large genotyping panels of over 100 nuclear genes coding for mitochondrial proteins (using next-generation sequencing platforms) are now commercially available in some countries at great cost savings compared with genotyping individual genes and might be considered as a cost-effective way to evaluate patients.

Treatment of respiratory chain disorders

Unfortunately, there is no ideal effective therapy for most patients with respiratory chain disorders, including those with liver failure and more slowly progressive liver disease. It is not clear that any currently available medical therapy significantly alters the course of severe disease; however, some patients have experienced improvement of neuromuscular symptoms with specific therapies. A recent Cochrane review of treatment strategies for mitochondrial disorders identified 12 studies that fulfilled the entry criteria [68]. Of these, eight were new studies. The comparability of the reviewed studies was extremely low because of differences in the specific diseases studied, differences in the therapeutic agents used, dosage, study design, and outcomes. There was no clear evidence supporting the use of any intervention in mitochondrial disorders. A recommendation was made to test novel agents in homogeneous study populations with clinically defined primary end-points.

Based on an understanding of the enzymatic and biochemical derangements, several treatment strategies have been proposed although not proven to be effective (Table 35.8). Acute metabolic acidosis is treated with the slow infusion of sodium bicarbonate intravenously, anemia or thrombocytopenia is treated with transfusions, and chronic pancreatic insufficiency may require the provision of exogenous pancreatic enzymes with meals. Acute liver failure is treated with balanced intravenous administration of dextrose and lipids, correction of acidosis, treatment of hyperammonemia, and attention to infectious complications. Chronic liver disease management may include the use of infant formula high in medium-chain triglycerides, a diet with at least 30–40% fat, cornstarch to prevent hypoglycemia, evaluation and supplementation with fat-soluble vitamins (if cholestatic), routine immunizations (including hepatitis A and B vaccines), and monitoring for and treating complications of portal hypertension. Other mitochondrial strategies include supplementation with mitochondrial cofactors, scavengers of oxygen free radicals, and mitochondrial energy substrates, as well as avoidance of drugs and conditions known to have a detrimental effect on the respiratory chain [2]. Seizure control should not include phenobarbital since it can inhibit OXPHOS. Valproic acid should likewise be avoided if possible in these patients because of its effects on respiration and fatty acid metabolism. Exercise is important in patients with muscle involvement. Besides improving strength, a decrease in the proportion of mutant mtDNA in muscle can be stimulated by exercise training. Even induction of muscle necrosis by drug therapy has been proposed as a means to enhance proliferation of myoblasts to attain muscle fibers with less mutated mtDNA.

Pharmacologic support

A variety of antioxidant compounds have been proposed as scavengers of electrons or oxygen free radicals, as promoters of electron transport, or as stimulators of mitochondrial respiration [69,70]. Coenzyme Q_{10} (ubiquinone) has been reported to result in sustained improvement in several patients with complex III deficiency and perhaps in complex IV deficiency. Coenzyme Q is the electron acceptor for complex I and complex II of the respiratory chain, receiving electrons from NADH via complex I and various feeder pathways including the TCA cycle and the beta-oxidation cycle via succinate and FADH through complex II and electron transport flavoprotein. Using an animal model of liver injury that employed endotoxin-induced intrahepatic lipid peroxidation, exogenously administered ubiquinone prevented the marked reduction in hepatic levels of endogenous coenzyme Q, α-tocopherol, and glutathione; suppressed lipid peroxidation; and increased the survival rate in endotoxemic mice. Similar effects of ubiquinone were seen in an animal model of liver ischemia–reperfusion injury. Coenzyme Q analogues have also been shown to promote respiration in isolated hepatic and brain mitochondria and hepatic mitochondrial coenzyme Q levels have been shown to decrease after several weeks of bile duct ligation in the rat. However, supplementation has not

Table 35.8 Proposed pharmacologic treatments for respiratory chain disorders

Treatment	Action	Dosage[a]
Electron acceptors and cofactors		
Coenzyme Q_{10}	Redox bypass of complex I; free radical scavenger (antioxidant)	Adult: 60–300 mg/day Ped: 3–5 mg/kg daily
Idebenone	Redox bypass of complex I; free radical scavenger (antioxidant)	Adult: 90–270 mg/day Ped: 5 mg/kg daily
Thiamine (vitamin B_1)	Cofactor of pyruvate dehydrogenase	Adult: 50–300 mg/day
Riboflavin (vitamin B_2)	Acts as flavin precursor for complexes I and II	Adult: 50–200 mg/day
Menadione (vitamin K_3)	Bypass complex III (with vitamin C)	Adult: 4–160 mg/day
Antioxidants		
Vitamin E (TPGS)	Antioxidant	Adult: 400–800 IU/day Ped: 25 IU/kg daily
Ascorbic acid (vitamin C)	Antioxidant	Adult: 2–4 g/day
Other mechanisms of action		
Succinate	Donates electrons directly to complex II	Adult: 6–16 g/day
Carnitine	Replace secondary carnitine deficiency	Adult: up to 3 g/day Ped: 50–100 mg/kg daily
Creatine monohydrate	Enhances muscle phosphocreatine	Adult: up to 10 g/day Ped: 0.1–0.2 g/kg daily
Dichloroacetate	Reduces lactic acidosis by enhancing pyruvate dehydrogenase activity	Adult: 25 mg/kg/day Ped: 25–50 mg/kg daily

TPGS: *d*-α-tocopheryl polyethylene glycol 1 000 succinate.
[a] Pediatric (Ped) doses are estimates and have *not* been subjected to clinical dosage trials.
Source: adapted from Gillis and Sokol, 2003 [16].

been attempted in humans with cholestasis to our knowledge. In mitochondrial myopathies or cardiomyopathies, occasional patients have shown dramatic improvement in muscle strength and cardiac function after coenzyme Q supplementation. There have now been numerous reports of patients with myopathy and cerebellar ataxia and primary deficiencies of coenzyme Q who responded very well to repletion with this substance. There is little reported experience using coenzyme Q in patients with mitochondrial hepatopathies.

Other antioxidants that have been administered to patients with respiratory chain defects include menadione (vitamin K_3), ascorbic acid, and vitamin E (Table 35.8). Sustained improvement in isolated patients with complex III deficiency has been reported using menadione or coenzyme Q. Vitamin E is incorporated into mitochondrial membranes when administered exogenously and is of theoretical but unproven benefit. Treatment with riboflavin has been associated with improvement in a small number of patients with complex II deficiency. Succinate has occasionally been given to patients with complex I deficiency since this substrate enters the respiratory chain via complex II. L-Carnitine has been used as therapy in patients with secondary carnitine deficiency, the purpose being to scavenge potentially toxic metabolites that accumulate because

of the inhibition of FAO. However, in some patients with electron transport complex abnormalities, carnitine has led to increased liver injury, presumably through increased electron flow and increased generation of oxygen free radicals. Therefore, L-carnitine supplementation in patients with mitochondrial hepatopathies should be used carefully. Dichloroacetate administration has been proposed to stimulate pyruvate dehydrogenase activity and has occasionally resulted in reduced levels of plasma lactate but has not resulted in a clear change of the natural history of respiratory chain disorders. Dichloroacetate has been reported to cause a reversible peripheral neuropathy. There is a great need for the development of more effective therapeutic options for affected patients but it is possible that a dysfunctional respiratory chain will be incompatible with life once liver failure develops.

Drugs and compounds that can inhibit the respiratory chain either directly or through effects on the TCA cycle or beta-oxidation should be avoided if there is high suspicion of a respiratory chain defect, and certainly after the diagnosis has been established. These drugs include valproate, barbiturates, salicylates, tetracycline, chloramphenicol, ibuprofen, amiodarone, linezolid, reverse transcriptase inhibitors, and the ingestion of alcohol. Ringer's lactate should not be infused because of poor handling of lactate by many patients and propofol should be avoided as an anesthetic agent as it can interfere with mitochondrial function.

Dietary treatment

A high-lipid, low-carbohydrate diet should be instituted in patients with complex I deficiency [70]. A high-glucose diet is a metabolic challenge for patients with an impaired respiratory chain and may have precipitated hepatic failure in patients with Pearson syndrome. Since glucose oxidation is largely aerobic in the liver, the provision of large amounts of dextrose to impaired hepatic mitochondria may result in increased lactate production and worsening acidosis and ketosis. Based on these considerations, the recommendation is to avoid a hypercaloric diet high in carbohydrates and parenteral infusions of solutions containing high concentrations of dextrose. However, oral uncooked cornstarch therapy may be needed to prevent hypoglycemia. Succinate (16 g/day), succinate-producing amino acids, or propionylcarnitine have occasionally been given to patients with complex I deficiency since these compounds enter the respiratory chain at complex II.

Liver transplantation

Although the presence of significant neuromuscular or cardiac involvement in respiratory chain disorders should preclude the use of liver transplantation, a number of patients with defects isolated to the liver have now successfully undergone liver transplantation with excellent long-term outcomes and no extrahepatic disease expression. The prerequisite for considering liver transplantation in this setting is the exclusion of significant extrahepatic disease [2,71]. This includes careful clinical and laboratory screening of potentially affected organ systems (kidneys, heart, muscle, CNS, pancreas), MRI or functional MRI of the brain, echocardiography, and the exclusion of depressed respiratory chain enzyme activity in muscle and skin fibroblasts. It is possible that post-transplant chimerism by which dendritic cells from the graft migrate into other tissues of the recipient could play a role in correcting the defect in extrahepatic tissues, as has been proposed in patients recipients who had glycogen storage disease type IV and Gaucher disease type I. However, in patients who have received liver transplants and had clinically unrecognized neurologic involvement prior to transplant, progressive neurologic symptoms occurred following transplantation. In a series of 11 patients who underwent liver transplantation for OXPHOS deficiencies before 7 months of age, only five were alive and well at follow-up between 5 months and 8 years after transplantation. Three of the six patients who died developed neurologic features only after liver transplantation. All of the patients who had liver failure and associated gastrointestinal disease died shortly after liver transplantation. To date, 38 reported use of liver transplantation in respiratory chain disorders could be obtained from the literature, among which 18 patients were surviving (47% survival rate) although with

relatively short follow-up reported. It should be assumed that these patients were carefully selected and that these results are perhaps the best case scenario. This survival rate is far below that expected in pediatric liver transplantation (80–90%). Seven patients with *DGUOK* deficiency with neurologic involvement all died within 24 months of transplantation. Therefore, when evaluating young children with fulminant liver failure for liver transplantation, it is essential to obtain historical documentation of typical neurologic symptoms characteristic of these disorders and of gastrointestinal symptoms; a complete family history; and a thorough clinical and biochemical evaluation of neuromuscular and cardiac function. It must be stressed to the family that the absence of extrahepatic involvement prior to transplantation does not guarantee that severe neurologic symptoms will not develop after transplantation. Patients with mutations in *POLG*, *DGUOK* (with neurologic features), and *MPV17* do not appear to fare well after liver transplantation because of invariable severe neurologic progressive disease.

Gene therapy and cell-based therapy

Somatic gene transfer therapy is being tested in a number of human genetic disorders, with limited success so far. Several groups of investigators are designing novel methods to attempt to correct the underlying mtDNA defects present in some patients with mitochondrial hepatopathies. One approach has used an inhibitor of mitochondrial oxidation in cultured cells to alter the ratio of mutant to wild-type mtDNA. Another uses a self-replicating copy of a normal gene sequence delivered into mitochondria in vitro. Another approach is to inhibit replication of mutant mtDNA without affecting wild-type mtDNA. The MITO-Porter system is a liposome-based carrier that allows efficient cytoplasmic transit and then mitochondrial macromolecule delivery into the mitochondrial matrix of a mix that contains the mtDNA pool for use in mitochondrial gene therapy or drugs for delivery via membrane fusion [72]. Still another approach is to salvage OXPHOS function in cells by importing tRNAs from cytosol into mitochondria in patients with tRNA mutations (mtDNA mutations). Finally, various in vitro approaches can be taken to prevent recurrence, such as using donor eggs for future pregnancies. Another possibility for the future is of nuclear transfer from a maternal egg and fertilization in a donor cytoplasm using paternal sperm. The feasibility of mtDNA replacement in human oocytes by spindle transfer spindle–chromosomal complex transfer has been demonstrated in vitro [73]. The technique potentially isolates and transplants the chromosomes from a patient's unfertilized oocyte into the cytoplasm of another enucleated egg, containing healthy mtDNA as well as other organelles, RNA, and proteins.

Prenatal diagnosis

The ability to accurately provide prenatal diagnosis of maternally inherited mtDNA disorders is hampered by our incomplete knowledge of the actual proportion of mutant mtDNA

Table 35.9 Comparison of clinical features of several primary mitochondrial hepatopathies

Disorder	Onset	Seizures	Plasma lactate	Lactate:pyruvate molar ratio	mtDNA	Complexes involved	Genes involved
Neonatal liver failure	Acute	±	↑	↑	Normal	IV, III, or I	*BCS1L* and *SCO2*
mtDNA depletion syndrome	Acute/ chronic	+	↑	↑	Depletion	I, III, IV	*MPV17, POLG, DGUOK, SUCLG1, TWINKLE*
Alpers– Huttenlocher sydrome	Insidious	++	Normal	Normal	Normal	I	*POLG*
Pearson syndrome	Insidious	–	Normal or ↑	Normal or ↑	Deletion	I, III	
Villous atrophy syndrome	Chronic	–	↑	↑	Rearrangements	III	
Navajo neurohepatopathy	Acute or chronic	–	–	Normal or ↑	Depletion	I, III, IV	*MPV17*

+, present sometimes; ++, present always; ±, occasionally present; –, not present; ↑ increased; mt, mitochondrial.
Source: with permission from Sokol and Treem, 1999 [75].

that is necessary to produce the disease phenotype. and the random distribution of mtDNA into different tissues [74]. Therefore, the demonstration of the heteroplasmic presence of a known mtDNA mutation or deletion in chorionic villi or amniotic cells of a progeny in an affected family does not yet have an adequate predictive value to accurately assign a disease phenotype to the fetus. For the nuclear-encoded gene mutations that have been identified in a proband (e.g. *POLG, MPV17, DGUOK*), it is possible to assess amniocytes or chorionic villi for nuclear DNA mutations. Others have attempted to measure respiratory chain enzyme activity and ATP synthesis in digitonin-permeabilized cultured chorionic villus cells. This method would be helpful only in disorders in which the defect has a multisystemic expression in different cell types that include fibroblasts, which is not the case in all infants and young children with hepatic involvement, since only 40–50% of these enzyme deficiencies are expressed in cultured fibroblasts. Currently, prenatal diagnosis is useful primarily in families affected by a respiratory chain defect caused by a known nuclear-encoded causative gene.

Conclusions

Mitochondrial hepatopathies are one of the newly recognized group of important liver disorders in childhood, particularly in infancy and in patients with liver failure. The identification of several secondary mitochondrial hepatopathies stresses the critical nature of mitochondrial function in the pathogenesis of liver injury and in the cellular processes of necrosis and apoptosis. Primary mitochondrial hepatopathies should be considered in any child with liver disease and neuromuscular involvement, multisystemic disease, lactic acidosis, onset prior to 2 years of age, or rapidly progressive disease, and when hepatic steatosis is the dominant histologic finding on liver biopsy. A comparison of salient features of six of the primary mitochondrial hepatopathies is given in Table 35.9. Diagnosis is shifting to genotyping likely causative genes, as more nuclear genes are identified, and next-generation sequencing of nuclear and mitochondrial gene panels in the near future. Treatments are currently not satisfactory; however, liver transplantation may be successful in selected patients with isolated liver involvement. The field of mitochondrial medicine is developing rapidly with hope for new therapies in coming years.

Website information

Additional information can be obtained from the following Internet websites.

Family support groups and information

United Mitochondrial Disease Foundation: www.umdf.org
International Mitochondrial Disease Network: www.imdn.org

Scientific information

Mitochondrial Interest Group: http://www.nih.gov/sigs/mito/
MitoDat – Mendelian Inheritance and the Mitochondrion: www.lecb.ncifcrf.gov/mitoDat/
Mitochondrial Research Society (MRS): www.lecb.ncifcrf.gov/~zullo/migDB/mrs.html
Childhood Liver Disease Research Network (ChiLDReN): http://childrennetwork.org

Acknowledgements

Supported in part by NIH grants U54-DK078377, UO1-DK062453 and UL1RR025780 (UL1TR000154).

References

1. Koopman WJH, Willems PHGM, Smeitink JAM. Monogenic mitochondrial disorders, *N Engl J Med* 2012;**366**:1132–1141.

2. Lee WS, Sokol RJ. Mitochondrial hepatopathies: advances in genetics and pathogenesis. *Hepatology* 2007;**45**:1555–1565.

3. Beal MF, Hyman BT, Koroshetz W. Do defects in mitochondrial energy metabolism underlie the pathology of neurodegenerative diseases? *Trends Neurosci* 1993;**16**:125–131.

4. Wong LJ. Molecular genetics of mitochondrial disorders. *Dev Disabil Res Rev* 2010;**16**:154–162.

5. Taanman JW. The mitochondrial genome: structure, transcription, translation and replication. *Biochim Biophys Acta* 1999;**1410**: 103–123.

6. Lightowlers RN, Chinnery PF, Turnbull DM, Howell N. Mammalian mitochondrial genetics: heredity, heteroplasmy and disease. *Trends Genet* 1997;**13**:450–455.

7. Pagliarini DJ, Calvo SE, Chang B, *et al.* A mitochondrial protein compendium elucidates complex I disease biology. *Cell* 2008;**134**:112–123.

8. Efremov RG, Sazanov LA. Respiratory complex I: "steam engine" of the cell? *Curr Opin Structural Biol* 2011;**21**: 532–540.

9. Holt IJ, Harding AE, Morgan-Hughes JA. Deletions of muscle mitochondrial DNA in patients with mitochondrial myopathies. *Nature* 1988;**331** (6158):717–719.

10. Wallace DC, Singh G, Lott MT, *et al.* Mitochondrial DNA mutation associated with Leber's hereditary optic neuropathy. *Science* 1988;**242** (4884):1427–1430.

11. Skladal D, Halliday J, Thorburn DR. Minimum birth prevalence of mitochondrial respiratory chain disorders in children. *Brain* 2003;**126** (Pt 8):1905–1912.

12. Majamaa K, Moilanen JS, Uimonen S, *et al.* Epidemiology of A3243G, the mutation for mitochondrial encephalomyopathy, lactic acidosis, and strokelike episodes: prevalence of themutation in an adult population. *Am J Hum Genet* 1998;**63**: 447–454.

13. Chinnery PF, Johnson MA, Wardell TM, *et al.* The epidemiology of pathogenic mitochondrial DNA mutations. *Ann Neurol* 2000;**48**: 188–193.

14. Uusimaa J, Remes AM, Rantala H, *et al.* Childhood encephalopathies and myopathies: a prospective study in a defined population to assess the frequency of mitochondrial disorders. *Pediatrics* 2000;**105**:598–603.

15. Darin N, Oldfors A, Moslemi AR, *et al.* The incidence of mitochondrial encephalomyopathies in childhood: clinical features and morphological, biochemical, and DNA anbormalities. *Ann Neurol* 2001;**49**:377–383.

16. Gillis LA, Sokol RJ. Gastrointestinal manifestations of mitochondrial disease. *Gastroenterol Clin North Am* 2003;**32**:789–817.

17. Wong LJ, Scaglia F, Graham BH, Craigen WJ. Current molecular diagnostic algorithm for mitochondrial disorders. *Mol Genet Metab* 2010;**100**:111–117.

18. Bindoff LA, Engelsen BA. Mitochondrial diseases and epilepsy. *Epilepsia* 2012;**53**(Suppl 4):92–97.

19. Wong LJ. Mitochondrial syndromes with leukoencephalopathies. *Semin Neurol* 2012;**32**:55–61.

20. Finsterer J. Inherited mitochondrial disorders. *Adv Exp Med Biol* 2012;**942**:187–213.

21. Treem WR, Sokol RJ. Disorders of the mitochondria. *Semin Liver Dis* 1998;**18**:237–253.

22. Leonard JV, Schapira AH. Mitochondrial respiratory chain disorders I: mitochondrial DNA defects. *Lancet* 2000;**355**:299–304.

23. Leonard JV, Schapira AH. Mitochondrial respiratory chain disorders II: neurodegenerative disorders and nuclear gene defects. *Lancet* 2000;**355**:389–394.

24. Fellman V, Kotarsky H. Mitochondrial hepatopathies in the newborn period. *Semin Fetal Neonatal Med* 2011;**16**: 222–228.

25. Dimmock DP, Zhang Q, Dionisi-Vici C, *et al.* Clinical and molecular features of mitochondrial DNA depletion due to mutations in deoxyguanosine kinase. *Hum Mutat* 2008;**29**:330–331.

26. Pronicka E, Weglewska-Jurkiewicz A, Taybert J, *et al.* Post mortem identification of deoxyguanosine kinase (*DGUOK*) gene mutations combined with impaired glucose homeostasis and iron overload features in four infants with severe progressive liver failure. *J Applied Genet* 2011;**52**:61–66.

27. Wong LJ, Naviaux RK, Brunetti-Pierri N, *et al.* Molecular and clinical genetics of mitochondrial diseases due to *POLG* mutations. *Hum Mutat* 2008;**29**: E150–E172.

28. El-Hattab AW, Scaglia F, Craigen WJ, Wong LJC. MPV17-related hepatocerebral mitochondrial DNA depletion syndrome. In Pagon RA, Bird TD, Dolan CR, Stephens K (eds.) *GeneReviews.* Seattle, WA: University of Washington, Seattle, 1993–.

29. Finsterer J, Zarrouk Mahjoub S. Mitochondrial toxicity of antiepileptic drugs and their tolerability in mitochondrial disorders. *Expert Opin Drug Metab Toxicol* 2012;**8**:71–79.

30. Milone M, Massie R. Polymerase gamma 1 mutations: clinical correlations. *The Neurologist* 2010;**16**:84–91.

31. Horvath R, Hudson G, Ferrari G, *et al.* Phenotypic spectrum associated with mutations of the mitochondrial polymerase gamma gene. *Brain* 2006;**129**:1674–1684.

32. Narkewicz MR, Sokol RJ, Beckwith B, *et al.* Liver involvement in Alpers disease. *J Pediatr* 1991;**119**:260–267.

33. Saneto RP, Lee IC, Koenig MK, *et al.* *POLG* DNA testing as an emerging standard of care before instituting valproic acid therapy for pediatric seizure disorders. *Seizure* 2010;**19**: 140–146.

34. Ferrari G, Lamantea E, Donati A, *et al.* Infantile hepatocerebral syndromes associated with mutations in the mitochondrial DNA polymerase-gammaA. *Brain* 2005;**128**(Pt 4): 723–731.

35. Nguyen KV, Sharief FS, Chan SS, Copeland WC, Naviaux RK. Molecular diagnosis of Alpers syndrome. *J Hepatol* 2006;**45**:108–116.

36. Hudson G, Chinnery PF. Mitochondrial DNA polymerase-gamma and human disease. *Hum Mol Genet.* 2006;**15**: R244–R252.

37. Pearson HA, Lobel JS, Kocoshis SA, *et al.* A new syndrome of refractory sideroblastic anemia with vacuolization of marrow precursors and exocrine

pancreatic dysfunction. *J Pediatr* 1979;**95**:976–984.

38. Morikawa Y, Matsuura N, Kakudo K, et al. Pearson's marrow/pancreas syndrome: a histological and genetic study. *Virchows Arch A Pathol Anat Histopathol* 1993;**423**:227–231.

39. Cormier-Daire V, Bonnefont JP, Rustin P, et al. Mitochondrial DNA rearrangements with onset as chronic diarrhea with villous atrophy. *J Pediatr* 1994;**124**:63–70.

40. Garone C, Tadesse S, Hirano M. Clinical and genetic spectrum of mitochondrial neurogastrointestinal encephalomyopathy. *Brain.* 2011;**134**:3326–3332.

41. Giordano C, d'Amati G. Evaluation of gastrointestinal mtDNA depletion in mitochondrial neurogastrointestinal encephalomyopathy (MNGIE). *Meth Mol Biol* 2011;**755**:223–232.

42. Hirano M, Garone C, Quinzii CM. CoQ10 deficiencies and MNGIE: two treatable mitochondrial disorders. *Biochim Biophys Acta* 2012:**1820**: 625–631.

43. Hirano M, Silvestri G, Blake DM, et al. Mitochondrial neurogastrointestinal encephalomyopathy (MNGIE): clinical, biochemical, and genetic features of an autosomal recessive mitochondrial disorder. *Neurology* 1994;**44**:721–727.

44. Hirano M, Vu TH. Defects of intergenomic communication: where do we stand? *Brain Pathol* 2000;**10**: 451–461.

45. Teitelbaum JE, Berde CB, Nurko S, et al. Diagnosis and management of MNGIE syndrome in children: case report and review of the literature. *J Pediatr Gastroenterol Nutr* 2002;**35**:377–383.

46. Giordano C, Sebastiani M, Plazzi G, et al. Mitochondrial neurogastrointestinal encephalomyopathy: evidence of mitochondrial DNA depletion in the small intestine. *Gastroenterology* 2006;**130**:893–901.

47. Holve S, Hu D, Shub M, Tyson RW, Sokol RJ. Liver disease in Navajo neuropathy. *J Pediatr* 1999;**135**: 482–493.

48. Karadimas CL, Vu TH, Holve SA, et al. Navajo neurohepatopathy is caused by a mutation in the *MPV17* gene. *Am J Hum Genet* 2006;**79**:544–548.

49. Spiekerkoetter U. Mitochondrial fatty acid oxidation disorders: clinical presentation of long-chain fatty acid oxidation defects before and after newborn screening. *J Inherit Metab Dis* 2010;**33**:527–532.

50. Enns GM, Bennett MJ, Hoppel CL, et al. Mitochondrial respiratory chain complex I deficiency with clinical and biochemical features of long-chain 3-hydroxyacyl-coenzyme A dehydrogenase deficiency. *J Pediatr* 2000;**136**:251–254.

51. Browning MF, Levy HL, Wilkins-Haug LE, Larson C, Shih VE. Fetal fatty acid oxidation defects and maternal liver disease in pregnancy. *Obstet Gynecol* 2006;**107**:115–120.

52. Partin JC. Reye's syndrome. In Suchy F (ed.) *Liver Disease in Children*. St. Louis, MO: Mosby, 1994, pp. 653–671.

53. Sternlieb I, Feldmann G. Effects of anticopper therapy on hepatocellular mitochondria in patients with Wilson's disease: an ultrastructural and stereological study. *Gastroenterology* 1976;**71**:457–461.

54. Sternlieb I. Mitochondrial and fatty changes in hepatocytes of patients with Wilson's disease. *Gastroenterology* 1968;**55**:354–367.

55. Mansouri A, Gaou I, Fromenty B, et al. Premature oxidative aging of hepatic mitochondrial DNA in Wilson's disease. *Gastroenterology* 1997;**113**: 599–605.

56. Scatena R. Mitochondria and drugs. *Adv Exp Med Biol* 2012;**942**:329–346.

57. Pessayre D, Fromenty B, Berson A, et al. Central role of mitochondria in drug-induced liver injury. *Drug Metab Rev* 2012;**44**:34–87.

58. Manzo-Avalos S, Saavedra-Molina A. Cellular and mitochondrial effects of alcohol consumption. *Int J Environ Res Public Health* 2010;**7**:4281–4304.

59. McKenzie R, Fried MW, Sallie R, et al. Hepatic failure and lactic acidosis due to fialuridine (FIAU), an investigational nucleoside analogue for chronic hepatitis B. *N Engl J Med* 1995;**333**:1099–1105.

60. Apostolova N, Blas-Garcia A, Esplugues JV. Mitochondrial interference by anti-HIV drugs: mechanisms beyond Pol-gamma inhibition. *Trends Pharmacol Sci* 2011;**32**:715–725.

61. Sokol RJ, Winklhofer-Roob BM, Devereaux MW, McKim JM Jr. Generation of hydroperoxides in isolated rat hepatocytes and hepatic mitochondria exposed to hydrophobic bile acids. *Gastroenterology* 1995;**109**:1249–1256.

62. Serviddio G, Sastre J, Bellanti F, Vina J, Vendemiale G, Altomare E. Mitochondrial involvement in non-alcoholic steatohepatitis. *Mol Aspects Med* 2008;**29**(1–2):22–35.

63. Munnich A, Rotig A, Chretien D, et al. Clinical presentation of mitochondrial disorders in childhood. *J Inherit Metab Dis* 1996;**19**:521–527.

64. Rustin P, Chretien D, Bourgeron T, et al. Biochemical and molecular investigations in respiratory chain deficiencies. *Clin Chim Acta* 1994;**228**:35–51.

65. Munnich A, Rotig A, Chretien D, et al. Clinical presentations and laboratory investigations in respiratory chain deficiency. *Eur J Pediatr* 1996;**155**: 262–274.

66. Friedman SD, Shaw DW, Ishak G, Gropman AL, Saneto RP. The use of neuroimaging in the diagnosis of mitochondrial disease. *Dev Disabil Res Reviews* 2010;**16**:129–135.

67. Zhang W, Cui H, Wong LJ. Comprehensive one-step molecular analyses of mitochondrial genome by massively parallel sequencing. *Clin Chem* 2012;**58**:1322–1331.

68. Pfeffer G, Majamaa K, Turnbull DM, Thorburn D, Chinnery PF. Treatment for mitochondrial disorders. *Cochrane Database Syst Rev* 2012;(4): CD004426.

69. Taylor RW, Chinnery PF, Clark KM, Lightowlers RN, Turnbull DM. Treatment of mitochondrial disease. *J Biogenet Biomemb* 1997;**29**:195–205.

70. Suomalainen A. Therapy for mitochondrial disorders: little proof, high research activity, some promise. *Semin Fetal Neonatal Med* 2011;**16**: 236–240.

71. Sokal EM, Sokol R, Cormier V, et al. Liver transplantation in mitochondrial respiratory chain disorders. *Eur J Pediatr* 1999;**158**(Suppl 2):S81–S84.

72. Yamada Y, Harashima H. Delivery of bioactive molecules to the mitochondrial genome using a membrane-fusing, liposome-based

carrier, DF-MITO-Porter. *Biomaterials* 2012;**33**:1589–1595.

73. Tachibana M, Amato P, Sparman M, *et al*. Towards germline gene therapy of inherited mitochondrial diseases. *Nature* 2013;**493**:627–631.

74. Bredenoord AL, Pennings G, Smeets HJ, de Wert G. Dealing with uncertainties: ethics of prenatal diagnosis and preimplantation genetic diagnosis to prevent mitochondrial disorders. *Hum Reprod Update* 2008;**14**:83–94.

75. Sokol RJ, Treem WR. Mitochondria and childhood liver diseases. *J Pediatr Gastroenterol Nutr* 1999;**28**:4–16.

Chapter

36

Non-alcoholic fatty liver disease in children

Rohit Kohli, Kevin E. Bove, and Stavra A. Xanthakos

Introduction

Non-alcoholic fatty liver disease (NAFLD) is now considered to be the most common cause of liver disease in both adults and children in the USA because of its strong association with the epidemic rates of obesity across all age groups. Originally considered predominantly to be a disease of developed countries with affluent and sedentary lifestyles, NAFLD has emerged in the last decade as a significant cause of liver disease worldwide, even in developing economies [1]. Increasing industrialization and commercial globalization in Asia, South America, and the Middle East have led to significant population shifts toward more western dietary habits and reduced energy expenditure, which, in turn, have increased the prevalence of overweight and obesity, and led to the identification of NAFLD as a common cause of liver disease [2].

While diverse conditions can lead to abnormal hepatic steatosis, defined as steatosis in >5% of hepatocytes, NAFLD is predominantly associated with excess adiposity, in particular central adiposity, and occurs in the absence of significant alcohol intake. It can be found in lean individuals but typically they too have significant visceral adiposity or severe insulin resistance syndromes, such as lipodystrophy [3].

The term NAFLD encompasses a spectrum of fatty liver disease, ranging from bland steatosis to steatohepatitis (referred to as non-alcoholic steatohepatitis (NASH)). Non-alcoholic steatohepatitis is a potentially progressive and clinically more serious form of NAFLD that occurs when hepatic steatosis triggers overt hepatocyte injury including ballooning degeneration and apoptosis, occurrence of lobular and/or portal inflammation, and the development of varying degrees of fibrosis. In large cohort studies of patients diagnosed with NAFLD, 75% usually have bland steatosis with minimal inflammation and/or isolated mild fibrosis but lacking definitive histopathological features of NASH. Depending on the cohort examined, bona-fide NASH appears to affect up to 25% of patients with NAFLD, and of these 10–20% may progress to severe fibrosis or cirrhosis [4,5]. Therefore, an estimated 2–5% of patients with NAFLD may progress to severe fibrosis or cirrhosis.

Because a relatively small percentage of patients with NAFLD develop clinically significant fibrosis, the public health impact of NAFLD is often vigorously debated. However, given the global rise of epidemic obesity, the increasing prevalence of NAFLD worldwide is likely to herald a significant increase in rates of end-stage liver disease and liver-related mortality in coming decades; this will place ever greater stress on an inadequate supply of livers for transplantation. In fact, the proportion of liver transplantation performed for NASH-related cirrhosis in the USA alone has increased six-fold since the end of the 1990s. The looming impact of the current pediatric burden of NASH on subsequent generations of adults with liver disease remains to be determined. In the absence of easily implemented, widely effective pharmacotherapy, pediatric NASH is likely to contribute to an increasing rate of end-stage liver disease in future generations. Although the consequences of hepatic steatosis, particularly when clinically silent in many individuals, may initially seem trivial in relationship to other pediatric liver diseases with more overt and acute complications during infancy and childhood, pediatric NASH rightly constitutes a significant public health burden whose prevention and treatment in childhood urgently need to be addressed.

Epidemiology: a worldwide problem

Determining an accurate population-based prevalence of the histological spectrum of NAFLD remains elusive, as a liver biopsy is required to distinguish between non-NASH NAFLD and NASH and is understandably implausible in epidemiological studies. The most robust population estimate of pediatric NAFLD prevalence in the USA is based on a 2006 analysis of specimens derived from autopsies of 742 children who suffered accidental death between 1993 and 2003 in San Diego County [6]. There was an overall prevalence of 13% for fatty liver, defined as ≥5% of hepatocytes containing macrovesicular fat, with the highest prevalence (17.3%) in adolescents aged 15–19 years. A disproportionately higher proportion of Hispanic (11.8%), Asian (10.2%), and white non-Hispanic children (8.6%) were affected compared with black non-Hispanic

Table 36.1 Epidemiological studies of non-alcoholic fatty liver disease prevalence in children

Study	No.	Cohort description	Definition of NAFLD	Prevalence estimates
USA (Schwimmer et al., 2006) [6]	742	Autopsy-based studies of children after accidental death in San Diego County	>5% macrovesicular steatosis	13% in cohort, 10% adjusted for BMI, age, gender, race
USA (Fraser et al., 2007) [8]	5586	NHANES 1999–2004, ages 12–19 years	ALT >30 U/L	8%
USA (Strauss et al., 2000) [9]	2450	NHANES 1988–1994, ages 12–18 years	ALT >30 U/L	3.2%
Iran (Alavian et al., 2009) [10]	966	School children, ages 7–18 years	Sonographic steatosis	7.1%
Korea (Park et al., 2005) [11]	1594	Korea National Health and Nutrition Examination Survey 1998, ages 10–19 years	ALT >40 U/L	3.2% overall; 3.6% boys, 2.8% girls
Japan (Tominaga et al., 1995) [12]	825	Northern Japanese children, 4–12 years	Sonographic steatosis	2.6%
China (Meng et al., 2011) [13]	1452	Beijing school children, 7–17 years	Sonographic steatosis	6.8% boys, 2.3% girls
Australia (Booth et al., 2008) [14]	500	Population sample of 15-year-old school children from Sydney	ALT >32 U/L for boys, >20 U/L for girls	9% for boys, 5.3% for girls

BMI, body mass index; NAFLD, non-alcoholic fatty liver disease; NHANES, National Health and Nutrition Examination Survey.

children (1.5%). In comparison, an estimated 31% of 2287 adult participants from the Dallas Heart Study were found to have abnormal hepatic steatosis by MR spectroscopy [7]. Similarly, a disproportionately higher proportion of Hispanic (45%) and white adults (33%) were affected than black adults (24%), although the prevalence of abnormal steatosis in black participants was much larger than that found in the pediatric study (1.5%). Of the pediatric autopsy-based cohort with fatty liver, 23% had NASH, yielding an overall prevalence of NASH of 3% [6]. Because a relatively small percentage of adults and children with fatty liver develop steatohepatitis, there is likely an underlying genetic susceptibility to developing liver injury in response to steatosis in some individuals, whereas others are able to tolerate even large deposits of fat in the liver without developing a significant inflammatory or fibrotic reaction.

As the regional San Diego adolescent population was disproportionately Hispanic compared with the general USA, the authors subsequently adjusted the autopsy-derived estimate of 13% for age, gender, race, and ethnicity, yielding an overall estimated 10% prevalence of pediatric fatty liver disease in the USA. While this is the only pediatric population estimate based on histology, there are also several other pediatric population-based studies using serum alanine aminotransferase (ALT) levels and/or sonography as a screening measure, summarized in Table 36.1; the prevalence of presumed NAFLD ranging from 2.6 to 8% in various countries, with the highest prevalence reported in the USA [8].

Limitations of using serum ALT to screen for NAFLD are numerous and significant, but because it is inexpensive, minimally invasive, and widely available, it is still the most commonly used both clinically and in research. Significant limitations include that serum ALT can be normal even in

the presence of significant NAFLD, nearly a quarter of children with histological NAFLD may have a normal serum ALT, and up to 60% of these may even have fibrosis [15]. Elevations of serum ALT are also not specific for NAFLD but can indicate a range of other possible causes of hepatitis, which need to be excluded before considering an abnormal value to be an indicator of NAFLD. The definition of abnormal ALT also varies widely across different laboratories and populations. Local reference ranges for ALT are often calculated using regional populations that were not screened for silent liver disease, such as viral hepatitis, or obesity/overweight. As a consequence, many laboratory ranges for abnormal are set high and may miss clinically significant liver disease. In adults, for example, an upper limit of normal for ALT (defined as ≥95th percentile) derived from lean healthy Italian males and females was found to be 30 U/L and 19 U/L, respectively. Similarly, the 95th percentile upper limit of normal for ALT in 982 metabolically normal, healthy weight adolescents aged 12–19 years in an National Health and Nutrition Examination Survey (NHANES) was found to be 25.8 U/L for boys and 22.1 U/L for girls, far below the upper limits of normal typically derived in regional clinical laboratories (range 30–90 U/L in a representative survey) [16]. In most previously published studies using ALT as a screen for NAFLD, the defined abnormal level has ranged from >30 U/L to >40 U/L, which may have led to under-reporting of true population-based prevalence of fatty liver. An important caveat of using lower thresholds for abnormal ALT in epidemiological studies is that it will improve the sensitivity for detection of NAFLD but lower the specificity for NASH. In adult women, using lower criteria (ALT >19 U/L versus ALT >30 U/L) to define abnormal levels did improve the sensitivity for NASH from 42% to 74% but lowered specificity from 80% to 42% [17]. Applying the biologically derived cut-offs for pediatric ALT values to cohorts of children with documented hepatitis B or C infection and NAFLD doubled sensitivity for NAFLD to 85–92%, while only moderately decreasing specificity from 92% to 80–85% [16].

Across all screening modalities, the prevalence of NAFLD is strongly associated with increasing obesity, with the San Diego County autopsy study demonstrating a seven-fold rise in NAFLD prevalence as obesity increased, from 5% in normal, to 16% in overweight, and to 38% in obese children [6]. Varying rates of abnormally elevated serum ALT have been detected in cohorts of obese children ranging from 10% to 25%. Higher estimates, approximately 40–50% prevalence, were found using ultrasonographic evidence of fatty liver as the screening method. Limited data exist on the prevalence of NAFLD in extremely obese children (body mass index (BMI) >99th percentile). Only 17% of over 16 000 extremely obese adolescents in a cohort of children and adolescents attending 111 weight management programs across Germany, Austria, and Switzerland had an ALT and/or aspartate aminotransferase (AST) >50 U/L, while 34 of 41 severely obese adolescents (83%; BMI >59 kg/m^2) undergoing bariatric surgery were found to have histologic NAFLD, with only 29% having abnormal liver enzymes, defined as ALT >45 U/L for males and >35 U/L for females [18].

Additional risk factors for NAFLD identified in multiple population-based as well as smaller cohort studies include increasing insulin resistance, Hispanic/Mexican-American ethnicity, male gender, and waist circumference [6]. In one cohort of 134 multiethnic obese children, Hispanic children tended to present with NAFLD at younger ages, with 17.5% of Hispanic boys first diagnosed at younger than 7 years of age. In addition, older age, elevated serum C-reactive protein and triglyceride levels were also positively associated with elevated serum ALT in a pediatric NHANES analysis. Many of these same clinical and demographic risk factors are also associated with increased histological severity or risk of fibrotic NASH in children, including older age, elevated triglyceride levels, Hispanic or Asian ethnicity, male gender, waist circumference, markers of insulin resistance, and elevated blood pressure [15,19,20]. Elevated fasting triglyceride and glucose levels, waist circumference, hypertension, and obesity are considered components of the metabolic syndrome. Of these, increased waist circumference was the only component independently associated with liver fibrosis in a cohort of 197 Caucasian children aged 3–19 years with biopsy-confirmed NAFLD in Italy [19]. However, obese children with the metabolic syndrome are five times as likely to have any spectrum of NAFLD compared with obese children lacking the metabolic syndrome. The association of features of the metabolic syndrome with histological severity of NAFLD in children, in particular fibrosis, is aligned with data in adults that also suggest that metabolic syndrome increases odds of having severe fibrosis by 3.5-fold. Both prevalence and severity of NAFLD appears to be decreased in black obese children, despite a high prevalence of obesity and other cardiovascular disease risk factors.

Risk of liver disease progression has been difficult to calculate accurately since estimation of fibrosis requires a liver biopsy, and large-scale prospective natural history studies with serial biopsy data in children and adults have not yet been published. However, a pooled analysis of 10 small case series in adults with longitudinal follow-up biopsies has estimated that up to 37% of adults with NASH may develop progressive fibrosis over a wide range of follow-up (1–21 years), with a smaller percentage (15–20%) developing severe fibrosis within a decade. Once cirrhosis develops, the risk of mortality does not appear to differ when compared with hepatitis C virus-associated cirrhosis [21]. Hepatocellular carcinoma can evolve from fibrotic NASH, even in the absence of cirrhosis in some cases but appears to occur less frequently than in hepatitis C virus-related liver disease [21,22]. Several small case series in children document that fibrosis progression can occur even during childhood, with progression to cirrhosis occurring in as short a time span as 2 years in some cases [23,24]. In adult series, potential clinical predictors of progression include more pronounced insulin resistance, progressive weight gain, age, and inflammation. Prognostic indicators in childhood remain unknown because of the small sample size of reported cases.

The overall impact of NAFLD on mortality remains unclear, with inconsistent results in adults and lack of any data in children. Initial studies in regional referral cohorts of adults suggested that NAFLD conferred a higher risk for overall mortality and liver-related mortality compared with reference general populations. In a community-based Minnesota study of 420 adults diagnosed with NAFLD between 1980 and 2000, predominantly by imaging studies, overall survival was lower than expected compared with the general population, with a standardized mortality ratio of 1.34 (95% confidence interval (CI), 1.003–1.760; $p = 0.03$) [5]. Liver disease was the third leading cause of death, occurring in 13% of those who died, compared with the 13th leading cause in the general population. The two leading causes of death were malignancy and ischemic heart disease (28% and 25% of the deceased, respectively). Independent risk factors for death were age, impaired fasting glucose, and cirrhosis, but the authors did not adjust for confounders despite the strong association of NAFLD with insulin resistance, central obesity, diabetes, and lipid abnormalities. In a study of 131 adults with biopsy-proven NAFLD from the Cleveland Clinic, 78 (59.5%) died over a median follow-up period of 18.5 years, with maximum follow-up of 28.5 years. The three most common causes of death were coronary artery disease, malignancy, and liver-related death. Those with NASH had a significantly higher liver-related mortality (17.5%) than those with non-NASH NAFLD (2.7%, $p = 0.005$). Independent predictors of liver-related death were histologic NASH at time of initial biopsy, diabetes mellitus type 2, older age at biopsy, lower serum albumin, and increased serum levels of alkaline phosphatase (all $p < 0.05$). Independent predictors of overall mortality were type 2 diabetes, older age at biopsy, lower serum albumin, and higher serum glucose.

While these regional cohort studies raise concern for a heightened risk of death in patients with NAFLD, and in particular for those with NASH, three of four national cohort studies in subjects drawn from NHANES III and using recommended stratified analysis methodology did not find an overall increased risk of all-cause mortality associated with NAFLD. Different cut-off values of abnormal ALT were used to define NAFLD in the studies and ultrasound was also used to define steatosis in a third, which accounts in part for different numbers of subjects. An analysis of 980 patients with suspected NAFLD and 6594 patients without NAFLD, with a mean of 8.7 years of follow-up, found no statistically significant increase in overall mortality for the entire cohort with NAFLD [25]. However, in a subgroup of patients aged 45–54 years, suspected NAFLD was associated with higher all-cause mortality (hazard ratio (HR), 4.40; 95% CI, 1.27–13.23) and cardiovascular mortality (HR, 8.15; 95% CI, 2.0–33.2), after adjusting for conventional cardiovascular disease risk factors. No statistically significant increase in overall mortality was associated with elevated serum ALT in overweight, although elevated ALT was associated with increased liver-related death [26]. The most recent analysis drawn from NHANES III, and stratifying patients into those with and without sonographic evidence of steatosis and those with and without increased liver enzymes, also found no statistically significant increased risk of death from all causes, cardiovascular disease, or liver disease. The lack of an impact of NAFLD on overall mortality has also been supported by a large cohort study of patients in Denmark. Limitations of all of these studies include a relatively short period of follow-up from time of initial diagnosis, and lack of biopsy data to differentiate between NASH and non-NASH NAFLD.

Even though the presence of presumed NAFLD does not appear to confer an increased risk of overall mortality, it remains clearly associated with features of the metabolic syndrome and may independently confer a higher risk of cardiovascular disease, including increased carotid intima media thickness in adults. Ominously, children with NAFLD also have a significantly higher prevalence of the metabolic syndrome than obese children without evidence of NAFLD (50% and 15%, respectively; $p < 0.001$). In 100 obese children with NAFLD confirmed by ultrasound and elevated liver enzymes with exclusion of other causes, flow-mediated dilation of the brachial artery was significantly impaired and carotid intima media thickness significantly greater than in 150 obese children without evidence of NAFLD [27]. Children with NAFLD had 2.25 times the risk of low percentage flow-mediated dilatation and two times the risk of increased carotid intima media thickness, after adjusting for age, gender, Tanner stage, and presence of metabolic syndrome [27]. The independent associations of carotid intima media thickness with NAFLD, BMI, waist circumference, and systolic blood pressure (all $p \leq 0.005$) were also confirmed in a population-based study of 642 adolescents aged 11–13 years in southern Italy [28]. The increased presence of these preclinical markers of atherosclerosis suggests that these children are likely to face high rates of cardiovascular events in the future, in accordance with adult data.

Pathogenesis

Given the global disease burden and accumulating epidemiological data since the early 1990s, the pathophysiology of NAFLD has been extensively investigated in both animal and human studies. While the factors that have fueled this epidemic, including our increasingly sedentary lifestyle and easy and cheaply available calorie-dense processed foods, are clear for all to see, it is the disproportionate morbidity across various clinical subgroups, races, and ethnicities that has energized moves to improve understanding of the pathogenic risk factors involved in NAFLD progression [23]. It is now clear that not all NAFLD is created equal. While steatosis alone has been associated with insulin resistance and type 2 diabetes, the presence of NASH at diagnosis has been linked to a higher risk of hastened progression, end-stage liver disease, and need for liver transplantation. Therefore, the primary focus of recent research into pathogenesis of NASH has been to distinguish between the various constituents of the NAFLD spectrum, including steatosis alone and more advanced NASH, and then to understand the key drivers of these differences.

Lipids and the non-alcoholic fatty liver disease spectrum

Puri *et al.* [29] first performed lipidomic analysis of the NAFLD spectrum in adults and reported that the mean triacylglycerol to diacylglycerol ratios were higher in NASH than in steatotic or normal livers (31, 26, and 7, respectively). There was also a similar stepwise increment in hepatic free cholesterol, which was significantly increased in NASH, while the free cholesterol to total phosphatidylcholine ratio increased progressively (0.34, 0.69, and 0.71, respectively) [29]. A follow-up study of plasma lipodomic profiles in adults revealed a stepwise increase in the lipoxygenase "HEPE" metabolites 5-(S)-, 8(S)-, and 15(S)-hydroxyeicosatetraenoic acid that characterized a progression from normal to steatosis to NASH. The level of 11(S)-hydroxyeicosatetraenoic acid, a non-enzymatic oxidation product of arachidonic (20:4) acid, was significantly increased in NASH alone. Parallel lipidomic analysis of murine and human liver tissues determined that mice maintained on a high-fat or high-fat high-carbohydrate diet provide a reproducible model of progressive liver disease. These studies demonstrated that lipid species may serve as markers of advanced liver disease and, importantly, marked increases in diacylglycerol species and oxidative stress markers such as oxidized coenzyme Q could be hallmarks of NASH with fibrosis [30]. There is now growing direct lipidomic data in children as well; suggesting increased total cholesterol, low density lipoprotein (LDL) cholesterol, and triglycerides in children with the NAFLD spectrum. There is also a correlation between worsening atherogenic profile and biopsy-proven NASH when compared with steatosis alone [31]. Similarly, a pilot study linked the increased intake of fructose to plasma oxidized LDL levels in children. The impact of dietary constituents on the NAFLD spectrum disorders is discussed in more detail below. These data together lead to the conclusion that oxidative stress-related liver injury, possibly through increased diacylglycerol species, is involved in progression of isolated steatosis to NASH.

Mitochondria and endoplasmic reticulum stress

It has now been well described that mitochondrial damage occurs in human NAFLD. Sanyal et al. [32] reported that there was loss of mitochondrial cristae and paracrystalline inclusions in 9 of 10 subjects with NASH, compared with 0 of 6 subjects with steatosis alone. Terminal deoxynucleotidyl transferase dUTP nick end labeling (TUNEL) detects DNA fragmentation; TUNEL-positive cells denoting cell death from apoptosis, potentially from mitochondrial injury, were significantly increased in liver biopsy specimens from patients with NASH compared with those simple steatosis and controls. Unexpectedly, TUNEL-positive cells were also greater in patients with NASH than in those with alcoholic hepatitis. Immunohistochemistry demonstrated active caspases 3 and 7 in NASH specimens, confirming the occurrence of apoptosis in this disease [33]. Further, this ongoing mitochondrial damage may be associated with reactive oxygen species release and progression of disease to more severe forms [34]. Endoplasmic reticulum stress associated with the unfolded protein response has also been shown to be more characteristic of liver biopsies from patients with NASH compared with those with normal liver histology or steatosis alone. Specifically, mRNA expression for C/EBP homologous protein (CHOP) and protein-content activated Janus-N kinase (known endoplasmic reticulum stress downstream elements) were increased in patients with NASH (Figure 36.1).

Genes and the non-alcoholic fatty liver disease spectrum

Multiple genome-wide associations and other genetic studies of adults have now validated the impact of genetic polymorphisms on disease severity and even heritability within the NAFLD spectrum. The gene that has the strongest association with NAFLD progression is PNPLA3, encoding the patatin-like phospholipase domain-containing protein 3 (acylglycerol O-acyltransferase). There is mounting evidence that polymorphisms in this gene modify the natural history of NAFLD in adults. Two recent meta-analyses concluded that the effect of the GG (I148M; rs738409) allele was to increase fat accumulation in the liver. Homozygosity GG increased necro-inflammatory histological scores (3.24-fold higher) and risk

of developing fibrosis (3.2-fold higher) when compared with CC homozygous individuals. Further, the same rs738409 GG genotype versus the CC genotype was associated with a 28% increase in serum ALT [36]. These disease-modifying PNPLA3 polymorphisms are most frequently found in the Hispanic population, a group at higher risk of NASH, and are significantly less common within the African-American population, who appear to be relatively protected from hepatic steatosis and NASH. These adult PNPLA3 data have now also been reproduced in pediatric cohorts. The prevalence of the G allele was found to be higher in a multiethnic cohort of obese children and adolescents with hepatic steatosis, as determined by MRI [37]. Another study from Italy, with 149 children with biopsy-proven NAFLD (6–13 years of age), reported the PNPLA3 rs738409 polymorphism to be associated with severity of steatosis, hepatocellular ballooning, lobular inflammation, and perivenular fibrosis [38].

Another gene that has been studied as a modifier of NAFLD progression is APOC3, encoding apolipoprotein C3. In a cohort of healthy young Asian-Indian men, carriers of the APOC3 variant alleles (C482T, T455C, or both) had a 38% rate of NAFLD, even though their mean BMI was <25, while none of the wild-type homozygotes had NAFLD [39]. The data regarding the influence of APOC3 polymorphisms are not that clear in children. A study of 455 obese children failed to find any association between the APOC3 gene variants and hepatic steatosis [37].

Similarly, genes regulating oxidative stress pathways have been implicated in studies in adult and pediatric NAFLD. A common non-synonymous polymorphism in SOD2, encoding an antioxidant superoxide dismutase 2 (C47T; rs4880) was found to be associated with more advanced fibrosis in NASH with an odds ratio of 1.56 [40]. In a study of 234 obese Taiwanese children, a variant (UGT1A1*6) in UGT1A1, encoding a UDP-glucuronosyltransferase, is associated with higher relative rates of plasma bilirubin levels and was protective against NAFLD [41].

Nutrigenomics

It is clear that nutritional intake influences the prevalence and outcomes of NAFLD, a disease closely linked to excess caloric intake and adiposity. As discussed above, there are genetic factors that can predispose an individual or particular ethnic group to worsening insults from similar or fewer nutritional mal-influences. It is, therefore, important to understand these nutrient insults and their mechanism of liver injury in the NAFLD spectrum.

A nutritional constituent that has received much attention and research is fructose. The impact of overall excess caloric intake is, of course, the underlying insult that produces obesity. An analysis of BMI, gender, calorie intake, and age-matched patients from the NASH clinical research network database (https://www.jhucct.com/nash) indicated that increased fructose consumption was associated with lower

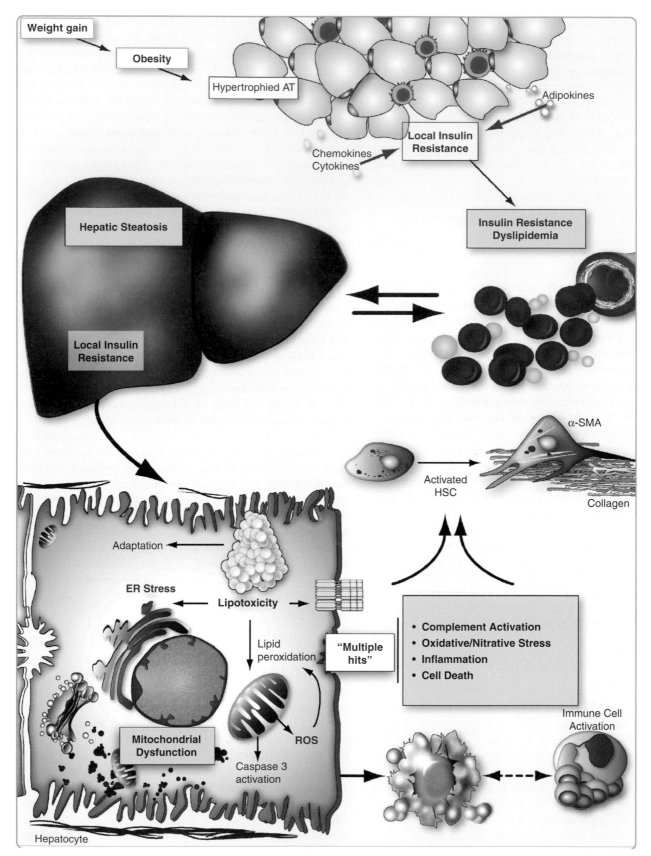

Figure 36.1 Pathogenesis of non-alcoholic fatty liver disease (NAFLD)–non-alcoholic steatohepatitis (NASH). Weight gain and obesity result in adipose tissue (AT) expansion and infiltration by macrophages with development of local insulin resistance and release of free fatty acids (FFA) into circulation.

steatosis grade and higher fibrosis stage [42]. A further study of children using the same database showed that uric acid, a surrogate for total fructose consumption, was significantly associated with biopsy-proven NASH [43]. Interestingly, this study did not report significant differences in overall energy consumed from fat, carbohydrates, and protein in children with steatosis alone or NASH. Therefore, fructose consumption itself seems to be an independent predictor of more severe disease (NASH) within the NAFLD spectrum.

Other than fructose, sugar-sweetened beverages as a whole have been linked to obesity in general and metabolic syndrome in particular through database studies such as NHANES [43]. Natural compounds have also been thought of as treatment options for NAFLD, as discussed below.

Nature versus nurture

Studies implicate both genetic and environmental influences on the progression and severity of NAFLD spectrum disorders. Initially a "two-hit" hypothesis had been proposed wherein the presence of steatosis was the first hit and then a "hypothesized" second hit would promote progression of the liver injury. This hypothesis was revised recently to now consider a "multiple parallel hit" hypothesis, which includes an understanding of the importance of "nature" and our genetic susceptibilities. We believe that this may be a more accurate portrayal of the pathogenesis of NAFLD spectrum disorders and, therefore, answers the conundrum as to why certain individuals with hepatic steatosis are protected from progressing to severe liver disease compared with others who are more predisposed to disease progression, fibrosis, cirrhosis, and liver-related morbidity [23].

Clinical diagnostic and prognostic tools

Clinically, the spectrum of NAFLD remains challenging to diagnose and monitor as it is often clinically silent with few overt signs and symptoms in children, even in patients with NASH. The most commonly reported symptoms in children are abdominal pain and fatigue [24]. In some cases, a complaint of abdominal pain prompts imaging studies that identify abnormal hepatic steatosis and lead to referral. The most common physical signs include obesity, in particular central adiposity, hepatomegaly, acanthosis nigricans, and splenomegaly [24]. However, NAFLD can also present in thin individuals with severe insulin resistance caused by lipodystrophy or in

individuals who have centralized obesity but an overall normal BMI [1,3]. In childhood, NAFLD presenting with overt jaundice and signs of end-stage liver disease is very rare, with one case report of an Hispanic girl aged 11 years who had grade 3 esophageal varices and cirrhotic NASH [24]. She subsequently underwent liver transplantation at age 20 years, which to our knowledge is the youngest reported case of the use of transplantation for NASH diagnosed in childhood. There have also been case reports of two children who developed cirrhosis at ages 10 and 14, with one child progressing to portal hypertension and variceal bleeding within 2 years of diagnosis.

Many patients with NAFLD are first identified by elevated ALT or AST found incidentally or during screening of an overweight and obese child for comorbid conditions. The American Academy of Pediatrics Expert Committee Recommendations Regarding the Prevention, Assessment and Treatment of Child and Adolescent Overweight and Obesity suggests that, in the current absence of evidence-based recommendations for screening, biannual screening of ALT and AST should begin at age 10 for children with BMI ≥95th percentile and in children with BMI of 85–94th percentile if other cardiovascular disease risk factors are present [44]. The degree of implementation of these screening recommendations among pediatric practitioners is not known. Further, after identification of hepatic steatosis on imaging studies or persistently elevated serum aminotransferases, subsequent referral patterns to pediatric gastroenterology and hepatology specialists are difficult to ascertain.

Associated medical conditions that appear to confer a higher risk of NAFLD include insulin resistance and diabetes mellitus type 2, polycystic ovarian syndrome, hypertriglyceridemia, hypothalamic obesity, lipodystrophy, and possibly obstructive sleep apnea. A thorough screening should be done in any patient diagnosed with NAFLD or NASH, as many children may be unaware that they have such concomitant illnesses as:

- viral hepatitis: hepatitis C
- autoimmune hepatitis
- storage diseases:
  - Wilson disease
  - hemochromatosis
- alcohol abuse
- metabolic diseases
  - glycogen storage diseases
  - abetalipoproteinemia and hypobetalipoproteinemia

Figure 36.1 (*cont.*) These events are thought to be critical for the development of hepatic steatosis, which, in turn, contributes to local hepatic insulin resistance. Early in the disease process, the liver adapts to excess FFA; however, over time, these adaptive mechanisms fail, resulting in lipotoxicity. Lipotoxicity can trigger multiple deleterious pathways in hepatocytes including endoplasmic reticulum (ER) stress, upregulation of death receptors, and mitochondrial dysfunction. As a consequence, there is increased production of a wide variety of reactive oxygen, nitrogen, and lipid species, which dysregulate multiple redox-sensitive signaling pathways leading to further increase in triglyceride accumulation. The ensuing disruption of mitochondrial function triggers caspase activation and cell death: key "hits" in the progression to NASH. In conjunction, release of reactive species from hepatocytes can trigger activation of immune cells and convert the normally quiescent stellate cells to a fibrosis-inducing cell. This combination of events that are critical for the progression from steatosis to steatohepatitis to fibrosis is present to different extents in the various animal models that were more commonly used to study NAFLD and NASH. HSC, hepatic stellate cells; ROS, reactive oxygen species; α-SMA, alpha-smooth muscle actin. (Reproduced with permission from Kohli *et al.*, 2011 [35].)

- lipodystrophy
- cystic fibrosis
- urea cycle disorders
- fatty acid transport and oxidation disorders
- carnitine deficiency
- oxidative phosphorylation disorders
- Reye syndrome
- medication toxicity:
  - glucocorticoids
  - high-dose estrogen
  - valproic acid
  - amiodarone
  - aspirin-induced Reye syndrome (postviral)
- parenteral nutrition
- collagen vascular disorders: juvenile rheumatoid arthritis (often medication induced)
- nutritional intake
  - malnutrition
  - starvation
  - kwashiorkor
  - malabsorptive disorders.

Identification often requires further specific therapy for these conditions.

Anthropometrics

The presence of metabolic syndrome is quite high in children with NAFLD, up to a 50–66% prevalence found in large single center cohort studies in both the USA and Italy [15]. Metabolic syndrome has been shown to be associated with central adiposity, and waist circumference has been found to be predictive of worsening and progression of obesity comorbidities. A study of 201 obese children in the context of NAFLD spectrum disorders found that increased waist–hip ratio was associated with elevated serum aminotransferases [45]. Higher metabolic and cardiovascular risks are associated with higher waist-to-height ratios in obese children [46]. The strongest evidence to date linking anthropometric measures and histological severity of NAFLD came from the work of Manco *et al.* [19], who have reported data from a study of 197 Caucasian children 3–19 years of age showing that increasing waist circumference correlated with biopsy-proven liver fibrosis. Nobili *et al.* [47] validated a combination of non-invasive markers and reported them collectively as the Pediatric NAFLD fibrosis index (PNFI) in 141 children with fibrosis on liver biopsy. They proposed a final model based on age, waist circumference, and triglycerides, in which a PNFI ≥9 had an area under the receiver operating characteristic (ROC) curve of 0.85 for the prediction of liver fibrosis, within their cohort (positive likelihood ratio, 28.6). Therefore, anthropometric measures may be useful as clinical discriminators individually or as part of expanded diagnostic panels to discriminate need for liver biopsy.

Routine laboratory tests

Routine hepatic laboratory measures (serum aminotransferases) have been used as primary screening tools to identify obese individuals at risk of NAFLD. Unfortunately, it became clear early on that these measures alone are grossly insensitive in identifying NAFLD spectrum disorders in children. Children with biopsy-proven NASH can have normal liver enzymes. Therefore, serum ALT alone cannot be taken as a reliable indicator of NAFLD/NASH. Further, repeated measures of ALT can fluctuate. In an analysis of randomized placebo-controlled therapeutic clinical trials of adults with NAFLD/NASH, it was shown that even placebo administration can be associated with a decrease in serum ALT [48]. The conclusion from this analysis of five randomized trials with 162 placebo-treated and 189 active-treatment patients was that serum ALT is not a reliable measure of treatment response. Patton *et al.* [49] examined components of routine laboratory tests predictive of NAFLD pattern and fibrosis severity but found them not to have adequate discriminate power to replace liver biopsy in evaluating pediatric NAFLD. They prospectively studied children enrolled in the NASH Clinical Research Network who underwent a liver biopsy and reviewed their clinical data. They identified 176 children and determined that an area under the ROC curve for a model with AST and ALT was 0.75 (95% CI, 0.66–0.84) and 0.74 (95% CI, 0.63–0.85) for distinguishing steatosis from advanced NASH and bridging fibrosis from lesser degrees of fibrosis, respectively. Similar correlations were seen with serum ALT and rising free fatty acid and triglyceride content in the liver as assessed by MRI in a study of obese adolescents.

Finally, as mentioned above, there is no standard, outcome-based reference range for serum ALT that is universally accepted by all laboratories, such as exists for abnormal lipid values in adults. Biologically derived, the 95th percentile ALT thresholds for healthy weight, metabolically normal, and liver disease-free adolescents participating in NHANES were found to be 22 U/L and 26 U/L for females and males, respectively, which suggests that regional laboratory reference ranges are often set too high [16]. However, using a biologically determined threshold as low as 22 U/L in girls and 26 U/L in boys to detect liver disease and initiate further testing has not yet undergone any cost-effectiveness analyses and may generate a barrage of unnecessary and expensive tests. Therefore, in our clinical practice, we routinely initiate additional screening for liver disease if ALT elevations are persistently >40 U/L – roughly 1.5 to 2 times the upper limit of normal suggested by the NHANES analysis – on at least two measurements 1 month apart. Some studies have also suggested that elevated serum AST and gamma-glutamyltransferase (GGT) correlate better with fibrosis and/or improvement after weight loss, but the significance of isolated mild serum AST and GGT elevations in the absence of elevated ALT is less certain [50]. When persistent elevations in ALT are identified, and in some contexts AST and GGT, it is important to exclude other potential causes of chronic hepatitis, including viral hepatitis (B, C and also A if indicated), autoimmune hepatitis, drug or alcohol injury, Wilson disease, hemochromatosis, and celiac disease through appropriate serological testing as well as by clinical history and physical examination. Basically, routine serum aminotransferases continue to guide practitioners in the evaluation of NAFLD but they cannot be used exclusively to screen and monitor progression across the NAFLD spectrum.

Research tests and panels

To address this lacuna in diagnosis, management, and monitoring, many investigators have attempted to develop unique tools to study and quantify changes within the NAFLD spectrum. These efforts have been tested in both adults and children, although a large section of this work has been led by pediatric hepatologists. One can speculate that this is driven by the increased perceived risk and cost of performing an invasive procedure such as a liver biopsy in a child. In 44 consecutive adults with suspected NAFLD at the time of liver biopsy, plasma cytokeratin-18 fragments (CK-18) were markedly increased in the patients with NASH [51]. A cut-off value of 395 U/L, calculated using the ROC curve approach, showed a specificity of 99.9%, a sensitivity of 85.7%, and positive and negative predictive values of 99.9% and 85.7%, respectively, for the diagnosis of NASH. Nobili *et al.* [47] used an enhanced liver fibrosis (ELF) test panel in a pediatric cohort. They analyzed 112 consecutive subjects that were likely to have NAFLD for levels of hyaluronic acid, N-terminal propeptide of type III collagen, and tissue inhibitor of metalloproteinase 1. The area under ROC curves/best possible ELF test cut-off values for the prediction of stages of fibrosis (1–3) were 0.92/9.28, 0.92/9.33, 0.90/9.54, 0.98/10.18, and 0.99/10.51, respectively, for "any" (≥1 stage), moderate–perisinusoidal (≥1b stage), moderate–portal/periportal (≥1c stage), significant (≥2 stage), or advanced (≥3 stage) [47]. The more anthropometric data-based PNFI and the ELF panel were tested in the same pediatric cohort and found to predict liver biopsy-proven fibrosis with an area under the ROC curves of 0.761 and 0.924, respectively, and 0.944 when combined [52]. Other tests, such as

assessing serum oxidized products of mitochondrial electron chain components, are currently under development [30]. These tests are not commercially available at present for use in routine patient care and require validation in larger cohorts of children in varied ethnic milieus before they can widely be adopted.

Imaging

In addition to the anthropometric and laboratory-based assessments outlined above, there are multiple imaging modalities available and under development that provide insight into the NAFLD spectrum disorders in children. Routine standard imaging such as ultrasound can identify moderate to significant hepatic steatosis. Ultrasound-based diagnostic criteria have been proposed for NAFLD. Unfortunately, beyond identifying steatosis, ultrasound alone cannot distinguish between the severity of the NAFLD spectrum, such as inflammation, and various stages of fibrosis. An important advancement in the use of sonographic imaging was the introduction of transient elastography (TE) technology. Ultrasound-based TE techniques have been tested in children with NAFLD spectrum disorders [53]. Values of at least 9 kPa have been shown to be associated with the presence of advanced fibrosis; values of 7–9 kPa were reported to predict fibrosis stages 1 or 2, but could not discriminate between these two stages. These findings have yet to be validated in larger cohorts, and interobserver variability and testing procedures for pediatric patients have still to be standardized.

Use of MR-based technologies has been established for fat quantification in children. The availability of these techniques has been helpful even for genetic studies where fat quantification by MR spectroscopy has been shown to correlate with deleterious genotypes for the single nucleotide polymorphism (rs738409), in *PNPLA3* in 85 obese youths [37]. Building from the ultrasound-based TE technology, a newer approach for the pediatric practitioner is MR-based elastography but this is still in a development stage. The premise is similar to ultrasound-based elastography but currently no pediatric norms or definitive data are available for NAFLD spectrum disorders. At our center, we have recently begun using this modality (Figure 36.2).

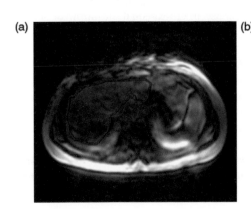
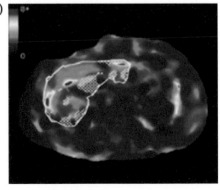

Figure 36.2 Magnetic resonance elastography. Images from a 14-year-old girl with body mass index of 28.13 kg/m² (97.51% for age) and mildly elevated liver enzymes (alanine aminotransferase 67 U/L, aspartate aminotransferase 30 U/L). (a) Axial T₂-weighted fat-saturation image. (b) Elastography image with increasing stiffness reflected by color spectrum 0–8. See intense 7–8 score in areas of the liver. (Images courtesy Daniel Podberesky MD and Suraj Serai PhD, Department of Radiology and Medical Imaging, Cincinnati Children's Hospital Medical Center, Cincinnati, OH, USA.)

Liver biopsy

Regardless of the initial screening modality, the liver biopsy remains the gold standard for diagnosis, staging, and prognosis for the NAFLD spectrum disorders. Long-term natural history and intervention studies continue to depend on this invasive technique to validate their results [50]. In five adult randomized placebo-controlled therapeutic trials for NASH, liver histological changes and a ≥2 point improvement were seen only in the therapeutic arms and not in the placebo arm [48]. Similarly, all studies attempting to validate novel biomarkers, imaging based or plasma based, rely on liver biopsy data for area under the curve and sensitivity/specificity calculations. Consequently, liver histology obtained by tissue biopsy continues to be the standard against which to test new diagnostic, prognostic, and therapeutic measures in NAFLD spectrum disorder studies. However, even this gold standard is hampered by limitations related to sampling error and intra- and inter-rater variability. In biopsies from 43 obese individuals undergoing bariatric procedures where the biopsies were obtained simultaneously from both the right and left lobes of the liver; the agreement for steatosis was 93%, for inflammation 74%, for fibrosis 98%, and for a NAFLD activity score ≥5 it was 93% [54]. Therefore, there is a clear limitation given the potential sampling error in this procedure particularly when quantifying inflammation.

In the absence of any consensus guidelines even among pediatric gastroenterologists and hepatologists on the appropriate use of liver biopsy in the evaluation and management of children with NAFLD, practice patterns vary considerably among different centers. Those opposed to routine liver biopsy often cite an unfavorable risk–benefit ratio, arguing that the chance of changing the diagnosis is low and that the lifestyle recommendations remain the same regardless of histological severity. However, increasing data are emerging about the severity of NAFLD spectrum in children and supporting the use of additional therapies for more aggressive and severe biopsy-proven NASH, as discussed under Treatment, below. Therefore, there may be a move toward more routine use of liver biopsy to help to stage and grade the disease and to evaluate risk for progression. Liver biopsy is also considered by some to be of even greater importance to definitively exclude other liver diseases, given the rise in pediatric obesity and greater potential for missing an overlap between NAFLD and a coexisting other liver disease, such as autoimmune hepatitis or Wilson disease. At our center, liver biopsy confirmation and staging is recommended where lifestyle management fails to significantly improve ALT elevations (and in some cases AST and GGT depending on clinical context) after a 3–6 month trial period (Figure 36.3).

The risk of liver biopsy, while not insignificant, remains low. In adults, the risk of death directly related to liver biopsy was approximately 1 in 10 000, or 0.0001, in an analysis of 61 187 adults undergoing liver biopsy in the National Health Service in the UK with only six episodes of major bleeding occurring per 1000 biopsies [55]. Liver biopsy mortality in children has not been estimated in any large-scale national study but has been estimated to be 0.6% from a retrospective study of 469 patients at our center; the three deaths in this cohort occurred in patients with cancer or bone marrow transplant, a subgroup also found to be at five-fold risk for significant bleeding requiring transfusion. Therefore, it is likely that the risk of liver biopsy in an otherwise healthy obese child is much lower than estimated by this study.

In respect to NAFLD, a valid and important consideration is whether there are increased risks and relevant safety data for liver biopsy in overweight and obese children. To our knowledge, there are no specific published analyses to date of risks of liver biopsy complications in large cohorts of obese or super-obese children with NAFLD/NASH. Ultrasound-guided liver biopsy was shown to be safe in a study of 120 biopsies from 67 children wherein the overall incidence of complications was reported at 5%, with only two patients requiring surgical intervention. Interventional radiology-based liver biopsies have also been reported. In a series of 249 children, 294 biopsies were carried out with a low incidence of complications, with only two instances of a more than 2 g/dL decrease in hemoglobin values following biopsy [56]. It is current practice at our center to use interventional radiology-based ultrasound-guided biopsies for our morbidly obese children.

Histopathology of non-alcoholic fatty liver disease and non-alcoholic steatohepatitis

Non-alcoholic fatty liver disease is a broad disease category based upon clinical, laboratory, and morphological criteria. Causes of hepatic steatosis, an essential element in NAFLD, are many and include poor nutrition, malabsorption, celiac disease, collagen vascular disease, hepatitis C virus, postviral epidemic Reye syndrome, parenteral alimentation, hypertriglyceridemia, various drugs such as corticosteroids, liver toxins, and metabolic diseases as different as cystic fibrosis, Wilson disease, fatty acid oxidation defects, urea cycle defects, and disorders of oxidative phosphorylation. The morphologic diagnosis of NASH depends on finding evidence of a necroinflammatory process in addition to steatosis. When ethanol abuse has been excluded, NASH typically is observed in liver biopsy performed because of unexpected elevation of serum aminotransferases in a patient with obesity and/or diabetes mellitus.

The pattern of hepatic steatosis in NASH typically is a mixture of macro- and microsteatosis. Helpful to the histopathologist is the knowledge that in many conditions with hepatic steatosis, particularly those encountered in the pediatric age group, inflammation and fibrosis are usually absent. The histologic changes that help to distinguish NASH as a subcategory of NAFLD are necroinflammatory features (Figure 36.4): inflammation, degenerative changes in hepatocytes, and fibrosis. The degenerative changes in hepatocytes

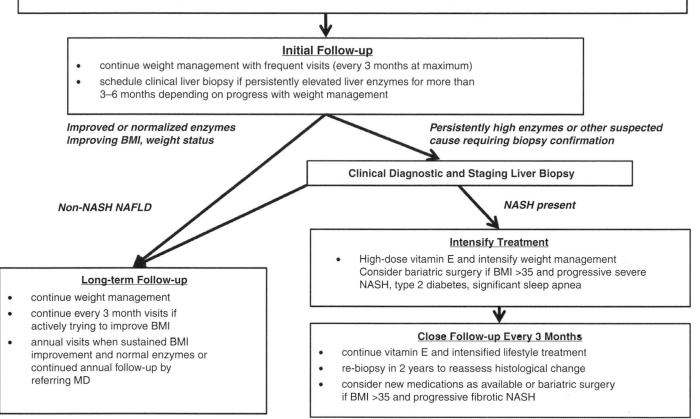

Figure 36.3 Non-alcoholic fatty liver disease (NAFLD) management algorithm. ALT, alanine aminotransferase (U/L); BMI, body mass index; MD, clinician; NASH, non-alcoholic steatohepatitis.

include ballooning, apoptosis, acidophil bodies, and presence of Mallory–Denk cytoplasmic bodies. Lobular inflammatory lesions in NASH tend to be small and multifocal; the lesions are composed of minute aggregates of mononuclear inflammatory cells, polymorphonuclear leukocytes, and Kupffer cells, presumed to be reacting to focal hepatocyte degeneration and necrosis, although the latter is not always apparent. Portal area infiltrates composed of mononuclear inflammatory cells are more common in children than in adults with NASH. The pattern of fibrosis in NASH tends to be pericellular with zone 3 predominance, but progressive fibrosis is often periportal as well. In aggregate, these light microscopic changes indicate persistent active hepatocyte injury associated with accumulation of fat and other regressive changes in hepatocytes, such as ballooning and Mallory–Denk bodies. The changes of NASH are potentially reversible and tend to diminish with treatment of the underlying condition. However, a significant proportion of patients with NAFLD progresses to end-stage liver disease.

The challenge continues to be identification of those at greatest risk.

Efforts to codify the histological features of NAFLD and their relative importance have focused on identifying degrees of severity of the liver lesion. Grading systems necessarily focus on the components of the cellular pathology but have also sought to create objective tools for measuring the effectiveness of therapy over time and to predict risk for progression. Matteoni *et al.* [4] advocated dividing NAFLD into four subtypes: steatosis alone, steatosis with lobular inflammation, steatosis with ballooning, and steatosis with Mallory–Denk bodies or fibrosis. The last two subtypes were suggested to be regarded as steatohepatitis. This approach minimized the presence of lobular inflammation alone but recognized ballooning, Mallory–Denk bodies, and fibrosis as features of a more significant inflammatory lesion with the potential for serious liver injury. Brunt *et al.* [57] proposed an evaluation system for NASH that separated fibrosis patterns from activity patterns,

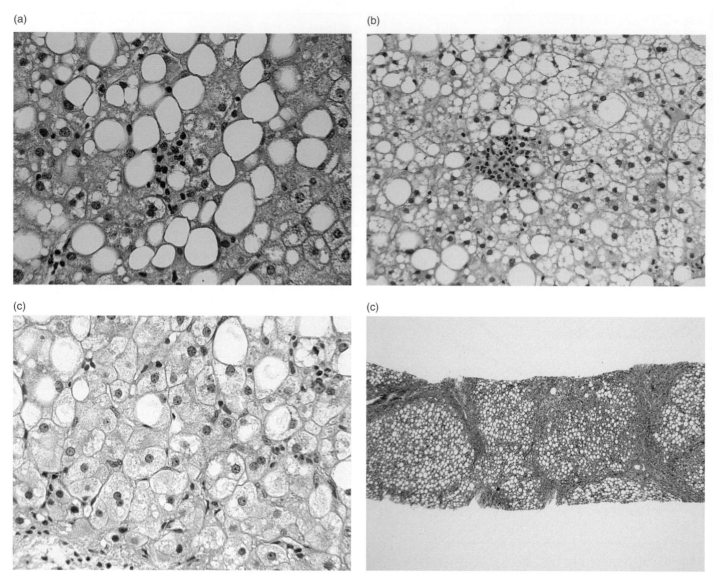

Figure 36.4 Histopathology of non-alcoholic fatty liver disease by light microscopy. (a) Steatohepatitis in a 17-year-old male with morbid obesity, diabetes mellitus, and insulin resistance. Distended clear hepatocytes contain lipid. A small cluster of intralobular mononuclear inflammatory cells is apparent. (Hematoxylin & eosin stain, original magnification ×160.) (b) Steatohepatitis in an 18-year-old male with morbid obesity, diabetes mellitus, and insulin resistance. Distended hepatocytes contain abundant macro- and microvesicular lipid. A prominent cluster of intralobular inflammatory cells contains a mixture of inflammatory cells including polymorphonuclear leukocytes. (Hematoxylin & eosin stain, original magnification ×250.) (c) Steatohepatitis in a 12-year-old boy with morbid obesity and diabetes mellitus. Balloon degeneration of hepatocytes is evident throughout this field. A minor focus of intralobular inflammation is at the upper right. (Hematoxylin & eosin stain, original magnification ×250.) (d) Chronic steatohepatitis in a 12-year-old boy with morbid obesity and diabetes mellitus. Prominent portal inflammation is accompanied by bridging portal fibrosis. (Trichrome stain, original magnification ×25.)

similar to common practice for many form of chronic hepatitis. Kleiner *et al.* [58] designed and validated a comprehensive composite histological scoring system for NASH intended for use in clinical trials to compare results in sequential biopsies in the NASH Clinical Research Network and also to aid in a standardized approach toward grading the activity and staging of NAFLD in natural history and clinical trial studies. The system comprises 14 histological features; four of these have semiquantitative scores: steatosis (range 0–3), lobular inflammation (0–3), hepatocellular ballooning (0–2), and fibrosis (0–4). The first three scores are summed together to yield a

NAFLD activity score (NAS; range 0–8). In the NASH Clinical Research Network validation study, most NAS ≥5 correlated with a pathological designation of NASH and NAS <3 with a designation of not-NAFLD. The authors emphasized that the scoring system should not replace the pathologist's diagnostic determination of steatohepatitis. This is particularly true for pediatric NASH, in which there was less interobserver agreement for scoring, most likely because features considered hallmarks of adult NASH (lobular inflammation and ballooning degeneration) are less pronounced, and isolated periportal fibrosis is more common. This system was not intended for routine use but unfortunately it has been adopted by many pathologists, with the implication that a high NAS indicates more definitive and significant NASH than a low score. Most recently, Brunt *et al.* [57] reported that the histopathological diagnosis of NASH and assignment of a NAS have distinct meanings and purposes that often do not coincide. Their data showed that liver biopsies with high NAS values may not meet criteria for NASH in a significant number of patients, and, conversely, those with low NAS values may have clear indicators for NASH.

Because lobular inflammation, ballooning degeneration, and perisinusoidal fibrosis are less prominent, and portal inflammation and periportal fibrosis more prominent, in children with NASH, some authors have proposed subdividing pediatric NASH into two types: type 1, or adult type, characterized by steatosis with more ballooning degeneration and/or perisinusoidal fibrosis and no portal features; and type 2, or pediatric type, marked by more portal inflammation and periportal steatosis/fibrosis [59]. In the original description of these subtypes in a regional southern Californian cohort aged 2–18 years, type 1 was found more often in white children and type 2 in children of Asian, Native American and Hispanic ethnicity; however, it is important to mention that the entire cohort was predominantly Hispanic, Asian, or Native American (83% of the cohort). Subsequently, a multicenter study of 130 children from four clinical centers across the USA and one center from Canada found that there was overlap of type 1 and type 2 NASH in 82% of the cohort [50]. Patients with significant fibrosis in this cohort were more likely to have higher lobular and portal inflammation scores, perisinusoidal fibrosis and a NAS >5. Therefore, the proposed pediatric subtypes remain of unknown generalizability and clinical significance.

Hepatocyte ultrastructural changes in NAFLD may be striking, particularly in those patients with NASH [32]. Excess smooth and rough endoplasmic reticulum is common, sinusoidal inflammatory cells are prevalent, and an array of focal changes in mitochondria includes variable, sometimes extreme, pleomorphism, matrix crystalloids, and megamitochondria (Figure 36.5). These changes are best interpreted as indicators of current organelle stress and are a rough measure of current disease activity; however, data are not available to determine if they specifically correlate with light microscopy findings or outcome.

Assessment of ballooning change is stated to be of critical importance to the diagnosis of NASH but is often problematical for the inexperienced (Figure 36.4). Unequivocal balloon cells are enlarged with pale, flocculant, sometimes vacuolated, cytoplasm and show qualities of degeneration that may or may not include Mallory–Denk bodies, which are rare in children. Ballooning is a continuum and imperfect examples are common in many cases of borderline NASH. Overzealous or overly cautious identification of ballooning could result in misinterpretation. One problem is that well-glycogenated hepatocytes containing lipid droplets, a common finding in NAFLD, are enlarged but not necessarily ballooned. So far, a specific histochemical stain or serum marker for the process of hepatocyte balloon degeneration with predictive value for outcome remains an elusive goal. In the meantime, it is agreed that histologically unequivocal NASH with associated fibrosis carries a significant risk for progressive liver disease and early mortality.

Treatment: existing options and future horizons

Attaining a healthy weight remains the optimal way to manage NAFLD and NASH, particularly in children, where end-stage liver disease remains rare and improvements with weight loss are more likely. Numerous studies in adults have shown that a weight loss of 5–10% can lead to significant metabolic improvements in serum insulin, glucose, lipids, and hepatic steatosis by imaging and even repeat histology in some studies [60]. Likewise, pediatric cohort studies have supported that a 5–10% decrease in baseline weight loss can result in significant improvement in serum aminotransferases and/or sonographic improvement in steatosis [24]. In one prospective study, 84 children with biopsy-confirmed NAFLD underwent a 1-year lifestyle advice and diet program; 57 of the 84 completed the program [61]. There was a mean decrease in BMI associated with significant improvement in AST, ALT, triglycerides, cholesterol, insulin, glucose levels, and the score on the Homeostasis Model of Assessment–Insulin Resistance (HOMA-IR) (all $p < 0.0001$). Those with the most significant improvement in ALT lost 5% or more of body weight. It was not reported how many children failed to improve weight or BMI, but 68% did not complete the 1 year program. Also the sustainability of the weight loss is not known. In a longitudinal follow-up study of 66 children diagnosed with NAFLD, 50 (76%) regained weight at time of last follow-up (mean, 6.4 years; range, 0.05–20.00) and in 46% serum aminotransferases increased back to the starting values [24]. However, a more intensive and standardized 1-year lifestyle intervention in 109 children reported a persistent positive effect at 1 and 2 years after the intervention. Serum aminotransferases improved and sonographic hepatic steatosis was reduced when compared with 51 children not participating in the intervention. The degree of overweight reduction was also associated with a decrease in NAFLD as measured by ultrasound.

Specific dietary recommendations have not been standardized but evidence from animal models and/or human studies suggest that high-fat diets, specifically saturated fats, and diets high in fructose may promote hepatic steatosis and fibrosis [30,42]. Studies in adults have shown that, short term, a low-carbohydrate diet can rapidly reduce intrahepatic triglyceride content measured by MR spectroscopy. Given that high sugar/fructose intake has been associated with increased severity of fibrosis, our program recommends avoiding added sugars and adheres to evidence-based recommendations to increase fruits and vegetables, reduce screen time, and increase activity (Figure 36.3). Ideally, this is achieved through a gradual

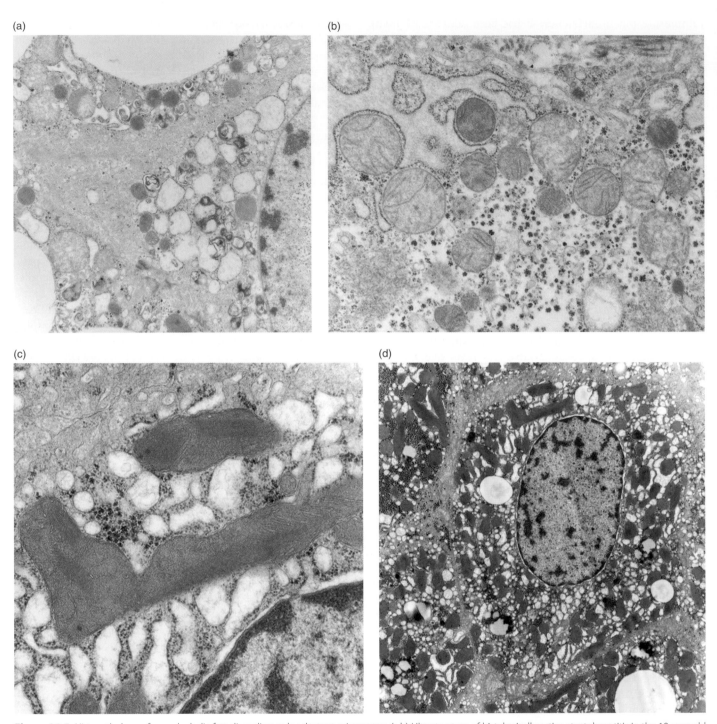

Figure 36.5 Histopathology of non-alcoholic fatty liver disease by electron microscopy. (a,b) Ultrastructure of histologically active steatohepatitis in the 18-year-old male in Figure 36.4b. (a) All hepatocytes showed show similar alterations including diffuse stress reactivity of smooth- and rough-surfaced endoplasmic reticulum and acute-appearing variable degenerative changes in mitochondria that included enlargement with matrix rarefaction, extremely prominent autophagic bodies, and numerous lipid vesicles of variable size. No mitochondrial matrix crystalloids were present (original magnification ×10 000). (b) Higher magnification of mitochondria shows regressive abnormalities in size, matrix density, and arrangements of cristae, but no matrix inclusions. The ill-defined cytoplasmic tangle of filaments at the lower left may be an early Mallory–Denk body (original magnification ×15 000). (c) Ultrastructure of steatohepatitis in an 18-year-old male with morbid obesity and minimally active steatohepatitis. All hepatocytes showed similar alterations including diffuse stress reactivity of smooth-surfaced endoplasmic reticulum (small evenly dispersed vesicles of uniform size), patches of dilated rough-surfaced endoplasmic reticulum, mildly pleomorphic mitochondria some of which are conspicuously misshapen, and a few scattered small lipid vesicles (original magnification ×8000). (d) Mitochondria in teenager show abnormalities of size, shape, and matrix inclusions commonly encountered in steatohepatitis as well as in unrelated disorders with secondary mitochondrial stress. Crystalloid matrix inclusions are apparent. Cisterns of endoplasmic reticulum are abnormally dilated (original magnification ×40 000).

reduction in excess caloric intake and an increase in physical activity so that changes are sustainable in the long term. Depending on patient readiness and family support, this can sometimes be achieved with intermittent, every 3–6 months, office visits and counseling, but for some patients it remains a struggle to make significant lifestyle changes, and more comprehensive weight management programs are necessary [62]. Such programs are ideally multidisciplinary, including physicians, nurses, nurse practitioners, registered dieticians, support group or social workers, psychologists, and frequent biweekly to monthly visits.

In the event that weight loss is not achieved or does not yield improvements or normalization of ALT or hepatic steatosis by imaging, proven pharmaceutical options for pediatric NAFLD remain limited because of a paucity of double-blind randomized controlled studies performed in children. In one randomized controlled study of lifestyle measures with or without added antioxidant therapy (alpha-tocopherol 600 IU/day plus ascorbic acid 500 mg/day for 24 months), a significant histologic improvement occurred in both groups, with the same proportion achieving the primary endpoint of improvement in NAS by ≥ 2 points [63]. A 2-year multicenter, randomized, double-blind controlled trial of vitamin E or metformin versus placebo was conducted for the treatment of biopsy-confirmed NAFLD in 173 children aged 8–17 years (the TONIC study) [64]. In this landmark study conducted with rigorous methodology and clearly defined outcomes, neither drug achieved the primary outcome, defined as a significant or sustained reduction in ALT compared with the placebo group. However, secondary analyses of patients with NASH showed that a higher proportion achieved resolution with vitamin E compared with placebo, mainly through histologic improvements in ballooning degeneration. This is in agreement with results from a larger randomized controlled trial of vitamin E in 247 adults without diabetes, who were randomized to pioglitazone 30 mg daily, a natural form of vitamin E 800 IU once daily, or placebo for 96 weeks [65]. The primary outcome in the adult trial was an improvement in histologic features of NASH and the sample size was accordingly larger. Vitamin E compared with placebo was associated with a higher rate of improvement in NASH (43% versus 19%; $p = 0.001$). Vitamin E resulted in a significant reduction in hepatic steatosis and lobular inflammation, but not in fibrosis. While pioglitazone also improved NASH, it did not reach significance compared with placebo (34% versus 19% ($p = 0.04$), with a Bonferroni adjusted $p < 0.025$ required because of the two planned primary comparisons). However, pioglitazone also improved steatosis and lobular inflammation significantly. Despite its demonstrated benefit for NASH, pioglitazone was associated with weight gain that did not resolve after discontinuing the drug. Further, pioglitazone is not approved for use in children.

Limitations of the TONIC study included that the primary outcome was change in serum ALT rather than histologic change. This was because there were no prior histology-based pilot studies in children to guide sample size calculations. Also, the oral metformin dose of 500 mg twice daily is significantly less than the dose typically aimed for in clinical practice (1000 mg twice daily) and was likely to have been inadequate as patients in this arm did not show an average improvement in HOMA-IR, fasting insulin, or glucose during the trial. Therefore it remains inconclusive whether metformin might provide some benefit for pediatric NASH, either alone or in combination with another agent such as vitamin E. In a randomized placebo-controlled study of 50 obese adolescents with lifestyle intervention plus either oral metformin 850 mg twice daily or placebo, liver ultrasound at 6 months showed a significant improvement over baseline in fatty liver prevalence and severity. Insulin sensitivity improved significantly in the metformin-treated group compared with placebo.

Long-term risks of taking high-dose vitamin E remain controversial. Several studies, including a recent systematic review and meta-analysis, have raised a concern for increased all-cause mortality associated with high-dose vitamin E in adults, whereas others have called these findings into question. A large-scale international study of healthy adult males receiving vitamin E, selenium, or both versus placebo suggested that vitamin E at 400 IU/day significantly increased the risk of prostate cancer compared with placebo, with an absolute increase in risk of 1.6/1000 person-years [66]. During the 2-year pediatric randomized control trial of vitamin E, no significant adverse events were noted related to vitamin E 800 IU daily, but the safety of indefinite lifelong usage of vitamin E in younger healthier subjects remains unknown. Further, only half of the patients with NASH responded in the trial, indicating that it is not a panacea for NASH. For this reason, our program prescribes the natural form of vitamin E only for patients with biopsy-proven NASH, as recommended by the TONIC study. Adherence should be assessed to help to interpret response and we strongly feel that repeat histological assessment should be performed after 2 years of treatment, so that vitamin E can be discontinued if no response has occurred and/or alternative therapy can be initiated. There are no guidelines as to whether and how long vitamin E should be continued in responders after a 2-year period.

Weight loss, antioxidants, and insulin sensitizers (metformin in children and thiazolidendiones in adults) have been the most extensively studied treatments for NAFLD and NASH [60]. Ursodeoxycholic acid, even at higher dosing ranges, has not been shown to improve NASH in randomized placebo-controlled trials in adults. Experimental therapies that have been shown to improve NASH histology in adults in small placebo-controlled randomized controlled trials include pentoxifylline, a downregulator of tumor necrosis factor-α; telmisartan, an angiotensin receptor blocker; and L-carnitine. Polyunsaturated fatty acids have also been shown to improve biochemical and radiological markers in a few pilot studies but are lacking data regarding histological outcomes. The NASH Clinical Research Network is planning to undertake another 1-year randomized controlled trial in children using cysteamine, a precursor of glutathione and a potent antioxidant, after a small pilot study in 11 children showed significant reductions in ALT at 24 weeks [67]. Combination therapy with promising agents targeting different mechanisms (e.g. insulin sensitizers plus antioxidants) has been inadequately studied but may be of potential benefit and worth exploring in future studies.

Bariatric surgery has been shown in several prospective and retrospective adult cohort studies and subsequent meta-analyses to be promising in the treatment of adult NASH, with reductions in steatosis. In a meta-analysis of 15 studies, comprising 766 paired liver biopsies in adults, the pooled proportion of patients with complete resolution of NASH was 69.5% (95% CI, 42.4–90.8), while there were even higher proportions of patients with improvement *or* resolution in steatosis (91.6% overall), steatohepatitis (81.3%), and fibrosis (65.5%). Yet the absence of randomized controlled trials precludes an unbiased assessment of weight-loss surgery as a superior therapy for NASH, particularly in patients with advanced fibrosis or cirrhosis [68]. A preliminary analysis of six adolescents with follow-up liver biopsies 5–22 months after gastric bypass reported that steatosis also resolved in five, with improvement in overall NAS in four. However, portal inflammation persisted in three and portal fibrosis developed in two [69]. On the strength of data in adults and in the absence of any strong pharmacological options for severe fibrotic NASH in adolescents, expert guidelines for bariatric surgery in adolescents consider "severe steatohepatitis" a reason to consider this modality in the morbidly obese adolescent. While it has not been clearly demonstrated that bariatric surgery is more effective for NASH than non-surgical weight loss with or without vitamin E in this age group, the preponderance of other significant comorbidities in these severely obese adolescents, including type 2 diabetes and obstructive sleep apnea, may make weight-loss surgery a reasonable option to achieve measurable improvement in several serious comorbid conditions.

Liver transplantation for end-stage liver disease related to NASH during childhood has not been reported to date in the medical literature, with the youngest reported transplant occurring at age 20 for pediatric NASH [24]. In adults, the proportion of liver transplants performed for NASH cirrhosis has increased six-fold from 1997–2003 to 2010, and it is now the fourth most common indication for transplant in adults. Reassuringly, 1-, 3-, and 5-year survival rates of patients receiving liver transplants for NASH-related end-stage liver disease appear superior to those receiving transplants for hepatocellular carcinoma, hepatitis C, alcoholic liver disease, acute hepatic necrosis, hemochromatosis, or cryptogenic liver disease. Recurrence of NAFLD and NASH after liver transplant has been reported in adults. Recurrence appears to be associated with higher pre- and post-transplant BMI and higher post-transplant serum triglycerides.

Conclusions

Clearly, progress has been made in both fundamental and germane understanding since NAFLD was first described over three decades ago. These important advances aside, NAFLD remains an ongoing challenge both for the clinician and the researcher. Distinct and large gaps exist in our knowledge base, including having only a rudimentary understanding of NAFLD pathogenesis and progression and our inability to diagnose stage, and monitor NAFLD noninvasively. A basic armamentarium is available to manage NAFLD. We now know that obesity-related liver disease is the *most prevalent liver disease* in children in the western world and also that NASH is currently positioned to become the *leading cause of liver transplantation* in adults. Therefore, pediatricians should advocate for and assist public health efforts to combat obesity and its comorbidities, including NAFLD. Clinicians treating children with gastroenterologic issues should aim to screen and identify those at risk for NAFLD, and physician–scientists must continue efforts to prevent liver disease in children stemming from the obesity epidemic.

References

1. Das K, Mukherjee PS, Ghosh A, *et al.* Nonobese population in a developing country has a high prevalence of nonalcoholic fatty liver and significant liver disease. *Hepatology* 2010;**51**:1593–1602.

2. Popkin BM, Adair LS, Ng SW. Global nutrition transition and the pandemic of obesity in developing countries. *Nutr Rev* 2012;**70**:3–21.

3. Semple RK, Savage DB, Cochran EK, Gorden P, O'Rahilly S. Genetic syndromes of severe insulin resistance. *Endocr Rev* 2011;**32**:498–514.

4. Matteoni CA, Younossi ZM, Gramlich T, *et al.* Nonalcoholic fatty liver disease: a spectrum of clinical and pathological severity. *Gastroenterology* 1999;**116**:1413–1419.

5. Adams LA, Lymp JF, ST Sauver, *et al.* The natural history of nonalcoholic fatty liver disease: a population-based cohort study. *Gastroenterology* 2005;**129**:113–121.

6. Schwimmer JB, Deutsch R, Kahen T, *et al.* Prevalence of fatty liver in children and adolescents. *Pediatrics* 2006;**118**:1388–1393.

7. Browning JD, Szczepaniak LS, Dobbins R, *et al.* Prevalence of hepatic steatosis in an urban population in the United States: impact of ethnicity. *Hepatology* 2004;**40**:1387–1395.

8. Fraser A, Longnecker MP, Lawlor DA. Prevalence of elevated alanine aminotransferase among US adolescents and associated factors: NHANES 1999–2004. *Gastroenterology* 2007;**133**:1814–1820.

9. Strauss RS, Barlow SE, Dietz WH. Prevalence of abnormal serum aminotransferase values in overweight and obese adolescents. *J Pediatr* 2000;**136**:727–733.

10. Alavian SM, Mohammad-Alizadeh AH, Esna-Ashari F, Ardalan G, Hajarizadeh B. Non-alcoholic fatty liver disease prevalence among school-aged children and adolescents in Iran and its association with biochemical and

anthropometric measures. *Liver Int* 2009;**29**:159–163.

11. Park HS, Han JH, Choi KM, Kim SM. Relation between elevated serum alanine aminotransferase and metabolic syndrome in Korean adolescents. *Am J Clin Nutr* 2005;**82**:1046–1051.

12. Tominaga K, Kurata J, Chen Y, *et al.* Prevalence of fatty liver in Japanese children and relationship to obesity: an epidemiological ultrasonographic survey. *Dig Dis Sci* 1995;**40**:2002–2209.

13. Meng L, Luo N, Mi J. Impacts of types and degree of obesity on non-alcoholic fatty liver disease and related dyslipidemia in Chinese school-age children? *Biomed Environ Sci* 2011;**24**:22–30.

14. Booth ML, George J, Denney-Wilson E, *et al.* The population prevalence of adverse concentrations and associations with adiposity of liver tests among Australian adolescents. *J Paediatr Child Health* 2008;**44**:686–691.

15. Manco M, Marcellini M, Devito R, *et al.* Metabolic syndrome and liver histology in paediatric non-alcoholic steatohepatitis. *Int J Obes* 2008;**32**:381–387.

16. Schwimmer JB, Dunn W, Norman GJ, *et al.* SAFETY study: alanine aminotransferase cutoff values are set too high for reliable detection of pediatric chronic liver disease. *Gastroenterology* 2010;**138**:1357–1364.

17. Kunde SS, Lazenby AJ, Clements RH, Abrams GA, *et al.* Spectrum of NAFLD and diagnostic implications of the proposed new normal range for serum ALT in obese women. *Hepatology* 2005;**42**:650–656.

18. Xanthakos S, Miles L, Bucuvalas J, *et al.* Histologic spectrum of nonalcoholic fatty liver disease in morbidly obese adolescents. *Clin Gastroenterol Hepatol* 2006;**4**:226–232.

19. Manco M, Bedogni G, Marcellini M, *et al.* Waist circumference correlates with liver fibrosis in children with non-alcoholic steatohepatitis. *Gut* 2008;**57**:1283–1287.

20. Schwimmer JB, Deutsch R, Rauch JB, *et al.* Obesity, insulin resistance, and other clinicopathological correlates of pediatric nonalcoholic fatty liver disease. *J Pediatr* 2003;**143**:500–505.

21. Bhala N, Angulo P, van der Poorten D, *et al.* The natural history of nonalcoholic fatty liver disease with advanced fibrosis or cirrhosis: an international collaborative study. *Hepatology* 2011;**54**:1208–1216.

22. Ascha MS, Hanouneh IA, Lopez R, *et al.* The incidence and risk factors of hepatocellular carcinoma in patients with nonalcoholic steatohepatitis. *Hepatology* 2010;**51**:1972–1978.

23. Kohli R, Boyd T, Lake K, *et al.* Rapid progression of NASH in childhood. *J Pediatr Gastroenterol Nutr* 2010;**50**:453–456.

24. Feldstein AE, Treeprasertsuk S, Sharatcharoenwitthay AP, *et al.* The natural history of nonalchololic fatty liver disease in children: a follow-up study for up to 20 years. *Hepatology* 2008;**48**(Suppl):335A.

25. Dunn W, Xu R, Wingard DL, *et al.* Suspected nonalcoholic fatty liver disease and mortality risk in a population-based cohort study. *Am J Gastroenterology* 2008;**103**:2263–2271.

26. Ruhl CE, Everhart JE. Determinants of the association of overweight with elevated serum alanine aminotransferase activity in the United States. *Gastroenterology* 2003;**124**:71–79.

27. Pacifico L, Anania C, Martino F, *et al.* Functional and morphological vascular changes in pediatric nonalcoholic fatty liver disease. *Hepatology* 2010;**52**:1643–1651.

28. Caserta CA, Pendino GM, Amante A, *et al.* Cardiovascular risk factors, nonalcoholic fatty liver disease, and carotid artery intima-media thickness in an adolescent population in southern Italy. *Am J Epidemiol* 2010;**171**:1195–1202.

29. Puri P, Wiest MM, Cheung O, *et al.* The plasma lipidomic signature of nonalcoholic steatohepatitis. *Hepatology* 2009;**50**:1827–1838.

30. Kohli R, Kirby M, Xanthakos SA, *et al.* High-fructose, medium chain trans fat diet induces liver fibrosis and elevates plasma coenzyme Q9 in a novel murine model of obesity and nonalcoholic steatohepatitis. *Hepatology* 2010;**52**:934–944.

31. Nobili V, Alkhouri N, Bartuli A, *et al.* Severity of liver injury and atherogenic lipid profile in children with nonalcoholic fatty liver disease. *Pediatr Res* 2010;**67**:665–670.

32. Sanyal AJ, Campbell-Sargent C, Mirshahi F, *et al.* Nonalcoholic steatohepatitis: association of insulin resistance and mitochondrial abnormalities. *Gastroenterology* 2001;**120**:1183–1192.

33. Feldstein AE, Canbay A, Angulo P, *et al.* Hepatocyte apoptosis and fas expression are prominent features of human nonalcoholic steatohepatitis. *Gastroenterology* 2003;**125**: 437–443.

34. Kohli R, Pan X, Malladi P, Wainwright MS, Whitington PF. Mitochondrial reactive oxygen species signal hepatocyte steatosis by regulating the phosphatidylinositol 3-kinase cell survival pathway. *J Biol Chem* 2007;**282**:21327–21336.

35. Kohli R, Feldstein AE. NASH animal models: Are we there yet? *J Hepatol* 2011;**55**:941–943.

36. Sookoian S, Pirola CJ. Meta-analysis of the influence of I148M variant of patatin-like phosp holipase domain containing 3 gene (*PNPLA3*) on the susceptibility and histological severity of nonalcoholic fatty liver disease. *Hepatology* 2011;**53**:1883–1894.

37. Santoro N, Kursawe R, D'Adamo E, *et al.* A common variant in the patatin-like phospholipase 3 gene (*PNPLA3*) is associated with fatty liver disease in obese children and adolescents. *Hepatology* 2010;**52**:1281–1290.

38. Valenti L, Alisi A, Galmozzi E, *et al.* I148M patatin-like phospholipase domain-containing 3 gene variant and severity of pediatric nonalcoholic fatty liver disease. *Hepatology* 2010;**52**:1274–1280.

39. Petersen KF, Dufour S, Hariri A, *et al.* Apolipoprotein C3 gene variants in nonalcoholic fatty liver disease. *N Engl J Med* 2010;**362**:1082–1089.

40. Al-Serri A, Anstee QM, Valenti L, *et al.* The *SOD2* C47T polymorphism influences NAFLD fibrosis severity: Evidence from case-control and intra-familial allele association studies. *J Hepatol* 2012;**56**:448–454.

41. Lin YC, Chang PF, Hu FC, Chang MH, Ni YH. Variants in the *UGT1A1* gene and the risk of pediatric nonalcoholic fatty liver disease. *Pediatrics* 2009;**124**: e1221–e1227.

42. Abdelmalek MF, Suzuki A, Guy C, *et al.* Increased fructose consumption is

associated with fibrosis severity in patients with nonalcoholic fatty liver disease. *Hepatology* 2010;**51**:1961–1971.

43. Welsh JA, Sharma A, Abramson JL, *et al.* Caloric sweetener consumption and dyslipidemia among US adults. *JAMA* 2010;**303**:1490–1497.

44. Barlow SE. Expert Committee recommendations regarding the prevention, assessment, and treatment of child and adolescent overweight and obesity: summary report. *Pediatrics* 2007;**120**(Suppl 1):S164–S192.

45. Lee TH, Kim WR, Benson JT, Therneau TM, Melton LJ, III. Serum aminotransferase activity and mortality risk in a United States community. *Hepatology* 2008;**47**:880–887.

46. Maffeis C, Banzato C, Talamini G. Waist-to-height ratio, a useful index to identify high metabolic risk in overweight children. *J Pediatr* 2008;**152**:207–213.

47. Nobili V, Alisi A, Vania A, *et al.* The pediatric NAFLD fibrosis index: a predictor of liver fibrosis in children with non-alcoholic fatty liver disease. *BMC Med* 2009;**7**:21.

48. Loomba R, Wesley R, Pucino F, *et al.* Placebo in nonalcoholic steatohepatitis: insight into natural history and implications for future clinical trials. *Clin Gastroenterol Hepatol* 2008;**6**:1243–1248.

49. Patton HM, Lavine JE, van Natta ML, *et al.* Clinical correlates of histopathology in pediatric nonalcoholic steatohepatitis. *Gastroenterology* 2008;**135**:1961–1971.

50. Carter-Kent C, Yerian LM, Brunt EM, *et al.* Nonalcoholic steatohepatitis in children: a multicenter clinicopathological study. *Hepatology* 2009;**50**:1113–1120.

51. Wieckowska A, Zein NN, Yerian LM, *et al.* In vivo assessment of liver cell apoptosis as a novel biomarker of disease severity in nonalcoholic fatty liver disease. *Hepatology* 2006;**44**:27–33.

52. Alkhouri N, Carter-Kent C, Lopez R, *et al.* A combination of the pediatric NAFLD fibrosis index and enhanced liver fibrosis test identifies children with fibrosis. *Clin Gastroenterol Hepatol* 2011;**9**:150–155.

53. Nobili V, Vizzutti F, Arena U, *et al.* Accuracy and reproducibility of transient elastography for the diagnosis of fibrosis in pediatric nonalcoholic steatohepatitis. *Hepatology* 2008;**48**:442–448.

54. Larson SP, Bowers SP, Palekar NA, *et al.* Histopathologic variability between the right and left lobes of the liver in morbidly obese patients undergoing Roux-en-Y bypass. *Clin Gastroenterol Hepatol* 2007;**5**:1329–1332.

55. West J, Card TR. Reduced mortality rates following elective percutaneous liver biopsies. *Gastroenterology* 2010;**139**:1230–1237.

56. Potter C, Hogan MJ, Henry-Kendjorsky K, Balint J, Barnard JA. Safety of pediatric percutaneous liver biopsy performed by interventional radiologists. *J Pediatr Gastroenterol Nutr* 2011;**53**:202–206.

57. Brunt EM, Kleiner DE, Wilson LA, Belt P, Neuschwander-Tetri BA. Nonalcoholic fatty liver disease (NAFLD) activity score and the histopathologic diagnosis in NAFLD: distinct clinicopathologic meanings. *Hepatology* 2011;**53**:810–820.

58. Kleiner DE, Brunt EM, Van Natta M, *et al.* Design and validation of a histological scoring system for nonalcoholic fatty liver disease. *Hepatology* 2005;**41**:1313–1321.

59. Schwimmer JB, Behling C, Newbury R, *et al.* Histopathology of pediatric nonalcoholic fatty liver disease. *Hepatology* 2005;**42**:641–649.

60. Musso G, Gambino R, Cassader M, Pagano G. A meta-analysis of randomized trials for the treatment of nonalcoholic fatty liver disease. *Hepatology* 2010;**52**:79–104.

61. Nobili V, Marcellini M, Devito R, *et al.* NAFLD in children: a prospective clinical-pathological study and effect of lifestyle advice. *Hepatology* 2006;**44**:458–465.

62. DeVore, S, Kohli R, Lake K, *et al.* A multidisciplinary clinical program is effective in stabilizing BMI and reducing ALT in pediatric patients with NAFLD. *J Pediatr Gastroenterol Nutr* 2013;**57**:119–123.

63. Nobili V, Manco M, Devito R, *et al.* Lifestyle intervention and antioxidant therapy in children with nonalcoholic fatty liver disease: a randomized, controlled trial. *Hepatology* 2008;**48**:119–128.

64. Lavine JE, Schwimmer JB, van Natta ML, *et al.* Effect of vitamin E or metformin for treatment of nonalcoholic fatty liver disease in children and adolescents: the TONIC randomized controlled trial. *JAMA* 2011;**305**:1659–1668.

65. Sanyal AJ, Chalasani N, Kowdley KV, *et al.* Pioglitazone, vitamin E, or placebo for nonalcoholic steatohepatitis. *N Engl J Med* 2010;**362**:1675–1685.

66. Klein EA, Thompson JR, Tangen CM, *et al.* Vitamin E and the risk of prostate cancer: the Selenium and Vitamin E Cancer Prevention Trial (SELECT). *JAMA* 2011;**306**:1549–1556.

67. Dohil R, Schmeltzer S, Cabrera BL, *et al.* Enteric-coated cysteamine for the treatment of paediatric non-alcoholic fatty liver disease. *Aliment Pharmacol Ther* 2011;**33**:1036–1044.

68. Chavez-Tapia NC, Tellez-Avila FI, Barrientos-Gutierrez T, *et al.* Bariatric surgery for non-alcoholic steatohepatitis in obese patients. *Cochrane Database Syst Rev* 2010;(**1**): CD007340.

69. Xanthakos SA, Miles L, Bove K, Inge T. Outcome of nonalcoholic fatty liver disease (NAFLD) in adolescents after bariatric surgery. *Obesity (Silver Spring)*, 2007;**15**(Suppl 1):A209.

37

Peroxisomal diseases

Paul A. Watkins and Kathleen B. Schwarz

Peroxisomal structure and function

General aspects of peroxisomes

Peroxisomes were first identified in renal proximal tubule cells by a Swedish graduate student in 1954. Initially called microbodies, these organelles were studied intensively by de Duve and coworkers. Because they contained enzymes that both produced (e.g. amino acid and urate oxidases) and degraded (e.g. catalase) hydrogen peroxide, de Duve proposed the name peroxisomes [1]. Microbodies found in some lower organisms and plants were named for the specialized functions that they carry out. For example, glyoxysomes of fungi and plants contain the five enzymes of the glyoxylate cycle and glycosomes house the enzymes of glycolysis in trypanosomes. While peroxisomes have been found in essentially all plant and animal cells with the exception of mature erythrocytes, they range in size from about 0.1 μm (microperoxisomes of intestine and brain) up to 1.0 μm (characteristic of hepatic and renal peroxisomes; range: 0.2–1.0 μm) (Figure 37.1).

A single lipid bilayer comprises the peroxisomal membrane. The organelle's matrix is finely granular, but microcrystalline cores of urate oxidase are present in the hepatic peroxisomes of some species (e.g. rats). No cores are found in human peroxisomes as humans lack urate oxidase. Unlike chloroplasts and mitochondria, peroxisomes contain no DNA although it has been speculated that all three organelles evolved from endosymbionts. Since the discovery of peroxisomes, numerous membrane proteins and matrix enzymes have been identified. Much research on peroxisomes has been fueled by the identification of patients whose cells lack either normal appearing organelles or one or more peroxisomal metabolic functions.

Biogenesis of peroxisomes

The processes involved in the de novo formation and division of peroxisomes have been intensively studied and debated for many years. Studies done primarily with yeast mutants and cells obtained from human patients with peroxisomal biogenesis disorders have substantially increased our understanding of the proteins and processes involved. Proteins required for peroxisome biogenesis are called peroxins and are encoded by *PEX* genes. Ma *et al.* [3] have reviewed peroxisome assembly.

It was initially thought that peroxisomes, like lysosomes, originated by budding from the endoplasmic reticulum. Because nearly all peroxisomal proteins are non-glycosylated, and because both peroxisomal matrix and membrane proteins are synthesized in the cytoplasm on free polyribosomes, an alternative hypothesis suggested that these organelles arose from fission of pre-existing peroxisomes. In this view, newly synthesized proteins destined for peroxisomes are post-translationally targeted to the organelle; following the import of both membrane and matrix proteins, peroxisomes grow in size and ultimately divide. This model did not, however, explain the origin of peroxisomal membrane lipids. Studies with yeast mutants led to a re-evaluation of the contribution of the endoplasmic reticulum to peroxisome biogenesis, and to new models for peroxisome maturation. In mammalian cells, the peroxisomal membrane protein **PEX16** is cotranslationally targeted to endoplasmic reticulum membranes. This, in turn, recruits other membrane proteins such as **PEX3** and **PEX19** prior to budding off as nascent peroxisomes.[1]

Peroxisomal matrix proteins are imported into the growing organelle by a complex process involving many peroxins. Two peroxins, **PEX5** and **PEX7**, have been identified as cytoplasmic receptors for proteins destined for entry into peroxisomes. Most matrix proteins are targeted by a tripeptide sequence, referred to as peroxisome targeting signal (PTS). The originally described PTS1 sequence, which binds to PEX5, is located at the C-terminus of a protein and consists of serine–lysine–leucine, but several conserved variants have subsequently been identified. A small number of peroxisomal enzymes enter the organelle via PTS2, a nine amino acid residue sequence near, but not at, the N-terminus with consensus (R/K)(L/V/I/Q)XX (L/V/I/H/Q) (L/S/G/A/K)X(H/Q)(L/A/F), where "X" is any

---

[1] Official National Center for Biotechnology Information (NCBI) names of genes and proteins are **bold** when they first appear in the text.

Liver Disease in Children, Fourth Edition, ed. Frederick J. Suchy, Ronald J. Sokol, and William F. Balistreri. Published by Cambridge University Press. © Cambridge University Press 2014.

(a) (b)

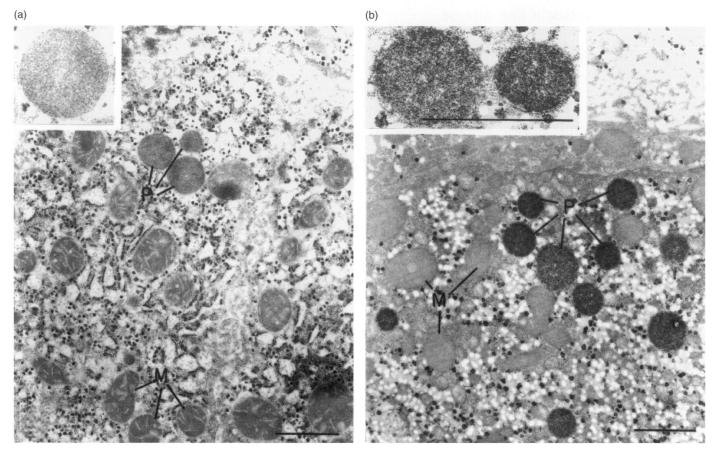

Figure 37.1 Human liver peroxisomes. Electron micrograph of normal human liver. (a) Peroxisomes (P) are readily distinguished from mitochondria (M) by their morphology. (b) Catalase cytochemistry revealing diaminobenzidine staining of peroxisomes. (Magnification ×16 000; bar, 1 μm; insets, magnification ×38 000.) (With permission from Lazarow *et al.*, 1985 [2].)

amino acid. PEX7 is the cytoplasmic receptor for PTS2-containing proteins. Some matrix proteins contain neither PTS1 nor PTS2, and it has been suggested that they enter the organelle either via an internal PTS, or by a "piggy-back" mechanism in which they bind to a PTS1-containing protein and concomitantly enter the peroxisome. Cytoplasmic PEX19 is thought to act as a receptor, as well as a chaperone, for peroxisomal membrane proteins. Peroxisome targeting signals for membrane proteins (mPTS) are less well defined than those for matrix proteins. No consensus sequences have been identified. Rather, the signal seems to involve a group of basic amino acids in an α-helical configuration adjacent to a hydrophobic domain.

Patients whose cells lack morphologically normal peroxisomal structures have a *disorder of peroxisome biogenesis* (reviewed by Steinberg *et al.* [4]). Skin fibroblasts from such patients may completely lack peroxisomes. More commonly, however, they have vesicular structures containing some peroxisomal membrane proteins. These cells either lack all matrix enzymes (peroxisomal "ghosts") or exhibit poor import of some matrix enzymes. Complementation analysis, in which fibroblasts from two different patients are chemically fused using polyethylene glycol prior to biochemical or

morphological analysis, revealed that multiple *PEX* gene products are necessary for the normal assembly of functional peroxisomes. Investigation of both human and yeast cells with defects in peroxisome biogenesis have led to the identification of more than 30 peroxins. Thirteen peroxins have been detected in humans, and mutations in at least 12 different *PEX* genes (complementation groups) have been described in patients. In addition to the *PEX* gene products already mentioned, other peroxins function as docking factors, components of import channels, or proteins necessary for receptor recycling.

Peroxisome proliferation

Treatment of rats or mice with clofibrate or any of a number of related hypolipidemic compounds results in hepatomegaly and a significant increase in the number of hepatic peroxisomes [5]. Synthesis of several hepatic peroxisomal enzymes is induced, particularly those involved in peroxisomal fatty acid beta-oxidation. Several other xenobiotic compounds (e.g. industrial phthalate ester plasticizers, herbicides, and organic solvents) have similar effects. Chemically induced peroxisome proliferation in rodents is also associated with a significantly increased incidence of hepatic neoplasia. Concerns that patients taking hypolipidemic drugs may have increased risk of cancer prompted intense investigation into the mechanism of action of peroxisome proliferators. The effects of these compounds are mediated by peroxisome proliferator activated receptors (PPARs), which are members of the steroid hormone family of nuclear receptors [6]. Three PPAR isoforms are known: PPARα, PPARδ (also called PPARβ or NUC1), and PPARγ. While tissue expression patterns for these isoforms differ, all three are found in liver. When activated by ligand binding, PPARs heterodimerize with the retinoid X receptor and bind to cis-acting peroxisome proliferator response elements to enhance gene transcription.

The mechanism of peroxisome proliferator-induced carcinogenesis is not thought to be via mutagenic or genotoxic properties of proliferators or their metabolites. Rather, the sustained induction of peroxisomal oxidases and the resulting increased generation of intracellular hydrogen peroxide may be responsible for initiation of neoplastic transformation. Interestingly, the induction of peroxisome proliferation and enzyme induction appears to be species specific. Chronic administration of hypolipidemic agents to humans and non-human primates does not cause peroxisome proliferation. Furthermore, there is no evidence linking long-term treatment of patients with lipid-lowering drugs to increased incidence of hepatic tumors.

Peroxisomal metabolic pathways

Peroxisomes carry out a significant number of vital catabolic and anabolic processes. Many of these pathways involve lipid metabolism, but the spectrum of peroxisomal metabolic function is diverse, including amino acid, purine, and polyamine metabolism. Degradation of very-long-chain fatty acids (VLCFA) and branched-chain fatty acids plus synthesis of ether-linked phospholipids, bile acids, docosahexaenoic acid, and isoprenoid compounds are among the different pathways of peroxisomal lipid metabolism.

Peroxisomal beta-oxidation

Degradation of dietary and stored fatty acids for energy production in humans and other higher organisms takes place in mitochondria. In lower organisms such as yeast, the oxidation of fatty acids is confined to peroxisomes. The recognition that mammalian peroxisomes also contain the enzymatic machinery for fatty acid beta-oxidation came to light in 1976 [7]. Shortly thereafter, three peroxisomal enzymes catalyzing the four reactions required to chain-shorten fatty acids were found in rat liver. These events marked the beginning of more than two decades of research into the metabolic functions carried out within peroxisomes.

The process by which fatty acids enter peroxisomes is not well characterized. Unlike the situation in mitochondria, carnitine is not known to be involved in this process. Peroxisomal membranes contain three members of the ATP-binding cassette subfamily D (ABCD1–ABCD3) of transmembrane proteins thought to be involved in membrane transport [8]. Coenzyme A (CoA) thioesters of VLCFA (containing 22 or more carbons) are thought to be transported into peroxisomes via ABCD1. Activation of the fatty acid to its CoA derivative would occur extraperoxisomally. Once inside peroxisomes, saturated, unbranched fatty acyl-CoAs are degraded by the sequential action of three peroxisomal enzymes: acyl-CoA oxidase (ACOX1), D-bifunctional protein (DBP; also known as multifunctional enzyme 2; encoded by HSD17B4), and 3-oxoacyl-CoA thiolase (ACAA1), yielding acetyl-CoA and an acyl-CoA shortened by two carbons (Figure 37.2). L-bifunctional protein (LBP; encoded by EHHADH), and SCPX thiolase (encoded by SCP2) can partially substitute for DBP and ACAA1, respectively. While the enzymatic reactions are similar, there are distinct differences between the mitochondrial and peroxisomal pathways. The first mitochondrial reaction is catalyzed by an FAD-containing dehydrogenase that donates its electrons to the respiratory chain. In contrast, ACOX1 (also an FAD enzyme) is coupled to the production of hydrogen peroxide from molecular oxygen. Peroxisomal DBP and LBP contain both enoyl-CoA hydratase and hydroxyacyl-CoA dehydrogenase activities. In mitochondria, these reactions are catalyzed by separate enzymes. Enoyl-CoA isomerase activity has also been attributed to LBP. Distinct mitochondrial and peroxisomal enzymes catalyze the thiolytic cleavage of 3-ketoacyl-CoAs.

The relative contribution of mitochondria to the oxidation of common long-chain fatty acids such as palmitic and oleic acids is considerably greater than that of peroxisomes, commensurate with coupling to energy production and ketogenesis in mitochondria. However, saturated VLCFA are catabolized only in peroxisomes. Dicarboxylic fatty acids, leukotrienes and other prostanoids, and certain polyunsaturated fatty acids are also partially degraded by this pathway. Studies with knockout mice have suggested that LBP is important in the degradation of dicarboxylic fatty acids [9].

The peroxisomal beta-oxidation pathway as described above is not capable of degrading 2-methyl-branched-chain fatty acids such as pristanic acid, the product of peroxisomal alpha-oxidation of phytanic acid (see below). These fatty acids are catabolized by a pathway consisting of branched-chain acyl-CoA oxidase (ACOX2), DBP, and SCPX thiolase (Figure 37.2). SCPX is a 58 kDa protein (encoded by SCP2) whose C-terminal 14 kDa is identical to sterol carrier protein 2 (SCP2) and whose N-terminal 44 kDa has thiolase activity. SCP2, originally thought to be involved in cholesterol movement in cells, may function in peroxisomes as an acyl-CoA-binding protein. Interestingly, the C-terminal portion of DBP has a high degree of homology to SCP2.

Additional peroxisomal enzymes required for fatty acid beta-oxidation include acyl-CoA synthetases for activating long-chain fatty acids and VLCFA, carnitine acetyltransferase, carnitine octanoyltransferase, α-methylacyl-CoA racemase (AMACR; see below), 2,4-dienoyl-CoA reductase, trans-2-enoyl-CoA reductase, and Δ(3,5),Δ(2,4)-dienoyl-CoA isomerase.

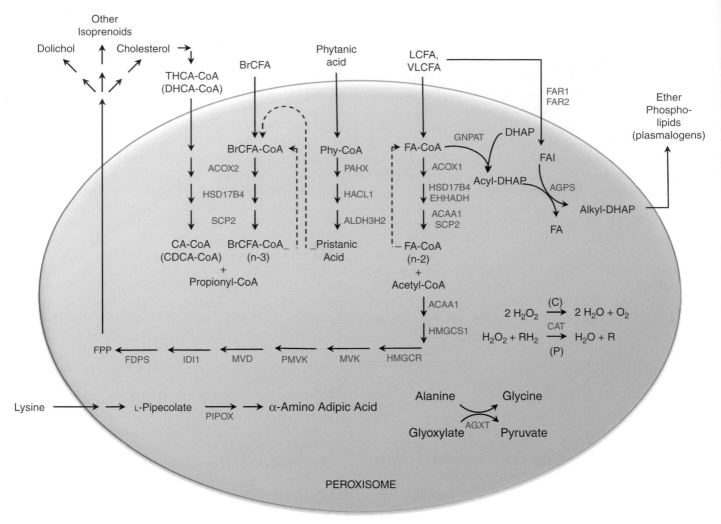

Figure 37.2 Overview of peroxisomal metabolic pathways. Peroxisomal pathways for the beta-oxidation of straight-chain and branched-chain fatty acids, the alpha-oxidation of phytanic acid, bile acid synthesis, ether phospholipid (plasmalogen) synthesis, cholesterol synthesis, pipecolic acid metabolism, glyoxylate detoxification, and hydrogen peroxide detoxification are outlined. Enzymes necessary for beta-oxidation of the coenzyme A derivatives (FA-CoA) of long-chain fatty acids (LCFA) and very-long-chain fatty acids (VLCFA) include acyl-CoA oxidase (ACOX1), D- or L-bifunctional protein (HSC17B4 and EEHADH, respectively), and 3-ketoacyl-CoA thiolase or the thiolase domain of sterol carrier protein X (ACAA1 and SCP2, respectively). The CoA derivatives of branched-chain fatty acids (BrCFA) undergo beta-oxidation by a separate but related group of enzymes that includes branched-chain acyl-CoA oxidase (ACOX2), HSD17B4, and SCP2. These enzymes also convert the CoA thioesters of the bile acid precursors tri- and dihydroxycholestanoic acids (THCA-CoA and DHCA-CoA, respectively) into the CoA derivatives of cholic acid (CA-CoA) and chenodeoxycholic acid (CDCA-CoA). The CoA derivative of phytanic acid (Phy-CoA) is converted to pristanic acid by the alpha-oxidation pathway, which includes the enzymes phytanoyl-CoA α-hydroxylase (PAHX), hydroxyphytanoyl-CoA lyase (HACL1) and aldehyde dehydrogenase (ALDH3H2). Pristanic acid is further metabolized by the branched-chain beta-oxidation pathway. Synthesis of ether phospholipids, including plasmalogens, requires two peroxisomal matrix enzymes: dihydroxyacetone (DHAP) acyltransferase (GNPAT) and alkyl-DHAP synthase (AGPS). The former catalyzes the acylation of DHAP and the latter the displacement of the fatty acid by a fatty alcohol (FAl). Fatty acyl-CoA reductases (FAR1, FAR2) on the peroxisomal membrane are involved in FAl production. Several enzymes involved in the cholesterol biosynthetic pathway between acetyl-CoA and farnesyl pyrophosphate (FPP) are peroxisomal, including thiolase (ACAA1), HMG-CoA synthase (HMGCS1), mevalonate kinase (MVK), phosphomevalonate kinase (PMVK), diphosphomevalonate decarboxylase (MVD), isopentenyl pyrophosphate isomerase 1 (IDI1), and farnesyl diphosphate synthase (FDPS). The peroxisomal enzyme L-pipecolic acid oxidase (PIPOX) degrades L-pipecolic acid, an intermediate in lysine catabolism. Glyoxylate produced by peroxisomal oxidases is detoxified by the alanine:glyoxylate aminotransferase (AGXT) reaction. Hydrogen peroxide generated by the numerous peroxisomal oxidases is detoxified by either the catalatic (C) or peroxidatic (P) activity of catalase (CAT). Peroxisomal enzymes for the activation (acyl-CoA synthetases) and transport of fatty acids are not shown.

Human diseases result from impaired peroxisomal fatty acid beta-oxidation. Patients with disorders of peroxisome biogenesis have defective beta-oxidation of both VLCFA and branched-chain fatty acids [4,10]. Other peroxisomal metabolic processes are also affected. In these disorders, the absence of normal peroxisomes results in mistargeting or cytoplasmic degradation of beta-oxidation enzymes. Most of these enzymes contain PTS1; however, ACAA1 is one of the few known

PTS2-containing proteins. Impaired beta-oxidation of VLCFA is also found in patients with deficiency of either ACOX1 or DBP, and in patients with X-linked adrenoleukodystrophy (*ABCD1* mutation). Branched-chain fatty acid metabolism and bile acid synthesis (see below) are normal in ACOX1 deficiency. Patients with DBP deficiency have decreased ability to degrade 2-methyl-branched-chain fatty acids and have impaired bile acid synthesis. However, it was not clear why these patients could not break down VLCFA normally, as they were initially thought to suffer from LBP deficiency. Only one patient had been reported to have deficiency of ACAA1, but subsequent analysis revealed that this patient had a mutation in *HSD17B4* but normal thiolase. A 45-year-old man with SCP2 deficiency was diagnosed in 2006. Documented deficiencies of LBP and branched-chain acyl-CoA oxidase have not been reported.

Since peroxisomes lack electron transport coupled to ATP synthesis, fatty acid oxidation in this organelle must serve another purpose. In some cases, the catabolic beta-oxidation pathways participate in biosynthesis processes. This is clearly the case for bile acid synthesis from cholesterol (see below). In addition, a requirement for peroxisomal beta-oxidation in the normal synthesis of docosahexaenoic acid (C22:6ω3) has been demonstrated [11]. The precursor of docosahexaenoic acid, eicosapentaenoic acid (C20:5ω3), undergoes two cycles of fatty acid elongation, forming C24:5ω3, followed by desaturation to yield C24:6ω3. The latter compound is then chain-shortened by one cycle of peroxisomal beta-oxidation, yielding docosahexaenoic acid. In other cases, it appears that a function of peroxisomal beta- and alpha-oxidation (below) is degradation of compounds that are toxic when present in excess: VLCFA, phytanic acid, and many xenobiotics fall into this category.

Peroxisomal alpha-oxidation

Fatty acids with 3-methyl branches cannot be degraded by beta-oxidation. Phytanic acid (3,7,11,15-tetramethylhexadecanoic acid), derived from the phytol side-chain of chlorophyll, is the most significant 3-methyl-branched fatty acid in the human diet. Phytanic acid is not synthesized by humans but rather is ingested in the diet primarily in the form of ruminant meats and fats (e.g. dairy products). Identification of this fatty acid as the compound that accumulated in plasma and tissues of patients with Refsum disease [12], which typically presents as an adult-onset neuropathy without significant liver disease, led to the discovery of the alpha-oxidation pathway. As shown schematically in Figure 37.2, phytanic acid is activated to its CoA thioester and then hydroxylated on C-2 in an oxygen-requiring dioxygenase reaction catalyzed by phytanoyl-CoA α-hydroxylase (**PAHX**). Hydroxyphytanoyl-CoA lyase then catalyzes the cleavage of α-hydroxyphytanoyl-CoA to pristanal, a branched-chain fatty aldehyde, and the C-1 metabolite formyl-CoA. The latter rapidly degrades to formate and CoA at neutral pH. Pristanal is then oxidized to pristanic acid (2,6,10,14-tetramethylpentadecanoic acid) via an aldehyde dehydrogenase. Pristanic acid must then be converted to its CoA derivative prior to subsequent metabolism, and it has been suggested that this reaction is catalyzed by peroxisomal very-long-chain acyl-CoA synthetase 1 [13]. The net result of alpha-oxidation is the decarboxylation of phytanic acid with shift of the position of the methyl group by one carbon, allowing further degradation of pristanoyl-CoA by the branched-chain peroxisomal beta-oxidation pathway.

PAHX, like ACAA1, is a PTS2-containing protein, whereas hydroxyphytanoyl-CoA lyase contains a PTS1. Because these matrix proteins are not properly targeted in disorders of peroxisome biogenesis, elevated plasma levels of phytanic acid and defective phytanic acid oxidation are observed. However, because phytanic acid is solely of dietary origin, plasma levels and total body burden in a given patient reflect both the patient's age and choice of food. In some children with defective peroxisome biogenesis, abnormal phytanic acid metabolism was the initial observation, prompting the name infantile Refsum disease (IRD). As discussed below, patients with peroxisome biogenesis disorders have multiple peroxisomal metabolic defects. The designation IRD is now used descriptively for those patients with a peroxisome biogenesis disorder and the longest survival.

Bile acid synthesis

Bile acid metabolism is covered extensively in Chapter 33 and will be addressed only briefly here, with particular emphasis on the role of peroxisomes. Bile acids are synthesized in the liver from cholesterol. This process requires shortening of the acyl side-chain of the sterol and was found to take place in peroxisomes (Figure 37.2) [10]. Hydroxylases and dehydrogenases located in the endoplasmic reticulum convert cholesterol into trihydroxycholestanoic acid (THCA) and dihydroxycholestanoic acid (DHCA). The side-chains of THCA and DHCA resemble 2-methyl-branched-chain fatty acids and must undergo a single cycle of beta-oxidation to produce the primary bile acids cholic acid and chenodeoxycholic acid, respectively. Activation of THCA and DHCA to their CoA derivatives is thought to occur mainly in the endoplasmic reticulum [13]. The mechanism for entry of these activated bile acid precursors into peroxisomes is not known. Both THCA-CoA and DHCA-CoA are converted to the correct stereoisomers via peroxisomal AMACR (see below) before being acted upon by the D-specific branched-chain beta-oxidation machinery. The products of beta-oxidation are the CoA derivatives of the primary bile acids. Peroxisomal bile acid-coenzyme A:amino acid *N*-acyltransferase then catalyzes the formation of glycine or taurine conjugates of cholic acid and chenodeoxycholic acid, which exit the peroxisome by a specific transporter.

As for many other peroxisomal metabolic processes, it was the observation of bile acid abnormalities in patients with peroxisome biogenesis disorders that helped to elucidate the complete bile acid biosynthetic pathway. Abnormal bile acid profiles are also found in DBP deficiency.

α-Methylacyl-CoA racemase

Stereoisomers of certain substrates and intermediates in the pathways of branched-chain fatty acid degradation and bile acid synthesis are found in nature. These include phytanic acid, pristanic acid, bile acid precursors, and other intermediates that contain asymmetric carbon centers [14]. The alpha-oxidation of phytanic acid produces both 2*R*- and 2*S*-stereoisomers of pristanic acid; however, the branched-chain acyl-CoA oxidase can only utilize 2S-isomers as substrates. These two stereoisomers of pristanic acid can be interconverted by AMACR, an enzyme found in both peroxisomes and mitochondria. The methyl groups on C-6 and C-10 of pristanic acid are also in the R-configuration, and thus require AMACR as this fatty acid is progressively shortened via several cycles of beta-oxidation.

The bile acid precursors THCA and DHCA are also normally found as both R- and S-stereoisomers. Because the carbon numbering system differs between fatty acids and sterols, it is C-25 in the bile acid precursors that is alpha to the carboxyl carbon in the side-chain. Similar to the situation that exists with pristanic acid, only the 25S-stereoisomers of THCA or DHCA are substrates for ACOX2 and can thus be converted into mature bile acids. As AMACR converts 25R- to 25S-stereoisomers, it facilitates utilization of R-isomers.

Ether lipid biosynthesis

Phospholipids containing an ether-linked alkyl or alkenyl chain on C-1 of glycerol instead of an ester-linked acyl group account for about 18% of membrane phospholipids [15]. The latter (alkenyl-containing) ether lipids are also known as plasmalogens. Peroxisomes contain three enzymes vital to ether lipid synthesis: acyl-CoA reductases, dihydroxyacetone (glycerone) phosphate acyltransferase and alkylglycerone phosphate synthase (Figure 37.2). Similar to the situation for bile acid synthesis, enzymes found in the endoplasmic reticulum are also required for complete synthesis of plasmalogens. The importance of ether phospholipids is illustrated by the severity of clinical symptoms in rhizomelic chondrodysplasia punctata (RCDP) [4]. Children with RCDP have profoundly disturbed ether lipid synthesis, shortening of proximal limbs, severely disturbed endochondral bone formation, and profound intellectual disability. The disorder is caused by defects in PEX7, the PTS2 receptor. Although dihydroxyacetone phosphate acyltransferase is targeted to peroxisomes by PTS1, alkylglycerone phosphate synthase is a PTS2-containing protein. As noted above, PAHX is a PTS2 protein; consequently, phytanic acid oxidation is also defective in RCDP. However, deficiency of dihydroxyacetone phosphate acyltransferase alone or alkylglycerone phosphate synthase alone results in the RCDP clinical phenotype [16], indicating that ether lipids are required for normal membrane function. Because peroxisomal matrix protein import is defective in the disorders of peroxisome biogenesis, ether phospholipid synthesis is impaired in these patients.

Cholesterol and isoprenoid biosynthesis

One of the first indications that peroxisomes play a role in isoprenoid synthesis came from immunoelectron micrographs showing that 3-hydroxy-3-methyl glutaryl-CoA reductase was present in the organelle [17]. Subsequent studies suggested that peroxisomes are involved in cholesterol and dolichol synthesis. Several enzymes in the cholesterol biosynthetic pathway between acetyl-CoA and farnesyl pyrophosphate have now

been detected in peroxisomes [18] (Figure 37.2), although some can also be found in the endoplasmic reticulum. However, studies in human skin fibroblasts from patients with peroxisome biogenesis disorders have raised questions regarding the significance of these observations. While the overall contribution of peroxisomes to cholesterol synthesis is not known with certainty, some patients with peroxisome biogenesis disorders were found to have decreased plasma cholesterol. Deficiency of the peroxisomal enzyme mevalonate kinase (**MVK**) results in mevalonic aciduria [19].

Peroxisomal amino acid metabolism

Peroxisomes contain several important enzymes of amino acid metabolism, particularly alanine:glyoxylate transaminase (**AGXT**) and L-pipecolate oxidase (**PIPOX**); AGXT is found only in the liver and catalyzes the transfer of the α-amino group of alanine to glyoxylate, yielding glycine and pyruvate as products (Figure 37.2). This peroxisomal enzyme is quantitatively important for degrading glyoxylate produced by two other peroxisomal enzymes, hydroxyacid oxidase (glycolate oxidase) 1 and D-amino acid oxidase. These two enzymes, which convert glycolate and glycine, respectively, to glyoxylate, are typical flavin-linked peroxisomal oxidases that utilize molecular oxygen and produce hydrogen peroxide. If not efficiently detoxified by the AGXT reaction, glyoxylate is further metabolized by glycolate oxidase to oxalate. Deficiency of AGXT occurs in primary hyperoxaluria type 1 (PH1), in which accumulation of oxalate leads to the formation of calcium oxalate kidney stones and renal failure [20]. The disease is often fatal unless liver or liver/kidney transplantation is performed. Although AGXT is targeted to peroxisomes via PTS1, a common polymorphism near the N-terminus of AGXT unmasks a weak mitochondrial targeting signal. In some patients with PH1, polymorphisms combined with additional mutations mistarget AGXT to mitochondria, thus blocking the enzyme's ability to detoxify glyoxylate.

L-Pipecolic acid is synthesized in humans as an intermediate in the minor pathway of lysine catabolism. The peroxisomal enzyme PIPOX is required for conversion of the imino acid pipecolic acid to Δ^1-piperideine-6-carboxylic acid. This is then converted to α-aminoadipic acid and ultimately to glutaric acid. Like other peroxisomal oxidases, L-pipecolic acid oxidase requires FAD and produces hydrogen peroxide. The enzyme is targeted to peroxisomes by PTS1 and so accumulation of L-pipecolic acid occurs in patients with peroxisome biogenesis disorders. Some of these patients were initially described as having hyperpipecolic acidemia but were subsequently found to have multiple peroxisomal biochemical abnormalities that place them in the Zellweger syndrome spectrum (see below). However, three children with hyperpipecolic acidemia but without other peroxisomal dysfunction were identified in 1999 [21]. No liver findings were noted in these patients. Mild elevations in plasma pipecolic acid are sometimes seen in DBP deficiency and Refsum disease. In addition, pipecolic acid levels are elevated in the mitochondrial disorder glutaric acidemia type 2 [22]. Only about 1% of lysine is degraded via pipecolic acid in the liver. A significantly greater proportion of lysine may be catabolized by this pathway in brain, and neurotoxicity of L-pipecolate has been suggested as contributing to the neurological problems in peroxisomal diseases.

Catalase

The most abundant enzyme in peroxisomes – and one of the most abundant proteins in liver – is catalase [1]. This enzyme plays a vital role in peroxisomal metabolism by decomposing hydrogen peroxide generated by peroxisomal oxidases (Figure 37.2). The catalase reaction proceeds via two mechanisms: a catalitic process ("C" in Figure 37.2) in which hydrogen peroxide is degraded to water and oxygen, and a peroxidatic process ("P" in Figure 37.2) in which a cosubstrate is oxidized by hydrogen peroxide. Unlike many peroxisomal enzymes, catalase remains active in the cytosol in the absence of normal peroxisomes. Assessing whether catalase is contained within organelles or free in the cytoplasm is useful for diagnosis of peroxisomal diseases [4]. Individuals who lack catalase (acatalasemia) are known but are either asymptomatic or have ulcerating oral lesions that are often gangrenous.

Biochemical and molecular abnormalities in peroxisomal disorders with liver involvement

Biochemical assays of peroxisomal metabolism and molecular diagnostic tools

Several assays have been developed to facilitate diagnosis of peroxisomal diseases. Plasma assays include quantification of VLCFAs, phytanic acid, L-pipecolate, and bile acid intermediates by gas chromatography or gas chromatography–mass spectrometry. Urinary pipecolate and oxalate can be measured. Ether lipids (plasmalogens) in erythrocyte membranes can be quantified. A skin biopsy and culture of fibroblasts are very useful for metabolic studies. The cellular oxidation of radiolabeled phytanic acid, VLCFAs, and pristanic acid utilizes the alpha-oxidation pathway and also both beta-oxidation pathways. Ether lipid synthesis can also be measured in fibroblasts. More specialized assays such as the subcellular distribution of catalase in fibroblasts, immunofluorescence analysis for peroxisomal proteins/enzymes, and capacity to metabolize the bile acid intermediate varanyl CoA have also facilitated diagnosis.

Wanders and Waterham pointed out that the three biochemical functions which are most useful in the laboratory diagnosis of peroxisomal diseases are beta-oxidation of fatty acids (e.g. VLCFA), biosynthesis of plasmalogens, and alpha-oxidation of phytanic acid [23]. Initial screening tests that address the first two of these functions, and that are capable of detecting a majority of patients with peroxisomal diseases, include measurement of plasma VLCFA levels and erythrocyte membrane plasmalogen levels. Peduto et al. [24] also

emphasized that elevations in plasma L-pipecolate levels, which are frequently measured in general metabolic screens, can raise suspicion of a peroxisomal disorder. While the urinary bile acid profile is characteristic in both the peroxisome biogenesis disorders and DBP deficiency [25], this assay is not as widely available as other diagnostic tests.

Moser and coworkers developed a liquid chromatography–tandem mass spectrometry method for newborn screening for X-linked adrenoleukodystrophy using dried blood spots [26]. This assay measures the VLCFA content (as hexacosanoic acid, C26:0) of lysophosphatidylcholine with a high degree of sensitivity and accuracy. The assay will also detect newborns with deficiencies of ACOX1 and DBP, and most peroxisome biogenesis disorders.

In addition to biochemical tests, DNA-based complementation analysis has been used to identify specific PEX gene defects in patients with peroxisome biogenesis disorders [27]. Suspected defects could then be confirmed by DNA mutation analysis. DNA testing for mutations in PEX genes, ABCD1, AGXT, and many other genes encoding peroxisomal enzymes is currently available (see www.genetests.org).

Disorders of peroxisome biogenesis

Peroxisome biogenesis disorders include the Zellweger syndrome spectrum and RCDP type 1 [4]. Zellweger syndrome spectrum includes infants and children with Zellweger syndrome, neonatal-onset adrenoleukodystrophy, and IRD. In these disorders, hepatic peroxisomes are generally absent or at least markedly decreased in number as a consequence of a deficiency of one of the PEX genes. Failure of peroxisomes to form normally results in a spectrum of biochemical abnormalities that reflect the different pathways present in the organelle (Table 37.1). Plasma VLCFA levels are elevated and fibroblast VLCFA oxidation is decreased. Plasma and urine pipecolate levels are elevated. Fibroblasts oxidize phytanic acid at a decreased rate and, depending on the age and diet of the patient, plasma phytanic acid levels can be elevated. Erythrocyte membrane plasmalogens are decreased and fibroblast ether lipid synthesis is defective. High plasma levels of the bile acid precursors DHCA and THCA are present. Catalase is free in the cytoplasm of fibroblasts. Conjugated hyperbilirubinemia is seen in patients with Zellweger syndrome spectrum. One patient with a PEX19 mutation was reported to have elevated liver enzymes along with both conjugated and unconjugated hyperbilirubinemia at 1 month of age [28].

Patients with RCDP type 1 differ biochemically from those with Zellweger syndrome spectrum. The former is caused by mutations in PEX7, encoding the PTS2 receptor. Only biochemical pathways that include enzymes targeted to the peroxisomal matrix via PTS2 are affected. These include alkylglycerone phosphate synthase and PAHX; consequently, impaired ether lipid synthesis and a decreased phytanic acid oxidation rate are the primary biochemical abnormalities. Although ACAA1 is also a PTS2-containing enzyme, VLCFA

Table 37.1 Biochemical defects in peroxisomal disorders

Test	Zellweger syndrome spectrum	Acyl-CoA oxidase deficiency	D-bifunctional protein deficiency	Rhizomelic chondrodysplasia punctata	Primary hyperoxaluria type 1	Mevalonate kinase deficiency
Plasma						
VLCFA	↑	↑	↑	N	N	N
Phytanic acid	N-↑	N	↑	↑	N	N
Pristanic acid	N-↑	N	↑	N	N	N
Bile acid precursors	↑	N	N-↑	N	N	N
Pipecolate	↑	N	N	N	N	N
Cholesterol	N-↓	N	N	N	N	N-↓
Urine						
Pipecolate	↑	N	N	N	N	N
Oxalate	N	N	N	N	↑	N
Erythrocyte membrane						
Plasmalogens	↓	N	N	↓	N	N
Fibroblast						
VLCFA beta-oxidation	↓	↓	↓	N	N	N
Pristanic beta-oxidation	↓	N	↓	N	N	N
Phytanic alpha-oxidation	↓	N	N-↓	↓	N	N
Ether lipid synthesis	↓	N	N	↓	N	N
Catalase distribution	C	P	P	P	P	P

NALD, neonatal adrenoleukodystrophy; IRD, infantile Refsum disease; VLCFA, very-long-chain fatty acids; N, normal; C, cytoplasmic catalase; P, peroxisomal catalase.

beta-oxidation is not typically affected in RCDP type 1, as SCP2 can substitute for ACAA1 in this pathway (Figure 37.2).

Deficiencies of individual peroxisomal enzymes

Clinically, distinction between patients with isolated deficiency of ACOX1 or DBP and those with Zellweger syndrome spectrum is difficult. Biochemical analyses can facilitate a correct diagnosis [4,10,23]. All of these patients have increased plasma VLCFA levels. Patients with DBP deficiency also have impaired branched-chain fatty acid metabolism and often accumulate bile acid precursors, whereas those with ACOX1 deficiency have normal branched-chain and bile acid metabolism. Unlike Zellweger syndrome spectrum disorders, plasmalogens are normal in these conditions and hepatic peroxisomes are present. However, in both ACOX1 and DBP deficiencies, hepatic peroxisomes are both decreased in number and are larger than normal.

The diagnostic hallmarks of PH1 (AGXT deficiency) include elevated oxalate and glycolate in urine and, occasionally, the presence of calcium oxalate crystals in liver [20]. The finding of at least a 50% decrease in AGXT activity in a liver biopsy confirms the diagnosis. Interestingly, excretion of oxalate and glycolate is not usually elevated in the peroxisome biogenesis disorders.

Large amounts of mevalonic acid are excreted by patients with mevalonic aciduria (MVK deficiency) [19]. Although decreased plasma cholesterol levels have been reported in patients with peroxisome biogenesis disorders, normal to slightly depressed levels are usually found in mevalonic aciduria.

Patients with elevated urine or plasma levels of pipecolic acid will generally have additional biochemical defects typical of Zellweger syndrome spectrum disorders. However, a small number of patients with isolated hyperpipecolic acidemia have now been described [21]. These patients had no overt liver disease in contrast to the patients with biogenesis defects.

Three of four patients with documented AMACR deficiency presented with increased plasma levels of both pristanic acid and the bile acid intermediates THCA and DHCA [29]. The fourth patient had increased amounts of THCA metabolites in urine but normal plasma pristanic acid levels [30]. Because phytanic acid (and therefore its alpha-oxidation product pristanic acid) is of dietary origin, its absence in plasma would not rule out racemase deficiency, particularly in very young children.

Clinical manifestations of peroxisomal disorders

With advances in molecular biology, the family of peroxisomal disorders has grown geometrically; the estimated cumulative incidence of these peroxisomal disorders is 1:25 000 [31]. All of the abnormalities described so far have been autosomal recessive with the exception of X-linked adrenoleukodystrophy. Parental consanguinity is common. One of the problems in attempting to classify peroxisomal disorders is that clinical syndromes have been linked to mutations in a variety of peroxisomal genes and there is a limited correlation between genotype and phenotype.

Two types of classification are generally used: disorders of peroxisomal biogenesis and disorders of single enzymes (Table 37.2). Those disorders in which some sort of hepatic involvement has been reported are noted in Table 37.2, and the various types of liver abnormality characteristic of those disorders are listed in Table 37.3. A brief summary of each of the peroxisomal disorders for which hepatic disease has been described will be presented as will a discussion of putative mechanisms underlying the liver disease, the approach to making a biochemical diagnosis (Table 37.1), and a suggested algorithm for the hepatologist who might encounter a child with one of these disorders.

Group 1: disorders of peroxisome biogenesis

Zellweger syndrome

Zellweger syndrome is a generalized peroxisomal biogenesis disorder and the phenotype is caused by mutations in any of several different genes involved in peroxisome biogenesis: **PEX1**, **PEX2**, *PEX3*, *PEX5*, **PEX6**, **PEX10**, **PEX12**, **PEX13**, **PEX14**, *PEX16*, *PEX19*, and **PEX26** [4]. Zellweger syndrome, neonatal adrenoleukodystrophy, and IRD constitute a spectrum of overlapping features the most severe of which is Zellweger syndrome and the least severe being IRD.

Zellweger syndrome is characterized by craniofacial abnormalities (wide anterior fontanelle, prominent forehead, anteverted nostrils, low nasal bridge, epicanthal folds, flattened philtrum and narrow upper lip, together with bilateral clinodactyly and talipes equinus varus). Severe neurologic abnormalities are characteristic, including hypotonia, areflexia, absent Moro response, profound intellectual disability, and seizures. Polycystic kidneys, cryptorchidism, and clitoromegaly have been noted. Poor sucking is usually noted in the newborn period and persists, leading to severe failure to thrive. Skeletal radiographs demonstrate stippled epiphyses, and dislocated hips are common. Cerebral ventricles may be dilated, and cerebral atrophy with an abnormal gyral pattern is

Table 37.2 Peroxisomal disorders

Group	Disorders
Group 1: biogenesis defects	Zellweger syndrome[a]
	Neonatal adrenoleukodystrophy[a]
	Infantile Refsum disease[a]
	Hyperpipecolic acidemia([a]?)
	Rhizomelic chondrodysplasia punctata type 1
Group 2: single enzyme/protein deficiencies	D-bifunctional protein deficiency[a]
	Acyl-CoA oxidase deficiency[a]
	Hyperoxaluria type 1 (alanine:glyoxylate aminotransferase deficiency)[a]
	Mevalonate kinase deficiency[a]
	Hyperpipecolic acidemia (L-pipecolate oxidase deficiency)
	X-linked adrenoleukodystrophy
	Rhizomelic chondrodysplasia punctata type 2 (dihydroxyacetone phosphate acyltransferase deficiency)
	Rhizomelic chondrodysplasia punctata type 3 (alkyl dihydroxyacetone phosphate synthase deficiency)
	Refsum disease (classic type; phytanoyl-CoA hydroxylase deficiency)
	Glutaric aciduria type 3 (glutaryl-CoA oxidase deficiency)

[a] Liver abnormalities.

Table 37.3 Hepatic abnormalities characteristic of certain peroxisomal disorders

Disorder	Hepato megaly	Hepatitis	Jaundice	Stones	Fibrosis
Zellweger syndrome	X		X	X	X
Neonatal adrenoleukodystrophy	X				
Infantile Refsum disease	X		X	X	
Hyperpipecolic acidemia	X				
Acyl Co-A oxidase deficiency		X			X
D-bifunctional enzyme deficiency	X	X			X
Primary hyperoxaluria type 1	X				
Mevalonate kinase deficiency	X		X		

characteristic as are neonatal seizures. The average age of death is 5 months (range 1 week to 18 months in one series).

All children with Zellweger syndrome have liver disease. In normal human fetal liver, peroxisomes are present as early as the sixth week of gestation, but in children with Zellweger syndrome, hepatic peroxisomes are still absent at mid-gestation. Hepatic abnormalities include hepatomegaly (which may be slight and inconsistent or marked and persistent) and conjugated hyperbilirubinemia in early infancy, possibly resulting from intrahepatic biliary dysgenesis. Occasionally, jaundice can be transient. Late in the first year of life, firm hepatomegaly with splenomegaly suggestive of cirrhosis and portal hypertension has been reported. Hepatic histology reveals excessive hepatic iron stores and a cholangiolar lesion characterized by tiny plugs of bile in the cholangioles, particularly in the periportal area [32]. Electron microscopy of liver reveals absent peroxisomes and, occasionally, mitochondrial abnormalities. Angulated secondary lysosomes may be present in Kupffer cells and hepatocytes. Renal peroxisomes are also absent. The liver disease and some of the clinical features in a patient with a novel *PEX14* mutation were particularly notable because of similarities with Alagille syndrome: infantile jaundice, facial dysmorphy, posterior embryotoxon, and hepatomegaly. Liver histology revealed bile duct paucity, cholestasis, arterial hyperplasia, very small branches of the vena portae, and parenchymal destruction [33]. One patient with a mutation in *PEX19* had a severe phenotype with epilepsy, hypotonia, liver enzyme abnormalities, jaundice, liver failure, multiple gallstones, and a renal tubular defect. Setchell *et al.* [34] postulated that administration of primary bile acid would be beneficial in improving liver function by downregulation in the synthesis of these abnormal acids. Accordingly, they administered cholic acid and chenodeoxycholic acid (each 100 mg/day) via the oral route to a 6-month-old boy with Zellweger syndrome. Biochemical indices of liver function improved as did the hepatic histology, coincident with a significant decrease in serum and urinary cholestanoic acids. However Keane *et al.* [35] have pointed out the hazards of bile acid administration to peroxisome-deficient mice, as well as some of the benefits, showing that the therapy simultaneously alleviated cholestasis and aggravated mitochondrial damage. Administration of dietary Lorenzo's oil (a synthetic oil containing trioleate and trierucate) and the ethyl ester of docosahexaenoic acid in four patients with Zellweger syndrome increased levels of docosahexaenoic acid in the patients' livers [36].

Neonatal adrenoleukodystrophy

Neonatal adrenoleukodystrophy is also a defect of peroxisomal biogenesis. The disorder is cause by mutations in *PEX5*, encoding PTS1, or in *PEX1, PEX6, PEX10, PEX12, PEX13,* or *PEX 26* [4]. Approximately 25% of affected children have some dysmorphic features; deafness is characteristic, psychomotor delay is progressive, and hypotonia is moderate as are seizures. Electroencephalography may show hypsarrhythmia. Cortical atrophy and micropolygyria may occur. The adrenals are small

with atrophic cortices. Hepatic peroxisomes are absent or greatly diminished. Survival is longer than it is in Zellweger syndrome, with some children surviving into the second decade. A few residual peroxisomes may be seen in the liver, and hepatomegaly is characteristic. In general, the liver disease is mild. An 11-year-old boy with intellectual disability and sensorineural deafness has been described in whom chronic liver disease was considered his major clinical problem.

Infantile Refsum disease

Infantile Refsum disease, also a disorder of peroxisomal biogenesis, is caused by mutations in *PEX1, PEX2, PEX6, PEX12,* or *PEX26* [4]. The syndrome is characterized clinically by dysmorphic features in approximately 25%, large anterior fontanelle, failure to thrive, feeding problems, and poor vision. Craniofacial abnormalities are milder than those in Zellweger syndrome and may not be noted until later in the first year of life. Reported abnormalities include round facies, flat occiput, high forehead, frontal bossing, epicanthal folds, telecanthus, depressed nasal bridge, small mouth, protruding tongue, low-set ears, and short neck. Hypotonia is present occasionally, although not as marked as in Zellweger syndrome, and peripheral reflexes are preserved. There is progressive psychomotor delay. Sensorineural deafness (100%) and rotary nystagmus have been reported along with pigmentary retinopathy (Leber congenital amaurosis). Genitourinary abnormalities reported, include bilateral vesicopelvicalyceal dilation and vesicourethral reflux.

Hepatomegaly is often observed. Other hepatobiliary abnormalities include isolated neonatal cholestasis without other organ system involvement. Cholelithiasis and mildly deranged liver function have been reported as early as 6 months of age. Liver disease may progress and become clinically significant in children who survive the first decade. Hepatic peroxisomes are absent or deficient, and defects in bile acid metabolism are similar to those characteristic of Zellweger syndrome. There is one report of successful hepatocyte transplantation in this disorder [37].

Hyperpipecolic academia

A deficiency of PIPOX leads to isolated hyperpipecolic acidemia [21] and it is postulated that several cases originally described as hyperpipecolic acidemia were probably unrecognized examples of Zellweger syndrome prior to the discovery of the multiple peroxisomal defects characteristic of that syndrome. Patients with PIPOX deficiency presented with hypotonia and enlarged fontanelles, psychomotor retardation, facial dysmorphism, and aggression. Liver disease was not mentioned in the one report of patients with the isolated enzyme deficiency.

Group 2: isolated peroxisomal enzyme deficiencies
D-bifunctional protein deficiency

D-bifunctional protein contains both D-3-hydroxyacyl-CoA hydratase and D-3-hydroxyacyl-CoA dehydrogenase activities. Both peroxisomal fatty acid beta-oxidation and conversion of bile acid precursors to mature bile acids is abnormal in patients with DBP deficiency. Patients are hypotonic with mild craniofacial dysmorphism, multifocal tonic-clonic seizures, and calcific stippling of certain joints. Hepatomegaly and hepatic dysfunction have been reported; one patient in our institution also had liver fibrosis (G. V. Raymond, personal communication). However the liver disease is milder than that observed in Zellweger syndrome.

Acyl-CoA oxidase deficiency

Patients with ACOX1 deficiency clinically resemble patients with neonatal adrenoleukodystrophy but differ in that their hepatic peroxisomes are not decreased in number. Clinical features include profound hypotonia and dysmorphic features, including hypertelorism, epicanthal folds, low nasal bridge, low-set ears, and polydactyly.

In a series of six patients with the disorder, hepatic abnormalities were not observed; however, liver fibrosis and elevated serum aminotransferases have been seen in two patients in our institution (G V Raymond, personal communication). Neither liver failure nor portal hypertension has been reported. Livers of mice with selective disruption of *ACOX1* have metabolic abnormalities including development of steatohepatitis, hepatocellular regeneration, and spontaneous peroxisome proliferation, which often resulted in hepatocellular carcinomas; these changes have not been reported in humans.

Primary hyperoxaluria type 1

Although PH1 is secondary to deficiency of AGXT, phenotypically the disorder is distinct from all other peroxisomal disorders. It is characterized by a continuous, high urinary oxalate excretion and progressive bilateral oxalate urolithiasis and nephrocalcinosis. There are no neurologic or craniofacial abnormalities. In the era before organ transplantation, death from renal failure occurred in childhood or early adulthood. Extrarenal deposits of calcium oxalate have been observed in skin, retina, and myocardium. We have observed massive hepatomegaly secondary to calcium oxalate deposits in the liver of a 20-year-old patient with the disorder.

Pyridoxine is a cofactor in the AGXT enzyme pathway and pyridoxine in doses of up to 200 mg/day has been shown to reduce and, in some cases, normalize urinary oxalate and glycolate excretion. However, there are numerous *AGXT* missense mutations that cause PH1; recent studies of the crystal structure of AGXT indicate that patients with some missense mutations are less likely to respond to pyridoxine therapy than others. Orthophosphate supplementation may prevent the progression of calcium oxalate stones and small doses of a thiazide diuretic may be useful [38].

Since the primary enzyme defect is in the liver, renal transplantation is unsuccessful because the donor kidney is injured by continuous deposits of calcium oxalate. Therefore, since the late 1980s, the recommended approach for patients with end-stage renal disease secondary to PH1 is to perform combined liver–kidney transplantation. One patient suffered from livedo reticularis, peripheral gangrene, and third-degree heart block secondary to calcium oxalate sludge; all of these manifestations resolved following liver transplantation. Bergstrahl *et al.* [39] have used the life-table method to analyze transplantation outcomes in PH1. Kidney plus liver had better kidney graft outcomes than kidney alone, with death-censored graft survival of 95% versus 56% at 3 years ($p = 0.011$). Whether simultaneous liver–kidney transplant is done (to provide maximal immunologic benefit) or sequential liver transplantation followed by kidney transplantation (which provides biochemical benefit) depends on many factors including disease staging, facilities, and access to deceased or living donors [40].

Successful early combined liver and en bloc kidney transplant from a 2-year-old donor to a 3-month-old infant with PH1 has been reported [41]. Cadaveric liver followed by living donor kidney transplantation is another approach to PH1 that has been successful [42]. Still another reported approach is sequential liver and kidney transplants from the same living donor [43]. Given that combined liver–kidney transplantation does not induce true catch-up growth in the majority of children with PH1 who receive a transplant when kidney failure has already resulted in growth stunting, consideration could be given to transplantation at an earlier age before severe growth failure has resulted from end-stage kidney disease [44].

Novel non-transplant approaches include restoration of defective enzymatic activity through the use of chemical chaperones and hepatocyte cell transplantation, or recombinant gene therapy for enzyme replacement [45]. *Oxalobacter formigenes* has been administered to nine patients with PH1 with the goal of using colonic degradation of endogenous oxalate to decrease urinary oxalate [46]. The treatment was at least partially successful. However, all of the above non-transplant therapeutic approaches remain experimental at the present time.

Primary hyperoxaluria type 1 is probably the only peroxisomal disorder in which percutaneous liver biopsy was always needed in the past to establish a definitive diagnosis, as AGXT is only found in liver, where it is largely confined to peroxisomes. In patients with the disorder, enzyme activity in liver ranged from 11 to 47% of control values; the degree of deficiency appears to be related to clinical severity and the amount of biochemical derangement. In the future, molecular testing may supplant liver biopsy as an initial diagnostic approach to this disorder.

Prenatal diagnosis is possible; successful methods include enzyme assay, immunoassay, and immunoelectron microscopy of fetal liver tissues (second trimester) and linkage and mutation analysis of DNA isolated from chorionic villus samples in the first trimester.

Mevalonate kinase deficiency

Mevalonic aciduria, the first recognized defect in the biosynthesis of cholesterol and isoprenoids, is secondary to deficiency of MVK. Patients may have failure to thrive, developmental delay, anemia, hepatosplenomegaly, cataracts, and dysmorphic facies. On occasion, patients lack significant neurologic abnormalities and the presentation may be that of neonatal cholestasis or it may mimic that of congenital infections or myelodysplastic syndromes, with severe anemia, petechiae, hepatosplenomegaly, leukocytosis, and recurrent febrile episodes predominating [47].

α-Methylacyl-CoA racemase deficiency

Documented AMACR deficiency has only been reported for four patients to date. Two adults presented with adult-onset sensory motor neuropathy [29]. An infant with Niemann–Pick C disease was diagnosed serendipitously; no symptoms could clearly be attributed to the racemase deficiency [29]. Another infant presented with vitamin K deficiency, severe cholestasis, and giant cell neonatal hepatitis [30]. The infant responded well to treatment with cholic acid and fat-soluble vitamin supplementation. At age 7 years, she was reportedly in good health. This infant had an older sibling who had died of vitamin K deficiency prior to the infant's diagnosis of racemase deficiency. The sibling's liver had been used as a donor liver for a pediatric liver transplant procedure. The recipient had a post-transplant liver biopsy that was significant for acute rejection, bile duct proliferation, and fibrosis. It was assumed that the older sibling had succumbed to racemase deficiency. The liver recipient was then treated with ursodeoxycholic acid and was reportedly doing well 8 years post-transplant.

A mouse model for this disorder was produced in 2004 [48]. Interestingly the knockout mice showed a 44-fold increase of C_{27} bile acid precursors and >50% decrease in primary (C_{24}) bile acids in bile, serum, and liver but did not develop liver disease until they were fed a diet supplemented with phytol, a source for branched-chain fatty acids. The authors, therefore, proposed elimination of dietary phytol for patients with this disorder.

X-linked adrenoleukodystrophy

Three newborn boys with profound neonatal hypotonia, subsequent failure to thrive, and cholestatic liver disease have been described [49]. Liver biopsies showed cholestatis that was both intracanalicular and ductal. All three infants died; their livers were small, cholestatic, and fibrotic at autopsy. The infants lacked adrenoleukodystrophy protein and gene deletions were identified that extended into the promoter region of *ABCD1* and the neighboring gene, *DXS1357E*. The authors proposed the term CADDS (contiguous ABCD1 DXS1357E deletion syndrome) to describe this syndrome.

Putative mechanisms for hepatic abnormalities

Although mechanisms underlying the hepatic abnormalities observed in the above list of peroxisomal disorders have not been clarified, some generalizations can be made. Those disorders characterized by abnormalities in the metabolism of bile acids are most frequently associated with hepatomegaly, cholestasis, and hepatic fibrosis, including the Zellweger–neonatal adrenoleukodystrophy–IRD spectrum and DBP deficiency. The experience of Setchell *et al.* [34] in ameliorating cholestasis and hepatic histology in a child with Zellweger syndrome by administration of primary bile acids suggests that, in at least some patients, the liver disease results from deficiency of primary bile acids and/or accumulation of toxic bile acid intermediates. In one patient with Zellweger syndrome, the biliary profile of cysteinyl-leukotrienes was markedly abnormal, with increased omega-oxidation metabolites of cysteinyl-leukotriene 4 and decreased amounts of a beta-oxidation metabolite of cysteinyl-leukotriene 3, suggesting that these abnormal metabolites might contribute to the liver disease [50]. A rat hepatoma cell line has been used to investigate potential toxicity of the C_{27} bile acid intermediates that accumulate in several peroxisomal disorders. When these cells were exposed to these compounds, cell viability decreased and a dose-dependent decrease in ATP synthesis by isolated mitochondria was observed as well as a dose-dependent stimulated of reactive oxygen species, which were implicated in the toxicity. In contrast to Zellweger syndrome, RCDP, in which severe bony abnormalities are characteristic, is not associated with either liver disease or abnormalities in bile acid metabolism.

The *Pex5* knockout mouse model has been used to study the ontogenesis of hepatic peroxisomes and hepatic disease in Zellweger syndrome. Functional peroxisomes are not detected by the diaminobenzidine method and catalase is mislocalized to the nucleus and cytoplasm [51]. Crystals of VLCFA accumulate in liver, and mitochondria are abnormal both structurally and functionally, suggesting that oxidative stress may play a role in the liver injury. A number of mice have been developed with different *Pex* genes knocked out. These mice have proved valuable in investigating the physiological importance of these genes not only in the development of the neurologic abnormalities but also in understanding the basis of the hepatomegaly and liver fibrosis characteristic of these disorders [52].

As noted in Figure 37.2, both ACOX1 and MVK are distantly involved in the peroxisomal metabolism of bile acids through generation of THCA and DHCA from cholesterol. This relationship and/or the microvesicular steatosis characteristic of the *Acox1* knockout mouse described above may be responsible for the hepatic abnormalities noted in some patients with one of these disorders. Mouse models with targeted disruption of PPARα or peroxisomal beta-oxidation enzymes have suggested a link between these deficiencies and the development of steatohepatitis [53]. Conversely mice with coordinated upregulation of genes controlling peroxisomal beta-oxidation are resistant to diet-induced hepatosteatosis.

Approach to laboratory diagnosis of peroxisomal diseases

If a peroxisome biogenesis disorder is suspected on clinical grounds, quantification of plasma VLCFA levels by gas chromatography is the most informative initial biochemical assay

(Table 37.1). In some laboratories, phytanic and pristanic acids can be quantified in the same analysis, although these may not be informative based on the age or diet of the patient. If elevated VLCFA levels are detected, a skin biopsy should be requested for measurement of ether phospholipid synthesis and phytanic acid oxidation. This is particularly helpful in distinguishing biogenesis disorders from DBP deficiency. Plasma and urine bile acid analysis, urine pipecolic acid concentration, and erythrocyte membrane plasmalogen levels provide additional evidence to support a diagnosis. Although liver involvement is not generally a feature of ACOX1 deficiency and RCDP, these analyses will distinguish these disorders from biogenesis disorders and DBP deficiency. Janzen *et al.* [54] have developed a method for rapid quantification of conjugated and unconjugated bile acids and C_{27} precursors in dried blood spots and small amounts of serum that is appropriate for screening newborns for both cholestatic hepatopathy and peroxisomal disorders and distinguishing between the two. DNA testing can provide a definitive diagnosis.

Presentation of patients with peroxisomal diseases to the hepatologist

In general, patients with peroxisomal disorders whose hepatic manifestations lead to consultation by a pediatric hepatologist would exhibit typical craniofacial and neurologic abnormalities, which should lead to analysis of plasma VLCFA as the first step. However, it should be emphasized that at least some patients with IRD have presented with neonatal cholestasis without obvious extrahepatic manifestations, so a diagnostic work-up for this disorder should be considered for unexplained neonatal cholestasis which fails to resolve. Given that more than 50 peroxisomal enzymes have been described, it is likely that new peroxisomal disorders will be described in the future, and unexplained neonatal cholestasis may be a feature. Finally, the pediatric hepatologist can play a key role in establishing a definitive diagnosis of PH1 by performing a percutaneous liver biopsy for enzyme analysis if mutation testing of lymphocyte DNA does not yield a diagnosis. The pediatric hepatologist could also play an important role in the management of a patient with PH1 by helping in decision making regarding the appropriateness of pre-emptive liver transplant or hepatorenal transplant.

Treatment of liver disease in patients with peroxisomal disorders

Although treatment options for peroxisomal diseases remain limited, Setchell *et al.* [34] demonstrated that the combination of cholic acid and chenodeoxycholic acid improved the liver disease of one patient with Zellweger syndrome. Maeda *et al.* [55] demonstrated that the use of chenodeoxycholic acid alone was deleterious but that the combination of this bile acid and ursodeoxycholic acid was beneficial. Docosahexaenoic acid has led to dramatic clinical and biochemical improvement in patients with Zellweger syndrome and IRD and slight biochemical improvement in a child with neonatal adrenoleukodystrophy [56]. However, a subsequent randomized, double-blind, placebo-controlled trial involving 48 patients found no difference in outcomes between docosahexaenoic acid treatment and placebo. As described in detail in the section on PH1, this peroxisomal disorder is the most amenable to treatment but the conventional treatment is heroic: liver–kidney transplantation. With progress in cell, molecular, and genetic therapies, it is realistic to hope that these techniques may one day be applied to more definitive therapies for children who suffer from peroxisomal disorders.

References

1. de Duve C, Baudhuin P. Peroxisomes (microbodies and related particles). *Physiol Rev* 1966;**46**:323–357.

2. Lazarow PB, Black V, Shio H, *et al.* Zellweger syndrome: biochemical and morphological studies on two patients treated with clofibrate. *Pediatric Res* 1985;**19**:1356–1364.

3. Ma C, Agrawal G, Subramani S. Peroxisome assembly: matrix and membrane protein biogenesis. *J Cell Biol* 2011;**193**:7–16.

4. Steinberg SJ, Dodt G, Raymond GV *et al.* Peroxisome biogenesis disorders. *Biochim Biophys Acta* 2006;**1763**: 1733–1748.

5. Lai DY. Rodent carcinogenicity of peroxisome proliferators and issues on human relevance. *J Environ Sci Health C Environ Carcinog Ecotoxicol Rev* 2004;**22**:37–55.

6. Varga T, Czimmerer Z, Nagy L. PPARs are a unique set of fatty acid regulated transcription factors controlling both lipid metabolism and inflammation. *Biochim Biophys Acta* 2011;**1812**: 1007–1022.

7. Lazarow PB, De Duve C. A fatty acyl-CoA oxidizing system in rat liver peroxisomes; enhancement by clofibrate, a hypolipidemic drug. *Proc Natl Acad Sci USA* 1976;**73**:2043–2046.

8. Kemp S, Theodoulou FL, Wanders RJ. Mammalian peroxisomal ABC transporters: from endogenous substrates to pathology and clinical significance. *Br J Pharmacol* 2011;**164**:1753–1766.

9. Dirkx R, Meyhi E, Asselberghs S, *et al.* Beta-oxidation in hepatocyte cultures from mice with peroxisomal gene knockouts. *Biochem Biophys Res Commun* 2007;**357**:718–723.

10. Wanders RJ, Ferdinandusse S, Brites P. *et al.* Peroxisomes, lipid metabolism and lipotoxicity. *Biochim Biophys Acta* 2010;**1801**: 272–280.

11. Moore SA, Hurt E, Yoder E, *et al.* Docosahexaenoic acid synthesis in human skin fibroblasts involves peroxisomal retroconversion of tetracosahexaenoic acid. *J Lipid Res* 1995;**36**:2433–2443.

12. Wanders RJ, Komen J, Ferdinandusse S. Phytanic acid metabolism in health and disease. *Biochim Biophys Acta* 2011;**1811**:498–507.

13. Watkins PA. Very-long-chain acyl-CoA synthetases. *J Biol Chem* 2008;**283**: 1773–1777.

14. Lloyd MD, Darley DJ, Wierzbicki AS. et al. Alpha-methylacyl-CoA racemase: an "obscure" metabolic enzyme takes centre stage. *FEBS J* 2008;**275**: 1089–1102.

15. Horrocks LA, Sharma M. Plasmalogens and *O*-alkyl glycerophospholipids. In Nawthorne JN, Ansell GB (eds.) *Phospholipids. New Comprehensive Biochemistry.* Amsterdam: Elsevier Biomedical, 1982, pp. 51–93.

16. Itzkovitz B, Jiralerspong S, Nimmo G, et al. Functional characterization of novel mutations in GNPAT and AGPS, causing rhizomelic chondrodysplasia punctata (RCDP) types 2 and 3. *Hum Mutat* 2012;**33**:189–197.

17. Keller GA, Barton MC, Shapiro DJ, et al. 3-Hydroxy-3-methylglutaryl-coenzyme A reductase is present in peroxisomes in normal rat liver cells. *Proc Natl Acad Sci USA* 1985;**82**:770–774.

18. Kovacs WJ, Olivier LM, Krisans SK. Central role of peroxisomes in isoprenoid biosynthesis. *Prog Lipid Res* 2002;**41**:369–391.

19. Bader-Meunier B, Florkin B, Sibilia J, et al. Mevalonate kinase deficiency: a survey of 50 patients. *Pediatrics* 2011;**128**:e152–e159.

20. Williams EL, Acquaviva C, Amoroso A, et al. Primary hyperoxaluria type 1: update and additional mutation analysis of the *AGXT* gene. *Hum Mutat* 2009;**30**:910–917.

21. Kerckaert I, Poll-The BT, Wanders RJA, et al. Hepatic peroxisomes in isolated hyperpipecolic acidaemia justify its classification as single peroxisomal enzyme deficiency. *J Inherit Metab Dis* 1999;**22**(Suppl 1):29.

22. Frerman FE, Goodman SI. Nuclear-encoded defects of the mitochondrial respiratory chain, including glutaric acidemia type II. In Scriver CR, Beaudet AL, Sly WS, Valle D (eds.) *The Metabolic and Molecular Bases of Inherited Disease.* New York: McGraw-Hill, 1995, pp. 1611–1629.

23. Wanders RJ, Waterham HR. Peroxisomal disorders I: biochemistry and genetics of peroxisome biogenesis disorders. *Clin Genet* 2005;**67**: 107–133.

24. Peduto A, Baumgartner MR, Verhoeven NM et al. Hyperpipecolic acidaemia: a diagnostic tool for peroxisomal disorders. *Mol Genet Metab* 2004;**82**:224–230.

25. Yousef IM, Perwaiz S, Lamireau T, et al. Urinary bile acid profile in children with inborn errors of bile acid metabolism and chronic cholestasis; Screening technique using Electrospray tandem mass-spectrometry (ES/MS/MS). *Med Sci Monit* 2003;**9**: MT21–31.

26. Hubbard WC, Moser AB, Tortorelli S, et al. Combined liquid chromatography-tandem mass spectrometry as an analytical method for high throughput screening for X-linked adrenoleukodystrophy and other peroxisomal disorders: preliminary findings. *Mol Genet Metab* 2006;**89**:185–187.

27. Ebberink MS, Mooijer PA, Gootjes J, et al. Genetic classification and mutational spectrum of more than 600 patients with a Zellweger syndrome spectrum disorder. *Hum Mutat* 2010;**32**:59–69.

28. Mohamed S, El-Meleagy E, Nasr A, et al. A mutation in *PEX19* causes a severe clinical phenotype in a patient with peroxisomal biogenesis disorder. *Am J Med Genet A* 2010;**152A**: 2318–2321.

29. Ferdinandusse S, Overmars H, Denis S, et al. Plasma analysis of di- and trihydroxycholestanoic acid diastereoisomers in peroxisomal alpha-methylacyl-CoA racemase deficiency. *J Lipid Res* 2001;**42**:137–141.

30. Van Veldhoven PP, Meyhi E, Squires RH, et al. Fibroblast studies documenting a case of peroxisomal 2-methylacyl-CoA racemase deficiency: possible link between racemase deficiency and malabsorption and vitamin K deficiency. *Eur J Clin Invest* 2001;**31**:714–722.

31. Roth KS. Peroxisomal disease: common ground for pediatrician, cell biologist, biochemist, pathologist, and neurologist. *Clin Pediatr* 1999; **38**:73–75.

32. Bove KE, Daugherty CC, Tyson W, et al. Bile acid synthetic defects and liver disease. *Pediatr Dev Pathol* 2000;**3**:1–16.

33. Huybrechts SJ, Van Veldhoven PP, Hoffman I, et al. Identification of a novel *PEX14* mutation in Zellweger syndrome. *J Med Genet* 2008;**45**: 376–383.

34. Setchell KD, Bragetti P, Zimmer-Nechemias L, et al. Oral bile acid treatment and the patient with Zellweger syndrome. *Hepatology* 1992; **15**:198–207.

35. Keane MH, Overmars H, Wikander TM, et al. Bile acid treatment alters hepatic disease and bile acid transport in peroxisome-deficient PEX2 Zellweger mice. *Hepatology* 2007;**45**:982–997.

36. Arai Y, Kitamura Y, Hayashi M, et al. Effect of dietary Lorenzo's oil and docosahexaenoic acid treatment for Zellweger syndrome. *Congenit Anom* 2008;**48**:180–182.

37. Dhawan A, Mitry RR, Hughes RD. Hepatocyte transplantation for liver-based metabolic disorders. *J Inherit Metab Dis* 2006;**29**:431–435.

38. Milliner DS, Eickholt JT, Bergstralh EJ et al. Results of long-term treatment with orthophosphate and pyridoxine in patients with primary hyperoxaluria. *N Engl J Med* 1994;**331**:1553–1558.

39. Bergstralh EJ, Monico CG, Lieske JC. et al. Transplantation outcomes in primary hyperoxaluria. *Am J Transplant* 2010;**10**:2493–2501.

40. Cochat P, Fargue S, Harambat J. Primary hyperoxaluria type 1: strategy for organ transplantation. *Curr Opin Organ Transplant* 2010;**15**: 590–593.

41. Heffron TG, Rodriguez J, Fasola CG. et al. Successful outcome after early combined liver and en bloc-kidney transplant in an infant with primary hyperoxaluria type 1: a case report. *Pediatr Transplant* 2009;**13**: 940–942.

42. Malla I, Lysy PA, Godefroid N, et al. Two-step transplantation for primary hyperoxaluria: cadaveric liver followed by living donor related kidney transplantation. *Pediatr Transplant* 2009;**13**:782–784.

43. Rosenblatt GS, Jenkins RD, Barry JM. Treatment of primary hyperoxaluria type 1 with sequential liver and kidney transplants from the same living donor. *Urology* 2006;**68**:427 e7–8.

44. Nissel R, Latta K, Gagnadoux MF, et al. Body growth after combined liver–kidney transplantation in children with primary hyperoxaluria type 1. *Transplantation* 2006;**82**:48–54.

45. Bobrowski AE, Langman CB. Hyperoxaluria and systemic oxalosis: current therapy and future directions. *Expert Opin Pharmacother* 2006;7:1887–1896.

46. Hoppe B, Beck BB, Milliner DS. The primary hyperoxalurias. *Kidney Int* 2009;**75**:1264–1271.

47. Hinson DD, Rogers ZR, Hoffmann GF *et al.* Hematological abnormalities and cholestatic liver disease in two patients with mevalonate kinase deficiency. *Am J Med Genet* 1998;**78**:408–412.

48. Savolainen K, Kotti TJ, Schmitz W, *et al.* A mouse model for {alpha}-methylacyl-CoA racemase deficiency: adjustment of bile acid synthesis and intolerance to dietary methyl-branched lipids. *Hum Mol Genet* 2004;**13**:955–965.

49. Corzo D, Gibson W, Johnson K, *et al.* Contiguous deletion of the X-Linked adrenoleukodystrophy gene (*ABCD1*) and *DXS1357E*: a novel neonatal phenotype similar to peroxisomal biogenesis disorders. *Am J Hum Genet* 2002;**70**:1520–1531.

50. Mayatepek E, Ferdinandusse S, Meissner T, *et al.* Analysis of cysteinyl leukotrienes and their metabolites in bile of patients with peroxisomal or mitochondrial beta-oxidation defects. *Clin Chim Acta* 2004;**345**:89–92.

51. Baumgart E, Vanhorebeek I, Grabenbauer M, *et al.* Mitochondrial alterations caused by defective peroxisomal biogenesis in a mouse model for Zellweger syndrome (*Pex5* knockout mouse). *Am J Pathol* 2001;**159**:1477–1494.

52. Baes M, Van Veldhoven PP. Generalised and conditional inactivation of *Pex* genes in mice. *Biochim Biophys Acta* 2006;**1763**: 1785–1793.

53. Reddy JK. Nonalcoholic steatosis and steatohepatitis. III. Peroxisomal beta-oxidation, PPARalpha, and steatohepatitis. *Am J Physiol Gastrointest Liver Physiol* 2001;**281**: G1333–G1339.

54. Janzen N, Sander S, Terhardt M, *et al.* Rapid quantification of conjugated and unconjugated bile acids and C_{27} precursors in dried blood spots and small volumes of serum. *J Lipid Res* 2010;**51**:1591–1598.

55. Maeda K, Kimura A, Yamato Y, *et al.* Oral bile acid treatment in two Japanese patients with Zellweger syndrome. *J Pediatr Gastroenterol Nutr* 2002;**35**:227–230.

56. Martinez M, Vazquez E, Garcia-Silva MT, *et al.* Therapeutic effects of docosahexaenoic acid ethyl ester in patients with generalized peroxisomal disorders. *Am J Clin Nutr* 2000;**71**:376S-385S.

Urea cycle disorders

38

Derek Wong and Stephen Cederbaum

Introduction

The urea cycle was first described in 1932 by Krebs and Henseleit [1] (Figure 38.1). The urea cycle disorders (UCD) result from defects in the metabolism of the extra nitrogen produced by the breakdown of protein and other nitrogen-containing molecules. The incidence of these disorders in the USA is estimated to be at least 1 in 25 000 births, but partial defects may make this number much higher.

This chapter discusses the clinical presentation, underlying molecular pathology, treatment options, and diagnostic testing for this group of diseases. The study of UCDs is of particular interest in gastroenterology because many acquired or genetic diseases of the liver have an impact on this cycle and the processing of ammonia and nitrogen. Many of the treatment strategies employed in treating patients with rare urea cycle defects are exportable to the larger community of patients with hyperammonemia.

Some basics of nitrogen metabolism

The bulk of the nitrogen that requires processing comes from removal of the amino group on amino acids during the process of oxidative breakdown. This occurs during normal metabolism and at a higher rate during times of caloric insufficiency or stress as a means of energy release during periods of negative nitrogen balance. The brain produces a significant amount of ammonia, which it must convert to glutamine for export through the addition of nitrogen, first to α-ketoglutarate to make glutamate, and then to glutamine with the addition of nitrogen.

Under normal conditions there are 30 µmol/L soluble ammonia and 200 mg/L urea nitrogen in blood. The conversion to urea in the liver is, therefore, a very efficient and mostly one-way process, with a net expenditure of one ATP per urea molecule produced. Once produced, the urea is excreted primarily via the kidneys (75%), where it is used as a concentrating agent. The remaining 25% is excreted into the gut

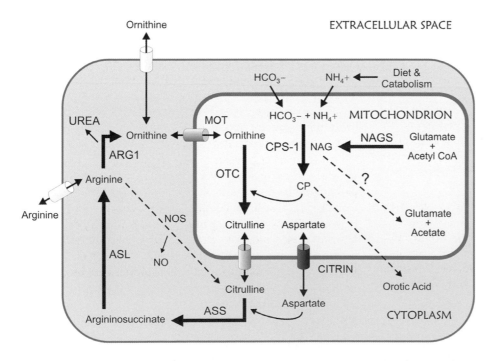

Figure 38.1 Diagram of the hepatic components of the urea cycle. NO, nitric oxide; NOS, nitric oxide synthase; CP, carbamoyl phosphate; CPS-1, carbamoyl phosphate synthetase 1; NAG, N-acetylglutamate; NAGS, N-acetylglutamate synthase; ASS, argininosuccinate synthase 1; ASL, argininosuccinate lyase; ARG1, arginase 1; MOT, mitochondrial ornithine transporter (hyperornithinemia–hyperammonemia–homocitrullinemia syndrome).

Table 38.1 Genes directly involved in the urea cycle and urea cycle disorders

Protein	Abbreviation	Gene symbol	Chromosome	Location
Carbamoyl phosphate synthetase 1	CPS	CPS1	2q34	Mitochondria
Ornithine transcarbamylase	OTC	OTC	Xp11.4	Mitochondria
Argininosuccinate synthase 1	ASS	ASS1	9q34.11	Cytoplasm
Argininosuccinate lyase	ASL	ASL	7q11.21	Cytoplasm
Arginase 1	ARG	ARG1	6q23.2	Cytoplasm
N-Acetylglutamate synthase	NAGS	NAGS	17q21.31	Mitochondria
Mitochondrial ornithine transporter (ornithine translocase)	MOT	SLC25A15	13q14.11	Mitochondrial membrane
Citrin	CITRIN	SLC25A13	7q21.3	Mitochondrial membrane

where bacteria can convert it into ammonia or use it to make their own amino acids or proteins. The remainder can then re-enter the body through the portal system. Ammonia levels in the portal vein normally are between 100 and 300 µmol/L, compared with 10–30 µmol/L in the general circulation.

Molecular aspects of the urea cycle

The urea cycle is the sole processing mechanism for waste nitrogen. As shown in Figure 38.1, the urea cycle is composed of five primary enzymes, one enzyme producing an essential cofactor, and two transporters moving molecules across the mitochondrial membrane (Table 38.1). Inborn errors of metabolism are associated with each step in the pathway and have been well described. The cycle has the interesting property of having a subset of the enzymes participate in another metabolic pathway, which produces arginine for anabolism and for the synthesis of nitric oxide. The urea cycle as a nitrogen clearance system is limited primarily to the human liver and to a lesser extent to the intestine, with carbamoyl phosphate synthetase and ornithine transcarbamylase limited exclusively to those tissues. The enzymes downstream that process citrulline into arginine are ubiquitous in their distribution. Functional changes in carbamoyl phosphate synthetase 1 (encoded by CPS1), the rate-limiting enzyme in the urea cycle, would have the greatest impact on cycle function from environmental stress.

A mutation in any gene may be severe enough to eliminate all enzymatic or transport activity or it may cause alteration in gene expression or the gene product that alters activity to a variable extent. The severity of symptoms in the latter case may be attenuated and be dependent on the degree of residual pathway function, sometimes causing illness only in circumstances of severe stress and catabolism.

Clinical presentation of urea cycle defects

The symptoms of urea cycle defects are primarily neurologic in origin. The acute disease presentation is brought about by cerebral edema, leading to neurocognitive dysfunction.

Elevations in ammonia are thought to have a direct effect on cerebral edema, whereas elevations in brain glutamine levels (a buffer for excess nitrogen) are thought to affect neurotransmission and perhaps the edema as well [2–6]. Depending on the age of the patient, the outward manifestations of cerebral edema can vary from nausea and vomiting, increased agitation, or somnolence to neurologic posturing as pressure is brought to bear on the brainstem. The closed space of the skull magnifies the effect of the swelling and unchecked progression will typically result in complete venous stasis or herniation of the brainstem. Without aggressive treatment, the prognosis for a patient with hyperammonemia and cerebral edema is poor. The exceptions to this clinical presentation are the disorders in the transporters (hyperornithinemia–hyperammonemia–homocitrullinemia (HHH) syndrome and citrin deficiency) and arginase deficiency, which are described separately. Although the inborn errors of urea cycle metabolism are being addressed in this chapter, it should be remembered that there are a number of conditions that affect the cycle which are not primarily genetic. In patients with a partial defect in the urea cycle, symptoms may not appear until a sufficiently stressful event occurs to unmask the deficit (Table 38.2).

An increasing number of reports describe liver failure in the early stages of some UCDs [7–9]. There are no consistent pathgnomonic findings on the histopathology of liver biopsies from patients with UCDs that are distinguishing, except for patients with defects in argininosuccinic acid lyase deficiency. Many of these patients develop significant hepatomegaly (often extending to the pelvis) with progressive fibrosis of the liver. On microscopic examination the hepatocytes may be pale and swollen [10].

Neonatal onset

Neonatal presentation typically is the result of a severe defect in urea cycle capacity. Although the stress and catabolism of the neonatal period creates an additional ammonia burden, there is clinical evidence that these patients will become

Table 38.2 Conditions that affect or stress urea cycle function

Functional stresses	Examples
Urea cycle enzymes	Deficiency
Damage to the liver (both chronic and acutely)	Chemical toxins, e.g. ethanol, industrial chemicals Infectious processes
Drug effects on the cycle	Direct interference with enzymes Valproic acid (Depakote) Chemotherapeutic drugs, particularly cyclophosphamide Massive cell lysis with chemotherapy
Damage or general disruption of hepatic function	Systemic antifungals Chemotherapy with hepatotoxic effects Acetaminophen
Other metabolic diseases	Organic acidemias (such as methylmalonic, propionic, etc.) Lysinuric protein intolerance Pyruvate carboxylase deficiency Fatty acid oxidation defects Galactosemia Tyrosinemia Glycogen storage disease
Transient hyperammonemia	In the newborn (premature infants)
Vascular bypass of the liver	With scarring or vascular bypass
Nitrogen overload of the system	Massive hemolysis (such as large bone fracture or trauma) Total parenteral nutrition Protein catabolism from starvation or bariatric surgery
Stress	Postpartum stress Heart–lung transplant
Renal disease	
Gastrointestinal	Bleeding

Table 38.3 Symptoms of newborns with urea cycle defects

Timescale	Symptoms
At birth	Normal appearance
Next 2–3 days (sometimes 1–2 weeks)	Hyperventilation (in the early stages) Feeding disruption (increases catabolism) Somnolence progressing to lethargy then coma Loss of thermoregulation (hypothermia) Neurologic posturing (from cerebral edema) Seizures

protein breakdown to overwhelm any residual ammonia detoxification capacity. As the cerebral edema and vascular stasis progresses the patient may develop hyperventilation, resulting in an elevation in the blood pH from respiratory alkalosis. As the pressure increases on the brainstem and CNS function fails, the patient's respiratory rate will decrease and eventually stop. A portion of patients will develop seizures of some form, although these can be difficult to detect in the context of decreasing CNS function. Unchecked, the patients will become comatose and eventually die from CNS failure, often compounded by brainstem herniation.

Delayed onset

Patients presenting with a delayed onset typically have some partial function in their urea cycle [12]. The onset of symptoms is a factor of their residual enzyme activity, diet, and environmental stressors (Table 38.4). These patients can manifest an acute hyperammonemic episode similar to that seen in the neonatal patients if they undergo a significant catabolic stress such as during an infection or after trauma. These episodes can occur anywhere from just outside the newborn period to late in life (sixth to seventh decade). Many of these patients will experience numerous mild hyperammonemic episodes, which can result in cumulative neurologic damage without an acute episode. It is unknown, but possible, that the chronic mild elevations of ammonia and glutamine affect neurologic development in these patients as well. The diagnosis is often delayed because the symptoms and signs can be quite subtle. As a probable result of mild hyperammonemia from dietary exposure, many of these patients subconsciously avoid protein in their diet, which can be an important historic clue. These patients can also have episodes triggered by drugs, which decrease urea cycle function such as valproic acid or chemotherapeutic agents [13–19]. Other reported triggers include postpartum stress, heart–lung transplant, short bowel, kidney disease, parenteral nutrition, gastrointestinal bleeding, and bariatric surgery [12].

hyperammonemic even under ideal conditions [11]. The difficulty with recognizing these patients is the similarity of these symptoms to other more common problems such as neonatal sepsis (Table 38.3). Infants with a UCD usually appear normal at birth but deteriorate as the ammonia, which is no longer filtered by the placenta, accumulates. This typically occurs within the first 48–72 hours of life, but may be delayed by 1–2 weeks. As they develop cerebral edema, they will feed poorly, become agitated and then progress to somnolence and lethargy. Most patients will develop some degree of dehydration from decreased intake. Although the decrease in oral intake will reduce the amount of dietary protein that can produce ammonia, the catabolism induced by poor intake and the stress of the neonatal period results in enough tissue

Table 38.4 Common clinical features of late-onset urea cycle defects

Features	Causes
Dramatic and rapid increase in nitrogen load	Trauma Rapid weight loss and autocatabolism Increase in protein turnover from intravenous steroids
Diet preference	Tend to avoid protein in diets
Behavioral or psychiatric illness	Often a history of behavioral or psychiatric illnesses Rapid deterioration of neurologic status Severe encephalopathy inconsistent with medical condition Usually involve defects in first part of urea cycle Evidence for cerebral edema by clinical examination or radiograph Seizures Decrease in oral intake leading up to decompensation

Classic urea cycle disorders

Patients with deficiencies of ornithine transcarbamylase, carbamoyl phosphate synthetase 1, N-acetylglutamate synthase, argininosuccinate synthase 1, and argininosuccinate lyase may be indistinguishable on a clinical basis, although studies are underway to identify differences in symptoms in individual disorders. The most frequent disorders as a percentage of all UCDs are ornithine transcarbamylase deficiency (55%), argininosuccinic acid synthase deficiency (27%), and carbamoyl phosphate synthase deficiency (14%) [20].

Ornithine transcarbamylase deficiency

Ornithine transcarbamylase deficiency is an X-linked disease with approximately 15% of carrier females manifesting overt symptoms of partial deficiency, particularly during pregnancy or other stressful events. Another fraction may have subtle symptoms but be undetected in the absence of a family history of more severe disease. The median age of presentation of females was 10 years [20].

Argininosuccinate lyase deficiency

Argininosuccinate lyase deficiency has more severe chronic symptoms than other disorders in this group, most likely because of the toxicity of argininosuccinic acid [21]. Patients with this deficiency have increased rates of developmental delay, seizure disorder, and other neurologic symptoms when compared to other UCDs. In addition, patients with argininosuccinate lyase deficiency may develop more severe liver disease with hepatic fibrosis and hypertension.

Ornithine translocase deficiency

The HHH syndrome is an autosomal recessive inherited disorder in ornithine translocase (mitochondrial ornithine transporter), resulting in diminished ornithine transport into the mitochondria. Ornithine accumulation in the cytoplasm results in high plasma ornithine concentrations, whereas reduced intramitochondrial ornithine causes impaired ureagenesis and orotic aciduria. The clinical symptoms are related to the hyperammonemia and resemble those of the UCDs. Homocitrulline is thought to originate from transcarbamoylation of lysine. Most patients have intermittent hyperammonemia accompanied by vomiting, lethargy, and, in extreme cases, coma. Chronic symptoms include impaired growth, intellectual disability, spasticity, and seizures. Adults are found with partial activity of the enzyme and symptoms of protein avoidance. Diagnosis may be complicated because plasma ornithine levels can normalize on a protein restricted diet.

Citrin deficiency (citrullinemia type 2)

Citrin is an aspartate glutamate transporter across the mitochondrial membrane. Citrin deficiency is more common in Japanese and other Asian populations but is now known worldwide. Citrin deficiency results in limitation of activity for the enzyme argininosuccinic acid synthase, which combines aspartate and citrulline to make argininosuccinic acid (Figure 38.1). Citrin deficiency may present with non-specific neonatal intrahepatic cholestasis that usually resolves after infancy [22]. Newborn screen may demonstrate hypergalactosemia, hypermethioninemia, and/or hyperphenylalaninemia in addition to increased citrulline. Children and adults often develop an aversion to carbohydrate-rich foods. Later presentations may include classic hyperammonemia, but older patients more often have neurologic symptoms including abnormal behaviors, delusions, and seizures [23,24]. Other complications include hyperlipidemia, hepatoma, and pancreatitis [24–27].

Arginase deficiency

Arginase deficiency is not typically characterized by rapid-onset hyperammonemia. These patients often present with progressive spasticity with greater severity in the lower limbs. They also develop seizures and gradually lose intellectual attainments. Growth is usually slow, and without therapy these patients usually do not reach normal adult height. Other symptoms that may present early in life include episodes of irritability, anorexia, and vomiting. Severe episodes of hyperammonemia are seen infrequently with this disorder but can be fatal. Treatment is similar to other UCDs.

Diagnosis

The first step in diagnosing UCDs is clinical suspicion. A blood ammonia is the first laboratory test to evaluate for a patient with a suspected UCD. Particular care should be taken in drawing blood for ammonia measurement because there is considerable variability depending on technique and handling. The clinician should remember that treatment should not be

Table 38.5 Diagnosis of urea cycle disorders

Deficiency diagnosis	Biochemical markers	Enzyme assay[a]	Newborn screening[b]
N-Acetylglutamate synthase	Orotic acid N-↓, Cit ↓	Liver	Low citrulline
Carbamoyl phosphate synthetase 1	Orotic acid N-↓, Cit ↓	Liver	Low citrulline
Ornithine transcarbamylase	Orotic acid ↑, Cit ↓	Liver	Low citrulline
Argininosuccinate synthase 1	Cit ↑, Arg N-↓	Fibroblasts, liver	High citrulline
Argininosuccinate lyase	Cit ↑, ASA ↑, Arg N-↓	Fibroblasts, liver, red blood cells	High citrulline
Arginase	Arg ↑	Red blood cells	High arginine
Mitochondrial ornithine transporter	Orn ↑, Homocit ↑	Fibroblasts	Unknown[c]
Citrin	Cit ↑, Thr/Ser ratio ↑	Fibroblasts	High citrulline (sometimes)

Arg, arginine; ASA, argininosuccinic acid; Cit, citrulline; Homocit, homocitrulline; N, normal; Orn, ornithine; Ser, serine; Thr, threonine.
[a] Not all enzyme assays may be available clinically.
[b] Newborn screening may have variable sensitivity and specificity in the urea cycle disorders, particularly N-acetylglutamate synthase, carbamoyl phosphate synthetase 1, and ornithine transcarbamylase deficiencies.
[c] In theory, hyperornithinemia–hyperammonemia–homocitrullinemia syndrome may have high ornithine on newborn screening, but no cases have been documented.

delayed in efforts to reach a final diagnosis and that later stages of treatment should be tailored to the specific disorder.

Laboratory data useful in the diagnosis of UCDs include plasma ammonia levels, pH, carbon dioxide, anion gap measurement, plasma amino acids, and urine organic acid analyses [28,29]. Both pH and carbon dioxide can vary with the degree of cerebral edema and hyper- or hypoventilation. In neonates, it should be remembered that the basal ammonia level is higher than that of adults, which typically is <35 μmol/L (100 μmol/L is often observed). An elevated plasma ammonia of 150 μmol/L or higher, associated with a normal anion gap and a normal blood glucose level, is a strong indication for the presence of a UCD.

Quantitative amino acid analysis can be used to evaluate these patients and arrive at a tentative diagnosis. Elevations or depressions of the intermediate amino-containing molecules arginine, citrulline, and argininosuccinate offer clues to the point of defect in the cycle. The amino acid profile in sick newborns without UCDs may show lower levels of arginine and citrulline and higher levels of glycine than in well children [29]. The levels of the nitrogen buffering amino acid glutamine will also be quite high and can serve as confirmation of the hyperammonemia. If a defect in N-acetylglutamate synthase, carbamoyl phosphate synthetase 1, or ornithine transcarbamylase is suspected, the presence of the organic acid orotic acid in the urine can help to establish the diagnosis. Orotic acid is produced when there is an overabundance of carbamoyl phosphate, which spills into the pyrimidine biosynthetic system.

As shown in Table 38.5, biochemical testing with measurement of plasma amino acids is critical in differentiating between the various forms of UCD. Although enzyme testing is an effective means of diagnosis, it has largely been supplanted in the USA by DNA sequence analysis. A frequently updated web resource for testing information can be found at the US National Institutes of Health (NIH)-sponsored site (http://www.geneclinics.org). The availability of tandem mass spectrometry for newborn screening has allowed early diagnosis of distal UCDs, although false negative results still occur. Newborn screening for proximal disorders such as ornithine transcarbamylase deficiency is difficult because of the lack of specificity and sensitivity of a low citrulline assay.

The differential diagnosis of patients with hyperammonemia includes other inborn errors of metabolism. Branched-chain organic acidemias cause anion gap acidosis and ketosis. Fatty acid oxidation disorders usually result in hypoketotic hypoglycemia. Pyruvate carboxylase deficiency causes lactic acidosis, decreased aspartate, and increased alanine. Lysinuric protein intolerance causes post prandial hyperammonemia with decreased plasma lysine, arginine, ornithine, and increased urine amino acids. Premature infants are susceptible to transient hyperammonemia of the newborn and may develop extremely high ammonia levels within 24 hours of birth, but with normal other biochemical parameters.

Treatment of urea cycle disorders

Box 38.1 provides an overview of urea cycle management. The proper treatment of these patients requires a highly coordinated team of specialists trained in caring for patients with inborn errors of metabolism. An NIH-sponsored website with links to experts in urea cycle management and treatment protocols, the Urea Cycle Disorders Consortium, is available (http://www.rarediseasesnetwork.org/ucdc).

Management of patients in a urea-cycle-based hyperammonemic coma is based on three interdependent principles: first, physical removal of the ammonia (and glutamine) by dialysis or some form of hemofiltration; second, reversal of the catabolic state through caloric supplementation and, in extreme cases, hormonal suppression (glucose/insulin drip); and third, pharmacologic scavenging of excess nitrogen.

Central venous access should be established and dialysis, if available, begun at the highest available flow rate [30]. Dialysis is effective for the removal of ammonia, and clearance is dependent on the flow through the dialysis circuit. In severe hyperammonemia, provision for hemofiltration should be made to follow the dialysis until the patient is stabilized and the catabolic state is reversed. Some patients will reaccumulate ammonia after their initial round of dialysis and may require additional periods of dialysis. Most patients will have a slight rise in ammonia after dialysis because removal by scavengers and the liver will not be as effective. This slight rise usually does not necessitate repeat dialysis. Peritoneal dialysis and particularly exchange transfusion are far less effective methods of ammonia removal and should be avoided.

Management of the catabolic state is often overlooked in its importance. Because the catabolism of protein stores is often the triggering event for hyperammonemia, the patient will not completely stabilize until it is reversed. Fluids, dextrose, and intravenous fat emulsions should be given to blunt the catabolic process. The patient should be assessed for dehydration and fluids replaced. Because these patients suffer from cerebral edema, care should be taken with overhydration. The nitrogen-scavenging drugs are usually administered

in a large volume of fluid, which should be taken into consideration. A regimen of 80 cal/kg daily is a reasonable goal. Although it is not common practice at all centers, the administration of insulin and glucose are useful in profound catabolic states. At the same time, protein should be *temporarily* removed from intake. Supplementation of arginine serves to replace arginine not produced by the urea cycle (in addition to the partial cycle function it can stimulate) and prevents its deficiency from causing additional protein catabolism. Refeeding the patient as soon as practical is useful because more calories can be administered this way. The use of essential amino acid formulations in feeding can reduce the amount of protein necessary to meet basic needs.

Emergency pharmacologic management (Table 38.6) with ammonia scavengers and arginine is initiated as soon as possible using the drug combination sodium phenylacetate/sodium benzoate (Ammonul; Ucyclyd Pharma, Baltimore, MD, USA), ideally while the dialysis is being arranged and the diagnostic workup is under way. Two agents are used in combination to trap nitrogen in excretable forms. Sodium benzoate combines with glycine to make hippurate, which is excreted by the kidneys (or removed in the dialysate), and sodium phenylacetate combines with glutamine to make phenacetylglutamine, which is also excreted in the urine [31,32]. The body replaces these amino acids using excess nitrogen. It is suspected that the removal of glutamine by phenylacetate has the additional benefit of removing a compound suspected of having a major role in the neurotoxicity of these disorders [4,33–37].

The first (loading) dose should be given over 90–120 minutes, with subsequent maintenance doses over 24 hours. After the initial loading phase and dialysis, the patients should be converted to the maintenance doses of the ammonia scavengers listed in the manufacturer's packaging insert. If the exact enzyme defect is known, the amount of arginine administered can be adjusted downward. If chronic therapy is warranted, the patient can then be switched to the oral prodrug of phenylacetate, phenylbutyrate (Buphenyl).

Box 38.1 Urea cycle management

Overall goals of therapy
1. Maximize protection of central nervous system
2. Physically remove large ammonia and glutamine load (dialysis)
3. Add pharmacologic agents to remove nitrogen
4. Treat catabolic state

Stages of management
1. Recognition
2. Emergency management and stabilization
3. Bulk ammonia removal and nitrogen scavenging
4. Stabilization (drug/diet)

Table 38.6 Recommended dosing of urea cycle drugs by diagnosis and size of the patient in acute treatment

Diagnosis	Dosing NaPA/NaBZ	10% Arginine	Dose delivered NaPA/NaBZ (each)	I 10% Arginine
Weight 0–20 kg				
CPS, OTC, NAGS deficiencies	2.5 mL/kg	2.0 mL/kg	250 mg/kg	200 mg/kg
ASS, ASL deficiencies, unknown	2.5 mL/kg	6.0 mL/kg	250 mg/kg	600 mg/kg
ARG deficiency	2.5 mL/kg	None	250 mg/kg	None
Weight >20 kg				
CPS, OTC, NAGS deficiencies	55 mL/m^2	2.0 mL/kg	5.5 g/m^2	4 g/m^2
ASS, ASL deficiencies, unknown	55 mL/m^2	6.0 mL/kg	5.5 g/m^2	12 g/m^2
ARG deficiency	55 mL/m^2	None	5.5 g/m^2	None

ARG, arginase; ASL, argininosuccinate lyase; ASS, argininosuccinate synthase 1; CPS, carbamoyl phosphate synthetase 1; NAGS, *N*-acetylglutamate synthase; NaPA/NaBZ, sodium phenylacetate/sodium benzoate; (Ammonul); OTC, ornithine transcarbamylase.

Arginine is also used in the acute phase of treatment of UCDs unless arginase deficiency is suspected. In addition to replenishing circulating amino acid levels, arginine can use those parts of the cycle not affected by genetic blocks and incorporate some nitrogen. N-Carbamyl-L-glutamate (Carbaglu, Orphan Europe, Paris, France) is a carbamoyl phosphate synthetase 1 activator and a structural analogue of N-acetylglutamate; it is indicated for treatment of N-acetylglutamate synthase deficiency [38]. Studies are anticipated to test the utility of these agents in carbamoyl phosphate synthetase 1 deficiency [39] and in branched-chain organic acidemias that inhibit carbamoyl phosphate synthetase 1. The dosages and administration of these drugs should only be done in consultation with an experienced specialist. A resource for finding these physicians and other treatment suggestions is the NIH-sponsored Urea Cycle Disorders Consortium (http://www.rarediseasesnetwork.org/ucdc).

Other treatment issues

The use of osmotic agents such as mannitol is not considered effective in treating the cerebral edema caused by hyperammonemia. In canines, opening the blood–brain barrier with mannitol resulted in cerebral edema by promoting the entry of ammonia into the brain fluid compartment [5,40]. Intravenous steroids and valproic acid should be avoided. Measures to reduce cerebral metabolism to protect the brain, such as head cooling, have been proposed, but their efficacy is untested. Antibiotics and a workup for sepsis are indicated to treat potential triggering events. Other measures include physiologic support (pressors, buffering agents to maintain pH and buffer arginine hydrochloride, etc.) and maintenance of renal output, particularly if ammonia scavengers are being used. Finally, it is imperative to reassess continuation of care after the initial phase of treatment.

Rapid response to the hyperammonemia improves outcome. Symptomatology centers around cerebral edema and pressure on the brainstem. The resulting decrease in cerebral blood flow plus prolonged seizures, when they occur, are poor prognostic factors. In adults, because the sutures of the skull are fused, sensitivity to hyperammonemia appears considerably greater than in children. Therefore, treatment should be aggressive and instituted at a lower ammonia concentration than in children. Electroencephalography should be performed because many of these patients develop continuous, albeit temporary, seizures. Evaluation of brainstem function and higher cortical function as well as cerebral blood flow studies are useful to assess outcome. The decision for continuation is based on baseline neurologic status, duration of the patient's coma, potential for recovery, and whether the patient is a candidate for liver transplantation. If the basic UCD is severe enough, then liver transplantation should be considered.

Diagnostic samples of DNA, liver, and skin should be obtained because they can be central in family counseling and future treatment issues.

Long-term management

Every effort should be made to avoid triggering events. In particular, intravenous steroids for asthma or use of valproic acid are contraindicated. Long-term diet modification with nutritional oversight is often necessary in patients with chronic episodes of hyperammonemia. Patients should also avoid dehydration, a particularly common occurrence among adults in connection with alcohol intake, hiking, and airline flights. Not all adults who recover from a hyperammonemic episode require chronic therapy with nitrogen scavengers, but they ought to be considered because many of these patients can become more brittle as time goes on. Special precautions must be taken to avoid catabolism during subsequent illness or surgery, as well as during any event resulting in significant bleeding or tissue damage.

Should psychiatric problems occur over the long term, care-givers should be alert to the possibility of hyperammonemia. In addition, many patients with citrullinemia type 2 in particular have presented with mental disturbance [23,24].

In recent years, liver transplantation has become the treatment of choice for many of the patients with more severe UCDs. The survival rate in larger series has been >90% [41], presumably because of the elimination of hyperammonemic crises. Although patients with UCDs who have undergone early transplantation have improved neurologic outcomes compared with those managed with medical therapy alone, patients are still significantly affected. One study showed an average developmental quotient of 69 for four children with transplantation prior to 1 year of age, presumably because of residual effects from their early metabolic crises [42]. Arginine remains an essential amino acid in some proximal urea cycle defects [43] and should be replaced based on achieving normal blood levels ≥4 hours after a therapeutic dose.

It is important to provide genetic counseling to assess risk to other family members.

Future directions

The Urea Cycle Disorders Consortium has led a long-term effort to study the pathophysiology and clinical outcome of patients with UCD. Early results from the Consortium's cross-sectional study have provided enough subjects to legitimize previous observations, such as increased morbidity in treated patients with argininosuccinate lyase deficiency, decreased branched-chain amino acid levels in phenylbutyrate-treated subjects, and increased glutamine levels in proximal disorders compared with distal disorders [44]. As of 2011, over 500 patients had been enrolled in the cross-sectional study. Both the Urea Cycle Disorders Consortium and the National Urea Cycle Disorder Foundation can provide information to interested patients and families. Both of these resources can be easily located on the Worldwide Web.

Newer imaging modalities are being studied as biomarkers of disease states. Use of ^{1}H MR spectroscopy has shown decreased myoinositol and increased glutamine in asymptomatic patients with normal MRI scans [45]. Diffusion tensor imaging detects subtle abnormalities in patients with partial ornithine transcarbamylase deficiency that may correlate with disease severity [46]. The role of secondary creatine deficiency in the pathogenesis of hyperammonemia-induced brain damage needs to be explored [47]. Finally, the use of liver cell transplantation as a bridge therapy until liver transplantation is an exciting area of research that will be studied during the next several years [48].

Conclusions

The urea cycle provides an excellent model for the understanding of inborn errors of metabolism. Defects throughout the cycle affect a variety of molecular mechanisms including catalytic enzymes, cofactor producers, and transport proteins. The timely diagnosis and treatment of these diseases directly affects the outcome of the patient, and awareness by the clinician is paramount. The promise of early detection by newborn screening, improved therapies, and the increased ability to detect brain abnormalities will have a substantial effect on the health of these individuals in the future.

Acknowledgements

The authors would like to acknowledge Marshall Summar, MD, and the Urea Cycle Disorders Consortium for grant aid.

References

1. Krebs HA, Henseleit K. Untersuchungen uber die harnstoffbildung im tierkorper. *Hoppe-Seyler Z Physiol Chem* 1932; **210**:325–332.

2. Batshaw ML. Hyperammonemia. *Curr Probl Pediatr* 1984;**14**:1–69.

3. Brusilow SW. Urea cycle disorders: clinical paradigm of hyperammonemic encephalopathy. *Prog Liver Dis* 1995;**13**:293–309.

4. Butterworth RF. Effects of hyperammonaemia on brain function. *J Inherit Metab Dis* 1998;**21**(Suppl 1):6–20.

5. Fujiwara M. Role of ammonia in the pathogenesis of brain edema. *Acta Medica Okayama* 1986;**40**:313–320.

6. Takahashi H, Koehler RC, Hirata T, *et al.* Restoration of cerebrovascular CO_2 responsivity by glutamine synthesis inhibition in hyperammonemic rats. *Circ Res* 1992;**71**:1220–1230.

7. Mustafa A, Clarke JT. Ornithine transcarbamoylase deficiency presenting with acute liver failure. *J Inherit Metab Dis* 2006;**29**:586.

8. Faghfoury H, Baruteau J, de Baulny HO, *et al.* Transient fulminant liver failure as an initial presentation in citrullinemia type I. *Mol Genet Metab* 2011;**102**:413–417.

9. Fecarotta S, Parenti G, Vajo P, *et al.* HHH syndrome (hyperornithinaemia, hyperammonaemia, homocitrullinuria), with fulminant hepatitis-like presentation. *J Inherit Metab Dis* 2006;**29**:186–189.

10. Mori T, Nagai K, Mori M, *et al.* Progressive liver fibrosis in late-onset argininosuccinate lyase deficiency. *Pediatr Dev Pathol* 2002;**5**:597–601.

11. Tuchman M, Mauer SM, Holzknecht RA, *et al.* Prospective versus clinical diagnosis and therapy of acute neonatal hyperammonaemia in two sisters with carbamoyl phosphate synthetase deficiency. *J Inherit Metab Dis* 1992;**15**:269–277.

12. Summar ML, Barr F, Dawling S, *et al.* Unmasked adult-onset urea cycle disorders in the critical care setting. *Crit Care Clin* 2005;**21**(Suppl 4):S1–S8.

13. Mitchell RB, Wagner JE, Karp JE, *et al.* Syndrome of idiopathic hyperammonemia after high-dose chemotherapy: review of nine cases [see comments]. *Am J Med* 1988;**85**:662–667.

14. Batshaw ML, Brusilow SW. Valproate-induced hyperammonemia. *Ann Neurol* 1982;**11**:319–321.

15. Bourrier P, Varache N, Alquier P, *et al.* [Cerebral edema with hyperammonemia in valpromide poisoning. Manifestation in an adult, of a partial deficit in type I carbamoylphosphate synthetase.] *Presse Med* 1988;**17**:2063–2066.

16. Castro-Gago M, Rodrigo-Saez E, Novo-Rodriguez I, *et al.* Hyper-aminoacidemia in epileptic children treated with valproic acid. *Childs Nerv Syst* 1990;**6**:434–436.

17. Elgudin L, Hall Y, Schubert D. Ammonia induced encephalopathy from valproic acid in a bipolar patient: case report. *Int J Psychiatry Med* 2003;**33**:91–96.

18. Kugoh T, Yamamoto M, Hosokawa K. Blood ammonia level during valproic acid therapy. *Jpn J Psychiatry Neurol* 1986;**40**:663–668.

19. Vainstein G, Korzets Z, Pomeranz A, Gadot N. Deepening coma in an epileptic patient: the missing link to the urea cycle. Hyperammonaemic metabolic encephalopathy. *Nephrol Dial Transplant* 2002;**17**:1351–1353.

20. Summar ML, Dobbelaere D, Bruslow S, Lee B. Diagnosis, symptoms, frequency and mortality of 260 patients with urea cycle disorders from a 21-year, multicentre study of acute hyperammonaemic episodes. *Acta Paediatr* 2008;**97**:1420–1425.

21. Erez A, Nagamani SC, Lee B. Argininosuccinate lyase deficiency: argininosuccinic aciduria and beyond. *Am J Med Genet* 2011;**157**:45–53.

22. Ohura, T, Kobayashi K, Tazawa Y, *et al.* Clinical pictures of 75 patients with neonatal intrahepatic cholestasis caused by citrin deficiency (NICCD). *J Inherit Metab Dis* 2007;**30**:139–144.

23. Saheki T, Kobayashi K. Mitochondrial aspartate glutamate carrier (citrin) deficiency as the cause of adult-onset type II citrullinemia (CTLN2) and idiopathic neonatal hepatitis (NICCD). *J Hum Genet* 2002;**47**:333–341.

24. Saheki T, Kobayashi K, Iijima M, *et al.* Adult-onset type II citrullinemia and idiopathic neonatal hepatitis caused by citrin deficiency: involvement of the aspartate glutamate carrier for urea synthesis and maintenance of the urea cycle. *Mol Genet Metab* 2004; **81**(Suppl 1): S20–S26.

25. Ben Shalom E, Kobayashi K, Shaag A, *et al.* Infantile citrullinemia caused by citrin deficiency with increased dibasic amino acids. *Mol Genet Metab* 2002;**77**:202–208.

26. Naito E, Ito M, Matsuura S, *et al.* Type II citrullinaemia (citrin deficiency) in a neonate with hypergalactosaemia detected by mass screening. *J Inherit Metab Dis* 2002;**25**:71–76.

27. Tamamori A, Okano Y, Ozaki H, *et al.* Neonatal intrahepatic cholestasis caused by citrin deficiency: severe hepatic dysfunction in an infant requiring liver transplantation. *Eur J Pediatr* 2002;**161**:609–613.

28. Steiner RD, Cederbaum SD. Laboratory evaluation of urea cycle disorders. *J Pediatr* 2001;**138**(Suppl 1):S21–S29.

29. Summar M. Current strategies for the management of neonatal urea cycle disorders. *J Pediatr* 2001;**138**(Suppl 1):S30–S39.

30. Summar M, Pietsch J, Deshpande J, Schulman G. Effective hemo-dialysis and hemofiltration driven by an extracorporeal membrane oxygenation pump in infants with hyperammonemia. *J Pediatr* 1996;**128**:379–382.

31. Batshaw ML. Sodium benzoate and arginine: alternative pathway therapy in inborn errors of urea synthesis. *Prog Clin Biol Res* 1983;**127**:69–83.

32. Batshaw ML, Brusilow SW. Evidence of lack of toxicity of sodium phenylacetate and sodium benzoate in treating urea cycle enzymopathies. *J Inherit Metab Dis* 1981;**4**:231.

33. Batshaw ML, Brusilow SW. Treatment of hyperammonemic coma caused by inborn errors of urea synthesis. *J Pediatr* 1980;**97**:893–900.

34. Brusilow SW, Valle DL, Batshaw M. New pathways of nitrogen excretion in inborn errors of urea synthesis. *Lancet* 1979;**2**:452–454.

35. Brusilow SW. Phenylacetylglutamine may replace urea as a vehicle for waste nitrogen excretion. *Pediatr Res* 1991;**29**:147–150.

36. Connelly A, Cross JH, Gadian DG, *et al.* Magnetic resonance spectroscopy shows increased brain glutamine in ornithine carbamoyl transferase deficiency. *Pediatr Res* 1993;**33**:77–81.

37. Willard-Mack CL, Koehler RC, Hirata T, *et al.* Inhibition of glutamine synthetase reduces ammonia-induced astrocyte swelling in rat. *Neuroscience* 1996;**71**:589–599.

38. Caldovic L, Morizono H, Yevgeny D, *et al.* Restoration of ureagenesis in *N*-acetylglutamate synthase deficiency by *N*-carbamylglutamate. *J Pediatr* 2004;**145**:552–554.

39. Kuchler G, Rabier D, Poggi-Travert F, et. al. Therapeutic use of carbamylglutamate in the case of carbamoyl-phosphate synthetase deficiency. *J Inherit Metab Dis* 1996;**19**:220–222.

40. Fujiwara M, Watanabe A, Shiota T, *et al.* Hyperammonemia-induced cytotoxic brain edema under osmotic opening of blood–brain barrier in dogs. *Res Exp Med* 1985;**185**:425–427.

41. Morioka D, Kasahara M, Takada Y, *et al.* Current role of liver transplantation for the treatment of urea cycle disorders: A review of the worldwide English literature and 13 cases at Kyoto University. *Liver Transplant* 2005;**11**:1332–1342.

42. Campeuau PM, Pivalezza PJ, Miller G, *et al.* Early orthotopic liver transplantation in urea cycle defects: Follow up of a developmental outcome study. *Mol Genet Metab* 2010;**100**:S84-S87.

43. Rabier D, Narcy C, Bardet J, *et al.* Arginine remains an essential amino acid after liver transplantation in urea cycle enzyme deficiencies. *J Inherit Metab Dis* 1991;**14**:277–280.

44. Tuchman M, Lee B, Lichter-Konecki U, *et al.* Cross-sectional multi-center study of patients with urea cycle disorders in the United States. *Mol Genet Metab* 2008;**94**:397–402.

45. Gropman AL, Fricke ST, Seltzer RR, *et al.* 1H MRS identifies symptomatic and asymptomatic subjects with partial ornithine transcarbamylase deficiency. *Mol Genet Metab* 2008;**95**:21–30.

46. Gropman AL, Gertz B, Shattuck K, *et al.* Diffusion tensor imaging detects areas of abnormal white matter microstructure in patients with partial ornithine transcarbamylase deficiency. *Am J Neuroradiol* 2010;**31**:1719–1723.

47. Braissant O. Ammonia toxicity to the brain: Effects on creatine metabolism and transport and protective roles of creatine. *Mol Genet Metab* 2010;**100**:S53–58.

48. Meyburg J, Das AM, Hoerster F, *et al.* One liver for four children: first clinical series of liver cell transplantation for severe neonatal urea cycle defects. *Transplantation* 2009;**87**:636–641.

Bacterial, parasitic, and fungal infections of the liver

Donald A. Novak, Gregory Y. Lauwers, and Richard L. Kradin

Introduction

Both systemic and local infections caused by bacterial, fungal, and parasitic agents may cause significant hepatic dysfunction. This chapter will attempt to delineate clinical syndromes caused by some of these organisms in the pediatric patient.

Bacterial infections

Associated liver disorders

Hyperbilirubinemia associated with sepsis

While jaundice in association with bacterial sepsis may occur in adults, it appears to be significantly more common during infancy. Historically, infections of the urinary tract predominate but sepsis originating from other sites may contribute [1]. Accordingly, Gram-negative bacilli, and particularly *Escherichia coli*, are responsible for the majority of cases, although Gram-positive organisms have been associated. Abnormal liver chemistries are found in approximately 50% of premature neonates with Gram-negative bacteremia [2]. Clinical and laboratory manifestations are primarily those of the underlying disease state. Hyperbilirubinemia may be marked, with the direct fraction predominant. Alkaline phosphatase levels are often elevated, while serum aminotransferases remain normal or minimally increased. Hepatic biopsy usually demonstrates canalicular cholestasis, with minimal evidence of hepatocyte damage or inflammatory response (Figure 39.1). On occasion, the biopsy may demonstrate prominent acute cholangitis with portal bile ductular proliferation, pathologic changes often seen in large bile duct obstruction. In these cases, the possibility of large duct obstruction must be excluded by ultrasound or endoscopic retrograde cholangiopancreatography (ERCP). Jaundice resolves with appropriate treatment of the underlying infection; duration of jaundice may vary from several days to several weeks. While the pathophysiology of sepsis-related cholestasis has not been fully elucidated, endotoxin, which is known to diminish bile flow and provoke cholestasis, may play a role. Other inflammatory mediators with potential roles include tumor necrosis factor, the leukotrienes, and interleukin-1. Fatty liver has also been reported in conjunction with Gram-negative sepsis [3].

Pyogenic hepatic abscess

Pyogenic liver abscess (PLA) continues to be a significant source of morbidity, if not mortality, in the pediatric population. Although early reports quoted an incidence of 3 in 100 000 hospital admissions (prior to 1977) [4]; recent studies have suggested an increasing rate of PLA, conditionally attributed to improved overall survival of immunocompromised patients. Current rates seem to be approximately 10–25 in 10 000 in the developed world, with higher rates noted in less developed nations [5]. Concomitantly, mortality has fallen from older estimates of 36% to 15% in recent series; mortality rates are higher in those with multiple abscesses [6]. Patients at risk include those with impaired host defenses; chronic granulomatous disease and leukemia are commonly

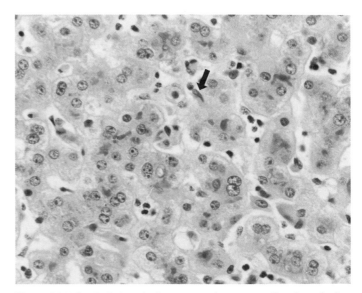

Figure 39.1 Sepsis. Perivenular hepatocytes demonstrate dilated canaliculi containing bile. The sinusoids contain a mixed inflammatory infiltrate associated with Kupffer cell hyperplasia.

Liver Disease in Children, Fourth Edition, ed. Frederick J. Suchy, Ronald J. Sokol, and William F. Balistreri. Published by Cambridge University Press. © Cambridge University Press 2014.

(a)

(b)

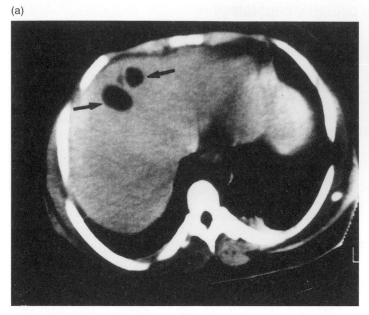
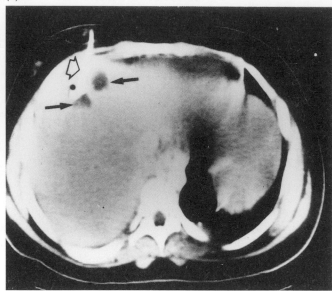

Figure 39.2 Pyogenic liver abcess by CT. (a) Before drainage showing abscess cavities (arrows). (b) After percutaneous drainage, with the open arrow indicating the drainage catheter.

noted in children. Approximately 50% of children with PLA are under the age of 6.

Clinical manifestations of PLA in children are non-specific but commonly include fever, abdominal pain, right upper quadrant tenderness and hepatomegaly [4]. Multiple abscesses, as well as those caused by gas-forming organisms, may present in a more fulminant manner. Ruptured abscesses presenting with abdominal pain and septic shock are also associated with higher mortality rates. Laboratory findings may include elevation of the erythrocyte sedimentation rate (ESR), leukocytosis, anemia, and hypoalbuminemia. Serum aminotransferase and bilirubin values may be variably elevated; in series of adult patients, serum alkaline phosphatase values are more reliably increased. Diagnosis of PLA is generally made via a high index of clinical suspicion in conjunction with appropriate imaging techniques. Approximately 75% of PLA are located in the right lobe of the liver. In a 1989 review of 109 children with PLA, CT and angiography were noted to be the most sensitive techniques, followed by ultrasound and radioisotope scanning [7]. Ultrasound, typically the first modality employed, with a sensitivity as high as 96% reported, may miss lesions in the dome of the liver. Lesion detection can also be made with MRI. All techniques presently available are hampered by a lack of specificity. As the differential diagnosis of intrahepatic cysts includes abscess caused by non-pyogenic organisms, congenital cysts, tumor with central necrosis and/or hemorrhage, as well as vascular malformation, specific diagnosis generally requires lesion aspiration with subsequent Gram stain and culture. In appropriate clinical situations, serology for hydatid disease and *Entamoeba histolytica* should be considered prior to aspiration. Percutaneous drainage under CT or ultrasound guidance is often feasible, particularly in the case of large,

solitary, superficial lesions (Figure 39.2). As opposed to adults, in whom Gram-negative bacilli predominate, *Staphylococcus aureus* is the predominant etiologic agent in children. This may reflect the significant number of immunocompromised patients in pediatric series of PLA. Enteric Gram-negative bacteria, predominantly *E. coli* and *Klebsiella* sp., account for approximately 31% of PLA in recent series, while anaerobic organisms are causative in at least 15% [8]. Other organisms found include *Nocardia asteroides*, *Streptococcus* sp., *Yersinia* sp., *Salmonella* sp., *Campylobacter jejuni*, *Pasturella multocida*, and *Legionella pneumophila*, among others to be discussed later in the chapter. Infections may be mixed. Tuberculosis is a rare cause of hepatic abscess as is actinomycosis; fungal and parasitic infections are described below [9].

The etiology of PLA is variable. Adult series demonstrate a preponderance of patients with pre-existing biliary tract disease, in whom PLA develops as a consequence of cholangitis. Traumatic injury to the liver may result in PLA, as may sepsis. Extension from contiguous sites of infection may occur. Predisposition by prior infection with *Toxocara canis* has also been hypothesized [10]. In children, altered host defenses seem to play an important role [11], as may portal vein bacteremia from intra-abdominal infectious processes (e.g. appendiceal abscess, abscess secondary to ingested foreign body, and inflammatory bowel disease). Occurrence of PLA has also been associated with the use of umbilical venous catheters in the newborn population. Approximately one-half of patients in adult series had no evident etiology.

Successful therapy of PLA is contingent upon rapid and accurate diagnostic efforts. Drainage and appropriate antibiotic coverage continue to be the mainstays of therapy. Initial antibiotic coverage should be broad spectrum, including agents effective against Gram-positive aerobes, Gram-negative bacilli, and anaerobic organisms. Subsequent therapy is dictated by culture results. Percutaneous drainage is indicated in those patients in whom lesions are accessible under CT or ultrasound guidance [12].

Catheters placed via these techniques are generally left in place until abscess collapse, usually 24–72 hours. Irrigation may be required. Alternatively, single or, if required, multiple discrete aspirations can be performed instead of leaving a catheter in place. Potential contraindications to these techniques include inaccessible lesions and ascites. Complications include peritonitis, formation of additional abscess collections, fistula formation, hepatic laceration, and hemorrhage. Patients in whom percutaneous drainage is not feasible, is not successful, or in whom an additional source of intra-abdominal infection (or biliary obstruction) exists, may require open drainage procedures.

Non-operative management may also play a role, primarily in patients with multiple abscesses. Success in this instance is more likely when abscesses are small. Duration of antibiotic therapy is variable. Treatment periods of 3–6 weeks are generally accepted. Prognosis is as denoted above but is worse in patients with multiple abscesses.

Cholangitis

Bacterial cholangitis, or infection of the biliary system, is a relatively uncommon event in pediatrics. At-risk patients are those with abnormalities of the biliary tract, particularly following hepatic portoenterostomy after a diagnosis of biliary atresia. Risk of cholangitis after the Kasai procedure is approximately 40–50% [13], with highest incidence occurring in the first 3 months after surgery. Late-onset cases have also been reported. Other conditions that may predispose to cholangitis include choledocholithiasis, choledochal cyst, and Caroli disease. Rarely, cholangitis in the absence of other risk factors may be noted.

The etiology of cholangitis is multifactorial. The normal biliary tract is sterile; the sphincter of Oddi aids in the prevention of bacterial reflux into the biliary tree from the duodenum. Destruction of this sphincter mechanism, as occurs in the Kasai procedure, may be associated with ascending bacterial colonization from the bowel. Indeed, patients in whom adequate bile drainage is attained after the Kasai procedure have a higher incidence of cholangitis than do those in whom surgery was unsuccessful. This illustrates the importance of direct contact between the biliary system and bowel flora in the pathogenesis of cholangitis. Biliary infection may also be produced via portal bacteremia. Conversely, the presence of bacteria in the bile is probably not sufficient to produce clinically significant cholangitis. It is likely that a combination of biliary obstruction and infected bile is required. In this regard, biliary parasites may play an important role.

Classically, the combination of right upper quadrant abdominal pain, fever, and jaundice (the Charcot triad) has been associated with the majority of adults with cholangitis.

Bowel sounds are generally present. Hypotension may be a presenting feature in under half of adults. Presenting clinical features in a series of children after the Kasai procedure included fever (100%), acholic stools or increase in serum bilirubin (68%), shock, and decrease in bile flow (43%) [13]. Associated laboratory findings include leukocytosis or leukopenia, elevated ESR, and, as noted, increased serum bilirubin. Other features often noted in series of adult patients include elevation of serum alkaline phosphatase and aminotransferases. Further diagnostic evaluation of the patient with suspected cholangitis should include bacteriologic cultures of the blood and urine. Blood cultures may provide the etiologic organism in approximately 50% of patients [13]. Initial imaging studies should include either ultrasonography or CT scanning to evaluate for (1) abscess formation associated with cholangitis, (2) presence of calculi, (3) presence of ductal dilation, or (4) other obstructing lesions including choledochal cyst or periportal mass. Magnetic resonance cholangiopancreatography (MRCP) may also be useful in selected patients [14]. Patients in whom culture results are negative, and in whom the clinical picture warrants it, should undergo a percutaneous hepatic biopsy, for both culture and histologic examination. Performed in the presence of normal coagulation parameters, this procedure has been shown to be relatively safe, and, at least in adult series, may be safely performed in the presence of ductal dilation. Hepatic culture was positive in 32 of 69 children with presumed cholangitis [13]. *E. coli* was the most frequently isolated pathogen (50% of first and second cholangitis episodes) in this and other studies. Other commonly isolated organisms include *Klebsiella* sp., enterococci, *Bacteroides* sp., *Enterobacter* sp., and *Pseudomonas* sp. Anaerobic organisms may also be isolated; mixed cultures are not uncommon. In approximately 30% of episodes, no bacterial agent is identified. Hepatic histologic changes may be useful in these cases. Pathologic alterations include infiltration of the portal triads, bile ductules, and ductule lumens with neutrophils. Portal edema may occur, as may changes consistent with biliary obstruction (Figure 39.3) [15].

Therapy of acute cholangitis includes careful attention to vital signs and perfusion status, providing adequate fluid resuscitation and pressure support if needed. The patient is made nil by mouth; nasogastric suction may be required in the presence of ileus. Toxic patients with evidence of biliary obstruction may require emergency intervention, endoscopic, percutaneous or, less commonly, operative. In most other patients, intervention should be withheld until after several days of antibiotic therapy and reduction of fever. Antibiotic therapy is initially given by the parenteral route. Choice of antibiotics is governed by sensitivities of common organisms, and the achievable serum and biliary antibiotic levels. Potential choices include intravenous ampicillin and sulbactam, third-generation cephalosporins (e.g. cefotaxime), or ampicillin in combination with an aminoglycoside. Alternatively, a broad-spectrum penicillin derivative with good biliary penetration (e.g. mezlocillin) may be utilized. The newer penicillin

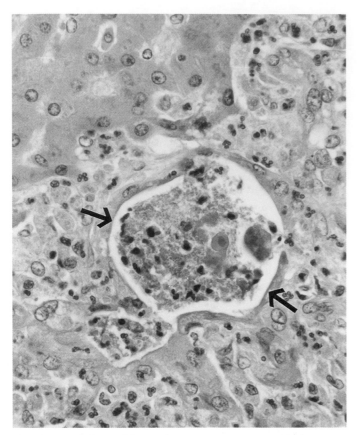

Figure 39.3 Cholangitis following hepatic portoenterostomy. The lumen of the bile duct is filled with acute inflammatory cells and necrotic debris. Neutrophils extend into the bile duct epithelium and surrounding portal tract stroma. The epithelium lining the bile duct is reactive and focally attenuated.

derivatives have the advantage of covering *Enterococcus* (was *Streptococcus*) *faecalis* as well as a variety of anaerobic organisms. Mezlocillin used alone has been prospectively compared with an ampicillin/gentamicin regimen in the treatment of cholangitis in adults and found to have a higher rate of cure in addition to a lower incidence of toxicity [16]. Ciprofloxacin has gained acceptance in the therapy of cholangitis in adults but its use in young children continues to be debated. Trimethoprim–sulfamethoxazole has also been utilized. Particularly ill patients may require addition of specific anaerobic coverage, as well as the use of other antibiotic combinations including piperacillin/tazobactam, ticarcillin/clavulanate, imipenem, or meropenem [17]. Duration of treatment is generally 21 days for severe disease.

Biliary decompression may be required in those patients with biliary obstruction. Initial data regarding site of obstruction may be garnered through use of spiral CT and/or MRCP [14]. Subsequently, ERCP and placement of nasobiliary drainage tubes after papillotomy and stone removal (if necessary) is performed. These procedures have now been safely performed in significant numbers of children [18]. Subsequent cholangiography may delineate the site of obstruction, allowing definitive therapy to be undertaken endoscopically in select cases.

Percutaneous cholangiography and decompression have also been advocated. Finally, surgical intervention may be required in some patients.

The prognosis of cholangitis in children has not been clearly delineated, but in one study of cholangitis after the Kasai procedure, the mortality rate was approximately 1% [13]. Mortality in adult series is considerably higher, presumably because of the higher incidence of malignant lesions and debilitated patients in these groups. Repeated episodes of cholangitis can result in the cessation or diminution of bile flow in those patients who have undergone successful Kasai procedures. Therefore, aggressive diagnostic and therapeutic efforts seem justified in this population.

Perihepatitis

First noted by Stajano in 1919, Fitz-Hugh (1934) [19] and Curtis (1930) [20] independently described the syndrome of perihepatitis associated with salpingitis that now bears their names. Generally noted in young women, symptoms include acute-onset, severe right upper quadrant pain, occasionally with radiation to the shoulder and back. Pain is intensified by the intake of breath or palpation of the abdomen. A friction rub may be present over the anterior liver surface. Fever may be present. The patient often has both a history of previous pelvic inflammatory disease and physical findings suggestive of same. Laboratory findings are non-specific but often include an elevated ESR. Serum aminotransferase levels are normal or minimally elevated. Abdominal CT may reveal hyperemia of the anterior liver surface. Laparoscopic (laparotomy) findings early in the course of perihepatitis include "violin string" adhesions between the hepatic capsule and the adjacent abdominal wall and diaphragm. Later findings consist of hemorrhagic spots and white fibrous plaques on the liver surface. The hepatic parenchyma does not appear involved. Diagnosis in the proper clinical situation is made via isolation of the causative microorganisms, *Neisseria gonorrhoeae* and/or *Chlamydia trachomatis* from the cervix, urethra or rectum, or, more commonly, via polymerase chain reaction (PCR) of an appropriately collected urine. The pathophysiology of perihepatitis associated with salpingitis remains uncertain. Postulated mechanisms include ascending infection from the genital tract to the perihepatic region, as well as spread via the bloodstream. Treatment is through eradication of the underlying infection with an appropriate antibiotic regimen.

The liver may also be involved in patients with gonococcal bacteremia; approximately 50% may have abnormalities of serum aminotransferase levels [21].

Specific bacterial infections
Cat scratch disease

Cat scratch disease, caused by pleomorphic Gram-negative bacteria identified as *Bartonella henselae*, typically consists of regional lymphadenitis following inoculation of the responsible agent, usually by a cat. Clinical manifestations may also include encephalitis, pneumonitis, arthritis, osteomyelitis, and neuroretinitis, among many others [22]. While hepatosplenomegaly and anicteric hepatitis had previously been reported in association with cat scratch disease, the association with hepatic and splenic abscesses was first noted in 1985 [23]. Affected patients often present with systemic symptoms including fever, chills, myalgia, malaise, and abdominal pain. Clinically evident adenopathy is generally but not universally present. Elevated ESR is frequently observed, while serum aminotransferases, bilirubin, and alkaline phosphatase levels are typically normal. Abdominal imaging studies, usually performed as part of an evaluation for fever of unknown origin, reveal multiple, small, hypodense lesions in the parenchyma of the liver and spleen (Figure 39.4). *B. henselae* antibody titers are characteristically elevated. At surgery, firm nodules are

noted. Biopsy often reveals necrotizing granulomatous hepatitis [23]. Organisms may be noted within the lesions (Figure 39.5). Direct confirmation of identity may be made through the demonstration of *B. henselae* DNA in the hepatic tissue via PCR. Differential diagnosis includes other causes of hepatic granulomas, including infection with a variety of bacterial, fungal, parasitic, and viral agents. In addition, neoplasms, hypersensitivity reactions, and sarcoidosis must be considered. In the absence of widely available culture techniques for the cat scratch bacilli, precise diagnosis in the proper clinical situation (e.g. lymphadenopathy, history of cat contact and/or scratch, and identification of inoculation site) necessitates elimination of other causes of granulomatous hepatitis.

Therapy in the immunocompetent host remains problematic but some authorities recommend parenteral antibiotic treatment, often gentamicin [24], for up to 3 weeks. Potentially effective oral therapy includes trimethoprim–sulfamethoxazole, rifampin, azithromycin dihydrate, and ciprofloxacin [24]. Corticosteroids have also been employed when there is persistent fever [22]. Recovery appears to be complete.

Typhoid hepatitis

Typhoid fever, most often caused by *Salmonella typhi* and *Salmonella paratyphi* (ser.) is a syndrome characterized by fever, headache, and abdominal pain. A relative bradycardia may be present. Subsequent findings may include pneumonia and encephalopathy. Intestinal perforation or bleeding may occur. Approximately 27% of patients have hepatomegaly [25], and 5–10% of patients will have clinical jaundice. Serum aminotransferases and alkaline phosphatase are mildly abnormal in 50% of cases. In one series, symptoms of hepatitis were present in 5% of patients [25]. A recent series demonstrated abnormal liver chemistries in 36% of patients with *Salmonella enteritidis* enterocolitis [26]. Hepatic biopsy findings are

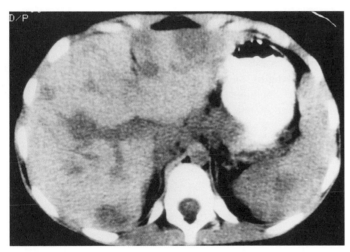

Figure 39.4 Cat scratch disease. CT of the liver and spleen shows multiple areas of low attenuation throughout the hepatic and splenic parenchyma.

(a)

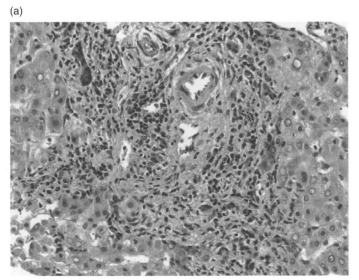

(b)

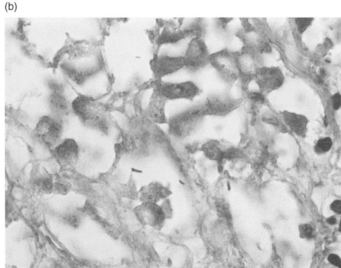

Figure 39.5 Cat-scratch disease. (a) Portal region showing non-specific chronic lymphocytic inflammation extending across the limiting plate of an adjacent hepatic lobule. (b) Several extracellular bacilli located within the collagenous matrix (Warthin–Starry silver stain).

relatively non-specific and include the presence of typhoid nodules (focal areas of hepatocyte necrosis surrounded by a mononuclear cell infiltrate), sinusoidal dilation, and mononuclear cell inflammation of portal tracts. Less-frequently noted were ballooning degeneration of hepatocytes, steatosis, and hepatic granulomata [27]. Typically, findings were noted in combination and could be found in biopsies from patients without hepatomegaly. Diagnosis is established via culture and/or serology. Hepatic abnormalities typically resolve with treatment of the underlying infection.

Brucellosis

Brucellosis, in humans generally attributable to *Brucella melitensis*, *B. abortus*, or *B. suis*, is an often prolonged illness characterized in children by fever, weight loss, malaise, arthralgia, back pain, and headache. Complications may include abscess formation, meningoencephalitis, pneumonitis, osteomyelitis, nephritis, and endocarditis. Infection is typically acquired via contact with infected animals or ingestion of contaminated milk products.

Hepatic involvement in brucellosis is relatively common. Approximately 25% of affected children have hepatosplenomegaly on physical examination [28] and 84% have abnormal hepatic enzyme studies [29]. Clinical jaundice is relatively infrequent, as is cholecystitis, either calculous or acalculous [30]. Common laboratory abnormalities in children include lymphocytosis and elevation of the ESR. Liver biopsy findings include portal inflammation and focal hepatocyte necrosis in 90% of patients [31], while non-caseating granuloma formation may be noted in up to 70% of patients, primarily within the first 100 days of illness. Diagnosis is made through history of possible exposure, culture and PCR of infected tissue, as well as by specific serology. Treatment is with tetracycline or doxycycline in conjunction with rifampin. Trimethoprim–sulfamethoxazole may be utilized in children under 9 years of age. In rare cases of hepatic abscess secondary to *Brucella* infection, surgery made be required in addition to medical therapy.

Tularemia

Caused by infection with *Francisella tularensis*, tularemia may occur in typhoidal or ulceroglandular forms. Infection is typically via exposure to infected mammalian vectors (e.g. rabbits, squirrels, dogs, cats) or through tick bites, although other more tangential methods of spread have been reported. Hepatic involvement appears to be relatively infrequent; however, one series reported abnormal liver tests in 58% [32]. Hepatomegaly, clinical hepatitis, and hepatic abscess formation have all been reported. Pathologic findings in tularemic hepatitis include focal coagulative necrosis with chronic inflammatory infiltrate. Diagnosis is via examination of serum *F. tularensis* titers and culture. Treatment is with streptomycin or aminoglycoside antibiotics. Ciprofloxacin and doxycycline may be indicated for mild disease [24].

Yersinia enterocolitica

Yersinia enterocolitica has been implicated in the development of hepatic abscesses in the setting of hemochromatosis in adults [33].

Toxic shock syndrome

Toxic shock syndrome is described as a complication of tampon use but is a consequence of bacterial infection generally attributable to staphylococcal and streptococcal species. In the former, staphylococcal toxin TSST-1 acts as a superantigen, causing a ctytokine storm via T-cell activation.

Diagnostic criteria include fever, diffuse macular rash with desquamation (primarily of palms and soles 1–2 weeks after disease onset), hypotension, involvement of three or more organ systems, including CNS, liver, kidney, muscles, gastrointestinal tract, and mucous membranes, plus negative workup for other potential causes. Hepatic involvement in toxic shock syndrome has been described by several investigators. Cholestasis, as delineated by elevated serum bile acid and bilirubin levels, has been noted in conjunction with elevated serum aminotransferases. Pathologic changes consistent with an acute cholangitis have been described [34]. Other observed alterations included portal inflammation and steatosis. Minimal intrahepatic cholestasis was noted. Hepatic abnormalities resolve with adequate anti-infective therapy, generally consisting of a beta-lactamase-resistant antistaphylococcal agent in conjunction with clindamycin, which inhibits bacterial protein synthesis [24].

Streptococcal infection

Infections with Group A β-hemolytic streptococci have long been associated with hepatic dysfunction. Jaundice has been reported as both an early and late complication of scarlet fever; the late-onset component may have reflected use of serum therapy in the early 1900s [35]. Early-onset jaundice was noted in association with hepatic tenderness and hepatomegaly. Pathologic findings include focal areas of hepatocyte necrosis, as well as portal inflammatory infiltrates consisting of polymorphonuclear leukocytes and lymphocytes. Streptococci may be noted in biopsy specimens [35,36]. The etiology of observed alterations is unclear but may involve direct infection versus toxin effect. Streptococcal infection has also been associated with fulminant hepatic failure.

Pneumococcal infections (*Streptococcus pneumoniae*), including those manifested as pneumonia, are also associated with a high incidence of hepatic enzyme abnormalities and, less frequently, jaundice [37]. Differential diagnosis of pneumonia associated with cholestasis must also include that caused by *Legionella* sp.

Listeriosis

Listeria monocytogenes is a Gram-positive bacillus that may be acquired transplacentally, perinatally, or via genital contact. Nosocomial and food-borne outbreaks have also been reported. Neonates, those with pre-existing hepatic disease (including hepatic transplantation), and immunosuppressed individuals are most at risk. The disorder is characterized by the formation of granulomas. In neonates, the liver is often diffusely involved. Hepatic involvement is noted less often in older individuals. Other clinical manifestations may include, depending upon age, respiratory distress, cardiac dysfunction, meningitis, endocarditis, and osteomyelitis. Diagnosis is made through the use of cultures. Treatment is generally undertaken with ampicillin in combination with gentamycin or other aminoglycosides [24].

Mycobacterial infections

Tuberculosis

Involvement of the liver in tuberculosis is well known. In congenital tuberculosis, the liver is often the primary site of infection, perhaps because of blood flow through the ductus venosus. In older patients, the liver is also frequently affected. Up to 75% of patients with extrapulmonary tuberculosis [38], as well as most patients with miliary tuberculosis, have hepatic involvement, as do smaller proportions of those with pulmonary involvement. Hepatic manifestations are heterogeneous; most common are small hepatic granulomas found in portal areas. Early granulomas are composed of lymphocytes and epithelioid cells; subsequently giant cell formation and necrosis may predominate. Lesions may reach 1–2 mm in size in miliary tuberculosis (Figure 39.6) [39]. Larger 1–2 cm tuberculomata may be seen, as may tuberculous hepatic abscesses, either in conjunction with an extrahepatic foci of infection or as a primary lesion. Biliary obstruction may occur as the result of perihilar adenopathy. Presenting symptoms typically depend upon the location of associated disease; most hepatic disease attributed to tuberculosis is asymptomatic. Congenital tuberculosis may present in the first 1 to 2 weeks of life with failure to thrive; hepatosplenomegaly and jaundice may be later manifestations. In older patients, weight loss, fever, and anorexia predominate; abdominal pain is sometimes present. Hepatomegaly is common; splenomegaly is less frequently appreciated. Jaundice may occur, as may ascites. Alkaline phosphatase levels are abnormal in approximately 75% of patients and aminotransferase levels in 35%. Plain film of the abdomen may reveal large, confluent, hepatic calcifications as well as calcifications along the course of the common bile duct. Liver CT may reveal abscess formation; ring enhancement may be present. It may also reveal the diffuse, small, low-density lesions typical of miliary tuberculosis. Duct dilation may be noted with CT or ultrasonography. Delineation of the site of ductal obstruction may require endoscopic retrograde cholangiography and/or percutaneous transhepatic cholangiography. Laparoscopy may be a highly specific means of diagnosing hepatic tuberculomata; visible lesions were found in 49 of 53 patients examined [40]. Diagnosis generally requires biopsy; both histology (with appropriate stains for acid-fast bacteria) and culture should be performed. Culture of other sites,

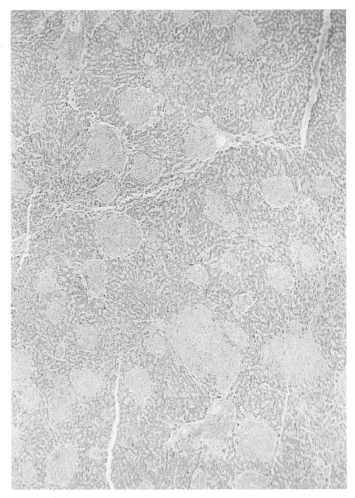

Figure 39.6 Miliary tuberculosis. Numerous oval epithelioid granulomas are scattered throughout the liver.

including gastric aspirate, sputum, and bone marrow, may be appropriate and PCR analysis may also be of use.

Treatment is that of active tuberculosis; for susceptible strains, 2 months of isoniazid, rifampin, and pyrazinamide daily, followed by 4 months of isoniazid and rifampin. Regimens include daily observed therapy during the intensive phase of treatment [41]. Early, aggressive therapy is of particular importance in congenital tuberculosis [42]. Abscesses may require percutaneous catheter placement and drainage; surgery is occasionally required. The prognosis of hepatic tuberculosis in children is unclear. The worst prognosis may be in neonatally acquired infection.

Mycobacterium avium complex

Mycobacterium avium complex has also been associated with liver disease, generally in the setting of profound immunodeficiency associated with advanced HIV infection. Liver disease generally occurs in the context of systemic disease. Elevated serum aminotransferases and alkaline phosphatase are frequently noted. Granulomas containing prominent foamy macrophages may be noted on liver biopsy: acid-fast bacilli

(a)

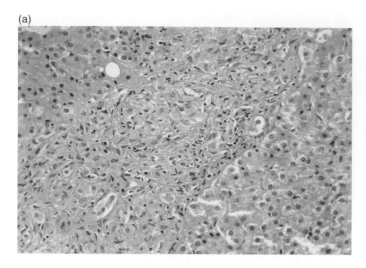

(b)

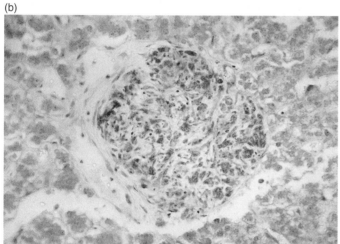

Figure 39.7 *Mycobacterium avium* complex. (a) Non-necrotizing epithelioid granuloma are formed of large foamy histiocytes. (b) Acid-fast bacillus stain demonstrates bacilli engulfed by histiocytes.

may be seen in some cases (Figure 39.7) [43]. Diagnosis of disseminated infection generally is made by culture of blood, sputum, or feces. Treatment is through the use of a combination of at least two drugs with antimycobacterial activity; ethambutol and clarithromycin are most often used. Prophylaxis with azithromycin or clarithromycin is recommended for HIV-infected patients with profound immunosuppression [44].

Actinomycosis

Actinomycosis is caused by *Actinomyces israelli*, a ubiquitous organism found worldwide. Part of normal human oral flora, *A. israelli* may also be responsible for infections of the cervico-facial, abdominal, and thoracic regions. Hepatic infection typically occurs via direct extension or portal vein seeding from other intra-abdominal foci of infection. Hepatic infection may be primary in 15% of cases [45]. Early hepatic infection may present non-specifically as hepatitis. Subsequent infection results in hepatic abscess formation. Advanced infection may also mimic hepatic neoplasia. Sinus formation is common and

may discourage attempts at percutaneous aspiration in suspected cases. Diagnosis is made by positive culture and demonstration of "sulfur" granules, diagnostic of actinomycosis. Therapy is with high-dose intravenous penicillin; subsequent oral therapy may include penicillin or tetracycline. Treatment for up to 1 year may be necessary [24]. Surgical resection of large lesions may be required.

Ehrlichioses

The ehrlichioses are a group of tick-borne diseases caused by bacteria of the genus *Ehrlichia*. These bacteria infect either human monocytes (*Ehrlichia chaffeensis*; transmitted by Lone Star ticks) or human granulocytes (human granulocyte ehrlichiosis agent; transmitted by *Ixodes scapularis* and *I. pacificus*). Symptoms include fever, headache, myalgia, and malaise. Complications include prolonged fever, shock, adult respiratory distress syndrome, mental status changes, pneumonitis, and rhabdomyolysis, among others. Approximately 70–90% of affected patients demonstrate abnormal serum aminotransferases, peaking on day 6–7 of illness at approximately 10 times normal values, and then decreasing slowly as the illness resolves. Immunosuppressed patients may have smaller increases in aminotransferases [46]. Liver pathology has been studied in a limited number of patients. Cholestasis, with neutrophilic infiltration of the bile duct epithelium suggesting bile duct obstruction, has been noted [47]. Sinusoidal monocytic infiltration has been a more common finding. Others note focal hepatic necrosis and/or ring granuloma formation. Diagnosis is made through serology and PCR. Treatment is generally undertaken with doxycycline [24]. Hepatic abnormalities resolve completely after therapy.

Syphilis

The liver is a common site of involvement in both congenital and secondary syphilis. Indeed, transfer of treponemes across the placenta into the fetal circulation presumably accounts for the widespread organ involvement noted in congenital syphilis. Symptomatic infants are often small for gestational age, with evidence of lymphadenopathy, hemolytic anemia, and thrombocytopenia. Bony abnormalities may occur in 80–90% of affected infants, while rash occurs in 40–60%. Other associated findings include neurologic disease, dental and ocular abnormalities, and nephrosis. Hepatic involvement is frequent, with hepatomegaly estimated to occur in 50–90% of symptomatic infants. Rarely, hepatic failure may occur [48]. Conjugated hyperbilirubinemia may also occur. Diagnosis is made through use of serology. Evaluation of the infant with findings suggestive of congenital syphilis should include serum VDRL (Venereal Disease Research Laboratory test), radiography of the long bones, and examination of cerebrospinal fluid. Hepatic biopsy is generally not required for diagnosis. Wright and Berry reviewed liver sections from 59 children who died of congenital syphilis in the preantibiotic period; 50 of the 59 sections were "histologically normal," but 41 were "heavily infiltrated with treponemes, so much that it appeared that there were more treponemes than liver" [49]. Conversely, specimens from children treated with penicillin often show histologic changes consisting of extramedullary hematopoiesis, parenchymal and portal inflammation, and occasional focal scarring, leading to the hypothesis that penicillin therapy may exacerbate syphilitic hepatitis. Nonetheless, penicillin remains the cornerstone of therapy for affected infants. Although syphilitic hepatitis may persist for weeks or months following treatment, the process generally resolves without sequelae.

Hepatic involvement is also a well-recognized consequence of secondary and tertiary syphilis. Approximately 50% of patients with secondary syphilis have hepatic enzyme abnormalities, while jaundice is significantly less common, occurring in 1–12% of affected patients. Serum alkaline phosphatase values are often disproportionately elevated. Biopsy findings are variable but may include areas of focal necrosis encircled by lymphocytes, neutrophils, and eosinophils. Granulomatous changes may be present, as may pericholangitis. In tertiary syphilis, gumma formation is noted. Resolution is typically complete following adequate treatment of the underlying infection.

Borreliosis

Lyme disease

Lyme disease is caused by *Borrelia burgdorferi*, a tick-borne spirochete. Acute signs and symptoms include erythema chronicum migrans, fever, malaise, headache, stiff neck, arthralgias, myalgias, and lymphadenopathy. Arthritis may be chronic. Hepatic involvement in humans has been described; 19–37% may have abnormal liver tests [50]. Symptoms consistent with hepatic dysfunction may be elicited and include nausea, vomiting, anorexia, and weight loss. Hepatomegaly and right upper quadrant pain may be noted. Liver biopsy in one patient revealed infiltration of sinusoids by neutrophils and mononuclear cells [51]. Microvesicular fat, Kupffer cell hyperplasia, ballooning hepatocytes, and increased hepatocyte mitotic activity were also noted. *B. burgdorferi* organisms were present in the biopsy specimen [51].

Diagnosis of Lyme disease requires a high index of suspicion on the part of the investigating physician. History of travel to affected areas, or of clinical signs/symptoms consistent with infection, must be elicited and appropriate serologic studies performed (enzyme-linked immunosorbent assay (ELISA) or indirect fluorescent antibody, followed by Western blotting if positive). Assessment with PCR may also be of use. Treatment of early disease is with doxycycline [24]; cefuroxime or amoxicillin may be used in children under 9 years of age. Parenteral therapy with ceftriaxone or penicillin V may be required in those patients with severe carditis, persistent arthritis, or meningitis. Chronic hepatitis has not been described with *B. burgdorferi* infection.

Borrelia recurrentis

Patients with *Borrelia recurrentis* infection are also known to have hepatic involvement. In a series of patients with louse-

borne disease, 62% were noted to have hepatic tenderness [52]. Patients may have mild elevation of serum aminotransferases; jaundice may also occur. Diagnosis is via examination of blood smears for *Borrelia*. Treatment with doxycycline, erythromycin, and penicillin may be effective, particularly if the diagnosis is made early in the disease course.

Leptospirosis

Leptospirosis is caused by one of several serotypes of *Leptospira interrogans*, a coiled, motile spirochete whose primary hosts include a variety of domestic and wild animals. At-risk individuals have traditionally included those exposed to cattle, hogs, horses, and rats. Exposure to blood, other body fluids, or fluids contaminated by urine from affected animals may result in disease transmission to humans. Disease in children has been attributed to canine exposure. After an incubation period of 4–20 days, one of two general disease patterns may occur. Approximately 90–95% of patients in adult series will remain anicteric and undergo an initial phase of disease lasting 4–9 days, marked by the presence of spirochetes in the peripheral circulation and characterized by fever, anorexia, abdominal pain, conjunctival erythema, lymphadenopathy, rash, and muscle tenderness. Headache and, less often, nuchal rigidity may occur. Approximately 50% of patients undergo a second period of fever, often marked by meningeal involvement, hepatitis, and, occasionally, endocarditis and myocarditis. In 5–10% of patients, there will be a more severe course, marked by significant jaundice, renal failure, hemorrhage, and vascular collapse, with death occurring in up to 40%. Children with leptospirosis suffer many of the signs and symptoms noted above. Hepatomegaly was seen in five of nine hospitalized children with leptospirosis; acalculous cholecystitis was also noted in five, serum bilirubin >1.2 mg/dL in seven, and elevated serum aminotransferase in six [53]. More recent series have confirmed these differences in presentation between children and adults. Also in contrast to data from adult series, severe disease in children is not limited to the icterohemmorhagiae serogroup of *L. interrogans*. Other abnormal laboratory findings may include elevated serum creatinine phosphokinase, leukocytosis, thrombocytopenia, and proteinuria. Serum prothrombin time may be elevated but generally normalizes in response to vitamin K administration.

The pathophysiology of leptospirosis-associated hepatic disease remains uncertain. Hepatic biopsy findings include edema, disorganization of liver cell plates, and multinucleated cells, reflecting hepatocyte proliferation(Figure 39.8). Erythrophagocytosis may be seen [54]. In approximately 10% of patients, small foci of hepatocellular necrosis may be present. Histologic alterations do not correlate with degree of jaundice. Diagnosis of leptospirosis may be made via culture of blood or cerebrospinal fluid during early stages of illness, and from urine subsequently. Serology (ELISA, microscopic agglutination test) and PCR may also be of use, because culture of this organism is often difficult. Although not diagnostic, darkfield examination of the urine may provide useful information.

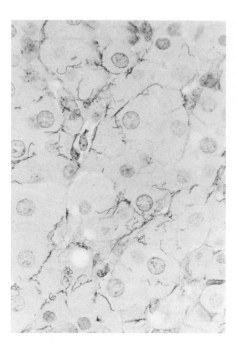

Figure 39.8
Leptospirosis. Numerous spirochetes are present. Detail of the spirochete coiling is somewhat obscured by the silver deposits in this silver impregnation-based stain (Warthin–Starry).

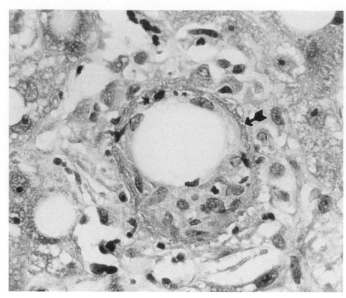

Figure 39.9 Q fever. Fibrinoid ring lesion containing a large, central lipid droplet surrounded by few inflammatory cells and encircled by a ring of fibrinoid material (arrow).

Treatment of affected individuals with parenteral penicillin appears most efficacious if initiated within the first few days of illness [24]; ceftriaxone, cefotaxime, and doxycycline are also of use. Doxycycline may serve as effective prophylaxis in high-risk individuals.

Rickettsial disease

Rocky Mountain spotted fever, the clinical syndrome associated with *Rickettsia rickettsii* infection, is characterized by fever; petechial rash beginning peripherally, spreading to the trunk, and often involving the palms and soles; and headache. Ticks serve as vectors for disease transmission. Hepatic involvement may occur; clinical manifestations include hepatomegaly and, rarely, jaundice. Pathologic changes noted at autopsy have consisted of portal triaditis, portal vasculitis, and erythrophagocytosis. Rickettsial organisms may be found in portal blood vessels and/or sinusoidal lining cells [55]. Diagnosis is via serology and high index of clinical suspicion. Treatment is with doxycycline.

Q fever

Q fever is caused by *Coxiella burnetti*, a proteobacteria, and is characterized by fever, headache, malaise, myalgia, and pneumonitis, although asymptomatic infection predominates in humans. Transmission occurs largely via inhalation of the *Coxiella* organism; this mode of transmission differs from rickettsiae, with which Q fever has been historically associated [56]. Animal hosts include cattle, sheep, goats, and rodents. Transmission may also occur through ingestion of contaminated milk.

Symptomatic infection in humans lasts 9–16 days, although acute infection may last up to 3 months. Chronic infection may occur, primarily in the form of Q fever

endocarditis and osteomyelitis. Hepatic involvement is frequent in acute Q fever. Specifically, 70–85% of patients are noted to have abnormal liver tests, and 11–65% are noted to have symptoms referable to hepatic involvement [57]. Hepatomegaly (16%) and hepatic tenderness may be present [56]. In one center, 42% of patients with Q fever presented with hepatitis in the absence of pulmonary symptoms [57]; 5% of patients present with jaundice. Although uncommon, hepatic failure secondary to Q fever has been documented in children.

Pathologic findings in the liver of patients with acute Q fever classically include fibrin ring granulomas, consisting of a central clear space surrounded by histiocytes and a fibrin ring (Figure 39.9). Early lesions may contain neutrophils, while giant cells are noted in later lesions [58]. Non-specific changes include steatosis, mononuclear infiltration of portal areas, and Kupffer cell hyperplasia. Fibrosis may rarely occur; hepatitis may rarely become chronic. Diagnosis is via detection of antibodies to phase I and II antigens of *C. burnetti*. Treatment is usually problematic because of the self-limited nature of most infections; however, doxycycline is efficacious; co-trimoxazole is recommended for children younger than 8 years of age.

Parasitic diseases of the liver

Entamoeba histolytica

Entamoeba histolytica, a protozoa distributed worldwide, is estimated to occur in the USA with an incidence of approximately 3–5%. Incidence may be higher in specific groups, including residents of group homes, male homosexuals, and immigrants from endemic areas. The organism is found in both trophozoite and cyst forms. Infection is fecal–oral passage of cysts; consequently infected children often live in crowded conditions marked by poor sanitation. After traversing the stomach, ingested cysts dissolve during passage through the small bowel and colon where, in the presence of colonic bacteria, they mature into trophozoites. Colonic infection may be asymptomatic or may manifest as invasive disease characterized by abdominal pain, bloody diarrhea, and the presence of "pipe stem" ulcers. The cecum and ascending colon tend to be most heavily involved. Hepatic disease occurs when trophozoites reach the liver, presumably via the portal vein, and are able to penetrate into the hepatic parenchyma, where, through the elaboration of proteolytic enzymes, abscess formation occurs (Figure 39.10). Subsequent spread of trophozoites to other organs, including brain, lung, heart, and spleen, has been described. In addition, local spread of amebic organisms may result in the presence of cutaneous ulcerations, most commonly noted in the perineal area in children.

Hepatic abscess formation is estimated to occur in 1–7% of children with invasive amebiasis. Children under 3 years of age seem to be most commonly affected; no male:female differential in incidence exists in this age group. Single or multiple cavities may be present; the right lobe of the liver is most commonly involved. The abscess cavity consists of a liquefied central area, surrounded by necrotic hepatic tissue. Ameba

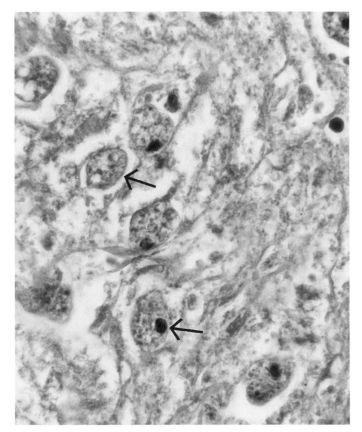

Figure 39.10 Amoebic abscess. Necrotic material surrounds numerous *Entamoeba histolytica* trophozoites (arrows). The trophozoites, which are oval eosinophilic organisms, contain a single nucleus ranging in size from 10 to 65 μm. The cytoplasm of the trophozoites is characteristically granular and vacuolated, and often contains phagocytosed erythrocytes.

may be noted in the necrotic tissue or in the adjacent hepatic parenchyma. Signs and symptoms of amebic abscess include fever, abdominal pain, abdominal distension, and tender hepatomegaly, but presentation in young children may be non-specific. Patients may present with an acute abdomen secondary to intraperitoneal abscess rupture. Free perforation into the peritoneal cavity is, however, less likely than slow leakage with intra-abdominal abscess formation. Other reported symptoms include dyspnea and productive cough, occasionally as a result of abscess rupture into the chest with formation of a hepatobronchial fistula. Patients in whom an intrahepatic amebic abscess has ruptured into the pericardium may present in shock. Jaundice is notably uncommon. History of a preceding diarrheal episode is present in less than 50% of patients; approximately 10% have dysentery concurrent with hepatic abscess. Routine laboratory examinations are of limited value in the diagnosis of hepatic amebic abscess. Serum aminotransferases are elevated in less than 25% of affected children, and serum alkaline phosphatase is generally normal in this age group [59]. Leukocytosis is common, as are elevated ESR and increased globulin fractions. Radiography of the chest may reveal right lower lobe infiltrates, pleural effusions, or elevation of the right or left hemidiaphragms. Hepatic scintigraphy has proven useful in adult series; a filling defect is noted corresponding to abscess location. As with pyogenic liver abscess, current imaging methods of choice would seem to be CT and/or ultrasonography. Examination of stools for trophozoites or cysts should be performed but is positive in less than 50% of patients with hepatic amebic abscess. Proctosigmoidoscopy and rectal biopsy may also be of use. Serologic testing for ameba is a useful diagnostic tool, particularly in areas which have relatively low incidences of amebic disease. Approximately 95% of patients with amebic liver abscess have positive enzyme immunoassays [59]. These studies remain positive for significant periods of time after acute infection. As a means of differentiation from pyogenic abscess, fine-needle aspiration of the abscess cavity is often required. Fluid obtained in this manner is reddish-brown in color and typically sterile. Examination of this "pus" yields amebic organisms in less than one-third of patients.

Therapy of amebic abscess consists primarily of the use of amebicidal agents, most often metronidazole 50 mg/kg per day in divided doses for 10 days, followed by a luminal amebicide such as iodoquinol or paromomycin. Nitazoxanide has been shown efficacious as a single agent in preliminary studies [60]. Surgical drainage is generally not required and mortality rates appear to be significantly higher when this is employed. Indications for surgical drainage include presentation with an acute abdomen as well as failure of other therapeutic measures. Percutaneous aspiration is more frequently utilized, although evidence of added efficacy to medical therapy alone is unclear [61]. Current indications include poor response to amebecidal therapy after 4–5 days, or as decompressive therapy in those patients in whom rupture of the abscess cavity, into the pleural, peritoneal, or pericardial cavities, seems imminent.

Repeated percutaneous aspirations in patients with amebic liver abscesses may significantly speed abscess resolution. Rupture of the abscess cavity is associated with significant mortality, approximately 30% die when rupture into the pericardium occurs. Conversely, mortality rates in adults with recognized, uncomplicated, hepatic amebic abscess are approximately 1%. Current pediatric mortality rates are unclear but may be significantly higher because of delays in diagnosis.

Echinococcal disease

Human infection with *Echinococcus granulosus* may occur after ingestion of ova excreted by infected dogs. Dogs generally acquire infection via consumption of sheep liver and/or intestine containing hydatid cysts. Scolices contained within the cysts then develop within the canine small intestine, maturing into adult tapeworms, 3–6 mm long. Rupture of the gravid proglottid releases 400–800 eggs, which are excreted in canine feces. Ingestion of eggs typically occurs after the handling of an infected dog or the drinking of contaminated water. The ingested embryo, after release from the egg in the duodenum, penetrates the intestinal mucosa and enters the portal circulation. Organisms may then lodge in the liver or lung of affected patients. Endemic areas include the Mediterranean basin, the Yukon territories, and parts of Africa, South America, Australia, and New Zealand, as well as sheep-rearing areas of the USA. Infection is common in childhood, although symptoms may not occur for many years. Although in adult series involvement of the liver occurs three times more frequently than the lung, involvement of the lung is noted frequently in children. Simultaneous involvement of the liver and lung may occur. Other sites of infection in approximately 10% of children include the brain, bones, genitourinary tract, eyes, spleen, and heart. Hepatic involvement is marked by the development of "cysts" within the hepatic parenchyma, most often within the right lobe. Typically, the cyst is surrounded by a fibrous capsule elaborated by the host. An acellular, hyalinized layer forms the exocyst, underlaid by a germinal layer. Extrusions of the germinal layer form brood capsules that contain protoscolices. Hydatid sand, composed of separated brood cysts and protoscolices, floats within the main cyst cavity. Septation may occur, as may formation of daughter cysts.

Symptoms of echinococcal cyst formation occur as a result of cyst growth and subsequent compression of surrounding tissues. Therefore, right upper quadrant pain and fullness may be the only presenting features. Jaundice may occur as a result of compression of the porta hepatis; cholangitis may arise secondary to cyst rupture into the biliary tract. Compression of hepatic veins by cysts may result in Budd–Chiari syndrome [62]. Rupture into the pericardial, peritoneal, or pleural cavities may occur. Other atypical presentations may also occur in children. Anaphylaxis may occur upon release of cyst fluid. Laboratory data are typically non-specific; elevation of serum alkaline phosphatase and aminotransferases may be noted. Eosinophilia may be present. Radiography of the abdomen may show calcification of the cyst wall in adults; this change is seldom apparent in children. Ultrasound is useful and can demonstrate the presence of hydatid sand as well as delineate septations and the presence of daughter cysts. The appearance may be difficult to differentiate from simple cysts or tumors. Lesions can be localized by CT and, preferably, MRI, and this also allows staging of lesions in most cases [63]. Endoscopic retrograde cholangiography may demonstrate involvement of the biliary tree by daughter cysts following rupture of the primary hepatic cyst. This complication appears to be less frequent in children than in adults. Definitive diagnosis rests upon demonstration of positive serology (ELISA) to *E. granulosus*, although false negative results may occur. Percutaneous aspiration for diagnostic purposes has generally not been recommended because of risks of anaphylaxis and dissemination; however, multiple reports of cyst drainage under CT, ultrasound, or laparoscopic guidance cast doubt on this dogma. In fact, although historically the primary treatment of hydatid disease has been surgical, with primary resection of peripheral and small lesions, currently PAIR (puncture, aspiration, injection with 95% ethanol or 20% NaCl for at least 15 minutes, followed by reaspiration of fluid) is the treatment of choice, combined with albendazole therapy both before and after PAIR therapy [63]. Large lesions require may still require cyst decompression, irrigation with scolicidal solutions, and, in some cases, omentoplasty [64]. Laparoscopic approaches have also been utilized successfully; care is taken to avoid peritoneal dissemination at surgery. Praziquantel may be utilized perioperatively. Daughter cysts in the biliary tree may be removed endoscopically after sphincterotomy [65]. In addition, utilizing ERCP, scolicidal agents have been infused into hepatic cysts that have ruptured into the biliary tract [66]. In unapproachable hepatic lesions, therapy with albendazole, 15 mg/kg daily for 1 to 6 months, has in some cases resulted in reduction in cyst size. Alaskan and Canadian patients infected with *E. granulosus* may have a more benign course.

Ascariasis

Human infection with the roundworm *Ascaris lumbricoides* is extremely common in tropical and temperate regions worldwide. Infection occurs via ingestion of embryonated eggs passed in human feces and deposited in soil, where development into the infective form occurs. As a result, incidence is highest among children and in areas with poor sanitation facilities. Ingested eggs hatch in the proximal small intestine. Larva penetrating the small bowel mucosa, are carried in the venous circulation to the lungs, and subsequently pass through the lungs and into the esophagus, once again reaching the small bowel where maturation takes place. Mild hepatic abnormalities may be associated with migrating larvae; dead larvae may stimulate granuloma formation. Most clinically relevant hepatic involvement, however, occurs when one or more adult worms pass thru the ampulla of Vater into the common bile duct. Worms may subsequently return to the duodenum or may infest the gallbladder and intrahepatic bile ducts. Obstruction of the pancreatic duct may also occur [67]. Symptoms of biliary ascariasis, notably more common in children than in adults, include (in uncomplicated cases) the acute onset of right upper quadrant pain (100%), vomiting (96%), history of worm infestation (64%), worm passage in stool or vomitus (50%), and fever (27%). Signs include right upper quadrant tenderness (100%), palpable gallbladder (11%), hepatomegaly (16%), and jaundice (2%) [68]. Complications of biliary ascariasis are infrequent but may occur in a higher percentage of affected adults (53%) than children (5%) [68]. Jaundice, hepatomegaly, and fever occur in higher proportions of complicated infestations. Death of ascarids within the common bile duct causes mucosal destruction and fibrosis, resulting in stricture and predisposing to stone formation. Death of worms in the intrahepatic bile ducts is associated with the release of eggs and the subsequent development of suppurative cholangitis and hepatic granuloma formation (Figure 39.11). Abscess formation may also occur; rupture of abscesses into the peritoneal or pleural cavities may then follow. Other reported complications include cholecystitis, perforation of the common bile duct, and pylephlebitis of the hepatic and/or portal veins.

Laboratory data in uncomplicated biliary ascariasis are frequently unrevealing, with normal serum aminotransferases noted in 90% of patients [68]. Hyperamylasemia may be present in approximately 25% of patients with common duct ascarids. Ultrasound may demonstrate the presence of ascarids in the common duct; abscess formation may be noted. Both CT and MRCP are useful. Definitive diagnosis may be made by demonstration of adult worms or ova in stool or vomitus. Panendoscopy may demonstrate the presence of ascarids in the duodenum, while endoscopic retrograde cholangiography allows demonstration of adult worms throughout the biliary tree. Therapy of biliary ascariasis in uncomplicated infections is expectant; antihelminthic therapy consists of albendazole, mebendazole, or ivermectin. Nitazoxanide is also efficacious

[24]. In resistant infections, endoscopic sphincterotomy with worm extraction may be effective [69]. Nasobiliary tube placement may allow instillation of antihelminthic agents into the biliary system. Worm removal has also been performed via the percutaneous, transhepatic route. Surgery may be required when hepatic abscess is present, as well as in the presence of common duct and gallbladder perforation.

Toxocariasis

Visceral larva migrans, caused by the nematode *Toxocara canis*, occurs worldwide. After ingestion by a dog, embryonated ova undergo a life cycle similar to that described above for *A. lumbricoides*. Additionally, fetal animals may be infected in utero via transplacental spread of the organism. Human infection typically results from ingestion of soil contaminated by embryonated ova. Infection is most common in children; average age is 2 years. Subsequent to ingestion, larvae penetrate the intestinal wall and migrate via lymphatics and the venous circulation to, most commonly, the liver and lung. Other affected organs include the eye, heart, and CNS. Symptoms include cough, wheezing, fever, pallor, and visual impairment. Hepatosplenomegaly, rales/wheezing, lymphadenopathy, and pruritic skin lesions may be present on physical examination. Marked eosinophilia and hyperglobulinemia are generally present, while routine biochemical indicators of hepatic injury are typically normal. Titers of isohemagglutinins to A and B blood group antigens are elevated. Serologic confirmation with an ELISA test is available and CT may demonstrate multiple low-density lesions, as might MRI. Early pathologic findings in the liver consist of larvae surrounded by eosinophils; later findings include granulomas composed of epithelioid cells, giant cells, lymphocytes, and fibroblasts [70]. Treatment entails the administration of albendazole or mebendazole but the efficacy of these regimens remains uncertain. Corticosteroids may be utilized concomitantly in children with pulmonary and/or ocular disease.

Capillariasis

Infection of the human liver by *Capillaria hepatica*, a nematode usually affecting rodents, cats, and dogs, is uncommon but may be associated with a spectrum of clinical findings similar to that noted for toxocariasis. Symptoms include fever, hepatomegaly, and eosinophilia in approximately 90% of affected patients. Diagnosis is generally made through the demonstration of organisms in percutaneous hepatic biopsy specimens. Treatment options include albendazole and mebendazole [24].

Schistosomiasis

Infection with *Schistosoma haematobium*, *S. mansoni*, or *S. japonicum* occurs in approximately 230 million people globally (World Health Organization data). The majority of these infections occur in the pediatric population. Both *S. mansoni* and *S. japonicum* are capable of causing hepatic disease; areas

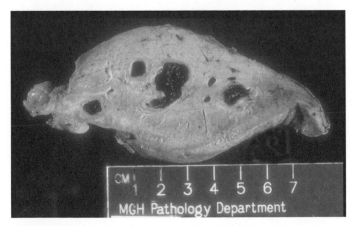

Figure 39.11 Oriental cholangitis secondary to infection by *Ascaris lumbricoides*. This section of the liver shows the characteristically cystically dilated bile ducts.

of endemicity include Africa, the Middle East, South America, and sections of the Caribbean basin for *S. mansoni*, while *S. japonicum* is noted predominantly in central and southeast Asia. *S. haematobium* primarily affects the urinary tract. Schistosomal organisms infect humans by direct penetration through the skin of cercariae, previously released from a snail host. After penetration, cercariae develop into schistosomulae and eventually migrate to the liver where, in intrahepatic portal venules, they mature and mate. Single mating pairs persist within the liver for an average of 4–7 years. The adult organisms then move within the portal venous system to branches of the inferior (*S. mansoni*) or superior (*S. japonicum*) mesenteric veins. Eggs subsequently produced may be excreted in feces or retained in tissue. Hepatic lesions are produced as a result of the hosts immunologic response to ova deposited in the portal venous system (Figure 39.12). Initial T helper 1 and subsequently T helper 2 responses to egg antigens result in the formation of granulomatous lesions which surround the ovum and are composed primarily of eosinophils, epithelioid cells, lymphocytes, and plasma cells [71]. Giant cells and fibrosis become prominent after death of the ovum. Pigment may be present. Destruction of small portal radicles occurs, presumably producing the presinusoidal portal hypertension characteristic of hepatosplenic

schistosomiasis. Fibrosis and thrombophlebitis of larger portal branches results in the "pipestem fibrosis" described by Symmers [72]. Approximately 10% of children infected with *S. mansoni* display hepatic disease with periportal fibrosis. True cirrhosis is generally not seen. Clinical manifestations of schistosomiasis are protean; distinct clinical syndromes are associated with each stage of infection. Hepatic disease is marked by hepatosplenomegaly; development of hepatic disease appears to correlate with severity of infestation. Symptoms of hepatic disease are few; patients may present with upper gastrointestinal bleeding from esophageal varices as the first sign of disease. Later signs may include edema and ascites. Laboratory abnormalities are also few; hypersplenism may result in anemia, thrombocytopenia, and leukopenia. Eosinophilia and hyperglobulinemia are often noted. Serum aminotransferases are generally not markedly elevated, while serum alkaline phosphatase may be increased. Serologic studies (ELISA) may be useful. Ultrasound allows detection and grading of periportal fibrosis, accurate measurement of liver and spleen size, and measurement of portal vein size, as well as detection of intra-abdominal varices. Both CT and MRI can indicate the presence of periportal fibrosis. Definitive diagnosis rests upon the isolation of schistosome eggs in stool or urine in *S. haematobium* infection. Rectal biopsy tissue may be

(a)

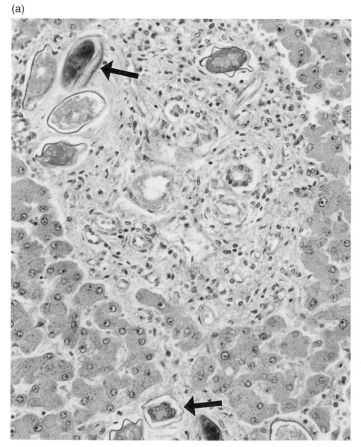

(b)

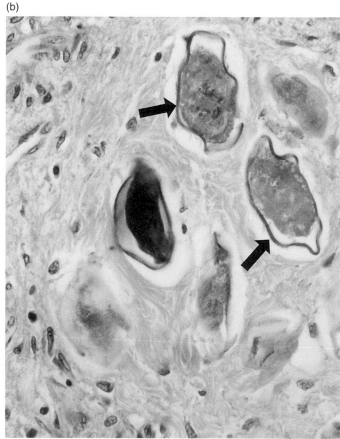

Figure 39.12 Schistosomiasis. Numerous eggs are present in the portal tracts (arrows), which are mildly expanded and fibrotic, a reaction to the presence of the eggs.

examined for the presence of eggs, as may hepatic biopsy specimens. Panendoscopy may be useful to establish the presence of varices. The pharmacologic treatment of choice is praziquantel, 40–60 mg/kg daily in divided doses. Oxamniquine may also be utilized in *S. mansoni* infections [24]. Trials of single-dose combined therapy with ivernectin, albendazole, and praziquantel have also shown promise [73]. Mild periportal fibrosis may resolve in children after effective therapy. Acute variceal hemorrhage is managed in the routine manner; chronic hemorrhage may require variceal banding or, in some cases, shunt placement.

Liver flukes

Clonorchis sinensis

Infection with *Clonorchis sinensis*, a 1–2.5 cm trematode, is endemic throughout the Far East, as is another fluke, *Opisthorchis* spp., which has similar symptoms and effects. The life cycle of these flukes begins when embryonated eggs are ingested by operculate snails. Development into cercariae occurs within this host; after subsequent release the cercariae penetrate fresh water fish and become encysted within their flesh. Ingestion of contaminated fish by humans allows release of metacercariae in the duodenum from whence they migrate through the ampulla and into the small bile ducts where they mature (Figure 39.13). The lifespan of adult flukes is 20–30 years. Perhaps as a result, most symptomatic patients are at least 30 years of age. Injury to the bile ducts occurs and is manifested by adenomatous proliferation and goblet cell hyperplasia [74]. Fibrosis occurs with chronic infection. Secondary bacterial infection with *E. coli* occurs frequently and predisposes to formation of hepatic abscesses (recurrent

pyogenic cholangitis). Calculi are common. Repeated episodes may result in biliary stricture and periportal fibrosis. Egg deposition may also be associated with the presence of giant cell reaction in the liver, as well as with portal granulomas. Development of cholangiocarcinoma may occur in those with long-standing disease. Symptoms of infection vary in intensity with worm load and duration of infection. Early or mild disease may be asymptomatic; more severe infections may be with fever, malaise, anorexia, jaundice, and hepatosplenomegaly. Later symptoms involve the consequences of portal hypertension and biliary obstruction. Laboratory findings in late disease include elevations of serum aminotransferases, alkaline phosphatase, and bilirubin. Hyperglobulinemia is frequent. Ultrasound and CT may reveal duct dilation; associated cholangiocarcinomas, stones, and/or abscesses may also be visualized. Direct visualization of the biliary system with ERCP allows delineation of ductal morphology, identification and extraction of calculi, and detection of *Clonorchis* eggs and worms via aspiration of bile. Percutaneous cholangiography may also be useful. Diagnosis may be made through stool examination, as well as through examination of bile. Therapy involves treatment with praziquantel, 75 mg/kg in three doses in 1 day. Pyogenic cholangitis must be treated with appropriate antibiotics. Endoscopic papillotomy and stone extraction, as well as insertion of endoprostheses, may be required. In long-standing recurrent pyogenic cholangitis, other surgical interventions may be required.

Fasciola hepatica

Fasciola hepatica is a trematode found worldwide; primary hosts include sheep and cattle. The life cycle is similar to that described for *Clonorchis*. Human infection occurs after ingesting contaminated aquatic plants (e.g. watercress). In the

(a)

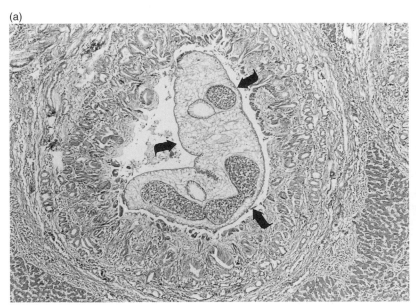

(b)

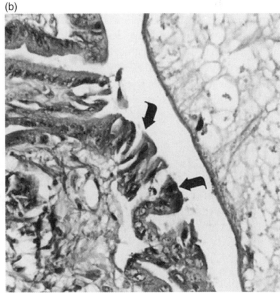

Figure 39.13 Clonorchiasis. (a) A dilated bile duct (arrows) contains an adult *Clonorchis sinensis*. (b) Associated atypical hyperplasia of the lining bile duct epithelium (arrows) is thought to be a premalignant epithelial process.

human, metacercariae penetrate the duodenal wall, traverse the peritoneal cavity, and subsequently penetrate the hepatic capsule. The organisms then migrate through the liver parenchyma until reaching the bile ducts, where they persist. Symptoms and pathologic changes, therefore, reflect not only biliary tract disease as in clonorchiasis but also parenchymal damage, manifested by the presence of necrotic microabscesses within the liver. Both sonography and CT may help to delineate these abnormalities [75]. Eosinophilia is common. Diagnosis rests upon serology and/or demonstration of ova in the stool. Endoscopic retrograde cholangiography may also be useful in the biliary phase of disease, both as a diagnostic (identification of eggs and intact flukes, visualization of flukes radiographically) and therapeutic (removal of flukes after sphincterotomy) measure [69]. Treatment is with triclabendazole 10 mg/kg given once. Because availability of this drug may be an issue, bithionol, 30–50 mg/kg on alternate days for 10–15 doses may also be used, as may nitazoxanide [24].

Leishmaniasis

Visceral leishmaniasis, or kala-azar, caused by *Leishmania donovani*, is endemic throughout the Mediterranean basin, as well as parts of Africa, South America, Russia, and China. Organisms are inoculated into humans via sandfly bites and are rapidly phagocytosed by dermal macrophages, where they proliferate. Rupture of infected macrophages allows organism spread to reticuloendothelial cells within the liver, spleen, bone marrow, lymph nodes, kidneys, and intestine. The hepatic lesion in older children and adults is characterized by Kupffer cell hyperplasia, many of which contain parasites. Portal tract infiltration with eosinophils, lymphocytes, and plasma cells may occur, as may granuloma formation. Fibrin ring granulomas have been reported [76]. Infants may demonstrate significant hepatocellular necrosis. Symptoms of infection include an incubation period of up to several months followed by fever, failure to thrive, anemia, hepatosplenomegaly, diarrhea, and bleeding diathesis. Hemophagocytic lymphohistiocytosis is a rare complication [77]. Laboratory data may reveal elevations of serum aminotransferase and alkaline phosphatase; hypoalbuminemia and prolongation of prothrombin times may be noted with more advanced disease. Bone marrow biopsy often demonstrates the presence of Leishman–Donovan bodies. Other diagnostic measures may include serology and PCR. Nodular hepatosplenic lesions may sometimes be seen by ultrasound or CT. Prognosis of untreated leishmaniasis is poor; liposomal amphotericin B 3 mg/kg daily on days 1–5, 14, and 21 is the drug of choice. Alternatives include stibogluconate sodium, meglumine antimonate and miltefosine [24]. Repeated treatment may be required.

Malaria

Malarial disease remains an important cause of morbidity and mortality throughout much of the world, occurring most frequently in tropical and subtropical climates. Deaths from malarial disease are most common in children between 1 and 5 years of age. Severe infection may also occur in neonates. Human infection with *Plasmodium falciparum*, *P. vivax*, *P. malariae*, and *P. ovale* is initiated after passage of sporozoites into the bloodstream at the time of the bite of an infected mosquito host. Sporozoites selectively invade hepatocytes, initiating the exoerythrocytic stage of development. Parasite division then occurs until rupture of the hepatocyte releases merozoites. Erythrocytes are then invaded. Spread of disease occurs upon the development of merozoites into micro- and macrogametes, which may be ingested by feeding mosquitos and reinitiate the malarial life cycle. Other methods of spread include transfusion and shared needles. Transplacental spread appears uncommon. Symptoms of malaria include fever, gastrointestinal complaints (nausea, vomiting, and diarrhea), headache, lethargy, myalgia, and delirium. Fever in children is often continuous. Neurologic complications, noted primarily with *P. falciparum*, include seizures and coma; renal failure may occur. Tender hepatosplenomegaly is often noted, as is jaundice. Hyperbilirubinemia commonly reflects hemolysis. Although sporadic patients may become significantly jaundiced with marked elevation of serum aminotransferase levels, milder alterations of these parameters are the norm [78]. Hepatic failure, at least as characterized by coagulopathy, is uncommon, although other clinical findings including encephalopathy, may be present. In jaundiced patients, pathologic findings include hepatocytes congestion, malarial pigment deposition, and inflammatory infiltrates [79]. At autopsy, the liver is noted to be congested and dark red/gray in color. Histologic findings include hypertrophied Kupffer cells containing red blood cells and malarial pigment. Sinusoids are congested with red blood cells. Portal tract infiltration by lymphocytes may occur in chronic infection. If shock has occurred, centrilobular necrosis may be present.

Diagnosis of malarial infection may be made via detection of malarial organisms in thin and thick peripheral blood smears prepared with Giemsa stain; PCR testing is also available. Treatment is initiated in most cases with chloroquine phosphate given orally, 10 mg/kg of the base (maximum dose 600 mg), followed by 5 mg/kg at 6 hours, 24 hours, and 48 hours [24]. Directly observed therapy is preferable. Quinidine hydrochloride is the parenteral drug of choice; however, significant side effects limit its use to emergency situations. Pyronaridine–artesunate shows promise for multiple malarial strains [80]. While relapse of disease may occur in individuals infected with *P. vivax* and *P. ovale*, hepatic abnormalities in treated patients typically resolve completely. While vaccine development shows promise [81], antimalarial chemoprophylaxis continues to be strongly recommended for travelers to endemic areas.

Fungal infections of the liver
Candidiasis

Hepatosplenic candidiasis occurs predominantly in neutropenic patients, primarily those receiving chemotherapy because of pre-existing malignancy. Infection of the liver and spleen may occur as a consequence of seeding during generalized fungemia. Symptoms in the neutropenic patient are non-specific; the diagnosis may be suspected in those patients in whom fever persists after the resolution of neutropenia. Fever occurs in approximately 85% of affected patients; other signs and symptoms include abdominal pain (57%), hepatomegaly (44%), and splenomegaly (43%). Serum alkaline phosphatase is generally elevated (60%) but bilirubin and aminotransferase are elevated less frequently. Leukocytosis is present in approximately 30% [82]. In approximately 90% of patients, CT will show early lesions as areas of variably enhancing diminished attenuation; MRI is similarly sensitive. Ultrasound is less sensitive but easily available; "bull's-eye" lesions are characteristic. Ultrasound remains a useful technique because of its portability and subsequent ease of repeated examinations. All techniques may miss small lesions. Given the toxicity of antifungal therapy, tissue diagnosis is often desirable. Percutaneous liver biopsy was able to confirm the diagnosis of hepatosplenic candidiasis in 70% of patients [82]. Laparoscopic and open liver biopsies are successful in higher proportions of patients; lesions are visible grossly as small yellow–white nodules throughout the liver. Early hepatic lesions are composed of pseudohyphae and yeast forms surrounded by neutrophils and an outer fibrous rim. Lesions progress to well-formed granulomas with giant cell change. Fungal organisms may be stained with periodic acid–Schiff or silver stains. Culture of lesions is positive in 60% of untreated patients but in only 30% of those receiving prior antifungal therapy. Blood cultures may also yield candidal organisms. Assays with PCR hold promise for the monitoring of therapy. Therapy in neutropenic patients is predicated upon the use of liposomal amphotericin B. Alternatively, echinocandins (caspofungin, micafungin, anidulafungin) may be used [83]. Fluconazole has been of use in the treatment of hepatosplenic candidiasis resistant to amphotericin B therapy and is of particular use in prophylaxis. It, or the echinocandins, should be the treatment of choice in stable non-neutropenic patients. Optimal duration of therapy is unclear; treatment regimens of several months may be required to produce radiologic resolution. Prognosis in children is difficult to assess given the multiple problems of most affected patients; survival rates of approximately 60% with amphotericin therapy have been described [82].

Trichosporon hepatitis

Trichosporon cutaneum has been rarely associated with granulomatous hepatitis in immunocompromised patients. Hepatic biopsy may reveal granulomas surrounding central areas of necrosis in which fungal organisms can be visualized. Prognosis has been poor in a very limited number of patients; very long treatment periods may be required [84].

Penicillium marneffei

Penicillium marneffei has been reported as a pathogen in immunocompromised patients, including children. Multisystem involvement is the rule but primary hepatic disease may also occur [85]. Patterns of disease within the liver include abscesses or, in immunocompromised patients, diffuse organ infiltration with yeast. A CT of the liver may reveal diffuse low-attenuation lesions. Definitive diagnosis is with culture or direct demonstration of organisms in biopsy specimens. Treatment is with a course of amphotericin B followed by itraconazole [24].

Coccidioidomycosis

Coccidioidomycosis, endemic in the southwestern USA as well as in parts of Mexico, Central and South America, is caused by the fungus *Coccidioides immitis*. Transmission is generally via inhalation of arthrospores; accordingly, pulmonary infection is most often seen. Perinatal transmission, although uncommon, has been described. Disseminated infection is most often noted in immunocompromised patients. Infected infants may also have a severe disease course but, as a rule, disseminated infection is less frequent in children than in adults. Hepatic involvement is estimated to occur in 25–60% of patients with disseminated disease [86]. The lungs are infected most frequently, followed by the spleen; other involved organs include the skin, meninges, bones, and genitourinary system [87]. Infection may begin with fever; often pulmonary symptomatology predominates. Less commonly, hepatic symptoms may predominate. Hepatomegaly may occur in conjunction with elevations in serum aminotransferase and, to a lesser degree, serum alkaline phosphatase. Clinically apparent jaundice is not common. Serology is often useful in patients with disseminated disease; in a literature review, 87% of patients had at least one positive serologic test. Liver biopsy may be diagnostic; normal-appearing hepatic parenchyma surrounds granuloma and giant cells containing spherules (stained with periodic acid–Schiff or methenamine silver) (Figure 39.14). Hepatic abscess formation has also been reported. Current treatment of disseminated disease is with oral itraconazole or fluconazole. Amphotericin B may be used for severe or non-responsive infection [24]. Prognosis for disseminated disease is relatively poor for immunocompromised patients and for patients who do not receive antifungal therapy.

Cryptococcosis

Cryptococcosis, associated with the fungal organism *Cryptococcus neoformans*, is responsible for human disease involving the lung, meninges, skin, and bones. The liver may be involved as part of disseminated disease; primary hepatic involvement may rarely occur. Gross examination of the liver reveals white nodules. Histologic features are those of granuloma surrounding fungal organisms. Cholangitis associated with cryptococci

(a)

(b)

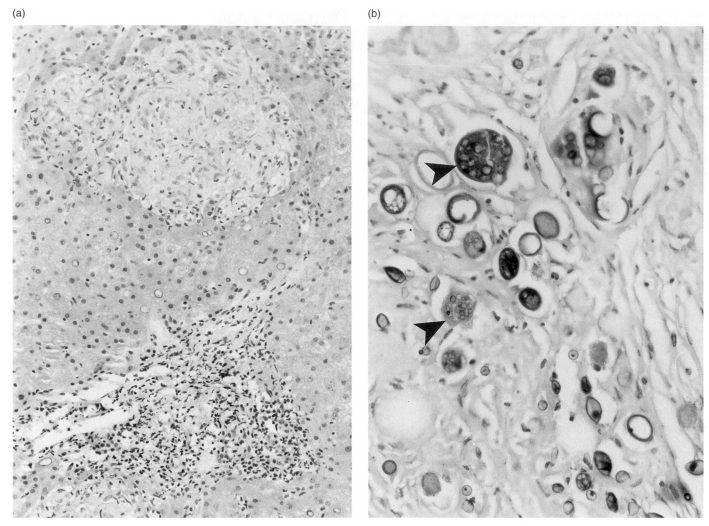

Figure 39.14 Coccidioidomycosis. (a) A lobular epithelioid granuloma is present containing numerous multinucleated giant cells. (b) Higher-power examination demonstrates numerous thick-walled spherules, ranging in size from 20 to 200 μm in diameter (arrowheads). Some of the spherules are filled with the characteristic endospores, ranging in size from 3 to 7 μm in diameter.

has also been described; ascending infection from the bowel was postulated. Diagnosis may be made by culture, microscopy, immunoassay, and, potentially, PCR. Therapy includes the use of amphotericin B in combination with fluorocytosine. Fluconazole, alone or in combination with flucytosine, may be useful in milder disease, although data are limited [24].

Histoplasmosis

Histoplasma capsulatum, the fungal agent responsible for histoplasmosis, is endemic in the Ohio and Mississippi river valleys in the USA. Inhalation of spores is the usual route of infection; the gastrointestinal tract may rarely act as the portal of entry. Approximately 50% of patients undergo asymptomatic infection. In symptomatic, immunocompetent patients, self-limited pulmonary infection is most common. Hepatic involvement occurs in conjunction with disseminated disease, although disease limited to the liver has been reported. Infants

may undergo a severe, acute form characterized by fever (90%), malaise (82%), cough (42%), weight loss (42%), diarrhea (32%), nausea or vomiting (26%), and an enlarged abdomen (13%) [88]. Marked hepatosplenomegaly is noted; lymphadenopathy and pulmonary findings are less constant. Laboratory findings include anemia, thrombocytopenia, and neutropenia. Jaundice may occur, as may mild to moderate elevations of serum aminotransferases and alkaline phosphatase. Subacute disseminated disease occurs less frequently in children and is associated with focal involvement of the intestine, adrenal glands, meninges, oropharyngeal cavity, or heart. Hepatomegaly is again common. Chronic disease is primarily noted in adults. Diagnosis may be made through the use of serology and the discovery of *Histoplasma* organisms in infected secretions or tissue. Hepatic biopsy may reveal Kupffer cells loaded with fungal spores, prominent in sinusoids and periportal areas, and often associated with compression and necrosis of adjacent hepatocytes. Kupffer cell infiltration

(a)

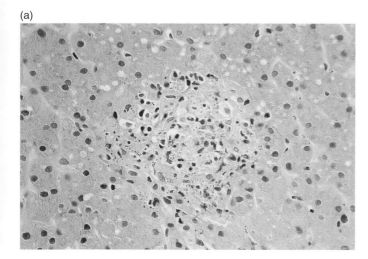

(b)

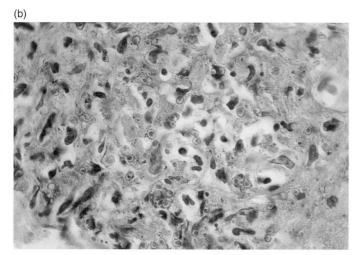

Figure 39.15 *Histoplasma capsulatum.* (a) Aggregated macrophages and Kupffer cells forming an ill-defined granuloma. (b) High-power magnification shows clustered fungi (periodic acid–Schiff–D stain).

of veins and arteries may be present. Granuloma formation is most commonly seen in chronic disease (Figure 39.15). Antifungal therapy is indicated in disseminated disease; untreated disseminated disease in infants is generally fatal. Amphotericin B and itraconazole have been employed as therapeutic agents [24].

Aspergillosis

A variety of *Aspergillus* species have been implicated in human disease. Pulmonary aspergillosis is the most frequent form of disease; disseminated disease most frequently occurs in immunocompromised individuals [89], although occurrence in infants, children, and immunocompetent adults has been reported. Organs involved include the lungs, brain, intestines, heart, kidneys, thyroid, pancreas, esophagus, and spleen. Hepatic involvement was noted in 5 of 32 patients in an autopsy series of patients with disseminated aspergillosis; four of these were hepatic transplant recipients [90]. Hepatic abscess formation may be noted; aspiration with cytology and culture may be useful in diagnosis. Granuloma formation has also been described. Voriconazole is the treatment of choice in invasive disease except in neonates, where high-dose amphotericin B is utilized [24]. Other alternatives include posaconazole, caspofungin, itraconazole, and amphotericin B.

Other fungal diseases

Other fungal diseases of the liver associated with disseminated infections, often in immunocompromised hosts, include mucormycosis and blastomycosis. Hepatic lesions in paracoccidioidomycosis occur primarily in generalized infections and include necrosis, granulomatous nodules, and portal fibrosis. Obstructive jaundice from compression of the common bile duct by infected lymph nodes has also been described.

References

1. Hamilton JR, Sato N. Jaundice associated with severe bacterial infection in young infants. *Pediatrics* 1963;**63**:121–132.

2. Shamir R, Maayan-Metzger A, Bujanover Y, *et al.* Liver enzyme abnormalities in Gram-negative bacteremia of premature infants. *Pediatr Infect Dis J* 2000;**19**:495–498.

3. Lanza JS, Rosato EL. Regulatory factors in the development of fatty infiltration of the liver during Gram-negative sepsis. *Metabolism* 1994;**43**:691–696.

4. Chusid MJ. Pyogenic hepatic abscess in infancy and childhood. *Pediatrics* 1978;**62**:554–559.

5. Mishra K, Basu S, Roychoudhury S, Kumar P. Liver abscess in children: an overview. *World J Pediatr* 2010;**6**: 210–216.

6. Chou FF, Sheen CS, Chen YS, Chen MC. Single and multiple pyogenic liver abscesses: clinical course, etiology, and results of treatment. *World J Surg* 1997;**21**:384–388.

7. Pineiro CV, Andres JM. Morbidity and mortality in children with pyogenic liver abscess. *Am J Dis Child* 1989;**143**:1424–1427.

8. Lederman ER, Crum NF. Pyogenic liver abscess with a focus on *Klebsiella pneumoniae* as a primary pathogen: an emerging disease with unique clinical characteristics. *Am J Gastroenterol* 2005;**100**:322–331.

9. Pelton SI, Kim JY, Kradin RL. Case records of the Massachusetts General Hospital. Case 27-2006. A 17-year-old boy with fever and lesions in the liver and spleen. *N Engl J Med* 2006;**355**: 941–948.

10. Rayes AA, Teixeira D, Serufo JC, *et al.* Human toxocariasis and pyogenic liver abscess: a possible association. *Am J Gastroenterol* 2001;**96**:563–566.

11. Muorah M, Hinds R, Verma A, *et al.* Liver abscesses in children: a single center experience in the developed world. *J Pediatr Gastroenterol Nutr* 2006;**42**:201–206.

12. Bari S, Sheikh KA, Malik AA, Wani RA, Naqash SH. Percutaneous aspiration versus open drainage of liver abscess in children. *Pediatr Surg Int* 2007;**23**:69–74.

13. Ecoffey C, Rothman E, Bernard O, *et al.* Bacterial cholangitis after surgery for biliary atresia. *J Pediatr* 1987;**111**(6 Pt 1):824–829.

14. Bornman PC, van Beljon JI, Krige JE. Management of cholangitis. *J Hepatobiliary Pancreat Surg* 2003;**10**:406–414.

15. Desmet DM. Cholestasis; extrahepatic obstruction and secondary biliary cirrhosis. In Macsween RNM, Anthony PP, Scheuer PJ (eds.) *Pathology of the Liver*. Edinburgh: Churchill Livingstone, 1979, pp. 272–305.

16. Gerecht WB, Henry NK, Hoffman WW, *et al.* Prospective randomized comparison of mezlocillin therapy alone with combined ampicillin and gentamicin therapy for patients with cholangitis. *Arch Intern Med* 1989;**149**:1279–1284.

17. Lee JG. Diagnosis and management of acute cholangitis. *Nat Rev Gastroent Hepatol* 2009;**6**:533–541.

18. Cheng CL, Fogel EL, Sherman S, *et al.* Diagnostic and therapeutic endoscopic retrograde cholangiopancreatography in children: a large series report. *J Pediatr Gastroenterol Nutr* 2005;**41**:445–453.

19. Fitz-Hugh T. Acute gonococcic peritonitis of the right upper quadrant in women. *JAMA* 1934;**102**:2094–2096.

20. Curtis AH. A cause of adhesions in the right upper quadrant. *JAMA* 1930;**94**:1221–1222.

21. Holmes KK, Counts GW, Beaty HN. Disseminated gonococcal infection. *Ann Intern Med* 1971;**74**:979–993.

22. Massei F, Gori L, Macchia P, Maggiore G. The expanded spectrum of bartonellosis in children. *Infect Dis Clin North Am* 2005;**19**:691–711.

23. Rocco VK, Roman RJ, Eigenbrodt EH. Cat scratch disease. Report of a case with hepatic lesions and a brief review of the literature. *Gastroenterology* 1985;**89**:1400–1406.

24. Pickering LK for the AAP Committee on Infectious Diseases. *Red Book*, 29th edn. Elk Grove Village, IL: American Academy of Pediatrics, 2012.

25. Ramachandran S, Godfrey JJ, Perera MV. Typhoid hepatitis. *JAMA* 1974;**230**:236–240.

26. Gonzalez-Quintela A, Campos J, Alende R, *et al.* Abnormalities in liver enzyme levels during *Salmonella enteritidis* enterocolitis. *Rev Esp Enferm Dig* 2004;**96**:559–562.

27. Mert A, Tabak F, Ozaras R, *et al.* Typhoid fever as a rare cause of hepatic, splenic, and bone marrow granulomas. *Intern Med* 2004;**43**:436–439.

28. Bolton JP, Darougar S. Perihepatitis. *Br Med Bull* 1983;**39**:159–162.

29. Lulu AR, Araj GF, Khateeb MI, *et al.* Human brucellosis in Kuwait: a prospective study of 400 cases. *Q J Med* 1988;**66**(249):39–54.

30. Al Otaibi FE. Acute acalculus cholecystitis and hepatitis caused by *Brucella melitensis*. *J Infect Dev Ctries* 2010;**4**:464–467.

31. Cervantes F, Bruguera M, Carbonell J, Force L, Webb S. Liver disease in brucellosis. A clinical and pathological study of 40 cases. *Postgrad Med J* 1982;**58**(680):346–350.

32. Evans ME, Gregory DW, Schaffner W, McGee ZA. Tularemia: a 30-year experience with 88 cases. *Medicine* 1985;**64**:251–269.

33. Crosbie J, Varma J, Mansfield J. *Yersinia enterocolitica* infection in a patient with hemachromatosis masquerading as proximal colon cancer with liver metastases: report of a case. *Dis Colon Rectum* 2005;**48**:390–392.

34. Ishak KG, Rogers WA. Cryptogenic acute cholangitis-association with toxic shock syndrome. *Am J Clin Pathol* 1981;**76**:619–626.

35. Fishbein WN. Jaundice as an early manifestation of scarlet fever. Report of three cases in adults and review of the literature. *Ann Intern Med* 1962;**57**:60–72.

36. Albrecht H. Bacterial and miscellaneous infections of the liver. In Zakim D, Boyer TD (eds.) *Hepatology*. Philadelphia, PA: Saunders, 2003, pp. 1109–1124.

37. Zimmerman HJ, Thomas LJ. The liver in pneumococcal pneumonia. Observations in 94 cases on liver function and jaundice in pneumonia. *J Lab Clin Med* 1950;**35**:556–567.

38. Korn RJ, Kellow WF, Heller P, *et al.* Hepatic involvement in extrapulmonary tuberculosis. *Am J Med* 1959;**27**:60–71.

39. Sharma S. Granulomatous diseases of the liver. In Zakim D, Boyer TD (eds.) *Hepatology*. Philadelphia, PA: Saunders, 2003, pp. 1317–1340.

40. Alvarez SZ, Carpio R. Hepatobiliary tuberculosis. *Dig Dis Sci* 1983;**28**:193–200.

41. Vijayasekaran D. Treatment of childhood tuberculosis. *Indian J Pediatr* 2011;**78**:443–448.

42. Patel S, DeSantis ER. Treatment of congenital tuberculosis. *Am J Health Syst Pharm* 2008;**65**:2027–2031.

43. Wilkins MJ, Lindley R, Dourakis SP, Goldin RD. Surgical pathology of the liver in HIV infection. *Histopathology* 1991;**18**:459–464.

44. Mofenson LM, Brady MT, Danner SP, *et al.* Guidelines for the Prevention and Treatment of Opportunistic Infections among HIV-exposed and HIV-infected children: recommendations from CDC, the National Institutes of Health, the HIV Medicine Association of the Infectious Diseases Society of America, the Pediatric Infectious Diseases Society, and the American Academy of Pediatrics. *MMWR Recomm Rep* 2009;**58**:1–166.

45. Jonas RB, Brasitus TA, Chowdhury L. Actinomycotic liver abscess. Case report and literature review. *Dig Dis Sci* 1987;**32**:1435–1437.

46. Thomas LD, Hongo I, Bloch KC, Tang YW, Dummer S. Human ehrlichiosis in transplant recipients. *Am J Transplant* 2007;**7**:1641–1647.

47. Sehdev AE, Dumler JS. Hepatic pathology in human monocytic ehrlichiosis. *Ehrlichia chaffeensis* infection. *Am J Clin Pathol* 2003;**119**:859–865.

48. Listernick R. Liver failure in a 2-day-old infant. *Pediatr Ann* 2004;**33**:10–14.

49. Wright DJ, Berry CL. Liver involvement in congenital syphilis. *Br J Vener Dis* 1974;**50**:241.

50. Nadelman RB, Nowakowski J, Forseter G, *et al.* The clinical spectrum of early Lyme borreliosis in patients with culture-confirmed erythema migrans. *Am J Med* 1996;**100**:502–508.

51. Schoen RT. Relapsing or reinfectious lyme hepatitis. *Hepatology* 1989;**9**:335–336.

52. Brown V, Larouze B, Desve G, *et al.* Clinical presentation of louse-borne relapsing fever among Ethiopian

refugees in northern Somalia. *Ann Trop Med Parasitol* 1988;**82**:499–502.

53. Wong ML, Kaplan S, Dunkle LM, Stechenberg BW, Feigin RD. Leptospirosis: a childhood disease. *J Pediatr* 1977;**90**:532–537.

54. Feigin RD, Anderson DC. Leptospirosis. In Feigin RD, Cherry JD, Demmler GJ, Kaplan S (eds.) *Textbook of Pediatric Infectious Diseases*. Philadelphia, PA: Saunders, 2004, pp. 1708–1722.

55. Adams JS, Walker DH. The liver in Rocky Mountain spotted fever. *Am J Clin Pathol* 1981;**75**:156–161.

56. Parker NR, Barralet JH, Bell AM. Q fever. *Lancet* 2006;**367**:679–688.

57. Domingo P, Orobitg J, Colomina J, Alvarez E, Cadafalch J. Liver involvement in acute Q fever. *Chest* 1988;**94**:895–896.

58. Westlake P, Price LM, Russell M, Kelly JK. The pathology of Q fever hepatitis. A case diagnosed by liver biopsy. *J Clin Gastroenterol* 1987;**9**:357–363.

59. Hotez PJ, Strickland AD. Amebiasis. In Feigin RD, Cherry JD, Demmler GJ, Kaplan S (eds.) *Textbook of Pediatric Infectious Diseases*. Philadelphia, PA: Saunders, 2004, pp. 2660–2669.

60. Rossignol JF, Kabil SM, El Gohary Y, Younis AM. Nitazoxanide in the treatment of amoebiasis. *Trans R Soc Trop Med Hyg* 2007;**101**:1025–1031.

61. Chavez-Tapia NC, Hernandez-Calleros J, Tellez-Avila FI, Torre A, Uribe M. Image-guided percutaneous procedure plus metronidazole versus metronidazole alone for uncomplicated amoebic liver abscess. *Cochrane Database Syst Rev* 2009;21.

62. Agarwal N, Kumar S. Budd–Chiari syndrome owing to liver hydatid disease: case report and review of the literature. *Ann Trop Paediatr* 2009;**29**:301–304.

63. Nunnari G. Hepatic echinococcosis: clinical and therapeutic aspects. *World J Gastroenterol* 2012;**18**:1448–1458.

64. Schipper HG, Kager PA. Diagnosis and treatment of hepatic echinococcosis: an overview. *Scand J Gastroenterol Suppl* 2004;**241**:50–55.

65. Sciume C, Geraci G, Pisello F, *et al.* Treatment of complications of hepatic hydatid disease by ERCP: our experience. *Ann Ital Chir* 2004;**75**:531–535.

66. Baraket O, Feki MN, Chaari M, *et al.* Hydatid cyst open in biliary tract: therapeutic approaches. Report of 22 cases. *J Visc Surg* 2011;**148**: e211–e216.

67. Krige J, Shaw J. Cholangitis and pancreatitis caused by biliary ascariasis. *Clin Gastroenterol Hepatol* 2009;**7**:A30.

68. Louw JH. Abdominal complications of ascariasis. *Surg Rounds* 1981;**4**:54–65.

69. Bektas M, Dokmeci A, Cinar K, *et al.* Endoscopic management of biliary parasitic diseases. *Dig Dis Sci* 2010;**55**:1472–1478.

70. Edington GM. Other viral and infectious diseases. In Macsween RNM, Anthony PP, Scheuer PJ (eds.) *Pathology of the Liver*. Edinburgh: Churchill Livingstone, 1979, pp. 192–220.

71. Bica I, Hamer DH, Stadecker MJ. Hepatic schistosomiasis. *Infect Dis Clin North Am* 2000;**14**:583–604.

72. Symmers W. Note on a new form of liver cirrhosis due to the presence of ova of *Bilharzia haematobium*. *J Pathol Bacteriol* 1903;**9**:237–239.

73. Namwanje H, Kabatereine N, Olsen A. A randomised controlled clinical trial on the safety of co-administration of albendazole, ivermectin and praziquantel in infected schoolchildren in Uganda. *Trans R Soc Trop Med Hyg* 2011;**105**:181–188.

74. Sun T. Pathology and immunology of *Clonorchis sinensis* infection of the liver. *Ann Clin Lab Sci* 1984;**14**:208–215.

75. Karahocagil MK, Akdeniz H, Sunnetcioglu M, *et al.* A familial outbreak of fascioliasis in Eastern Anatolia: a report with review of literature. *Acta Trop* 2011;**118**:177–183.

76. Moreno A, Marazuela M, Yebra M, *et al.* Hepatic fibrin-ring granulomas in visceral leishmaniasis. *Gastroenterology* 1988;**95**:1123–1126.

77. Rajagopala S, Dutta U, Chandra KS, *et al.* Visceral leishmaniasis associated hemophagocytic lymphohistiocytosis: case report and systematic review. *J Infect* 2008;**56**:381–388.

78. Tangpukdee N, Thanachartwet V, Krudsood S, *et al.* Minor liver profile dysfunctions in *Plasmodium vivax*, *P. malaria* and *P. ovale* patients and normalization after treatment. *Korean J Parasitol* 2006;**44**:295–302.

79. Kochar DK, Singh P, Agarwal P, *et al.* Malarial hepatitis. *J Assoc Physicians India* 2003;**51**:1069–1072.

80. Poravuth Y, Socheat D, Rueangweerayut R, *et al.* Pyronaridine-artesunate versus chloroquine in patients with acute *Plasmodium vivax* malaria: a randomized, double-blind, non-inferiority trial. *PLOS One* 2011;**6**: e14501.

81. Epstein JE, Tewari K, Lyke KE, *et al.* Live attenuated malaria vaccine designed to protect through hepatic CD8(+) T cell immunity. *Science* 2011;**334**(6055):475–480.

82. Thaler M, Pastakia B, Shawker TH, O'Leary T, Pizzo PA. Hepatic candidiasis in cancer patients: the evolving picture of the syndrome. *Ann Intern Med* 1988;**108**:88–100.

83. Aikawa N, Kusachi S, Oda S, Takesue Y, Tanaka H. Clinical effects of micafungin, a novel echinocandin antifungal agent, on systemic fungal infections in surgery, emergency, and intensive-care medicine: evaluation using the AKOTT algorithm. *J Infect Chemother* 2009;**15**:219–227.

84. Meyer MH, Letscher-Bru V, Waller J, *et al.* Chronic disseminated *Trichosporon asahii* infection in a leukemic child. *Clin Infect Dis* 2002;**35**: e22–e25.

85. Kantipong P, Panich V, Pongsurachet V, Watt G. Hepatic penicilliosis in patients without skin lesions. *Clin Infect Dis* 1998;**26**:1215–1217.

86. Keckich DW, Blair JE, Vikram HR. Coccidioides fungemia in six patients, with a review of the literature. *Mycopathologia* 2010;**170**: 107–115.

87. Smith G, Hoover S, Sobonya R, Klotz SA. Abdominal and pelvic coccidioidomycosis. *Am J Med Sci* 2011;**341**:308–311.

88. Troillet N, Llor J, Kuchler H, Deleze G, Praz G. Disseminated histoplasmosis in an adopted infant from El Salvador. *Eur J Pediatr* 1996;**155**:474–476.

89. Hasan RA, Abuhammour W. Invasive aspergillosis in children with hematologic malignancies. *Paediatr Drugs* 2006;**8**:15–24.

90. Boon AP, O'Brien D, Adams DH. 10 year review of invasive aspergillosis detected at necropsy. *J Clin Pathol* 1991;**44**:452–454.

Systemic disease and the liver

Kathleen M. Campbell

Introduction

The liver is the largest parenchymal organ in the body and has the most complicated circulation of any organ, with dual afferent blood supply from the portal vein and hepatic artery. Although the liver mass accounts for only 2.5% of adult body weight, it receives nearly 25% of the resting cardiac output and at any given time contains 10–15% of total body blood volume. In addition to serving as an important blood volume reservoir, the liver is also a complex metabolic organ with important functions in biosynthesis, immunity, metabolism, and clearance. By virtue of its size, multiple metabolic functions, and prominent position in the circulatory system, the liver is frequently involved, either as an accomplice or as an innocent bystander, in a range of systemic, circulatory, and inflammatory disorders. This chapter reviews hepatic involvement in common childhood systemic diseases.

Hepatic dysfunction in the intensive care unit

Hepatic dysfunction, primarily manifest as jaundice, is a common occurrence in the intensive care unit, affecting up to one-third of non-cirrhotic adults [1]. The causes of "intensive care unit jaundice" are multifactorial and may reflect increased bilirubin production (hemolysis, gastrointestinal bleeding, and resorption of hematomas), decreased intrahepatic bilirubin processing (shock, pharmacologic effects, use of total parenteral nutrition), and/or decreased bilirubin excretion (sepsis, biliary obstruction). Severe shock (that requiring significant pressor support), sepsis, use of mechanical ventilation (positive end-expiratory pressure ventilation), and major surgery are independent risk factors for hepatic dysfunction in critically ill patients [1]. In low-flow and hypoxic states, the liver is at particular risk because selective splanchnic vasoconstriction will result in decreased inflow via the portal vein. Normally the hepatic artery buffer response can partially compensate for decreased portal flow; however, this is an energy-dependent process and becomes markedly less efficient with severe or prolonged hypoperfusion [2]. In addition, high-dose systemic vasopressors (dopamine, epinephrine, and norepinephrine) reduce total liver blood flow by up to 50% and decrease the ratio of hepatic oxygen supply to consumption, delivering a second hit to the liver.

The association between hepatic dysfunction and mechanical ventilation can be ascribed to the impact of positive inspiratory pressure and positive end-expiratory pressure on portal vein and hepatic artery hemodynamics, increased right-sided heart pressure, and increased intrahepatic resistance [3].

In addition to direct effects on hepatic blood flow and metabolism, all of the above mechanisms of liver injury simultaneously activate the inflammatory cascade, which itself has multiple effects on hepatic function.

Infection

Systemic infection, even in the absence of shock, is frequently associated with hepatic dysfunction. The pattern of hepatic dysfunction is predominately a cholestatic one, with serum bilirubin levels elevated out of proportion to changes in other biochemical markers. In fact, a rising conjugated bilirubin level may be the first indication of infection in an at-risk patient. Sepsis-associated cholestasis is classically thought of in the context of Gram-negative bacteremia. While lipopolysaccharide (i.e. endotoxin), the macromolecule derived from Gram-negative bacterial cell walls, is a potent initiator of local and systemic inflammation, cholestasis in association with systemic infection can be triggered by any infectious or inflammatory state.

In the setting of systemic infection, the liver participates as both a perpetrator and a victim. The immediate response of the liver to an acute inflammatory state, including infection, is the increased production and release of a group of circulating proteins known as acute phase proteins, the goal of which is to prepare the organism to minimize tissue damage, promote tissue repair, isolate and neutralize invading pathogens, and prevent further pathogen entry. These proteins include fibrinogen, C-reactive protein, complement factors C3 and C9, haptoglobin, ceruloplasmin, α_2-macroglobulin, CD14, α_1-antichymotrypsin, α_1-cysteine proteinase inhibitor, α_1-antitrypsin, and lipopolysaccharide-binding protein. This

Liver Disease in Children, Fourth Edition, ed. Frederick J. Suchy, Ronald J. Sokol, and William F. Balistreri. Published by Cambridge University Press. © Cambridge University Press 2014.

acute phase response is initiated when injury at an extrahepatic site prompts local monocytes, macrophages, and other immunologically active cells to release proinflammatory cytokines, including interleukin (IL)-1, IL-6, and tumor necrosis factor-α (TNFα) [4]. Within the liver itself, Kupffer cells, the resident macrophages, play a critical role in protecting the organism by scavenging endotoxin from the portal circulation. However, in the process, these cells themselves become a major source of proinflammatory cytokines that can mediate hepatocellular injury. These cytokines activate the STAT3/NF-κB signaling pathways within hepatocytes, resulting in increased transcription of acute phase proteins. These circulating acute phase proteins are responsible for the clinical phenomena that accompany systemic infection/inflammation in adults, including leukocytosis, fever, altered consciousness, changes in lipid metabolism, decreased gluconeogenesis, cachexia, insulin resistance, and muscle weakness.

The importance of this cascade in the control of systemic infection/inflammation is illustrated in several animal models in which production of acute phase proteins is blocked. For example, with hepatocyte-specific deletion of gp130, the signaling receptor of the IL-6 proinflammatory family of cytokines, mortality is significantly increased in a mouse model of polymicrobial sepsis, despite normal bacterial clearance [5]. The same is true in STAT-3 knockout mice, which experienced significantly higher mortality and demonstrated decreased levels of acute phase proteins than control littermates after cecal ligation and puncture-induced peritonitis [6]. Unfortunately, the same proinflammatory cytokines that activate the protective arm of the acute phase response simultaneously inhibit hepatocyte and cholangiocyte transport mechanisms, including the sodium-dependent bile salt transporter and the multispecific organic anion transporter 2 at the hepatocyte basolateral membrane, and the bile salt export pump, which transports monovalent bile acids, and the conjugate export pump, which transports divalent bile acids, at the canalicular membrane [7]. The end-result is stagnation of bile flow and cholestasis.

Alterations in the hepatic microvasculature also contribute to sepsis-associated cholestasis. The release of potent vasoconstrictors and physical obstruction of the hepatic sinusoids by inflammatory cells and fibrinous microthrombi lead to endothelial cell damage and hepatocyte necrosis. Circulation to the biliary tract, dependent on the most distal branches of the hepatic arterial tree, is particularly sensitive to altered intrahepatic blood flow.

Another component of the innate immune system, the neutrophil, plays a central role in the inflammatory response to systemic infection. Once neutrophils are activated, they disseminate throughout the body and can become sequestered in the capillary networks of internal organs, such as the liver. Within the liver, neutrophils can contribute to significant hepatocellular damage; however, they may also play a protective role. Sequestration of neutrophils within liver sinusoids may enhance bacterial trapping and clearance during sepsis, thus limiting the spread of infection, albeit at a cost to the liver itself [8].

As a rule, hepatic dysfunction associated with infection is reversible and does not progress to liver failure with coagulopathy and/or encephalopathy. The presence of hepatic dysfunction has little prognostic significance; the prognosis is that of the underlying disease and therapy should be directed at aggressively treating the primary infection and providing support for the circulatory and other organ systems.

Heart disease and circulatory failure

Hepatic dysfunction occurs frequently in children with disorders of acute or chronic circulatory compromise. Hypoxic liver injury can occur in association with congestive heart failure, pericardial tamponade, hypovolemic or septic shock, cardiorespiratory arrest, asphyxia, prolonged seizures, heatstroke, or cardiopulmonary bypass. Occasionally, the clinical presentation is severe enough to resemble fulminant hepatic failure.

The liver is unique in possessing an afferent dual blood supply, with two-thirds of hepatic blood flow made up of partially deoxygenated blood rich in nutrients and hormones arriving from the abdominal organs via the low-pressure, low-resistance portal venous system, and the remainder being well-oxygenated blood delivered via the high-pressure, high-resistance hepatic artery. Of these two systems, only the hepatic artery supplies the major bile ducts, making the biliary tree particularly susceptible to altered hepatic arterial flow. As blood enters the liver through the portal triad (zone 1) and flows through the sinusoids (zone 2) to the central vein (zone 3), the concentrations of oxygen and other nutrients decrease. This oxygen-tension gradient in the hepatic lobule accounts for the increased susceptibility of pericentral hepatocytes (zone 3) to necrosis associated with hypoxia or poor perfusion.

Regulation of hepatic blood flow occurs not only through classic arterial autoregulation (the constrictive response of an artery in the setting of increased arterial pressure), but also through the hepatic arterial buffer response. This unique mechanism represents the ability of the hepatic artery to produce compensatory flow changes in response to changes in portal venous flow. These flow changes depend on the concentration of adenosine in the space of Mall, the small fluid-filled space surrounding the terminal branches of the hepatic artery and portal vein. The secretion of adenosine into the space of Mall occurs at a constant rate, while the washout of adenosine through the portal venules is dependent on portal flow. When portal vein flow is reduced, the concentration of adenosine increases, leading to dilatation of the hepatic artery. Adenosine also activates sensory nerves in the space of Mall and initiates renal fluid retention (hepatorenal reflex), thus increasing circulating blood volume [9].

The endothelium-derived relaxing factor nitric oxide also plays a role in modulating the hepatic microcirculation in both health and disease. Nitric oxide acts as a potent vasodilator in the hepatic arterial circulation but exerts only a minor effect on the portal venous bed [10].

Clinically, ischemic hepatopathy is characterized by a marked and rapid elevation of serum aminotransferases within 48 hours of the initial insult. Although some definitions require serum aminotransferases of at least 20 times the upper limit of normal, ischemic hepatopathy has been histologically confirmed in patients with enzyme levels well below this limit [11]. Classically, serum aminotransferase concentrations may reach 5000–10 000 IU/L, while alkaline phosphatase levels are usually normal. Serum levels of creatinine, lactate, and lactate dehydrogenase are often increased. Hepatomegaly, jaundice, and coagulopathy may be present [11]. The course of hypoxic liver injury is self-limited if the underlying circulatory disturbance is corrected. The half-life of aspartate aminotransferase and alanine aminotransferase (ALT) in serum is 17 to 24 hours. Serum concentrations can be expected to decrease by at least 50% within 72 hours of the insult and return to normal within 11 days if perfusion and oxygenation are restored and urine output is normal [12].

The histology in hypoxic liver injury is marked by centrilobular necrosis with preservation of the periportal zone. Prognosis of hypoxic liver injury depends on the underlying disease and therapy should be directed toward restoring adequate blood flow and oxygenation while addressing the underlying cause of hemodynamic instability.

Patients with chronic liver congestion are particularly susceptible to hypoxic liver injury when perfusion is compromised. Many reports document the classic clinical and histologic picture of hypoxic liver injury in patients with chronic congestive heart disease and an acute event leading to decreased perfusion, sometimes without an obvious or significant decrease in systolic blood pressure [11]. This increased propensity is likely the result of a combination of insults: decreased cardiac output, which may lead to chronic recurrent subclinical hypoxic events; splanchnic vasoconstriction from activation of the renin–angiotensin system, which may further decrease hepatic arterial blood flow; increased sinusoidal pressure; and endotoxemia promoted by ischemic and/or congested bowel [11].

In addition to facilitating the development of classical hypoxic liver injury with markedly elevated serum aminotransferases and centrilobular necrosis, chronic hepatic congestion is itself associated with a distinct liver lesion marked by a spectrum of fibrotic changes ranging from mild sinusoidal fibrosis to the appearance of broad fibrous septa to frank cirrhosis (cardiac cirrhosis) [13]. Although most frequently described in association with right-sided heart failure, this lesion can also complicate ischemic heart disease, restrictive lung disease, constrictive pericarditis, pericardial effusion, and any other entity resulting in elevated central venous pressure. Clinically, chronic passive congestion may be silent. Biochemical abnormalities may have an insidious onset, with a profile that is predominantly cholestatic, with elevations in serum gamma-glutamyltransferase (GGT) and alkaline phosphatase

levels out of proportion to elevations in serum aminotransferases. In a study of over 1000 adults with heart failure, cholestatic markers correlated with indices of right-sided heart failure, and serum gamma-glutamyltransferase and alkaline phosphatase levels predicted death or heart transplantation, suggesting that these may serve as biomarkers of heart failure in relevant populations [14].

In children, the most common causes of heart failure are likely to be congenital heart diseases. Among these, anomalies such as pulmonary atresia, ventricular septal defect, and transposition of the great arteries may lead to pulmonary hypertension and chronic passive liver congestion. In addition, as new approaches for surgical and medical management of congenital heart lesions have increased the long-term survival of infants with critical complex heart disease, the long-term impact of these therapies is becoming obvious. One example is the presence of liver disease in patients with the Fontan circulation. This palliative procedure, used in patients with single ventricle physiology, re-establishes normal systemic oxygen saturation by directly routing systemic venous return to the pulmonary arterial system. Unfortunately, it is associated with both acute and chronic liver dysfunction. Acute dysfunction, usually around the surgery itself, represents classic hypoxic liver injury related to hypoperfusion, while long-term liver dysfunction may reflect a combination of chronic passive congestion and decreased cardiac index [15]. While most patients with a Fontan circulation are asymptomatic from a liver disease perspective and have only mild biochemical abnormalities (elevated gamma-glutamyltransferase of 40–60%), they are at significant risk for ongoing liver fibrosis/cirrhosis [16]. Up to 46% of adolescent and adult Fontan survivors have MRI evidence of significant liver fibrosis, and several cases of hepatocellular carcinoma have been reported in long-term Fontan survivors [17].

Hepatic venous outflow obstruction

Effective obstruction of hepatic venous outflow can occur at several levels. When the obstruction is at the level of the hepatic sinusoids it is termed veno-occlusive disease (VOD; discussed below). Obstruction at the level of the heart is termed chronic passive congestion (discussed above), while obstruction to outflow at any level from the small hepatic veins to the junction of the inferior vena cava (IVC) with the right atrium constitutes Budd–Chiari syndrome. Budd–Chiari syndrome can be classified as primary when there is intraluminal obstruction by a thrombus or web, or secondary when there is extrinsic compression by an abscess, cyst or tumor.

While membranous obstruction of the hepatic veins or IVC is a common cause of Budd–Chiari syndrome in Africa and Asia, and has been described in children as well as adults, the most common cause of Budd–Chiari syndrome in western countries is hepatic vein thrombosis [18]. Thrombosis of the hepatic veins, or, less commonly, the IVC can occur in relation to prothrombotic disorders, antifibrinolytic disorders, local endothelial cell damage, or some combination of these factors. Prothrombotic disorders in turn can be classified as either genetic or acquired.

The most common causes of inherited thrombophilia relevant to Budd–Chiari syndrome are the gain of function mutations in factor V Leiden (leading to activated protein C resistance) and prothrombin (leading to excessive prothrombin generation), and loss of anticoagulant function through protein C, protein S, or antithrombin deficiencies [19]. The reported prevalence of one or more of these inherited defects in patients with Budd–Chiari syndrome is variable, and often both inherited and acquired risk factors coexist. In addition, serum levels of protein C, protein S, and antithrombin can be difficult to interpret in patients with existing thrombosis, as acquired deficiencies, related to the thrombosis or secondary effects, are common.

Hyperhomocysteinemia, frequently resulting from a polymorphism in *MHTR* (677TT), encoding methylene tetrahydrofolate reductase, may also be a risk factor for Budd–Chiari syndrome. However, like deficiencies of the natural anticoagulants, homocysteine level in patients with existing thrombosis and secondary liver disease can be hard to interpret [19].

Theoretically, antifibrinolytic disorders might also potentiate the development of Budd–Chiari syndrome. While increased plasma levels of plasminogen activator inhibitor 1 and decreased levels of thrombin-activatable fibrinolysis inhibitor, plasmin inhibitor, and apolipoprotein A1 have been described in patients with Budd–Chiari syndrome, the genetic basis for these differences is not yet understood [20].

The most common acquired cause of thrombophilia is myeloproliferative disorder. Although rare, thrombocythemia, polycythemia, and thrombocytosis may all occur in children and may be associated with a risk for venous thrombosis. In adults, mutations in *JAK2*, encoding the JAK2 tyrosine kinase, have been associated with both myeloproliferative disorder and Budd–Chiari syndrome, although the mechanism by which these mutations contribute to a prothrombotic tendency is not yet known [21]. The association between myeloproliferative disorders and *JAK2* mutations is so strong that the mutation itself may serve as a marker for occult or evolving myelodysplasia [21].

Other acquired risk factors for Budd–Chiari syndrome include the presence of anti-phospholipid and anti-cardiolipin antibodies, often associated with rheumatologic conditions; other chronic inflammatory states such as Behçet disease, pregnancy, and the peripartum period; and use of oral contraceptives. Each of these factors, genetic and/or acquired, is unlikely to lead to Budd–Chiari syndrome individually. In many cases, multiple thrombophilic risk factors have been identified in a percentage of patients, and in those for whom only one risk factor was evident, and as yet unidentified predisposition may be at play.

Budd–Chiari syndrome most often presents as chronic obstruction with hepatomegaly, ascites, abdominal distension, and abdominal pain. Often, abdominal and chest wall collaterals are prominent and distended, and serum aminotransferase and bilirubin levels are only minimally to moderately elevated [22]. Unlike adults, children may have only firm hepatomegaly and ascites may be absent. The histology of chronic Budd–Chiari syndrome is microscopically indistinguishable from chronic passive congestion and VOD, with zone 3 congestion, necrosis, and fibrosis [22]. A liver biopsy can help to define the chronicity of the obstruction and provide clues regarding the prognosis: cirrhosis and the presence of portal hypertension are associated with poor outcomes. Regardless of the site of hepatic outflow obstruction, the end effect on the liver is the same. The key to diagnosis is in the clinical scenario and not the histologic picture.

Acute Budd–Chiari syndrome can present with similar clinical findings but is more likely to include jaundice and coagulopathy. Acute congestion with massive centrilobular necrosis and fulminant hepatic failure is occasionally the presenting scenario of hepatic venous outflow obstruction, particularly if it occurs in the setting of pre-existing chronic liver disease.

The first step in evaluation of a patient with suspected hepatic venous outflow obstruction is pulsed Doppler ultrasonography of the hepatic vessels and IVC. When this modality is used by experienced practitioners, the presence of specific findings in the hepatic or caval veins, such as stenosis, thrombosis, fibrotic cord, or insufficient recanalization of the vessel, along with caudate lobe hypertrophy, can identify Budd–Chiari syndrome with a high specificity [23]. Cross-sectional imaging is the second line of investigation in patients with non-diagnostic ultrasonography, with MRI being the procedure of choice. In addition to allowing more complete visualization of the IVC along the entire course, MRI and CT allow better visualization and anatomic orientation of the mesenteric and portal vasculature for therapeutic planning. Both CT and MRI can also reveal a range of morphologic and attenuation changes in the hepatic parenchyma, from the classic fan-shaped enhancement of the caudate lobe and central liver to parenchymal changes consistent with cirrhosis [24]. With improvements in cross-sectional imaging, hepatic venography is rarely required for the diagnosis of Budd–Chiari syndrome and tends to be used only in those situations where an interventional radiologic therapy can be offered.

Therapy for Budd–Chiari syndrome ranges from supportive medical management of complications to liver transplantation, and depends on the site and chronicity of the obstruction, the degree of liver dysfunction, and, in children, the size of the patient. Initial therapy is conservative, emphasizing diuresis, treatment of predisposing factors, and prophylactic anticoagulation to decrease the risk of additional thromboses. In patients with long-standing obstruction and evidence of either portal hypertension or synthetic dysfunction, early evaluation for liver transplantation may be the most appropriate and expedient course. In all other cases, acute or chronic, the focus is on removing or bypassing the obstruction and re-establishing normal portal and hepatic vein pressures.

While directed thrombolytic therapy of hepatic vein/IVC thrombosis has been reported, the role in managing children, either primarily or as adjunctive therapy, is not defined. Percutaneous transluminal angioplasty with stent placement has also been described in children and is a mainstay of therapy in adults [25]. Transjugular intrahepatic portosystemic shunting is the most common interventional radiology procedure employed for Budd–Chiari syndrome in adults, and there is growing experience using this technology in small children [26]. However, open surgical procedures, including thrombosis or web resection with pericardial patch grafting, and mesocaval, splenocaval, splenoatrial, and splenojugular shunts are still commonly employed in both children and adults. Liver transplantation remains the salvage therapy for patients with inadequate response to shunting procedures or recurrent shunt thrombosis. Importantly, in patients with underlying thrombophilia, long-term anticoagulation is necessary to prevent recurrence post-transplant.

Hematologic disorders

Hemoglobinopathies

Hepatobiliary disorders are common in children with hemoglobinopathies and can be related to effects of the hematologic disease itself, or complications of therapy. The most commonly encountered hemoglobinopathy is sickle cell anemia. The acute vaso-occlusive crises that characterize this disease involve the liver in up to 39% of patients. This involvement varies from acute painful hepatomegaly to a mixed cholestatic and hepatocellular picture with minimal overt symptoms. Acute sickle cell hepatic crisis is found in 10% of patients admitted for painful crisis and presents clinically with right upper quadrant pain, fever, elevated white blood cell count, and variable increases in serum aminotransferases and bilirubin [27].

Acute hepatic sequestration is a relatively uncommon complication of sickle cell disease in which sickled erythrocytes obstruct the hepatic sinusoids and become trapped in the liver. Clinically, it presents with right upper quadrant pain, hepatomegaly, jaundice, and a fall in hemoglobin [28]. Treatment is identical to that required for splenic sequestration, with special attention to hemoglobin and hemodynamics, as the sequestered erythrocytes may not be destroyed and, on return to the systemic circulation, may lead to hypervolemia, congestive heart failure, and cerebral hemorrhage.

A rare, but potentially fatal complication of sickle cell disease is sickle cell intrahepatic cholestasis, also termed sickle cell hepatopathy. This condition is thought to represent a severe form of sickle cell hepatic crisis in which intrahepatic sickling of erythrocytes leads to sludging and congestion of hepatic vascular beds, followed by tissue ischemia, widespread microscopic infarctions, and, in severe cases, liver synthetic dysfunction. Sickle cell hepatopathy is differentiated from the more common hepatic crisis by the presence of significant hyperbilirubinemia, with the conjugated fraction exceeding 50% of the total bilirubin [28]. While there are no standard diagnostic criteria, one group has proposed that, in the absence of viral hepatitis, extrahepatic obstruction or hepatic sequestration, a threshold serum bilirubin level of >13 mg/dL is diagnostic. Up to 50% of patients who meet this criterion can present with coagulopathy and/or encephalopathy. For this subgroup, the prognosis is poor. Treatment of sickle cell hepatopathy consists of supportive therapy and exchange transfusion, which should be promptly initiated in patients with severe hepatic dysfunction [29].

Patients with sickle cell disease can develop cirrhosis even in the absence of other causes of chronic liver disease. It is hypothesized that repeated microvascular occlusion, focal necrosis, and scarring lead to stellate cell activation and progressive fibrosis. In addition, two-thirds of patients who develop cirrhosis, and one-third of all patients with sickle cell disease, have evidence of a second liver disorder that might lead to fibrosis and that likely potentiates liver damage. The most common of these are viral hepatitis and secondary hemosiderosis, both related to chronic transfusion therapy.

Although historically viral hepatitis, particularly with hepatitis C virus, was a major cause of transfusion-related hepatitis, the implementation of universal screening of blood products in the early 1990s has practically eliminated blood transfusion as a mode of transmission, particularly in developed countries. However, the increased use of transfusion therapy to prevent stroke in children with sickle cell disease, and the heavier transfusion requirements for patients with thalassemia, have increased the risks of transfusion-associated hemosiderosis. Aggressive monitoring of iron levels, both in the blood and in the liver, and institution of chelation therapy are now the standard of care for patients with hemoglobinopathies who require transfusions.

Other unusual hepatic lesions noted in sickle cell anemia are hepatic vein thrombosis, focal nodular hyperplasia, and hepatic abscesses. Impaired hepatic microcirculation may cause areas of infarction, which then act as a nidus for infection. Microinfarcts in the gastrointestinal epithelium increase intestinal permeability and allow translocation of enteric organisms while splenic dysfunction impedes clearance of bacteria.

Coagulation disorders

Historically, the hepatic complications in patients with hemophilia and other coagulation disorders were caused by transfusion-acquired hepatotropic viruses. The use of recombinant products and improved screening of the blood supply has decreased this exposure, while routine administration of hepatitis A and B vaccines have decreased the consequences of exposure. In the modern era, non-alcoholic fatty liver disease (NAFLD) may replace chronic viral infection as the most common cause of liver injury in children with hemophilia [30].

Leukemia and lymphoma

Hepatomegaly, jaundice, and asymptomatic elevated serum aminotransferases frequently occur in patients with lymphoma, leukemia, and intra-abdominal solid tumors. The processes that contribute to these hepatic abnormalities are multiple, including tumor infiltration, intrahepatic or extrahepatic biliary obstruction, and hepatotoxic drugs.

Acute lymphoblastic leukemia is the most common hematologic malignancy in childhood and is frequently associated with hepatic involvement. At the time of diagnosis, 34% of patients have abnormal liver biochemistries and almost 50% have hepatosplenomegaly. After initiation of treatment, most hepatic abnormalities in patients with acute lymphoblastic leukemia result from medication toxicity. Methotrexate and 6-mercaptopurine/thioguanine are mainstays of the treatment protocols and have well-characterized hepatotoxicity. One study of 243 children with acute lymphoblastic leukemia receiving oral methotrexate therapy found that two-thirds had an abnormal serum ALT at some point during treatment, and 17.6% had one or more serum ALT values >720 IU/L [31]. In spite of this, and with no modification of therapy in the presence of elevated ALT, only 16% of patients maintained an abnormal ALT after therapy was complete [31]. Liver histology, by comparison, tells a different story. Histologic evaluation of 27 children shortly after completion of chemotherapy, which included both methotrexate and 6-mercaptopurine, found abnormal pathology in all patients, with fatty changes in 93%, iron accumulation in 70%, and mild fibrosis in 11% [32]. On long-term follow-up, 5–13% of 6-thioguanine recipients have non-cirrhotic portal hypertension caused by periportal liver fibrosis or nodular regenerative hyperplasia [33].

Hepatosplenomegaly is also common in acute non-lymphocytic leukemia and chronic myeloid leukemia. The chemotherapeutic agents used for these disorders are generally not recognized as significant hepatotoxins; however, with the advent of prolonged tyrosine kinase inhibitor therapy as an alternative to bone marrow transplant in chronic myelogenous leukemia, long-term hepatic complications may emerge [34].

Pediatric lymphomas can also be associated with a variety of hepatic complications. In children with stage IV, or disseminated, Hodgkin lymphoma, the liver is the most common extralymphatic site of involvement, with infiltration in over 50% of patients. In rare cases, Hodgkin lymphoma is associated with severe liver dysfunction and may even present as fulminant hepatic failure. Idiopathic cholestasis and vanishing bile duct syndrome have both been reported in association with Hodgkin lymphoma, and occur in the absence of infiltrative liver disease. The pathophysiologic basis of both is postulated to be a paraneoplastic process, with release of a cholestatic substance, potentially an autoreactive antibody, from the tumor cells themselves [35]. While the prognosis of Hodgkin-associated vanishing bile duct syndrome is generally thought to be worse than Hodgkin-associated intrahepatic cholestasis, both conditions have been reported to resolve with prompt treatment of the underlying lymphoma [35]. Unfortunately, treatment is complicated and options limited in the setting of significant cholestasis or overt liver dysfunction.

Non-Hodgkin lymphoma can also be associated with vanishing bile duct syndrome, fulminant liver failure, and an acute hepatitis presentation; however, obstructive jaundice is a more common hepatic complication of non-Hodgkin disease in children [36].

Additional hepatic complications in patients with hematologic malignancies include exposure to non-chemotherapy hepatotoxic medications, radiation therapy, and opportunistic infections. Pediatric cancer survivors, of both hematologic and solid tumors, may develop focal nodular hyperplasia even in the absence of 6-thioguanine exposure. Focal nodular hyperplasia may present with either complications of portal hypertension or a liver mass, which must be differentiated from recurrent malignancy.

Allogeneic stem cell transplantation

Hepatic complications are common in children undergoing stem cell transplant and can be classified based on etiology (primary disease, chemotherapeutic regimen, other drug-induced liver injury, infectious, vascular, parenteral nutrition-associated, immunologic), or by timing related to SCT (pretransplant, early post-transplant, late post-transplant). A structured approach is necessary when evaluating the patient with hepatic injury following SCT, with the primary goal of identifying conditions amenable to therapy. Because of the complex clinical and treatment scenarios of these patients, more than one pathologic process is frequently operant.

Liver disease prior to stem cell transplantation

The indications for SCT in children are multiple, varied, and expanding. Many of the immunodeficiency syndromes for which SCT is indicated are associated with liver disease independent of SCT, for example sclerosing cholangitis associated with lymphohistiocytic syndromes and hyper-IgM syndrome, and chronic hepatic and biliary tract infections associated with severe combined immunodeficiency and chronic granulomatous disease. Other indications for pediatric SCT, such as blood dyscrasias and relapsed leukemia/lymphoma, may be associated with hepatic complications such as chronic viral hepatitis, drug-induced liver injury, and iron overload. Identification of pre-existing conditions, regardless of their etiology, and optimization of liver health is crucial prior to SCT. Patients with chronic liver disease, and even well-compensated cirrhosis, are at higher risk for severe hepatic complications following SCT.

Veno-occlusive disease

Veno-oclusive disease, or sinusoidal obstruction syndrome, is a clinical diagnosis defined by the presence of hyperbilirubinemia, tender hepatomegaly, and sudden weight gain related to fluid accumulation, in the appropriate clinical setting. It is

Table 40.1 Causes of veno-occlusive disease

Cause	Examples
Foods	Pyrrolizidine alkaloids found in plants such as ragwort and groundsel Nitrosamines
Drugs	Gemtuzumab ozogamicin 6-Thioguanine Urethane 6-Mercaptopurine Actinomycin D Dacarbazine Vincristine Oxaliplatin Azathioprine Cyclophosphamide Busulfan Carmustine Cytosine arabinoside Indicine N-oxide Cysteamine Estrogens
Other chemicals	Arsenic Polysorbate
Radiation	Chemoradiation
Disease	Hepatic veno-occlusive disease with immunodeficiency (autosomal recessive, SP110 mutations)

caused by toxic injury to the sinusoidal epithelial cells, leading to their detachment and embolization in the central area of the hepatic lobule with consequent outflow obstruction. In VOD, concentric narrowing of the terminal hepatic venules occurs without associated abnormalities of the larger hepatic veins or the inferior vena cava. While VOD can occur in a variety of settings, currently the most common is in association with high-dose myeloablative conditioning therapy for SCT [37] (Table 40.1).

The incidence of VOD is variable, depending upon the degree of pre-existing liver disease, the conditioning regimen employed, and, potentially, the presence of genetic polymorphisms affecting drug metabolism. An analysis of 135 published reports from 1979 to 2007 found an overall mean incidence of VOD of 13.7% [38]. In a single, large, adult center, the incidence of VOD during the 1990s was 38% in patients who received cyclophosphamide and total body radiation and 12% in patients who received cyclophosphamide and oral busulfan [37]. Unfortunately, there are no data available on overall incidence rates in pediatric SCT centers.

The clinical course of VOD is variable. Typically, it begins with increase in liver size, right upper quadrant tenderness, and insidious weight gain within 10–20 days of SCT in those receiving cyclophosphamide-containing regimens, and up to 30 days after treatment with other regimens. Jaundice follows within 4–10 days [37]. Clinical ascites develops in 50% of patients with VOD; abdominal pain and encephalopathy may also develop. Abdominal ultrasound, including pulsed Doppler analysis of the hepatic and portal vessels, can support the diagnosis of VOD and exclude other causes of hepatomegaly and jaundice. In particular, it is critical to distinguish VOD from pericardial disease and right-sided heart failure, as these conditions share the same mechanism of hepatic injury and may present with identical symptoms. Unfortunately, no specific ultrasound parameters in children are as useful as the clinical criteria. Ultrasound findings suggestive of VOD include reversal of portal venous flow, attenuation of hepatic venous flow, gallbladder wall edema, and increased resistive indices in the hepatic artery. In addition, although a variety of laboratory abnormalities have been described in VOD, none seems to add diagnostic or prognostic significance beyond that of the clinical triad of weight gain, jaundice, and hepatomegaly.

The gold standard for diagnosis of VOD is measurement of the wedged hepatic venous pressure gradient. A gradient >10 mmHg is highly specific for VOD [39]. Early histologic changes in VOD may be patchy and include dilatation of the sinusoids and extravasation of red blood cells into the perisinusoidal space, particularly in zone 3. Perivenular hepatocytes may atrophy and necrose, leading to fragmented hepatocyte cords. The later stages of VOD are characterized by collagenization of the sinusoids and a variable degree of obstruction of venular lumens. These late changes are correlated with severity and outcome [37].

The injury to endothelial cells and hepatocytes in zone 3 provides insight into the pathogenesis of VOD. The increased risk for development of VOD after total body irradiation is well documented. Injury to the radiosensitive endothelial cells results in passive congestion and decreased venous outflow, thereby compromising clearance of potentially cytotoxic drugs and their metabolites. Nutritional deficiencies or exposure to drugs that alter the function of the cytochrome P450 system may further compromise the cytoprotective mechanisms of hepatocytes. Because hepatocytes in zone 3 play a central role in the metabolism of antineoplastic drugs, they are more susceptible to disorders associated with altered drug clearance and metabolism. Gene polymorphisms affecting glutathione S-transferase, necessary for busulfan metabolism, and the cytochrome P450 system, necessary for cyclophosphamide metabolism, have both been associated with VOD. If clinicians could further stratify risk for VOD based on pharmacogenetic profiles, mitigation of post-transplant complications might be possible.

Treatment of VOD is largely supportive and should focus on maintaining intravascular volume while minimizing accumulation of extravascular fluid. Serial therapeutic paracentesis may be necessary to prevent respiratory compromise and provide comfort. Sodium restriction and diuretics are generally required to manage fluid accumulation; however, volume depletion must be avoided to prevent compromise of hepatic and renal blood flow.

A variety of therapeutic strategies designed to prevent or treat VOD have been utilized in single centers and small populations. Continuous heparin infusion, tissue plasminogen activator, antithrombin III, fresh frozen plasma, *N*-acetylcysteine, prostaglandin E, and glutamine have been reported in various combinations and with various outcomes. Demonstration of survival benefit in randomized controlled trials is necessary before these agents can be recommended, particularly in children. However, data on the benefit of prophylactic ursodeoxycholic acid (UDCA) support wide use as an ancillary agent in pediatric SCT. Two modestly sized randomized trials of prophylactic UDCA showed a decreased incidence of VOD in treated patients compared with those who received placebo (40% versus 15% in one trial and 18.5% versus 3% in the other), while a third study, which failed to identify a difference in the incidence of VOD, found a significantly better 1-year survival rate in patients who received UDCA (71% versus 55%) [40]. A systematic review of clinical trials using prophylactic UDCA, including those mentioned above, found a beneficial effect on both the incidence of VOD and on transplant-related mortality [40]. Although these conclusions may be limited by the unclear distinction between VOD and other hepatic complications identified in the various studies, the potential benefit of UDCA, and favorable side effect profile, support its common use in children following SCT.

Another promising agent for the prevention and treatment of VOD is defibrotide, a mixture of porcine oilgodeoxyribonucleotides. Although the exact mechanism of action against VOD is unclear, defibrotide is known to have anti-inflammatory, antithrombotic, and profibrinolytic effects without systemic anticoagulant effects. After initial hopeful reports about the use of defibrotide as therapy for severe VOD, a large, pediatric, randomized controlled trial from Europe was conducted. In this study, which included 356 children with SCT, those who received prophylactic defibrotide had a statistically significant decreased incidence of VOD at 30 days after SCT (11% versus 20% in per-protocol analysis). Treated patients also had a decreased incidence of graft-versus-host disease (GVHD) and renal failure than control subjects, with no increased incidence of adverse events [41]. Although additional studies to replicate these findings and define the role of defibrotide in treatment of existing VOD are necessary, results to date suggest that it may be the most useful therapy available.

More than 70% of patients with VOD will recover spontaneously with appropriate supportive management [37]. Poor prognosis is associated with higher total serum bilirubin at any given point in time, rapid weight gain early after SCT, renal failure, and multiorgan system failure [38].

Graft-versus-host disease

Aside from primary disease relapse, GVHD is the most serious cause of morbidity and mortality following SCT. While GVHD has been described in patients after solid organ transplantation, in infants receiving intrauterine and exchange transfusions for hemolytic disease, and in immunocompromised patients receiving non-irradiated blood products, the most frequent setting is in recipients of SCT. Acute GVHD develops when the graft contains immunocompetent T-cells, the recipient is sufficiently immunocompromised such that he/she is unable to reject the transplanted cells, and the recipient expresses tissue antigens not present in the donor [42]. Given these criteria for the development of GVHD, it is no surprise that transplant from an unrelated donor and increased donor–recipient HLA mismatch are risk factors for GVHD.

Acute GVHD, by classical definition, occurs in the first 100 days after SCT, and it affects 26–52% of SCT recipients. The target organs are skin, intestine, and liver; *isolated* hepatic involvement, while reported, is rare. Initial clinical features of hepatic GVHD include elevated serum alkaline phosphatase and gamma-glutamyltransferase, hepatomegaly, and jaundice. The grade of GVHD (0–IV) correlates with the increasing serum bilirubin level, with grade III or IV associated with a markedly decreased survival compared with grades 0–II. Across all grades, initial liver involvement is an independent risk factor for non-relapse mortality [43].

The diagnosis of acute hepatic GVHD is frequently made on clinical grounds, particularly when there is evidence of skin and/or gastrointestinal tract involvement; however, the differential diagnosis for cholestasis in a STC recipient is broad and includes not only VOD and GVHD but also drug-induced liver disease, opportunistic infection, and parenteral nutrition-associated liver disease. Therefore, in the absence of classic findings of GVHD, or with a poor response to GVHD therapy, liver biopsy may be necessary to confirm the diagnosis. One study of adults with SCT who died with hyperbilirubinemia demonstrated that liver GVHD was significantly overdiagnosed when only clinical criteria were employed: only 50% of the patients diagnosed with GVHD based on clinical criteria were found to have histologic evidence of GVHD [44]. However, before proceeding with liver biopsy, the clinical information to be gained must be weighed against the risk, as complication rates as high as 27% have been reported in pediatric SCT recipients [45].

The characteristic histologic findings of GVHD involve the small bile ducts. Bile duct damage, atypia, and pericholangitis are sensitive histologic markers for acute hepatic GVHD, while endotheliitis of the portal or central veins and lymphocytic portal inflammation can also be seen. Unlike other epithelial cell lines, apoptotic bile duct cells are infrequent. While hepatic GVHD typically presents as a cholestatic syndrome, a *hepatitic* form of GVHD has been described, characterized biochemically by sudden and marked elevation of serum aminotransferase levels and histologically by marked lobular hepatitis and necro-inflammation in addition to classic bile duct injury. These histological abnormalities may be difficult to distinguish from drug-associated liver injury and viral hepatitis.

Chronic GVHD (arbitrarily defined as presenting after day 100 following SCT) has a broader spectrum of presentation and may manifest as asymptomatic biochemical changes, progressive cholestatic disease, or acute hepatocellular injury (hepatitic GVHD) [37]. The histologic findings may be identical to acute GVHD, but there is a higher likelihood of encountering chronic changes, including bile ductular proliferation, bridging fibrosis, and, eventually, vanishing bile duct syndrome [46].

Prevention of GVHD is the first approach to management. Strategies among centers vary widely but may include a combination of the following medications and treatments: tacrolimus, cyclosporine, prednisone, mycophenolate moffetil, methotrexate, polyclonal antibody preparations, and use of donor T-cell depletion. Treatment of established acute GVHD requires augmented immunosuppression. The options for therapy have broadened over the years as the armamentarium of immunosuppressive agents has expanded. Standard primary therapy is with corticosteroids but this is effective in only 30–50% of patients [42]. Options for steroid-resistant GVHD include polyclonal and monoclonal anti-lymphocyte antibody preparations, anti-TNF antibodies, anti-IL2 receptor antibodies, sirolimus, and denileukin difitox (a novel immunotoxin that binds to the IL-2 receptor) [47].

Chronic hepatic GVHD is less amenable to immunosuppressive therapy: 10% of patients require more than 5 years of therapy and 40% of patients die without resolution of hepatic GVHD [37]. Because of this poor response, the risks of immunosuppression must be weighed against the potential benefits of therapy. The only liver-specific therapy is UDCA, which results in improvements in serum biochemistry and pruritus. There are no data as to the impact on histology or long-term outcome. For patients with severe GVHD resulting in chronic cholestasis and/or cirrhosis, liver transplantation may be an option, with published 1- and 5-year survival rates of 72.4% and 62.9%, respectively, in a mixed pediatric/adult population [48].

Other complications of stem cell transplantation

In addition to the specific complications discussed above, children with SCT are at risk for the same hepatic complications as other chronic-disease populations, including viral hepatitis, iron overload, and drug-induced liver injury. In addition, emerging data suggest that there is a significant incidence of fatty liver disease and insulin resistance in adult survivors of pediatric SCT. Interestingly, this appears to be associated with pre-SCT cranial radiotherapy rather than with obesity [49].

Collagen vascular disease

Hepatomegaly, splenomegaly, biochemical abnormalities, and/or histologic changes are commonly found in the setting of the various collagen vascular disorders. The hepatic involvement may be a primary manifestation of the disease itself, related to immune-mediated injury, or secondary to drug toxicity or fatty infiltration.

Juvenile idiopathic arthritis

Hepatomegaly and splenomegaly are common in children with juvenile idiopathic arthritis (JIA), affecting 10–15% at some point in time and occurring more frequently in those with systemic JIA (Still disease). Asymptomatic elevations in serum aminotransferases unrelated to muscle injury may occur from the collagen disease itself, in which case the elevations are usually sporadic, correlate with disease activity, and rarely lead to progressive liver injury. In these cases, liver biopsy may reveal non-specific portal inflammation, periportal fibrosis, and Kupffer cell hyperplasia [50]. Other, specific causes of liver dysfunction in patients with JIA include drug toxicity (41% of those with liver dysfunction), fatty liver (6%), viral hepatitis (1–2%), primary biliary cirrhosis (4%), and autoimmune hepatitis (1–2%) [51]. The distinction between classic autoimmune hepatitis and hepatitis related to the collagen disease itself is an important one, and requires demonstration of pathognomonic histologic features, as patients with autoimmune hepatitis may have extrahepatic manifestations resembling JIA, and patients with JIA may be overdiagnosed with autoimmune hepatitis based on scoring systems alone.

The most common cause of liver abnormalities in patients with JIA is drug toxicity. Aspirin causes a dose-related reversible hepatotoxic reaction that often recurs with rechallenge and is usually asymptomatic and detected only because of mild increases in serum aminotransferases. Liver biopsy reveals a mononuclear cell infiltrate of the portal tracts without significant hepatocellular necrosis. Although rare, there is a higher incidence of Reye syndrome in patients with JIA than in the general population; any patient with a rheumatologic disorder taking aspirin who develops vomiting or neurologic symptoms should be evaluated promptly for this complication.

Non-steroidal anti-inflammatory drugs have largely replaced aspirin in the treatment of JIA and carry a much lower risk of hepatotoxicity. Even so, treatment-related hepatobiliary adverse events occur in approximately 1% of patients treated with ibuprofen and celecoxib, and 4% of patients treated with diclofenac [52]. The risk is higher for patients with rheumatoid arthritis than for those with osteoarthritis, and may be increased by coinfection with hepatitis C virus or concomitant exposure to other hepatotoxic drugs. In the current era, use of parenteral gold therapy, the earliest treatment for rheumatoid arthritis, is exceedingly rare in children. However, in the past it was associated with a number of severe hepatotoxic reactions, including consumptive coagulopathy with liver failure, and fulminant hepatic necrosis. Biologic therapy for the treatment of JIA has become mainstream. Options include anti-TNFα therapy (etanercept, adalimumab, infliximab), costimulatory blockade (abatacept), and IL-1 and IL-6 blockade (anakinra, tocilizumab). With all of these agents, elevation of serum aminotransferases requires dose adjustment or medication discontinuation, although this is rare.

Methotrexate has long been a front-line disease-modifying antirheumatic drug used in the treatment of refractory JIA.

There are two forms of hepatotoxicity associated with methotrexate: (1) benign, acute, transient elevation of serum aminotransferases; and (2) indolent, silent hepatic fibrosis that can progress to cirrhosis. Despite initial data from adults suggesting a significant incidence of methotrexate-induced fibrosis in patients on long-term methotrexate therapy, recent data from both adult and pediatric studies are reassuring. Transient increases in serum aminotransferases are seen in only 15% of patients receiving methotrexate, and although liver biopsies may show minor, non-specific histologic changes, fibrosis or cirrhosis is rare [53]. More advanced hepatic injury is associated with additional risk factors in both children and adults, including alcohol consumption, viral hepatitis, obesity or the metabolic syndrome, and concomitant use of additional hepatotoxic drugs. Many studies have shown that serial biochemical abnormalities are significantly associated with the presence of liver fibrosis, highlighting the need for laboratory monitoring in methotrexate-treated patients [53].

The histopathologic changes caused by methotrexate are well described and are graded using the Roenigk classification. The earliest features are ultrastructural and include lysosomal and mitochondrial injury, bile duct damage, and stellate cell hyperplasia. Other lesions include variable periportal inflammation, marked macrovesicular steatosis, zone 3 lesions, hepatocyte nuclear pleomorphism, and Kupffer cell hyperplasia. The fibrosis associated with methotrexate is periportal with extension into the parenchyma in a "chicken-wire" pattern [54].

Persistent hepatosplenomegaly and/or marked biochemical abnormalities in a patient with JIA should raise concern for one of the clearly defined syndromes associated with rheumatologic conditions, specifically Felty syndrome, amyloidosis, and macrophage activation syndrome. Felty syndrome consists of the triad of neutropenia, splenomegaly, and rheumatoid arthritis. Two-thirds of patients have hepatomegaly and over half have abnormal liver function tests. The primary histologic lesion is sinusoidal inflammation, which may progress to nodular regenerative hyperplasia and portal hypertension [50]. Long-standing rheumatoid arthritis is the most common cause of secondary amyloidosis. Although this may present with persistent hepatomegaly or biochemical abnormalities, the gastrointestinal tract and the kidney are more frequently involved.

Severe hepatocellular dysfunction in the setting of JIA is most likely to occur with macrophage activation syndrome, a rare and frequently fatal complication of rheumatologic and other systemic inflammatory disorders. Macrophage activation syndrome is generally viewed as an acquired form of hemophagocytic lymphohistiocytosis and results from uncontrolled proliferation and activation of T-lymphocytes and macrophages. As in hemophagocytic lymphohistiocytosis, deranged liver function, manifest by markedly elevated serum aminotransferases and conjugated bilirubin levels, coagulopathy, and/or hepatosplenomegaly, is common in macrophage activation syndrome [55]. Prompt recognition of macrophage activation syndrome is vital so that appropriate immunosuppression can be initiated.

Systemic lupus erythematosus

The incidence and spectrum of liver involvement in patients with systemic lupus erythematosus (SLE) is similar to that found in JIA, although the distribution is somewhat different. More than one-third of patients with SLE have some elevation in serum aminotransferase or gamma-glutamyltransferase levels, while 40% have clinically detectable hepatomegaly [56]. As in JIA, a number of patients with SLE have drug-induced liver injury (32%) or primary liver involvement with the collagen vascular disease itself (lupus-associated hepatitis; 5%). However, in contrast to JIA, patients with SLE and liver dysfunction have a higher incidence of fatty liver (17%) and autoimmune hepatitis (10%) [51]. Distinguishing between lupus-associated hepatitis and classic autoimmune hepatitis has important prognostic and therapeutic implications, as lupus-associated hepatitis has a more benign course with rare need for targeted therapy. The histologic features of lupus-associated hepatitis are less dramatic than classic autoimmune hepatitis, with mild lobular inflammation and no piecemeal necrosis. The presence of anti-ribosomal P antibody may also be a distinguishing feature, as it is present in 69% of patients with lupus-associated hepatitis and is rare with classic autoimmune hepatitis [57].

A variety of additional specific liver diseases have been described in patients with SLE, including primary sclerosing cholangitis, autoimmune sclerosing cholangitis, primary biliary cirrhosis, granulomatous hepatitis, viral hepatitis, and nodular regenerative hyperplasia. Portal vein thrombosis, Budd–Chiari syndrome, and hepatic VOD can also occur in the setting of SLE, usually because of the coexistence of the antiphospholipid syndrome [57].

The liver may be involved in neonatal lupus, which is most often characterized by congenital heart block, dermatitis, and hematologic abnormalities. The disorder is transient and is the result of transplacental passage of maternal anti-Ro and anti-La antibodies that invade affected tissues. Liver manifestations can be found in 15–25% of patients with neonatal lupus and consist of three patterns: liver failure occurring at birth or in utero, conjugated hyperbilirubinemia with little or no aminotransferase elevation that occurs in the first few weeks of life, and transient and asymptomatic aminotransferase elevation with normal conjugated bilirubin levels that occurs at several months of life. The cholestasis and serum aminotransferase elevation resolve spontaneously over the course of months. Liver pathology in neonatal lupus is variable based on the clinical presentation. In neonates with early-onset liver failure, histologic findings often resemble neonatal iron storage disease, while those with more benign presentations have a gamut of histology ranging from neonatal giant cell hepatitis to a biliary atresia-like lesion with large bile duct obstruction and portal fibrosis with a mixed portal inflammatory component.

Miscellaneous disorders

Sjögren syndrome, scleroderma, dermatomyositis, mixed connective tissue disease, and Behçet disease may all be associated with liver dysfunction of varying incidence. In Sjögren syndrome, liver involvement is common; 36–44% of patients have abnormal serum biochemistry and of those with a definitive liver diagnosis, primary biliary cirrhosis (with or without anti-mitochondrial antibodies) is the most common [51]. In contrast, liver involvement is rare in scleroderma, although 15–25% of patients have positive liver autoantibodies. As with Sjögren syndrome, the most common liver diagnosis is primary biliary cirrhosis.

Dermatomyositis does not have prominent hepatic manifestations but it may initially be mistaken for liver disease because of elevated serum aminotransferases secondary to rhabdomyolysis. A history of proximal muscle weakness and an elevated serum creatine phosphokinase point to the correct diagnosis. Interestingly, Behçet disease and mixed connective tissue disease are rarely associated with autoimmune hepatitis or primary biliary cirrhosis. Instead, liver dysfunction associated with these disorders is more likely to be related to fatty liver or drug toxicity [51]. Although venous thromboembolism is less likely in this group of disorders than in JIA or SLE, it is a reported cause of Budd–Chiari syndrome, particularly in patients with Behçet disease.

A spectrum of hepatobiliary abnormalities have been reported in Kawasaki disease, including hydrops of the gallbladder, hepatomegaly, elevated serum aminotransferases, and clinical jaundice. The mechanism of liver involvement in Kawasaki disease is likely a combination of generalized vasculitis of small/medium arteries and hepatic congestion secondary to heart dysfunction. Hepatobiliary disease is not a significant cause of morbidity or mortality in patients with Kawasaki disease and responds well to treatment with intravenous immunoglobulin. However, abnormal liver biochemistry, particularly conjugated bilirubin, may be an indication for intravenous immunoglobulin-resistant disease [58].

Endocrine disorders

Hypopituitarism

Although the mechanisms are not well characterized, pituitary hormones, particularly adrenocorticotropic hormone and thyroid-stimulating hormone, play a role in the regulation of bile acid secretion and bile flow. The absence of pituitary hormones, either singly or in combination, is frequently associated with hepatobiliary manifestations, particularly in neonates. Congenital hypopituitarism is the most common form of pituitary dysfunction in neonates and can be caused by a variety of single gene disorders and genetic syndromes, many of which are associated with midline, ocular, and/or genital defects. The most common form of congenital hypopituitarism is the syndrome of septo-optic dysplasia, a heterogeneous condition with a reported incidence of 1 in 10 000. Septo-optic dysplasia is defined by the presence of two or more of the following: (1) unilateral (12%) or bilateral (88%) optic nerve hypoplasia, (2) midline forebrain defects such as agenesis of

the corpus callosum or absent septum pellucidum, and (3) pituitary hypoplasia with variable hypopituitarism. Approximately 30% of patients manifest the complete triad, while 62% have some degree of hypopituitarism and 60% have an absent septum pellucidum [59]. Classically, septo-optic dysplasia presents in the neonatal period with hypoglycemia, roving eye movements, and cholestasis. The cholestasis associated with pituitary hormone deficiency is mild and non-progressive and usually resolves within 6–10 weeks with appropriate treatment of the endocrine disorder(s).

Adrenal disorders

Congenital defects in adrenocorticoid hormone production and secretion can cause mild cholestasis in neonates and in adults may be associated with asymptomatic elevated serum aminotransferases. However, excess of adrenocorticoid hormones, whether exogenous or endogenous, is far more likely to be associated with hepatic complications. Many patients with Cushing syndrome meet the definition for the metabolic syndrome and are at risk for the hepatic complications of this syndrome.

Thyroid disorders

Thyroid hormones have both primary and secondary effects on the liver. Primary effects include the stimulation of bile salt-independent bile flow, likely via modulation of the activity of the Na^+/K^+-ATPase on the canalicular membrane, while secondary effects are related to thyroid hormone-induced changes in lipid metabolism, adiposity, metabolic rate, and cardiac function. Liver injury associated with the hyperthyroid state is common and may present with a hepatocellular or a cholestatic pattern. Abnormalities in serum aminotransferases are reported in 27–37% of patients with hyperthyroidism. The mechanism seems to be relative hypoxia in the perivenular regions caused by an increase in hepatic oxygen demand without an appropriate increase in hepatic blood flow. While in most patients this liver injury is self-limited, progression of liver disease, and even fulminant hepatic failure, has been reported in patients with thyrotoxicosis. In these instances, severe injury is likely precipitated by high-output heart failure [60]. A cholestatic pattern is less likely in hyperthyroidism, with elevated gamma-glutamyltransferase and bilirubin levels reported in 17% and 5% of patients, respectively. Overt jaundice is rare and usually indicates secondary complications (heart failure, malnutrition, sepsis) or underlying liver disease. With appropriate treatment, the liver dysfunction associated with hyperthyroidism is reversible, although several of the medications used to treat the disease have hepatotoxic side effects of their own [60].

Reversible abnormalities of liver function are also common in hypothyroidism. In addition to reductions in bile salt-independent bile flow, the activity of bilirubin UDP-glucuronyltransferase is decreased, resulting in a reduction in bilirubin excretion [60]. The end effect is often mild jaundice, with mixed conjugated and unconjugated hyperbilirubinemia. Increasing reports that overt and subclinical hypothyroidism are risk factors for NAFLD and the metabolic syndrome suggest that NAFLD may be an equally common manifestation of liver disease in hypothyroidism [61]. Less common manifestations of hypothyroidism that may involve the liver, and can mimic liver failure, are myxedema ascites (peritoneal fluid with a high protein content with a low serum–ascites albumin gradient) and myxedema coma.

There is an association between autoimmune thyroid disease and primary autoimmune liver disease. Any patient with one manifestation of autoimmune disease may develop symptoms in another organ at any time, routine screening is recommended.

Diabetes mellitus

Evidence of liver dysfunction may be found in up to one-third of patients with diabetes. The spectrum of histopathologic lesions includes increased hepatocyte glycogen, hyalin deposition, steatosis, and fibrosis leading to cirrhosis. Although the most common manifestation of liver disease in diabetes is NAFLD, Mauriac syndrome is the complication most unique to children. This syndrome is characterized by severe growth failure, hepatomegaly, pubertal delay, and Cushingoid features in children with uncontrolled type 1 diabetes. The histologic findings resemble those seen in glycogen storage disease, with mild to marked glycogen accumulation in hepatocytes. While Mauriac syndrome has become less common with the availability of long-acting insulin preparations and increased attention to glycemic control, it is still encountered today [62].

Nutritional disorders

The most common nutrition-related liver disease is NAFLD, which is discussed in Chapter 36; however, there are a variety of other nutritional disorders in children in which the liver is affected. These include global nutritional deficiencies, individual nutrient deficiencies and excesses, nutrition-related gastrointestinal disease, and use of dietary supplements.

Celiac disease

Liver dysfunction is one of the recognized extra-intestinal manifestations of celiac disease, and can be found in 15–55% of patients. A variety of hepatic abnormalities have been reported, including asymptomatic elevated serum aminotransferases, NAFLD, the spectrum of autoimmune liver diseases, fulminant liver failure, and cryptogenic cirrhosis. The most common of these is elevated serum aminotransferases, which can be found in up to 25% of children at presentation and may be the indication for evaluation. In fact, some reports suggest that as many as 10% of all patients referred for evaluation of asymptomatic increased aminotransferases have unrecognized celiac disease [63].

The most common histologic abnormality in celiac disease is non-specific hepatitis with mild periportal inflammation, Kupffer cell hyperplasia, focal ductular proliferation, minimal steatosis, and absence of chronic changes. The mechanism of this liver injury is not well defined. Hypotheses include increased intestinal permeability, systemic auto immunity, mucosal damage and inflammation, malnutrition, and intestinal bacterial overgrowth with secondary entry of toxins, antigens and inflammatory mediators into the portal circulation [64]. Regardless, both serum and histologic abnormalities improve with a gluten-free diet, usually within 6 months. If a patient does not respond to a gluten free diet within 1 year, other causes of liver disease should be sought and excluded.

Malnutrition

While malnutrition is frequently a significant complication of advanced liver disease, liver dysfunction is rarely a serious complication of malnutrition. Both kwashiorkor (protein–calorie malnutrition) and marasmus (total caloric deprivation) are associated with metabolic changes that promote hepatic steatosis. In early caloric deprivation, glycogen stores are depleted and the body shifts to the use of ketones as fuel. Insulin levels decrease and hydrocortisone levels increase, stimulating skeletal muscle proteolysis. As caloric restriction progresses, elevated serum growth hormone and increased sympathetic nervous system activity cause a shift in energy metabolism from proteolysis to lipolysis. Lipid metabolism is altered, partly through a decrease in the number of peroxisomes in hepatocytes and depleted intracellular carnitine. Free fatty acids mobilized from adipose tissue are transported to the liver and hepatic fat content increases [65]. Malnutrition also leads to functional immunodeficiency, increasing the risk of infection, which leads to further metabolic stress, creating a vicious cycle.

Significant hepatomegaly is more common in kwashiorkor, a syndrome induced by inadequate protein intake with or without adequate caloric intake. The constellation of clinical features seen in kwashiorkor also includes apathy, edema, and characteristic skin and hair lesions. The liver is characterized by massive steatosis. In developing countries, kwashiorkor usually occurs after weaning and with the introduction of the native diet in toddlers; however, it has been described in non-poverty situations, usually from the use of inappropriate milk substitutes in infants.

Hepatic abnormalities have been reported in patients with eating disorders. Up to 25% of adolescent females with anorexia nervosa have elevated serum alanine aminotransferases; these levels correlate inversely with body mass index and percent body fat [66]. Asymptomatic elevated liver cell numbers have also been reported in patients with bulimia. A coagulopathy caused by vitamin K deficiency without any evidence of liver disease has been reported rarely in patients with bulimia.

The liver manifestations of nutritional deficiencies are rapidly reversed with treatment of the underlying nutritional disorders. Chronic liver disease has not been reported.

Dietary supplements

The use of alternative and complementary therapies such as herbal medicines, homeopathy, and vitamin therapy is increasingly common, particularly in western societies. While these compounds may be applied to children, particularly those with chronic disorders, for their purported healing benefits, they are most often used for weight loss or muscle building. For this reason, dietary supplements are most likely to be encountered in adolescents. A wide variety of agents have been implicated, including *Camellia sinensis* (green tea extracts), *Cassia angustifolia* (senna), *Morinda citrifolia* (noni juice), *Ephedra sinica* (Ma huang), *Teucrium chamaedrys* (Germander), Onshidou-Genbi-Kounou and Chaso (Japanese herbals), and usnic acid [67]. In addition, hepatotoxicity has been reported in a number of commercially available dietary supplements that contain multiple ingredients whose potential hepatotoxic properties are unclear. Hepatic injury caused by hypervitaminosis A has been recognized for decades. Manifestations include asymptomatic elevation of serum liver enzymes, cholestasis, non-cirrhotic portal hypertension, progressive fibrosis, and even cirrhosis. Young age may predispose certain individuals to develop vitamin A hepatotoxicity at doses as low as 20 000 IU/day. Hepatotoxicity is mediated by the dose-dependent effect of retinoids on hepatic stellate cells [67].

Miscellaneous disorders

Sarcoidosis

Sarcoidosis, which is rare in childhood, is a multisystem, chronic granulomatous disorder of unclear etiology. The pathologic feature is the presence of non-caseating epithelioid cell granulomas, which primarily affect the lungs and the lymphatics but may also be present in other tissues. Asymptomatic liver test abnormalities are found in 35% of patients with sarcoidosis, and splenomegaly and/or hepatomegaly are found in 5–21%. Up to 70% of patients have liver granulomas incidentally noted at the time of autopsy [68]. True granulomatous hepatitis is found in 15–50% of patients and a minority of these may progress to portal hypertension and end-stage liver disease [69]. The hepatic lesion in sarcoidosis can be cholestatic (resembling primary biliary cirrhosis or primary sclerosing cholangitis), necro-inflammatory (resembling viral infection or drug reaction), or vascular (presenting sinusoidal dilatation or nodular regenerative hyperplasia). Portal hypertension can result not only from hepatic fibrosis but also from portal vein or hepatic vein thrombosis in granulomatous phlebitis [68].

Sarcoidosis may be seen in association with such systemic disorders as Crohn disease, celiac disease, amyloidosis, lymphoma, thyroiditis, and Addison disease. Systemic steroids are the mainstay of treatment for sarcoidosis, although the optimal dosage, duration of therapy, and likelihood of liver response remain uncertain.

Amyloidosis

Amyloidosis is the syndrome that results when a variety of insoluble misfolded proteins are deposited in organs, leading to end-organ damage. Typically this occurs in one of two settings: clonal plasma cell disorders with overproduction of immunoglobulin light chain, or uncontrolled chronic inflammatory states with overproduction of serum amyloid, an acute phase reactant produced in the liver. The most frequently affected organs are the spleen, kidney, heart, and liver. The usual hepatic presentation is hepatomegaly and/or elevated alkaline phosphatase with well-preserved hepatic function. In adults, amyloidosis is associated with chronic infections or inflammatory states such as rheumatoid arthritis and tuberculosis. In children, amyloidosis is rare. The most common causes are tuberculosis, JIA, cystic fibrosis, and familial Mediterranean fever. Amyloidosis should be suspected in any patient with a chronic inflammatory disorder who develops hepatomegaly and proteinuria; diagnosis can be confirmed by rectal or kidney biopsy.

Congenital disorders of glycosylation

The congenital disorders of glycosylation (CDG) are a growing class of multisystem disorders characterized physiologically by defects in the synthesis and attachment of glycans to proteins and lipids. Many forms of CDG are recognizable by transferrin isoelectric focusing, which displays two distinct abnormal patterns based on altered *N*-glycosylation. More recently, disorders of *O*-glycosylation and glycolipid glycosylation are being identified via linkage analyses in affected families and application of advanced gene sequencing techniques [70].

Most of the CDGs include prominent neurologic symptoms and significant dysmorphism, in addition to involvement of a variety of extrahepatic organs, including the heart, immune system, skeletal system, skin, intestines, and the coagulation cascade (both prothrombotic tendencies and coagulopathy). However, not all organs present simultaneously, and liver disease may be the first and only symptom. A broad spectrum of hepatic abnormalities has been described in the CDG, ranging from elevated serum aminotransferases to cirrhosis to coagulopathy (Table 40.2).

Phosphomannomutase II deficiency is the most common CDG, with a type 1 pattern on transferrin isoelectric focusing. Liver involvement may include hepatomegaly, elevated serum aminotransferases, and/or coagulation defects [70].

Phosphomannose isomerase deficiency has little neurologic involvement and is primarily a liver and intestinal disorder with abnormal coagulation, protein-losing enteropathy, recurrent thromboses, liver disease and hypoglycemia [71]. It is the only treatable CDG, frequently responding to enteral mannose therapy.

Table 40.2 Congenital disorders of glycosylation with liver involvement

Type	Gene	Enzyme deficiency	Clinical features
Defects in N-glycosylation			
Ia (PMM2-CDG)	PMM2	Phosphomannomutase II	Mental retardation, hypotonia, inverted nipples, lipodystrophy, cerebellar hypoplasia, stroke-like episodes, seizures, hepatomegaly, steatosis, fibrosis
Ib (MPI-CDG)	MPI	Phosphomannose isomerase	Hepatic fibrosis, hypoglycemia, coagulopathy, protein-losing enteropathy
Ic (ALG6-CDG)	ALG6	Dol-P-Glc: Man(9)-GlcNAc(2)-P-P-Dol glucosyltransferase (glucosyltransferase I)	Mental retardation, hypotonia, esotropia, seizures, hepatomegaly
If (MPDU1-CDG)	MPDU1	Lec35 (Man-P-Dol utilization 1)	Severe developmental delay, hypotonia, seizures, failure to thrive, cortical blindness, hepatosplenomegaly, knee and ankle contractures
Ih (ALG8-CDG)	ALG8	Dol-P-Glc:Glc(1)-Man(9)-GlcNAc(2)-P-P-Dol glucosyltransferase (glucosyltransferase II)	Hypoalbuminemia, protein-losing enteropathy, hepatomegaly, renal disease, CNS dysfunction, coagulation factor defects
Ii (ALG2-CDG)	ALG2	GDP-Man:Man(1)-GlcNAc(2)-P-P-Dol mannosyltransferase (mannosyltransferase II)	Mental retardation, intractable seizures, iris coloboma, hepatomegaly, coagulopathy
Ik (ALG1-CDG)	ALG1	GDP-Man: GlcNAc2-P-P-Dol mannosyltransferase (mannosyltransferase I)	Microcephaly, intractable seizures, coagulation abnormalities, hypotonia, hepatosplenomegaly, immune defects
Il (ALG9-CDG)	ALG9	Dol-P-Man:Man(6)- and Man(8)-GlcNAc(2)-P-P-Dol mannosyltransferase (mannosyltransferase VII–IX)	Hepatomegaly, microcephaly, hypotonia, seizures, cystic renal disease
IIb (GLS1-CDG)	GLS1	Glucosidase I	Hypotonia, seizures, hepatomegaly, hepatic fibrosis, steatosis, bile duct proliferation
IId (B4GALT1-CDG)	B4GALT1	β-1,4-Galactosyltransferases	Diarrhea, dysmorphic features, hepatomegaly, mild hepatopathy, coagulation defects
Combined defects in N- and O-glycosylation			
IIe (COG7-CDG)	COG7	Conserved oligomeric Golgi complex subunit 7	Hepatomegaly, progressive jaundice, hypotonia, intractable seizures, recurrent infections, cardiac failure
IIh (COG1-CDG)	COG1	Conserved oligomeric Golgi complex subunit 1	Hepatosplenomegaly, hypotonia, growth retardation, microcephaly, mild mental retardation
Defects in lipid glycosylation			
Amish infantile epilepsy (SIAT9-CDG)	SIAT9	Lactosylceramide α-2,3 sialyltransferase (GM3 synthase)	Failure to thrive, intractable seizures, developmental delay, hepatosplenomegaly

The histologic lesion in CDG is variable. In children with phosphomannomutase II deficiency, hepatocytes may appear swollen with steatosis, expansion of portal tracts, and bridging fibrosis. Electron microscopy may show lysosomal inclusions. In children with phosphomannomutase deficiency, the picture resembles congenital hepatic fibrosis with hamartomatous collections of bile ducts and slight steatosis [72]. As identification of new glycosylation defects, their physiologic consequences and the diagnostic approach expands, the CDG should be considered in any patient presenting with explained liver dysfunction.

References
1. Brienza N, Dalfino L, Cinnella G, *et al.* Jaundice in critical illness: promoting factors of a concealed reality. *Intensive Care Med* 2006;**32**:267–274.

2. Jakob SM, Tenhunen JJ, Laitinen S, *et al.* Effects of systemic arterial hypoperfusion on splanchnic hemodynamics and hepatic arterial buffer response in pigs. *Am J Physiol Gastrointest Liver Physiol* 2001;**280**: G819–G827.

3. Brienza N, Revelly JP, Ayuse T, Robotham JL. Effects of PEEP on liver arterial and venous blood flows. *Am*

J Respir Crit Care Med 1995;**152**: 504–510.

4. Parker GA, Picut CA. Immune functioning in nonlymphoid organs: the liver. *Toxicol Pathol* 2012;**40**:237–247.

5. Sander LE, Sackett SD, Dierssen U, *et al.* Hepatic acute-phase proteins control innate immune responses during infection by promoting myeloid-derived suppressor cell function. *J Exp Med* 2010;**207**: 1453–1464.

6. Sakamori R, Takehara T, Ohnishi C, *et al.* Signal transducer and activator of transcription 3 signaling within hepatocytes attenuates systemic inflammatory response and lethality in septic mice. *Hepatology* 2007;**46**: 1564–1573.

7. Geier A, Fickert P, Trauner M. Mechanisms of disease: mechanisms and clinical implications of cholestasis in sepsis. *Nat Clin Pract Gastroenterol Hepatol* 2006;**3**:574–585.

8. McDonald B, Kubes P. Neutrophils and intravascular immunity in the liver during infection and sterile inflammation. *Toxicol Pathol* 2012;**40**:157–165.

9. Lautt WW. Regulatory processes interacting to maintain hepatic blood flow constancy: Vascular compliance, hepatic arterial buffer response, hepatorenal reflex, liver regeneration, escape from vasoconstriction. *Hepatol Res* 2007;**37**:891–903.

10. Vollmar B, Menger MD. The hepatic microcirculation: mechanistic contributions and therapeutic targets in liver injury and repair. *Physiol Rev* 2009;**89**:1269–1339.

11. Ebert EC. Hypoxic liver injury. *Mayo Clin Proc* 2006;**81**:1232–1236.

12. Peltenburg HG, Hermens WT, Willems GM, Flendrig JG, Schmidt E. Estimation of the fractional catabolic rate constants for the elimination of cytosolic liver enzymes from plasma. *Hepatology* 1989;**10**:833–839.

13. Arcidi JM Jr., Moore GW, Hutchins GM. Hepatic morphology in cardiac dysfunction: a clinicopathologic study of 1000 subjects at autopsy. *Am J Pathol* 1981;**104**:159–166.

14. Poelzl G, Ess M, Mussner-Seeber C, *et al.* Liver dysfunction in chronic heart failure: prevalence, characteristics and prognostic significance. *Eur J Clin Invest* 2012;**42**:153–163.

15. Camposilvan S, Milanesi O, Stellin G, *et al.* Liver and cardiac function in the long term after Fontan operation. *Ann Thorac Surg* 2008;**86**:177–182.

16. Wu FM, Ukomadu C, Odze RD, *et al.* Liver disease in the patient with Fontan circulation. *Congenit Heart Dis* 2011;**6**:190–201.

17. Pike NA, Evangelista LS, Doering LV, *et al.* Clinical profile of the adolescent/adult Fontan survivor. *Congenit Heart Dis* 2011;**6**:9–17.

18. Chen H, Cheng Y, Ning S, Chen Y. Budd–Chiari syndrome caused by multiple membranous obstruction of the inferior vena cava in a young man. *Ann Vasc Surg* 2011;**25**:1139 e5–7.

19. Shetty S, Ghosh K. Thrombophilic dimension of Budd–Chiari syndrome and portal venous thrombosis: a concise review. *Thromb Res* 2011;**127**:505–512.

20. Hoekstra J, Guimaraes AH, Leebeek FW, *et al.* Impaired fibrinolysis as a risk factor for Budd–Chiari syndrome. *Blood* 2010;**115**:388–395.

21. Goulding C, Uttenthal B, Foroni L, *et al.* The JAK2(V617F) tyrosine kinase mutation identifies clinically latent myeloproliferative disorders in patients presenting with hepatic or portal vein thrombosis. *Int J Lab Hematol* 2008;**30**:415–419.

22. Singh V, Sinha SK, Nain CK, *et al.* Budd–Chiari syndrome: our experience of 71 patients. *J Gastroenterol Hepatol* 2000;**15**:550–554.

23. Boozari B, Bahr MJ, Kubicka S, *et al.* Ultrasonography in patients with Budd–Chiari syndrome: diagnostic signs and prognostic implications. *J Hepatol* 2008;**49**:572–580.

24. Wang L, Lu JP, Wang F, Liu Q, Wang J. Diagnosis of Budd–Chiari syndrome: three-dimensional dynamic contrast enhanced magnetic resonance angiography. *Abdom Imaging* 2011;**36**:399–406.

25. Nagral A, Hasija RP, Marar S, Nabi F. Budd–Chiari syndrome in children: experience with therapeutic radiological intervention. *J Pediatr Gastroenterol Nutr* 2010;**50**:74–78.

26. Di Giorgio A, Agazzi R, Alberti D, Colledan M, D'Antiga L. Feasibility and efficacy of transjugular intrahepatic porto-systemic shunt (TIPS) in children. *J Pediatr Gastroenterol Nutr* 2012;**54**:594–600.

27. Koskinas J, Manesis EK, Zacharakis GH, *et al.* Liver involvement in acute vaso-occlusive crisis of sickle cell disease: prevalence and predisposing factors. *Scand J Gastroenterol* 2007;**42**:499–507.

28. Ebert EC, Nagar M, Hagspiel KD. Gastrointestinal and hepatic complications of sickle cell disease. *Clin Gastroenterol Hepatol* 2010;**8**:483–9; quiz e70.

29. Ahn H, Li CS, Wang W. Sickle cell hepatopathy: clinical presentation, treatment, and outcome in pediatric and adult patients. *Pediatr Blood Cancer* 2005;**45**:184–190.

30. Revel-Vilk S, Komvilaisak P, Blanchette V, *et al.* The changing face of hepatitis in boys with haemophilia associated with increased prevalence of obesity. *Haemophilia* 2011;**17**:689–694.

31. Farrow AC, Buchanan GR, Zwiener RJ, Bowman WP, Winick NJ. Serum aminotransferase elevation during and following treatment of childhood acute lymphoblastic leukemia. *J Clin Oncol* 1997;**15**:1560–1566.

32. Halonen P, Mattila J, Ruuska T, Salo MK, Makipernaa A. Liver histology after current intensified therapy for childhood acute lymphoblastic leukemia: microvesicular fatty change and siderosis are the main findings. *Med Pediatr Oncol* 2003;**40**: 148–154.

33. Rawat D, Gillett PM, Devadason D, Wilson DC, McKiernan PJ. Long-term follow-up of children with 6-thioguanine-related chronic hepatoxicity following treatment for acute lymphoblastic leukaemia. *J Pediatr Gastroenterol Nutr* 2011;**53**:478–479.

34. Suttorp M, Yaniv I, Schultz KR. Controversies in the treatment of CML in children and adolescents: TKIs versus BMT? *Biol Blood Marrow Transplant* 2011;**17**:S115–S122.

35. Ballonoff A, Kavanagh B, Nash R, *et al.* Hodgkin lymphoma-related vanishing bile duct syndrome and idiopathic cholestasis: statistical analysis of all published cases and literature review. *Acta Oncol* 2008;**47**:962–970.

36. Ghosh I, Bakhshi S. Jaundice as a presenting manifestation of pediatric non-Hodgkin lymphoma: etiology, management, and outcome. *J Pediatr Hematol Oncol* 2010;**32**:e131–e135.

37. McDonald GB. Hepatobiliary complications of hematopoietic cell transplantation, 40 years on. *Hepatology* 2010;**51**:1450–1460.

38. Coppell JA, Richardson PG, Soiffer R, *et al.* Hepatic veno-occlusive disease following stem cell transplantation: incidence, clinical course, and outcome. *Biol Blood Marrow Transplant* 2010;**16**:157–168.

39. Shulman HM, Gooley T, Dudley MD, *et al.* Utility of transvenous liver biopsies and wedged hepatic venous pressure measurements in sixty marrow transplant recipients. *Transplantation* 1995;**59**:1015–1022.

40. Tay J, Tinmouth A, Fergusson D, Huebsch L, Allan DS. Systematic review of controlled clinical trials on the use of ursodeoxycholic acid for the prevention of hepatic veno-occlusive disease in hematopoietic stem cell transplantation. *Biol Blood Marrow Transplant* 2007;**13**:206–217.

41. Corbacioglu S, Cesaro S, Faraci M, *et al.* Defibrotide for prophylaxis of hepatic veno-occlusive disease in paediatric haemopoietic stem-cell transplantation: an open-label, phase 3, randomised controlled trial. *Lancet* 2012;**379**: 1301–1309.

42. Pidala J. Graft-vs-host disease following allogeneic hematopoietic cell transplantation. *Cancer Control* 2011;**18**:268–276.

43. Robin M, Porcher R, de Castro R, *et al.* Initial liver involvement in acute GVHD is predictive for nonrelapse mortality. *Transplantation* 2009;**88**:1131–1136.

44. Kagoya Y, Takahashi T, Nannya Y, *et al.* Hyperbilirubinemia after hematopoietic stem cell transplantation: comparison of clinical and pathologic findings in 41 autopsied cases. *Clin Transplant* 2011;**25**:e552–e557.

45. Oshrine B, Lehmann LE, Duncan CN. Safety and utility of liver biopsy after pediatric hematopoietic stem cell transplantation. *J Pediatr Hematol Oncol* 2011;**33**:e92–e97.

46. Shulman HM, Kleiner D, Lee SJ, *et al.* Histopathologic diagnosis of chronic graft-versus-host disease: National Institutes of Health Consensus Development Project on Criteria for Clinical Trials in Chronic Graft-versus-Host Disease: II. Pathology Working Group Report. *Biol Blood Marrow Transplant* 2006;**12**:31–47.

47. Choi SW, Levine JE, Ferrara JL. Pathogenesis and management of graft-versus-host disease. *Immunol Allergy Clin North Am* 2010;**30**:75–101.

48. Barshes NR, Myers GD, Lee D, *et al.* Liver transplantation for severe hepatic graft-versus-host disease. An analysis of aggregate survival data. *Liver Transplant* 2005;**11**:525–531.

49. Tomita Y, Ishiguro H, Yasuda Y, *et al.* High incidence of fatty liver and insulin resistance in long-term adult survivors of childhood SCT. *Bone Marrow Transplant* 2011;**46**:416–425.

50. Ebert EC, Hagspiel KD. Gastrointestinal and hepatic manifestations of rheumatoid arthritis. *Dig Dis Sci* 2011;**56**:295–302.

51. Takahashi A, Abe K, Yokokawa J, *et al.* Clinical features of liver dysfunction in collagen diseases. *Hepatol Res* 2010;**40**:1092–1097.

52. Soni P, Shell B, Cawkwell G, Li C, Ma H. The hepatic safety and tolerability of the cyclooxygenase-2 selective NSAID celecoxib: pooled analysis of 41 randomized controlled trials. *Current Med Res Opin* 2009;**25**:1841–1851.

53. Hashkes PJ, Balistreri WF, Bove KE, Ballard ET, Passo MH. The relationship of hepatotoxic risk factors and liver histology in methotrexate therapy for juvenile rheumatoid arthritis. *J Pediatr* 1999;**134**:47–52.

54. Kaplowitz N, DeLeve LD. *Drug-induced Liver Disease*, 2nd edn. New York: Informa Healthcare, 2007.

55. Shimizu M, Yokoyama T, Yamada K, *et al.* Distinct cytokine profiles of systemic-onset juvenile idiopathic arthritis-associated macrophage activation syndrome with particular emphasis on the role of interleukin-18 in its pathogenesis. *Rheumatology* 2010;**49**:1645–1653.

56. Ebert EC, Hagspiel KD. Gastrointestinal and hepatic manifestations of systemic lupus erythematosus. *J Clin Gastroenterol* 2011;**45**:436–441.

57. Schlenker C, Halterman T, Kowdley KV. Rheumatologic disease and the liver. *Clin Liver Dis* 2011;**15**:153–164.

58. Eladawy M, Dominguez SR, Anderson MS, Glode MP. Abnormal liver panel in acute Kawasaki disease. *Pediatr Infect Dis J* 2011;**30**:141–144.

59. Alatzoglou KS, Dattani MT. Genetic forms of hypopituitarism and their manifestation in the neonatal period. *Early Hum Dev* 2009;**85**:705–712.

60. Malik R, Hodgson H. The relationship between the thyroid gland and the liver. *Q J Med* 2002;**95**:559–569.

61. Chung GE, Kim D, Kim W, *et al.* Non-alcoholic fatty liver disease across the spectrum of hypothyroidism. *J Hepatol* 2012.

62. Elder CJ, Natarajan A. Mauriac syndrome: a modern reality. *J Pediatr Endocrinol Metab* 2010;**23**:311–313.

63. Bardella MT, Vecchi M, Conte D, *et al.* Chronic unexplained hypertransaminasemia may be caused by occult celiac disease. *Hepatology* 1999;**29**:654–657.

64. Mounajjed T, Oxentenko A, Shmidt E, Smyrk T. The liver in celiac disease: clinical manifestations, histologic features, and response to gluten-free diet in 30 patients. *Am J Clin Pathol* 2011;**136**:128–137.

65. Finn PF, Dice JF. Proteolytic and lipolytic responses to starvation. *Nutrition* 2006;**22**:830–844.

66. Fong HF, Divasta AD, Difabio D, *et al.* Prevalence and predictors of abnormal liver enzymes in young women with anorexia nervosa. *J Pediatr* 2008;**153**:247–253.

67. Stickel F, Kessebohm K, Weimann R, Seitz HK. Review of liver injury associated with dietary supplements. *Liver Int* 2011;**31**:595–605.

68. Dulai PS, Rothstein RI. Disseminated sarcoidosis presenting as granulomatous gastritis: a clinical review of the gastrointestinal and hepatic manifestations of sarcoidosis. *J Clin Gastroenterol* 2012.

69. Cremers J, Drent M, Driessen A, *et al.* Liver-test abnormalities in sarcoidosis. *Eur J Gastroenterol Hepatol* 2012;**24**:17–24.

70. Hennet T. Diseases of glycosylation beyond classical congenital disorders of glycosylation. *Biochim Biophys Acta* 2012;**1820**:1306–1317.

71. Theodore M, Morava E. Congenital disorders of glycosylation: sweet news. *Curr Opin Pediatr* 2011;**23**:581–587.

72. Damen G, de Klerk H, Huijmans J, den Hollander J, Sinaasappel M. Gastrointestinal and other clinical manifestations in 17 children with congenital disorders of glycosylation type Ia, Ib, and Ic. *J Pediatr Gastroenterol Nutr* 2004;**38**:282–287.

Ronen Arnon, Maureen M. Jonas, Antonio R. Perez-Atayde, and Frederick J. Suchy

Introduction

Fibrocystic liver disease refers to a heterogeneous group of disorders that share some pathophysiologic and clinical features but have important differences. Cystic dilatation of intrahepatic bile duct structures and variable degrees of portal fibrosis are the hallmarks of fibrocystic liver disease. In most instances, there are morphologic abnormalities in the kidneys and pancreas that parallel those of the liver. For this reason, and to appreciate more thoroughly the shared pathogenesis and implications for organogenesis, fibrocystic liver disease and corresponding renal counterparts are discussed together.

It has been recognized for centuries that hepatic and renal cysts are seen in the same individuals [1], although it has not always been accepted that they are manifestations of the same diseases. The older literature contains confusing descriptive classifications of fibrocystic diseases, with imprecise and overlapping definitions. Even now, attempts at describing clinical and radiographic features, prognosis, natural history, and treatment are somewhat hampered by reliance on these descriptive reports. However, much of the molecular basis for these disorders has been elucidated, and clinical diagnoses are being modified using more exact genetic criteria. The current consensus is that genetic determinants of differentiation and development of renal tubules and biliary structures result in a broad spectrum of congenital abnormalities grouped under the heading of fibrocystic liver and kidney disease.

Embryologic development of the liver has been discussed in Chapter 1 and will not be fully reviewed here. However, to understand this group of developmental disorders, it is necessary to review the stages of formation of the macroscopic and microscopic biliary tree. At about the eighth week of gestation, precursor cells that lie adjacent to the hilar portal vein vessels dramatically increase production of cytokeratin. This sleeve-like layer of cells duplicates and extends toward the periphery along small intrahepatic portal vein branches. The resultant double-layered sleeve of cytokeratin-rich cells that are separated by a slit- or plate-like lumen has been designated as the ductal plate.

The ductal plate undergoes progressive remodeling from 12 weeks of gestation into the postnatal period. This process begins at the hilum and proceeds toward the periphery. As shown in Figure 41.1, short segments of the double-layered sleeve dilate to form tubules. As they form, individual bile ductules are incorporated into the periportal mesenchyme around the portal vein branches. These developing bile ductules consistently express cytokeratin 19 and begin expressing cytokeratin 7 as well as other markers of differentiated biliary epithelia by 20 weeks of gestation. In contrast, precursor cells that are not associated with the differentiating ductal plate and bile ductules lose cytokeratin 19 expression. These cells maintain cytokeratin 8 and 18 production and eventually give rise to hepatocytes.

Biliary differentiation involves a series of interactions between the mesenchyme surrounding the portal vein branches and the ductal plate epithelia. As a result, the ductal plate is induced to form bile ducts, which are incorporated into the portal mesenchyme. The non-tubular elements of the ductal plate involute. This remodeling of the ductal plate leads to the formation of the intrahepatic biliary tree. The largest bile ducts are formed first, followed by segmental, interlobular, and finally the smallest ductules. Arrest or derangement in remodeling leads to the persistence of primitive bile duct configurations, or to what Jorgensen termed ductal plate malformation (DPM) [2]. The occurrence of DPM at different generations of the developing biliary tree gives rise to different clinicopathologic entities. Defects in ductal plate remodeling are typically accompanied by portal vein branching abnormalities [3].

Fibrocystic diseases of the liver are most often accompanied by cystic disorders of the kidney, as listed in Table 41.1. Much of the work elucidating the pathogenesis of these disorders has been done using animal models, cell systems, and clinical material from affected kidneys. Therefore, it is important to understand renal tubular development and how it parallels biliary development. Nephron formation begins about the eighth week of gestation, as the ureteric bud branches induce the mesenchymal cells to begin a series of stereotypical changes. The induced mesenchyme forms cap-like aggregates

Table 41.1 Renal disorders associated with fibropolycystic liver diseases

Fibropolycystic liver disease	Associated renal disorder
Congenital hepatic fibrosis	Autosomal recessive polycystic kidney disease[a] Autosomal dominant polycystic kidney disease Cystic renal dysplasia Nephronophthisis
Caroli syndrome	Autosomal recessive polycystic kidney disease[a] Autosomal dominant polycystic kidney disease
Caroli disease	Autosomal recessive polycystic kidney disease
Von Meyenburg complexes (isolated)	?
Von Meyenburg complexes with congenital hepatic fibrosis or Caroli syndrome	Autosomal recessive polycystic kidney disease
Von Meyenburg complexes with polycystic liver disease	Autosomal dominant polycystic kidney disease
Polycystic liver disease	Autosomal dominant polycystic kidney disease[a]

[a] Most common associated disorder.

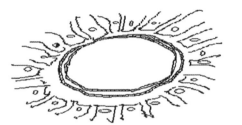 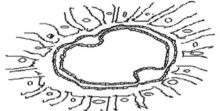 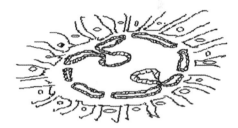

Figure 41.1 Schematic representation of the primordial ductal plate remodeling. The two layers of cells are originally separated by a slit-like lumen. Segments of the lumen dilate to form tubules, which eventually become bile ducts, incorporated into the portal tract mesenchyme. The remainder of the ductal plate involutes.

over the advancing ureteric bud branches, which then become vesicular as they undergo a mesenchymal to epithelial transformation, polarize, and form a lumen. These vesicular structures then elongate to form S-shaped tubules. The lower portion of each tubule gives rise to the glomerular capsule and the remainder to the proximal and distal tubules. In a reciprocal fashion, the ureteric bud continues to divide, and its terminal branches differentiate into the collecting ducts. Nephrogenesis proceeds in a centripetal pattern, from the inner cortex to the periphery, and is completed by 34 weeks of gestation.

Osathanondh and Potter [4] morphologically classified the tubular abnormalities that occur in different polycystic kidney diseases. In autosomal recessive polycystic kidney disease (ARPKD), the cystic lesion involves fusiform dilatations, 1–8 mm in size, of the terminal collecting duct branches. The extent of collecting duct involvement varies inversely with age at presentation. In affected fetuses and neonates, 90% of the collecting tubules are dilated compared with 10% in adolescents. In comparison, in autosomal dominant polycystic kidney disease (ADPKD), cysts may develop in any nephron segment or in the collecting duct, but on average they involve only 1% of the nephron population [5]. These cysts most often develop in childhood but have been detected in a fetus as early as 16 weeks of gestation. They are clinically silent until the third or fourth decade of life.

Solitary non-parasitic cyst of the liver

Solitary non-parasitic cysts resemble the cysts seen in fibrocystic diseases in that they are developmental rather than neoplastic in origin and are lined by simple cuboidal or columnar biliary-type epithelium (Figure 41.2). The surrounding hepatic parenchyma displays secondary atrophy, portal fibrosis, and bile duct proliferation. However, the cysts are not associated with DPM and are not seen in association with renal, pancreatic, or other cysts. Most are unilocular and do not have any clinical manifestations. When they are symptomatic, the most common presentation is that of an upper abdominal mass, although rupture, infection, or hemorrhage also may occur. Asymptomatic simple cysts do not require treatment and can be monitored by ultrasound. Intervention is only necessary if there is progressive enlargement, symptoms, or if imaging characteristics cause diagnostic uncertainty [6].

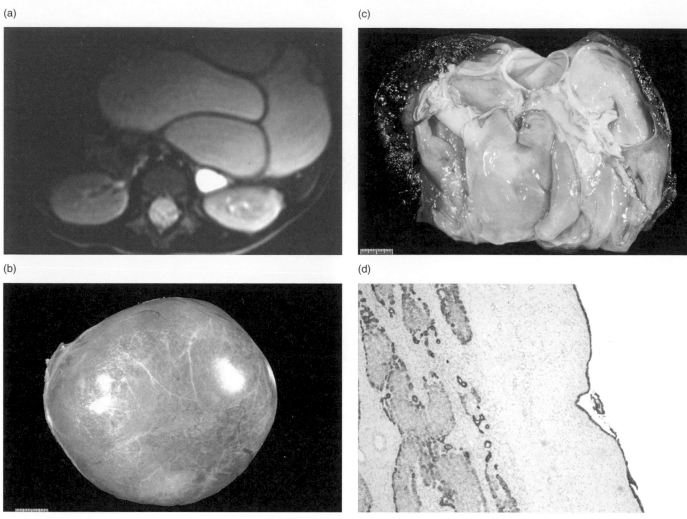

Figure 41.2 Solitary non-parasitic liver cyst. (a) CT demonstrating large multiloculated hepatic cyst. (b) External gross appearance of the resected cyst showing smooth, shiny surface. (c) Cut surface of the cyst demonstrating loculations. (d) Microscopically, the cyst wall is lined by AE1 cytokeratin-positive biliary epithelium. The outer part of the cyst wall contains atrophic hepatic parenchyma with portal bile duct proliferation and fibrosis.

Congenital hepatic fibrosis

A hereditary disorder characterized by hepatic fibrosis, portal hypertension, and renal cystic disease was described and called congenital hepatic fibrosis (CHF) [7]. Typically, CHF is associated with ARPKD. Some investigators considered CHF and ARPKD a single disorder with a wide spectrum of manifestations, whereas others argued that they are two distinct entities that share phenotypically similar biliary lesions: ARPKD is described more frequently in neonates and infants, in whom the renal lesion is clinically more severe, whereas CHF is more commonly seen in older children and adolescents, in whom the renal involvement may be minimal [8]. However, the identification of the gene for ARPKD, *PKHD1* (polycystic kidney and hepatic disease 1) [9,10], has provided proof that at least most ARPKD with CHF is genetically homogeneous. Using a technique for rapid screening of *PKDH1* in ARPKD pedigrees, the detection rate of mutations was 85% in severely affected patients, 41.9% in moderate

ARPKD, and 32.1% in adults with CHF or Caroli disease [11]. *PKHD1* encodes fibrocystin/polyductin. Recent studies have demonstrated that fibrocystin/polyductin is localized to primary cilia and suggest a causative role for this organelle in cystic renal disease [12].

Although CHF is most commonly seen in association with ARPKD, it has been reported as an isolated entity as well as with ADPKD and nephronophthisis [13]. In three families with CHF and ADPKD, pathogenic *PKD1* mutations were found in all eight affected patients. Portal hypertension was the main manifestation of CHF; hepatocellular function was preserved and liver enzymes were largely normal.

Presence of CHF also has been described in a variety of other rare conditions or syndromes, as listed in Table 41.2. In some of these syndromes, cystic disease of the pancreas is also observed. In most pedigrees, CHF is transmitted as an autosomal recessive trait. Although some reports cite a higher incidence in males, this observation remains controversial. The overall incidence of CHF is unknown. For purposes of

Table 41.2 Hepatic fibrocystic syndromes

Disease	Inheritance	Gene (protein product)	Renal disease	Liver disease	Associated features
Autosomal recessive polycystic kidney disease	AR	*PKHD1* (fibrocystin)	Cystic dilatation of collecting tubule	DPM, CHF, Caroli disease	
Autosomal dominant polycystic kidney disease	AD	*PKD1* (polycystin 1), *PKD2* (polycystin 2)	Cysts from all portions of tubule	DPM, CHF, and Caroli disease rarely	Liver cysts derived from but not connected to bile ducts; intracranial and aortic aneurysms; mitral valve prolapse and other cardiac valvular defects; pancreatic cysts; colonic diverticula, inguinal hernias
Autosomal dominant polycystic liver disease	AD	*PRKCSH* (hepatocystin), *SEC36*	None	Cysts arising from biliary microhamartomas and periductal glands, rarely CHF	Less commonly share some of the extrarenal manifestations observed in ADPKD
Nephronophthisis type 3	AR	*NPHP3* (nephrocystin-3)	Cysts at corticomedullary junction	CHF	Tapetoretinal degeneration
Jeune syndrome	AR	Loci 12p, 15q13; *IFT8* (intraflagellar transport protein)	Cystic renal tubular dysplasia	CHF, Caroli disease	Short stature, skeletal dysplasia, small thorax, limb shortness, polydactyly, pelvic abnormalities
Joubert syndrome	AR	*AH11* (jouberin), *HPHP1*, *NPHP1-4-8* (apical surface), *NPHP5-6* (centrosomes)	Cystic dysplasia, nephronophthisis	CHF	Dysgenesis of cerebellum, Dandy–Walker malformation, cardiac defects
Coach syndrome (overlap with Joubert syndrome)	AR	*MKS3*, *CC2D2A*, *RPGRIP1L*	Cystic dysplasia	CHF	Cerebellar vermis hypoplasia, oligophrenia (developmental delay/mental retardation), ataxia, coloboma
Meckel–Gruber syndrome	AR	*MKS1*, *TMEM67*, *TMEM216*, *CEP290*, *CC2D2A*, *RPGRIP1L*, *B9D1*, *B9D2* (involved with function of cilia)	Corticomedullary cysts	DPM	CNS malformations, cardiac defects, polydactyly
Bardet–Biedl syndrome	AR triallelic	*BBS1–8* (eight genes; M390R mutation)	Cystic dysplasia, nephronophthisis	CHF	Retinal degeneration, obesity, limb deformities, hypogonadism
Oral-facial-digital syndrome type 1	X-linked	*OFD1* (centrosomal protein localized at the basal bodies at the origin of primary cilia)	Multiple renal medullary and cortical macrocysts	Dilatations of the intrahepatic bile ducts, CHF	Oral clefts, hamartomas or cysts of the tongue, digital anomalies, pancreatic cysts
Ivemark syndrome	AR	–	Cystic dysplasia	CHF, Caroli disease	Pancreatic fibrosis, situs inversus, polysplenia, cardiac and CNS anomalies
Congenital disorder of glycosylation-Ib	AR	*PMI* (phosphomannose isomerase)	None	DPM, CHF	Chronic diarrhea, protein-losing enteropthy, coagulapathy

ADPKD, autosomal dominant polycystic kidney disease; AD, autosomal dominant; AR, autosomal recessive; CHF, congenital hepatic fibrosis; CNS, central nervous system; DPM, ductal plate malformation.

discussion, a descriptive approach is taken here; this section focuses on the biliary lesion, and the renal tubular lesion is reviewed in the discussion of ARPKD.

Pathology

The liver of patients with CHF appears grossly speckled with gray–white bands of fibrous tissue identifiable to the naked eye (Figure 41.3a,b). Microscopically, CHF is characterized by islands of normal liver that are separated by broad and narrow septa of dense, mature fibrous tissue. The fibrous tissue contains elongated or cystic spaces lined by regular biliary epithelium which represent cross-sections of the hollow structures comprising the DPM (Figure 41.3c).

Prominent bands of mature fibrous tissue connect adjacent portal triads. Although the periportal fibrous is marked, the associated inflammatory cell infiltration of the portal area is usually mild. Portal vein branches often appear reduced in size and number, and the sparsity of venous channels may account in part for portal hypertension. The hepatic lesions of CHF tend to become more prominent with time, but the rate of progression is variable. The fibrosis may increase secondary of recurrent episodes of cholangitis. The fibrosis of CHF can be differentiated from cirrhosis, in which there is nodular regeneration, often inflammation and necrosis and there is no presence of biliary channels. The portal tracts in CHF are expanded by mature collagenous tissue, which forms interportal bridges that initially do not disrupt the acinar architecture and explains the absence of hepatocellular dysfunction. Progressive liver synthetic dysfunction may be related to recurrent episodes of ascending cholangitis.

Clinical manifestations

The onset of signs and symptoms is variable, ranging from early childhood to the fifth or sixth decade of life, but most patients are diagnosed during adolescence or young adulthood

(a)

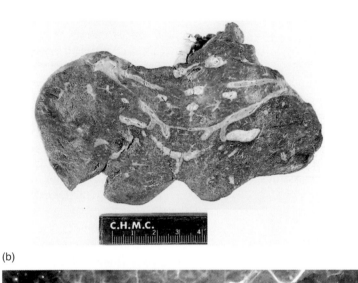

(b)

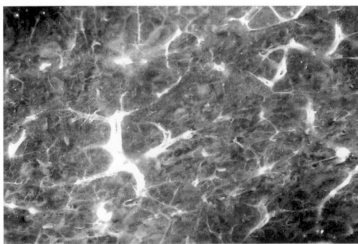

(c)

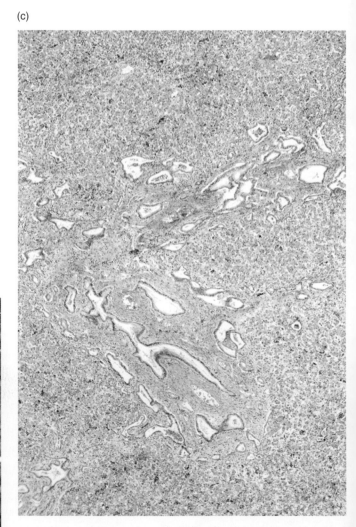

Figure 41.3 Congenital hepatic fibrosis. (a,b) Gross liver specimen demonstrating the prominent gray–white bands of fibrous tissue. (c) Microscopic section demonstrating dilated irregularly branching bile ducts, ductal plate malformation, and prominent portal fibrosis.

Table 41.3 Manifestations of congenital hepatic fibrosis

Type	Manifestations	Laboratory findings
Portal Hypertensive	Splenomegaly Varices, normal liver function, normal growth	Thrombocytopenia Neutropenia ± elevated alkaline phosphatase
Cholangitic	Cholestasis, recurrent cholangitis, hepatic dysfunction, poor growth	Elevated alkaline phosphatase ± elevated bilirubin
Mixed	Mixed	All of the above
Latent	None	None

There are four clinical forms of CHF (Table 41.3): (1) portal hypertensive CHF, which is the most common; (2) cholangitic; (3) mixed; and (4) latent.

Portal hypertensive form

The clinical manifestations of patients with portal hypertensive CHF are usually recurrent upper gastrointestinal hemorrhage from ruptured esophageal varices, splenomegaly, and hypersplenism. These episodes have been described as early as 19 months of age [14], although they are more commonly seen in older children. The pathogenesis of development of portal hypertension has been attributed to the compression of portal vein radicles in the fibrous bands and to an anomaly in the branching pattern of the portal vein, giving rise to hypoplastic and involutive branches [7]. Although all individuals with CHF have DPM detectable by liver biopsy at birth, abnormal liver echogenicity and splenomegaly may not be detectable during early childhood because portal fibrosis and portal hypertension are time-dependent pathologies that develop and progress with age. The severity and rate of progression of CHF and its complications vary widely even within the same family, which makes prognostication difficult [15].

Cholangitic form

Patients with cholangitic CHF have an abnormal intra- and extrahepatic biliary tree. The main manifestations are cholestasis and recurrent episodes of cholangitis, which can lead to sepsis, liver dysfunction, and poor growth. Biliary stone formation and cholangiocarcinoma can develop at a relatively young age [16].

Other complications

Pulmonary hypertension (portopulmonary hypertension) and vascular shunts in the pulmonary parenchyma (hepatopulmonary syndrome) are complications of portal hypertension that can be rarely seen in CHF. Ascites and encephalopathy are less common in CHF than in cirrhosis.

Laboratory findings

In patients with CHF uncomplicated by either portal hypertension or cholangitis, the laboratory evaluation is usually unremarkable. Serum aminotransferase and bilirubin levels are characteristically normal. Bilirubin, gamma glutamyltransferase, and alkaline phosphatase can be elevated during episodes of cholangitis. Thrombocytopenia and neutropenia is seen in patients with portal hypertension and hypersplenism. Urea and creatinine levels may be elevated in patients with renal involvement.

Physical examination

Jaundice may be seen in patients with cholangitis or with deterioration of liver function. Abdominal distension can be present. The liver is enlarged and firm with a prominent left lobe and the spleen is enlarged in patients with portal hypertension.

Diagnosis

The diagnosis of CHF can be suspected in patients with liver and renal disease, supported by imaging findings and confirmed on the basis of mutation analysis [14]. Mutations in ARPKD/CHF are distributed throughout *PKHD1*, and polymorphisms are common. The current mutation detection rate is 80–85%. There is marked allelic heterogeneity, and most affected patients appear to be compound heterozygotes. Prenatal diagnosis of ARPKD/CHF, on the basis of haplotype analysis and on mutation analysis, has been performed [17]. Liver biopsy can provide further characteristic findings of CHF, but its routine use is rarely required particularly in those with fibrocystic renal disease, because the diagnosis can be established on clinical findings alone. Liver biopsy may be reserved for patients with equivocal findings.

Imaging

Diagnosis of CHF is suggested by ultrasound, CT, or MRI of the abdomen. Sonographically, the liver has a patchy pattern of increased echogenicity. Sonographic evaluation should include Doppler flow studies of the portal vasculature looking for evidence of portal hypertension, such as reversal of portal flow or splenomegaly. Ultrasound can demonstrate dilated ducts that often contain sludge and stones. In addition, small branches of the portal vein are often seen within the dilated ducts, each of which appears as a small, echogenic dot in the non-dependent part of the dilated duct ("central dot sign") [18]. Imaging with CT and/or MRI are used for clarification and confirmation of the ultrasound findings and for demonstration of the extent of the disease. They provide a more complete assessment of blood flow and the entire biliary ductal system (magnetic resonance cholangiopancreatography (MRCP)). They also provide better tissue characterization and thus improve differentiation between fibrocystic liver diseases and polycystic liver disease (PLD). Endoscopic retrograde cholangiopancreatography and percutaneous transhepatic cholangiography are invasive procedures with risk of complications and are generally reserved for patients who need therapeutic intervention.

Differential diagnosis of congenital hepatic fibrosis

It is easy to confuse CHF with cirrhosis because of the extensive fibrosis seen on biopsy and the portal hypertension seen in CHF. Patients with CHF usually have preserved hepatic synthetic function and the pathologic findings in biopsies from these patients differ from those in biopsies of patients with cirrhosis (see Pathology). Diseases of the bile ducts that can lead to cirrhosis include primary sclerosing cholangitis. As CHF can have cholangitis, the bile duct strictures and dilations often seen in primary sclerosing cholangitis may be mistaken for the dilated extrahepatic bile ducts of CHF and even the intrahepatic cysts of CHF. Non-cirrhotic portal hypertension creating a nodular regenerative hyperplasia may be more difficult to distinguish from CHF than cirrhotic portal hypertension and relies on medical history, physical examination, laboratory testing, and imaging. Liver biopsy is often needed to identify intrahepatic causes of non-cirrhotic portal hypertension. Cysts in the liver, especially when few and small, may be a normal variant. The hepatic cysts seen in autosomal dominant PLD (ADPLD) are not typically associated with CHF and can be distinguished from cysts associated with CHF by the large number of cysts and the extent of involvement of the hepatic parenchyma.

Therapy

Therapy depends on the type of CHF and the clinical manifestation of the disease. It is mainly supportive and it is directed toward treating biliary tract infection and the complications of portal hypertension. Antibiotic therapy is indicated for ascending cholangitis. Although evidence is lacking, antibiotic prophylaxis for recurrent cholangitis is sometimes used in individuals who have had cholangitis [19]. The treatment of biliary stones depends on their location, number, and size. Care is best provided in a tertiary care facility with expertise in managing biliary stones. Although there are theoretical reasons why choleretics such as ursodeoxycholate may impede the development of abnormalities of the bile ducts, or even fibrosis, this has not been proven. The management of portal hypertension in children lacks an evidenced-based approach. Some centers proceed with primary prophylaxis with a nonselective beta-blocker for large varices identified by surveillance endoscopy. Variceal bleeding can be treated endoscopically by sclerotherapy or band ligation. The liver function in CHF is usually well preserved for prolonged periods, and a selective shunting procedure can provide relief from the complications of portal hypertension. A surgical shunt would also be a strong consideration in an individual with large varices that have never bled if appropriate expert care is not available for emergency management of variceal bleeding [20]. Liver

transplantation is indicated in patients with end-stage liver disease or recurrent uncontrolled cholangitis. Shneider et al. [19] have discussed the special issues in the decision making regarding liver transplantation in children with liver disease (CHF or Caroli syndrome) and ARPKD. Clearcut indications for combined liver and kidney transplantation in ARPKD included the combination of renal failure and either cholangitis or refractory complications of portal hypertension (including significant hepatopulmonary syndrome).

Surveillance

Decreased growth rate of children with CHF should be investigated as it is less likely to be the result of portal hypertension than of other associated problems, such as reduced renal function in patients with ARPKD. Extrapolating from studies in adults with cirrhosis, children with CHF may be screened for esophageal varices particularly when the platelet count decreases significantly over time or prior to interventions such as renal transplantation [21]. Small varices warrant a repeat esophagogastroduodenoscopy in a year. If no varices are identified, esophagogastroduodenoscopy should be repeated within 2–3 years. The appropriate frequency of surveillance imaging is not well defined and depends on disease severity.

For individuals with mild disease, ultrasound examination every 2 years would be adequate; for those with more severe disease, an annual ultrasound examination could enable adequate monitoring of disease progression. No data on surveillance for cholangiocarcinoma or hepatocellular carcinoma in this setting are available.

Genetic counseling

Once the diagnosis of CHF has been established in a proband, a family history focusing on hepatorenal fibrocystic disease, CHF/Caroli syndrome, liver or kidney disease of unknown etiology can be used to determine the inheritance pattern in an individual with CHF. If an autosomal recessive syndrome is not identified in the proband and/or the findings and/or family history suggest autosomal dominant inheritance, then ultrasound examination of parents and siblings to evaluate for the presence of asymptomatic kidney and/or liver disease characteristic of ADPKD is useful [20]. Other evaluations, including kidney function tests, and genetic testing may be useful to establish the specific hepatorenal fibrocystic disease associated with CHF based on the abnormalities identified on family history and physical examination.

Autosomal recessive polycystic kidney disease

Autosomal recessive polycystic kidney disease was once referred to as infantile polycystic disease. However, it has since been recognized in adults. It is estimated to occur in 1 in 6000–40 000 live births. Although ARPKD includes a spectrum of clinical and histopathologic manifestations, there are two constant features: (1) biliary tract abnormalities arising from DPM

(a) (b) (c)

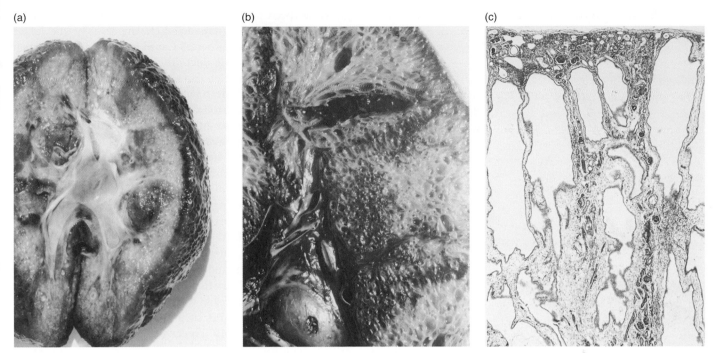

Figure 41.4 Autosomal recessive polycystic kidney disease. (a,b) The cut surface of the kidney demonstrates innumerable small opalescent cysts of fairly uniform size. (c) Microscopically, the cysts represent cystically dilated collecting ducts, arranged perpendicularly to the capsule.

and (2) fusiform dilatation of the renal collecting ducts. In 1971, Blythe and Ockenden [8] proposed subclassification into four genetic types based on age at presentation and severity of renal disease. However, variations in disease manifestations among siblings have been noted, suggesting that these distinctions are merely descriptive and do not represent different genetic subsets. So far, all cases studied have mapped to the *PKHD1* locus, at 6p21-p12. Whether isolated CHF without ARPKD also maps to this locus is not yet known. Fibrocystin/polyductin is the product of *PKHD1* [9,10].

In affected infants, the kidneys retain their natural shape and are massively enlarged. Macroscopically, the renal surface is studded with small opalescent cysts representing the fusiform dilatation of the collecting ducts (Figure 41.4a,b). Microscopically, the dilated collecting ducts are arrayed at right angles to the capsule, and the corticomedullary junction is obscured (Figure 41.4c). In contrast, the glomeruli and other nephron segments appear normal. With time, progressive interstitial fibrosis develops, resulting in a progressive decline of renal function. The hepatic lesion in ARPKD includes enlarged, irregularly fibrotic portal areas that contain tortuous and large bile ducts associated with persistence of the ductal plate. These histopathologic findings are indistinguishable from those of isolated CHF [14]. If the process leads to macroscopic dilatation of the intrahepatic biliary tree, it will fall into the category of Caroli syndrome (Figure 41.5). Clinically, just as in isolated CHF, the severity of the hepatic lesion varies inversely with age.

Hematemesis and melena herald the development of esophageal varices. Typically, children present with variceal bleeding at ages 5 to 13 years, but it has been reported in

infants [14]. The children may have firm hepatomegaly and splenomegaly in addition to nephromegaly. Blood urea nitrogen and serum creatinine values vary with the severity of renal involvement. Hepatic synthetic function, bilirubin, and aminotransferase values are generally normal. Anemia, leukopenia, and thrombocytopenia suggest associated hypersplenism. Although the disease phenotype is quite variable, many children have some degree of coexistent portal hypertension and chronic renal failure. The diagnosis is suggested by the clinical presentation and radiologic studies.

In the infant, ultrasound reveals massive, hyperechoic kidneys with loss of the corticomedullary junction and a variably enlarged, echogenic liver. In older children, kidney size and echogenicity are more variable, and macroscopic cysts may be evident. The liver findings by ultrasound, including Doppler studies, CT, and MRI are described in the earlier discussion on CHF. Definitive diagnosis may require renal and liver biopsies, but the diagnosis can be inferred from histology in one organ and typical sonographic findings.

Treatment for the hepatic lesions in ARPKD is the same as that described for CHF. The patients are at risk for ascending cholangitis with associated sepsis and hepatic failure; unexplained or prolonged fever may warrant diagnostic liver biopsy and culture. Although portal hypertension can be managed successfully and hepatic synthetic function is generally well preserved in ARPKD, liver transplant may be warranted in patients with chronic cholangitis. Many patients with ARPKD die in the perinatal period or during infancy from renal failure or pulmonary insufficiency. A long-term outcome study of neonatal survivors with ARPKD reported 1- and 5-year patient

(a)

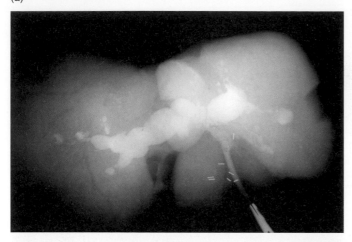

(b)

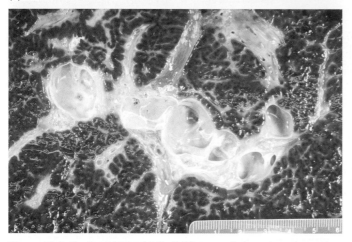

Figure 41.5 Caroli syndrome. (a) Cholangiogram of a hepatic explant with marked dilatation of the intrahepatic biliary tree. (b) Cut surface of the same liver showing both the cystic dilatation of the biliary tree and the fibrous bands throughout the liver consistent with congenital hepatic fibrosis.

survival rates of 85 and 82%, respectively, and renal survival at 5, 10, 20 years of 86, 71, 42%, respectively [22].

Caroli disease and Caroli syndrome

Caroli described two forms of congenital dilatation of the intrahepatic biliary tree associated with renal cystic disease [23]. In the more common type, the portal tract lesion is the ductal plate malformation typical of CHF. This entity is now referred to as Caroli syndrome. The second, much rarer type is characterized by pure ductal ectasia and is now called Caroli disease. These entities are more common in females. Both conditions are transmitted in an autosomal recessive fashion and are associated with ARPKD or, very rarely, with ADPKD [24]. Most choledochal cysts are not related to Caroli disease or syndrome, but predominant extrahepatic bile duct disease was found in four patients with ARPKD who underwent MRCP. All four patients had portal hypertension, although liver biochemistries did not suggest biliary disease [25].

It has been postulated that Caroli disease results from an arrest in ductal plate remodeling at the level of the larger intrahepatic bile ducts whereas Caroli syndrome results when the full spectrum of bile duct differentiation is affected, such that the smaller interlobular ducts are involved and CHF develops. Because some reports describe changes limited to the left hepatic lobe, Caroli disease has been described in some classification schemes as either diffuse or localized.

Presenting signs and symptoms include intermittent abdominal pain and hepatomegaly. Steatorrhea has been described. In Caroli syndrome, because the lesion of CHF is also present, evidence of portal hypertension is common and usually precedes cholangitis. In both Caroli disease and syndrome, ductal ectasia predisposes to bile stagnation, with consequent sludge and stone formation and risk of infection.

The age of presentation of Caroli syndrome is highly variable. Renal symptoms and cholestasis present in infancy, while cholangitis and manifestations of portal hypertension are more likely presenting features in early childhood. Diagnosis is confirmed by imaging studies such as abdominal CT, ultrasound (Figure 41.6a) and MR cholangiography (Figure 41.6b,c), which demonstrate irregular cystic dilatation of the large, proximal intrahepatic bile ducts.

Liver biopsy is rarely required to make the diagnosis of Caroli disease or syndrome. The pathologic findings of Caroli disease may show ectasia of the larger intrahepatic ducts with features of cholangitis. Intrahepatic bile duct ectasia and proliferation with severe periportal fibrosis are the pathological features of the CHF component of Caroli syndrome.

The differential diagnosis of Caroli syndrome and disease includes primary sclerosing cholangitis, recurrent pyogenic cholangitis, obstructive biliary dilatation, PLD, and choledochal cyst. The ductal dilatation in primary sclerosing cholangitis is usually isolated and fusiform in opposition to the characteristic saccular dilatation of Caroli syndrome and disease. It may be difficult to differentiate between PLD and Caroli syndrome, as in both diseases the patients can have hepatic and renal cysts. However, the hepatic cysts of PLD do not communicate with the usually normal bile ducts and portal hypertension is rare in PLD. Cholangitis, cholelithiasis, biliary abscess, septicemia, and cholangiocarcinoma are all potential complications of Caroli syndrome and disease. The increased risk of cholangiocarcinoma in these patients has been postulated to occur because of prolonged exposure of the ductal epithelia to high concentrations of unconjugated secondary bile acids and probably to recurrent cholangitis. Liver failure secondary to recurrent cholangitis or biliary cirrhosis, liver abscesses or complications of portal hypertension increase the mortality rate of these patients.

Therapy for Caroli syndrome is similar to that for CHF. Infection is managed with antibiotics and, in severe, localized disease, lobectomy of the affected lobe. In fact, partial hepatectomy also has been shown to be effective if the biliary lesion is predominantly confined to a discrete area [26]. Recently, Lendoire *et al.* [27] reported the long-term outcome of surgical

(a)

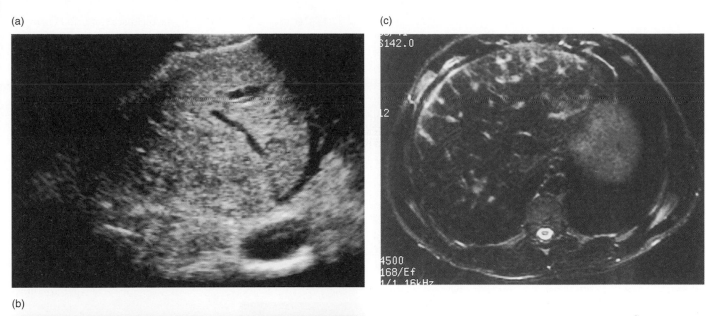

(b)

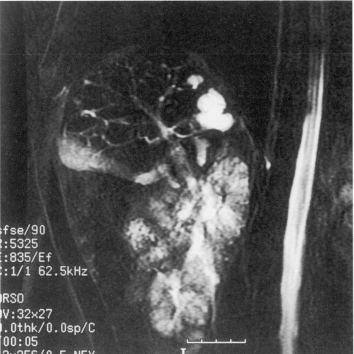

(c)

Figure 41.6 Radiographic findings in Caroli syndrome. (a) Ultrasound of the liver demonstrating a large posterior cyst and a prominently dilated intrahepatic bile duct. The hepatic echotexture is coarse and heterogeneous. (b) MR cholangiogram, coronal oblique view, in the same patient, demonstrating the cysts noted on ultrasound as well as more diffuse involvement of the intrahepatic bile ducts. (c) The composite transverse section provides even more detail about the extent of intrahepatic bile duct dilatation.

treatment of 24 adults with Caroli disease. They concluded that surgical resection was the best curative option in unilateral disease providing long-term survival free of symptoms and complications. Liver transplantation is recommended for bilobar disease with progressive decompensation of liver function and complications of portal hypertension or in the case of recurrent cholangitis and a suspicion of cholangiocarcinoma. Liver transplant may be indicated in infants as well. Kim *et al.* [28] described recently a 7-month-old infant with Caroli disease who underwent a successful liver transplantation for recurrent cholangitis and cirrhosis. Special issues exist in the decision making process regarding liver transplantation in

children with ARPKD. Indications for combined liver and kidney transplantation in ARPKD include the combination of renal failure and either recurrent cholangitis or refractory complications of portal hypertension [19]. Millwala *et al.* [29] published a study based on United Network for Organ Sharing data on 104 patients with Caroli disease/Caroli syndrome who received transplants between 1987 and 2006. They showed excellent patient and graft survival similar to, or better than, that of patients receiving transplants for other causes. The overall 1-, 3-, and 5-year graft survival rates (79.9%, 72.4%, and 72.4%, respectively) and patient survival rates (86.3%, 78.4%, and 77%, respectively) were excellent. For eight patients

(a)

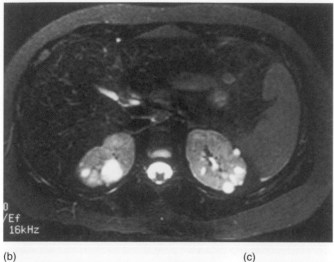

(b)

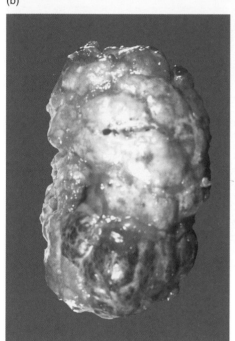

(c)

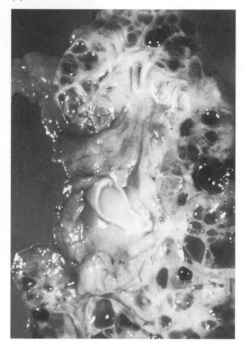

Figure 41.7 Autosomal dominant polycystic kidney disease. (a) MRI demonstrates the variability in size and distribution of the renal cysts, and the normal liver and biliary tree. There is a tiny hepatic cyst in the left lobe (tiny white dot) that does not appear connected to the biliary tree. (b) Resected kidney has multiple cysts deforming the capsule and obscuring the normal contour. (c) The cut surface demonstrates variable size and distribution of the cysts.

who received a combined liver/kidney transplantation, the 1-year patient and graft survival was 100%. Millwala *et al.* [29] have proposed an algorithm for evaluation and medical and surgical management of Caroli disease.

Autosomal dominant polycystic kidney disease

Bristowe [1] first described the association between hepatic and renal cysts in adults in 1856. Initially, this disorder was termed adult polycystic disease; subsequently, the nomenclature was changed to reflect the mode of genetic transmission. Autosomal dominant polycystic kidney disease occurs in 1 in 400–1000 individuals. It is the most common hereditary renal abnormality, affecting over 500 000 individuals in the USA; it accounts for 10% of all cases of end-stage renal disease [30].

Approximately 10% of patients with ADPKD will not have a positive family history of ADPKD and are presumed to have a new genetic mutation.

Like ARPKD, ADPKD is characterized by renal and hepatic cysts, but ADPKD is often associated with other visceral anomalies as well. These include intracranial and aortic aneurysms, mitral valve prolapse and other cardiac valvular defects, pancreatic cysts, colonic diverticula, and inguinal hernias [5]. ADPKD is rarely associated with CHF or Caroli syndrome; the more typical hepatic manifestation of ADPKD is PLD.

The kidneys in ADPKD contain numerous cysts of varying size in an irregular distribution, resulting in enlargement and distortion (Figure 41.7). In young children, the cysts are smaller and have a tendency to cluster; they occasionally involve the glomeruli as well as the collecting system. The kidneys of older children and adults have the more conventional findings of irregularly sized cysts distributed throughout the entire organ, with normal intervening renal parenchyma.

The symptomatic onset of ADPKD varies but is usually after age 40. Complications include systemic hypertension, hematuria, proteinuria, and pyelonephritis. In approximately 50% of patients with ADPKD, the renal lesion progresses to end-stage renal disease [5,30]. Infection, hemorrhage, and rupture can occur in both renal and hepatic cysts.

Generally, laboratory tests are of little diagnostic value. Elevations in blood urea nitrogen and serum creatinine, as well as diminution of urinary concentrating ability, are related directly to the severity of renal involvement. Serum alkaline phosphatase is elevated in 10–20% of patients, whereas serum aminotransferases and bilirubin values are usually normal. Diagnosis requires a careful family history, assessment of clinical symptoms and signs, and imaging techniques, such as ultrasonography or CT of the abdomen; MRI is a useful diagnostic modality to identify cyst infection, hemorrhage, or calcification. Renal ultrasound is normal in about 20% of patients at 20 years of age. In families in whom ADPKD has been identified, genetic linkage testing can be used to determine whether at-risk individuals are carrying the disease gene.

Mutation in one of two genes, *PKD1* or *PKD2*, lead to ADPKD, with *PKD1* mutations accounting for approximately 85% of cases. It is a very large, complex gene (46 exons) located on chromosome 16p13. It encodes the protein polycystin 1, which is a large membrane-bound protein with receptor-like properties that interacts with polycystin 2, the protein product of *PKD2*. Polycystin 1 is found throughout the body, including abdominal organs (kidneys, liver, pancreas), as well heart and vasculature. Its widespread presence helps to explain the multi-organ system phenotype. *PKD2* is a smaller gene (15 exons) located on chromosome 4q21-q23 and its mutations account for only 15% of ADPKD. Its product, polycystin 2, is a cation channel that modulates the concentration of intracellular calcium, an important determinant of several downstream signaling processes [31]. The polycystin 1/polycystin 2 complexes have a major influence on cell proliferation, adhesion, apoptosis, cell matrix interactions, differentiation, tubular patterning, and cell polarity. Therefore, it is expected that cell structure and function are severely disturbed in ADPKD, resulting in the formation of cysts. The characterization of the proteins altered in ADPKD further support the central role of the cilium in the pathogenesis of PKD [32,33]. Patients who have ADPKD are heterozygotes with one mutant and one wild-type allele. Therefore, it is proposed that a first-hit occurs with a germline mutation in *PKD1* or *PKD2* and that another somatic mutation in the wild-type allele is required to initiate cyst formation [34]. Hepatic cysts are present in about 50% of patients with ADPKD who have renal failure. Hepatic cysts increase in number and size with age but are uncommon in patients younger than 16 years of age [35]. Hepatic cystogenesis is influenced by estrogen, with the largest cysts observed in women who have been pregnant or who have used estrogens.

Hepatic cysts in ADPKD are derived from, but are not in continuity with, the biliary tract. There is little information on the effect of the type or position of mutations on the extent of hepatic cystic disease [36].

Treatment

Most patients with liver cysts do not need treatment. Patients with severe symptomatic disease require interventions to reduce cyst volume and hepatic size. The choice of procedure (percutaneous cyst aspiration with or without sclerosis, laparoscopic cyst fenestration, combined liver resection and cyst fenestration, and liver transplantation) is dictated by the anatomy and distribution of the cysts.

Combined percutaneous cyst drainage and antibiotic treatment provide the best treatment results for hepatic cyst infections. Long-term oral antibiotic suppression or prophylaxis is indicated for relapsing or recurrent infection. Fluoroquinolones and trimethoprim–sulfamethoxazole are effective against the typical infecting organisms and have good penetration into the biliary tree and cysts [37].

Von Meyenburg complexes (biliary microhamartomas)

Von Meyenburg complexes are microscopic lesions in the liver characterized by a discrete round or irregular-shaped cluster of small, often dilated bile ductules embedded in dense fibrous stroma. They also have been called biliary microhamartomas and may be found incidentally in otherwise histologically normal liver specimens. The ductular lumens within a complex are interconnecting. Often von Meyenburg complexes are seen in livers affected with CHF, Caroli syndrome, or PLD; in fact, they are suspected of being the cause of the last. From an embryologic perspective, these complexes appear to result from ductal plate malformation of the most peripheral interlobular bile ducts. The predominantly accepted hypothesis is that the ductal structures of von Meyenburg complexes originally communicated with the developing biliary tree but became separated through progressive dilatation, kinking, and surrounding fibrosis [38]. Although von Meyenburg complexes are common and generally asymptomatic, cholangiocarcinoma in association with these lesions have been reported in adults [39]. A possible preoperative imaging diagnosis of von Meyenburg complexes seems to depend on the size of the bile duct structure in each hamartoma. Although MRCP seems to be the best imaging tool [40], the diagnosis requires a careful histological examination showing cystic dilatation of bile ducts embedded in a fibrous stroma with no signs of malignancies.

Polycystic liver disease

Autosomal dominant PLD is a distinct clinical and genetic entity in which multiple bile duct-derived cysts develop and are unassociated with cystic kidney disease. Liver cysts arise from the dilatation of biliary microhamartomas (von

Meyenburg complexes) and from peribiliary glands. Cysts are rarely identified in children. The reported incidence of ADPLD is less than 0.01%. Patients are often asymptomatic, even with large cysts.

The liver cysts in PLD are usually macroscopic and vary in diameter, although they are rarely larger than 10 cm. They contain clear or blood-tinged fluid. The cysts tend to be distributed in or closely associated with the portal tracts, and the lining epithelia have a biliary phenotype. These hepatic cysts arise from progressive dilatation of the ductules in von Meyenburg complexes and they do not communicate with the biliary tree. Clinical manifestations include abdominal pain, abdominal mass, hepatomegaly, cyst infection with abscess formation, compression and obstruction of the biliary tree, cyst rupture, and bleeding. In extreme cases, hepatic replacement with resultant hepatic insufficiency may occur (Figure 41.8). In some instances, there are no symptoms at all, and the cysts are discovered incidentally by abdominal imaging or at autopsy.

There are no specific laboratory test abnormalities of ADPLD, and generally the liver synthetic function is maintained during all stages of the disease.

Management of PLD is somewhat controversial and often requires a combination of medical and surgical approaches. In many instances, no treatment is necessary. Somatostatin analogues have been used and were found to be effective reducing the volume of polycystic liver [41]. Another new medical option being evaluated is the use of mTOR inhibitors (sirolimus) that in animal models reduce the progression of cyst size. When cysts become infected, antibiotics alone are often ineffective and they should be used in conjunction with a percutaneous drainage procedure. For relief of pain or biliary compression, surgical approaches have included transhepatic fenestration (aspiration and surgical deroofing of the cyst) or a combination of fenestration and resection procedures. Fenestration also may be accomplished laparoscopically and provides symptomatic relief and reduction of liver size in some patients [42].

Hoevenaren *et al.* [43] have compared the clinical features of patients with isolated PLD with those of patients with polycystic liver and ADPKD. Patients with isolated PLD had greater numbers and larger sizes of liver cysts but had less associated morbidities than patients with ADPKD. Liver cyst decompressions were performed more frequently in patients with isolated PLD; however, serious hepatic complications, sufficient to require consideration of liver transplantation, were more frequent in patients with ADPKD. Liver transplantation is the only curative therapeutic options in patients with severe PLD. It is indicated in patients with extremely disabling symptoms that lead to a seriously decreased quality of life and in patients with complications of chronic liver disease such as portal hypertension [44].

Two genes have been associated with ADPLD, *PRKCSH* and *SEC63*, which encode the β-subunit of glucosidase II (also called hepatocystin) and SEC63, respectively [45].

(a)

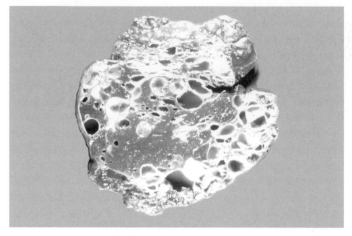

(b)

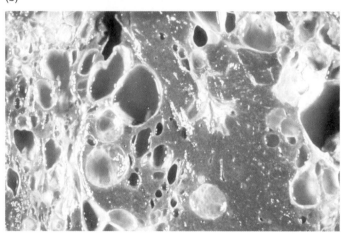

Figure 41.8 Polycystic liver disease. (a) The liver contains numerous cysts of varying size. The parenchyma appears compressed. (b) Close-up view shows thin-walled cysts, some containing mucoid clear fluid.

Hepatocystin is an acidic phosphoprotein known to be a substrate for protein kinase C and is involved in the proper folding and maturation of glycoproteins. It is localized to the endoplasmic reticulum. SEC63 is a component of the protein translocation machinery in the endoplasmic reticulum. It is uncertain how these proteins, which are involved in regulation of glycosylation in the endoplasmic reticulum and possibly signal transduction, lead to the formation of hepatic cysts. However, a related observation is that one of the congenital disorders of glycosylation (CDG-Ib) is associated with a liver pathology reminiscent of CHF [46]. Therefore, glycosylated proteins are in some way important for maintaining the normal structure and function of the biliary tree. Recently, Jenssen *et al.* [47] found secondary, somatic mutations (second hits) in more than 76% of liver cyst epithelia among patients with ADPLD who had a heterozygous germline mutation in *PRKCSH*. They concluded that ADPLD is recessive at the cellular level, and loss of functional hepatocystin is an important step in cystogenesis.

Pathogenesis and animal models

Much of the work elucidating pathogenesis and genetic control of development of the liver and kidney has been done by studying humans and animals with genetic cystic renal disorders. The genetic information is summarized in Table 41.4. Three working hypotheses have been proposed to account for renal cyst development: (1) tubule obstruction, (2) defective basement membrane assembly, or (3) dysregulated epithelial proliferation. The weight of the experimental evidence from human and animal model studies suggests that dysregulated epithelial proliferation is of major importance [48]. Experimental evidence for the role of epithelial hyperplasia in renal cyst development includes: increased growth potential of cyst-derived epithelial cells, detection of epidermal growth factor in renal cyst fluid, and overexpression with apical mislocation of epidermal growth factor receptor in cystic kidneys. Animal studies have confirmed that transforming growth factor-α and epidermal growth factor are cystogenic in murine organ culture and that mice that overproduce transforming growth factor-α develop cystic kidneys. Experimental manipulation of epidermal growth factor receptor activity affects cyst development in vivo.

Tubular fluid hypersecretion is also observed in cyst development and has been attributed to the immature pattern of Na$^+$/K$^+$-ATPase distribution, with apical rather than basolateral expression of this enzyme, in cyst epithelia from both humans and mice.

Pathogenesis and identification of genetic influences on cyst development in the kidney and liver has been elucidated with murine models. The *Cpk* mouse mutant develops ARPKD and death from renal failure in the first weeks of life. The heterozygote has been noted to develop hepatic cysts. Abnormally elevated expression of the proto-oncogenes c-*Myc*, c-*Fos*, and c-Ki-*Ras* has been demonstrated in cystic kidneys from *cpk*$^{+/+}$ mice; this proto-oncogene expression far exceeds the extent of cell proliferation.

The intrinsic proliferative capacity of *Cpk* cystic cells and ADPKD cystic cells in mice is essentially the same as that of normal controls [49]. On the basis of these observations, it has been proposed that the elevated proto-oncogene expression reflects a maturational arrest in renal tubuloepithelial differentiation, which in turn leads to cyst formation [48]. In other words, cystic renal epithelia are unable to differentiate terminally, and their continued proliferation, albeit at a normal rate, results in cyst formation. Several other lines of evidence support this hypothesis. As discussed, in human ADPKD and ARPKD cystic epithelia, as well as *Cpk*$^{+/+}$ mice renal cysts, there are abnormalities in the membrane localization of the Na$^+$/K$^+$-ATPase and the epidermal growth factor receptor, consistent with a less differentiated cell phenotype. Another spontaneous mutation in mice, *Bpk*, results in the development of both massively enlarged kidneys with cysts and proliferative bile duct dilatation. The observation that the biliary epithelial hyperplasia in this animal was stimulated by epidermal growth factor provided additional evidence for the role of this system [50].

A novel animal model in which the responsible gene has been identified and characterized is the insertional transgenic *Ift88*^{Tg737Rpw} mutation, now called ORPK mouse. This mouse develops renal and hepatobiliary pathology similar to that seen in ARPKD/CHF. The mutant *Tg737* gene has been mapped to the mouse chromosome 14, and its human homologue to human chromosome 13. Although this location eliminates the possibility that this is the gene for human ARPKD/CHF, studies of the encoded protein have greatly added to understanding of its possible functions, as well as its interactions with other implicated gene products, such as polycystin 1. Of special interest to the understanding of the hepatic lesion is the model in which the renal disease is differentially corrected by experimental expression of the cloned wild-type complementary DNA (cDNA). These animals do not have the kidney disease but continue to have functional and histologic liver abnormalities. Liver epithelial

Table 41.4 Genetics of fibropolycystic liver and kidney disease

Fibrocystic disease	Incidence	Onset of symptoms	Gene (loci)	Gene product	Function of gene product
CHF (isolated)	Unknown	Childhood	Unknown	Unknown	Unknown
ARPKD with CHF	1/6000 to 1/40 000	Infancy	*PKHD1* (6p21-p12)	Fibrocystin	Unknown
ADPKD ± PLD	1/400 to 1/1000	Adulthood	*PKD1* (chromosome 16)	Polycystin 1	Cell–cell or cell–matrix interactions
			PKD2 (chromosome 4)	Polycystin 2	?Channel protein
			Other	Unknown	Ligand for polycystin 1 or 2?
PLD (isolated)	Unknown	Adulthood	*PRKCSH*	Hepatocystin	Subunit of glucosidase II
PLD		Adulthood	*SEC63*	Sec63	Protein translocation

CHF, congenital hepatic fibrosis; ARPKD, autosomal recessive polycystic kidney disease; ADPKD, autosomal dominant polycystic kidney disease; PLD, polycystic liver disease.

(a)

(c)

(b)

(d)

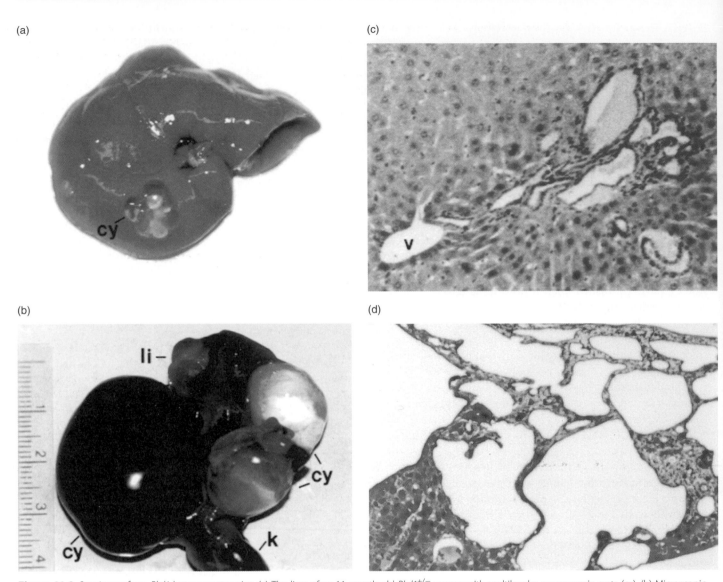

Figure 41.9 Specimens from *Pkd1* heterozygote mice. (a) The liver of an 11-month-old *Pkd1*$^{+/-}$ mouse with multilocular macroscopic cysts (cy). (b) Microscopic section of the liver reveals ductal plate malformation and cystic bile duct dilatation. (c) En bloc resection of the liver (li) and right kidney (ki). The liver contains many large cysts (cy). The kidneys are unremarkable. (d) Microscopic section of this liver reveals multiple back-to-back cysts.

cell lines from both wild-type and the mutant ORPK mice have been isolated and studied. The epithelial cells have morphologic and immunologic characteristics of oval cells, which are felt to be pluripotent hepatic stem cells of primitive bile duct origin. These characteristics include an immature pattern of gene expression and rapid proliferation. In culture, the cells give rise to dysplastic ductular structures. Transfection of the mutant cell line with wild-type *Tg737* cDNA decreases the proliferation rate, indicating that this gene controls proliferation and differentiation of oval cells into normal mature biliary epithelium. Further evidence for this role is the characterization of *Tg737* as a hepatic tumor suppressor gene [51].

The exact molecular pathogenesis of ADPKD is being elucidated. There are at least three genotypes resulting in virtually indistinguishable phenotypes.

A major advance in the understanding of the pathogenesis of cystic diseases has been the identification and characterization of the gene products of the best studied ADPKD genes, *PKD1* and *PKD2*. *PKD1* is the gene responsible for most cases of ADPKD. Targeted deletion of exon 34 in *Pkd1*, the mouse homologue of this gene, results in renal cysts and perinatal death in homozygotes. *Pkd1* heterozygote mice progressively develop renal and hepatic cysts (Figure 41.9). Hepatic cysts are observed in 27% of mice aged 9–14 months and 87% of older mice [52]. Human *PKD1* had been localized to chromosome 16, but the specific gene was elusive until a contiguous gene deletion was recognized in a family affected by both ADPKD and tuberous sclerosis. One family member had only tuberous sclerosis, and genetic analysis revealed the site of the translocation that disconnected the two disorders, allowing exact localization of *PKD1*. Its product, polycystin 1, has 4304 amino acid residues, a large extracellular domain, a membrane-spanning region, and a short intracellular region. The intracellular C-terminus has been demonstrated to interact with polycystin 2.

The physicochemical characteristics of polycystin 1 suggest that it is likely involved in cell–cell or cell–matrix interactions. Polycystin 1 has been localized to renal tubular epithelia, hepatic bile ductules, pancreatic ducts, and cerebral blood vessels, tissues known to be affected in ADPKD. Expression of polycystin is greater in fetal than adult tissue. When the immature cyst epithelia from patients with ADPKD were studied, overproduction of polycystin 1 was detected. In addition, monoclonality of the epithelial cells in a cyst has been demonstrated. Because ADPKD is a germline mutation but cyst development is sporadic and focal (in a patient or in a family), it has been postulated that a "second hit" injury to the normal allele is necessary to permit proliferation and cyst development. These second hits, which are obviously frequent given the manifestations of ADPKD, occur at the somatic level, explaining the phenotypic variability.

The gene product of *PKD2*, polycystin 2, is probably a channel protein, possibly a calcium channel signal. The demonstration of the interaction of polycystins 1 and 2 indicates that the phenotypic expression of ADPKD results from an abnormality in either gene, causing disruption of this interaction and subsequent abnormal regulation of the epithelial development. Loss of function of either protein results in the tubular cells reverting to a less differentiated state, which is more prone to proliferation. It has been postulated that the small proportion of ADPKD families without either the *PKD1* or *PKD2* mutations have an abnormality in the ligand or an intracellular partner of polycystins 1 or 2.

The primary cilium is a specialized sensory organelle that senses fluid flow and is found in many types of epithelial cell. Recent evidence indicates that polycystin 1 and polycystin 2 mediate the sensory process in the primary cilia of renal tubular cells [53]. Support for this putative mechanism of action is provided by the finding that the homologue in the ORPK mouse model of PKD is also localized to the primary cilium [54].

The affected gene in ARPKD is *PKDH1*. Twenty-nine mutations and 40 mutant alleles have been identified [9,10]. Mutations are scattered throughout the gene, and most *PKHD1* mutations are unique to single families. *PKDH1* is expressed during development of kidney, lung, liver, and CNS. Fibrocystin, the product of *PKDH1*, acts as a membrane-associated protein affiliated with the primary cilia in renal epithelial cells of mice and humans. This localization at the apical domain of polarized epithelial cells suggests that fibrocystin, like polycystin 1 and 2, may be involved in tubulogenesis or maintenance of duct-lumen architecture.

As yet, similar studies have not been conducted on human biliary tissues. However, disruption of *Pkhd1*, the rat homologue associated with the polycystic kidney rat model, results in abnormal ciliary morphology in biliary epithelium. Therefore, the observations in the kidney may perhaps be extended to the DPM model, with abnormalities in primary cilia function responsible for defective differentiation in both tissues. A number of researchers have hypothesized that DPM arise from an arrest in the terminal differentiation of the ductal plate epithelia. This hypothesis is entirely consistent with various single gene mutations in fibrocystin causing a spectrum of disease phenotype.

Disease progression in the human polycystic kidney diseases and the CHF/Caroli spectrum are all associated with variable degrees of necrotizing inflammation and fibrosis. In the liver, Desmet [3] postulated that one or more fetal antigens that are expressed on the immature biliary epithelium trigger an autoimmune response. In many cases, there is no apparent inflammation in the liver, so that the stimulus for the vigorous fibrogenesis is not known. Recently, studies in tissue homogenates from CHF liver samples demonstrated higher levels of thrombospondin 1 and transforming growth factor-β_1 compared with normal livers [55]. These cytokines are secreted by stellate cells, the most significant source of collagen in pathologic hepatic processes such as cirrhosis. The role of non-inflammatory stellate cell activation in the pathogenesis of fibrocystic liver disease requires further study.

A proposed maturational arrest in renal and biliary tubuloepithelial differentiation could serve as a single unifying hypothesis to explain the spectrum of disease phenotypes, the development of renal cysts, and the fibrosis associated with disease progression in ARPKD, CHF, and Caroli disease. However, although attractive, this construct is imperfect because it does not adequately address several issues in ADPKD and PLD: the less-abundant fibrosis, the temporal disparity between renal and liver cyst formation, and the variable disease course in affected infants versus affected adults. Some of these discrepancies might be explained by the type of mutations identified. More precise formulation requires further work in both the human diseases and animal models to identify the genetic factors controlling renal tubular and biliary differentiation and growth. With these molecular tools, the pathogenic mechanisms operative in this spectrum of disease may be further unraveled.

Raynaud *et al.* [56] have evaluated how DPMs develop in three mouse models, namely mice with livers deficient in hepatocyte nuclear factor (HNF) 6, HNF1b, or cystin-1 (the *Cpk* mutation leading to congenital polycystic kidney in mice). Human liver from a patient with a *HNF1B/TCF2* mutation, and from fetuses affected with ARPKD were also analyzed. They found that DPM and cyst formation in *Cpk* mice and human ARPKD results from dysmorphogenesis affecting the parenchymal and portal sides of developing ducts with normal differentiation but perturbed apicobasal polarity.

References

1. Bristowe C. Cystic disease of the liver associated with a similar disease of the kidneys. *Trans Pathol Soc Lond* 1856;7:229–234.

2. Jorgensen MJ. The ductal plate malformation. *Acta Pathol Microbiol Immunol Scand Suppl A* 1977;**257**:1–88.

3. Desmet VJ. Congenital diseases of intrahepatic bile ducts: variations on the theme "ductal plate malformation." *Hepatology* 1992;**16**:1069–1083.

4. Osathanondh V, Potter EL. Development of the human kidney as shown by microdissection. *Arch Pathol* 1963;**76**:277–302.

5. Gabow PA. Autosomal dominant polycystic kidney disease. *N Engl J Med* 1993;**329**:332–342.

6. Rogers TN, Woodley H, Ramsden W, Wyatt JI, Stringer MD. Solitary liver cysts in children: not always so simple. *J Pediatr Surg* 2007;**42**:333–339.

7. Kerr DNS, Harrison CV, Sherlock S, et al. Congenital hepatic fibrosis. *Q J Med* 1961;**30**:91–117.

8. Blythe H, Ockenden BG. Polycystic disease of the kidneys and liver presenting in childhood. *J Med Genet* 1971;**8**:257–284.

9. Onuchic LF, Furu L, Nagasaka Y, et al. PKHD1, the polycystic kidney and hepatic disease 1 gene, encodes a novel large protein containing multiple immunogloulin-like plexin-transcription-factor domains and parallel beta-helix 1 repeats. *Am J Hum Genet* 2002;**70**:1305–1317.

10. Ward CJ, Hogan MC, Rossetti S, et al. The gene mutated in autosomal recessive polycystic kidney disease encodes a large, receptor-like protein. *Nat Genet* 2002;**30**:259–269.

11. Rossetti S, Torra R, Coto E, et al. A complete mutation screen of PKHD1 in autosomal-recessive polycystic kidney disease (ARPKD) pedigrees. *Kidney Int* 2003;**64**:391–403.

12. Bergmann C, Senderek J, Windelen E, et al. Clinical consequences of PKHD1 mutations in 164 patients with autosomal-recessive polycystic kidney disease (ARPKD). *Kidney Int* 2005;**67**:829–848.

13. O'Brien K, Font-Montgomery E, Lukose L, et al: Congenital hepatic fibrosis and portal hypertension in autosomal dominant polycystic kidney disease. *J Pediatr Gastroenterol Nutr* 2012;**54**:83–89.

14. Srinath A, Shneider BL. Congenital hepatic fibrosis and autosomal recessive polycystic kidney disease: an analytic review of the literature. *J Pediatr Gastroenterol Nutr* 2012;**54**:580–587.

15. Adeva M, El-Youssef M, Rossetti S, et al. Clinical and molecular characterization defines a broadened spectrum of autosomal recessive polycystic kidney disease (ARPKD). *Medicine* 2006;**85**:1–21.

16. Summerfield JA, Nagafuchi Y, Sherlock S, et al. Hepatobiliary fibropolycystic disease: a clinical and histological review of 51 patients. *J Hepatol* 1986;**2**:141–156.

17. Zerres K, Senderek J, Rudnik-Schöneborn S, et al. New options for prenatal diagnosis in autosomal recessive polycystic kidney disease by mutation analysis of the *PKHD1* gene. *Clin Genet* 2004:**66**:53–57.

18. Akhan O, Karaosmanoğlu AD, Ergen B. Imaging findings in congenital hepatic fibrosis. *Eur J Radiol* 2007;**61**:18–24.

19. Shneider BL, Magid MS. Liver disease in autosomal recessive polycystic kidney disease. *Pediatr Transplant* 2005;**9**:634–639.

20. Gunay-Aygun M, Gahl WA, Heller T. Congenital hepatic fibrosis overview. In Pagon RA, Bird TD, Dolan CR, Stephens K (eds.) GeneReviews. Seattle, WA: University of Washington, Seattle, 1993–.

21. Garcia-Tsao G, Sanyal AJ, Grace ND et al. Prevention and management of gastroesophageal varices and variceal hemorrhage in cirrhosis. *Am J Gastroenterol* 2007;**102**:2086–2102.

22. Bergmann C, Senderek J, Windelen E, et al. Clinical consequences of PKHD1 mutations in 164 patients with autosomal-recessive polycystic kidney disease (ARPKD). *Kidney Int* 2005;**67**:829–848.

23. Caroli J, Couinaud C, Soupault R, et al. Une affection nouvelle, sans doute congénitale, des voies biliaires: la dilatation cystique unilobaire des canaux hépatiques. *Sem Hop Paris* 1958;**34**:136–142.

24. Jordan D, Harpaz N, Thung SN. Caroli's disease and adult polycystic kidney disease: a rarely recognized association. *Liver* 1989;**9**:30–35.

25. Goilav B, Norton KI, Satlin LM et al: Predominant extrahepatic biliary disease in autosomal recessive polycystic kidney disease: a new association. *Pediatr Transplant* 2006;**10**:294–298.

26. Raymond M-J, Huguet C, Danan G, et al. Partial hepatectomy in the treatment of Caroli's disease. *Dig Dis Sci* 1984;**29**:367–370.

27. Lendoire JC, Raffin G, Grondona J, et al. Caroli's disease: report of surgical options and long-term outcome of patients treated in argentina. multicenter study. *J Gastrointest Surg* 2011;**15**:1814–1819.

28. Kim RD, Book L, Haafiz A, et al. Liver transplantation in a 7-month-old girl with Caroli's disease. *J Pediatr Surg* 2011;**46**:1638–1641.

29. Millwala F, Segev DL, Thuluvath PJ. Caroli's disease and outcomes after liver transplantation. *Liver Transplant* 2008;**14**:11–17.

30. Welling LW, Grantham JJ. Cystic and developmental diseases of the kidney. In Brenner BM, Rector FC Jr (eds.) *The Kidney.* Philadelphia, PA: Saunders, 1991, pp. 33–36.

31. Macrae Dell K. The spectrum of polycystic kidney disease in children. *Adv Chronic Kidney Dis* 2011;**18**: 339–347.

32. Zhou J. Polycystins and primary cilia: primers for cell cycle progression. *Annu Rev Physiol* 2009:**71**:83–113.

33. Gascue C, Katsanis N, Badano JL. Cystic diseases of the kidney: ciliary dysfunction and cystogenic mechanisms. *Pediatr Nephrol* 2011;**26**:1181–1195.

34. Wilson PD. Polycystic kidney disease: new understanding in the pathogenesis. *Int J Biochem Cell Biol* 2004;**36**: 1868–1873.

35. D'Agata ID, Jonas MM, Perez-Atayde AR, et al. Combined cystic disease of the liver and kidney. *Semin Liver Dis* 1994;**14**:215–228.

36. Gunay-Aygun M. Liver and kidney disease in ciliopathies. *Am J Med Genet C Semin Med Genet* 2009;**151C**:296–306.

37. Torres VE, Harris PC, Pirson Y. Autosomal dominant polycystic kidney disease. *Lancet* 2007;**369**:1287–1301.

38. Desmet VJ. Ludwig symposium on biliary disorders: part I. Pathogenesis of ductal plate abnormalities. *Mayo Clin Proc* 1998;**73**:80–89.

39. Burns CD, Kuhns JG, Wieman TJ. Cholangiocarcinoma in association with multiple biliary microhamartomas. *Arch Path Lab Med* 1990;**114**:1287–1289.

40. Nagano Y, Matsuo K, Gorai K, *et al.* Bile duct hamartomas (von Mayenburg complexes) mimicking liver metastases from bile duct cancer: MRC findings. *World J Gastroenterol* 2006;**12**: 1321–1323.

41. van Keimpema L, Nevens F, Vanslembrouck R, *et al.* Lanreotide reduces the volume of polycystic liver: a randomized, double-blind, placebo-controlled trial. *Gastroenterology* 2009;**137**:1661–1668.

42. Kabbej M, Sauvanet A, Chauveau D, *et al.* Laparoscopic fenestration in polycystic liver disease. *Brit J Surg* 1996;**83**:1697–1701.

43. Hoevenaren IA, Wester R, Schrier RW, *et al.* Polycystic liver: clinical characteristics of patients with isolated polycystic liver disease compared with patients with polycystic liver and autosomal dominant polycystic kidney disease. *Liver Int* 2008;**28**:264–270.

44. Drenth JP, Chrispijn M, Nagorney DM, *et al.* Medical and surgical treatment options for polycystic liver disease. *Hepatology* 2010;**52**:2223–2230.

45. Drenth JP, Tahvanainen E, te Morsche RH, *et al.* Abnormal hepatocystin caused by truncating *PRKCSH* mutations leads to autosomal dominant polycystic liver disease. *Hepatology* 2004;**39**:924–931.

46. Jaeken J, Matthijs G, Saudubray J-M, *et al.* Phosphomannose isomerase deficiency: a carbohydrate-deficient glycoprotein syndrome with hepatic: intestinal presentation. *Am J Hum Genet* 1998;**62**:1535–1539.

47. Janssen MJ, Waanders E, Te Morsche RH, *et al.* Secondary, somatic mutations might promote cyst formation in patients with autosomal dominant polycystic liver disease. *Gastroenterology* 2011;**141**:2056–2063.

48. Calvet JP. Polycystic kidney disease: primary extracellular matrix abnormality or defective cellular differentiation? *Kidney Int* 1993;**43**:101–108.

49. Carone FA, Nakanura S, Schumacher BS, *et al.* Cyst-derived cells do not exhibit accelerated growth or features of transformed cells in vitro. *Kidney Int* 1989;**35**:1351–1357.

50. Nauta J, Sweeney WE, Rutledge JC, *et al.* Biliary epithelial cells from mice with congenital polycystic kidney disease are hyperresponsive to epidermal growth factor. *Pediatr Res* 1995;**37**:755–763.

51. Isfort RJ, Cody DB, Doersen CJ, *et al.* The tetratricopeptide repeat containing *Tg737* gene is a liver neoplasia tumor suppressor gene. *Oncogene* 1997;**15**:1797–1803.

52. Lu W, Fan X, Basora N, *et al.* Late onset of renal and hepatic cysts in Pkd1-targeted heterozygotes. *Nat Genet* 1999;**21**:160–161.

53. Nauli SM, Alenghat FJ, Luo Y, *et al.* Polycystins 1 and 2 mediate mechanosensation in the primary cilium of kidney cells. *Nat Genet* 2003;**33**:129–137.

54. Pazour GJ, Dickert BL, Vucica Y, *et al. Chlamydomonas* IFT88 and its mouse homologue, polycystic kidney disease gene *tg737*, are required for assembly of cilia and flagella. *J Cell Biol* 2000;**151**:709–718.

55. El-Youssef M, Mu Y, Huang L, *et al.* Increased expression of transforming growth factor-β_1 and thrombospondin-1 in congenital hepatic fibrosis: possible role of the hepatic stellate cell. *J Pediatr Gastroenterol Nutr* 1999;**28**:386–392.

56. Raynaud P, Tate J, Callens CA *et al.* Classification of ductal plate malformations based on distinct pathogenic mechanisms of biliary dysmorphogenesis. *Hepatology* 2011;**53**:1959–1966.

42

Tumors of the liver

Dolores López-Terrada and Milton J. Finegold

Introduction

The rarity and diversity of liver tumors in children means that no one medical center or group of physicians has adequate experience to deliver optimal care to every patient. Hence cooperative study groups have been essential in establishing diagnostic criteria, identifying prognostic factors, assembling new biologically important molecular data, and introducing and evaluating chemotherapy and other treatments.

The most significant development related to liver tumors in children since the third edition of this text was published [1] is the creation of an international consortium (European Société Internationale d'Oncologie Pédiatrique–Epithelial Liver Tumor Study International Society of Pediatric Oncologie (SIOPEL)) to gather epidemiologic, clinical, pathologic, and therapeutic data from existing national and regional registries [2]. The first report from the transplant arm of this group, PLUTO (Pediatric Liver Unresectable Tumor Observatory), in 2010 included 70 patients enrolled in the first 3 years from 36 centers in 17 countries [3]. As of January 2012, the PLUTO database had registered 170 patients, of whom 158 had received primary transplants: 127 with hepatoblastoma (HB), and 26 with hepatocellular carcinoma (HCC).

The clinical presentation of the vast majority of liver tumors in children is an asymptomatic palpable mass. The liver's functional capacity is rarely compromised by underlying cirrhosis. Most malignancies are large and may be difficult to excise without prior chemotherapy. Involvement of the perihilar segments or intrahepatic dissemination may necessitate transplantation. The vascularity of the liver and ready access of cancer cells to hepatic veins make pulmonary metastasis at presentation relatively common. Therefore, knowledge of precursor conditions and screening can be life saving.

Approximately two-thirds of all liver masses occurring in children are malignant. Twenty separate series totaling 1972 primary benign and malignant liver tumors in children from 1956 to 2001 included HB (37%), HCC (21%), benign vascular

Table 42.1 Hepatic tumors in childhood

Primary tumors	No. (%)
Hepatoblastoma	737 (37)
Hepatocellular carcinoma	422 (21)
Adenoma	50 (2.5)
Focal nodular hyperplasia	94 (5)
Benign vascular tumors	190 (15)
Mesenchymal hamartoma	133 (7)
Sarcoma (embryonal, angio, rhabdo)	156 (8)
Other	90 (4)

Data from Weinberg and Finegold, 1983 [4] and Stocker, 2001 [5].

tumors (15%), mesenchymal hamartomas and sarcomas (8%), adenomas and focal nodular hyperplasia (7.5%), and other tumors (4%) [4,5] (Table 42.1).

Epidemiology

Approximately 1.1% of all childhood tumors in the USA are malignant liver tumors according to the Surveillance, Epidemiology, and End Results (SEER) program of cancer registries, with an annual incidence rate of 1.8 per 1 000 000 children younger than 15 years [6]. Of 123 children registered with malignant liver tumors in 2000, 80% had HB and they accounted for 91% of the primary hepatic malignancies in children younger than 5 years [7]. Primary liver tumors accounted for 6–8% of congenital tumors in 265 neoplasms discovered within 30 days of birth [1].

The mean age at diagnosis was 19 months and the median age was 16 months in the Pediatric Oncology Group (POG) series of 106 HB accrued on biologic studies, similar to findings in other studies [7]. Only 5% occurred in children older than 4 years. Although rarely, HB has been reported in adults. It is slightly more common in males with a reported male: female ratio of 1.4–2.0:1 [7].

Liver Disease in Children, Fourth Edition, ed. Frederick J. Suchy, Ronald J. Sokol, and William F. Balistreri. Published by Cambridge University Press. © Cambridge University Press 2014.

Table 42.2 Constitutional genetic syndromes leading to liver tumors

Disease	Tumor type	Chromosome location	Gene
Familial adenomatous polyposis	HB, HCC, adenoma, biliary adenoma	5q21.22	*APC* (adenomatous polyposis coli)
Beckwith–Wiedemann syndrome	HB, vascular lesions–hemangioendothelioma	11p15.5	Cluster of genes, *P57KIP2*
Li–Fraumeni syndrome	HB, undifferentiated sarcoma	17p13	*TP53*:others
Trisomy 18	HB	18	–
Glycogen storage diseases types I–IV	HB, HCC, adenoma	Several	–
Hereditary tyrosinemia, type 1	HCC	15q23–25	*FAH* (encoding fumarylacetoacetate hydrolase)
Alagille syndrome	HCC, cholangiocarcinoma	20p12	*JAGGED1*
Other familial cholestatic syndromes	HCC, cholangiocarcinoma	18q21–22:2q24	*ATP8B1* (encoding FIC1), *ABCB11* (encoded bile salt export protein)
Neurofibromatosis	HCC, malignant schwannoma, angiosarcoma	17q11.2	*NF1*
Ataxia telangiectasia	HCC	11q22–23	*ATM* (ataxia telangiectasia mutated)
Fanconi anemia	HCC, fibrolamellar carcinoma, adenoma	1q42:3p,20q13.2–13.3:others	*FAA*, *FAC* (Fanconi anemia complementation group A and C) others (20%)
Tuberous sclerosis	Angiomyolipoma	9q34:16p13	*TSC1*, *TSC2* (tuberous sclerosis complex 1 and 2)
Simpson–Golabi–Behmel syndrome	HB and others (Wilms)	Xq26:Xp22	*GPC3* (encoding glypican 3)

HB, hepatoblastoma; HCC, hepatocellular carcinoma.

Data from several sources have shown an increase in the number of cases of HB since the 1970s. In the SEER data comparing the periods 1973–1977 with 1993–1997, rates per million for HB increased from 0.6 to 1.2, and for pediatric HCC they decreased (0.45 to 0.29) [7]. In the period 1979–1981, liver cancers represented 2% of all cancers in infants younger than 1 year, whereas a decade later, liver cancers increased to 4% of all cancers in infants.

A higher incidence of malignant liver tumors in children has been seen in Africa and Asia, where hepatitis B virus (HBV) infection is common. It is not surprising that almost all of the tumors are HCC because this tumor has been most closely correlated with hepatitis viral infection. Perinatally acquired HBV has also been demonstrated to have integrated into the genome in tumors from children with no clinical signs of present or past HBV infection. It is encouraging that aggressive immunization programs against hepatitis viruses have resulted in a decrease in the number of cases [8].

Hepatocellular carcinoma occurs primarily after age 10 years and is the most common hepatic malignancy of adolescence. In children 15–19 years of age, HCC accounted for 87% of all malignant liver tumors, although 12.8% occurred in children under age 5 years [7]. Patients with the fibrolamellar variant of HCC are more likely to be over 10 years of age [9].

Etiology

The causes of most liver tumors, similar to other types of childhood cancer, are unknown: HB occurs in association with several well-described cancer genetic syndromes (Table 42.2). The strong association of HB with prematurity may account for part of the observed increase in HB overall, as survival rates continue to increase among very small premature infants. In Japan, HB account for 58% of all malignancies occurring in surviving premature infants who weighed <1000 g at birth [1]. The Japanese Children's Cancer Registry data revealed that 15 of 303 (5%) cases of HB between 1985 and 1995 occurred in postpremature infants weighing <1500 g. The relative risk for infants weighing <1000 g at birth was 15.64 compared with 2.53 for infants weighing 1000–1499 g and 1.21 for infants weighing 2000–2499 g. These data have been widely confirmed, with a relative risk of 56.9% in New York State from 1985 to 2001 [10]. They indicate the need to determine the specific factors related to prematurity that contribute to hepatic tumorigenesis, as well as the need for surveillance of the survivors of extreme prematurity. Of all pediatric cancers, only retinoblastoma and non-astrocytic gliomas had a slightly increased relative risk in a US cohort of many thousand premature infants surviving to age [11], suggesting that a role of the liver in metabolism and handling of endogenous hormones and exogenous toxins while growing rapidly makes it particularly vulnerable to early birth. To date, no differences have been found in age of onset or histopathologic type of HB in small prematures versus term births.

Several studies have explored relationships between perinatal and maternal factors other than congenital syndromes and low birth weight and HB. One study documented a potential link with maternal pre-eclampsia and eclampsia [12]. Environmental factors have also been implicated in HB. An association with certain occupational exposures in fathers of children with HB has been reported [1]. These include excess exposures to metals such as in welding and soldering fumes (odds ratio, 8.0), petroleum products, and paints (odds ratio, 3.7). A prenatal exposure to acetaminophen in combination with petroleum products has also been noted in association with HB. Parental cigarette smoking has also been reported to be associated with an increased risk of developing HB, doubled if both parents smoked relative to neither parent smoking. A slightly increased risk was found in the New York study for mothers younger than 20 years of age, smokers, presumed use of infertility treatment, and higher maternal body mass index [10]. Cirrhosis following parenteral nutrition in infancy has been associated with the development of HCC in childhood [1]. Understanding the role that parenteral nutrition, which is clearly life saving for many premature infants, plays in the observed increase in the subsequent development of liver cancer in premature infants will await additional epidemiologic and pathophysiologic studies.

Constitutional genetic and metabolic abnormalities

Associations of liver tumors in children with genetic syndromes are summarized in Table 42.2.

Beckwith–Wiedemann syndrome (BWS) is caused by genetic abnormalities in chromosomal region 11p15 and a risk of diverse intra-abdominal embryonal tumors. The National Cancer Institute's BWS Support Group data indicate a relative risk of HB as 2280, higher than that for other embryonal tumors, including Wilms tumor [1]. The recognition of physical stigmata of BWS in an infant prompts surveillance for detection for embryonal tumors using serial abdominal sonography and serum α-fetoprotein (AFP) measurements, and this has proven beneficial to early resection. Vascular proliferations and mesenchymal hamartoma in the liver are also observed in BWS and have been misdiagnosed as HB because of serum AFP elevation (Figure 42.1). A significantly higher risk of neoplasia was recently reported in association with certain molecular subtypes of BWS, particularly patients with uniparental disomy and imprinting control element defects [1]. Patients with hemihypertrophy carry a higher risk of developing HB, which has also been reported in association with other overgrowth syndromes, particularly the Simpson–Golabi–Behmel syndrome, an X-linked overgrowth syndrome caused by deletions in GPC3, encoding glypican 3 [13].

The association of HB with familial adenomatous polyposis was first reported in 1982. This syndrome is caused by germline mutation of the gene APC (adenomatous polyposis coli). There is an estimated relative risk of 800 of HB in children in families with familial adenomatous polyposis compared with the general population [1]. In 50 children with apparently sporadic HB, five were found to have a constitutional mutation in APC [14]. Rare somatic mutation of APC have also been identified in HB, much less common than CTNNB1 mutations (gene encoding β-catenin), found in a majority of sporadic HBs. The interaction of APC protein and β-catenin, and relevance of the canonical WNT pathway activation in the pathogenesis of HB, are discussed later in this chapter. There are no definitive differences in age range, histologic type, or outcome in HB associated with familial adenomatous polyposis. Familial adenomatous polyposis has also been implicated in the pathogenesis of some hepatocellular adenoma, HCC, and fibrolamellar carcinoma, suggesting that mutated APC may confer a general low-level predisposition to tumorigenesis in the liver dependent on other environmental or developmental factors.

Children with hereditary tyrosinemia type I (fumarylacetoacetate hydrolase deficiency) have a very high incidence of HCC, which has been dramatically reduced by blocking the accumulation of toxic metabolites [15]. Glycogen storage diseases are also associated with the development of adenomas (Figure 42.2a,b) and occasionally HCC [15], and HCC and cholangiocarcinomas have been observed in patients with the Alagille syndrome and other familial cholestatic syndromes (Figure 42.2c–f) [16]. Many but not all of these are also associated with liver dysfunction and cirrhosis of the liver. The chronic cholestasis resulting from extrahepatic biliary atresia has preceded both HCC and HB in children. A 2-year-old child with HB and progressive familial intrahepatic cholestasis has also been documented [17]. We have seen three cases of HB in 2-year-old children with autosomal recessive polycystic kidney disease.

Diverse liver tumors have been reported in association with trisomy 18, neurofibromatosis, tuberous sclerosis, and ataxia–telangiectasia [1]. Hepatic tumors occurring in patients with Fanconi anemia who are treated with anabolic steroids demonstrate how a genetic defect in DNA repair coupled with an exogenous agent may contribute to the development of neoplasia. In some cases, tumor regression has been observed with the withdrawal of steroids.

Clinical presentation

The typical age of presentation of the various hepatic tumors, both benign and malignant, is shown in Table 42.3. Yolk sac tumors, primary endocrine neoplasms, and inflammatory myofibroblastic tumors are very rare and occur in adults more often than children. Most liver tumors present with an asymptomatic abdominal mass. Abdominal pain, weight loss, anorexia, nausea, and vomiting may be present, particularly in

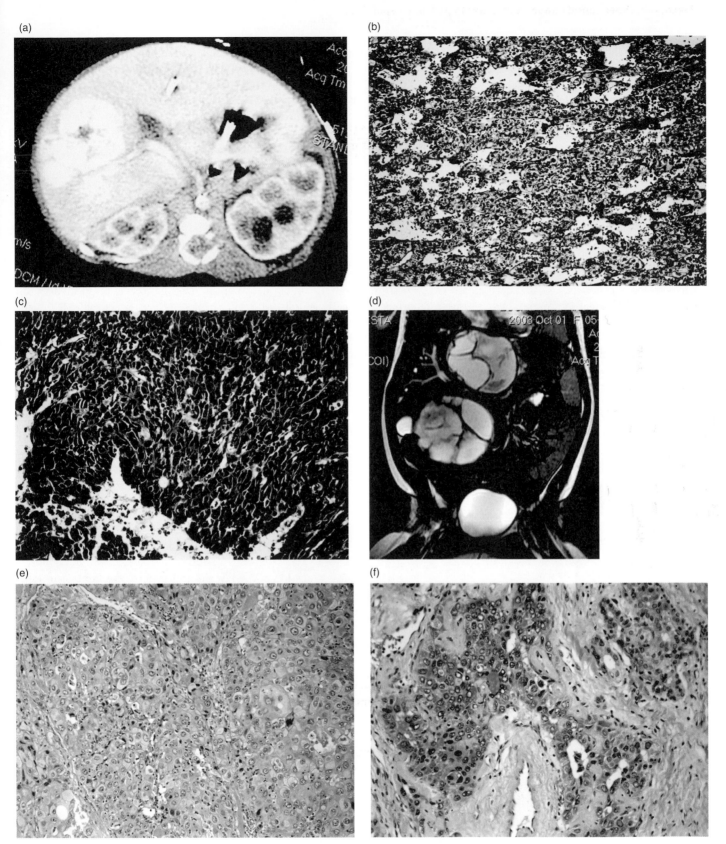

Figure 42.1 Hepatic tumors in Beckwith–Wiedemann syndrome. (a) CT at 1 week of age shows large enhancing mass and prominent hepatic artery. (b) Hemangioma with cavernous channels. No hepatocellular neoplasia. (c) Embryonal hepatoblastoma in an 8-month-old infant was detected by screening and cured by surgery and adjuvant chemotherapy. (d) Multicystic mass in the liver was biopsied at 1 month of age. It consisted of loose myxoid stroma blending with host parenchyma and contained a few clusters of immature hepatocytes and bile ducts as in (c). The serum α-fetoprotein at 1 year was 1306 ng/mL and MR imaging showed multiple heterogeneous masses (contributed by Dr. Stacey Berry, Banner Desert Medical Center, Mesa, AZ, USA). (e) Hepatocarcinoma in a resection from a child aged 3 years revealed diverse histology. The mesenchymal hamartoma had persistent biliary cysts embedded in a collagenous stroma. There were foci of small poorly differentiated cells with high nuclear-cytoplasmic ratio typical of embryonal hepatoblastoma, as in (c). Much larger, more pleomorphic and actively dividing cells are typical of hepatocarcinoma. (f) Cholangiocarcinoma. Neoplastic ductal elements representing a cholangiocarcinoma were also present. Review of the original biopsy revealed fetal hepatoblastoma.

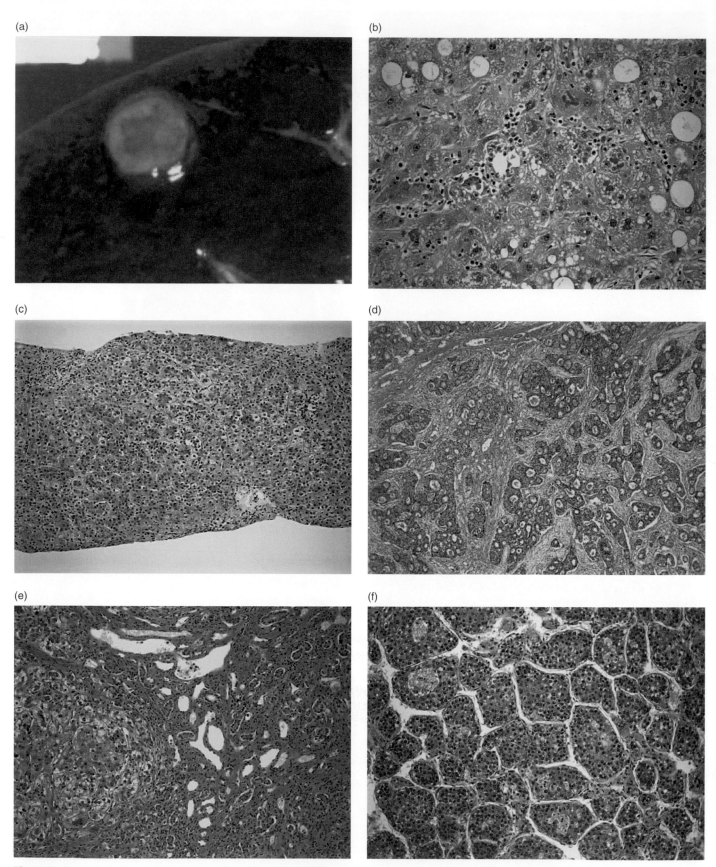

Figure 42.2 Metabolic diseases leading to neoplasia. (a) Adenoma in autopsy liver of a 12-year-old child with glycogen storage disease type IA (GSD-IA, glucose-6-phosphatase deficiency). (b) Adenoma in GSD-IA has "alcoholic hepatitis"-like histology with fat, Mallory bodies, and inflammation. (c) Alagille syndrome. Biopsy at 4 months of age showed bland cholestasis and paucity of the bile ducts. (d) Cholangiocarcinoma at age 8 years. (e) Biliary cirrhosis at age 29 months secondary to bile salt excretory protein deficiency (progressive familial intrahepatic cholestasis type 2). (f) Hepatocarcinoma found in explant.

Table 42.3 Neoplasia of the liver in children according to usual age of presentation

Age	Benign	Malignant	
		Primary	**Metastatic/systemic**
Infancy (0–1 year)	Hemangioendothelioma	Hepatoblastoma (small cell)	Langerhans cell histiocytosis
	Mesenchymal hamartoma	Rhabdoid tumor	Megakaryoblastic leukemia
	Teratoma	Yolk sac tumor	Metastatic neuroblastoma
Early childhood (1–3 years)	Hemangioendothelioma	Hepatoblastoma	Wilms
	Mesenchymal hamartoma	Rhabdomyosarcoma	Pancreaticoblastoma
	Inflammatory myofibroblastic tumor		
Later childhood (3–10 years)	Angiomyolipoma	Hepatocellular carcinoma, "transitional" hepatoblastoma[a]	Desmoplastic intra-abdominal small round cell tumor
	Adenoma	Embryonal (undifferentiated) sarcoma	
		Angiosarcoma	
		Nested stromal epithelial tumor	
Adolescence (10–16 years)	Adenoma (focal nodular hyperplasia)	Hepatocellular carcinoma[a] (fibrolamellar)	Hodgkin lymphoma
	Biliary cystadenoma	Leiomyosarcoma	
		Nested stromal epithelial tumor	

[a] Prokurat et al. [18] described a group of hepatocellular tumors of older children and adolescents, with an aggressive histopathology and clinical behavior, proposing the term, transitional liver cell tumors to denote these lesions.

advanced disease. Jaundice is rare and usually a symptom of extensive disease or hilar growth of any neoplasm with compression of the major bile ducts, such as inflammatory myofibroblastic tumor at the hilum or rhabdomyosarcoma, which arises in close association with larger ducts. Infants with hemangioendothelioma or hemangiomas associated with arteriovenous malformations may present with signs and symptoms of congestive heart failure [19]. In infants, diffuse hepatomegaly may occur secondary to transient myeloproliferative disorders or megakaryoblastic leukemia. In severe organ dysfunction, even the former may require chemotherapy. Disseminated neuroblastoma may also present as hepatic masses, as can Wilm's tumor.

Clinical symptoms of precocious puberty result from secretion of human β-chorionic gonadotropin or testosterone. The prognosis for seven children with HCC producing β-chorionic gonadotropin in Japan was very poor, with only one survivor. Cushing syndrome caused by adrenocorticotropic hormone-secreting hepatic malignancies with a distinctive nested pattern has been seen in four girls and one boy aged 11 and 12 years [19]. Large liver hemangiomas can be associated with profound hypothyroidism. Hypertension secondary to a renin-secreting mixed HB has been reported.

Liver enzymes and bilirubin are usually normal or only mildly elevated. A mild and normochromic normocytic anemia is common. Thrombocytosis occurs in approximately 50–80% of patients with HB and is probably related to thrombopoietin production by the tumor [19]. Mild coagulation abnormalities in children with malignant liver tumors are not unusual and a picture of a consumptive coagulopathy is sometimes associated with vascular malformations or a kaposiform hemangio-endothelioma (Kasabach–Merritt phenomenon).

Methods of diagnosis

Assessment of a liver tumor often begins with diagnostic imaging by plain film or ultrasound, which reveals a right upper quadrant mass. Calcifications are seen only in a minority of patients and are non-specific and plain films are of very limited value in characterizing hepatic masses. Increased echogenicity is suggestive of malignant disease, and the diagnostic yield is increased when accompanied by Doppler flow studies to assess tumor vascularity. However, ultrasound is not adequate to definitively establish resectability [20]. To define the extent of disease accurately, CT is used (Figure 42.3a). Particularly in infants, none of the imaging techniques currently available has 100% specificity. Of 26 children under age 3 months, six were inappropriately treated in the German cooperative liver tumor study because of imaging misinterpretations. Use of MRI with enhancement may provide additional information and reduce exposure of young children to ionizing radiation (Figure 42.3b) [20]. Typical imaging features for HCC are early arterial enhancement and possibly an isodense appearance compared with the surrounding liver in

(a)

(b)

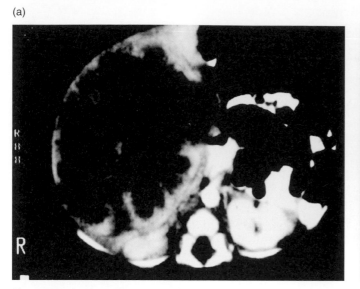

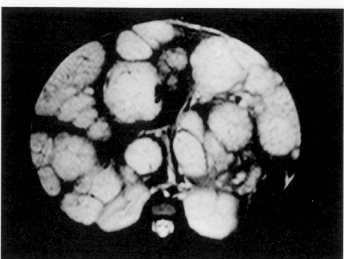

Figure 42.3 Imaging of liver tumors. (a) CT is used to demonstrate resectability of liver tumors. This patient was asymptomatic except for hepatomegaly at 5 days of age. Hepatoblastoma was resectable. (b) T_1-weighted MRI of multifocal hemangioendothelioma shows marked contrast enhancement after gadolinium (see Figure 42.15b).

the venous and delayed phases of four-phase multidetector CT (the non-contrast, arterial, venous, and delayed phases) or in dynamic contrast-enhanced MRI. These radiologic findings are related to increased vascularity of the tumor, supplied by the hepatic artery. For recurrent or metastatic HB, positron emission CT with [^{18}F]-fluorodeoxyglucose has proved to be more sensitive than MRI or CT [21]. Intrahepatic vascular dissemination of HCC is more common than for HB (Figure 42.4a), but both neoplasms have this propensity (Figure 42.4b). The most common site for metastases is the lung (Figure 42.4c), whereas metastases to the brain have been reported but are extremely rare. Therefore, CT imaging of the chest, abdomen, and pelvis is essential. When bone lesions are reported, it is unclear whether these represent true metastases or areas of osteopenia, and bone marrow involvement has only very rarely been observed.

Serum AFP is markedly elevated in more than 90% of patients with HB and in two-thirds of those with HCC [1]. It is also elevated in germ cell tumors with yolk sac components, a few of which arise in the liver. The major protein produced by the fetal liver, AFP is produced in large amounts in the newborn. In the normal term infant, serum AFP level can be as high as 100 000 ng/mL or greater. The half-life of AFP is 5–7 days and it falls throughout the first several months of life (Table 42.4). By age 1 year, the serum AFP is <10 ng/mL. However, it remains elevated in two genetic diseases that lead to HCC: heredity tyrosinemia type I and ataxia-telangiectasia. In BWS, it serves, along with periodic abdominal ultrasound, to detect the early onset of HB. In infants younger than 1 year with HB, it may initially be difficult to distinguish the contribution to elevated AFP from reactive, normal liver from that of malignant tumor. However, serum AFP is a useful tumor marker to assess response to therapy as well as to monitor for disease recurrence [1]. After a complete resection, serum

AFP levels should decline and approach normal ranges within several days to weeks (Table 42.5). Failure to do so indicates residual disease.

α-Fetoprotein is usually normal with small cell undifferentiated HB and infantile rhabdoid tumor, the fibrolamellar variant of HCC, as well as in most benign liver tumors. However, significantly elevated AFP has been reported in patients with infantile hemangioendothelioma and mesenchymal hamartoma, which has misled clinicians into treating for HB without confirmatory diagnostic biopsy [1,22]. When serum AFP was combined with ultrasonography to screen high-risk adults in China, a 5-year survival rate of 62.7% was achieved in those with HCC ≤5 cm in diameter versus larger ones, which had a 37.1% rate. Des-γ-carboxyprothrombin level in the serum is a marker of advanced HCC, and higher levels before transplantation indicate a poor prognosis.

The potential clinical use of glypican 3 oncofetal protein (GPC3) as a second diagnostic marker for HCC and HB has been reported recently. Glypican 3, a heparan sulfate proteoglycan anchored to the membrane, is expressed at markedly elevated levels in HCC, HB, and fetal liver but is undetectable in normal hepatocytes and non-malignant liver disease; however, it may also be present in embryonal sarcoma and mesenchymal hamartoma of the liver [23]. Various studies have demonstrated that glypican 3 could be used as a serologic test for the diagnosis of patients with HCC and recommended simultaneous measurement of both glypican 3 and AFP for HCC screening for improved sensitivity.

Staging

The conventional staging system for HB used by the US Children's Oncology Group (COG) is shown in Table 42.6. Stage I is defined as a tumor completely resected at

(a)

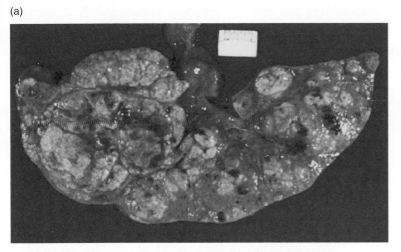

(b)

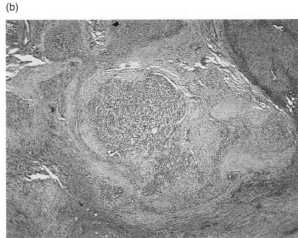

(c)

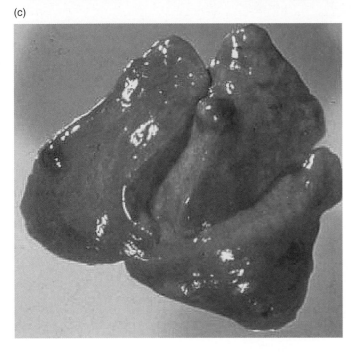

Figure 42.4 Dissemination of hepatic neoplasms. (a) Hepatocellular carcinoma in an 8-year-old child with perinatally acquired hepatitis B infection. (b) Embryonal hepatoblastoma in hepatic vein. (c) Stage IV hepatoblastoma with pulmonary metastases. This is the usual reason for treatment failure, but some patients have been saved by resection.

diagnosis. Stage II refers to resection with microscopic residual disease. Stage III indicates gross residual disease, including involvement of local lymph nodes and inability to resect the primary tumor. Stage IV tumors are those with distant metastases. In the most recent COG study (P9645; from 1999 to 2001), 44 of the 153 registered cases of HB (29%) were stages I and II, and 5 (3.4%) were stage I with "favorable" histology not requiring chemotherapy [1]. Only 15 (10%) were stage IV, with lung disease at diagnosis, versus 20% in the 1990–1994 SIOPEL-1 study [2]. In the US intergroup series, HCC was amenable to primary resection only 17% of the time but seven of the eight children with stage I disease were 5-year survivors.

The staging system developed by SIOPEL is based on the number of liver segments involved [25] (Figure 42.5). This pretreatment classification scheme (PRETEXT) is intended to

determine resectability by ultrasonography and CT preoperatively. This system divides the liver into four sectors: an anterior and a posterior sector on the right and a medial and a lateral sector on the left. Staging groups are assigned according to tumor extension within the liver as well as the presence or absence of involvement of the hepatic vein, portal vein, regional lymph nodes, or distant metastases. When the PRETEXT stage preoperatively was compared with the pathologic examination of specimens resected following chemotherapy, there was only 51% agreement, with 37% of 91 specimens overstaged by imaging and four patients with positive resection margins that were missed [25]. The current COG study of HB stratifies patients according the postsurgical staging system but will also attempt to validate the PRETEXT staging system with respect to tumor resectability and outcome [24].

Table 42.4 Physiologic serum α-fetoprotein levels

Age	Mean ± SD (ng/mL)
Premature	134 734 ± 41 444
Newborn	48 406 ± 34 718
Newborn to 2 weeks	33 113 ± 32 503
Newborn to 1 mo	9452 ± 12 610
2 months	323 ± 278
3 months	88 ± 87
4 months	74 ± 56
5 months	46.5 ± 19
6 months	12.5 ± 9.8
7 months	9.7 ± 7.1
8 months	8.5 ± 5.5

Table 42.6 Staging of hepatoblastoma by the Children's Oncology Group

Stage	
I	Favorable histology: completely resected with pure fetal histologic pattern and low mitotic index (<2/10 high-power fields) (stratum 1)
	Other histology: completely resected tumors with a histologic picture other than pure fetal with low mitotic index (stratum 2)
II	Grossly resected tumors with evidence of microscopic residual Resected tumors with preoperative (intraoperative) rupture (stratum 2)
III	Unresectable tumors: considered by the surgeon not to be resectable without undue risk to the patient Lymph node involvement is considered to constitute stage III disease and may require evaluation with a second laparotomy after initial courses of chemotherapy (stratum 3)
IV	Tumors with a measurable metastatic disease to lungs or other organs (stratum 3)

Children's Oncology Group [24].

Pathology

A protocol for the examination of HB specimens published by the College of American Pathologists in 2007 offers guidance relevant to all pediatric liver tumors [26]. It emphasizes the need to obtain fresh frozen samples of tumor and host liver, before and after chemotherapy, to facilitate molecular investigations for new treatments. A primary hepatic neoplasm, whether benign or malignant, is typically an expansile solitary mass (Figure 42.6). Multiple lesions are found in some hemangiomas and hemangioendotheliomas, adenomas, HCC, and rarely HB. Encapsulation is limited to some adenomas, although

Table 42.5 Estimated number of days for elevated α-fetoprotein to decline to normal levels (<10 ng/mL)

Initial level (ng/mL)	Time (days) for decline with presumed half-lives		
	5 days	7 days	10 days
10	5	7	10
20	10	14	20
40	15	21	30
80	20	28	40
160	25	35	50
320	30	42	60
640	35	49	70
1280	40	56	80
2560	45	63	90
5120	50	70	100
10 240	55	77	110
20 480	60	84	120

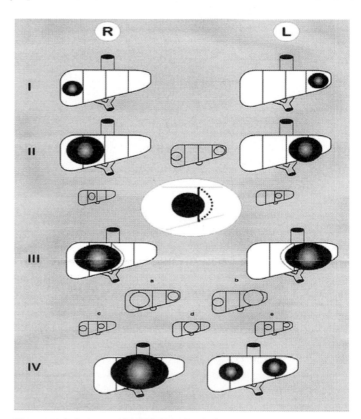

Figure 42.5 Staging in the PRETEXT scheme for preoperative evaluation of extent of tumor in the liver.

pseudocapsules secondary to compressive atrophy of the adjacent parenchyma can be deceptive with respect to an operative margin. Spontaneous focal necrosis of the rapidly growing HB is common, and many of these have large

(a)

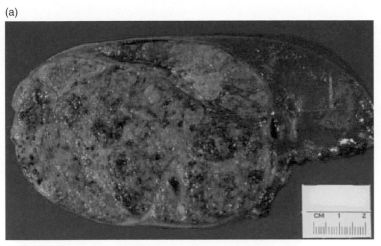

(b)

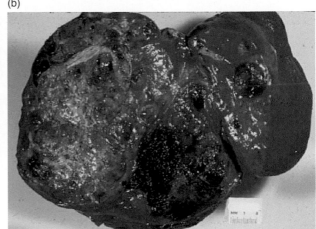

(c)

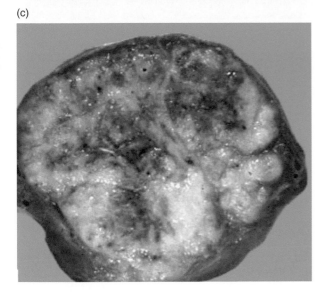

Figure 42.6 Gross appearance of hepatoblastoma. (a) Most of this tumor was composed of well-differentiated fetal hepatoblasts, and tan-brown like normal liver. (b) Mixed hepatoblastoma with embryonal, fetal, and mesenchymal tissues, with hemorrhage and necrosis. (c) Small cell undifferentiated hepatoblastoma is sarcoma-like, fleshy, moist and gray–white.

telangiectatic vessels, both of which account for highly diverse images and Doppler patterns and may lead to erroneous diagnosis, particularly in infants, when the serum AFP level does not reflect the expected values [25]. Metastatic spread of HB and HCC occurs via hepatic veins to the lungs and secondarily to the brain (Figure 42.4). Intravascular dissemination is frequent, but current chemotherapy can successfully eradicate tumor confined to the liver and even some that have metastasized [2].

Hepatoblastomas arise from precursors of mature hepatocytes and most tumors display many histologic patterns reflecting diverse stages of differentiation (Table 42.7). Embryonal histology is most common and resembles the histology of the liver at 6–8 weeks of gestation (Figure 42.7a,b). Well-differentiated neoplastic fetal hepatocytes may be virtually indistinguishable in cytologic and architectural growth pattern from the normal fetal liver (Figure 42.7c). The cytoplasm is often rich in glycogen and sometimes contains neutral fats. Nuclear–cytoplasmic ratio is typically slightly higher than non-neoplastic host hepatocytes. Cholangioblastic, or ductular,

differentiation (Figure 42.7d) has been reported, and this rare occurrence suggests origin from a precursor cell.

Hepatoblastomas may contain undifferentiated small cells that coexpress cytokeratin and vimentin, reflecting neither epithelial nor stromal differentiation (Figure 42.8). Whether the small undifferentiated cell is equivalent to a "stem" cell or the "oval" cell of the rodent liver is controversial [1]. Diverse immunohistochemical markers have led investigators to opposite conclusions. Rarely, the entire HB is composed of only one cell type; 2.0% of the 377 cases reviewed for the POG and COG from 1986 to 2005 that could be resected without chemotherapy (stages I and II) were small cell undifferentiated, whereas 3.4% were pure well-differentiated fetal with minimal mitotic activity (Table 42.8). The remainder were mixtures of diverse epithelial cells in varying proportions and of cells intermediate among the broad categories, with either discrete nodules of a single cell type or intimate intermingling of diverse cytologies (Figure 42.8b). This feature makes it difficult to predict behavior on the basis of a small biopsy of an unresectable tumor, and chemotherapy affects the diverse

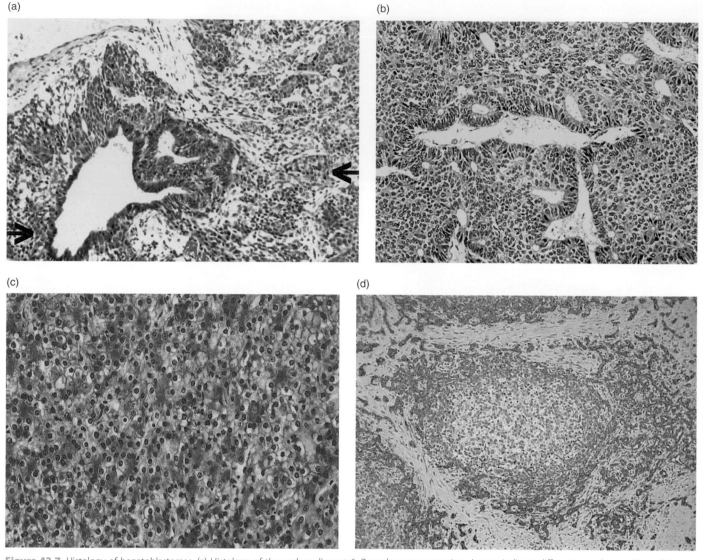

Figure 42.7 Histology of hepatoblastomas. (a) Histology of the embryo liver at 6–7 weeks postconception. Arrows indicate differentiating hepatoblasts. (b) Embryonal hepatoblastoma. Mimicry of the stages of development is the basis for tumor designations. A continuum between tumor types is, therefore, typical of hepatoblastoma. (c) Pure fetal hepatoblastoma. The uniformity of these mature mitotically inactive cells growing in a normal cord-like manner may make them difficult to distinguish from normal hepatocytes in aspirates or small biopsies. The greater nuclear/cytoplasm is helpful, as is immunohistochemistry (Figure 42.11). (d) Cholangioblastic hepatoblastoma. Cytokeratin 7 is stained in the proliferative bile ductular cells while hepatoblasts are unstained.

components differently. Well-differentiated fetal cells having significant mitotic activity (>2 in 10 high-power microscopic fields; Figure 42.9) very rarely occur in "pure" form except in small biopsies of stages III and IV tumor. They have been referred to as "crowded" fetal cells because glycogen content is usually less and the proportion of an image occupied by nuclei is consequently increased [1]. Fifteen percent of HB is classified as "mixed" because of stromal derivatives, particularly osteoid-like protein deposits, occasional rhabdomyoblasts, and, even more rarely, chondroid elements (Figure 42.10a). The osteoid-like foci become more prevalent following chemotherapy when the embryonal cells are often eradicated (Figure 42.10b) [28]. The efficacy of cis-platinum-based chemotherapy often makes it difficult to determine the

persistence of viable HB in resection specimens, for which immunohistochemistry for β-catenin and glypican 3 can be very helpful (Figure 42.11).

The designation "teratoid" is used for 3% of HB where some cells reflecting neural or neural crest origin are present. These include glial cells, neurons, and melanocytes (Figure 42.10c). True teratomas arising in the liver of infants have a full range of tissues from all embryonic germ layers, including brain-like and extraembryonal derivatives such as yolk sac and trophoblastic cells. Sometimes the distinction can be difficult when histology is the only available diagnostic tool (Figure 42.10d).

Rarely, enteroendocrine derivatives containing chromogranin and diverse hormones, such as gastrin, serotonin, or

Table 42.7 Classification of hepatoblastoma

Major categories	Epithelial
	Fetal, well differentiated (mitotically inactive, diploid)
	Crowded fetal (mitotically active)
	Embryonal
	Macrotrabecular
	Small cell undifferentiated
	Rhabdoid
	Mixed
	Osteoid stroma
	Undifferentiated mesenchymal-blastemal
Minor components	Ductal (cholangioblastic)
	Keratinizing squamous epithelium
	Intestinal glandular epithelium
	Neuroid–melanocytic (teratoid)
	Rhabdomyoblastic
	Chondroid

Table 42.8 Pediatric liver tumors by stage and histology

Tumor	Stage (No. (%))				Total
	I	II	III	IV	
Pure fetal	13 (3.7)		26	9	48 (14)
Fetal and embryonal	58	10	102	48	218 (64)
Small cell undifferentiated	1		6	1	8 (2)
Mixed epithelial/stomal	12		35	8	55 (16)
Teratoid	3	1	7	1	12 (3)
Rhabdoid			1	1	2 (0.5)
Totals	87 (25)	11 (3)	177 (52)	68 (20)	343

Pediatric and Children's Oncology Group, 1986–2005

somatostatin, are found in mixed HB and even more rarely as pure primary hepatic tumors. Small squamous pearls are frequent in mixed and teratoid tumors. Very rarely, glandular or ductal forms resembling the embryonal intestine or fetal bile ducts are found. Primary rhabdoid tumor of the liver has yet to be included among those reported to have deletions or mutations in the *hSNF5/INI1* tumor suppressor gene, as seen in CNS and renal and soft tissue primaries [29]. Expression of *WT1*, normally expressed in fetal kidney and mesoderm, has been reported in rhabdoid tumors, suggesting the potential role of WT1 in the process of mesodermal cells acquiring epithelial characteristics. Rhabdoid tumors share the coexpression of intermediate filaments with small cell undifferentiated HB, the onset in infancy, and poor prognosis (Figure 42.8c) [27,30]. A t(8;13) translocation has recently been documented in a malignant rhabdoid tumor of the liver. Although the name rhabdoid suggests a relationship to skeletal muscle, these tumors do not contain muscle proteins. True rhabdomyoblasts may be components of HB (Figure 42.10d) and there are full-fledged primary embryonal rhabdomyosarcomas of the liver that arise in close association to biliary epithelium, often having a polypoid growth pattern and causing obstructive jaundice.

When HB cells with either fetal or embryonal cytology grow in trabeculae of 20–100 or more cells rather than in the cords of 2–4 cells of the fetal liver, the pattern is called macrotrabecular. In our series, 18% of HB samples contained macrotrabecular foci, and one-third were stage IV at presentation [1]. This aggressive behavior may reflect the fact that such histology can be indistinguishable from HCC when it

occurs in pure form (Figure 42.12) [18]. Malignant tumors that have features of both HB and HCC have been observed in seven children with perinatally acquired HBV in our practice.

Hepatocarcinomas in children do not differ histologically from those in adults. The fibrolamellar variant (Figure 42.13a) occurs more commonly in adolescents and young adults. The presence of a central scar with radiating fibrous bands between tumor masses may suggests benign focal nodular hyperplasia (Figure 42.13b,c), but the histology is characteristic and the large atypical neoplastic cells are readily distinguished (Figure 42.13d). Unlike most hepatocarcinomas, fibrolamellar carcinomas arise in otherwise normal livers and for that reason are more readily resected and in many series have a higher rate of cure. However, children with fibrolamellar hepatocarcinomas do not have a more favorable prognosis and do not respond any differently to therapy from patients with typical HCC at the same stage [9]. Cholangiocarcinomas may occur in older children with antecedent cystic or cholestatic disease (Figure 42.2d). Like most adenocarcinomas, they are very resistant to treatment.

Solitary benign bile duct cysts are amenable to surgical excision. Twenty-nine children with a new variant of mixed tumor of the liver, the nested-stromal epithelial tumor, have been reported [19]; 18 were females aged 2–33 years, with 13 younger than 20 years at diagnosis. This tumor has a distinctive pattern of epithelial nests in a spindle-cell stroma, often with calcification or ossification, and a close association with bland-appearing bile ducts is observed (Figure 42.14). Five patients had a recurrence and one developed lung metastases a year after resection [31]. One patient had a Wilm tumor of the kidney following liver resection and others have had minor developmental genitourinary malformations. Six patients had clinical manifestations of Cushing syndrome, with immunochemical localization of adrenocorticotropic hormone in epithelial nests in some (Figure 42.14d).

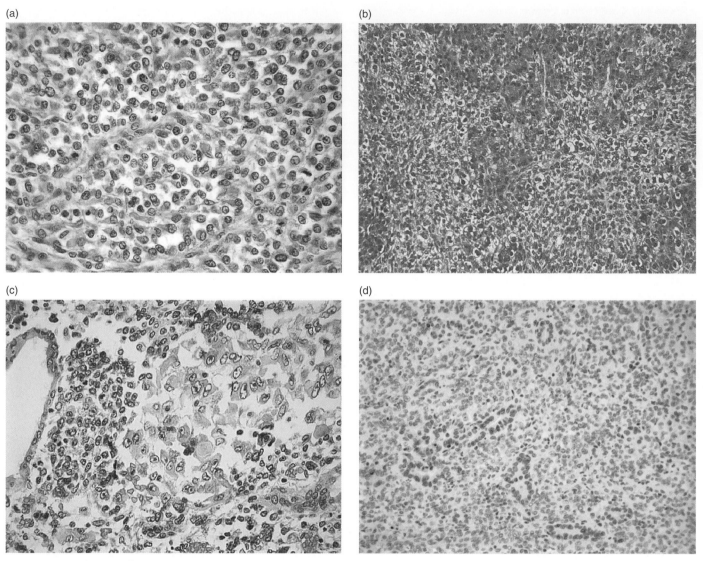

Figure 42.8 Small cell undifferentiated hepatoblastoma (SCU) and rhabdoid tumor. (a) When the proportion of these cells is high or they are the only component, they are usually found in infants and fail to respond to standard chemotherapy [27]. (b) Typically, small cells and fetal or embryonal hepatoblastoma are haphazardly intermingled so that small biopsies may not be representative of a large neoplasm's constituents. (c) Intimate association of SCU and rhabdoid tumor in an otherwise typical hepatoblastoma in a 7-month-old infant. Cells of both histotypes express cytokeratin and vimentin, intermediate filaments reflecting mesodermal–epithelial transition. (d) Nuclear expression of *INI* (ASMARC B1) is lost in rhabdoid tumors and the small cell hepatoblastomas of infancy. The entrapped bile ducts are positive. When otherwise indistinguishable cells are part of a typically pleomorphic hepatoblastoma as in (b), they are almost always positively stained.

Infantile hemangioendotheliomas (hemangiomas) are benign vascular tumors of the liver composed of thin vascular channels lined by a single layer of bland-appearing endothelial cells, which occur almost exclusively during the first year of life, sometimes associated with cutaneous and placental lesions. They are probably under-reported but accounted for more than 17% of all liver tumors in children and 40% of the benign tumors in the combined series (Table 42.1). They may be single or multicentric, well demarcated, or infiltrative (Figure 42.15a,b). Single lesions are usually self-resolving or cured by surgical resection. However, some of these tumors are large, multifocal, or present with clinical complications such as congestive heart failure or coagulopathy. The latter symptoms suggest the presence of an arteriovenous malformation (Figure 42.15c). These proliferative vascular lesions can be difficult to distinguish clinically and pathologically in an infant liver. They occurred with equal frequency in a 33-year period in Cincinnati [32]. In that series, hemangioendotheliomas occurred only in females, and all nine had positive expression of glucose transporter 1 on endothelial cells (Figure 42.15d). The proliferative capillaries associated with arteriovenous malformation were uniformly negative for glucose transporter 1. The only patient with concurrent angiosarcoma was a 5.5-year-old child with hemangioendothelioma. Highly proliferative vasoformative endothelium can be relatively avascular and deceptive by imaging, as well as worrisome with respect to aggressiveness (Figure 42.15e).

Epithelioid hemangioendotheliomas are rare neoplasms of intermediate malignant potential observed starting from the

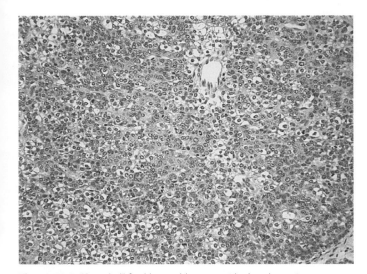

Figure 42.9 "Crowded" fetal hepatoblastoma with abundant mitoses. Whether stage I–II tumors with this or embryonal histology could have their postexcision adjuvant chemotherapy reduced or eliminated, as with the well-differentiated fetal tumors with minimal mitoses, is being evaluated in the current Children's Oncology Group trial [24].

(a)

second decade [33]. Often multinodular, they may be difficult to distinguish from metastatic adenocarcinoma because of their infiltrating growth in a fibrous stroma. Immunostains for CD34, CD31, and factor VIII serve to identify them (Figure 42.15f).

Angiosarcomas are rare and usually arise de novo, but a few have been reported in children as young as 4 and 5 years following biopsy or excision of benign hemangiomatous hamartomas in infancy or simultaneously in livers containing hemangioendotheliomas [19]. These highly infiltrative lesions disseminate widely within the liver (Figure 42.16) and metastasize to lungs and lymph nodes.

Undifferentiated, or embryonal, sarcomas present in children aged 6–10 years, usually de novo. However, at least seven cases have been described subsequent to or contemporaneous with a benign infantile mass lesion, the mesenchymal hamartoma [34]. These sarcomas generally present as large expansile masses but infiltrate the adjacent parenchyma widely, sparing bile ducts, and spread via veins through the liver and to the lungs (Figure 42.17). Many of them contain

(b)

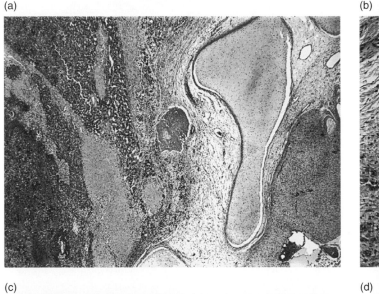

(c)

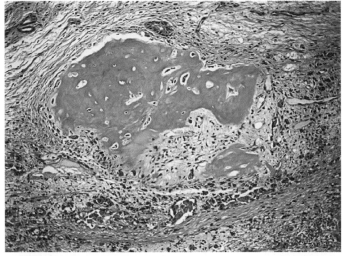

(d)

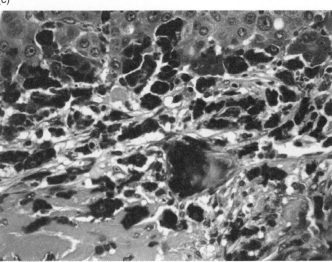

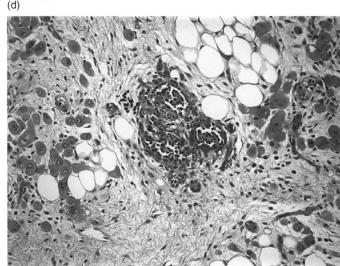

Figure 42.10 Mixed hepatoblastoma. (a) True bone and cartilage may be found. (b) Bone formation in mixed hepatoblastoma. It is particularly abundant following chemotherapy. (c) Melanocytes along with glia and other neural derivatives that invoke the designation "teratoid." (d) When organoid differentiation occurs, as with this fetal kidney, the question of true teratoma arises. The primitive glomeruli and tubules are surrounded by fetal rhabdomyoblasts.

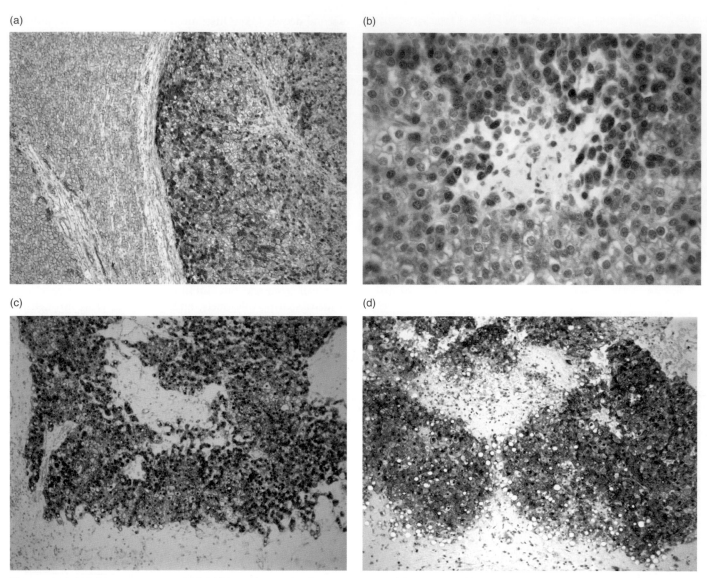

Figure 42.11 Helpful immunostaining. (a) Fetal hepatoblastoma has β-catenin staining of the nuclei in addition to the plasma membranes, just as in normal hepatocytes on the left. (b) In less mature cells, the protein is abundant in the cytoplasm, and in embryonal cells it is present in nuclei, where it contributes to the expression of several WNT pathway genes. The difference can be exploited in evaluation of a stage I tumor for chemotherapy. (c) Following chemotherapy, nuclear β-catenin can identify persistent cancer cells. (d) Glypican 3 in the cytoplasm is likewise very valuable for this purpose.

diverse elements displaying maturation of mesenchymal derivatives, including vessels, pericytes, smooth muscle, lipomatous and fibrohistiocytic features, in addition to large bizarre cells with irregular processes and multiple cytoplasmic globular inclusions containing secretory proteins such as α_1-antitrypsin (Figure 42.17c).

Mesenchymal hamartomas arise mainly in infants as typically single expansile masses composed of cystic spaces lined by either biliary epithelium or endothelial cells in a loose myxoid stroma (Figure 42.18). They may contain hemangiomatous foci, rarely leading to congestive failure and possibly reflecting origin from a vascular accident in utero that focally interfered with hepatocyte differentiation and growth (Figure 42.18d) [1]. Another hamartoma of the liver is the angiomyolipoma, a feature of tuberous sclerosis. There have been a few examples

in children, not all of whom have had confirmed tuberous sclerosis [1]. This is most often a tumor of adult females and can be difficult to distinguish from hepatocarcinoma on imaging and in fine-needle aspirates. The antibody to homatropine methylbromide, which stains the adipocytes and myoblasts of the hamartoma but not hepatocytes, has proved useful in the examination of fine-needle aspirates and biopsies. Two with aggressive behavior in children have been reported recently.

Hepatocellular adenoma is a benign tumor occurring in older children and adolescents that may prove problematic on imaging and in fine-needle aspiration cytology [2]. The increased incidence and hemorrhaging seen when oral contraception was first introduced have subsided with reduction of the estrogen content. Adenomas consist of nodular

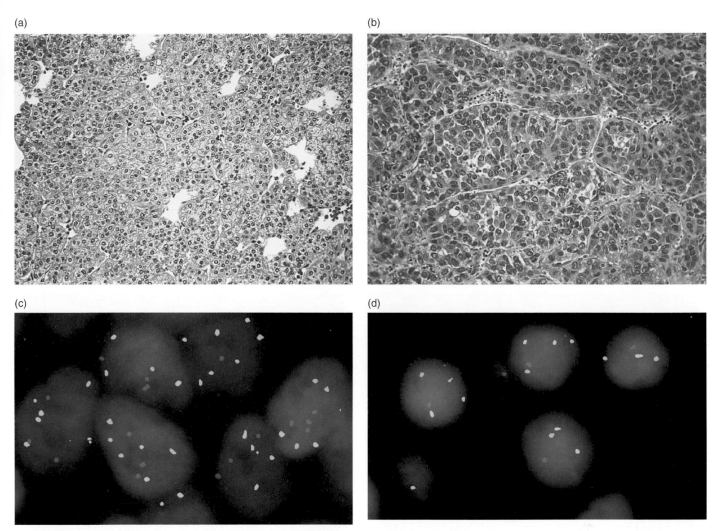

Figure 42.12 Distinguishing hepatoblastoma and hepatocellular carcinoma. (a,b) Macrotrabecular growth patterns can make hepatoblastoma (a) and hepatocellular carcinoma (b) difficult to distinguish, particularly in fine-needle aspirates or small biopsy samples. In some children, even as young as 2 years, both neoplasms are present simultaneously, or sequentially following chemotherapy. In older children and adolescents with aggressive tumors, the term "transitional liver cell tumor" has been applied [18]. (c,d) Fluorescent in situ hybridization (FISH) analysis of macrotrabecular hepatoblastoma (c) using chromosomes 2 (aqua), 8 (green), and 20 (orange) enumeration probes, demonstrating trisomies of chromosomes 2 and 20, and of macrotrabecular hepatocellular carcinoma (d) demonstrating chromosomes 2 and 20 monosomies.

proliferation of hepatocytes in cords having no relationship to portal tracts and have a pushing border with the surrounding liver (Figure 42.2a). Adenomas may acquire fibrous capsules and some may have steatosis and even features of alcoholic hepatitis (Figure 42.2b). They may be difficult to distinguish from well-differentiated carcinoma, so immunohistochemistry (Figure 42.11) and molecular analyses can be decisive [35]. Bioulac-Sage and colleagues have separated hepatocellular adenomas in adults into two classes, based on 135 resected specimens. "Inflammatory" adenomas expressed serum amyloid A and C-reactive protein immunohistochemically, whereas those failing to express liver fatty acid-binding protein were presumed to have mutations in *HNFA* (encoding hepatocyte nuclear factor-α), either constitutionally or in the tumors. Only those with mutations of *CTNNB1* (encoding β-catenin) progressed to or were associated with HCC [35]. This study

had only a few younger patients with underlying glycogenosis or other predisposing conditions. A few cases of carcinoma arising in young adults with glycogen storage disease have been particularly confusing because even when these patients have multiple tumors, most are benign. [15]. Focal nodular hyperplasia is typically a single large mass in an otherwise healthy liver characterized by central scarring that radiates between multiple nodules of regenerating parenchyma (Figure 42.12b,c). Unlike the adenoma, bile ducts are present in distorted portal tracts and these lesions are not neoplastic or preneoplastic. They are sometimes associated with primary perfusion anomalies and with adenomas [19].

The relative infrequency of liver tumors in children means that few centers care for more than one or two malignant examples each year. Therefore, it is not surprising that 10.6% of 123 biopsies submitted for pathology review in a US

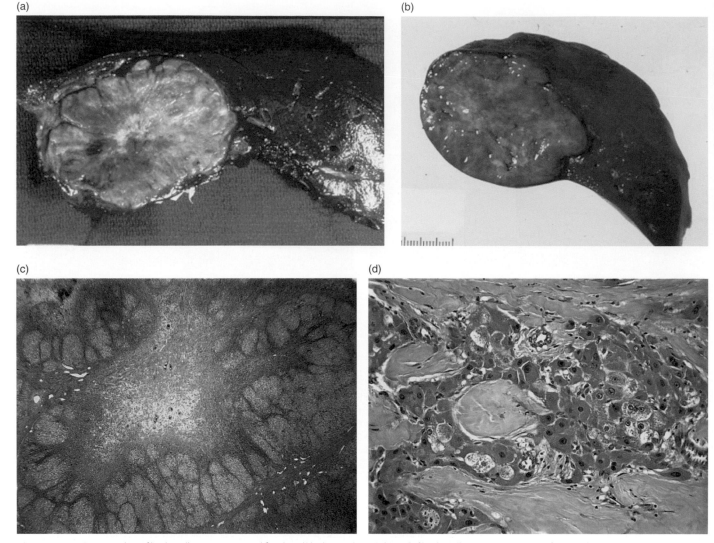

Figure 42.13 Distinguishing fibrolamellar carcinoma and focal nodular hyperplasia. (a,b) Both fibrolamellar carcinoma (a) and focal nodular hyperplasia (b) can have a central depression caused by scarring and occur in a non-cirrhotic host liver. (c) The hepatocytes surrounding a central scar in focal nodular hyperplasia are normal in appearance. (d) Histologically differentiating these is simple in that the large hypereosinophilic hepatocytes in the carcinoma are typically embedded in a dense fibrocollagenous stroma.

intergroup study were incorrectly interpreted. Among the errors were neuroblastoma, Wilms tumor, and choriocarcinoma [1]. Intra-abdominal desmoplastic small cell tumors and pancreaticoblastomas metastatic to the liver have also been misinterpreted as primary hepatic malignancies.

Acquired genetic abnormalities, hepatoblastoma, and other pediatric liver changes in tumors

Hepatoblastoma

Several acquired genetic abnormalities, molecular and epigenetic changes, have been reported in sporadic HBs [1]. Chromosomal abnormalities can be detected by conventional cytogenetic analysis in approximately half of HBs studied, with trisomies of chromosomes 2, 8, and 20 being the most frequent, followed by unbalanced translocations. A recurrent t(1;4)(q12; q34), translocation, and other translocations involving the long arm of chromosome 1 (1q), have been documented in a significant proportion of patients [36,37]. Genomic profiling studies, such as comparative genomic hybridization, have confirmed these abnormalities and suggest that gains of chromosomes 8, 20, and 2q24 region may be associated with an adverse prognosis [38,39]. Further studies will be needed to determine the importance of a number of amplified genes mapped to these chromosomal regions, such as *PLAG1*, which is located on chromosome 8q11.2-q13, the overexpression of which has been speculated to be responsible for upregulation of insulin-like growth factor 2 (IGF-2 (somatomedin A)) [40].

A better understanding of the oncogenic mechanisms responsible for HB comes from studies of normal liver

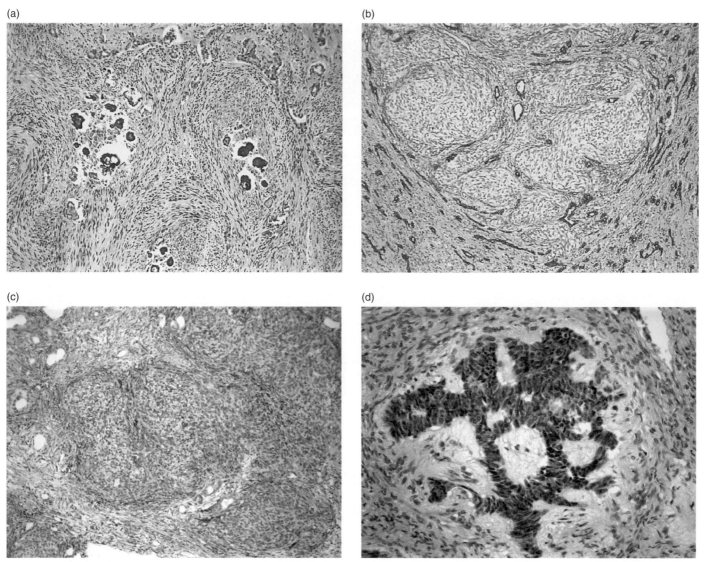

Figure 42.14 Nested stromal–epithelial tumor. (a) Epithelial nests within fibrous stroma. Some may calcify or ossify. The behavior of these tumors is difficult to predict with only 29 reported cases, but they grow very slowly, often to very large size, and may rarely metastasize. (b) Cytokeratin 7 staining reveals the intimate association of bile ductules and the neoplastic cells. This suggests a possible origin from an endocrine precursor. (c) Smooth muscle actin highlights the stromal component. (d) Adrenocorticotropic hormone is demonstrable in the epithelioid nests of females with Cushing syndrome.

development, as well as from understanding the oncogenic mechanisms responsible for other liver tumors [41].

Acquired genetic changes in HB may be shared by other embryonal tumors. An important tumor suppressor gene or growth factor gene located at 11p15.5 appears to be a factor in the development of embryonal tumors, and it is generally assumed but not proved that the critical gene lost is the same gene that is responsible for BWS. *p57KIP2* at 11p15.5 is a regulator of cellular proliferation and has been shown to be mutated in some families with BWS. Although not mutated, *p57K1P2* may be aberrantly expressed in HB. Another gene at that locus, *IGF2*, is preferentially expressed from the father in normal tissue. The parental allele-specific expression is variable in tumor tissue. *H19*, also at 11p15.5, shows the opposite pattern of expression of parental alleles, although the role of

this non-expressing gene in tumorigenesis is unclear. When losses of genetic material at 11p15.5 occur, the losses are always of maternal origin. This suggests that the loss of imprinting of genes, or differential function depending on parental origin, may have a role in the pathogenesis of HB. In HB that does not demonstrate loss of heterozygosity at 11p15.5, the differential expression of genes is lost, with expression from both parental alleles. Promoter-specific imprinting of *IGF2* has been demonstrated in HB and fetal human liver, and correlation between methylation changes in *IGF2* P3 promoter and expression has been observed in primary tumors and HB cell lines. Another gene located on 11p15.5 is *BWR1A*, encoding a transmembrane transporter, highly expressed in liver, paternally imprinted, and found to be mutated in a rhabdomyosarcoma cell line, making it a possible

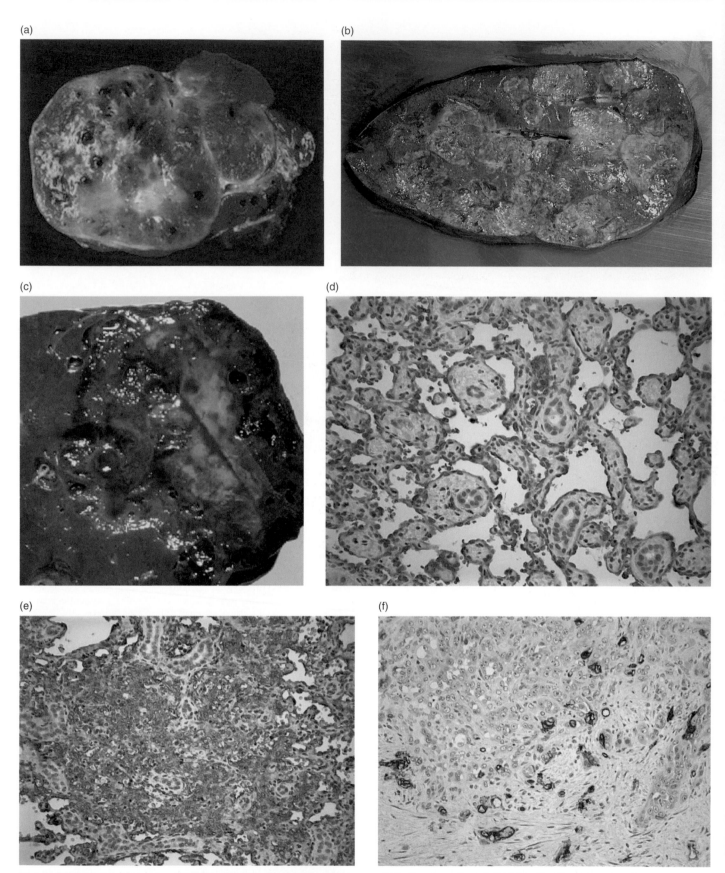

(a)

(b)

(c)

(d)

(e)

(f)

Figure 42.15 Angiomatous lesions in infancy. (a) Solitary hemangioma/hemangioendothelioma in a 5-month-old infant. The designation is used interchangeably. (b) Multicentric hemangioendothelioma in 5-month-old infant (see Figure 42.3b). (c) Arteriovenous malformation in a 3-week-old infant. (d) Immunohistochemical staining for glucose transporter 1 is uniformly positive in the endothelium of hemangioendothelioma and negative in the vessels of an arteriovenous malformation. (e) The active proliferation and infiltration of vasoformative-positive cells as shown with CD34 correlates with the extensive dissemination of the Dehner type 2 hemangioendothelioma. (f) Epithelioid hemangioendothelioma in a 15 year old. Distinguishing this infiltrating pseudoglandular pattern from metastatic carcinoma is difficult without immunohistochemical stains for endothelium.

(a)

(b)

(c)

(d)

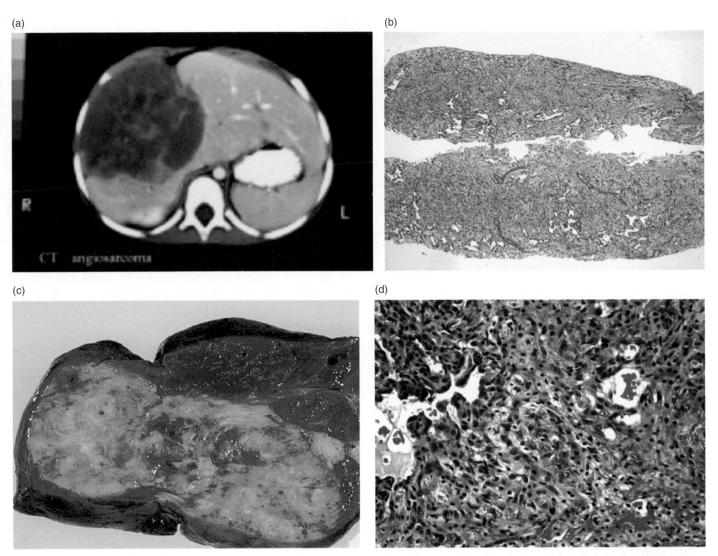

Figure 42.16 Angiosarcoma. (a) CT scan of a 4-year-old child with an asymptomatic mass. (b) Biopsy showed hemangioendothelioma but was suspicious for malignancy. (c) Resection was performed following chemotherapy. (d) The neoplastic cells infiltrate aggressively and only rarely form vascular channels.

tumor suppressor gene in HB. No mutations but allelic loss and reduced expression of *BWR1A* have been found in HB.

Glypican 3, a heparan sulfate proteoglycan possibly binding IGF-2, is overproduced in Wilms tumor and HB, suggesting a growth-promoting activity. Altered gene expression of other members of the IGF-binding proteins indicates that the IGF axis is seriously disturbed in these tumors.

A few cases of HB have occurred in infants with trisomy 18, but that trisomy is not a feature of sporadic tumors. Likewise, cytogenetically detectable chromosomal aberrations of chromosome 11p15, the locus for BWS, or 5q, the locus for *APC*, have not been reported in sporadic cases of HB. Acquired mutations of *APC* have been reported in several cases of HB and have not been reported in other embryonal tumors. Recent studies have focused on abnormalities of β-catenin, whose degradation is regulated by a adenomatous polyposis coli (APC)-dependent proteasomal degradation pathway. *CTNNB1* is more commonly altered in HB than is

APC. A German study has shown that 48% of HB have mutations of *CTNNB1*. Nuclear localization of β-catenin in HB, particularly in more aggressive tumors, is different from that of normal hepatocytes and well-differentiated fetal HB, which have only plasma membrane localization (Figure 42.18), and it correlates with shorter survival of these patients.

López-Terrada *et al.* [1] investigated the status of the canonical WNT signaling pathway in a subset of HBs and correlated the findings with histologic subtype, β-catenin immunostaining, and mutation status of *CTNNB1*. All tumors with embryonal–small cell histology showed point mutations in exon 3, deletions within or confined to exon 3, or no *CTNNB1* mutations. By contrast, HB with pure fetal epithelial histology demonstrated predominantly large deletions of *CTNNB1* including the entire exon 3 and most of exon 4. Immunohistochemistry demonstrated a correlation between the presence of *CTNNB1* mutations confined to exon 3 and increased nuclear translocation of β-catenin, particularly in the

(a)

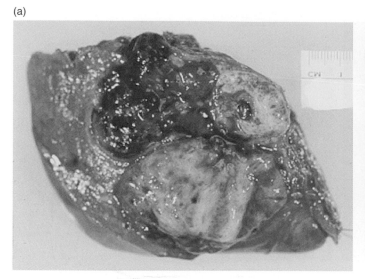

(b)

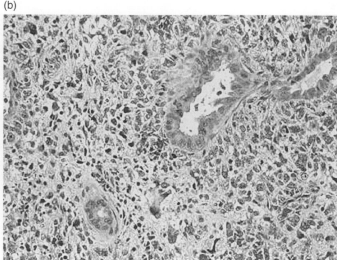

(c)

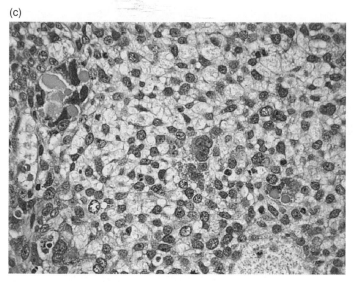

Figure 42.17 Undifferentiated or embryonal sarcoma. (a) Growth to a large size is typical because of the liver's enormous reserve. (b) Sarcomas infiltrate diffusely, sparing bile ducts. (c) Large eosinophilic cytoplasmic droplets of protein are common and help with the diagnosis.

higher-grade tumor components, whereas HBs with large *CTNNB1* deletions showed nuclear translocation of β-catenin confined to a much smaller proportion of tumor cells or only the normal staining of cell plasma membranes. Mutations confined to exon 3 maintain the β-catenin interaction domain for B-cell CLL/lymphoma 9 (BCL9), an interaction essential for transcription of *WNT* target genes and appear to facilitate the more aggressive phenotype seen in embryonal and small cell HB. By contrast, large deletions including the BCL9-interaction domain, although still resulting in decreased proteosomal degradation of β-catenin, would not be as capable of facilitating canonical *WNT* target gene expression as wild-type *CTNNB1*.

Signaling in the WNT pathway is necessary for differentiation, development, zonation, and metabolism [42]. Mutations in *CTNNB1* mutations involving the ubiquitination domain of β-catenin have been reported in several cancers, including chemically induced liver tumors, a subset of benign hepatic tumors, and HCCs. An increased incidence of HB is seen in

children in familial adenomatous polyposis (FAP) families, caused by germline mutations in *APC*, a critical gene in the WNT pathway. Acquired somatic mutations of *APC* also have rarely been reported in sporadic HB, but *CTNNB1* mutations appear much more prevalent in these tumors, and have been detected in 50–90% of patients tested [2]. Mutations of other canonical *WNT* genes have also rarely been reported. As a result of these mutations, the canonical WNT pathway is activated in a majority of HBs, representing a major hallmark of HB, and a useful diagnostic marker [43]. Ueda and colleagues [44] recently reported WNT activation in a small subset of HBs with wild-type β-catenin, associated with high expression levels of *TERT* (encoding telomerase reverse transcriptase), chemoresistance, and poor prognosis.

Signal activation of the WNT pathway has also been demonstrated as a late event in BWS-associated HB involving 11p15.5 uniparental isodisomy. Several studies have explored the contribution of additional WNT pathway molecules to hepatocarcinogenesis and indicate that, in addition to the

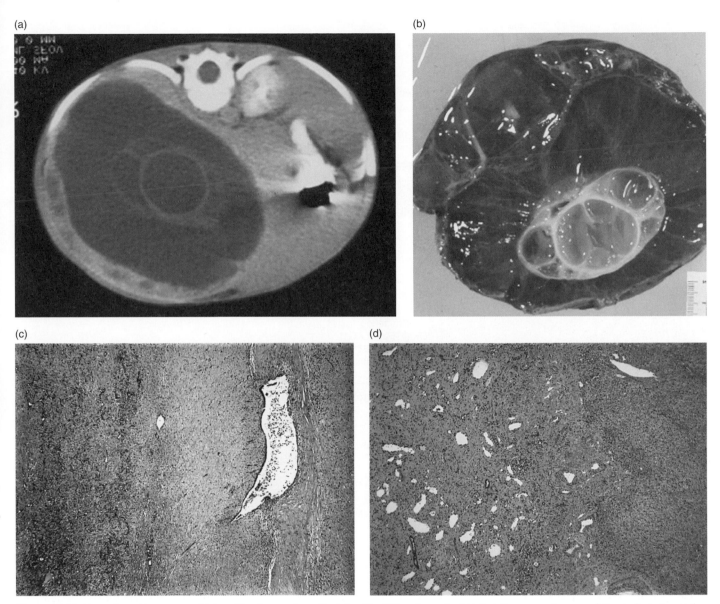

Figure 42.18 Mesenchymal hamartoma. (a) A multicystic mass is readily defined by CT in a 4-month-old infant. The apparent encapsulation is deceptive, and marsupialization is no longer suitable in view of the potential for sarcomatous growth. (b) A cut section of the resected specimen. (c) Cysts are lined by biliary epithelium or lymphatic endothelium. The stroma is myxomatous. (d) Frequently vascular proliferation is also present at the border with the host liver and hypercirculation has rarely been symptomatic, simulating hemangiomas.

CTNNB1 and *APC* mutations, *AXIN1* and *AXIN2* mutations and sequence variations appear to be important in 10% of HCC and HB (Figure 42.19). Dickkopf-1, an antagonist of wingless/WNT signaling pathway, is expressed in most HBs and Wilms tumors analyzed but is only rarely and weakly detectable in HCC and absent in normal liver and other tumor types. Elevated expression of mRNA for nine WNT pathway antagonists in HB has been described.

Investigation of potential nuclear targets associated with β-catenin/WNT signaling and potential β-catenin-binding partners has identified a correlation between deletions and mutations of *CTNNB1*, overexpression of the target genes *CCND1* (encoding cyclin D1) and *FN1* (encoding fibronectin 1), and

poorly differentiated histology in childhood HB. Overexpression of cyclin D1 and CDK4 proteins might play an important role in the tumorigenesis of HB, and high *CCND1* expression may be related with worse prognosis. An association between a *CCND1* polymorphism and the age of onset of HB has been reported, similar to what was demonstrated in FAP families and colorectal cancer.

Sonic Hedgehog (Shh) is another developmental pathway important in liver regeneration that is implicated in cancer, including HCC [45]. Increased transcription of *GLI1* (glioma-associated oncogene homolog 1) and *PTCH1* (Patched), methylation of the promoter of *HHIP* (encoding Hh-interacting protein), and a strong inhibitory effect on proliferation by

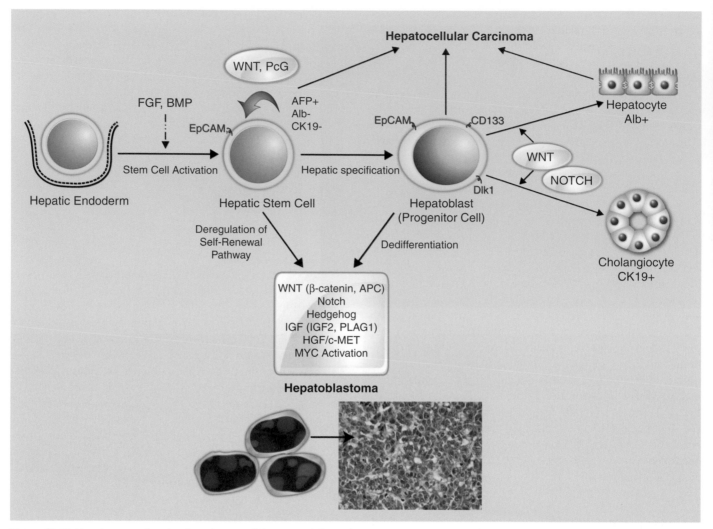

Figure 42.19 Hepatic stem cell and pediatric hepatocellular tumors. Relevant hepatic stem markers and signaling pathways involved in liver development, hepatoblast, hepatocyte, and cholangioblast differentiation. Postulated cellular origins of hepatoblastoma (and hepatocellular carcinoma), and main dysregulated pathways and genes reportedly involved in hepatoblastoma pathogenesis. AFP, α-fetoprotein; APC, anaphase-promoting complex; BMP, bone morphogenetic protein; EpCAM, epithelial cell adhesion molecule, FGF, fibroblast growth factor; IGF, insulin-like growth factor; HGF, hepatocyte growth factor; PcG, polycomb group proteins.

blocking Hh signaling have been reported using HB cells lines. However, a recent study failed to identify *PTCH1* mutations in a series of HBs [46]. Increased Shh, Patched, and glioma-associated oncogene homolog 1 has also been detected by immunohistochemical analysis in HB specimens [47].

The NOTCH pathway, involved in stem cell self-renewal, differentiation, and cholangiocytic lineage differentiation, is also aberrantly activated in some cancers, including HB [48]. *DLK1* encodes a NOTCH ligand (delta-like protein/preadipocyte factor 1/fetal antigen 1 or DLK/Pref1) that is highly produced in the mouse embryo and in bipotential transit amplifying oval cells; it is also upregulated in hepatocellular tumors, including HCC and HB, and is considered a potential therapeutic target for HB. NOTCH2 overproduction has been recently reported in HB [48].

Activation of the IGF axis and abnormal expression of molecules in this pathway also appears to be important in HB pathogenesis [49] and have been proposed as HB therapeutic targets. *IGF2* is an imprinted gene located on chromosome 11p15.5 [50] that regulates downstream phosphatidylinositol 3′-kinase or mitogen-activated protein kinase activation. Epigenetic changes of *IGF2* have been associated with BWS, Silver–Russell syndrome, Wilms tumors, rhabdomyosarcoma, and HB. Preferential induction of the mitogen-activated protein kinase pathway signaling was reported in aggressive histologic epithelial HB subtypes [51]. Hartmann and colleagues identified strong immunohistochemical staining for phosphorylated (p)-AKT and its targets p-glycogen synthase kinase 3β and p-mTOR in most HB tumors studied; as well as a *PIK3CA* mutation (encoding a catalytic subunit of phosphatidylinositol 3′-kinase) in one HB [52]. In addition, increased serum levels of hepatocyte growth factor (HGF) have been observed in patients with HB at the time of diagnosis and is proposed to be at least partly responsible for tumor progression. In a recently published study, HGF/c-MET-related activation of β-catenin was reported in a proportion of wild-type *CTNNB1* tumors [53]. Hence, HGF and its receptor c-MET are also candidates for targeted therapy in these tumors [54].

Hepatoblastomas are considered to derive from developmentally primitive liver pluripotent stem cells (hepatoblasts), which are defined by their ability to differentiate into multiple cell lineages and self-renew, and are responsible for organogenesis and organ regeneration. Signaling pathways involved in stem cell maintenance and proliferation include developmental and cancer-related pathways such as those dysregulated in HB, and discussed above. Heterogeneity seen in these tumors may be explained either by ongoing mutagenesis or by their origin from cancer stem cells arrested at different developmental stages and able to give rise to diverse forms of cancer, or by a combination of both (Figure 42.19) [55]. Molecular profiling of HCC has resulted in the recognition of stem cell signatures and characteristic profiles associated with response to therapy and survival. As in other tumor types, HCCs with the cancer stem cell profile had worse prognosis [56]. Expression profiling analysis has also been reported in limited numbers of HBs by several groups. Nagata and colleagues [57] identified 26 differentially expressed genes in HBs compared with adjacent liver tissue, including four located on the 1q21 chromosomal region (*ETV3, TPR, CD34*, and *NR1I3*), and other genes encoding cell division and growth regulators (*IGF2* and *IGFBP4*). A second study analyzed gene expression patterns and genomic alterations in HB, HCC, and adjacent liver and identified six genes (*IGF2, FN1, DLK1, TGFB1, MALAT1,* and *MIG6*) differentially overexpressed in HB [58].

Other abnormalities of cell cycle genes in HB include inactivation and transcriptional repression by hypermethylation of p16 and differential p27 protein expression patterns that correlate with the degree of histologic differentiation and mitotic activity of these tumors. Likewise, more production of expression of transforming growth factor-α, a potent stimulator of cell proliferation in the liver and in liver tumors, can be detected in better differentiated HB tumor cells, suggesting that the less-differentiated embryonal cells do not depend on growth stimulation provided by this cytokine.

FAS, a death receptor, and its ligand are coproduced in HB in vivo, but some inhibitors of FAS-mediated apoptosis are also expressed in these tumors, suggesting that it is probably the action of inhibitory molecules of the FAS pathway that allows the tumor cells of HB to avoid apoptosis.

Overproduction of telomerase, an enzyme related to cellular immortality, regulated by the expression of *TERT* (encoding telomerase reverse transcriptase), has been associated with poor outcome in patients with HB (Table 42.8).

Profiling of RNA and microRNA in HB identified two prognostically relevant groups of HBs characterized by a 16 gene signature, featuring 8q/2p gains and MYC signaling upregulation [39,59]. Both HB subclasses demonstrated

canonical WNT activation, but with distinctive expression of hepatic stem/progenitor markers in immature, embryonal HB. Profiling of microRNA in HBs and HCCs demonstrated that MYC-driven reprogramming of microRNA expression contributes to an aggressive hepatic progenitor cell tumor phenotype, and revealed a four-microRNA signature that may be useful to stratify patients with HB. These data suggest that new therapies targeting liver cancer stem cells may offer great promise in the future for the treatment of a subset of patients with HB.

Other hepatic tumors

Many studies of adult HCC and its precursors have demonstrated complex and heterogeneous genetic or chromosomal abnormalities, some involving the p53 and retinoblastoma families of proteins, and the WNT pathways [1]. In contrast to HB with a few characteristic chromosomal changes, HCC harbor multiple diverse chromosomal abnormalities, predominantly losses, with increased chromosomal instability in tumors associated with HBV infection. Alterations common to HB and HCC include gain of chromosomes 1q, 8q, and 17q, and loss of 4q. Another important common feature shared by the two tumor types is the frequent activation of WNT/β-catenin signaling by stabilizing mutations of *CTNNB1*. Some HCC is associated with underlying metabolic and chronic cholestatic disease, such as tyrosinemia or total parenteral nutrition [15]. However, pediatric HCCs are most often diagnosed in children without underlying cirrhosis, hepatitis, or known toxic exposures, so the underlying mechanisms of transformation of adult and pediatric HCC are likely to be different.

Mesenchymal hamartoma and embryonal sarcoma of the liver

Karyotypic analysis demonstrated the presence of chromosomal rearrangements involving the 19q13.4 locus in primary embryonal sarcomas of the liver as well as in a subset of mesenchymal hamartomas. Several cases of coexistent embryonal sarcoma and mesenchymal hamartoma, one with documented chromosome 19p abnormalities [34], have been reported, raising the possibility of a putative pathogenic relationship and suggesting a genetic link between these two rare hepatic lesions.

Vascular tumors

Studies regarding the genetics of pediatric malignant vascular tumors of the liver are limited. A single case of infantile hemangioendothelioma of the liver carried an interstitial deletion of chromosome 6q [19]. Inactivation of *P16*, most commonly by promoter methylation, is a frequent event in angiosarcomas of the liver [19]. Mutations of *P53* have also been described but are an uncommon event in sporadic hepatic angiosarcomas.

Table 42.9 Prognostic factors in hepatoblastoma

	Unfavorable outcome	Favorable outcome
Clinical		
Liver involvement	Multiple lobes	One lobe
Growth pattern	Multifocal	Unifocal
Vascular invasion	Present	Absent
Metastases	Distant metastases	Localized disease
Serum α-fetoprotein (ng/mL)	≤100 or >1 000 000	100–1 000 000
Serum α-fetoprotein decline	Slow	Rapid
Histopathology		
Differentiation	Undifferentiated small cell	Pure fetal, low mitotic activity
Genetic/molecular		
Ploidy	Aneuploidy	Diploidy
Chromosomal gains	+8q, +20	–
β-Catenin	Nuclear	Membranous/cytoplasmic
Cyclin-dependent kinase inhibitor 1B	Low	High
PLK1 oncogene expression	High	Low
Cyclin D1	High	Low
Telomerase	High	Low
Hedgehog activation (Gli)	High	Low
Expression profile	Stem/progenitor (Myc)	"Perivenous" gene expression
MicroRNA signature	Stem cell-like (Myc)	–
MicroRNA-492	Upregulated (metastases)	–

A novel t(1;3)(p36.3;q25) translocation resulting in a *WWTR1–CAMTA1* gene fusion has been recently described in epithelioid hemangioendothelioma [60], including two patients with liver involvment, but none in children.

Other rare genetic and molecular abnormalities associated with other uncommon pediatric liver tumors, such as inflammatory myofibroblastic tumor, angiomyolipoma, rhabdomyosarcoma, or rhabdoid tumors, have been described [61].

Karyotypic analysis demonstrated the presence of chromosomal rearrangements involving the 19q13.4 locus in primary embryonal sarcomas of the liver as well as in a subset of mesenchymal hamartomas. Two cases of coexistent embryonal sarcoma and mesenchymal hamartoma, one with documented chromosome 19p abnormalities, have been reported, raising the possibility of a putative pathogenic relationship and suggesting a genetic link between these two rare hepatic lesions.

Prognostic considerations

Surgical excision is essential to cure primary liver neoplasms [2]. Gross venous tumor extension, distant metastatic disease, and multifocality are bad prognostic signs (Table 42.9). Precocious puberty implies a poor outcome. The rapid decline of AFP levels in children with HB has been shown to correlate with better outcome. Both exceptionally low (<100 mg/mL) and exceptionally high (>1 000 000 mg/mL) values are associated with worse prognosis [2].

Histopathological differences in HB are important to assess prognosis and direct therapy but they cannot be fully evaluated from biopsies, which may be not representative particularly of tumors in young children. Well-differentiated, pure fetal HB with low mitotic rates can be treated with resection alone, while HB with a large proportion of undifferentiated small cells is associated with an unfavorable outcome [27]. Regrettably only 3.4% of stage I and II cases in the POG series over 20 years fell into the "favorable histology" resectable category, but all patients were cured without chemotherapy [62]. DNA ploidy pattern analysis has demonstrated an association between aneuploidy and significantly poorer prognosis in HB. Other genetic markers of prognostic relevance in HB include chromosomal gains on 8q and 20 and associated nuclear localization of β-catenin. An evaluation of 29 samples from patients with HB showed that primary well-differentiated fetal tumors without mitotic activity are strongly p27/Kip1 positive, while the vast majority of small undifferentiated cell components are p27 negative, as are the fetal cells that survive chemotherapy [1]. Whether these factors remain prognostically significant when highly active chemotherapy is administered is currently not clear.

Other molecular markers reported to be associated with poor prognosis in HB include high levels of telomerase activity, *PLK1* oncogene and overproduction of cyclin D1 (Table 42.9). Activation of developmental pathways, such as NOTCH [48,63] and Hedgehog [64], has also been correlated with the prognosis of these tumors.

Recent expression and microRNA profiling studies have identified a HB stem cell-like profile associated with MYC activation and poor prognosis [39,59], as well as gene signatures that have been proposed for patient stratification (see above). Currently, there is no routine clinical use of expression signatures, microRNA markers, and any of the other aforementioned molecular genetic alterations as prognostic indicators for HB. Ongoing molecular genetic studies, including different histological types, and careful clinical correlation may reveal prognostic markers and possible targets for therapy.

Treatment

Surgery, either as the initial approach or after chemotherapy has rendered the tumor resectable, is the mainstay of the treatment for HB. Patients with unresectable tumors are candidates for orthotopic liver transplantation. Although only 25–30% of all HB are resectable at the time of diagnosis, cisplatin-based chemotherapy has markedly increased the number of patients who can be rendered disease free through tumor resection after initial chemotherapy and has increased the cure rate from 25–30% (in the 1980s) to the currently achieved event-free survival of 75–80% or higher. Hepatocellular carcinoma does not respond well to chemotherapy or radiotherapy and surgical resection is the only curative modality. Unfortunately, less than 30% of all HCCs are resectable. The SIOPEL group used a pretreatment staging system for HB (PRETEXT, Figure 42.5) and found only one patient with stage I and 14 patients with stage II among their 40 enrolled patients, whereas the American COG used a postsurgical staging system that revealed eight patients with stage I (completely resected with microscopically negative margins) and none with stage II (completely resected but microscopically positive margins) among 46 enrolled children.

Surgery

The potential resectability of a tumor is assessed by Doppler ultrasonography, CT, or MRI, including delineation of the arterial and venous vascular supply. Intraoperative ultrasonography can offer further clarification. Resection is curative for most of the benign liver tumors, including the hepatic adenomas and mesenchymal hamartomas, where the risk for recurrences after resection alone is minimal [22]. Marsupialization of cystic mesenchymal hamartomas is no longer recommended because of the potential for the presence of sarcomatous

components or transformation [34]. Features that prevent primary surgical resection include bilobar disease, involvement of the porta hepatitis, or tumor extension into the inferior vena cava and the right atrium [2]. With the possible exception of infants with hepatic hemangioendotheliomas with characteristic imaging features (Figure 42.3b), a biopsy is necessary to establish the diagnosis in tumors that cannot be primarily resected. For primary rhabdomyosarcomas or lymphomas of the liver, chemotherapy is the initial primary approach, including drug delivery via retrograde biliary endoscopy [65]; however, for other tumors, surgeons and oncologists in the USA believe that an attempt at primary resection should be made [24]. An adequate biopsy will distinguish among HB, HCC, or other, more rare, lesions, including metastases. The presence of lung metastases generally dictates chemotherapy before hepatic resection, but aggressive treatment, including resection of lung lesions, can be life saving [2]. The controversy with respect to the role of preoperative chemotherapy (initial biopsy only) versus primary resection of the liver tumor between the COG and European groups should be resolved with a newly formed collaboration (see below). In the SIOPEL-1 study, primary surgery was performed only for patients with PRETEXT group I tumors (tumor confined to left lateral sector or right posterior section) [25]. In all other cases, resection was attempted after four to six cycles of cisplatin-based chemotherapy, including the resection of any lung metastases. In that study, biopsy was found to be a safe procedure, and preoperative chemotherapy made large tumors easier to resect [25]. The COG position favoring efforts at primary surgery is based on (1) 3–4% of stage I HB does not require chemotherapy (well-differentiated, pure fetal histology with low mitotic rate; Table 42.8), (2) the small subgroup of tumors with a significant fraction of small undifferentiated cells does not respond to current chemotherapy, and (3) about 4% of suspected HB turns out to be benign lesions or metastases, making upfront chemotherapy without at least an attempt at resection undesirable [24]. In two older studies performed by COG and its predecessor POG, major surgical complications (hemorrhage or bile duct injuries) were significantly more common after chemotherapy than after primary resection (COG, 25% versus 8%; POG, 23% versus 0%), but advances in imaging and surgical technique have minimized these issues [2].

Surgical resection usually involves hepatic lobectomy or trisegmentectomy. Porta hepatis dissection and division of hepatic ligamentous attachments to examine the vessels is required to ensure that resection is possible. Extension of the tumor into the diaphragm or other adjacent organs is not considered a sign of unresectability as contiguous organs may be resected en bloc for cure. Lymph nodes at the porta hepatitis need to be sampled, and celiac and para-aortic lymph nodes should be inspected and sampled if macroscopically suspicious. Liver biopsies along the margin of resection should be subjected to frozen section examination if there is any question of tumoral infiltration. Pulmonary metastases should be removed at the time of resection if possible because this appears to improve survival rates. Although an aggressive attitude toward total resection is encouraged to avoid the immunosuppression required after transplantation, this is often complicated by the limited hepatic reserve of the patient with HCC, who may also suffer from cirrhosis or infectious hepatitis.

A comparison of 1000 patients (mainly adults) who underwent hepatectomy for small HCC (<5 cm in diameter) with 1366 patients with large tumors showed a higher complete resection rate (93.6% versus 55.7%) for patients with smaller tumors [66]. More than 80% of the resections in the first group were considered curative, compared with only 61% in the group with tumors larger than 5 cm. It is not surprising that this translated into improved 5-year survival rates of 63% versus 37%. Hence, close follow-up and screening of children with known precursors is essential.

Chemotherapy

Combination chemotherapy has been extremely effective for most cancers in children, including HB [1]. The most effective drug has been cisplatinum, an alkylating agent, in combination with vincristine, which disrupts microtubules, and 5-fluorouracil, an antimetabolite, or doxorubicin, which produces DNA strand breaks. Irinotecan and etoposide are topoisomerase inhibitors that show promising activity but need to be studied further.

The COG compared the cisplatin, vincristine, and fluorouracil combination with cisplatinum and continuous infusion doxorubicin in HB and did not demonstrate any statistically significant differences. Patients with stage I, II, or resectable stage III did very well, with 5-year event-free survival rates of 91%, 100%, and 83%, respectively; patients with unresectable or metastatic disease had only an event-free survival of 50% and 10%, respectively. Avoiding doxorubicin cardiotoxicity made the former regimen the preferred standard in the USA for standard-risk HB [24]. For high-risk cases, as defined by PRETEXT IV, vascular invasion, intra-abdominal extension, distant metastases, or low serum AFP, SIOPEL was able to achieve event-free survival of 57% and 69%, respectively, and overall survival of 56% and 62%, respectively, for those with metastases [67]. In Japan, the combination of cisplatinum and adriamycin was able to improve the 5-year survival (cure rate) of stage IV HB from 0% in 1982–1990 to 57% for 1991–1997.

The US National Cancer Institute website [68] lists 23 protocols for HB as of January 2012. There are two active phase III studies: the current COG trial began in November 2008 and offers a combination of chemotherapy, surgery, and transplantation, depending on stage and histology [24] (see Table 42.6). The primary outcome measures are disease-free and overall survival and a secondary measure is the feasibility of referral for liver transplantation. The other open trial is for sodium thiosulfate as a means of preventing ototoxicity of cis-platinum now that amifostine has been found ineffective.

Protocols in phase I and II trials for refractory or recurrent solid tumors in children include (1) monoclonal antibody cixutumumab versus inhibitors of IGF-1 receptor, (2) the selective aurora A kinase inhibitor MLN8237 (alisertib), (3) the mTOR inhibitor sirolimus, in combination with etoposide and cyclophosphamide, (4) LDE 225 (Novartis), which blocks the Hedgehog signaling pathway, and (5) sorafenib and TCR 105 as antiangiogenesis agents. These are the first attempts at therapy of HB based on emerging knowledge of molecular pathways to neoplasia.

Other combinations of chemotherapy have lately cured some angiosarcomas and embryonal sarcomas, but HCC remains resistant. In a SIOPEL study, 37 children with HCC received preoperative chemotherapy with doxorubicin and cisplatinum. They had a disease-free survival rate of 28% after undergoing complete resection of the tumor. Event-free survival was 23% at 2 years and 17% at 5 years, but none of the patients who did not respond to preoperative chemotherapy survived [2]. Similar results were found in the COG study in which the 46 patients were enrolled and randomized to receive either cisplatinum, vincristine, and fluorouracil or cisplatinum and continuous infusion doxorubicin. Children with initially resectable tumors had a 5-year survival of 88% compared with patients who had stage III or IV disease (8% and 0%, respectively), but there was no difference between the two treatment regimens. The outcomes were no different for fibrolamellar carcinomas of comparable stage in the COG study or other studies [9]. Some promising results with intratumoral and other therapies for HCC in adults may prove useful in children as well.

Benign vascular tumors have a mortality of 30–80% when they cause a consumptive coagulopathy or congestive heart failure [19]. Large liver hemangiomas can cause severe hypothyroidism because of high levels of type 3 iodothyronine deiodinase activity in the hemangioma tissue. About 30% of hemangiomas respond rapidly to corticosteroids, given orally at a daily dose of 2–3 mg/kg (rarely 4–5 mg/kg) for 4–6 weeks, followed by a slow taper over 9–12 months, but 40% of hemangiomas will show only a partial response and the remaining 30% do not respond. Life-threatening hemangiomas that do not respond to corticosteroid therapy within 2 weeks should be considered for treatment with recombinant interferon-alfa (2–3 MU/m² body surface area) given subcutaneously every day for 9–12 months. The most worrisome side effects are spastic diplegia, sometimes persisting even after discontinuation of interferon therapy, and rarely hypothyroidism, caused by the formation of antithyroid antibodies. Corticosteroid treatment of infantile hemangiomas has been replaced by propranolol with great success [69]. Unresectable liver hemangiomas that are unresponsive to propranolol, steroids, or interferon may need to be treated with chemotherapy (vincristine, cyclophosphamide, or both) or transplantation.

Angiosarcoma of the liver is a rare but very aggressive tumor. A few patients have been cured by surgery and multidrug chemotherapy (including doxorubicin and cisplatinum).

A positive trend is being observed in the treatment of embryonal sarcomas [1] and peribiliary rhabdomyosarcoma. With typical soft tissue sarcoma protocols, including cisplatinum, doxorubicin (adriamycin)-type drugs, actinomycin, and etoposide or ifosphamide, all children with localized and resectable rhabdomyosarcoma were cured, and 70% of the original 17 are long-term survivors [1].

All current chemotherapy regimens have substantial toxicities. Neutropenia occurs in about half of the patients receiving the standard regimen of vincristine, 5-fluorouracil, and cisplatinum, whereas other hematologic toxicities are uncommon [1]. Ototoxicity occurs in approximately 30–40% of all patients treated with cisplatinum, some significant enough to warrant hearing aids. Clinical trials with sodium thiosulfate are ongoing in an effort to mitigate it.

Liver transplantation

Surgeons who are experienced in transplantation, aided by skilled radiologists, strive to resect whenever circumstances permit [70]. But if initial chemotherapy fails to permit resection, transplantation is an effective treatment for patients with unresectable tumors confined to the liver. A recent review of the worldwide experience included 147 patients [71]. Overall survival 10 years after liver transplant was 82% for the 106 children who underwent a "primary" liver transplant and 30% for the 41 children who underwent "rescue" liver transplant after previous partial hepatectomies failed to eradicate fully the HB. Other experiences in Cincinnati and Pittsburgh support the contention that transplantation offers a better outcome than maximal surgery in the form of trisegmentectomy; five of five patients with primary orthotopic liver transplant and two-thirds with rescue transplant were cured versus four of eight with surgery in this series. In Pittsburgh, an 83% 5-year survival rate was achieved by orthotopic liver transplantion, and this was not compromised by venous invasion, lymph nodes metastases, or contiguous spread [72].

A small series of 19 children with HCC who underwent liver transplantation showed similar results, with 1-, 3-, and 5-year survival rates of 79%, 68%, and 63%, respectively. An analysis of 135 children with HB and 41 with HCC in the US United Network for Organ Sharing (UNOS) database from 1987 to 2004 revealed approximately equal benefits of orthotopic liver transplantation at 1, 5, and 10 years (79%, 69%, and 66%, respectively, for HB; 86%, 63%, and 58%, respectively, for HCC) [70]. However, a shortage of donor livers and the fact that many patients present with metastatic disease limits the feasibility of transplantation.

Radiation therapy

Radiation has had a limited role in the treatment of liver cancers. It has occasionally been used in Europe as an adjunct treatment for unresectable HB but is unlikely to be included in any treatment protocols because liver tolerance for radiation is relatively low and the risk for intra-abdominal complications may be increased with this modality. Radiation has been used with limited success in adults with small, non-metastatic HCC. Using local radiotherapy, an objective response was observed in 106 of 158 (67.1%) patients. Patients treated with >50 Gy had a measurable response in 77.1%. Survival rates at 1 and 2 years after radiotherapy were 41.8% and 19.9%, respectively, with a median survival time of 10 months. Conformal radiotherapy may increase the efficacy and decrease the toxicity in the future.

Other modalities

Radiotherapy has also been used in conjunction with transcatheter arterial chemoembolization (TACE) in adults with unresectable HCC and appears to confer additional benefits. A study of 76 patients with large unresectable HCC who were treated with TACE followed by external-beam irradiation were compared with a cohort of 89 patients with large HCC who underwent TACE alone during the same period. The objective response rate in the TACE plus irradiation group was higher than that in the TACE alone group (47.4% versus 28.1%, $p < 0.05$). The overall survival rates in TACE plus irradiation group (64.0%, 28.6%, and 19.3% at 1, 3, and 5 years, respectively) were significantly higher than those in TACE alone group (39.9%, 9.5%, and 7.2%, respectively; $p = 0.0001$) [73]. This and other image-guided locoregional treatments such as cryoablation for HCC in adults have proven to have limited success [74] and have not been applied to children, except in instances of disseminated disease or compromise of other organs from underlying syndromic conditions.

Two studies have been reported using arterial chemoembolization in children with HB with mixed results. In Japan, six of eight children were free of disease for a mean of 50 months following resection. In the USA, six patients with HB received hepatic arterial chemoembolization with cisplatin and doxorubicin every 2–4 weeks until their tumors became surgically resectable or they showed signs of disease progression [62]. All patients had previously received systemic chemotherapy, and all six patients showed a partial response to the embolization treatment. However, four patients subsequently died of progressive disease; one developed a recurrence that was again treated with embolization, and another underwent orthotopic liver transplantation. The latter two patients were still alive 33 and 31 months later.

Interferon-alfa has been used for the treatment of HBV and hepatitis C infections, common in patients with HCC. Recombinant interferon-alfa also has an enhancing effect on the cytotoxicity of fluoropyrimidines, including the frequently used 5-fluorouracil. Leung et al. [75] reported prolonged survival in patients who received treatment with intravenous cisplatin, doxorubicin, 5-fluorouracil, and subcutaneously administered interferon-alfa, with a median survival of 7–8 months compared with a historical control of 2–3 months. An even longer median survival of 19.5 months was achieved by using a combination of systemic continuous fluorouracil combined with subcutaneous interferon-alfa given three times per week [76]. However, in this study fewer patients had cirrhosis (only 56% compared with 83.2% in the study of Leung *et al.*), more patients had a negative hepatitis serology (40% versus <10%), and the nine patients (21%) had the fibrolamellar variant of HCC. Combining interferon-alfa2b with surgery was effective for epithelial hemangioendothelioma as well.

Future prospects

Disseminated HB and unresectable HCC have an unsatisfactory prognosis. Screening of patients at increased risk for liver tumors is currently successful in detecting small and confined tumors for children with tyrosinemia and the BWS. It should be extended to include premature babies of very low birth weight, FAP family members, patients with glycogenoses, and chronic cholestatic syndromes, including biliary atresia and recipients of long-term parenteral nutrition.

More studies to enhance safety of efficacious treatments are needed. α-Fetoprotein is elevated in most patients with HB and many with HCC and, therefore, has been explored as a potential marker in imaging studies; it may lend itself to use for targeting antibody-mediated therapy [77].

Side effects, particularly ototoxicity, are common in children receiving cisplatin-based therapies. Oxaliplatin, a newer platinum agent with a more favorable toxicity profile, is being considered as a possible active agent against recurrent HB. Preclinical studies have shown oxaliplatin to be synergistic with fluorouracil and SN-38, the active metabolite of irinotecan. The COG has studied the role of amifostine as a chemoprotectant agent but did not see any protection against ototoxicity associated with the platinum agents.

The issue of multidrug resistance in patients with advanced or recurrent HB is being investigated. Increased expression of *MDR1* (encoding the multidrug resistance protein 1 (P-glycoprotein)) results in an accelerated removal of chemotherapeutic agents from the cell's interior. Inhibitors of P-glycoprotein are currently undergoing phase I trials, but their role in the treatment of HB has not yet been established.

Both HCC and HB are highly vascular neoplasms, and thus antiangiogenic approaches for this tumor are being tested.

Cyclooxygenase-2 (COX-2) is overproduced in many malignant tumors and has angiogenic activity through the increased production of vascular endothelial growth factor and prostaglandins, as well as through activation of matrix metalloproteinases, a constellation that facilitates invasion. Future treatment protocols may include a cyclooxygenase-2 inhibitor, angiostatin, or even antiangiogenic gene therapy. Thalidomide's antiangiogenic actions are being evaluated in combination with other agents, but its neurotoxicity is a serious problem. It has been effective in a patient with epithelioid hemangioendothelioma [78]. The success of imatinib, a tyrosine kinase inhibitor, in treating chronic myelogenous leukemia and gastrointestinal stromal tumors prompts the hope that unraveling the complexities of cancer stem cells and signaling pathways (as described above), such as β-catenin–WNT in HB, will provide points of attack for molecular therapies specific to particular neoplasms, particularly those arising from abnormalities in morphogenesis like HB.

Liver transplantation has become more acceptable, particularly with the growing availability of living donor donations. The several questions that remain in regard to the appropriate selection of patients, timing, and pre- and post-transplant chemotherapy are being studied by COG and SIOPEL [2]. The remarkable advances in treatment of rare tumors such as HB have only been possible through the multicenter collaboration of several groups (SIOPEL, COG, the German and Japanese liver tumor study groups). Continued cooperation regarding the development of new treatment modalities, as well as investigations of pathology and pathogenesis and of preventive and screening efforts, should further improve the medical response to these rare malignancies. Pathologists from Argentina, England, France Germany, Italy, Japan, and the USA convened in March 2011 at a COG-sponsored meeting to establish a working group. Each submitted and reviewed selected examples that were distributed electronically in advance. SIOPEL sponsored a second session in Paris in October 2011. By creating a common classification and database, their knowledge and experience will be continuously available for the prospective international collaborative studies of new treatments in the future.

References

1. López-Terrada D, Finegold, MJ. Tumors of the liver. In Suchy F, Sokol, RJ, Balistrieri, WF (eds.). *Liver Disease in Children* 3rd edn. Cambridge, UK: Cambridge University Press, 2008 pp. 943–974.

2. Meyers R, Aronson, DC, von Schweinitz D, Zimmermann A, Malogolowkin MH. Pediatric liver tumors. In Poplack PPD (ed.). *Principles and Practice of Pediatric Oncology*, 6th edn. Philadelphia,

   PA: Lippincott, Williams & Wilkins, 2011, pp. 838–860.

3. Otte JB, Meyers R. PLUTO first report. *Pediatr Transplant* 2010;**14**: 830–835.

4. Weinberg AG, Finegold MJ. Primary hepatic tumors of childhood. *Hum Pathol* 1983;**14**:512–537.

5. Stocker JT. Hepatic tumors in children. In Suchy FJ (ed.) *Liver Disease in Children*, 2nd edn. Philadelphia: Lippincott, Williams & Wilkins, 2001, pp. 915–948.

6. National Cancer Institute. *SEER Cancer Statistics Review, 1975–2007*. Bethesda, MD: National Cancer Institute, 2007 (http://seer.cancer.gov/csr/1975_2007/, accessed 22 July 2013).

7. Darbari A, Sabin KM, Shapiro CN, Schwarz KB. Epidemiology of primary hepatic malignancies in US children. *Hepatology* 2003;**38**: 560–566.

8. Chang MH. Cancer prevention by vaccination against hepatitis B. *Rec Results Cancer Res* 2009;**181**:85–94.

9. Katzenstein HM, Krailo MD, Malogolowkin MH, *et al.* Fibrolamellar hepatocellular carcinoma in children and adolescents. *Cancer* 2003;**97**: 2006–2012.

10. McLaughlin CC, Baptiste MS, Schymura MJ, Nasca PC, Zdeb MS. Maternal and infant birth characteristics and hepatoblastoma. *Am J Epidemiol.* 2006;**163**:818–828.

11. Spector LG, Puumala SE, Carozza SE, *et al.* Cancer risk among children with very low birth weights. *Pediatrics* 2009;**124**:96–104.

12. Ansell P, Mitchell CD, Roman E, *et al.* Relationships between perinatal and maternal characteristics and hepatoblastoma: a report from the UKCCS. *Eur J Cancer* 2005;**41**:741–748.

13. Li M, Shuman C, Fei YL, *et al.* GPC3 mutation analysis in a spectrum of patients with overgrowth expands the phenotype of Simpson–Golabi–Behmel syndrome. *Am J Med Genet* 2001;**102**:161–168.

14. Aretz S, Koch A, Uhlhaas S, *et al.* Should children at risk for familial adenomatous polyposis be screened for hepatoblastoma and children with apparently sporadic hepatoblastoma be screened for *APC* germline mutations? *Pediatr Blood Cancer* 2006;**47**:811–818.

15. Roy A, Finegold MJ. Hepatic neoplasia and metabolic diseases in children. *Clin Liver Dis* 2010;**14**:731–746.

16. Evason K, Bove KE, Finegold MJ, *et al.* Morphologic findings in progressive familial intrahepatic cholestasis 2 (PFIC2): correlation with genetic and immunohistochemical studies. *Am J Surg Pathol* 2011;**35**:687–696.

17. Richter A, Grabhorn E, Schulz A, *et al.* Hepatoblastoma in a child with progressive familial intrahepatic cholestasis. *Pediatr Transplant* 2005;**9**:805–808.

18. Prokurat A, Kluge P, Kosciesza A, *et al.* Transitional liver cell tumors (TLCT) in older children and adolescents: a novel group of aggressive hepatic tumors expressing beta-catenin. *Med Pediatr Oncol* 2002;**39**:510–518.

19. Hadzic N, Finegold MJ. Liver neoplasia in children. *Clin Liver Dis* 2011;**15**: 443–462.

20. McCarville MB, Kao SC. Imaging recommendations for malignant liver neoplasms in children. *Pediatr Blood Cancer* 2006;**46**:2–7.

21. Philip I, Shun A, McCowage G, Howman-Giles R. Positron emission tomography in recurrent hepatoblastoma. *Pediatr Surg Int* 2005;**21**:341–345.

22. Boman F, Bossard C, Fabre M, *et al.* Mesenchymal hamartomas of the liver may be associated with increased serum alpha foetoprotein concentrations and mimic hepatoblastomas. *Eur J Pediatr Surg* 2004;**14**:63–66.

23. Levy M, Trivedi A, Zhang J, *et al.* Expression of glypican-3 in undifferentiated embryonal sarcoma and mesenchymal hamartoma of the liver. *Hum Pathol* 2011 Sep 19.

24. Children's Oncology Group. Website. (http://www.childrensoncologygroup. org, accessed 24 July 2013).

25. Aronson DC, Schnater JM, Staalman CR, *et al.* Predictive value of the pretreatment extent of disease system in hepatoblastoma: results from the International Society of Pediatric Oncology Liver Tumor Study Group SIOPEL-1 study. *J Clin Oncol* 2005;**23**:1245–1252.

26. Finegold MJ, Lopez-Terrada DH, Bowen J, Washington MK, Qualman SJ. Protocol for the examination of specimens from pediatric patients with hepatoblastoma. *Arch Pathol Lab Med* 2007;**131**:520–529.

27. Wang LL, Filippi RZ, Zurakowski D, *et al.* Effects of neoadjuvant chemotherapy on hepatoblastoma: a morphologic and immunohistochemical study. *Am J Surg Pathol* 2010;**34**:287–299.

28. Biegel JA, Tan L, Zhang F, *et al.* Alterations of the *hSNF5/INI1* gene in central nervous system atypical teratoid/rhabdoid tumors and renal and extrarenal rhabdoid tumors. *Clin Cancer Res* 2002;**8**:3461–3467.

29. Trobaugh-Lotrario AD, Tomlinson GE, Finegold MJ, Gore L, Feusner JH. Small cell undifferentiated variant of hepatoblastoma: adverse clinical and molecular features similar to rhabdoid tumors. *Pediatr Blood Cancer* 2009;**52**:328–334.

30. Trobaugh-Lotrario AD, Finegold MJ, Feusner JH. Rhabdoid tumors of the liver: rare, aggressive, and poorly responsive to standard cytotoxic chemotherapy. *Pediatr Blood Cancer* 2011;**57**:423–428.

31. Grazi GL, Vetrone G, d'Errico A, *et al.* Nested stromal–epithelial tumor (NSET) of the liver: a case report of an extremely rare tumor. *Pathol Res Pract* 2010;**206**:282–286.

32. Mo JQ, Dimashkieh HH, Bove KE. GLUT1 endothelial reactivity distinguishes hepatic infantile hemangioma from congenital hepatic vascular malformation with associated capillary proliferation. *Hum Pathol* 2004;**35**:200–209.

33. Adler B, Naheedy J, Yeager N, Nicol K, Klamar J. Multifocal epithelioid hemangioendothelioma in a 16-year-old boy. *Pediatr Radiol* 2005;**35**: 1014–1018.

34. Shehata BM, Gupta NA, Katzenstein HM, *et al.* Undifferentiated embryonal sarcoma of the liver is associated with mesenchymal hamartoma and multiple chromosomal abnormalities: a review of eleven cases. *Pediatr Dev Pathol* 2011;**14**:111–116.

35. Bioulac-Sage P, Laumonier H, Sa Cunha A, Balabaud C. Hepatocellular adenomas. *Liver Int* 2009;**29**:142.

36. Schneider NR, Cooley LD, Finegold MJ, Douglass EC, Tomlinson GE. The first recurring chromosome translocation in hepatoblastoma: der(4)t(1;4)(q12;q34). *Genes Chromosomes Cancer* 1997;**19**:291–294.

37. Tomlinson GE, Douglass EC, Pollock BH, Finegold MJ, Schneider NR. Cytogenetic evaluation of a large series of hepatoblastomas: numerical abnormalities with recurring aberrations involving 1q12-q21. *Genes Chromosomes Cancer* 2005;**44**:177–184.

38. Suzuki M, Kato M, Yuyan C, *et al.* Whole-genome profiling of chromosomal aberrations in hepatoblastoma using high-density single-nucleotide polymorphism genotyping microarrays. *Cancer Sci* 2008;**99**:564–570.

39. Cairo S, Armengol C, De Reynies A, *et al.* Hepatic stem-like phenotype and interplay of Wnt/beta-catenin and Myc signaling in aggressive childhood liver cancer. *Cancer Cell* 2008;**14**:471–484.

40. Zatkova A, Rouillard JM, Hartmann W, *et al.* Amplification and overexpression of the IGF2 regulator PLAG1 in hepatoblastoma. *Genes Chromosomes Cancer* 2004;**39**:126–137.

41. Rountree CB, Mishra L, Willenbring H. Stem cells in liver diseases and cancer:

recent advances on the path to new therapies. *Hepatology* 2012;**55**: 298–306.

42. Thompson MD, Monga SP. WNT/ beta-catenin signaling in liver health and disease. *Hepatology* 2007;**45**: 1298–1305.

43. Armengol C, Cairo S, Fabre M, Buendia MA. Wnt signaling and hepatocarcinogenesis: the hepatoblastoma model. *Int J Biochem Cell Biol* 2011;**43**:265–270.

44. Ueda Y, Hiyama E, Kamimatsuse A, *et al.* Wnt signaling and telomerase activation of hepatoblastoma: correlation with chemosensitivity and surgical resectability. *J Pediatr Surg* 2011;**46**:2221–2227.

45. Huang S, He J, Zhang X, *et al.* Activation of the hedgehog pathway in human hepatocellular carcinomas. *Carcinogenesis.* 2006;**27**:1334–1340.

46. Chavan RS, Patel KU, Roy A, *et al.* Mutations of *PTCH1, MLL2,* and *MLL3* are not frequent events in hepatoblastoma. *Pediatr Blood Cancer* 2012;**58**:1006–1007.

47. Eichenmuller M, Gruner I, Hagl B, *et al.* Blocking the hedgehog pathway inhibits hepatoblastoma growth. *Hepatology* 2009;**49**:482–490.

48. Litten JB, Chen TT, Schultz R, *et al.* Activated NOTCH2 is overexpressed in hepatoblastomas: an immunohistochemical study. *Pediatr Dev Pathol* 2011;**14**:378–383.

49. Gray SG, Eriksson T, Ekstrom C, *et al.* Altered expression of members of the IGF-axis in hepatoblastomas. *Br J Cancer* 2000;**82**:1561–1567.

50. Prawitt D, Enklaar T, Gartner-Rupprecht B, *et al.* Microdeletion and IGF2 loss of imprinting in a cascade causing Beckwith–Wiedemann syndrome with Wilms' tumor. *Nat Genet* 2005;**37**:785–786; author reply 6–7.

51. Adesina AM, Lopez-Terrada D, Wong KK, *et al.* Gene expression profiling reveals signatures characterizing histologic subtypes of hepatoblastoma and global deregulation in cell growth and survival pathways. *Hum Pathol* 2009;**40**:843–853.

52. Hartmann W, Kuchler J, Koch A, *et al.* Activation of phosphatidylinositol-3'-kinase/AKT signaling is essential in hepatoblastoma survival. *Clin Cancer Res* 2009;**15**:4538–4545.

53. Purcell R, Childs M, Maibach R, *et al.* HGF/c-Met related activation of beta-catenin in hepatoblastoma. *J Exp Clin Cancer Res* 2011;**30**:96.

54. Grotegut S, Kappler R, Tarimoradi S, *et al.* Hepatocyte growth factor protects hepatoblastoma cells from chemotherapy-induced apoptosis by AKT activation. *Int J Oncol* 2010;**36**:1261–1267.

55. Marquardt JU, Factor VM, Thorgeirsson SS. Epigenetic regulation of cancer stem cells in liver cancer: current concepts and clinical implications. *J Hepatol* 2010;**53**: 568–577.

56. Lee JS, Heo J, Libbrecht L,*et al.* A novel prognostic subtype of human hepatocellular carcinoma derived from hepatic progenitor cells. *Nat Med* 2006;**12**:410–416.

57. Nagata T, Takahashi Y, Ishii Y, *et al.* Transcriptional profiling in hepatoblastomas using high-density oligonucleotide DNA array. *Cancer Genet Cytogenet* 2003;**145**:152–160.

58. Luo JH, Ren B, Keryanov S, *et al.* Transcriptomic and genomic analysis of human hepatocellular carcinomas and hepatoblastomas. *Hepatology* 2006;**44**:1012–1024.

59. Cairo S, Wang Y, de Reynies A, *et al.* Stem cell-like micro-RNA signature driven by Myc in aggressive liver cancer. *Proc Natl Acad Sci USA* 2010;**107**:20471–20476.

60. Errani C, Zhang L, Sung YS, *et al.* A novel *WWTR1–CAMTA1* gene fusion is a consistent abnormality in epithelioid hemangioendothelioma of different anatomic sites. *Genes Chromosomes Cancer* 2011;**50**:644–653.

61. Zimmermann A, Lopez-Terrada D. Pathology of Pediatric Liver Tumors. In Zimmermann A, Perilongo G, Malogolowkin MH, Von Schweinitz D (eds.) *Pediatric Liver Tumors.* Berlin: Springer, 2011, pp. 83–112.

62. Malogolowkin MH, Katzenstein HM, Krailo M, *et al.* Complete surgical resection is curative for children with hepatoblastoma with pure fetal histology. A report From the Children's Oncology Group. *J Clin Oncol* 2011;**29**:3301–3306.

63. Lopez-Terrada D, Gunaratne PH, Adesina AM, *et al.* Histologic subtypes of hepatoblastoma are characterized by differential canonical Wnt and Notch

pathway activation in DLK[+] precursors. *Hum Pathol* 2009;**40**:783–794.

64. Li YC, Deng YH, Guo ZH, *et al.* Prognostic value of hedgehog signal component expressions in hepatoblastoma patients. *Eur J Med Res* 2010;**15**:468–474.

65. Himes RW, Raijman I, Finegold MJ, Russell HV, Fishman DS. Diagnostic and therapeutic role of endoscopic retrograde cholangiopancreatography in biliary rhabdomyosarcoma. *World J Gastroenterol* 2008;**14**: 4823–4825.

66. Zhou XD, Tang ZY, Yang BH, *et al.* Experience of 1000 patients who underwent hepatectomy for small hepatocellular carcinoma. *Cancer* 2001;**91**:1479–1486.

67. Zsiros J, Maibach R, Shafford E, *et al.* Successful treatment of childhood high-risk hepatoblastoma with dose-intensive multiagent chemotherapy and surgery: final results of the SIOPEL-3HR study. *J Clin Oncol* 2010;**28**: 2584–2590.

68. US National Cancer Institute. *Protocols for Hepatoblastoma.* Bethesda, MD: US National Cancer Institute, 2012 (http:// clinicaltrials.gov/ct2/results? term=hepatoblastoma&pg=1. Accessed 24 July 2013).

69. Mazereeuw-Hautier J, Hoeger PH, Benlahrech S, *et al.* Efficacy of propranolol in hepatic infantile hemangiomas with diffuse neonatal hemangiomatosis. *J Pediatr* 2010;**157**:340–342.

70. Finegold MJ, Egler RA, Goss JA, *et al.* Liver tumors: pediatric population. *Liver Transplant* 2008;**14**:1545–1556.

71. Otte JB, Pritchard J, Aronson DC, *et al.* Liver transplantation for hepatoblastoma: results from the International Society of Pediatric Oncology (SIOP) study SIOPEL-1 and review of the world experience. *Pediatr Blood Cancer* 2004;**42**:74–83.

72. Reyes JD, Carr B, Dvorchik I, *et al.* Liver transplantation and chemotherapy for hepatoblastoma and hepatocellular cancer in childhood and adolescence. *J Pediatr* 2000;**136**: 795–804.

73. Guo WJ, Yu EX, Liu LM, *et al.* Comparison between chemoembolization combined with radiotherapy and chemoembolization alone for large hepatocellular

carcinoma. *World J Gastroenterol* 2003;**9**:1697–1701.

74. Guimaraes M, Uflacker R. Locoregional therapy for hepatocellular carcinoma. *Clin Liver Dis* 2011;**15**: 395–421.

75. Leung TW, Tang AM, Zee B, *et al.* Factors predicting response and survival in 149 patients with unresectable hepatocellular carcinoma treated by combination cisplatin, interferon-alpha, doxorubicin and 5-fluorouracil chemotherapy. *Cancer* 2002;**94**:421–427.

76. Patt YZ, Hassan MM, Lozano RD, *et al.* Phase II trial of systemic continuous fluorouracil and subcutaneous recombinant interferon alfa-2b for treatment of hepatocellular carcinoma. *J Clin Oncol* 2003;**21**:421–427.

77. Bei R, Mizejewski GJ. Alpha fetoprotein is more than a hepatocellular cancer biomarker: from spontaneous immune response in cancer patients to the development of an AFP-based cancer vaccine. *Curr Mol Med* 2011;**11**: 564–581.

78. Mascarenhas RC, Sanghvi AN, Friedlander L, *et al.* Thalidomide inhibits the growth and progression of hepatic epithelioid hemangioendothelioma. *Oncology* 2004;**67**:471–475.

Liver transplantation in children: indications and surgical aspects

M. Kyle Jensen, Maria H. Alonso, Jaimie D. Nathan, Frederick C. Ryckman, Gregory M. Tiao, and William F. Balistreri

Introduction

Liver transplantation has become the standard of care for end-stage liver disease in children and successful outcomes are now achieved in the vast majority of transplant recipients. Progressive improvement has occurred through better pre-operative care of patients with liver disease, improved operative techniques that has allowed the donor pool to expand, and improved immunosuppression strategies to prevent rejection while avoiding complications of over-immunosuppression. The success of the past, however, has also bred unique challenges for the future. With the increasing number of liver transplant candidates, improved donor awareness and organ availability must occur. A delicate balance between the risks assumed by living donors and the needs of their children must be struck. The increasing numbers of surviving patients present unique challenges and complications related to lifelong immunosuppression. The future success of pediatric liver transplantation will require appreciation of the increasingly complex care needs of this population and a national focus on donor organ shortages.

The evaluation process

Collective experience suggests that the progression of chronic liver disease is not linear, but rather exponential, suggesting that early warning signs of hepatic compromise, such as deteriorating synthetic function or refractory nutritional failure should lead to prompt evaluation. In children with acute liver failure (ALF) or rapidly progressive decompensation of chronic disease, aggressive critical care intervention is essential to maintain all other physiologic systems until a suitable donor organ becomes available.

The primary aim of a transplant evaluation is to identify candidates for whom liver transplantation is the optimal treatment. Patients should be considered for transplant evaluation as soon as they are diagnosed with any disease known to progress to liver failure. This includes patients with biliary atresia who remain jaundiced after hepatoportoenterostomy, or individuals with metabolic conditions that cannot be controlled by diet or other therapy. Patients who present with acute hepatitis, even with mild coagulopathy, should be considered for transfer early in their course. As a general rule, it is better to contact the transplant center early and often regarding patient status so that transfer can be made before the patient's condition deteriorates. Timely referral for transplantation must occur before the expected progressive deterioration associated with liver disease, and before life-threatening complications, or contraindications to transplantation, occur.

There are a number of key questions that should be answered with each transplant evaluation.

- Will liver transplantation improve both short-term and long-term survival compared with no transplantation?
- Will the transplantation improve quality of life?
- Is there irreversible and progressive non-hepatic disease that will negate the effects of liver transplantation on outcome?
- Is liver transplantation futile?
- Is there psychosocial support sufficient to optimize outcome?

Additional goals of the evaluation include ensuring that medical and surgical management is optimized and that an effective pretransplant care plan is developed. This includes identifying non-hepatic complications of liver disease that might adversely affect the operative and postoperative outcome. Malnourished patients should have their nutritional intake optimized through the use of nasoenteric feeding tubes and/or high-calorie formulae. Medications should be adjusted to treat encephalopathy, ascites, or other complications of liver disease as needed. Prophylaxis for bacterial peritonitis or recurrent cholangitis should also be administered when indicated.

Immune status related to prior viral exposures and routine childhood immunizations should be assessed. Immunizations, particularly attenuated live viruses, and preventive dental care should also be administered if time permits.

The patient and family should also be educated regarding expectations when placed on the waiting list. The family

Liver Disease in Children, Fourth Edition, ed. Frederick J. Suchy, Ronald J. Sokol, and William F. Balistreri. Published by Cambridge University Press. © Cambridge University Press 2014.

should be informed as to the expected course after transplantation, as well as possible complications that may result. It is also beneficial to discuss the indications for living related liver transplantation, such as the survival benefit in younger patients, and the risk to the donors, who are often the parents.

Further evaluation from a psychosocial standpoint is critical. An appropriate support system (i.e. two caregivers) is needed; other challenges such as financial stressors, barriers to learning, or unrealistic expectations by either the parents or patient, all of which could impact the child's care and outcome, should be identified. Older patients should also be encouraged to ask questions and if possible should provide assent to the operation. It is prudent to begin educating adolescent or preteenage patients regarding medication adherence as well as alcohol or other substance avoidance.

Indications and contraindications to liver transplantation

The most common clinical presentations prompting transplant evaluation in children can be classified as (1) cholestatic liver disease, (2) chronic liver disease with extrahepatic complications, (3) metabolic disease correctable with liver replacement, (4) acute liver failure, and (5) unresectable liver tumors, including vascular malformations which may lead to progressive heart failure. Table 43.1 reviews the primary diagnoses leading to liver transplantation in children.

Absolute contraindications to transplantation include (1) primary extrahepatic unresectable malignancy, (2) progressive terminal non-hepatic disease, (3) uncontrolled systemic sepsis, and (4) irreversible neurologic injury. Relative contraindications to transplantation which must be individually evaluated and addressed include: (1) acquired immunodeficiency syndrome (many centers also consider HIV-positive serology a contraindication), (2) advanced or partially treated systemic infection, (3) advanced hepatic encephalopathy (grade IV), (4) severe psychosocial abnormalities including substance abuse, (5) malignancy metastatic to the liver, and (6) metastatic liver tumors unresponsive to chemotherapy.

Primary liver diseases leading to liver transplantation

Cholestatic syndromes

Children with biliary atresia constitute approximately 50% of the pediatric liver transplant population. Portoenterostomy (the Kasai procedure) should be the primary surgical intervention for all infants with biliary atresia unless the initial presentation is late in infancy (>120 days of age), the liver biopsy shows advanced cirrhosis, or the clinical course is unfavorable. In these rare patients, primary liver transplantation is indicated [2]. Approximately 15–20% of patients with biliary atresia may not require liver transplantation [3]. The sequential use of the Kasai procedure and liver transplantation optimizes overall survival and organ utilization [4].

Clinical failure of the Kasai procedure can be manifest by various combinations of complications such as recurrent bacterial cholangitis, progressive portal hypertension with refractory ascites or variceal bleeding, malnutrition, and/or progressive hepatic synthetic failure. Approximately 50% of all infants with biliary atresia will have these complications and will require liver transplant within the first 2 years of life. Even children with the successful establishment of biliary drainage and normalization of serum bilirubin levels post-Kasai may develop progressive cirrhosis with portal hypertension, hypersplenism, variceal hemorrhage, and ascites formation. These complications typically lead to liver transplantation after the child is over 2 years of age.

An additional non-hepatic complication in patients with biliary atresia, as well as any other form of chronic liver disease, with or without portal hypertension is hepatopulmonary syndrome, which can even occur in patients with stable liver synthetic function. Subtle clinical changes such as exercise intolerance, decreased energy, a decline in room air oxygen saturations, clubbing of the fingers, or spider telangiectasias should prompt screening for hepatopulmonary syndrome with arterial blood gas or echocardiography. Children with hepatopulmonary syndrome should undergo liver transplantation to avoid progressive hypoxia or later fixed pulmonary hypertension.

Other cholestatic conditions, such as progressive familial intrahepatic cholestasis or Alagille syndrome may cause cirrhosis with synthetic liver dysfunction and/or portal hypertension causing variceal bleeding. In children afflicted with these conditions, indications for transplant include intractable pruritus, xanthomata, marked osteodystrophy with recurrent fractures recalcitrant to medical therapy, or, rarely, hepatocellular carcinoma [5].

Hepatic-based metabolic disease

A leading indication for liver transplantation in children is hepatic-based metabolic disease (see the relevant chapters for additional information on these disorders). In these patients, liver transplantation is not only life saving but also accomplishes phenotypic and functional cure of the disease. Liver replacement to correct the metabolic defect should be considered before other organ systems are affected or the consequences of the defect result in irreversible quality-of-life compromises or complications that would prove to be contraindications to transplantation. For example, patients with urea cycle defects who have repetitive hyperammonemic crises sustain significant neurologic injury with resulting developmental disability. Early transplantation allows the potential for neurologic protection and recovery with preservation of neurologic function and quality of life. The use of living donors who are heterozygous carriers of urea cycle defects has been successful and allows planned early transplantation [6].

Table 43.1 Primary diagnosis for liver transplantation: studies of Pediatric Liver Transplant (SPLIT) Registry 1995 through May, 2007 and Cincinnati Children's Hospital Medical Center (CCHMC) through December, 2010

	SPLIT	CCHMC
Total number	2702	418
Cholestatic		
Biliary atresia	1116	173
Alagille syndrome	76	12
Primary sclerosing cholangitis	67	10
Total parenteral nutrition-induced	48	6
Familial cholestasis/cirrhosis (i.e. FIC1)	40	4
Idiopathic cholestasis/cirrhosis	28	4
Neonatal hepatitis	28	2
Biliary strictures	3	0
Other	51	0
Total	1457 (53.9%)	211 (50.5%)
Metabolic disease		
α_1-Antitrypsin deficiency	82	33
Urea cycle defects	67	14
Cystic fibrosis	42	3
Wilson disease	31	3
Tyrosinemia	31	7
Glycogen storage disease	21	5
Crigler–Najjar syndrome	18	0
Neonatal hemochromatosis	16	2
Primary hyperoxaluria	8	4
Inborn error of bile acid metabolism	3	0
Other	86	0
Total	405 (15.0%)	71 (16.9%)
Acute liver failure		
Unknown etiology	291	51
Autoimmune hepatitis	43	3
Acute hepatitis A	3	0
Acute hepatitis B	1	0
Acute hepatitis C	0	0
Subacute hepatitis B	1	0
Subacute hepatitis C	4	0
Subacute acute liver failure	10	0
Other	26	1
Total	379 (14.0%)	55 (13.1%)

Table 43.1 (*cont.*)

	SPLIT	CCHMC
Cirrhosis/end-stage liver disease		
Autoimmune hepatitis/cirrhosis	84	12
Unknown	49	1
Neonatal hepatitis/cirrhosis	14	3
Hepatitis B cirrhosis	0	0
Hepatitis C cirrhosis	14	1
Other	21	16
Total	182 (6.7%)	33 (7.8%)
Tumor		
Hepatoblastoma	128	23
Hepatocellular carcinoma	21	2
Hemangioendothelioma	18	2
Other	13	4
Total	180 (6.7%)	31 (7.4%)
Other		
Congenital hepatic fibrosis	16	1
Budd–Chiari syndrome	13	1
Other	50	9
Total	79 (2.9%)	11 (2.6%)
Toxicity		
Drug induced	11	6
Accidental overdose	6	0
Attempted suicide	2	0
Other	1	0
Total	20 (0.7%)	6 (1.4%)

Source: Studies of Pediatric Liver Transplantation Consortium, 2007 [1] and Cincinnati Children's Hospital Medical Center.

Patients with tyrosinemia historically had a high risk of developing liver failure or hepatocellular carcinoma, requiring liver transplantation before extrahepatic spread of the tumor occurred. Currently, nitisinone (2-(2-nitro-4-trifluoromethyl-benzoyl)-1, 3-cyclohexanedione) is considered to be first-line therapy for tyrosinemia. Nitisinone, through inhibition of 4-hydroxyphenylpyruvate oxidase, prevents dysplasia and hepatocellular carcinoma, thus obviating the need for liver transplantation.

Neonatal hemochromatosis (also known as neonatal iron storage disease or congenital alloimmune hepatitis) presents a challenge in diagnosis and management [7]. Most patients present at birth or within weeks of birth with ALF with decompensated cirrhosis but lesser elevation of liver enzymes. Diagnosis is made by MRI demonstration of extrahepatic iron deposition or by buccal biopsy demonstrating hemosiderin deposition within the salivary glands. The use of exchange transfusion and intravenous immunoglobulin therapy has shown promise by increasing survival and reducing the need for liver transplantation [8]. Of the patients who do respond to medical therapies, hypoglycemia often improves within 24 hours of starting treatment, although coagulopathy does not normalize for several weeks.

Acute liver failure

Patients who develop ALF without recognized antecedent liver disease present diagnostic and prognostic difficulties. Rapid clinical deterioration frequently makes establishment of a primary diagnosis impossible before the need for urgent transplantation. The most common cause of ALF in children is a presumed yet unidentified viral illness; this is followed in relative incidence by drug toxicity, toxin exposure, and previously unrecognized metabolic disease. In infants, causes of ALF such as neonatal hemochromatosis or mitochondrial diseases must be considered.

Mitochondrial respiratory chain abnormalities, representing disorders in the electron transport proteins, present as ALF or as progressive liver disease with sudden decompensation [9]. Mitochondrial diseases are particularly important to recognize during the evaluation process, if possible, as they represent multiorgan progressive diseases that may not become evident until after liver transplantation. Special attention should be given to patients with *DGUOK* mutations (encoding deoxyguanosine kinase), the most common type of mitochondrial DNA depletion associated with a hepatocerebral phenotype. Current literature would suggest that these individuals may be considered for transplantation if they do not manifest any neurologic abnormalities; however, if abnormalities such as developmental delay or nystagmus are present, liver transplantation is not an option since it does not improve survival in this population [10]. A thorough evaluation of commonly affected, high-energy utilizing organs (CNS, cardiac or skeletal muscle, etc.) must be carried out. In patients with multisystem involvement, albeit mild, transplantation is not curative nor indicated. Additionally, patients with valproic acid-induced ALF are not transplant candidates as 1-year survival is significantly lower in this cohort of patients, even without a clear diagnosis of mitochondrial disease [11].

Patients may also present with congenital or acquired hemophagocytic lymphohistiocytosis-induced ALF. The acquired form may be triggered by infection such as Epstein–Barr virus in an immunocompromised host. In children who have hemophagocytic lymphohistiocytosis, inappropriate macrophage and natural killer cell activation causes severe hepatocyte injury. The primary treatment is hematologic, rather than organ replacement, as recurrence in the allograft has been shown to occur [12].

Selection of patients with ALF as candidates for transplantation is difficult as the natural history of each specific etiology is not clearly established. The King's College Institute of Liver Studies has developed a scoring system for children with ALF, stratifying their risk [13]. Factors predictive of poor outcome included international normalized ratio (INR) >4, serum bilirubin >235 µmol/L (13.8 mg/dL), age <2 years, and white blood cell count $>9 \times 10^9/\mu L$. Sensitivity and predictive ability increase when multiple factors are present. Similarly, poor prognostic factors in other independent studies include the time to onset of encephalopathy >7 days, prothrombin time >55 seconds, alanine aminotransferase <2384 IU/L on admission, grade 4 encephalopathy, infants <1 year, or the need for dialysis [14,15]. Although these criteria are helpful, careful observation for progression and clinical change is most valuable.

The role of liver biopsy is limited in ALF as these patients have marked coagulopathy, necessitating a transjugular or open approach. Sampling error may also limit the accuracy of diagnosis or prognosis. When autoimmune hepatitis is considered, however, biopsy may be helpful as individual patients may respond to immunosuppression.

Although the initial degree of encephalopathy is not predictive of the need for transplantation, progressive and increasing encephalopathy is associated with a high mortality without transplantation (grade I–II, 44%; grade III–IV, 78%) [12]. When candidates undergo transplantation before the development of irreversible neurologic abnormalities, survival is greatly improved [16]. Patients who undergo liver transplantation or recover spontaneously from ALF, however, may have suboptimal neurologic outcomes. Failure to maintain adequate cerebral perfusion pressure (mean blood pressure minus intracranial pressure, >50 mmHg; intracranial pressure, <20 mmHg) has been associated with very poor neurologic recovery post-transplantation [16].

For short-term stabilization, repetitive courses of plasmapheresis may ameliorate the clinical manifestations of ALF. Daily exchanges of volume equal to the extracellular volume (20% of body weight) are undertaken. Replacement fluids include fresh frozen plasma, platelets, and cryoprecipitate as needed. This will lead to temporary correction of coagulopathy and biochemical improvement. Plasmapheresis is also beneficial in preventing fluid overload, which can result from factor replacement alone. Neurologic improvement is common but not sustained. There is no evidence that plasmapheresis enhances native liver recovery. Daily repetitive courses are helpful, but ultimately, transplantation is the only effective treatment modality.

Malignancy

Outcomes for children who underwent liver transplant for liver tumors were initially poor. More recent experience has documented the efficacy of liver transplantation in a subset of patients with hepatoblastoma and has established transplantation as an integral part of the treatment strategy for these children [17].

In children who present with hepatoblastoma, complete surgical resection of the primary liver lesion remains the most crucial intervention required to achieve long-term survival. Adjuvant chemotherapy and conventional resection should be employed when feasible; however, some children have lesions that remain unresectable and complete hepatectomy with transplantation serves as the only option to achieve complete resection. Attempts at heroic resection are ill-advised as the survival rate in "rescue transplants" is inferior [17]. In these children, transplantation is best undertaken before completing chemotherapy, so that the final one or two cycles of chemotherapy can be given after successful liver transplantation.

Unlike the adult population, the frequency of hepatocellular carcinoma in the pediatric population is low; therefore, the experience in the application of liver transplantation in the pediatric population for this indication is limited. In patients whose disease is confined to the liver or who have no underlying metabolic liver disease, the use of liver transplantation is indicated. Chemotherapy alone does not appear to offer a survival advantage unless complete tumor resection is also offered. Although no specific criteria for transplant candidacy are established for children with hepatocellular carcinoma, adult criteria include patients with tumors classified as T1 or T2 utilizing the revised Milan criteria [18]. Table 43.2 describes how tumor size, the presence of metastases, and lymph node involvement impact eligibility for liver transplantation. Alternative criteria including the University of California San Francisco criteria have been proposed in order to render more patients eligible for liver transplantation, but these criteria have not been widely adopted [19].

Cystic fibrosis

Prolonged survival of patients with cystic fibrosis has increased consideration of selected individuals for liver transplantation. Liver disease occurs in up to one-third of all children with cystic fibrosis, and significant portal hypertension develops in approximately 10% [20]. Direct management of portal hypertensive variceal bleeding by variceal banding and portosystemic shunting allows prolonged survival, but in patients with hepatic synthetic decompensation, liver transplantation may be considered. Combined liver–lung transplantation has been performed for patients with pulmonary compromise (forced expiratory volume in 1 second (FEV$_1$) <50%) and, because of the increased mortality rate without transplantation, exception points are available for patients with FEV$_1$ <40% according to US United Network for Organ Sharing policy on liver allocation in patients with cystic fibrosis [21]. Postoperative long-term survival is compromised primarily by cardiopulmonary events, but the increased risk of polymicrobial or fungal sepsis also impacts survival.

Retransplantation

In children, the majority of retransplantation occurs because of acute allograft demise caused by vascular complications or primary non-function; chronic rejection and biliary complications are less common indications. The overall incidence of retransplantation ranges from 3% to 20%. Although the technical complexity of liver transplantation in children increases with allografts modified by surgical size reduction, the incidence of retransplantation is similar when primary whole organ allografts are compared with primary reduced-size allografts. Special attention should be paid to the renal function in these patients as well as their increased risk of bleeding and bowel injury during the repeat operation. Recent studies suggest patients who weigh <20 kg, are hospitalized in the intensive care unit at the time of transplant, or have total bilirubin >19.7 mg/dL have the worst survival rates after retransplantation [22].

Prioritization

In the early 1980s, the Organ Procurement and Transplantation Network (OPTN) was established by the US Government to develop a system to distribute organs in an equitable fashion. Amount of time accrued on the pretransplant waiting list and severity of illness, as expressed by patient location (home, hospital, intensive care unit), were the primary factors used to stratify patients. In 1996, the Child–Turcotte–Pugh (CTP) scoring system was adopted as a means of stratifying patients based on disease severity. This system utilized the serum total bilirubin, albumin, and INR, the presence of ascites, and the presence of hepatic encephalopathy as a means of stratifying patients into three categories based on survival rates. With only three categories, however, waiting time again became a dominant factor in organ allocation. Later studies demonstrated that in this system, waiting time had no relationship to risk of death, except for urgent status 1 patients, leading to dissatisfaction with the existing system [23].

A re-evaluation of this system by the Health Resources and Services Administration in 1998 established the "Final Rule," requiring allocation policies to be based on sound medical judgment using defined criteria to achieve the best use of donated organs and avoid wasting of organs [24]. Using

Table 43.2 Milan criteria for hepatocellular carcinoma

Classification	Definition	Liver transplant candidate[a]
T1	1 nodule <2 cm	Yes
T2	1 nodule 2–5 cm, or 2–3 nodules, all <3 cm	Yes
T3	1 nodule >5 cm, or 2–3 nodules, one >3 cm	No
T4	>4 nodules, any size	No

[a] Any patients with nodal involvement or metastatic disease as well as gross intrahepatic portal or hepatic vein involvement detected by CT, MRI, or ultrasound are excluded from transplantation.
Source: adapted from Hertl and Cosimi, 2005 [18].

Box 43.1   The MELD/PELD calculations

MELD formula

$$MELD\ score = 0.957 \times Log_e\ creatinine\ (mg/dL)$$
$$+ 0.378 \times Log_e\ bilirubin\ (mg/dL)$$
$$+ 1.120 \times Log_e\ INR$$
$$+ 0.643$$

PELD formula

$$PELD\ score = 0.480 \times Log_e\ bilirubin\ (mg/dL)$$
$$+ 1.857 \times Log_e\ INR$$
$$- 0.687 \times Log_e\ albumin\ (g/dL)$$
$$+ 0.436\ if\ the\ patient\ is\ less\ than\ 1\ year\ old$$
$$+ 0.667\ if\ the\ patient\ has\ growth$$
$$failure\ (\leq 2SD)$$

Scores for patients listed for liver transplantation before the patient's first birthday continue to include the value assigned for age (<12 months) until the patient reaches the age of 24 months.

For both formulae, the score is multiplied by 10 and rounded to the nearest whole number. Laboratory values <1.0 are set to 1.0 for the purposes of the score calculations.

Box 43.2   Criteria for listing patients as status 1

1. Acute liver failure with encephalopathy and one of the following:
   - ventilator dependence
   - dialysis or continuous venovenous hemofiltration (CVVH) or continuous venovenous dialysis (CVVD)
   - INR >2.0
2. Primary non-function of a transplanted liver within 7 days of implantation
3. Hepatic artery thrombosis within 14 days of transplantation
4. Acute decompensated Wilson disease
5. Chronic liver disease with PELD/MELD >25 and one of the following:
   - on a mechanical ventilator
   - gastrointestinal bleeding requiring at least 30 mL/kg of red blood cell replacement within the previous 24 hours, or candidates also on the intestine list needing at least 10 mL/kg of red blood cell replacement within the previous 24 hours
   - renal failure or renal insufficiency defined as requiring dialysis or continuous CVVH or continuous CVVD
   - Glasgow coma score <10 within 48 hours of the listing/extension.

knowledge gained from the Mayo End-Stage Liver Disease model, the Model for End-Stage Liver Disease (MELD) was established for adults, based on three biochemical values: serum creatinine, serum bilirubin, and INR. Using similar information derived from the Studies of Pediatric Liver Transplantation (SPLIT), the Pediatric End-Stage Liver Disease (PELD), a pediatric-specific scoring system, was adopted in 2002. The PELD score is based on total bilirubin, INR, serum albumin, age <1 year, and growth failure (either height or weight two standard deviations below normal). The details of these scoring algorithms are shown in Box 43.1.

Initial evaluation of this scoring system showed excellent ability to predict 3-month mortality while on the waiting list [25]. The effect of this matching system has been to slightly increase the percentage of children and adults who receive a deceased donor organ and decrease the rate of death or removal from the waiting list. The preferential policies to direct pediatric organs (donors <18 years of age) to pediatric recipients and status 1 (emergency transplantation) priority were maintained. Furthermore, patients with urea cycle defects or organic acidemias receive a PELD score of 30 for 30 days, after which time, if they have not received a transplant, their score increases to a status 1B. In similar fashion, currently, children with unresectable hepatoblastoma are listed with a PELD score of 30 for 30 days, which then increases to status 1B if they have not yet been transplanted. Additional criteria for listing a patient as status 1A or 1B are listed in Box 43.2.

This scoring system is dynamic and requires that patients' clinical status, including laboratory values and nutrition, be assessed periodically. As the biochemical values or patient condition changes, so does individual MELD/PELD score. At a minimum, laboratory tests should be repeated and the patient's score recalculated every 7 days for status 1, every 14 days for MELD/PELD score >25, monthly if 18–25, every 90 days for 11–17, and annually if <10.

Additional "exception" points may be awarded for specific risk factors not represented by the MELD/PELD equations, such as hepatopulmonary or portopulmonary syndrome, urea cycle defects, hepatic neoplasms, cystic fibrosis, primary hyperoxaluria, or amyloidosis. Although the PELD system improved numerical quantification of candidates and removed waiting time from the scoring equation, the PELD score has not proven to be a successful predictor of 30-day or long-term outcome following transplantation [26]. A rapid increase in the PELD score while awaiting donor availability may identify patients with accelerated deterioration and increased postoperative risk.

Initial concerns that identification and transplantation of "sicker patients first" would lead to decreased survival have not proved correct. In a review of the first year of PELD utilization, allograft and patient survival remained unchanged from the prior allocation system [25]. Of greater concern is the perceived failure of the PELD system to quantify candidate risk appropriately, as the majority of infants and children allocated organs have achieved a PELD score sufficient for transplantation through special exception points or status 1 [27]. Additional studies have shown that MELD/PELD scores can be improved upon if hyponatremia is considered in the scoring calculation [28]. Further modeling and analysis will allow this system to be modified to reflect identified predictive factors and continually improve access and equity to all potential recipients.

Outcomes on the waiting list

Once a child is listed, the goal is to optimize the patient's clinical status through improved nutrition, as well as monitoring and treating complications that arise because of the underlying liver disease. The patient should also be monitored for changes that will increase the PELD/MELD score or preclude transplantation should an organ become available. Once listed, 82% of patients will receive a transplant within 12 months in the USA, with 54% occurring during the first 3 months on the waiting list. The SPLIT data demonstrated that nearly 75% of status 1 patients receive a transplant while at this highest priority, while a proportion will clinically improve and be moved from status 1 to traditional MELD/PELD scoring, and 2% recover and are removed from the waiting list without transplantation.

Unfortunately, not all patients receive an allograft, and a small number will die prior to undergoing transplantation, including nearly 6% of patients listed as status 1 [1]. Children with hyponatremia are among those at increased risk of pretransplant mortality [28]. Among SPLIT participants through 2007, 4% of all patients awaiting their first transplant died without a transplant. Table 43.3 shows details of these patients; the highest risk of pretransplant mortality occurred in patients younger than 1 year of age and those with growth failure, ALF, or who were hospitalized. A higher PELD score also correlated with an increased risk of dying. The primary cause of death was cardiopulmonary or multiorgan failure, with renal failure and infection contributing in many patients.

Donor organ options and selection

The limited availability of pediatric donor organs and an increasing waiting list population has stimulated the development of innovative surgical procedures to increase donor options. Whole organ transplantation, replacing the recipient's liver with a size-matched liver, remains the primary goal for most children and teenagers. The limited supply of size-matched organs and the increased early complications associated with whole organ transplantation using infant donors has led to the development of reduced-size transplantation, transplanting only the left lobe (Couinaud segments 2, 3, 4), or left lateral segment (segments 2, 3) from a deceased donor liver. The rapid expansion of the waiting list population called into question the wisdom of shifting these donors into pediatric recipients as older patients suffered increased mortality while awaiting transplantation. However, the success of the operative techniques perfected through performing reduced-size transplantation has allowed the development of both split-liver transplantation, in which a single liver is used to transplant two recipients, and living-donor transplantation (Figure 43.1).

Several factors must be considered when donor options are evaluated for specific patients.

Table 43.3 Deaths while on waiting list awaiting first liver transplant

	No.	Deaths (% died)	3-month probability of death
Total	3389	135 (4%)	3.7
Age at listing (years)			
0–1	1419	85 (6.0)	6.0
1–5	787	24 (3.0)	3.0
5–13	678	8 (1.2)	0.5
>13	490	18 (3.7)	2.5
Primary diagnosis			
Biliary atresia	1330	38 (2.9)	2.2
Other cholestatic disease	455	25 (5.5)	4.8
Acute liver failure	460	20 (4.3)	13.6
a_1-Antitrypsin deficiency	101	2 (2.0)	1.1
Other metabolic	411	23 (5.6)	4.4
Cirrhosis	270	9 (3.3)	3.1
Other	362	18 (5.0)	3.7
Growth status at listing			
Height or weight z-score >2.0	2116	64 (3.0)	2.5
Height or weight z-score <2.0	1194	70 (5.9)	5.7
Patient status			
Intensive care unit	601	44 (7.3)	20.6
Hospitalized, not intensive care	554	37 (6.7)	7.2
Not hospitalized	2158	49 (2.3)	1.3
PELD/MELD score at listing			
<0	655	6 (0.9)	0.0
0–10	736	9 (1.2)	0.5
10–20	790	27 (3.4)	3.0
>20	859	75 (8.7)	15.2

PELD/MELD, Pediatric End-Stage Liver Disease/Model for End-Stage Liver Disease.
Source: Studies of Pediatric Liver Transplantation Consortium, 2007 [1]

Hepatocellular mass

The selection of a donor organ or segment with an appropriate parenchymal mass for adequate function is critical to success. Unfortunately, the minimal hepatic mass necessary for recovery is not clearly established. Any calculation must take into account the temporary loss of function caused by the donor's primary injury or illness and comorbidity, as well as the possibility of preservation damage, early acute rejection, or technical problems. Because preservation injury is greater in deceased donors, the hepatic mass needed using a whole, reduced-size, or split-liver

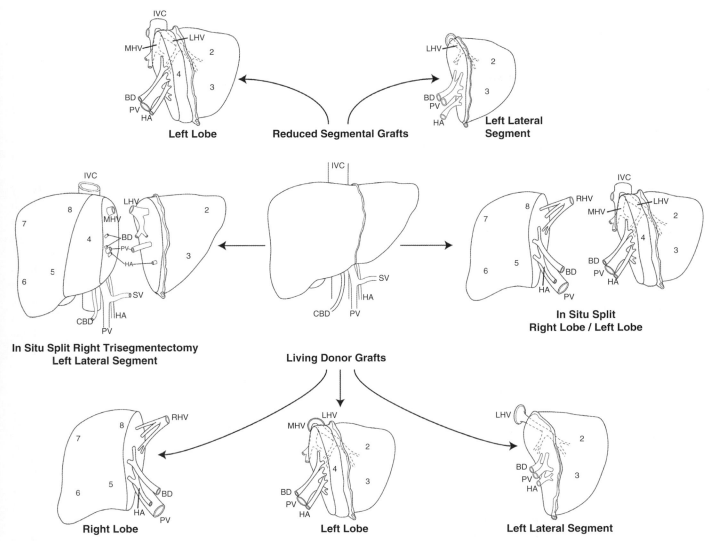

Figure 43.1 Schematic diagram of reduced-sized allografts, living donor, and split-liver transplants. Anatomic subdivisions as described by Couinaud. BD, bile duct; PV, portal vein; HA, hepatic artery; IVC, inferior vena cava; MHV, RHV, LHV, middle right and left hepatic vein, respectively; CBD, common bile duct; SV, splenic vein.

allograft should be greater than the calculated mass necessary using a living donor liver segment. The normal liver volume in a child can be calculated using the following formula: estimated liver volume = $706.2 \times$ body surface area $(m^2) + 2.4$ [29]. A donor weight range of 15–20% above or below that of the recipient is usually appropriate for whole organ donors, taking into consideration body habitus and factors that would increase recipient abdominal size such as ascites, hepatosplenomegaly, and others. When selecting donor segments, transplantation of at least 40–50% of this ideal calculated estimated liver volume is recommended [30]. Estimates of the donor allograft to recipient body weight ratio may prove to be the most accurate predictor of adequate allograft volume. A minimum allograft fraction of 1% recipient body mass is sufficient [24]. A donor allograft to recipient body weight ratio of 1–3% is optimal; where it is <0.7%, overall allograft and patient survival are compromised. In extreme cases in which small-for-size allografts are used, excessive portal flow can lead to hemorrhagic necrosis of the allograft.

Large-for-size allografts (donor allograft to recipient body weight ratio >5%) have a better relative outcome compared with small allografts but still show compromised survival [31].

Donor organ stability

The initial success of liver transplantation is closely related to the stability and quality of the donor. Assessment of donor organ suitability is primarily undertaken by evaluating clinical information and static biochemical tests. Clinical factors of concern include donor age, the reason and length of hospitalization, suffering from potential sepsis, or the use of excessive vasoconstricting inotropic agents for hemodynamic instability.

Recently, a Donor Risk Index was developed, which showed that donor age beyond 40 years (and particularly >60 years), donation after cardiac death, and split/reduced grafts were strongly associated with graft failure. Also significant, but with less impact were cerebrovascular accident or "other" cause of brain death when compared with trauma or anoxia. African-American donors and short donor height were also significantly associated with graft failure. Compared with an "ideal" donor, these factors increased the risk of graft failure by 19–53%. While most recipients in this study were over 18 years of age, children younger than 10 years were found to have received organs from donors with a Donor Risk Index of 0.332, corresponding to a 33.2% increase in the risk of graft failure [32].

Static biochemical tests (liver enzymes, coagulation profile) identify pre-existing functional abnormalities or the consequences of organ trauma but do not serve as good benchmarks of functional capability to differentiate acceptable from poor donor allografts. Electrolyte disturbances, such as metabolic acidosis (bicarbonate <18 mEq/L) and hypernatremia, and deteriorating trends identify increased risk [33]. Although marginal donor organs can be used as whole allografts, particularly when ischemic time is limited, they have proven to be very high risk when used as donors for reduced-size or split-liver allografts. Suggested criteria for identifying these critical "ideal" split-liver donors are shown in Table 43.4. Children can serve as excellent split-liver donors, with results comparable to those achieved using adult donors. Special concern for allocation of adequate hepatic mass and biliary and vascular structures for both split-liver recipients is critical for recipient recovery and should be part of the initial donor evaluation and decision to split. Any decrement in donor organ function adversely affects this hepatic mass calculation and must be considered in the final allocation of segments. Donor liver biopsy at the time of organ harvest, or during evaluation in liver donors, is helpful in questionable cases to identify pre-existing liver disease or donor liver steatosis. Livers with >30% macrovesicular steatosis are associated with increased risk of allograft loss, and those livers with >20% macrovesicular steatosis also have an increased risk, particularly if prolonged cold ischemia time occurs [34]. The transplant team must undertake the difficult process of balancing the stability and quality of the donor organ with the risk and health status of the potential recipient(s).

Age of donor

As seen in the Donor Risk Index, donor age affects the long-term results of pediatric liver transplantation. When the UNOS database was analyzed, survival analysis showed a

Table 43.4 Suggested criteria for identifying "split-liver" deceased donors

Donor characteristic	Ideal donor for split liver
Age	10–50 years
Serum sodium	<150 mEq/L
Hemodynamics	≤1 vasopressor
Cardiac arrest	<30 minutes (prefer no arrest)
Hospital stay	<5 days
Aspartate and alanine aminotransferases	<5× upper limit of normal range (<250 mg/dL)

3-year allograft survival rate of 81% for pediatric recipients of pediatric (<18 years of age) livers compared with 63% if livers were used from donors aged 18 years or older. In contrast, in multivariate analysis, the odds of allograft failure were reduced to 0.66 if pediatric recipients received livers from pediatric-aged donors while the odds of allograft failure for adults did not depend on donor age [35]. Additionally, the Mount Sinai Hospital adult series showed that adult (>18 years age) recipients of pediatric donor organs had an increased risk of hepatic artery thrombosis and poor function compared with recipients of adult donors, an effect that increased with increasing donor-to-recipient size discrepancy [36]. This was confirmed in the Mayo Clinic series, in which the 1-year allograft survival rate in adult transplant recipients receiving allografts from donors younger than 12 years of age was 64.3% compared with 87.5% when the donor was 12–18 years of age [37]. The main cause of allograft loss was again vascular complications. Because the outcome of small pediatric donor livers in adult recipients is poor, and small pediatric donors are the only source of life-saving organs for the infant recipient, the use of small pediatric donor livers in adults should be avoided.

Living donor selection

A similar critical element of living donor transplantation is the proper evaluation and selection of the donor, usually a parent or first-degree relative. Donors should be 18–55 years of age, have an ABO compatible blood type, and have no acute or chronic medical condition. Significant efforts are made to recognize potential donors who have thrombophilic tendency or risk factors, because pulmonary emboli have resulted in fatal complications in several donors. A history of thrombosis, significant varicosities, body mass index >30, or homozygous protein S, protein C, or factor V Leiden mutation all should exclude living donation [37]. In addition to the medical risks mentioned above, UNOS policies are in place to ensure that donor well-being is the primary focus of living-related donation. This includes having an independent donor advocate team and several well-defined goals:

- to determine if the potential donor is suitable after medical, psychosocial and radiologic evaluation
- to educate the potential donor regarding the risks and benefits of donation
- to provide counseling and support for the donor regarding family, disability, intellectual, emotional and other pressures
- to determine that the decision is without coercion
- to provide opportunities for the donor to "opt out" at any time.

At each transplant center, defined processes must be established to address each goal.

Following a satisfactory medical and psychological examination by a physician not directly involved with the transplant program, vascular imaging (MR, CT, or conventional angiography) is undertaken to assess the hepatic arterial anatomy, excluding potential donors with multiple or intrahepatic arteries to segments 2 and 3. Experience has shown that when donors are deemed unacceptable, 90% were rejected on the basis of history, physical examination, laboratory screening, and ABO type. Only 10% were excluded following angiography. Donor safety has been excellent in all series, with a mortality rate of up to 0.5%. Morbidity, however, is much higher with nearly one-third of all donors experiencing complications, most of which were minor without permanent sequelae, although a small proportion (approximately 0.1%) of living donors have subsequently been listed for liver transplantation themselves [38].

Ethical issues

The ethical issues that arise when using this large variety of surgically reduced allografts are complex [39]. Although different liver tranplants – whole organ, reduced size, split liver, living donor – all have similar survival and complication profiles in experienced centers, a significant "learning curve" exists in the complex donor and recipient operations. Maximizing the number of available donor organs cannot justify compromising patient safety or survival. The ethical obligation to maximize available organs must be balanced by clear and concise discussions at the time of evaluation with patients and families regarding risks, center experience, and success with these technically complex allografts. Parents and patients must maintain the right to refuse offered organs without risk of decreased access. Surgeons and hepatologists must be responsible for the moral stewardship of precious donor organs.

Donor liver procurement and liver transplantation

Whole organ procurement is now a well-described procedure. The principles of minimal mobilization to define vascular structures, in situ perfusion with 4°C preservation solution, and sequential en-bloc recovery of organs yield good allograft preservation. When reduction hepatectomy is needed for reduced-size allografts, this is accomplished following en-bloc recovery. The operative techniques for this reduction are well described [40]. Modifications of these procedures with in situ division of liver parenchyma form the basis for living donor and split-liver donor procedures.

Split-liver techniques involve the preparation of two allografts from a single donor [41]. In most cases, the extended right lobe allograft (segments 4–8) is used in an adult or large child, and the left lateral segment allograft (segments 2 and 3) is transplanted into a small recipient (Figure 43.1). Generally, the celiac trunk remains with the left lateral segment allograft and the main portal vein and the common hepatic duct remain with the extended right lobe allograft [42]. Conventional

techniques for transplanting the respective allografts with preservation of the native inferior vena cava are used. The use of in situ parenchymal division for left lateral segment recovery [43], as during living donor liver procurement, is our preferred method for split-liver donor preparation at the present time, although comparable results using ex vivo division have also been achieved [41].

Alternative transplant procedures

Resection of the left lobe of the native liver followed by auxiliary partial orthotopic transplantation (APOLT) of a left lateral segment allograft has been successfully undertaken for patients with metabolic disease (urea cycle abnormalities, Crigler–Najjar syndrome), ALF, and as a "bridge" with small-for-size syndrome. Although technically feasible, success (i.e. patient survival, native liver regeneration, and immunosuppression withdrawal leading to allograft removal) with APOLT is far from assured. Biliary complications, the need for re-transplantation, and the incidence of acute cellular rejection are increased in APOLT recipients, while survival is decreased compared with conventional transplantation. Patients with ALF have the least predictable success and patients with metabolic disease seemingly enjoy better outcomes. Further experience with APOLT has been more optimistic but the role of APOLT continues to be defined [44]. Isolated hepatocyte transplantation has also been used in an attempt to provide neurologic protection while awaiting organ acquisition or spontaneous recovery [45]. Ongoing research is required before this approach is more widely adopted and practiced.

Technical aspects

The technical details of pediatric liver transplant procedures are well described [46,47]. However, the following concepts deserve emphasis.

1. The most underestimated portion of this complex operative procedure entails the removal of the native liver. Multiple prior operations or revisions for biliary atresia, or multiple episodes of spontaneous bacterial peritonitis lead to extensive vascularized adhesions and scarring. These increase the risk of intestinal perforation and bleeding at transplantation.

2. Optimal arterial inflow is essential for donor liver recovery. When the native hepatic artery is <4–5 mm in diameter, implantation of the donor celiac axis directly on to the infrarenal aorta is preferred. When adequate length is lacking, a donor iliac arterial vascular interposition graft is used to accomplish this anastomosis. Access to the infrarenal aorta is provided by mobilizing the right colon and duodenum. Experience with microvascular reconstruction techniques for the hepatic artery, using both operating microscope and high-power 6× loupes, have been shown to be successful techniques in the setting of extremely fine arterial anastomoses [48,49].

3. Allograft outflow must be unimpeded. This is particularly important in "piggyback" implantation to the native inferior vena cava in small children, where a confluence of all three hepatic venous orifices achieves wide and effective outflow. Addition of a longitudinal incision in the anterior wall of the inferior vena cava augments the size of the outflow and provides stability to the allograft in the right upper abdomen [50]. Impaired outflow leads to allograft swelling, increased vascular resistance, and subsequent inflow thrombosis.

4. Immediate postoperative and daily Doppler ultrasound studies will assist in recognizing correctable blood flow abnormalities before allograft compromise.

5. Bile duct reconstruction as an end-to-side choledochojejunostomy into an isoperistaltic Roux-en-Y jejunal limb is our preference in young recipients or those with primary biliary pathology. Older children without primary biliary pathology can undergo direct stent-free choledochal reconstruction.

6. When closing the abdomen, increased intra-abdominal pressure should be avoided. In many cases, avoidance of fascial closure and the use of mobilized skin flaps and running monofilament skin closure is advisable. Musculofascial abdominal wall closure can be completed approximately 1 week postoperatively at which time long-term intravenous access can also be established, providing future vascular access for immunosuppression monitoring and biochemistry surveillance. Most allografts assume a suitable position within the abdomen at the time of closure.

Left lateral segment and living donor allografts are at great risk for hepatic venous obstruction if the left hepatic vein experiences any torsion. Clear discussion of these needs with the family before transplantation decreases the anxiety associated with reoperation and facilitates postoperative decision making.

Postoperative care of liver transplant recipients is discussed in Chapter 44.

Conclusions

Liver transplantation has evolved from an experimental procedure used in desperate conditions to the state of the art therapy for most patients with end-stage liver disease. The wide variety of surgical options developed to increase donor availability in pediatric transplantation have both improved survival and decreased waiting list mortality. However, the ideal implementation of the higher potential risk options such as split-liver and living donor transplantation require their use in candidates with satisfactory stability. Early referral of the potential recipient allows timely evaluation of potential living donors, or suitable time for acquisition of a deceased donor organ. Meticulous operative management and improved postoperative care have combined to offer excellent long-term survival and quality of life in pediatric recipients. The continued development of future options such as hepatocellular transplantation, gene therapy for hereditary diseases affecting the liver, and improved immunosuppressive management should yield greater success for the future.

References

1. Studies of Pediatric Liver Transplantation Consortium. *Annual Report 2007*. Rockville, MD: Emmes, 2007.

2. Kasai M, Mochizuki I, Ohkohchi N, *et al*. Surgical limitation for biliary atresia: indication for liver transplantation. *J Pediatr Surg* 1989;**24**:851–854.

3. Altman RP, Lilly JR, Greenfeld J, *et al*. A multivariable risk factor analysis of the portoenterostomy (Kasai) procedure for biliary atresia: twenty-five years of experience from two centers. *Ann Surg* 1997;**226**:348–353; discussion 353–355.

4. Otte JB, de Ville de Goyet J, Reding R, *et al*. Sequential treatment of biliary atresia with Kasai portoenterostomy and liver transplantation: a review. *Hepatology* 1994;**20**:41S–48S.

5. Englert C, Grabhorn E, Burdelski M, Ganschow R. Liver transplantation in children with Alagille syndrome: indications and outcome. *Pediatr Transplant* 2006;**10**:154–158.

6. Morioka D, Kasahara M, Takada Y, *et al*. Current role of liver transplantation for the treatment of urea cycle disorders: a review of the worldwide English literature and 13 cases at Kyoto University. *Liver Transplant* 2005;**11**:1332–1342.

7. Whitington PF. Neonatal hemochromatosis: a congenital alloimmune hepatitis. *Semin Liver Dis* 2007;**27**:243–250.

8. Rand EB, Karpen SJ, Kelly S, *et al*. Treatment of neonatal hemochromatosis with exchange transfusion and intravenous immunoglobulin. *J Pediatr* 2009;**155**:566–571.

9. Lee WS, Sokol RJ. Liver disease in mitochondrial disorders. *Semin Liver Dis* 2007;**27**:259–273.

10. Dimmock DP, Dunn JK, Feigenbaum A, *et al*. Abnormal neurological features predict poor survival and should preclude liver transplantation in patients with deoxyguanosine kinase deficiency. *Liver Transplant* 2008;**14**:1480–1485.

11. Mindikoglu AL, King D, Magder LS, *et al*. Valproic acid-associated acute liver failure in children: case report and analysis of liver transplantation outcomes in the United States. *J Pediatr* 2011;**158**:802–807.

12. McClean P, Davison SM. Neonatal liver failure. *Semin Neonatol* 2003;**8**:393–401.

13. Dhawan A, Cheeseman P, Mieli-Vergani G. Approaches to acute liver failure in children. *Pediatr Transplant* 2004;**8**:584–588.

14. Lee WS, McKiernan P, Kelly DA. Etiology, outcome and prognostic indicators of childhood fulminant hepatic failure in the United Kingdom. *J Pediatr Gastroenterol Nutr* 2005;**40**:575–581.

15. Baliga P, Alvarez S, Lindblad A, Zeng L. Posttransplant survival in pediatric fulminant hepatic failure: the SPLIT

experience. *Liver Transplant* 2004;**10**:1364–1371.

16. Rivera-Penera T, Moreno J, Skaff C, *et al*. Delayed encephalopathy in fulminant hepatic failure in the pediatric population and the role of liver transplantation. *J Pediatr Gastroenterol Nutr* 1997;**24**: 128–134.

17. Otte JB, Pritchard J, Aronson DC, *et al*. Liver transplantation for hepatoblastoma: results from the International Society of Pediatric Oncology (SIOP) study SIOPEL-1 and review of the world experience. *Pediatr Blood Cancer* 2004;**42**:74–83.

18. Hertl M, Cosimi AB. Liver transplantation for malignancy. *Oncologist* 2005;**10**:269–281.

19. Yao FY, Ferrell L, Bass NM, *et al*. Liver transplantation for hepatocellular carcinoma: comparison of the proposed UCSF criteria with the Milan criteria and the Pittsburgh modified TNM criteria. *Liver Transplant* 2002;**8**: 765–774.

20. Lu BR, Esquivel CO. A review of abdominal organ transplantation in cystic fibrosis. *Pediatr Transplant* 2010;**14**:954–960.

21. Organ Procurement and Transplantation Network. *Policies. Organ Distribution: Allocation of Livers*. Bethesda, MD: US Health Resources and Services Administration, Department of Health & Human Services, 2013 (http://optn.transplant. hrsa.gov/policiesAndBylaws/policies. asp, accessed 26 July 2013).

22. Lao OB, Dick AA, Healey PJ, *et al*. Identifying the futile pediatric liver re-transplant in the PELD era. *Pediatr Transplant* 2010;**14**:1019–1029.

23. Freeman RB Jr., Edwards EB. Liver transplant waiting time does not correlate with waiting list mortality: implications for liver allocation policy. *Liver Transplant* 2000;**6**:543–552.

24. Organ Procurement and Transplantation Network. Final rule with comment period. *Fed Regist* 1998;**63**:16296–16338.

25. Freeman RB Jr., Wiesner RH, Roberts JP, *et al*. Improving liver allocation: MELD and PELD. *Am J Transplant* 2004;4(Suppl 9):114–131.

26. Barshes NR, Lee TC, Udell IW, *et al*. The pediatric end-stage liver disease

(PELD) model as a predictor of survival benefit and posttransplant survival in pediatric liver transplant recipients *Liver Transplant* 2006;**12**: 475–480.

27. Shneider BL, Suchy FJ, Emre S. National and regional analysis of exceptions to the pediatric end-stage liver disease scoring system (2003–2004). *Liver Transplant* 2006; **12**:40–45.

28. Carey RG, Bucuvalas JC, Balistreri WF, *et al*. Hyponatremia increases mortality in pediatric patients listed for liver transplantation. *Pediatr Transplant* 2010;**14**:115–120.

29. Urata K, Kawasaki S, Matsunami H, *et al*. Calculation of child and adult standard liver volume for liver transplantation. *Hepatology* 1995;**21**:1317–1321.

30. Dahm F, Georgiev P, Clavien PA. Small-for-size syndrome after partial liver transplantation: definition, mechanisms of disease and clinical implications. *Am J Transplant* 2005;**5**:2605–2610.

31. Morimoto T, Ichimiya M, Tanaka A, *et al*. Guidelines for donor selection and an overview of the donor operation in living related liver transplantation. *Transplant Int* 1996;**9**:208–213.

32. Feng S, Goodrich NP, Bragg-Gresham JL, *et al*. Characteristics Associated with graft failure: the concept of a donor risk index. *Am J Transplant* 2006;**6**: 783–790.

33. Cuende N, Miranda B, Cañón JF, *et al*. Donor characteristics associated with liver graft survival. *Transplantation* 2005;**79**:1445–1452.

34. Spitzer AL, Lao OB, Dick AA, *et al*. The biopsied donor liver: incorporating macrosteatosis into high-risk donor assessment. *Liver Transplant* 2010;**16**:874–884.

35. McDiarmid SV, Davies DB, Edwards EB. Improved graft survival of pediatric liver recipients transplanted with pediatric-aged liver donors. *Transplantation* 2000;**70**:1283–1291.

36. Emre S, Soejima Y, Altaca G, *et al*. Safety and risk of using pediatric donor livers in adult liver transplantation. *Liver Transplant* 2001;7:41–47.

37. Yasutomi M, Harmsmen S, Innocenti F, *et al*. Outcome of the use of pediatric

donor livers in adult recipients. *Liver Transplant* 2001;7:38–40.

38. Burdelski MM, Rogiers X. What lessons have we learned in pediatric liver transplantation? *J Hepatol* 2005;**42**:28–33.

39. Organ Procurement and Transplantation Network. *Guidance for the Medical Evaluation of Potential Living Liver Donors*. Bethesda, MD: US Health Resources and Services Administration, Department of Health & Human Services, 2013 (http://optn. transplant.hrsa.gov/Content Documents/Guidance_Medical EvaluationPotentialLivingLiverDonors. pdf, accessed 26 July 2013).

40. Vulchev A, Roberts JP, Stock PG. Ethical issues in split versus whole liver transplantation. *Am J Transplant* 2004;**4**:1737–1740.

41. Ryckman FC, Flake AW, Fisher RA, *et al*. Segmental orthotopic hepatic transplantation as a means to improve patient survival and diminish waiting-list mortality. *J Pediatr Surg* 1991;**26**:422–427; discussion 427–428.

42. Renz JF, Yersiz H, Reichert PR, *et al*. Split-liver transplantation: a review. *Am J Transplant* 2003;**3**:1323–1335.

43. Lee TC, Barshes NR, Washburn WK, *et al*. Split-liver transplantation using the left lateral segment: a collaborative sharing experience between two distant centers. *Am J Transplant* 2005;**5**: 1646–1651.

44. Faraj W, Dar F, Bartlett A, *et al*. Auxiliary liver transplantation for acute liver failure in children. *Ann Surg* 2010;**251**:351–356.

45. Strom S, Fisher R. Hepatocyte transplantation: new possibilities for therapy. *Gastroenterology* 2003;**124**:568–571.

46. Ryckman FC, Fisher RA, Pedersen SH, Balistreri WF. Liver transplantation in children. *Semin Pediatr Surg* 1992;**1**:162–172.

47. Otte JB, de Ville de Goyet J, Sokal E, *et al*. Size reduction of the donor liver is a safe way to alleviate the shortage of size-matched organs in pediatric liver transplantation. *Ann Surg* 1990;**211**:146–157.

48. Inomoto T, Nishizawa F, Sasaki H, *et al*. Experiences of 120 microsurgical reconstructions of hepatic artery in

living related liver transplantation. *Surgery* 1996;**119**:20–26.

49. Guarrera JV, Sinha P, Lobritto SJ, *et al*. Microvascular hepatic artery anastomosis in pediatric segmental liver transplantation: microscope vs loupe. *Transplant Int* 2004;**17**: 585–588.

50. Tannuri U, Mello ES, Carnevale FC, *et al*. Hepatic venous reconstruction in pediatric living-related donor liver transplantation: experience of a single center. *Pediatr Transplant* 2005;**9**: 293–298.

Chapter 44

Liver transplantation in children: post-transplant care

Estella M. Alonso and Riccardo A. Superina

Introduction

Management in the early postoperative period requires the coordinated efforts of the transplant team and the pediatric intensive care staff. Patients with end-stage liver disease undergoing liver transplantation require meticulous medical care in the immediate postoperative period to assure adequate perfusion of the graft and avoid exacerbation of injury to other organ systems. Care should be guided by attention to the pretransplant physiologic state, which might include advanced portal hypertension and compromise to other organ systems, such as seen in hepatorenal or hepatopulmonary syndrome. Specifics of the transplant procedure including information regarding blood loss, challenging vascular anastomosis, and graft function following reperfusion are also essential considerations in the management plan.

General principles of early postoperative management

General aspects of the surgical procedure and common intra-operative complications are reviewed in Chapter 43. It is not uncommon for recipients to experience blood loss and replacement that exceeds their estimated blood volume and which can result in third-space fluid losses and pulmonary edema. Likewise, placement of a graft that exceeds the mass of the explanted liver can increase intra-abdominal pressure and impede ventilation. Management of fluid and cardiovascular support to maintain graft perfusion but limit pulmonary complications can be challenging. Monitoring of changes in arterial blood pressure and central venous pressure can detect acute intra-abdominal hemorrhage or vasodilatation caused by cytokine release related to allograft necrosis or systemic infection. The overwhelming majority of children remain intubated during the first to 12 to 24 hours following the procedure even when they have not had evidence of pre-existing lung disease. Likewise, many receive ionotropic support during the anhepatic and postperfusion phases of the procedure, which is gradually tapered off following abdominal closure. Cardiac function may be depressed during the procedure because of the circulation of cytokines and of lactic acid released from the graft at reperfusion and it may not be restored to normal until the metabolic function of the liver is re-established. One of the classic hallmarks of primary non-function of the graft is cardiovascular instability and persistent lactic acidosis. Although many patients are relatively fluid overloaded at the conclusion of the procedure, efforts are not made to encourage diuresis until at least 24 to 36 hours following the procedure because of concerns regarding hypoperfusion of the graft resulting from a sudden drop in intravascular volume and blood pressure. Some degree of diuresis occurs spontaneously on the second and third postoperative day provided the patient does not have intrinsic renal injury or advanced pretransplant hepatorenal syndrome.

Patients typically receive prophylactic antibiotics for 24–72 hours to prevent common postoperative bacterial infections including wound infections. In fact, the rate of wound infections following liver transplantation in children is low, typically <8% in most studies [1]. In situations where there is increased risk for postoperative intra-abdominal abscess, such as inadvertent enterostomies during surgical dissection or hepatic abscess in the explant, antibiotics should be extended and tailored to suspected organisms. Patients that are naive to cytomegalovirus (CMV) and Epstein–Barr virus (EBV) are at risk to contract these infections via passenger lymphocytes in the transplanted graft. Recipients who have had prior infection with these latent viruses are at risk to develop reactivation of the infection, resulting in clinical illness when exposed to immunosuppressive agents. To prevent symptomatic cytomegalovirus infection in the immediate postoperative period, most centers use antiviral prophylaxis with either ganciclovir or vangancyclovir. The method (intravenous versus oral) and the duration for therapy varies, but a common approach is to administer 14 days of intravenous therapy followed by 10–12 weeks of oral therapy. Antiviral therapy is intensified or restarted if patients develop clinically relevant cytomegalovirus disease.

It is also common for patients to receive some form of anticoagulation therapy to reduce the risk of vessel

Liver Disease in Children, Fourth Edition, ed. Frederick J. Suchy, Ronald J. Sokol, and William F. Balistreri. Published by Cambridge University Press. © Cambridge University Press 2014.

thrombosis. In a recent survey conducted through the Studies of Pediatric Liver Transplantation (SPLIT) Registry, over 50% of centers reported using continuous heparin infusion during the first postoperative week, followed by 3–6 months of an antiplatelet agents such as low-dose aspirin. Heparin infusions were typically not titrated to a target partial thromboplastin time as in treatment of deep venous thrombosis, and they were discontinued in the setting of excessive postoperative bleeding.

Patients generally receive some initial immunosuppression in the operating room, usually steroids, and chronic immunosuppressive treatment is started 12–24 hours after surgery. A detailed discussion of immunosuppression protocols and agents is included below. In patients with significant alterations in renal function prior to transplant, renal-sparing protocols that rely on antibody therapy during the first few postoperative days and delayed calcineurin inhibitor (CNI) exposure until later in the first week may be effective in preserving long-term renal function.

Early graft function as judged by coagulation parameters and clearance of bilirubin should improve steadily following reperfusion of the graft. When this improvement is not observed, graft injury resulting from ischemia–reperfusion injury or vessel thrombosis should be suspected. Screening of liver perfusion by Doppler ultrasound during the first postoperative days may identify vessel thrombosis prior to graft injury, allowing expedient thrombectomy and preventing graft injury. Ischemia–reperfusion injury is more common in extended criteria grafts and when there has been prolonged cold or warm ischemia time. Patients receiving technical variant grafts may display rising serum aminotransferases in the first 24 hours, likely released from hepatocyte injury near the cut surface as a result of marginal blood supply in that area. This elevation does not reflect global injury to the graft and is not usually associated with prolonged coagulopathy. Bilirubin levels that stall or begin to rise during the first 5 days after surgery are more likely to be an indication of a biliary leak, either "cut-edge" or anastomotic, than of acute rejection. Changes in the color of effluent from abdominal drains may herald this complication. Screening ultrasound to detect biliary leaks during this early period is rarely helpful since residual hematomas and ascites collections following the surgical procedure obscure the field; CT examination may be more revealing.

Immunosuppression

The introduction of CNIs as immunosuppressive agents in the 1980s was pivotal to successful liver transplantation in both adults and children. Most pediatric liver transplant centers use an immunosuppressive protocol that couples a CNI (usually tacrolimus) with steroids and a cell cycle inhibitor, such as azathioprine or mycophenolic acid. The mechanism of action of these agents, side effects, and drug interactions are detailed in a recent review [2]. Although the addition of an antimetabolite may not be essential in the first few weeks to months, its

Table 44.1 Pediatric liver transplant immunosuppression management

(a) Tacrolimus (calcineurin inhibitor)

Time post-transplant	Goal tacrolimus levels (ng/mL)
Post-transplant	
Months 1–3	10–12
Months 3–8	8–10
Months 8–18	5–8
Beyond 18 months	3–5
After late rejection	
Months 1–3	10–12
Months 3–4	8–12
Months 4–8	8–10
Months 8–18	5–8
Beyond 18 months	3–5

(b) Suggested steroid withdrawal schedule[a]

Time post-transplant	Daily steroid dosage (mg/kg)
Months 1–3	0.3
Months 3–4	0.2
Months 4–5	0.1
Months 5–6	0.05
Months 6	0.05 every other day for 2 weeks then STOP

[a] With normal laboratory tests; excludes patients with recent or ongoing rejection and/or patients with diagnosis of autoimmune liver disease.

(c) Cyclosporine serum goals post-transplant

Time post-transplant	Goal trough level (ng/mL)	Goal 2-hour peak level (ng/mL)
Months 1–3	250–300	800–1200
Months 3–8	200–250	600–1000
Months 8–18	150–200	400–800
Beyond 18 months	50–150	200–600

use may facilitate steroid withdrawal or avoidance. Table 44.1 summarizes a representative immunosuppression protocol including a timeline for target CNI levels during the first post-transplant year. Induction with monoclonal antibody therapy, although popular in the 1990s, is now used sparingly since the risk of graft loss to rejection in liver transplantation frequently does not outweigh the increased risk of

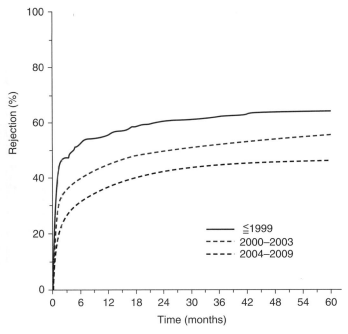

Figure 44.1 Incidence of first rejection for patients in the Studies of Pediatric Liver Transplantation Registry depicted by era of transplant. Total sample 3152 patients.

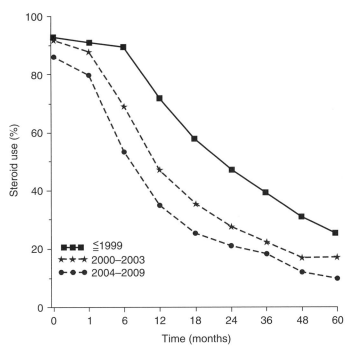

Figure 44.2 Post-transplant steroid use in the Studies of Pediatric Liver Transplantation Registry by year of transplant. Note the percentage of patients that remain on steroids in long-term follow-up has decreased over time. Patients who had a retransplant after 1 month are excluded.

opportunistic infection and malignancy posed by these agents. Although acute rejection is common following liver transplantation, with an incidence of 20–40% in children (Figure 44.1), a single episode of acute rejection does not appear to increase the risk of graft loss [3]. Therefore, most protocols in pediatric liver transplantation are aimed at achieving a low rate of immunosuppression-related complications while accepting some episodes of early acute rejection [4]. Discontinuation of steroids during the first 6–12 months is now routine in many programs (Figure 44.2). Approaches that individualize immunosuppression regimens to reduce toxicity based on individual patient risk factors are becoming more popular, for example the use of induction therapy with delayed CNI exposure in patients with pretransplant renal insufficiency/failure. Strategies of immunosuppression in pediatric solid organ transplantation have been the focus of several excellent reviews that highlight the mechanism of action and side effect profiles of commonly used agents [2].

Diagnosis and treatment of rejection

Acute rejection most commonly occurs during the first 2–6 weeks following transplantation or during periods of diminished immunosuppression exposure as a result of non-adherence or malabsorption. The histologic pattern of rejection includes several key elements (Figure 44.3), and grading of the severity of rejection is based upon histologic injury and liver functional impairment. First-line therapy generally includes steroid boluses, but episodes related to diminished immunosuppression exposure may respond to increasing levels of CNI. In early acute rejection, over 60% of patients

will respond to bolus intravenous solumedrol (10–20 mg/kg over 3–5 successive days), as judged by improvement in serum liver enzymes and direct bilirubin levels [5]. It is important to confirm suspected episodes of rejection histologically since multiple other causes of graft injury including CMV and EBV infection may mimic the clinical signs of rejection. However, histologic evaluation of response to augmented immunosuppression therapy is usually reserved for patients with suboptimal clinical response. In the setting of severe acute rejection, a Rejection Activity Index score of ≥7, or steroid-resistant rejection associated with significant graft dysfunction, therapy with an anti-lymphocyte preparation may be necessary.

Long-term maintenance of immunosuppression and tolerance

Follow-up studies of long-term survivors of liver transplantation reveal that patients require less immunosuppression as time elapses from transplant and that many display acceptable graft function while on monotherapy with a CNI: approximately 65% at both 5 years and 10 years [6,7]. Minimization of CNI exposure with reduction to once daily dosing may also be well tolerated by those without evidence of chronic inflammation on biopsy [8]. A smaller fraction, up to 20–40%, may even have operational tolerance as defined by normal or nearly normal graft histology after complete withdrawal of immunosuppression. Much of this experience has been reported in small groups of patients that were withdrawn from

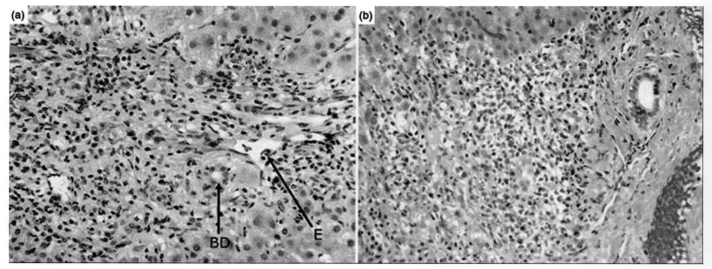

Figure 44.3 Post-transplant rejection. (a) Acute cellular rejection. Portal tract containing a dense lymphocytic infiltrate. The infiltrate fills the entire portal tract, with spillover of lymphocytes into the periportal (zone 1) hepatic parenchyma, in a pattern of interface hepatitis. The bile duct (BD) shows infiltration of the epithelium by several lymphocytes. The portal vein shows endothelial infiltration (E), also by lymphocytes. (b) Development of de novo autoimmune hepatitis. The portal tract also contains a dense lymphocytic infiltrate, with prominent interface hepatitis (upper left). However, the bile duct and the endothelium of the portal vein are spared by the infiltrate (right side of the image). (Hematoxylin & eosin stain, original resolution of both images ×200.)

immunosuppression because of life-threatening complications such as post-transplant lymphoproliferative disorder or progressive renal insufficiency. However, recently reported results of a multicenter trial to withdraw immunosuppression in living-related donor recipients have shown that 60% of these carefully selected patients fulfilled the definition of operational tolerance by maintaining normal graft function while off immunosuppression therapy for at least 1 year [9]. Patients most likely to tolerate immunosuppression withdrawal include those with normal liver enzymes and graft histology at baseline. However, in the subset of patients that did develop mild acute rejection, the process was easily reversible with enhanced immunosuppression. Experimental protocols to develop immune-based screening tools to optimize selection of patients for immunosuppression withdrawal are underway.

Infectious complications

The success of liver transplantation depends not only upon maintaining graft function but also upon the effective prevention and treatment of infectious complications. Since the early 1980s, infectious complications have been one of the most prominent causes of post-transplant mortality, with a recent SPLIT study showing infection is the most commonly implicated cause of death even in long-term follow-up [10].

Early infections

Approximately one-third of patients develop a bacterial infection within the first 30 days after liver transplantation [10]. These infections are predominantly caused by aerobic enteric Gram-negative organisms and frequently have an intra-abdominal focus. Enterococci and staphylococci are also

commonly isolated. The spectrum of bacterial isolates depend both upon the institution and patient colonization, but infection by anaerobic bacteria is uncommon. An important exception is in the setting of ischemic necrosis of the graft, and in this situation empiric antibiotic regimens should include anaerobic coverage. Fungal infections are far less common, documented in only 8% of patients within this same time frame. Intra-abdominal fungal infections are more common in the setting of bowel perforation or prolonged exposure to steroids in the pretransplant period [11].

Factors associated with an increased risk of early bacterial or fungal infection include age <12 months and receiving a technical variant graft. Increased risk in the setting of segmental grafts is likely related to surgical complications, particularly those involving the biliary tree. The risk of early bacterial and fungal infection appears to be falling with advancing experience, being 41% in patients in the SPLIT cohort of transplant recipients prior to 2002 and 32% in more recent experience.

Serious viral infections, including CMV, EBV, and adenovirus, typically present at a later time point in postoperative recovery: CMV disease occurs in 6%, with half presenting within the first 30 days [10]. The manifestations depend upon whether the infection is primary or a reactivation. Patient who have positive serologies supporting a previous infection prior to transplant can develop reactivation within the first few postoperative weeks if antiviral prophylaxis is not given. Symptoms tend to be milder in reactivation, but multisystem disease can occur. Manifestations of CMV disease, either reactivation or primary infection, commonly include fever, diarrhea, and elevation of liver enzymes. Less commonly, patients can develop a bilateral pneumonia. A high index of suspicion must be maintained because patients can develop severe disease quickly. Early treatment with ganciclovir can circumvent multisystem injury.

In contrast, most EBV disease occurs after 30 days post-transplant. Patients who are seronegative for EBV at transplant and acquire a primary infection while on T-cell immunosuppression are at increased risk to develop post-transplant lymphoproliferative disease. Increasing experience with immunosuppression protocols has helped to reduce the incidence of this disorder, which is now reported to be <3% during the first 15 months. The disease can present at any interval after transplant but is most common when levels of immunosuppression are relatively high. Post-transplant lymphoproliferative disease in the liver transplant recipient frequently presents as bulky adenopathy in the head and neck region and in the intra-abdominal or retroperitoneal area. Discrete lung lesions and ulceration in the small and/or large colon are also commonly observed. Presentation of gastrointestinal lesions typically includes chronic diarrhea and low serum albumin secondary to mild protein-losing enteropathy. Treatment strategies include reduction or elimination of CNIs when possible and rituximab, a monoclonal anti-CD20 antibody.

Pneumocystis jiroveci infection is also of concern during the first postoperative year. Prophylactic regimens of oral trimethoprim–sulfamethoxazole are fairly standard for the first 12 months. This and other opportunistic infections are rarely seen outside of setting of intense immunosuppression, such as antibody therapy for resistant rejection. The immunomodulatory impact of recent viral infection with CMV may also increase infection risk.

Infections in long-term follow-up

Bacterial infections presenting after the recovery from the transplant procedure are more commonly community acquired and can include bacterial pneumonia, urinary tract infection, and invasive pneumococcal disease. Recipients of solid organ transplants appear to be at higher risk for invasive pneumococcal disease than the general pediatric population and should be immunized appropriately [12]. Isolation of enteric bacteria from blood culture should raise the strong suspicion of biliary tract obstruction, as described below. Common viral pathogens such as respiratory syncytial virus and rotavirus can cause exaggerated infections in transplant recipients particularly when acquired during periods of intensified immunosuppression. Community exposure to varicella with subsequent infection can also result in a more severe course. Patients with evidence of acute varicella should be treated with intravenous acyclovir to prevent disseminated disease.

Evaluation of the febrile patient

The approach to a febrile episode in a liver transplant recipient varies by the interval from transplant and the level of immunosuppression. Patients who are within the first few postoperative weeks require a comprehensive search for blood-borne pathogens and intra-abdominal sources. This evaluation should include assessment of EBV and CMV viral load, even in patients who have been receiving prophylaxis. Evaluation for respiratory infection can be guided by the presence of respiratory symptoms. Gastroenteritis, either hospital or community acquired, is also likely to be associated with typical symptoms. Patients with central access are managed with empiric antibiotics while awaiting blood culture results, even if a plausible source other than the line is identified. Central catheter infections are relatively uncommon, and isolation of enteric organisms from central line cultures should prompt evaluation for an intra-abdominal or biliary source. Acute rejection rarely causes significant fever ($\geq$38.5°C (101.5°F)) but it can be associated with persistent low-grade fever over several days. Patients who are receiving intensified immunosuppression for treatment of acute rejection are at higher risk for reactivation of both EBV and CMV and it should be recognized that tissue infections may not always result in recovery of virus from the blood.

In intermediate and long-term follow-up, the differential also includes community-acquired infections. It is not uncommon for transplant recipients to have exaggerated and prolonged viral infections, even years after transplantation when immunosuppressive levels are relatively low. Late biliary strictures are also an important cause of unexplained fever and can result in positive blood cultures for enteric organism even when liver enzymes are normal. The more common scenario however, is a patient who has had intermittent elevation of cholestatic markers, with or without a history of acholic stools, who presents with high fever and a septic appearance. When fever occurs immediately after a percutaneous liver biopsy, chronic biliary obstruction with subclinical cholangitis is almost always the cause.

Selection of empiric antibiotic coverage should be designed to cover enteric organisms and skin flora if the patient has central access. Attention to a history of isolation of resistant organisms such as vancomycin-resistant enterococci or extended-spectrum beta-lactamase-producing species should also guide choices. Short-term empiric CMV therapy may also be warranted in patients with the appropriate clinical symptoms while confirmatory tissue samples are obtained. Isolated fever has been associated with CMV viremia, even in long-term follow-up, and therapy with intravenous ganciclovir is appropriate in these patients, even without evidence of tissue invasion.

Evaluation of graft dysfunction

The differential diagnosis of graft dysfunction varies with interval from transplant. Primary non-function of the allograft is a devastating problem that occurs in approximately 1–3% of patients and which is usually suspected even prior to abdominal closure. Grafts that are ultimately classified as having primary non-function typically do not exhibit appropriate reperfusion, despite patent vessels, and do not produce bile during the later operative phase. These grafts develop progressive ischemic necrosis, and liver synthetic function is severely compromised. Expedient retransplantation is necessary for patient survival. Causes of less-severe early graft injury include ischemia reperfusion injury (1–5 days) and postsurgical complications such as vascular thrombosis and biliary tract obstruction. Ischemia–reperfusion injury and hepatic arterial thrombosis (HAT) can both cause a similar pattern of moderate to severe early graft injury, which includes high aminotransferases and rising bilirubin. Timely diagnosis of HAT can allow thrombectomy before significant graft injury occurs. Acute rejection can present as early as 5 days after transplantation but most frequently presents between 1 to 6 weeks. For this reason, immunosuppression protocols are aimed at achieving the highest levels of suppression within this timeframe. Small-for-size syndrome is also an important cause of graft dysfunction within the first few weeks. Transplantation of an organ that is less than 0.8% of the patient's weight may result in a constellation of problems, including prolonged coagulopathy, increasing cholestasis, and signs of ongoing portal hypertension. Portal vessels in the smaller organ are unable to accommodate the rate of portal blood flow, which is proportional to patient size.

In long-term follow-up, the etiology of graft injury is more diverse. Acute rejection, vascular thrombosis, and biliary obstruction are still observed, but chronic inflammatory injury independent of these problems is also observed. Routine surveillance of graft histology in long-term follow-up has not been universally adopted, but programs that have implemented such screening suggest that chronic hepatitis is common in long-term survivors, even in those with normal liver enzymes.

Screening strategies

Although there is little consensus on the optimal interval, routine screening of serum liver enzymes and bilirubin levels is universal across all liver transplantation programs. In addition, several studies have observed that graft histology may be significantly abnormal even in the face of normal liver enzymes, leading to biopsy screening protocols at some centers. Screening protocols for graft imaging are even less standardized.

Serum liver enzymes, bilirubin, and coagulation are usually monitored daily in the first 7–10 days following transplantation. The pattern of alteration guides further evaluation of complications that might warrant surgical intervention. As the likelihood of vascular thrombosis and bile leak diminish during the second post-transplant week, monitoring is shifted to a twice or three times per week schedule to allow early diagnosis of acute rejection. As patients complete their first post-transplant month, rejection becomes less likely and monitoring is gradually tapered from a weekly to a once monthly schedule at 8–12 weeks. Some programs continue to monitor at monthly intervals even after the first post-transplant year,

while others shift to a quarterly schedule. A survey of centers included in the SPLIT Registry conducted in 2009 revealed that the majority of centers monitor no less than every 3 months, even in stable patients. Such monitoring allows not only assessment of serum liver enzymes, which may reflect subclinical liver injury, but also assessment of the relationship between liver enzymes and CNI levels. Some manipulation of CNI dosing to achieve normalized liver enzyme levels is acceptable, particularly in patients with a history of rejection. However, significant enzyme elevation (>3–4× baseline) and any rise in serum direct bilirubin should prompt graft biopsy since the pattern of enzyme elevation can be identical across a wide differential for graft injury.

Annual graft Doppler ultrasound assessments of the hepatic artery and portal vein are performed at some centers. Graft imaging is an obvious requirement when assessing new-onset graft dysfunction since biliary obstruction and vascular thrombosis can occur at any interval. It is helpful to exclude bile duct dilatation prior to percutaneous liver biopsy, since the risk of bile leak may be increased in the setting of biliary obstruction and it is essential to confirm hepatic arterial patency before planning percutaneous intervention for biliary obstruction. An increase in spleen size associated with a fall in platelet count may be an important sign of hepatic outflow obstruction or portal vein stenosis, which can be successfully treated with balloon angioplasty if diagnosed early. When laboratory tests are normal, the merits of screening ultrasound are less clear. Progressive fibrosis of the biliary jejunal anastomosis causing partial obstruction and bile duct dilatation can be diagnosed on ultrasound, allowing effectively percutaneous interventions before the obstruction causes graft injury or leads to cholangitis. Late hepatic arterial loss with resulting ischemic cholangiopathy is less amenable to therapy, but earlier diagnosis may help to set expectation for impending problems.

Graft injury and common complications
Hepatic arterial thrombosis

The incidence of HAT varies from 2 to 15% and the frequency of occurrence is related to the size of the recipient and donor vessels, the age of the recipient, and the quality of the donor organ [13,14]. The loss of the hepatic arterial flow to the newly transplanted organ can present in a variety of ways. In stable recipients who have received good-quality organs, the thrombosis may be asymptomatic initially and present with liver enzyme elevations of a minor to moderate degree a few days after the actual thrombotic event. In other patients, HAT may present with massive necrosis of hepatocytes, impressive serum aminotransferase elevation of >5000 IU/L, and signs of liver failure such as acidosis, uncorrectable and severe coagulopathy, and hemodynamic instability requiring vasopressors to support arterial blood pressure. Presentation may also be with early biliary complications such as bile leaks and bile duct necrosis. Since the bile ducts derive their blood supply exclusively from the hepatic artery, early bile leaks from the extrahepatic ducts and development of intrahepatic bile collections (bilomas) may be the chief symptoms even if the damage to hepatocytes is minor and liver synthetic function is not affected.

Ultrasound monitoring of the newly transplanted graft on postoperative day 1 is done chiefly to ensure the integrity of the arterial and venous flow to the liver. Early revascularization of the hepatic artery may be attempted when the thrombosis occurs on postoperative day 1 and is not accompanied by signs of graft damage. Revascularization is often successful in preventing subsequent graft damage [15]. However, even with successful restitution of arterial flow, chronic bile duct damage may present weeks or months after the transplant, with biliary sepsis secondary to stricture formation in the biliary tree. Strictures may occur at the anastomosis and be amenable to dilatation or surgical correction, or they may be multiple and located throughout the liver and require retransplantation [16].

Early postoperative HAT that is not successfully corrected usually requires early retransplantation in all patients. It may also occur later after transplantation and may present with signs of biliary sepsis or bile duct strictures in cholestatic enzymes. In patients with late presentation of HAT, therapeutic decisions are based chiefly on the severity of the damage to the graft and whether correction of the damaged ducts can be accomplished to the extent that long-term good-quality survival can be sustained. Revascularization in the late-onset HAT is not usually possible surgically nor can it reverse the damage that has already been well established in the graft.

Since HAT may have such devastating consequences, measures are taken to prevent this from happening. Meticulous technique must be used in the anastomosis of the two arterial segments from the donor and recipient. In vessels that are <3 mm in diameter, interrupted 8-0 prolene is used. In larger vessels in infant liver transplants, running or interrupted 7-0 prolene is used. Vessels are prepared for anastomosis by insuring that the intima is not damaged in any way, either in the preparation of the vessels or in the performance of the anastomosis. Operating microscopes have been used in the past, but in general, these are not necessary if 4.5× surgical loupes are used.

After the anastomosis, flow probes are used to determine the blood volume of flow through the anastomosis. As mentioned above, low-dose anticoagulation with heparin is commonly used and antiplatelet agents such as aspirin are started when the child resumes oral intake. Full therapeutic anticoagulation is used postoperatively only when the recipient is believed to be at increased risk for HAT. Ultrasound monitoring on the first postoperative day is always done for a baseline evaluation of flow and resistive index, and it is then ordered on an as-needed basis for the duration of the hospital stay of the recipient.

Recipients of live donor liver have a very low incidence of HAT. The excellent quality of the graft and the short preservation time results in a low resistance to blood flow through the graft and is thought to reduce the risk of HAT. The risk of HAT is increased in small graft weight to recipient weight ratios (≤1%), organs from small (<5 kg) donors, organs with complex donor arterial anatomy such as replaced right hepatic arteries that require more complicated reconstructions than usual, and in grafts from marginal donors.

Portal vein thrombosis/stenosis

The portal vein supplies the liver with 80% of its blood supply and 50% of the oxygen supply. Despite this, portal vein thrombosis (PVT) after transplantation is usually asymptomatic and is most frequently diagnosed on routine postoperative ultrasound monitoring.

Unlike HAT, where technical factors may not play a dominant role in the etiology of the thrombosis, acute post-transplant PVT is often technical in origin and can be corrected with revision of the anastomosis and improvement of mechanical factors that may be contributing to impaired flow [17].

Postoperative ultrasound is very sensitive and accurate in the determination of PVT. Clinical signs may be very subtle and not helpful in detecting portal vein flow problems. Liver enzyme elevation is not a feature of PVT. There may be a slight base deficit with a low serum bicarbonate, which is in contrast to the metabolic alkalosis that is often seen in the immediate post-transplant period. More commonly, PVT is seen in the technical variant transplants such as split-liver and live donor transplants. It is also more common when the recipient portal vein is hypoplastic or atretic and requires reconstruction with an interposition vein graft. In these situations, the portal vein ends up being longer than with whole liver transplants and takes a more meandering course as it lies horizontally across the inferior vena cava before coursing upward to a subphrenic location where it is anastomosed usually to a very short segment of donor vein. Care must be taken during the transplant to orient the vein properly in order to avoid twisting. Careful attention should also be directed to the anastomosis between the recipient vein, which may be quite small in diameter (<5 mm), and a donor vessel that is normal adult diameter.

If portal vein flow is not easily detected by ultrasound on the first postoperative day, the patient should be immediately re-explored. In re-exploration for PVT, it is usually not enough to simply remove the clot. The anastomosis must usually be undone, and the graft flushed with heparin and tissue plasminogen activator to clear microthrombi from the portal circulation. The recipient vein is usually also cleared both mechanically and with heparin, and the anastomosis is redone in an attempt to correct what may have been a technical issue contributing to poor flow after the first anastomosis. If the recipient portal vein is unusable, a jump graft formed from a deceased donor vein may be required from the superior mesenteric vein of the recipient to the donor portal vein. Infants with biliary atresia often develop hypoplasia and atresia of their extrahepatic portal veins, which may render them inadequate to revascularize the new liver with mesenteric blood.

These babies often require replacement of their entire portal vein with donor vein, or a jump graft from the superior mesenteric vein.

Early PVT, if left uncorrected, will usually result in the symptoms of portal hypertension over the course of the ensuing months and years, including the development of esophageal and gastric varices and hypersplenism. Chronic portal hypertension may also result from the gradual stenosis and ultimate occlusion of the extrahepatic portal vein. This is more common in technical variant transplants than with whole liver transplants. Frequent and regular monitoring of the transplanted liver's vasculature along with careful physical examination looking for splenic enlargement accompanied by thrombocytopenia may allow for successful radiological intervention to correct a stenosis. Percutaneous balloon dilatation of a venous stricture, anastomotic or otherwise, may restore mesenteric venous pressures to near normal [18]. In older children with larger veins, endovascular stenting may allow for permanent correction of a recurrent venous stricture. Stenting in smaller children is contraindicated because of the fixed nature of the stent, which will not expand to allow for the increasing venous flow that accompanies the growth of the child.

The meso-Rex bypass was first used in the setting of PVT after transplant of whole livers. This operation accesses the intrahepatic left portal vein within the recessus of Rex where the vein is still patent [19]. A vein graft is brought from the superior mesenteric vein to the intrahepatic portal vein and can successfully re-establish mesenteric flow to the liver. Unfortunately, when this technique is applied to PVT in technical variant grafts, it may be difficult or impossible to work with the remnant of the donor left portal vein. This is because the left portal vein stump may be located within the hepatic parenchyma, the Roux-en-Y loop to the bile duct lies over whatever remains of the donor left portal vein, and the distance between the superior mesenteric vein and the donor left portal vein is longer than what it may be in a whole liver. The Roux loop usually develops into a source of mesenteric venous blood for the graft through the development of spontaneous venous collaterals between the bowel and the bile duct. These collaterals, if taken down, may exacerbate the symptoms of portal hypertension. If the meso-Rex bypass cannot be attempted, a distal splenorenal shunt can be successfully used to palliate the symptoms of portal hypertension. Unfortunately, children with chronic portal vein stenosis or thrombosis after transplantation may ultimately require retransplantation to completely reverse their symptoms of intractable bleeding from intestinal varices.

Hepatic outflow obstruction

Hepatic outflow obstruction is fortunately the least common of all the vascular problems that can occur after liver transplantation. This complication has been reported more commonly following technical variant grafts [20]. The orientation of a segment 2 or 3 graft may cause twisting of the hepatic venous anastomosis, resulting in impaired hepatic venous drainage. We have also encountered rare anomalies in the donor whereby segments 2 and 3 drain primarily through intrahepatic venous communications into the middle hepatic vein and outflow occlusion occurs immediately after reperfusion. Outflow problems may also occur after retransplantation when the previous suprahepatic vena cava anastomosis may constrict outflow from the new liver.

Acute venous obstruction may cause severe damage to the graft and require retransplantation. Serum liver enzyme elevation is caused by centrilobular necrosis of hepatocytes. Doppler ultrasound examination of the graft may clearly show impaired flow through the hepatic veins and loss of normal phasicity, and reversal of flow in the portal vein usually indicates venous outflow problems. Chronic venous outflow obstruction may be more subtle and present with symptoms of portal hypertension including ascites, esophageal and gastric varices, and lower body edema. The liver is usually greatly enlarged. In the acute phase early after transplantation, outflow obstruction is very difficult to manage since any attempts at revising the venous anastomosis may be accompanied by warm ischemia of an already damaged graft. Repositioning of an acutely misaligned anastomosis by turning the orientation of the liver may help. Otherwise, retransplantation may be necessary. Chronic venous outflow obstruction may be corrected by percutaneous balloon dilatation of a venous stricture. The stricture typically occurs cephalad to the anastomosis and can be treated with a stent that bridges the stenosis by going from the vena cava above the liver into the hepatic vein, if the graft has a single vein, or into one of the hepatic veins in the case of a whole liver transplant. A gradient across the stenosis should be measured before and after the dilatation to ensure that the dilatation or stenting has had the desired effect. Repeated dilatation over years may be necessary to keep strictures from reforming. Chronic venous obstruction may ultimately cause scarring, synthetic failure, and necessitate retransplantation. Any patient with chronic venous outflow obstruction or repeated thrombosis merits a study of the coagulation system to exclude a hypercoagulable condition.

Biliary complications

Biliary leaks are predominantly an early postsurgical problem as described in Chapter 43. Visible bile in peritoneal drains and/or expanding fluid collections near the biliary anastomosis or cut edge of the liver in association with rising bilirubin and fever are classic signs. Cut edge leaks frequently resolve spontaneously unless an additional segmental bile duct has been missed in the original anastomosis. Some surgical teams perform "back table" cholangiography to avoid missing such ducts. Management of a leak from a major duct or at the anastomotic site almost always requires a surgical approach. Conservative management with local drainage and broad-spectrum antibiotics may be attempted if patients have comorbidities that make re-exploration risky.

Biliary obstruction caused by stricture and stone formation either at the anastomotic site or higher in the biliary tree is a common problem after liver transplantation, particularly in patients who have received a technical variant graft. Symptomatic biliary strictures most frequently occur within the first post-transplant year but can occur even in the second decade after liver transplantation [21]. The incidence of biliary strictures varies across studies, but most accept a rate that approaches 30% in technical variant grafts particularly when follow-up exceeds 12 months [22]. The signs and symptoms of biliary obstruction in the liver transplant recipient can be highly variable and many patients display only subtle symptoms. Bilirubin and liver enzymes, including cholestatic enzymes, may be normal until the patient develops secondary cholangitis or the ducts become completed occluded by stones. A history of intermittent pale stools and fluctuating serum liver enzymes is highly suspicious for this problem.

In addition to technical variant grafts, other risk factors include ischemic injury to the biliary system, either from the prolonged cold ischemia time or hepatic arterial insufficiency, CMV infection, and recurrent inflammatory disease such as primary sclerosing cholangitis. Strictures are classified as either anastomotic, limited to the area of the biliary enteric anastomosis, or intrahepatic. Some patients develop both. Anastomotic strictures are usually the result of scar formation, local ischemia, or technical issues. Intrahepatic strictures are frequently the result of global ischemic injury and have a high recurrence rate that frequently necessitates retransplantation [23]. Strictures from ischemic cholangiopathy typically presents earlier, 3–12 months following surgery, and are characterized by multiple strictures in second- and third-order ducts. In segment grafts, one segment may have normal-appearing ducts while the other, which may have had more compromise in blood flow, will exhibit multiple beaded ducts. Stone formation is frequently seen at narrow areas, and chronic bacterial colonization leading to acute cholangitis is also commonly observed.

Intrahepatic strictures have also been associated with immunological injury such as chronic rejection and recurrent or de novo primary sclerosing cholangitis.

Compromised hepatic arterial circulation should always be suspected in the setting of biliary strictures, but strictures can develop even in the setting of normal flow in the larger hepatic arterial branches. When arterial flow is inadequate, balloon dilatation and/or surgical intervention are rarely successful and could place the patient at risk for biliary perforation and resulting intra-abdominal infection. Since the majority of biliary anastomoses in pediatric liver transplantation are still performed by construction of a Roux-en-Y, the option of endoscopic evaluation and treatment is limited. The most commonly used diagnostic modalities include ultrasound, CT, and percutaneous cholangiography. In many instances, biliary obstruction does not result in biliary dilatation that can be detected on ultrasound or CT. Likewise, the sensitivity of magnetic resonance cholangiopancreatography evaluation for biliary obstruction in pediatric liver transplantation recipients does not appear to be as high as that in adults, where the sensitivity exceeds 90% [23]. In the setting of high clinical suspicion, a percutaneous cholangiogram should be obtained, even if radiographic studies are negative. Percutaneous balloon dilatation followed by temporary stent placement can be successful in treating both isolated anastomotic strictures and intrahepatic strictures, although this is much more effective for strictures involving only the anastomosis [21,24] (Figure 44.4).

Chronic graft hepatitis/de novo autoimmune hepatitis

It has been increasingly recognized that liver transplantation recipients can develop a pattern of chronic hepatitis, unrelated to chronic viral infection or typical features of rejection, that can lead to significant graft injury. Single-center experiences with protocol liver biopsies in long-term follow-up have revealed that the majority of pediatric recipients develop fibrosis over time, in many cases associated with chronic inflammatory changes. Despite any pretransplant evidence of autoimmune disease, many patients with these chronic inflammatory changes have positive autoantibodies similar to those found in patients with a primary diagnosis of autoimmune hepatitis, and so have been described as having "de novo" autoimmune hepatitis. There is general disagreement as to whether this form of chronic graft hepatitis has similar pathogenesis to primary autoimmune hepatitis, but all agree that left untreated these changes can lead to significant irreversible graft injury. The prevalence of this problem appears to be approximately 5–10% in pediatric liver transplant recipients [25], and differing prevalence across studies is dependent upon the method of case ascertainment. Many patients present with elevated serum liver enzymes detected at the time of routine screening. Liver biopsies performed for clinical causes reveal a pattern of interface hepatitis and variable degrees of fibrosis. Plasma cells are prominent feature in the inflammatory infiltrate. Serum antibodies including anti-nuclear antibodies and anti-smooth muscle antibodies are positive and serum IgG is frequently elevated. Occasionally, interface hepatitis will be seen on surveillance biopsies in the setting of normal serum liver enzymes. In these cases, elevations of autoantibodies and/ or serum IgG may also be detected. Elevation of serum antibodies in pediatric liver transplantation recipients have not proven to be an appropriate screening method for this graft injury, since elevated levels do not strongly predict histology injury [26]. The most common approach to management is reinstitution of steroid therapy. Many descriptions include a regimen of steroids and an antimetabolite such as azathioprine. Most patients respond well to steroid therapy, but many relapse when it is discontinued. Investigations of the immunologic phenotype in this disorder suggest that patients with this problem are relatively overimmunosuppressed and have significant alternations in regulatory T-cell function. Therefore, novel approaches such as reduction of T-cell immunosuppression coupled with agents such as sirolimus may be successful strategies to treat this injury while still preventing rejection.

(a)

(b)

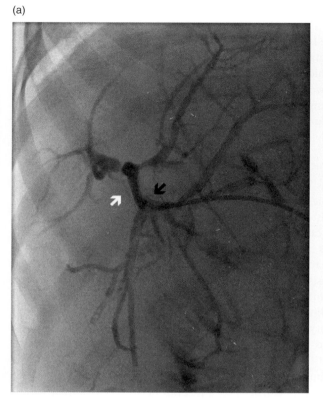
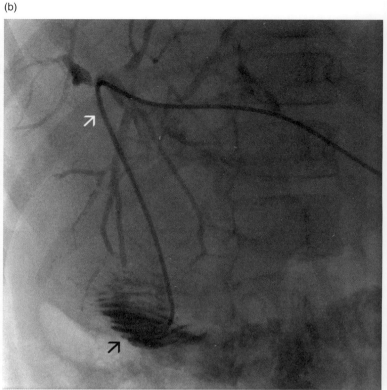

Figure 44.4 Images of a biliary structure obtained during percutaneous transhepatic cholangiography in a patient with a reduced size liver transplant. (a) A catheter (black arrow) is positioned in the left hepatic duct with a thin and faint line of contrast (white arrow) delineating a long segment stricture of the extrahepatic bile duct. (b) The catheter (white arrow) has now been advanced past the strictured bile duct into the duodenum (black arrow).

Long-term outcomes

Patient and graft survival

Many larger pediatric liver transplant programs are reporting 1-year adjusted patient and graft survival rates that exceed 95% and 90%, respectively. Comparing these outcomes by era of transplant shows that survival statistics have improved slightly over the past 5–7 years, more dramatically over the past 10–15 years. Most patient deaths and graft losses occur within the first 3 months following the procedure (Figure 44.5). Results of a recent analysis of risk factors associated with patient and graft loss conducted through the SPLIT Registry are illustrated in Table 44.2 [17]. Post-transplant complications were associated with the highest relative risks, with reoperation for any cause associated with an 11-fold increase in risk for death or graft loss. However, reoperation is a common occurrence in up to one-third of infants receiving technical variant graft requiring unplanned re-exploration within the first 30 days (unpublished SPLIT data). Technical variant grafts were independently associated with lower outcomes, but the hazard ratios were less pronounced when reoperation was added to the model.

Recent UNOS data on pediatric liver transplant recipients younger than 12 years of age have also suggested better immediate postoperative survival in whole graft recipients, but by 1 year, adjusted patient and allograft survivals were similar

regardless of the type (whole liver, deceased donor segmental, or living donor) [27]. Outcomes have also been reported to vary by primary disease, with biliary atresia associated with the lowest risk. However, in multivariate analysis this association is not upheld.

Although the slopes of patient and graft survival curves diminish in intermediate and long-term follow-up, there is still a gradual fall to 10-year survival and beyond. An analysis of the causes of patient death and graft loss in patients that survived the first post-transplant year implicated infections as the most common cause for late patient mortality [28]. In that analysis, 45% of patient deaths were attributed to the aggregated diagnoses of sepsis, multisystem organ failure, and post-transplant lymphoproliferative disease. Recurrent malignancy caused 18% of late deaths and rejection was implicated in only 3%. Conversely, rejection was the most common cause, 49%, of late graft loss in long-term follow-up.

Retransplantation

Patient and graft survivals after retransplantation are approximately 10% less than following primary transplantation. Indications for retransplantation vary by interval from transplant, but vascular complications account for a significant proportion: 47% at less than 30 days and 26% at >30 days [29]. Patient survival following early retransplantation is typically lower than when retransplant is performed after the first

Table 44.2 SPLIT patient survival: multivariate analysis of 2982 recipients of first liver transplantation for risk of poor survival

Factor	Comparison	Reference	Hazard ratio	Overall *p* value
Organ type				0.0299
	Liver		1.61	
	Cadaver reduced	Whole	1.83	
	Cadaver split		1.48	
Status at transplant				0.0001
	Intubated		3.02	
	Intensive care not intubated	Home	2.32	
	Hospitalized		1.73	
Primary immunosuppression				0.012
	Cyclosporine	Tacrolimus	1.43	
	Other		2.3	
Blood use (100 mL)	Yes	No	1.02	0.011
Septicemia within 30 days	Yes	No	2.99	<0.0001
Hepatic arterial thrombosis within 6 months	Yes	No	2.02	0.002
Portal vein thrombosis within 6 months	Yes	No	1.88	0.011
Retransplant of liver within 6 months	Yes	No	3.65	<0.0001
Reoperations within 30 days	Yes	No	10.57	<0.0001

Source: adapted with permission from McDiarmid *et al.*, 2011 [17].

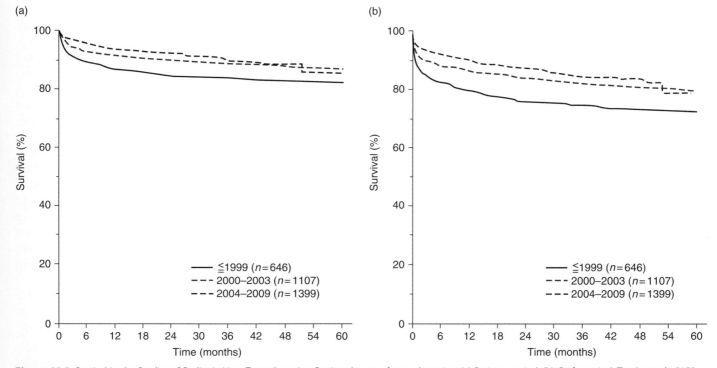

Figure 44.5 Survival in the Studies of Pediatric Liver Transplantation Registry by era of transplantation. (a) Patient survival. (b) Graft survival. Total sample 3152 patients undergoing first liver transplantation.

30 days, but this difference is likely because of the ongoing comorbidities that complicate care during the first few post-transplant weeks. Additional risk factors for patient mortality following retransplantation include donor age, use of a technical variant graft, and elevated international normalized ratio.

Chronic comorbidities

Chronic exposure to immunosuppression can cause progressive injury to multiple organ systems. Each agent has its own unique injury profile. Toxicity related to CNIs is of highest interest since most patients receive these medications for decades. Known side effects include diabetes, neurotoxicity, and acute and chronic renal injury.

The most common toxicity associated with CNI exposure is renal injury. Signs of this injury range from mild hypertension to overt renal insufficiency, which develops in a small minority of long-term survivors. Acute nephrotoxicity is secondary to afferent arteriolar vasoconstriction and reduce renal plasma flow and is dose related. Systemic hypertension is a common manifestation of this acute injury. Analysis of unpublished SPLIT data revealed that 42 of 149 children aged 5 years or older (28%) were hypertensive by age-, gender-, and height-adjusted standards at 6 months after liver transplant. This percentage was fairly constant over the first 2 years, but fell to <20% at 3 years. In longer term follow-up, the prevalence of elevated blood pressure was similar, ranging from 21% at the 5-year and 27% at the 10-year follow-up visit. Over half of these patients had elevated blood pressure at a subsequent follow-up visit, suggesting that the problem was not transient [30]. Chronic renal insufficiency is a common problem seen in long-term follow-up, with approximately 15% of patients having a measured glomerular filtration rate <90 mL/min per $1.73 \, m^2$ at ≥ 5 years following transplant [31]. The chronic renal injury is associated with structural changes in the kidney that include arteriolopathy and tubulointerstitial fibrosis. Many patients have a progressive decline in glomerular filtration rate, with limited reversibility even if CNI use is discontinued.

Diabetes mellitus is also a well-known complication associated with CNI use. Between 5 and 15% of patients develop diabetes, with the incidence varying by age and CNI exposure. Tacrolimus exposure is accepted as a risk factor that is significantly potentiated by concomitant exposure to steroids. Neurologic complications associated with CNI use are also reported in a significant subset of patients. Up to 10% of children may experience a seizure in the post-transplant period. Seizures are usually associated with posterior reversible encephalopathy syndrome. Seizures can be heralded by headache and vision changes and usually occur during the first few weeks of CNI exposure and are observed in the setting of either high or appropriate blood levels. They frequently require short-term anticonvulsant therapy, but patients without other neurologic injury rarely develop a chronic seizure disorder. Migraine headaches and tremors are also common and likely under-reported complications that are dose related.

Growth and development

Growth failure is a common finding in children with cirrhosis awaiting liver transplantation. The causes are multidimensional and include malnutrition in fat malabsorption, abnormal nitrogen metabolism, and increased energy expenditure. Children with cirrhosis have also been demonstrated to have growth hormone resistance [32]. Following successful liver transplantation and nutritional restitution, growth hormone and insulin-like growth factor 1 levels return to normal and the rate of linear growth improves [33]. However, catch-up growth is usually not observed until the second year following liver transplantation and may not be complete in many patients even years after transplantation [34,35]. Catch-up proceeds through intermediate follow-up after transplant (2–3 years) and then plateaus, leaving up to 25% of these patients with heights that are below the 5th percentile for age in long-term follow-up. A recent multivariate analysis of patients included in the SPLIT Registry revealed that linear growth impairment (<10th percentile) was more likely in patients with metabolic diseases, which included a diverse group ranging from α_1-antitrypsin deficiency to urea cycle defects (odds ratio, 4.4) and in those receiving steroids beyond the first 18 months post-transplant (odds ratio, 3.02). Higher percentiles for weight (odds ratio, 0.80) and height (odds ratio, 0.62) at liver transplantation were protective [34]. Prolonged steroid exposure was also associated with less catch-up growth. However, the strongest predictors of catch-up growth following liver transplantation were weight and height z-scores at transplant. Patients with lower weight percentiles exhibit less growth acceleration, suggesting that complications of malnutrition must be reversed before catch-up growth is achievable. Conversely, patients with lower height percentiles at transplant exhibited more linear growth acceleration in early follow-up. Previous reports examining the relationships between pre- and post-transplant growth have been inconclusive, with some authors demonstrating pretransplant growth failure to have a positive impact [35,36] and others demonstrating a negative impact [37]. Experience from the SPLIT Registry suggests both observations may be valid. Children with more severe growth arrest prior to transplant require the most catch-up growth to recover, and without other limitations, the acceleration of their post-transplant linear growth may be more pronounced than that of patients with closer to normal growth patterns prior to transplant. However, even with an above-average degree of catch-up growth following transplant, patients with the lowest height percentiles at transplant would be less likely to achieve normal percentiles post-transplant. Therefore, catch-up growth occurs, but is incomplete.

Improvements in growth have been achieved with steroid withdrawal or discontinuation and by supplemental use of recombinant human growth hormone therapy [38,39]. Recombinant growth hormone treatment response has been sustained in the second and third treatment years without advancing the bone age beyond chronological age, suggesting that prolonged therapy could be considered without a negative impact on duration of linear growth and adult height potential [40]. However, these measures may not be enough to improve final height since up to 50% of recipients have a final adult height which is 1.3 SD lower than their genetic potential [41]. Of note, patients with some diagnoses (e.g. Alagille syndrome) may not have improved growth despite these measures [42,43].

Chronic liver disease during childhood impairs neurodevelopmental processes in both infants and older children. Measurement of neurocognitive function at different ages following liver transplant has identified cognitive delay as a prevalent problem in this population. The onset of liver disease in infancy is believed to be a particularly important risk factor for neurocognitive delay. Infants with metabolic diseases, including those characterized by hyperammonemic crises such as urea cycle defects and tyrosinemia, can have significant neurologic damage. Several publications validate that early therapy, which may include liver transplantation to prevent these crises, can substantially reduce or eliminate this risk [44]. More commonly, liver disease in infancy is caused by biliary atresia or other forms of biliary cirrhosis. These infants typically experience advanced malnutrition, with growth arrest and profound muscle weakness prior to transplantation. Observational studies of these infants have revealed that although many maintain mental and motor development which is within the low average range before transplant their function drops significantly during the transplant process [45]. Delayed developmental recovery is associated with prolonged hospitalization and more advanced malnourishment prior to transplant. There are few studies that compare neurocognitive function before and after liver transplantation in children, but all support the concept that many patients have delays that persist even after successful physical rehabilitation [46–51]. The primary focus of studies so far has been evaluation of intelligence and academic achievement. Various groups have demonstrated severely impaired intellectual ability in 10–15% of recipients, with newer studies reporting slightly better outcomes. There also appears to be a significant increase in the prevalence of mild to moderate intellectual delay and learning disabilities in these patients. Several studies suggest a differential impairment of language, and verbal skills being more impaired [50]; hearing loss has been documented in up to 15%. This constellation of problems may interfere with school performance. In fact, approximately 30% of transplant recipients requires special educational services, even in long-term follow-up after transplantation [47]. Risk factors for these lower educational outcomes are not entirely clear, but prolonged hospitalization during the transplant process and growth arrest prior to transplant are commonly implicated. The need for special education services before transplant is also a strong predictor of ongoing needs in the post-transplant period.

Early results of a longitudinal, multicenter study measuring intelligence, academic achievement, and executive function in pediatric liver transplant recipients who received transplants at age 5 years or younger have identified that patients with cognitive delay can be identified as early as age 5–7 years [51]. Mild to moderate delay was demonstrated in 28% of this cohort at this early age and testing results 2 years later revealed that few had improvement in scores. Executive functions, which include organizational skills, multitasking and behavior regulation, was also delayed in this group, with the delays being more noticeable in the classroom than at home. Preliminary risk factor analysis suggests that demographic and socioeconomic indicators and peritransplant medical variables make a moderate contribution to lower outcomes, with problems experienced in long-term follow-up playing a smaller role.

Health-related quality of life has been the focus of several studies in pediatric liver transplant recipients. These studies have all had similar results, suggesting that these children have lower physical and psychosocial function than their healthy peers and with functional outcomes that are similar to children with other chronic pediatric medical conditions [47,52–55]. A recent SPLIT study of over 800 recipients revealed that psychosocial function was more compromised than physical function and that the aspect with the strongest influence on psychosocial health was school function [47]. Emotional and social domains were relatively preserved. Function at school can be impacted not only by cognitive impairment but also by loss of time in school. A large survey of children included in the SPLIT Registry revealed that one-third of the group had missed more than 10 days of school the previous year and 18% had missed more than 20 days. School absence was more common in older participants and children with shorter intervals from liver transplantation [46]. Results of single-center studies of behavioral adjustment and psychiatric outcomes following pediatric liver transplantation have been variable but do not suggest an increased prevalence of depression and anxiety disorders in this population. However, up to 16% of adolescents have reported symptoms consistent with post-traumatic stress disorder [56]. Parents of pediatric liver transplantation recipients also report symptoms of post-traumatic stress disorder plus significant levels of their own stress and anxiety related to the child's medical condition [52,57–59]. Family function has also been studied in this population [57]; although the overall level of family function appears similar to non-clinical groups, parents of older transplant recipients (>5 years) reported higher levels of stress that were influenced by demographic variables, such as parental employment status and education level.

The early postoperative period following pediatric liver transplantation can include multiple problems related to the challenges of performing segmental liver transplantation and the rehabilitation of children with advanced malnutrition. Immunosuppressive practices have evolved over time to embrace a strategy that minimizes immunosuppression exposure to reduce infection and cancer risk. The current expectation for pediatric liver transplant recipients is that they can survive many decades with their original graft. Careful attention to minimize immunosuppression exposure should reduce their risk of infection and medication-related comorbidities. Unfortunately, chronic allograft dysfunction is not uncommon, even when patients are meticulously managed, and many recipients report health states that reflect a disease burden that is similar to children with other chronic diseases. Future directions in the field should include continued efforts to perform transplantation prior to advanced malnutrition and failure of growth and development and to improve understanding of the determinants of chronic comorbidities in ultra-long-term follow-up.

References

1. Iinuma Y, Senda K, Fujihara N, *et al.* Surgical site infection in living-donor liver transplant recipients: a prospective study. *Transplantation* 2004;78: 704–709.

2. Urschel S, Altamirano-Diaz LA, West LJ. Immunosuppression armamentarium in 2010:mechanistic and clinical considerations. *Pediatr Clin North Am* 2010;57:433–457.

3. Wiesner RH, Demetris AJ, Belle SH, *et al.* Acute hepatic allograft rejection: incidence, risk factors, and impact on outcome. *Hepatology* 1998;28: 638–645.

4. Feng S. Long-term management of immunosuppression after pediatric liver transplantation: is minimization or withdrawal desirable or possible or both? *Curr Opin Organ Transplant* 2008;13:506–512.

5. Alonso EM, Piper JB, Echols G, Thistlethwaite JR, Whitington PF. Allograft rejection in pediatric recipients of living related liver transplants. *Hepatology* 1996;23:40–43.

6. Ng V, Alonso E, Bucuvalas J, *et al.* Health status of children alive 10 years after pediatric liver transplantation performed in the US and Canada: report of SPLIT experience. *J Pediatr* 2012;160:820–826.

7. Ng VL, Fecteau A, Shepherd R, *et al.* Outcomes of 5-year survivors of pediatric liver transplantation: report on 461 children from a North American multicenter registry. *Pediatrics* 2008;122:e1128–e1135.

8. Ekong UD, Bhagat H, Alonso EM. Once daily calcineurin inhibitor monotherapy in pediatric liver transplantation. *Am J Transplant* 2010;10:883–888.

9. Feng S, Ekong UD, Lobritto SJ, *et al.* Complete immunosuppression withdrawal and subsequent allograft function among pediatric recipients of parental living donor liver transplants. *JAMA* 2012;307:283–293.

10. Shepherd RW, Turmelle Y, Nadler M, *et al.* Risk factors for rejection and infection in pediatric liver transplantation. *Am J Transplant* 2008;8:396–403.

11. Gladdy R, Richardson S, Davies H, Superina R. Candida infection in pediatric liver transplant recipients. *Liver Transplant Surg* 1999;5:16–24.

12. Tran L, Hebert D, Dipchand A, *et al.* Invasive pneumococcal disease in pediatric organ transplant recipients: a high-risk population. *Pediatr Transplant* 2005;9:183–186.

13. Bekker J, Ploem S, de Jong KP. Early hepatic artery thrombosis after liver transplantation: a systematic review of the incidence, outcome and risk factors. *Am J Transplant* 2009;9:746–757.

14. Duffy JP, Hong JC, Farmer DG, *et al.* Vascular complications of orthotopic liver transplantation: experience in more than 4200 patients. *J Am Coll Surgeons.* 2009;208:896–903; discussion 5.

15. Caicedo J, Sher D, Alonso E, *et al.* Outcome of urgent revascularization in children with early hepatic artery thrombosis following liver transplantation. *Am J Transplant* 2005;5(Suppl 11):201.

16. Stringer MD, Marshall MM, Muiesan P, *et al.* Survival and outcome after hepatic artery thrombosis complicating pediatric liver transplantation. *J Pediatr Surg* 2001;36:888–891.

17. McDiarmid SV, Anand R, Martz K, Millis MJ, Mazariegos G. A multivariate analysis of pre-, peri-, and post-transplant factors affecting outcome after pediatric liver transplantation. *Ann Surg* 2011;254:145–154.

18. Perkins JD. Percutaneous transhepatic balloon dilation for portal venous stenosis. *Liver Transplant* 2006;12: 321–322.

19. de Ville de Goyet J, Gibbs P, Clapuyt P, *et al.* Original extrahilar approach for hepatic portal revascularization and relief of extrahepatic portal hypertension related to later portal vein thrombosis after pediatric liver transplantation. Long term results. *Transplantation* 1996;62:71–75.

20. Sakamoto S, Egawa H, Kanazawa H, *et al.* Hepatic venous outflow obstruction in pediatric living donor liver transplantation using left-sided lobe grafts: Kyoto University experience. *Liver Transplant* 2010;16:1207–1214.

21. Sunku B, Salvalaggio PRO, Donaldson JS, *et al.* Outcomes and risk factors for failure of radiologic treatment of biliary strictures in pediatric liver transplantation recipients. *Liver Transplant* 2006;12:821–826.

22. Anderson CD, Turmelle YP, Darcy M, *et al.* Biliary strictures in pediatric liver transplant recipients: early diagnosis and treatment results in excellent graft outcomes. *Pediatr Transplant* 2010;14:358–363.

23. Ayoub WS, Esquivel CO, Martin P. Biliary complications following liver transplantation. *Digest Dis Sci* 2010;55:1540–1546.

24. Miraglia R, Maruzzelli L, Caruso S, *et al.* Percutaneous management of biliary strictures after pediatric liver transplantation. *Cardiovasc Intervent Radiol* 2008;31:993–998.

25. Hubscher S. What does the long-term liver allograft look like for the pediatric recipient? *Liver Transplant* 2009;15 (Suppl 2):S19–S24.

26. Avitzur Y, Ngan BY, Lao M, Fecteau A, Ng VL. Prospective evaluation of the prevalence and clinical significance of positive autoantibodies after pediatric liver transplantation. *J Pediatr Gastroenterol Nutr* 2007;45:222–227.

27. Becker NS, Barshes NR, Aloia TA, *et al.* Analysis of recent pediatric orthotopic liver transplantation outcomes indicates that allograft type is no longer a predictor of survivals. *Liver Transplant* 2008;14:1125–1132.

28. Soltys KA, Mazariegos GV, Squires RH, *et al.* Late graft loss or death in pediatric

liver transplantation: an analysis of the SPLIT database. *Am J Transplant* 2007;7:2165–2171.

29. Ng V, Anand R, Martz K, Fecteau A. Liver retransplantation in children: a SPLIT database analysis of outcome and predictive factors for survival. *Am J Transplant* 2008;8: 386–395.

30. McLin VA, Anand R, Daniels SR, Yin W, Alonso EM. Blood pressure elevation in long-term survivors of pediatric liver transplantation. *Am J Transplant* 2012;12:183–190.

31. Campbell K, Ng V, Martin S, *et al.* Glomerular filtration rate following pediatric liver transplantation: the SPLIT experience. *Am J Transplant* 2010;10:2673–2682.

32. Maes M, Sokal E, Otte J. Growth factors in children with end-stage liver disease before and after liver transplantation: a review. *Pediatr Transplant* 1997;1: 171–175.

33. Sarna S, Laine J, Sipila I, Koistinen R, Holmberg C. Differences in linear growth and cortisol production between liver and renal transplant recipients on similar immunosuppression. *Transplantation* 1995;60:656–661.

34. Alonso EM, Shepherd R, Martz KL, Yin W, Anand R, Group SR. Linear growth patterns in prepubertal children following liver transplantation. *Am J Transplant* 2009;9:1389–1397.

35. McDiarmid S, JA G, DeSilva P, *et al.* Factors affecting growth after pediatric liver transplantation. *Transplantation* 1999;67:404–411.

36. Bartosh S, Thomas S, Sutton M, Brady L, Whitington P. Linear growth after pediatric liver transplantation. *J Pediatr* 1999;135:624–631.

37. Viner R, Forton J, Col T, *et al.* Growth of long term survivors of liver transplantation. *Arch Dis Child* 1999;80:235–240.

38. Sarna S, Sipila I, Ronnholm K, Koistinen R, Holmberg C. Recombinant human growth hormone improves growth in children receiving glucocorticoid treatment after liver

transplantation. *J Clin Endocrinol Metab* 1996;81:1476–1482.

39. Reding R. Steroid withdrawal in liver transplantation: benefits, risks, and unanswered questions. *Transplantation* 2000;70:405–410.

40. Puustinen L, Jalanko H, Holmberg C, Merenmies J. Recombinant human growth hormone treatment after liver transplantation in childhood: the 5-year outcome. *Transplantation* 2005;79: 1241–1246.

41. Scheenstra R, Gerver WJ, Odink RJ, *et al.* Growth and final height after liver transplantation during childhood. *J Pediatr Gastroenterol Nutr* 2008;47:165–171.

42. Lykavieris P, Hadchouel M, Chardot C, Bernard O. Outcome of liver disease in children with Alagille syndrome: a study of 163 patients. *Gut* 2001;49:431–435.

43. Quiros-Tejeira RE, Ament ME, Heyman MB, *et al.* Does liver transplantation affect growth pattern in Alagille syndrome? *Liver Transplant* 2000;6:582–587.

44. Campeau PM, Pivalizza PJ, Miller G, *et al.* Early orthotopic liver transplantation in urea cycle defects: follow up of a developmental outcome study. *Mol Genet Metab* 2010; 100(Suppl 1):S84–S87.

45. Wayman K, Cox K, Esquivel C. Neurodevelopmental outcome of young children with extrahepatic biliary atresia 1 year after liver transplantation. *J Pediatr* 1997;131:894–898.

46. Gilmour S, Adkins R, Liddell GA, Jhangri G, Robertson CM. Assessment of psychoeducational outcomes after pediatric liver transplant. *Am J Transplant* 2009;9:294–300.

47. Gilmour S, Sorenson L, Anand R, Yin W, Alonso E. School outcomes in children registered in the Studies of Pediatric Liver Transplantation (SPLIT) consortium. *Liver Transplant* 2010; 16:1041–1048.

48. Gritti A, Di Sarno AM, Comito M, *et al.* Psychological impact of liver transplantation on children's inner worlds. *Pediatr Transplant* 2001;5:37–43.

49. Kaller T, Schulz K, Sander K, *et al.* Cognitive abilities in children after liver transplantation. *Transplantation* 2005;79:1252–1256.

50. Krull K, Fuchs C, Yurk H, Boone P, Alonso E. Neurocognitive outcome in pediatric liver transplant recipients. *Pediatr Transplant* 2003;7:111–118.

51. Sorensen L, Neighbors K, Martz K, *et al.* Cognitive and academic outcomes after pediatric liver transplatation: Functional Outcomes Group (FOG) results. *Am J Transplant* 2011;11: 303–311.

52. Bucuvalas JC, Britto M, Krug S, *et al.* Health-related quality of life in pediatric liver transplant recipients: A single-center study. *Liver Transplant* 2003;9:62–71.

53. Cole CR, Bucuvalas JC, Hornung RW, *et al.* Impact of liver transplantation on HRQOL in children less than 5 years old. *Pediatr Transplant* 2004;8:222–227.

54. Sundaram SS, Landgraf JM, Neighbors K, Cohn RA, Alonso EM. Adolescent health-related quality of life following liver and kidney transplantation. *Am J Transplant* 2007;7:982–989.

55. Taylor RM, Franck LS, Gibson F, Donaldson N, Dhawan A. Study of the factors affecting health-related quality of life in adolescents after liver transplantation. *Am J Transplant* 2009;9:1179–1188.

56. Mintzer LL, Stuber ML, Seacord D, *et al.* Traumatic stress symptoms in adolescent organ transplant recipients. *Pediatrics* 2005;115:1640–1644.

57. Alonso EM. Growth and developmental considerations in pediatric liver transplantation. *Liver Transplant* 2008;14:585–591.

58. Alonso EM, Neighbors K, Mattson C, *et al.* Functional outcomes of pediatric liver transplantation. *J Pediatr Gastroenterol Nutr* 2003;37:155–160.

59. Young GS, Mintzer LL, Seacord D, *et al.* Symptoms of posttraumatic stress disorder in parents of transplant recipients: incidence, severity, and related factors. *Pediatrics* 2003; 111(6 Pt 1):e725–e731.

Index

Note: page numbers with suffix '*f*' refer to figures and those with suffix '*t*' refer to tables; chemicals listed under the main name, not the prefix such as Greek letter.